The Biology of
Cholesterol and
Related Steroids

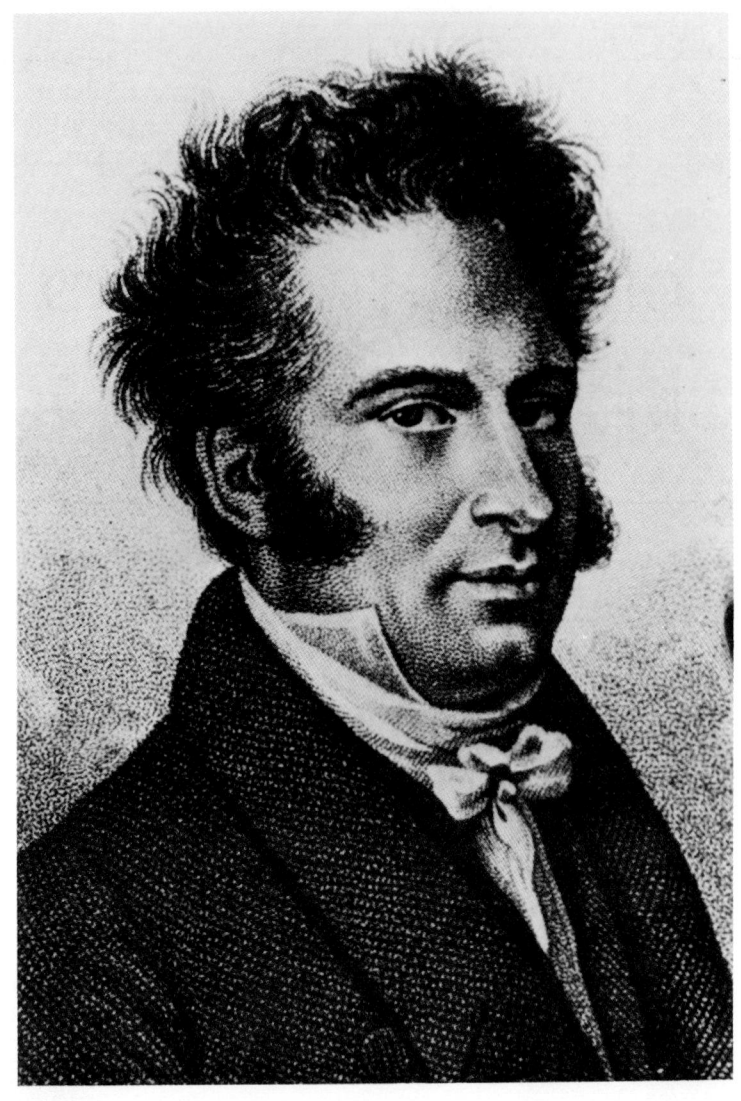

Michel Eugène Chevreul (1786–1889). This portrait was engraved by Ambroise Tardieu in 1825. (Reproduced by kind permission of Madame Florkin).

THE BIOLOGY OF CHOLESTEROL AND RELATED STEROIDS

N. B. Myant DM, FRCP

*Director, MRC Lipid Metabolism Unit,
Hammersmith Hospital, London*

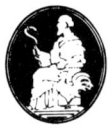

William Heinemann Medical Books Ltd
London

To A.A-B.
A.M.M.
J.H.
N.E.
P.A.

First published 1981
© N B Myant 1981

ISBN 0 433 22880 6

Filmset in 'Monophoto' Baskerville
by Eta Services (Typesetters) Ltd., Beccles, Suffolk
Printed and bound in Great Britain by R. J. Acford Ltd, Chichester

Contents

	Page
Preface	vii
Acknowledgements	x
Partial List of Abbreviations	xii
Conversion Table	xiv

Chapter

1	Chemistry	1
2	Analysis of Sterols and Related Steroids	53
3	The Distribution of Sterols and Related Steroids in Nature	123
4	The Biosynthesis of Sterols	161
5	The Metabolism of Cholesterol	227
6	Developmental Aspects of Cholesterol Metabolism	299
7	Sterols in Biological Membranes	315
8	Cholesterol Synthesis in Animal Tissues	339
9	Sterol Metabolism in Isolated Cells	397
10	Cholesterol Metabolism in the Whole Body	447

11	The Plasma Cholesterol: Composition and Metabolism	505
12	The Epidemiology of the Plasma Cholesterol	569
13	Cholesterol and Atherosclerosis	603
14	Disorders of Cholesterol Metabolism: Introduction	669
15	Disorders of Cholesterol Metabolism: The Hyperlipoproteinaemias	689
16	Disorders of Cholesterol Metabolism: The Hypolipoproteinaemias	773
17	Sterol Storage Diseases	817
18	Cholesterol Gallstones: Plasma Cholesterol in Liver Disease	853
	Index	889

Preface

In this book I have tried to assemble as much as possible of the information likely to be needed by anyone beginning to study sterols in relation to living organisms. I hope the book will also be useful to those already working on steroid biology, whatever their scientific background or particular interests within this general field. As the title implies, the main emphasis is on cholesterol and other steroids of animal tissues. This reflects my own interest and experience, essentially those of someone concerned to apply biochemistry and cell biology to clinical problems. Selected aspects of the distribution and metabolism of plant steroids are dealt with in the earlier chapters, though not in any depth; for a comprehensive account of these topics the reader should consult the monograph by Nes and McKean (1977).

To make the book as self-contained as possible I begin with a chapter covering those aspects of the chemistry of sterols that the reader I have in mind may wish to know about (a more detailed account, with numerous references to modern methodology, will be found in Gibbons *et al.*, 1982). This chapter should be read first, since it explains both the system of nomenclature used throughout the book and the stereochemistry of steroids, to which so much of the nomenclature refers. Although the remaining chapters were written to be read in sequence, most of them can stand on their own as independent essays or reviews, the subject matter becoming more clinical in the later chapters.

The historical section in Chapter 1 need be read only by those with an interest in the foundations on which current knowledge of steroid structure is based. This highly condensed account was included partly as an expression of admiration for the organic chemists whose work, continued over a period of more than 100 years (roughly from 1816 to 1954), culminated in the elucidation of the absolute configuration of cholesterol. The history of any branch of science written as a catalogue of completed discoveries can make dull reading and is usually of little value to the practising scientist, but attempts to recapture the mixture of undirected gropings, brilliant insights and pure luck that underlies a period of rapid progress in science can be very worthwhile. Anyone doubting this should read Judson's (1979) enthralling account of the beginnings of molecular biology. In a much smaller way, in Chapter 4, I discuss the development of ideas behind the unravelling of the biosynthetic pathway from small molecules to sterols, and in one or two other places I have adopted a similar approach where this helps to clarify a complex question. Those who prefer to have no history at all can ignore these passages without loss of continuity. However, it is worth noting that a knowledge of the background to a particular discovery helps to show how science really works, rather than how it is thought to work by non-scientists who write about the history or philosophy of science. This latter view is encapsulated in a story told by one of our most eminent philosophers, a classical scholar by training. It was suggested to him that in order to prepare himself for writing about science he should go to the Clarendon Laboratory and listen to the clicking of a Geiger counter.

It should not be necessary to refer here to the need for balance and objectivity in the sifting of evidence, something that has been taken for granted by the scientific community for about 300 years. Nevertheless, it is a fact that the very word 'cholesterol' tends to arouse emotional reactions that cloud rational judgement. This is apparent in the newspapers, on television, in day-to-day conversation and even in discussion among scientists. The reason for this state of affairs is, of course, the link thought to exist between cholesterol and a disease so serious and so widespread that it is difficult not to feel strongly about it. My own standpoint on cholesterol in relation to ischaemic heart disease is explained in Chapter 13 (which will probably displease both sides). I accept the plasma lipid hypothesis as a basis for action—that is, I believe that most people who are known to have hyperlipidaemia should be treated. But I have an open mind on the diet-heart question; the reader will have to work hard to find out what I think about the eating of eggs by healthy people.

With regard to the atherosclerosis problem in general, I see no advantage in adopting an evangelistic approach, since the question will ultimately be settled by the methods of science. It seems to me that those engaged in the current controversy should try to emulate Darwin, one of whose many endearing traits was a horror of being unfair to his opponents. In his autobiography he records that he kept a special notebook for facts that went against his theory because he found that he tended to forget them (Darwin, 1888). If in the discussion of atherosclerosis I have left out any significant evidence on either side of the argument, this is certainly not deliberate.

I think I owe readers some explanation for having attempted to deal with a subject that cuts across so many scientific disciplines. My main excuse is the belief that in the one-author textbook it is possible to achieve a unity of content, style and point of view not possible in a book written by many people, however strong-minded the editor. On the other hand, the single author cannot be expected to digest the enormous pool of knowledge at the disposal of a group of experts. I am well aware that there is hardly a paragraph in this book that could not have been written with more authority by someone else. An even greater disadvantage to the single author, as I discovered when it was too late to turn back, is the matter of time. In a field that is expanding very rapidly, new facts and new ideas accumulate so quickly that someone who can only write one chapter at a time is apt to get left behind. Chapters 2, 9 and 11 are beginning to look a little faded before they have even appeared in print and I have no doubt that by the time the next book on cholesterol is published several minor revolutions will have forced us to change many of our ideas in unforeseeable ways. The new instruments we are now learning to use may look like museum pieces, we may be using a new language, not based on the ultracentrifuge, for talking about lipoproteins and perhaps—who knows?—somebody will have cloned the DNA coding for pro-LDL-receptor.

London, N. B. Myant
July, 1980

REFERENCES

Darwin, F. *The Life and Letters of Charles Darwin*, including an autobiographical chapter. Edited by his son, Francis Darwin, Vol. 1. John Murray, London, 1888.
Gibbons, G. F., Mitropoulos, K. A. and Myant, N. B. *The Biochemistry of Cholesterol*. Elsevier, Amsterdam, 1982.
Judson, H. F. *The Eighth Day of Creation. Makers of the Revolution in Biology*. Simon and Schuster, New York, 1979.
Nes, W. R. and McKean, M. L. *Biochemistry of Steroids and Other Isopentenoids*. University Park Press, Baltimore, 1977.

Acknowledgements

I could not have written this book without the incalculable benefit of discussion and argument with each of my collaborators with whom I have worked on cholesterol or bile acids:

A. Angel	J. Iliffe	D. Reichl
S. Balasubramaniam	B. L. Knight	L. A. Simons
M. S. Brown	B. Lewis	J. Slack
H. A. Eder	A. A. Magide	A. K. Soutar
K. Fletcher	M. Mancini	M. Suzuki
G. F. Gibbons	K. A. Mitropoulos	G. R. Thompson
J. L. Goldstein	C. D. Moutafis	
I. M. Hais	C. M. Press	

I am also grateful to the following for their expert criticisms of sections of the book in draft:

E. H. Ahrens	L. J. Goad	G. Popják
V. S. Chadwick	S. M. Grundy	J. Slack
W. E. Connor	G. M. Murphy	A. K. Soutar
G. F. Gibbons	K. R. Norum	J. S. Wigglesworth

and to my wife, without whose influence there would have been more redundant verbiage in the text.

Among those listed above I owe a special debt to Howard Eder for more than twenty years of friendship; to Geoffrey Gibbons for always finding time to share his knowledge of the biochemistry of steroids with me; to Ivo Hais, who taught me the elements of stereochemistry during the unforgettable days of the Cuban nuclear missile crisis in 1962; and to Joan Slack, my genetics mentor. I also wish to thank George Popják for his stimulus and encouragement when I began to work on cholesterol. I also thank Dorothy Buyers and Jean De Luca for secretarial help, including the typing of numerous drafts, Katarzyna

Glynn for the diagrams and formulae, and Miss Read and her staff of the Wellcome Library (Royal Postgraduate Medical School) for their unfailing helpfulness. Finally, I thank the Medical Research Council for allowing me and my colleagues in the Lipid Metabolism Unit the greatest possible scientific freedom; throughout almost all my working life this admirable institution has paid me to do what I most enjoy doing.

'The wheel has come full circle'

Raymond Greene, who asked me to write a general text on cholesterol for Heinemann Medical Books, has been very patient throughout what must have seemed an unduly long gestation period (a good deal longer than that of an elephant); I now understand why people who write longish books often acknowledge the help they have had from their publishers. In retrospect, it now seems fitting that it was also Raymond Greene who referred A.A-B. (see Chapter 15) to Barry Lewis and myself in 1963 and thus initiated my continuing interest in familial hypercholesterolaemia, the disease that figures prominently in much of this book.

Partial List of Abbreviations

Å	Ångström unit $= 10^{-8}$ cm; 10 Å $= 1$ mµ $= 10^{-7}$ cm; 10^4 Å $= 1$ µ
ACAT	Acyl-CoA:cholesterol O-acyltransferase
ACR	Absolute catabolic rate
$[\alpha]_D$	Specific rotation for light of the sodium D line measured under specified conditions, usually with chloroform as solvent
CAMP	Cyclic AMP (adenosine 3′,5′-cyclic phosphate)
CD	Circular dichroism
CESD	Cholesteryl ester storage disease
CHD	1,2-Cyclohexanedione (not 'coronary heart disease')
CTX	Cerebrotendinous xanthomatosis
EC	Enzyme Commission; an enzyme is designated by a systematic name and number according to rules laid down by the Enzyme Commission of the International Union of Biochemistry (see Enzyme Nomenclature, Recommendations (1978) of the Nomenclature Committee of the International Union of Biochemistry, Academic Press, New York, 1979)
EHC	Enterohepatic circulation
ESR	Electron spin resonance
FCR	Fractional catabolic rate
FH	Familial hypercholesterolaemia
FPP	Farnesyl pyrophosphate
GLC	Gas-liquid chromatography
HDL	High-density lipoprotein
HMG	β-Hydroxy-β-methylglutar-ate (or -yl)
IDL	Intermediate-density lipoprotein
IHD	Ischaemic heart disease

IR	Infrared
LCAT	Lecithin:cholesterol acyltransferase
LDL	Low-density lipoprotein
m.p.	Melting point
MS	Mass spectrometer
MVA	Mevalonic acid
NMR	Nuclear magnetic resonance
ORD	Optical rotatory dispersion
PP	Pyrophosphate
P/S ratio	The ratio of polyunsaturated (2 or more double bonds) to saturated fatty acids
R_f	The distance run by a substance divided by the distance run by the solvent in a chromatographic system
R_T **(also RRT)**	Relative retention time of a substance on GLC, defined as the time between injection of the sample and the peak maximum, relative to that of a reference compound (usually 5α-cholestane for sterols)
S_f	Flotation rate in the ultracentrifuge measured under specified conditions
SMC	Smooth-muscle cells
T_c	Phase transition temperature
TLC	Thin-layer chromatography
TMS	Trimethylsilyl
UV	Ultraviolet
VLDL	Very-low-density lipoprotein

Conversion table for cholesterol concentration
(mg/100 ml ≡ mmol/l)

mg/100 ml	mmol/l	mg/100 ml	mmol/l
170	4.39	310	8.01
180	4.65	320	8.27
190	4.91	330	8.53
200	5.17	340	8.79
210	5.43	350	9.04
220	5.68	360	9.30
230	5.94	370	9.56
240	6.20	380	9.82
250	6.46	390	10.08
260	6.72	400	10.34
270	6.98	450	11.63
280	7.23	500	12.92
290	7.49	600	15.51
300	7.75	700	18.09

Chapter 1

Chemistry

1	THE DISCOVERY OF CHOLESTEROL AND PLANT STEROLS	3
2	DEFINITIONS	4
2.1	Steroid and sterol	4
2.2	Some stereochemical terms	4
2.2.1	Stereoisomerism	5
2.2.2	Configuration	6
2.2.3	Prochirality and chirality	6
2.2.4	A brief diversion on chirality in nature	9
2.2.5	Conformation	10
2.2.6	Relative and absolute configuration	11
3	RULES FOR STEROID NOMENCLATURE	11
3.1	The need for a system	11
3.2	Numbering of carbon atoms	12
3.3	Configuration	13
3.4	The side-chain	13
3.5	The sequence-rule procedure	15
3.6	A disadvantage of the R/S system	20
3.7	Parent steroids	20
3.8	The language of steroid nomenclature	24
3.9	Trivial names	27
3.10	Nomenclature of isotopically labelled steroids	28
4	THE CONFORMATION OF THE STEROID RING SYSTEM	29
5	THE STEREOCHEMISTRY OF CHOLESTEROL . . .	32
6	HISTORY OF THE ELUCIDATION OF STEROID STRUCTURE AND CONFIGURATION	34
6.1	Early history	34
6.2	Background to later history	34
6.3	The functional groups and the side-chain	35
6.4	The four steroid rings	36
6.5	Configuration	38

2   The Biology of Cholesterol and Related Steroids

7	SOME PHYSICAL AND CHEMICAL PROPERTIES	41
7.1	Physical constants	41
7.2	Liquid crystal formation	42
7.3	Some chemical reactions of cholesterol	43
7.3.1	Formation of digitonides	43
7.3.2	Formation of a dibromide	45
7.3.3	Oxidation by molecular oxygen	45
7.3.4	Colour reactions of sterols	46
7.3.4.1	The Liebermann-Burchard reaction	46
7.3.4.2	The Lifschütz reaction	47
7.3.4.3	Other colour reactions	48
7.3.4.4	Mechanism of colour reactions	48

Chemistry

1 THE DISCOVERY OF CHOLESTEROL AND PLANT STEROLS

The study of gallstones during the latter half of the eighteenth century led to the discovery that the major constituent of most human gallstones is a white crystalline substance soluble in alcohol and ether. Chevreul (1816) named this substance *cholestérine* (Gr. *chole*, bile; *stereos*, solid) but the name cholesterol was adopted by French and English workers when Berthelot (1859) showed that cholesterine was an alcohol. By the 1840's the compound now known as cholesterol had been shown to be a normal constituent of many animal tissues and in 1843 Vogel showed that it was present in the atheromatous lesions of human arteries. In the early years of the present century relatively simple colorimetric and gravimetric methods were developed for the assay of cholesterol in plasma and tissues. The availability of these methods for routine work opened the way for the study of cholesterol by clinicians, pathologists and epidemiologists and is largely responsible for the fact that, in relation to human health and disease, we now have so much more information about cholesterol than about other lipids.

Substances closely resembling cholesterol began to be isolated from fungi and green plants several decades after the discovery and characterization of cholesterol. The first unequivocal report of such a substance was that of Tanret (1889), who isolated a cholesterol-like crystalline compound from rye seeds infected with ergot and called it *ergostérine* (now called *ergosterol*). In 1906, Windaus and Hauth isolated from Calabar beans (*Physostigma venenosum*) a substance, similar to cholesterol, which they designated *stigmasterin*. Since then, a great many other 'sterols' have been isolated from the non-saponifiable fraction obtained from various parts of plants. Some of these are mentioned in Chapter 3.

2 DEFINITIONS

2.1 Steroid and sterol

Many substances present in animals and plants, including those with such diverse biological functions as bile acids, sex hormones and the sapogenins, are related structurally to cholesterol. All these substances have a nucleus containing the four-ringed carbon skeleton of cyclopentenophenanthrene (**1.1**) and are known as *steroids*. The general structural formula for the steroids, including the designation of the four rings, is shown in (**1.2**). R_1 and R_2 are usually methyl groups and R_3 is usually a side-chain. However, in some steroids R_1 is absent (as in oestrone), in others R_2 is modified (as in aldosterone) and in some there is no side-chain.

The term *sterol* is used with different shades of meaning by different writers and cannot be defined precisely. Most commonly it refers to any unsaponifiable steroid alcohol with an aliphatic side-chain of 8–10 carbon atoms and a hydroxyl group at C-3. The word may be prefixed, as in *hydroxysterol* (any sterol with one or more hydroxyl groups additional to that at C-3) and *phytosterol* (sterols present in plants). The term *stenol* usually refers to sterols with one or more nuclear double bonds, and *stanol* to their saturated homologues. Tetracyclic triterpenoids, C_{30} compounds containing the steroid ring system with two additional methyl groups at C-4 and one additional methyl at C-14 (see (**1.3**) for numbering of carbon atoms), are now included within the term *steroid* and may be regarded as 4,4,14-trimethyl steroids.

As a consequence of their mode of biogenesis, naturally occurring steroids usually have the configurations at C-8, 9, 10, 13, 14 and 17 shown in (**1.17**). However, the term may legitimately be extended to include natural or chemically-synthesized compounds containing the steroid ring system but with different stereochemistry at one or more of these centres of asymmetry. In the nomenclature of these atypical steroids, the abnormal configuration must be specified (see Section 3.7).

2.2 Some stereochemical terms

Certain aspects of the stereochemistry of organic molecules are of fundamental importance in the biogenesis and metabolism of cholesterol and other steroids. A brief discussion of some of the relevant terms used in this and later chapters may therefore be helpful to the non-specialist. The main features of the stereochemistry of steroids can be understood fairly easily from diagrams in which the steroid ring system is represented as a flat structure and groups lying above or below the plane of the paper are shown by drawing the

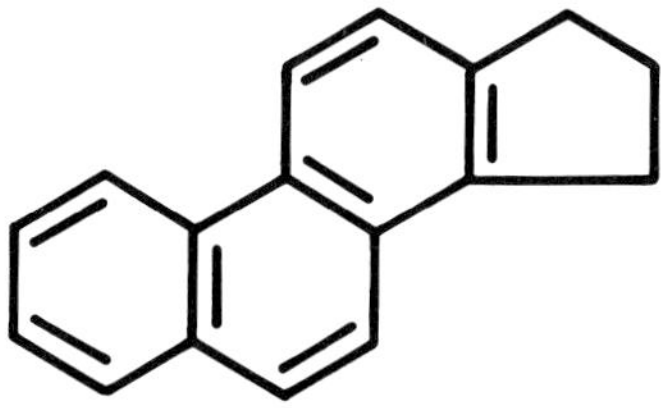

(1.1)

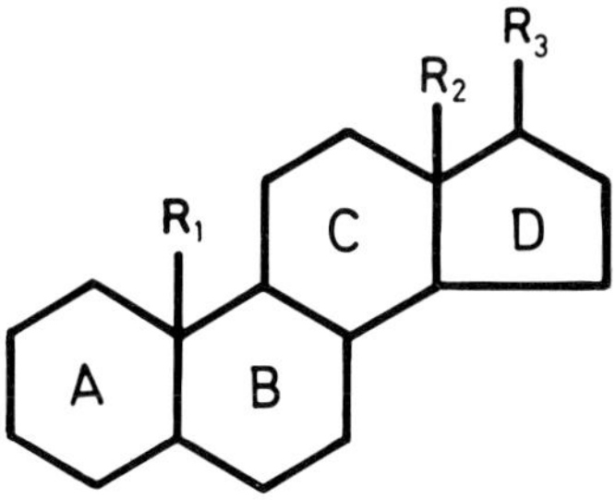

(1.2)

bonds in the way described below. However, the arrangements in space of atoms or groups attached to asymmetric or prochiral centres (see below) may be difficult to appreciate from projections drawn on paper, but become immediately obvious when viewed in a three-dimensional model. Stereochemical relationships can often be demonstrated with everyday objects such as bread pellets and matchsticks or tooth picks. But anyone with a serious interest in the biology of cholesterol would do well to build a model of the molecule with one of the sets available commercially, such as the Dreiding Stereomodels (Büchi, Switzerland) or the Orbit Molecular Building System (RJM Exports Ltd., Oxford, U.K.), and to study it carefully until he or she becomes familiar with all the details of its stereochemistry.

2.2.1 Stereoisomerism

The constitution of a molecule of a given molecular formula defines the sequential arrangement of its atoms. Hence, constitutional isomers have the same molecular formula but different constitutions. A constitutional formula is drawn in two dimensions without regard to the direction of bonds above or below the plane of the paper. Thus:

$$CH_3-CH(OH)-CH_3 \quad \text{and} \quad CH_3-CH_2-CH_2OH$$

are constitutional isomers. Molecules which have the same

constitution but differ in the spatial arrangement of their atoms are known as *stereoisomers*. 5α-Cholestane (**1.21**), for example, is a stereoisomer of 5β-cholestane (**1.22**) but deoxycholic acid is a constitutional isomer of chenodeoxycholic acid.

2.2.2 Configuration

The term *configuration* refers to the arrangement in space of the atoms of a molecule of a given constitution, without regard to differences in spatial arrangement that can be brought about without breaking bonds and re-forming them in a different way. Thus, the configuration of 5α-cholestane is different from that of its *configurational isomer* 5β-cholestane, since a 5α-hydrogen atom cannot be converted into a 5β-hydrogen atom without breaking a bond and re-forming it. The boat and chair forms of cyclohexane (Fig. 1), on the other hand, have the same configuration (see *conformation*).

The term configuration may also be used to denote the spatial arrangement of a particular atom or group in a molecule of a given stereochemical formula. For example, the hydroxyl group at C-3 of lithocholic acid is said to be in α configuration.

In stereochemical formulae, the configuration of an atom or group lying above the plane of the paper is shown by drawing the bond as a thick line (━━) or as a wedge (◢), the broad end of the wedge representing the end of the bond nearer to the observer. The configuration of an atom or group lying below the plane of the paper is shown by drawing the bond as a broken line (----). If the configuration is not known the bond is drawn as a wavy line (∼).

2.2.3 Prochirality and chirality

In order to define *prochirality*, the term 'chiral' must first be considered. If a molecule cannot be superimposed on its own mirror image it is said to be *chiral*, or to possess *chirality* (Gr. *cheir*, a hand), i.e. it may be considered to have a left-hand and a right-hand side which can always be recognized, however the molecule is placed in space. If a molecule can be superimposed on its own mirror image it is said to be *achiral*. The simplest example of a chiral molecule is one in which a carbon atom (C) is attached to four different atoms or groups (*abde*); thus, A cannot be superimposed on its own mirror image (B):

Since a molecule of this form has no element of symmetry, it is said to be *asymmetric* and the carbon atom attached to the four ligands is said to lie at a chiral or asymmetric centre. All asymmetric molecules are optically active and exist in mirror-image forms known as enantiomorphs (enantiomers) (Gr. *enantios*, opposite; *morphi*, shape), e.g. A is the enantiomer of B. Enantiomers rotate the plane of polarized light in equal but opposite directions; in all other respects their physical and chemical properties are similar. A mixture of equal parts of a pair of enantiomers is optically inactive and is called a racemic mixture or a racemate.

A given molecule may have more than one chiral centre. For example, there are eight in cholesterol (carbon atoms 3, 8, 9, 10, 13, 14, 17 and 20), giving a total of 256 (2^8) possible stereoisomers by the van't Hoff rule. If a molecule has two or more chiral centres it can exist in stereoisomeric forms that are not mirror images of one another. Isomers related in this way are termed *diastereomers* or *diastereoisomers*. In the case of cholesterol, for example, only the sterol with the opposite configuration at *each* of the eight chiral centres is the enantiomer of cholesterol. All the other 254 possible stereoisomers are its diastereomers. [Note that for reasons we need not go into here the terms chiral and asymmetric, as applied to molecules or objects, are not quite synonymous (see Hart, 1975)].

A molecule of the form Ca_1a_2bd, where a_1, a_2, b and d are atoms or groups attached to a carbon atom and a_1 and a_2 are identical, is achiral, since it can be superimposed on its own mirror image:

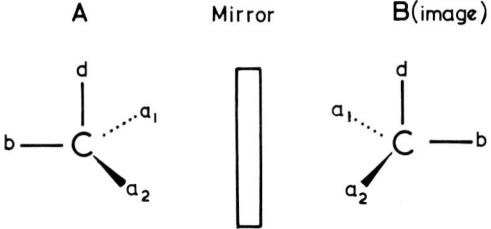

However, although a_1 and a_2 are identical, they are not geometrically equivalent. This can be appreciated by imagining a model of the molecule with b to the rear. In whatever way the model is placed in space, the ligand a_1 in A will always be clockwise with respect to d and a_2 will always be anticlockwise. If either a_1 or a_2 is replaced by a fourth ligand, e, the molecule becomes chiral, the absolute configuration of the chiral molecule depending upon which of the two a ligands is replaced. Hence, a molecule of the form Ca_1a_2bd is said to be *prochiral* and to possess a prochiral centre. The term prochiral may also be used to refer to the atom at the centre of a prochiral group or molecule; a prochiral carbon atom is sometimes called a *meso* carbon atom. A given molecule may have more than one prochiral centre.

For example, there are three in mevalonic acid (carbon atoms 2, 4 and 5). A prochiral molecule exists in only one configuration. Hence, there is no enantiomer of Ca_1a_2bd, where a_1 and a_2 are identical. In the following examples the carbon atom marked with an asterisk is prochiral:

$$HO-\overset{CH_3}{\underset{H}{\overset{|}{*C}}}\cdots H \qquad \text{Ethyl alcohol}$$

$$HO-\overset{COOH}{\underset{CH_2\,COOH}{\overset{|}{*C}}}\cdots CH_2\,COOH \qquad \text{Citric acid}$$

$$R-\overset{H}{\underset{CH_3}{\overset{|}{*C}}}\cdots CH_3 \qquad \text{Cholesterol}$$

(*C is C-25; the two methyl groups are C-26 and C-27; R is the remainder of the molecule)

The above is an attempt to explain prochirality in terms of structures in which the prochiral centre is a carbon atom. A more general definition of prochirality is given in the review by Hanson (1966). The great importance of prochiral carbon atoms in biochemistry is due to the fact that enzymes 'recognize' the non-equivalence of the two identical groups or atoms of a prochiral structure. Hence, every enzymic reaction involving one of the pair of identical atoms or groups linked to a prochiral centre is stereospecific. For example, if one of the two identical a groups in a compound Ca_1a_2bd is replaced enzymically by e, the product will consists almost exclusively of molecules having only one of the two possible configurations (*either* Ca_1bde or Ca_2bde, depending upon the particular enzyme catalyzing the reaction).

A word or two about the relation between prochirality and symmetry may help to clear up a common misunderstanding. The discovery that enzymes distinguish between the two halves of an apparently symmetrical molecule, such as citric acid, at first caused some surprise. It was said that enzymes behave asymmetrically towards symmetrical substrates. However, a prochiral structure is not truly symmetrical, since it has no plane through which it can be bisected into identical halves. A plane passing through the prochiral C atom, the methyl group and the hydroxyl group of ethyl alcohol would divide the molecule into two equal halves, but they would be mirror images of one another that would not be superimposable. In technical terms, a molecule which is achiral but which cannot be divided into superimposable halves is *non-dissymmetric*.

Note that many household objects are prochiral and one usually has little difficulty in distinguishing between the two sides of such objects. For example, a cup with one handle is prochiral. It is superimposable on its own mirror image, but the two halves obtained by bisecting it through the handle could not be made from the same mould. With the handle as a frame of reference, one could point to the side from which a right-handed person would drink.

2.2.4 A brief diversion on chirality in nature

> 'What can more resemble my hand than its image in a looking glass? Yet I cannot put such a hand as I see in the glass in place of the original.'
>
> Immanuel Kant (1724–1804)

The existence of chirality or 'handedness' in nature has been a source of wonder and interest to many artists and scientists since the Renaissance and must, indeed, have been recognized, if unconsciously, by the earliest artists who succeeded in representing chiral structures such as human hands. Leonardo da Vinci, Velázquez, Louis Pasteur and Lord Kelvin and, in our own time, the sculptor Michael Ayrton (see Ayrton, 1978), were but a few of those who have been fascinated by the relation between chiral objects and their enantiomers. However, not all great artists have had an infallible sense of chirality. In Rembrandt's famous 'The Anatomy Lesson of Dr. Tulp' the muscle insertions of the left arm of the corpse are, in fact, those of a right arm; in other words, the corpse in Rembrandt's painting is a diastereomer of a real one.

Although throughout this book we are concerned with chirality only at the molecular level, as implied above, enantiomers are observable in the macroscopic world about us. Our own hands and feet are enantiomeric. At an even higher level of organization, some degree of functional or structural mirror imaging is present in about a quarter of all separate one-egg twins, depending upon the amount of asymmetry that has developed in the embryo before the twinning division occurs, and in Siamese twins mirror imaging may be almost complete (Newman, 1942).

Chirality at the molecular level is a property of all living matter and is a consequence of the fact that the tetravalent carbon atom is a constituent of organic molecules. But this does not explain why a particular one of the two possible enantiomers of a given chiral organic molecule is universally present throughout nature in nearly every known instance. Why, for example, should the cholesterol present in all animal and plant tissues be the enantiomer we know it to be, rather than its mirror image, whose physical and chemical properties are the same and are therefore equally capable of fulfilling the biological functions of cholesterol? From a mechanistic point of view the answer lies in the stereo-specificities of the enzymes catalyzing the stereochemical reactions involved in the biosynthesis of cholesterol (Popják and Cornforth, 1966). But this fails to explain why, in evolutionary terms, the one rather than the other enantiomer has appeared in nature. The answer to the more general question is very relevant to the problem of the origin of life. Some would say that it was a matter of chance as to which configuration was selected in the earliest chiral molecules. Another possibility is that configuration was determined by the 'handedness' of a physical agent, such as plane-polarized UV irradiation, concerned in the non-biological formation of primitive organic molecules. In passing, it is interesting to note that according to a Canon of the Church of England the deity is not chiral; 'God doesn't have ... a right side and a left side', he is reported as saying (Cross, 1977).

2.2.5 Conformation

The term *conformation*, as used in stereochemistry, expresses the fact that the atoms of a molecule of given configuration may exist in different spatial arrangements. Roughly speaking, a change in the conformation of a molecule may be defined as any change in its shape that can be brought about by rotating, bending or stretching bonds without breaking them.

Examples:

(1) Cholesterol can exist in an infinite number of conformations by rotation of the bonds joining the carbon atoms of the backbone of the side-chain. Some of these conformations are more stable than others, but their interconversion requires little energy. Hence, a solution of cholesterol contains an equilibrium mixture of molecules with side-chains in different conformations.

(2) The ring of cyclohexane (C_6H_{12}) can exist in two relatively stable conformations, one resembling a boat (boat form) and the other resembling a chair (chair form). For a discussion of these conformations in relation to the steroid ring system, see p. 30.

Note that although it is useful to distinguish between conformation and configuration, the distinction is not absolute. In general, changes in conformation (as defined above) require only small activation energies, whereas changes in configuration require large activation energies. Hence, the physical separation of conformational isomers is usually difficult or impossible because the isomers are so readily interconvertible, whereas the separation of configurational isomers is in principle always possible. However, there are borderline cases where a change in conformation requires considerable energy of activation, e.g. when steric hindrance is present. The decision as to whether the change is one of conformation or configuration may then be arbitrary.

2.2.6 Relative and absolute configuration

The *relative configuration* of a molecule of a given constitution defines the spatial arrangement of its atoms or groups relative to each other or to the corresponding atoms or groups in a molecule of a different compound. The *absolute configuration* of a molecule defines the absolute spatial arrangement of its atoms or groups when the orientation of the molecule is specified. One may have complete knowledge of the relative configuration at each asymmetric centre of a molecule without knowing its absolute configuration. For example, the configuration at each asymmetric centre of cholesterol, relative to that of the hydroxyl group at C-3, was established before the absolute configuration at any centre had been deduced. Until then, the designation of the C-3 hydroxyl group as β was arbitrary (though correct by chance) and hence it was not known whether the steric formula shown at (**1.29**) was a correct representation of the cholesterol molecule itself or of its mirror image.

3 RULES FOR STEROID NOMENCLATURE

3.1 The need for a system

A few steroids may be referred to without ambiguity by trivial names. The word 'cholesterol', for example, denotes a unique substance of definite molecular constitution and stereochemistry, different from all of its isomers. For the great majority of steroids, however, a descriptive system of nomenclature, capable of extension to all possible steroids, is required. Such a system must provide a set of rules by which the three-dimensional structure of any steroid can be represented diagrammatically in two dimensions and a 'language' for denoting any steroid, including its absolute configuration when this is known, in spoken or written communication. What is needed is analogous to an alphabet from which an almost infinite number of words can be constructed. With minor exceptions, the rules for nomenclature of steroids mentioned in this book follow the 'Definitive Rules for Nomenclature of Steroids' formulated jointly by the International Union of Pure and Applied Chemistry (IUPAC) and the International Union of Biochemistry (IUB). These rules are known as the *IUPAC-IUB 1971 Definitive Rules for Steroid Nomenclature* (see 'IUPAC-IUB Rules' in list of references at the end of this chapter). The following is a brief summary of those IUPAC-IUB rules that apply to cholesterol and related steroids. The earlier convention for notation of the side-chain is also described, since this is still used in many books and journals.

3.2 Numbering of carbon atoms

Formulae of the steroid ring system projected on to the plane of the paper are oriented with ring D in the position shown in (**1.2**). The numbering of the carbon atoms in steroids is shown in the structural formula (**1.3**).

(**1.3**)

If one or more carbon atoms is not present (e.g. C-28 and C-29 are not present in cholesterol) the numbering of the remaining carbons is unchanged. If one of the two methyl groups attached to C-25 is substituted, it is denoted C-26; e.g. 26-hydroxycholesterol (not 27-hydroxycholesterol). This last rule, though convenient, has the disadvantage that C-25 is a prochiral carbon and therefore the two terminal methyl groups are not geometrically equivalent; one is *pro-R* and the other is *pro-S* (see the sequence-rule procedure, Section 3.5, and IUPAC-IUB (1971) formulae (56) and (57) for the method of drawing *R* and *S* configurations at C-25). See Chapter 5, Section 1.2.4 for discussion of this. In (**1.3**) the carbon atom at each angle is assumed to be linked to as many hydrogen atoms as are needed to satisfy its valency of four, and the strokes at C-10, -13, -20, -25 and -28 denote methyl groups.

Note: According to the IUPAC-IUB rules, all hydrogen atoms and methyl groups at ring junctions (-5, -8, -10, -13 and -14) must always be shown as H or CH$_3$ (or Me). This rule is not generally followed and is ignored in this book (as in **1.3**), except in certain special cases.

3.3 Configuration

Rules for depicting the configuration of bonds lying above or below the plane of the paper have already been stated on p. 6. When the steroid formula is oriented as in (**1.3**), groups or atoms attached to the ring system are denoted β if they lie above the plane of the paper or α if they lie below the plane of the paper. If their configuration is not known they are denoted ξ.

3.4 The side-chain

Free rotation of single bonds in the steroid side-chain raises difficulties with regard to its nomenclature. The configuration of C-20 in relation to C-17 is denoted by the α/β/ξ convention applicable to any substituent attached to a ring carbon atom. In the older literature, the configuration of substituents at C-20 in steroids of the pregnane series (see Parent steroids) is specified by orienting the side-chain with the C-21 methyl group to the rear (below the plane of the paper). A substituent to the right is then denoted α and a substituent to the left is denoted β, as in (**1.4**).

By analogy, this convention can be extended to longer side-chains. The C-17 to C-20 bond is rotated so that the longest part of the side-chain is to the rear. A substituent at C-20 is then denoted α if it lies to the right and β if it lies to the left. Thus, the C-21 methyl group shown in the partial formula of cholesterol (**1.5**) is β.

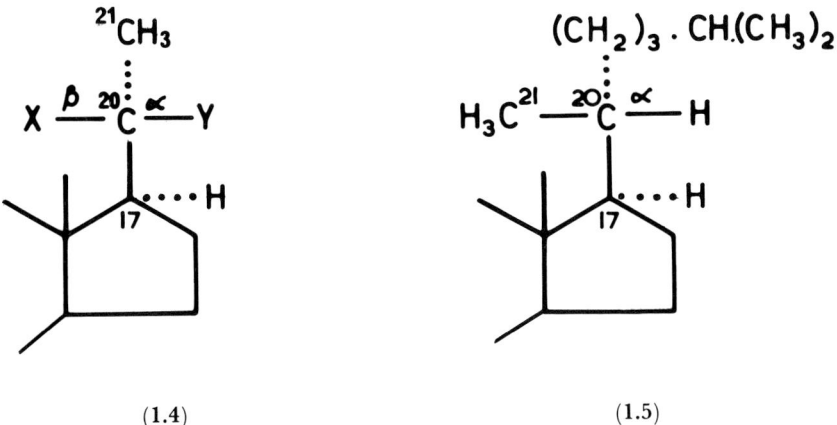

(1.4)   (1.5)

14 The Biology of Cholesterol and Related Steroids

Further extension to substituents at C-22, -23 and -24 is also possible if the side-chain is projected onto the plane of the paper with the longest carbon chain extended up and to the rear according to the Fischer projection. Substituents are then denoted α if they lie to the right and β if they lie to the left. For example, the methyl group attached to C-24 of ergosterol (partial formula (**1.6**)) is β and the ethyl group attached to C-24 of stigmasterol (partial formula (**1.7**)) is α.

(1.6)   (1.7)

The method now generally used for depicting the configuration of atoms or groups attached to asymmetric carbon atoms in the sterol side-chain is to draw the side-chain as a projection on paper, folded either as in (**1.8**) or as in (**1.9**), and to denote the configuration of substituents above or below the plane of the paper, respectively, by wedges or broken lines. Note that the 180° rotation of the C-23–C-24 bond in (**1.8**) to give the folding shown in (**1.9**) reverses the positions of the hydrogen and methyl group at C-24.

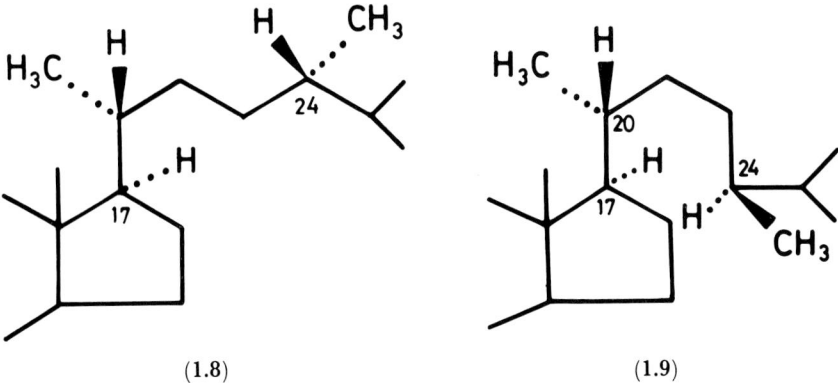

(1.8) (1.9)

3.5 The sequence-rule procedure

Although the older convention for nomenclature of the sterol side-chain has been described in the previous section, the IUPAC-IUB recommend that this convention should be superseded by the *sequence-rule procedure*. This recommendation is now accepted by most chemical and biochemical journals and is generally followed in this book, except that the α/β system is retained for denoting the stereochemistry at C-20 in derivatives of pregnane and in one or two other instances where the older system is more convenient.

The sequence-rule procedure, proposed by Cahn, Ingold and Prelog (1966), is a convention for specifying the configuration of substituents at an asymmetric centre. Its advantage over alternative conventions is that it can be applied without ambiguity to any asymmetric centre and that, with slight modification (Hanson, 1966), it can be used to designate each of the two similar atoms or groups attached to a prochiral carbon atom. Its use in steroid chemistry therefore brings the nomenclature of the stereochemistry of steroids into line with the system used in other branches of chemistry. Only the main outlines of the sequence-rule procedure are described here. For a full account of all the rules the reader should consult the paper by Cahn *et al.* (1966) or the simplified description given by Cahn (1964). Prelog, in his Nobel lecture (Prelog, 1976), also has discussed the problem of devising a universally applicable system of stereochemical nomenclature.

The procedure is carried out in two stages and should be envisaged in terms of a three-dimensional model. The atoms linked directly to the asymmetric centre are given an *order of priority* (or precedence), by applying a series of rules in a definite sequence. When the order of priority has been established, the model is oriented with the atom of lowest priority to the rear. If the order of priority of the remaining

16 The Biology of Cholesterol and Related Steroids

three atoms decreases in a clockwise direction, the configuration is denoted *R* (L. *Rectus*, right). If it decreases in an anticlockwise direction, the configuration is denoted *S* (L. *Sinister*, left). There are four sequence rules, but only the first two need be considered here:

(1) High atomic number precedes low atomic number.
(2) High atomic weight precedes low atomic weight.

A simple example will illustrate the main principles of the procedure. Suppose that a carbon atom is linked to four different atoms, *a*, *b*, *d* and *e*, and that the order of atomic numbers is $a > b > d > e$. Models of the two enantiomers would be viewed with *e* to the rear and the two possible configurations would be as shown, the arrangement on the right in each pair being obtained by rotation of the model around the C-*a* axis through 90° to bring *e* below the plane of the paper:

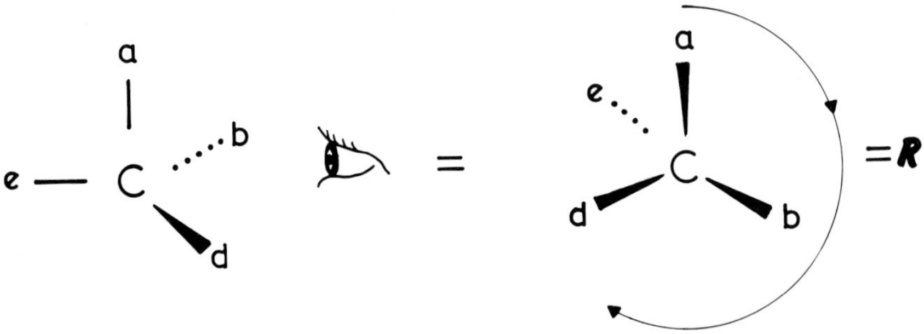

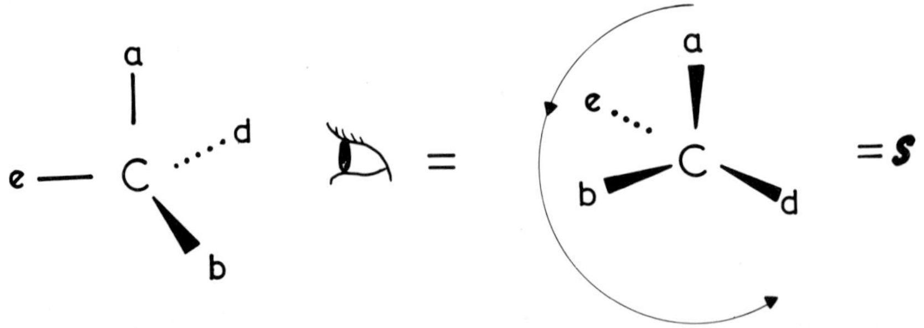

In many cases, two or more of the atoms linked to the asymmetric centre are identical. Priority between identical atoms may then be decided by considering the atoms to which these, in turn, are linked. If priority still cannot be decided, the next atoms in the chain are considered, this process being repeated until a decision is reached.

Examples:

(1) In the compound $CH_2OH.*CH.CH_3$ with Cl on the *C, the order of priority of atoms linked to the asymmetric carbon atom (*C) is

$$Cl > \genfrac{}{}{0pt}{}{CH_2OH}{CH_3} > H$$

The CH_2OH group has priority over CH_3 because of the oxygen atom. Therefore the two possible configurations are:

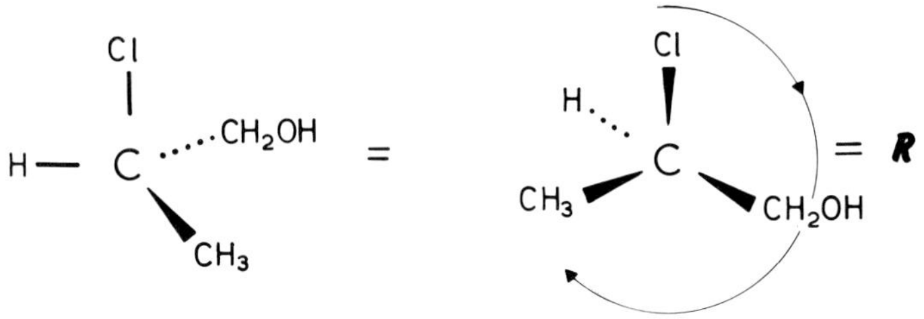

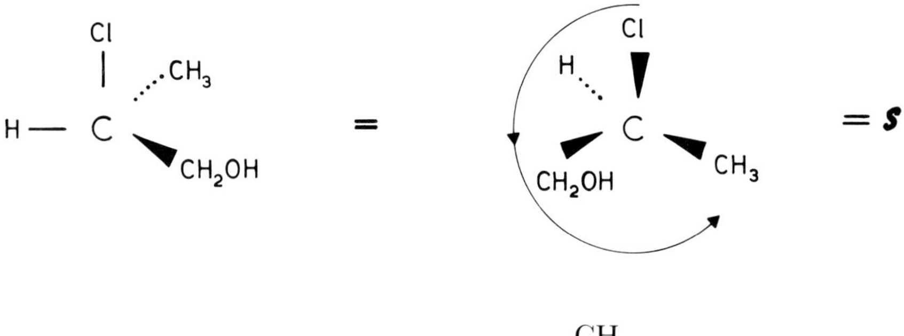

[Figure: Two pairs of stereochemical representations showing configurations labeled $= R$ and $= S$]

(2) In mevalonic acid $\underset{(5)}{CH_2OH}.\underset{(4)}{CH_2}.\overset{\overset{CH_3}{|}}{\underset{(3)}{*COH}}.\underset{(2)}{CH_2}.\underset{(1)}{COOH}$, the order of priority of atoms linked to the asymmetric carbon atom (C-3) is

$$O > \genfrac{}{}{0pt}{}{CH_2.COOH}{CH_2.CH_2OH} > CH_3$$

18 The Biology of Cholesterol and Related Steroids

To determine which of the two CH_2 groups (C-2 and C-4) has priority, we consider the next carbon atom to which each is directly linked. Since COOH has two oxygen atoms it has priority over CH_2OH. Therefore the R configuration is

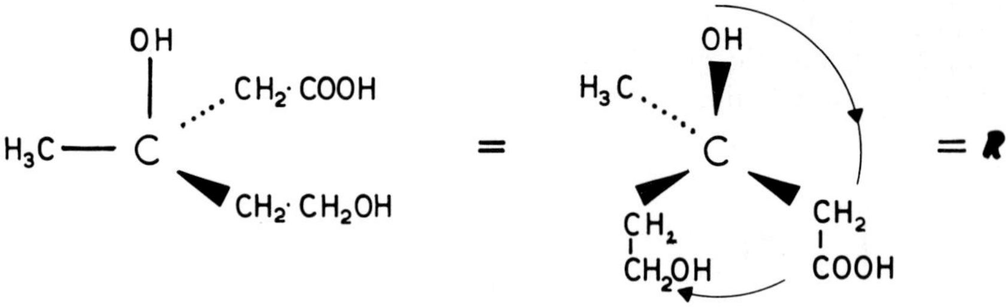

(3) In the α/β notation for substituents in the side-chain of cholesterol, the methyl group attached to the asymmetric carbon atom (C-20) is β. To specify the configuration at C-20 in the R/S notation, we project the structure formed by C-20 and its adjacent carbon atoms on to the plane of the paper as follows:

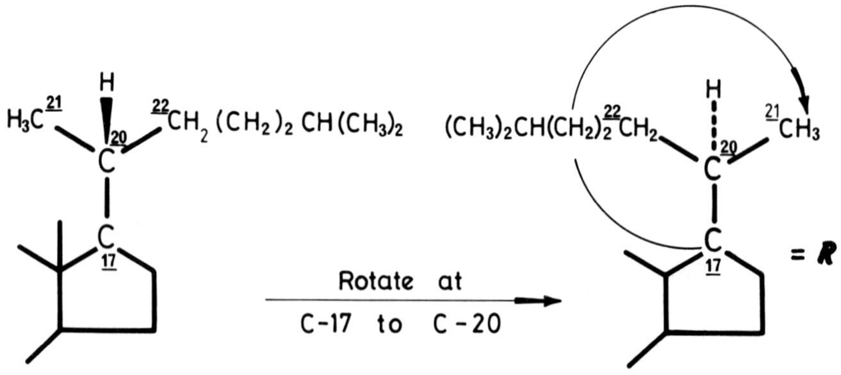

C-17 is linked distally to two carbon atoms and therefore has priority over C-22. C-22 is linked distally to one carbon atom and therefore has priority over C-21. Therefore the order of priority is C-17 > C-22 > C-21 and the configuration at C-20 is R.

By similar reasoning it may be shown that the configuration at C-24 in ergostanol is S.

The R/S notation for specifying configuration may also be extended to prochiral centres. An atom or group a_1 at a prochiral centre Ca_1a_2bd, where a_1 and a_2 are identical, is designated *pro-R* (or *pro-S*) if the centre acquires R (or S) configuration when the priority of a_1 is raised above that of a_2 *without changing its priority relative to b and d.*

Examples:

(1) If the hydrogen atom denoted H_R in ethyl alcohol (**1.10**) is replaced by deuterium, the configuration of the asymmetric molecule so produced is R, since rule 2 of the sequence-rule procedure states that higher atomic weight precedes lower atomic weight. Therefore H_R is the *pro-R* hydrogen. Similarly, H_S is the *pro-S* hydrogen:

(1.10)

(2) In citric acid (**1.11**) the group containing the carbon atom *C is the *pro-R* $CH_2 \cdot COOH$ group, because the asymmetric molecule formed by replacing H_2 by D_2 is R:

(1.11)

Note that if *C is replaced by ^{14}C, the configuration of the molecule becomes S because ^{14}C has priority over ^{12}C; hence the need for the restriction in the italicized part of the definition of *pro-R/S* given above.

(3) In $(3R)$-mevalonic acid (**1.12**) the hydrogen atom denoted H_R at C-5 is the '*pro-R* hydrogen at C-5'.

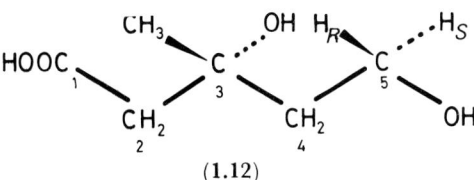

(1.12)

If H_R were replaced by tritium, the radioactive molecule so produced would have an additional centre of asymmetry at C-5 and would be designated $(3R, 5R)$-$[5\text{-}^3H_1]$mevalonic acid. Note that if C-4 in (**1.12**) were replaced by ^{14}C, the configuration of the molecule would still be $3R$. This is so because, although ^{14}C has higher atomic weight than ^{12}C, application of rule 1 of the sequence-rule procedure gives priority to C-2 over C-4. In general, isotopic substitution determines the assignment of R/S configuration at an asymmetric centre only when it is the sole cause of asymmetry (as in the isotopic substitution of the *pro-R* hydrogen at C-5 of mevalonic acid by tritium).

3.6 A disadvantage of the R/S system

The R/S system for denoting the configuration at a chiral centre has the minor drawback that the designation at a given centre may be changed by a change in other parts of the molecule. For example, assignment of the configuration at C-3 of hydroxymethylglutaryl-CoA (HMG-CoA) is changed when HMG-CoA is reduced to mevalonic acid in the biosynthesis of cholesterol (see p. 187). In the natural enantiomer of HMG-CoA the configuration at C-3 is S, but when the —CO.SCoA group at C-5 of HMG-CoA is reduced to the —CH_2OH group of mevalonic acid, C-5 loses priority to C-1 and the configuration at C-3 becomes R. The change is, of course, only a nominal one and does not involve any change in the spatial relations of the four groups attached to C-3. Another example concerns the effect of a double bond on the configuration at C-24 of the sterol side-chain. The side-chains of β-sitosterol (**1.13**) and stigmasterol (**1.14**) both have an ethyl group at C-24 in α configuration according to the old terminology. However, while β-sitosterol is $24R$, stigmasterol is $24S$ because the Δ^{22} double bond gives precedence to C-23 over C-25. By similar reasoning ergostanol (**1.15**) is $24S$ and ergosterol (**1.16**) is $24R$, although both have the 24β configuration.

Despite such problems as these in the application of the R/S system (see, also, Arigoni and Eliel, 1969), the advantages of the sequence-rule procedure far outweigh its disadvantages as a component of a language for transmitting complete three-dimensional information about a compound containing any number of asymmetric centres. With the help of models and a little practice, the R/S system of notation is not difficult to learn. Its invention was a landmark in the history of chemical nomenclature and it is now used in almost all the relevant current textbooks and journals, and in catalogues of labelled and unlabelled compounds.

3.7 Parent steroids

The language of steroid nomenclature is based on the names used for a small number of parent or stem compounds from which all other steroids are considered to be derived structurally. Any steroid may

Chemistry 21

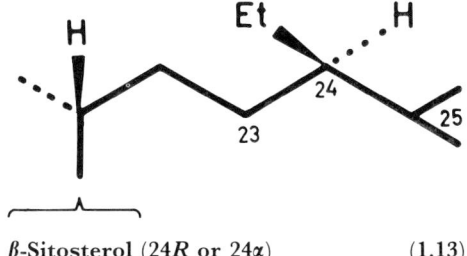

β-Sitosterol (24R or 24α)   (1.13)

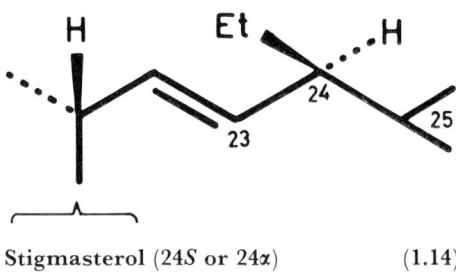

Stigmasterol (24S or 24α)   (1.14)

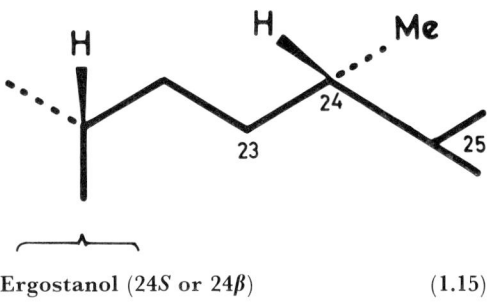

Ergostanol (24S or 24β)   (1.15)

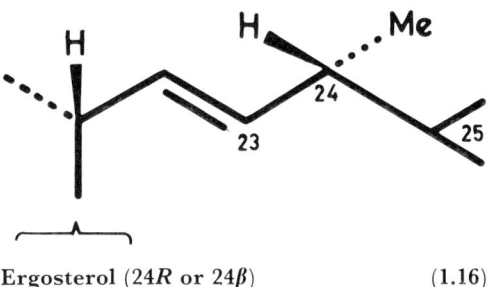

Ergosterol (24R or 24β)   (1.16)

22 The Biology of Cholesterol and Related Steroids

then be given a systematic name by inflexion of the stem name and addition of affixes to denote modifications to the parent steroid. Each parent compound contains a steroid ring system in which the configuration at all asymmetric centres except C-5 is implied. For the nomenclature of atypical steroids in which the configuration at one or more centres of asymmetry differs from that shown in (**1.19**), see IUPAC-IUB (1971). Most of the steroids closely related biologically to cholesterol are structural derivatives of one or other of the four stem compounds:

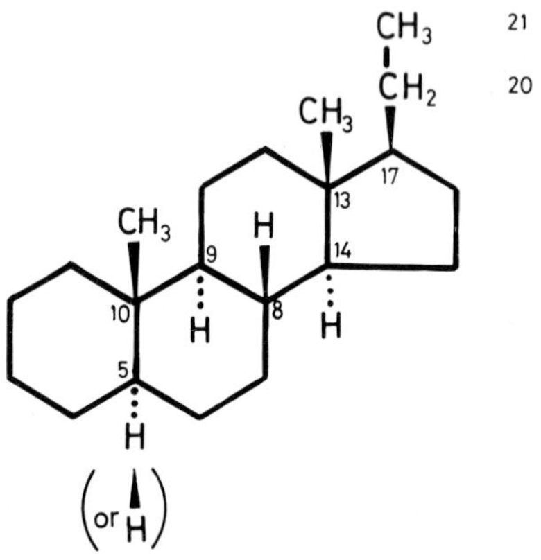

Pregnane (1.17)

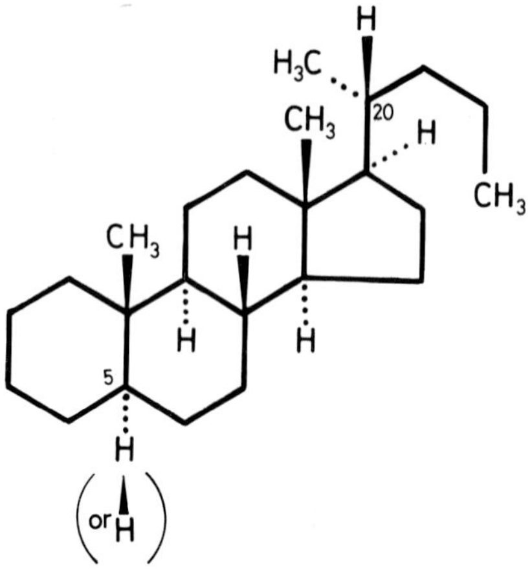

Cholane (1.18)

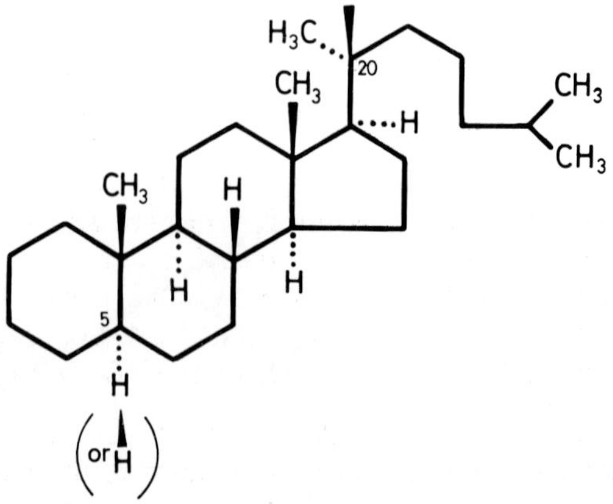

Cholestane (1.19)

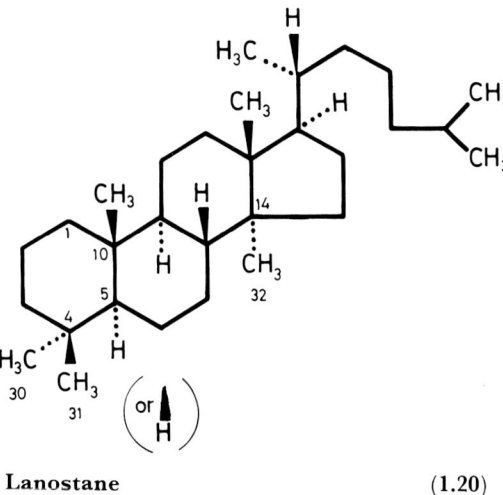

Lanostane (1.20)

The formulae of all the parent steroids, including those of spirostans, azasteroids, cardenolides and other steroids with a heterocyclic side-chain, will be found in IUPAC-IUB (1971).

The following points should be noted in relation to the above parent compounds:

(1) In all four, the configuration of the methyl groups at C-10 and C-13, and of the side-chain at C-17, is β.

(2) In all four, the configuration of the hydrogen or methyl group at C-9 and C-14 is α and of the hydrogen atom at C-8 is β.

(3) The configuration at C-20 in cholane, cholestane and lanostane is R (i.e., the C-21 methyl group is β, according to the α/β system for nomenclature of the side-chain exemplified in (**1.5**)).

(4) In lanostane the three additional methyl groups are numbered 30 (4α), 31 (4β) and 32 (14α).

(5) The configuration of the hydrogen atom at C-5 may be α or β. This isomerism gives rise to two series of steroids derived from each of the four parent steroids. In the 5β series the methyl group at C-10 and the hydrogen atom at C-5 are oriented on the same side of the ring system and the A/B ring junction is therefore *cis*. In the 5α series the C-5 hydrogen atom and the C-10 methyl group are on opposite sides of the ring system and the A/B ring junction is *trans*. In both series of steroids the B/C and C/D ring junctions are *trans* except in the cardiac aglycones and toad poisons, in which the C/D ring junction is *cis*.

Various abbreviated forms of the complete stereochemical formula of a steroid are commonly used. For example, in many journals the methyl groups are not shown as CH_3, the configurations at C-10, C-13 and C-17 are not specified and the hydrogen atoms at C-8, C-9 and

24 The Biology of Cholesterol and Related Steroids

C-14 are omitted. In such formulae, all the configurations shown in (**1.17**), (**1.18**), (**1.19**) and (**1.20**), as well as the R configuration at C-20, are implied. Thus 5α- and 5β-cholestane may be represented by (**1.21**) and (**1.22**), respectively.

5α-Cholestane   (**1.21**)

5β-Cholestane   (**1.22**)

3.8 The language of steroid nomenclature

Unsaturation is denoted by changing the terminal 'ane' of the parent hydrocarbon to 'ene', 'adiene', 'triene', etc., for one, two, three, etc., double bonds. The position of a double bond is indicated by inserting the number of the carbon atom with the lower number of the pair linked by the double bond. If the double bond links two carbon atoms not consecutively numbered, both numbers are inserted. For example, (**1.23**) is cholesta-5,8(14)-diene.

Note that double bonds are no longer indicated by Δ in systematic names, but Δ may be used in a general sense, e.g. 'a Δ^5-steroid'.

Substituents are denoted by prefixes or suffixes. When a suffix is added to the name of the parent hydrocarbon, the terminal *e* of 'ane', 'ene', etc., is omitted before a vowel or the letter *y*. Table 1.1 lists some of the commoner affixes used in the nomenclature of steroids.

Chemistry 25

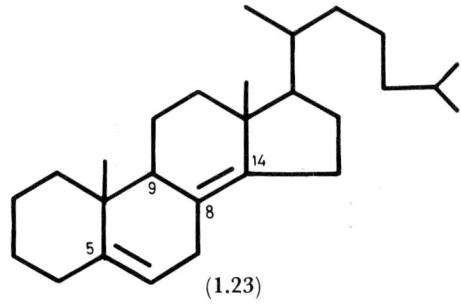

(1.23)

Table 1.1
Some affixes used in the systematic nomenclature of steroids

Substituent	Prefix	Suffix
Acetate, CH₃.COO	acetoxy	yl acetate
Carbonyl, C:O	oxo (not keto)	one
Carboxylic acid, .CO₂H	carboxy	oic acid
		(sometimes ic acid)
Epoxide, —O—	epoxy	—
Hydroxyl, .OH	hydroxy	ol
Amine, .NH₂	amino	amine

Only one suffix should be used in a systematic name. If more than one affix is required, the suffix should be chosen according to the following decreasing order of preference: carboxylic acid, ester, aldehyde, ketone, alcohol. The position of the substituent and, when applicable, its configuration, are denoted by a carbon number and Greek letter before the affix. The configuration of a substituent attached to a carbon atom in the side-chain, if known, is denoted by a prefix including the number of the carbon atom and the letter *R* or *S* (e.g., (24*S*)-).

The following examples illustrate some of the above rules:

5α-Cholestan-3β-ol   (1.24)

26 The Biology of Cholesterol and Related Steroids

5α-Cholestane-3β,7α-diol (1.25)

3β,7α-Dihydroxy-5α-cholest-8(14)-en-26-oic acid (1.26)

3β,7α-Dihydroxy-12-oxo-5α-cholest-8-en-26-oic acid (1.27)

3β,7α,24-Trihydroxycholest-5-en-12-one (1.28)

(If the configuration of the 24-hydroxyl group were known to be S, the systematic name of (**1.28**) would be $(24S)$-$3\beta,7\alpha,24$-trihydroxycholest-5-en-12-one).

3.9 Trivial names

Trivial names may be used for many steroids. However, apart from the few exceptions which cannot give rise to ambiguity, the systematic name should always be given with the first reference to the compound. Some journals permit modification of certain trivial names by prefixes indicating the addition or removal of substituents, provided that the position and, when relevant, the configuration are indicated, e.g. 7α-hydroxycholesterol, 7-dehydrocholesterol, 26-hydroxycholesterol. The prefix *deoxy* (or *desoxy*) is used to denote replacement of a hydroxyl group by a hydrogen atom, e.g. deoxycholic acid (see p. 235). The prefix *allo* (Gr. *allos*, change) is used to denote 5α configuration in steroids which usually have the 5β configuration, e.g. allolithocholic acid (see p. 241). The prefix *epi* is used to denote the inversion of a substituent, usually a hydroxyl group, from its usual configuration, e.g. epicoprostanol (5β-cholestan-

Table 1.2
Trivial names of some steroids

Trivial name	Systematic name
Agnosterol	*4,4,14-Trimethyl-5α-cholesta-7,9(11),24-trien-3β-ol
Cholanic acid	5β-Cholan-24-oic acid
Cholestane	5α-Cholestane
Cholestanol	5α-Cholestan-3β-ol
Cholestanone	5α-Cholestan-3-one
Cholesterol	Cholest-5-en-3β-ol
Cholic acid (and see Chapter 5 for other bile acids)	$3\alpha,7\alpha,12\alpha$-Trihydroxy-5β-cholan-24-oic acid
Coprostane	5β-Cholestane
Coprostanol (also coprosterol)	5β-Cholestan-3β-ol
Coprostanone	5β-Cholestan-3-one
7-Dehydrocholesterol	Cholesta-5,7-dien-3β-ol
Desmosterol	Cholesta-5,24-dien-3β-ol
Epicholestanol	5α-Cholestan-3α-ol
Epicoprostanol	5β-Cholestan-3α-ol
7α-Hydroxycholesterol	Cholest-5-ene-$3\beta,7\alpha$-diol
Lanosterol	*4,4,14-Trimethyl-5α-cholesta-8,24-dien-3β-ol
Lathosterol	5α-Cholest-7-en-3β-ol
Methostenol (also lophenol)	4α-Methyl-5α-cholest-8-en-3β-ol
Zymosterol	5α-Cholesta-8,24-dien-3β-ol

* Note that lanosterol and its derivatives may also be regarded as derivatives of a parent steroid lanostane (IUPAC-IUB, 1971, formula (27)) containing two methyl groups at C-4 and one α-methyl group at C-14 of cholestane. Thus, lanosterol may be called 5α-lanosta-8,24-dien-3β-ol.

28 The Biology of Cholesterol and Related Steroids

3α-ol). *Epimerization* refers to the conversion of a compound to its epi-isomer.

Table 1.2 lists some trivial names that are to be found in the older literature or are still in use. Many others are mentioned in later chapters of this book, particularly in the sections dealing with plant steroids, bile acids and corticosteroids. Trivial names, provided that they stand for well-defined substances, play a necessary though limited role in the language of steroid chemistry and biochemistry. For a steroid, such as cholesterol, that is frequently referred to or is biologically important, the trivial name may continue in use after its structure has been elucidated to the point where it can be given a systematic name.

3.10 Nomenclature of isotopically labelled steroids

The system most generally used for designating isotopically labelled steroids (and other organic compounds) is that known as the 'square-brackets-preceding' system, in which the symbol for the isotope is placed within square brackets before the name for the part of the molecule containing the label, e.g. [^{3}H]cholesterol; cholesteryl[^{14}C]oleate; [^{3}H]cholesteryl oleate; [^{3}H]cholesteryl-[^{14}C]oleate. For details, including punctuation, see IUPAC (1977).

Note that a specimen of a compound with multiple labelling can often be prepared either by mixing specimens of the singly-labelled compounds or by a biological or chemical synthesis which results in the presence of labelling at more than one position in a given molecule. Thus, a specimen of [^{3}H]cholesteryl[^{14}C]oleate prepared by mixing [^{3}H]cholesteryl oleate with cholesteryl[^{14}C]oleate would contain no doubly-labelled molecules, whereas a specimen synthesized from [^{3}H]cholesterol and [^{14}C]oleic acid would consist of a mixture of unlabelled molecules, molecules containing one or other of the two labels and a very small proportion of molecules containing both labels. In the latter case, the proportions of each class of molecule in the mixture can be deduced from the specific activities of the [^{3}H]cholesterol and the [^{14}C]oleic acid used in the synthesis.

The positions of isotopic labelling are designated by Arabic numbers placed before the symbol for the isotopic element, e.g. [4-^{14}C]cholesterol; [1,4-^{14}C]cholesterol (cholesterol labelled in positions 1 and 4). The configuration of the label in steroids or other compounds labelled stereospecifically with tritium or deuterium is indicated by Greek letters or by the *R/S* system, e.g. [7α-^{3}H]cholesterol; [4-^{14}C; 6β,7α-^{3}H$_2$]cholesterol (cholesterol labelled with ^{14}C at position 4 and with tritium at positions 6β and 7α); (2*R*, 3*R*, 4*S*)-[2-^{14}C; 2,4-^{3}H$_2$]mevalonic acid (3*R*-mevalonic acid labelled with ^{14}C at position 2 and with the *pro-R* hydrogen at C-2 and the *pro-*

S hydrogen at C-4 replaced by tritium). Note that the chemically synthesized [^{14}C]cholesterol designated [26-^{14}C]cholesterol is labelled at C-26 and C-27 and should be designated [26(27)-^{14}C]cholesterol.

The letter U, as in [U-^{14}C]glucose, denotes more or less uniform labelling at all positions. The letter G, as in [G-^{3}H]cholesterol, indicates that the label is present at most of the possible positions but is not uniform. The letter n or N (standing for 'nominal') placed after the Arabic number denoting the position of an isotopic label indicates that the label is expected to be predominantly at that position. For example, [7α(n)-^{3}H]cholesterol refers to cholesterol which, from its method of preparation, is expected to contain its tritium predominantly but not exclusively in the 7α position. If 95% or more of the label is present at a single position, the compound is considered to be specifically labelled. For further details and for methods of determining the position and configuration of the tritium in labelled compounds see the catalogue of radiochemicals supplied by The Radiochemical Centre, Amersham, U.K. and the review by Chambers *et al.* (1978).

4 THE CONFORMATION OF THE STEROID RING SYSTEM

The three-dimensional shape of the steroid ring system can best be appreciated by first considering cyclohexane (C_6H_{12}). The cyclohexane ring can exist in two relatively stable conformations, one resembling a boat (boat form) and the other resembling a chair (chair form). Models of a cyclohexane molecule in the two conformations are shown in Fig. 1.1. Inspection of Fig. 1.1 shows that in both models half of

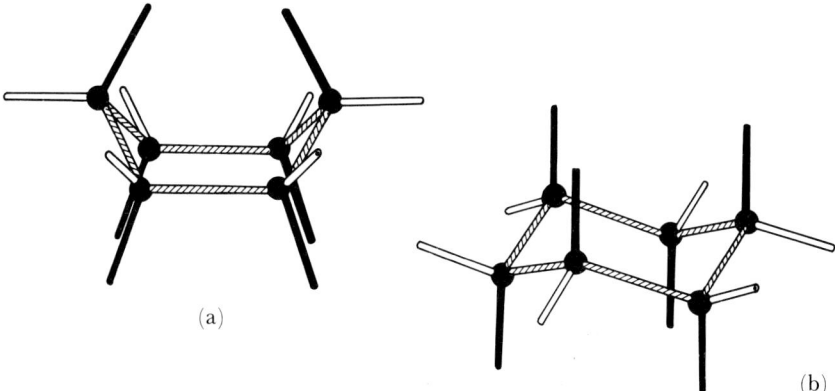

Figure 1.1
Models of the cyclohexane ring in boat (a) and chair (b) conformation. White, equatorial; black, axial.

30   The Biology of Cholesterol and Related Steroids

the twelve C—H bonds lie roughly in the general plane of the ring (*equatorial, e*) and half lie roughly at right angles to this plane (*axial, a*).

In the steroid nucleus, rings A, B and C are usually in the more stable chair form in both the 5α and the 5β series, but the angle between the planes of rings A and B is influenced by the configuration of the hydrogen atom at C-5. Perspective formulae of the 5α and 5β steroid ring systems, and the conformations (whether *e* or *a*) of the hydrogen atoms or methyl groups attached to the rings, are shown in Figs. 1.2 and 1.3. The conformations at C-6, 7, 8, 9, 11, 12, 13, 14, 15, 16 and 17 are the same in the 5α and 5β series, but the conformations with respect to ring A at C-1, 2, 3, 4 and 10 are different. For example, a β substituent at C-3 is equatorial in the 5α series, but is axial in the 5β

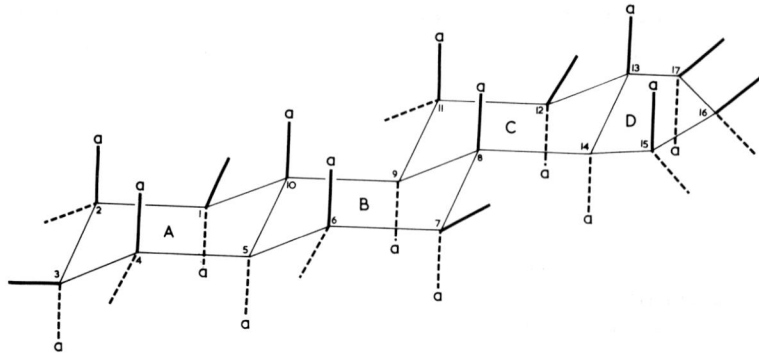

Figure 1.2
Projection of the steroid ring system with *trans* A/B ring fusion (5α hydrogen) to show axial (a) or equatorial orientation of substituents.

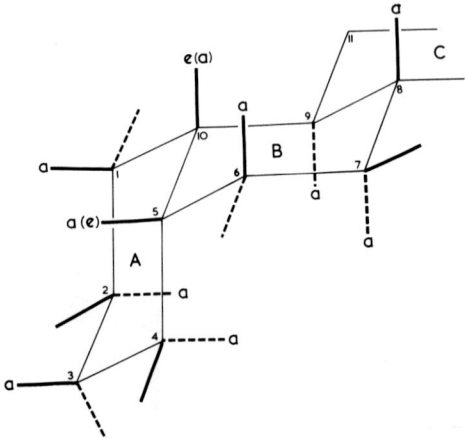

Figure 1.3
Projection of the steroid ring system with *cis* A/B ring fusion (5β hydrogen) to show axial (a) or equatorial orientation of substituents.

series. The conformations of α and β substituents at the carbon atoms of the ring system in the 5α and 5β cholestane series are shown in Table 1.3.

The conformation of a substituent in the steroid nucleus has a considerable influence on its stability and reactivity. Since adjacent axial groups are closer to each other than are adjacent equatorial groups, and therefore repel each other more strongly, a substituent is usually more stable if it is equatorial than if it is axial. Reactions depending upon the accessibility of a nuclear substituent, such as hydrolysis of an ester, or acylation of a hydroxyl group, are generally more rapid if the substituent is equatorial. The conformation of substituents also influences the behaviour of steroids during adsorption or partition chromatography, and may significantly limit or facilitate the chromatographic separation of isomers. Equatorial hydroxyl groups are more strongly adsorbed than axial hydroxyl groups, and in some cases this effect outweights the effect of the

Table 1.3

The conformation of substituents at C-1 to C-17 of the steroid ring system with A/B trans (5α) and A/B cis (5β) fusion. This Table should be read in conjunction with *Figs. 1.2 and 1.3*

Carbon atoms	A/B trans α position	A/B trans β position	A/B cis α position	A/B cis β position
1	ax	eq	eq	ax
2	eq	ax	ax	eq
3	ax	eq	eq	ax
4	eq	ax	ax	eq
5	ax	—	—	ax(A),eq(B)
10	—	ax	—	eq(A),ax(B)

Carbon atoms	A/B trans and A/B cis β position	A/B trans and A/B cis α position
6	eq	ax
7	ax	eq
8	—	ax
9	ax	—
11	eq	ax
12	ax	eq
13	—	ax
14	ax	—
15	eq	ax
17	ax	eq

Note: In the A/B *cis* configuration (Fig. 1.3), the planes of the A and B rings are at right angles so that substituents at C-5 and C-10 are axial with respect to one ring and equatorial with respect to the other. As shown in Fig. 1.2, substituents at C-16 are neither axial nor equatorial with respect to ring D.

32 The Biology of Cholesterol and Related Steroids

configuration of the A/B ring-junction. For example, 5β bile acids (*cis*-A/B-fusion) are in general less strongly adsorbed, and therefore have faster mobility, than their 5α isomers (*trans*-A/B-fusion); but allolithocholic acid, a 5α bile acid in which the 3α-hydroxyl group is axial (see Fig. 1.2), has faster mobility than lithocholic acid, the 5β isomer in which the 3α -hydroxyl group is equatorial (see Fig. 1.3). For a comprehensive account of the influence of conformation on the chemical reactions of steroids see Gibbons *et al.* (1982).

5   THE STEREOCHEMISTRY OF CHOLESTEROL

Cholesterol ($C_{27}H_{45}OH$) is cholest-5-en-3β-ol. The main features of its stereochemistry, some of which have already been referred to, are shown in (**1.29**).

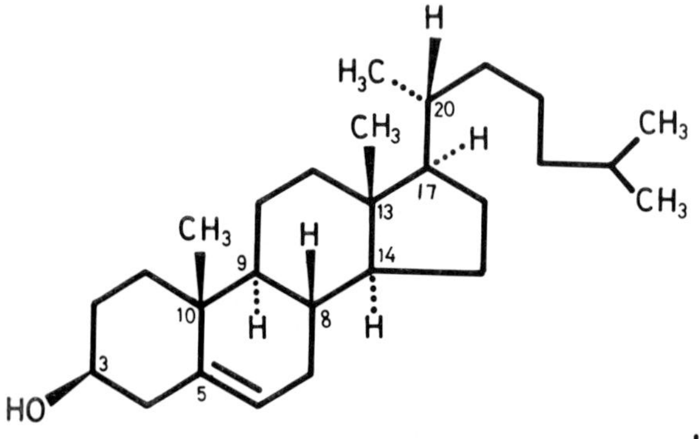

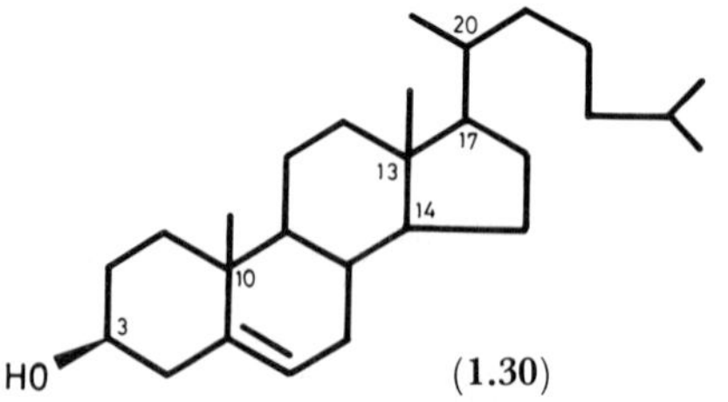

The following points should be noted:

(1)   The angular methyl groups at C-10 and C-13, the hydrogen atom at C-8 and the side-chain at C-17 are in β configuration.
(2)   The hydrogen atoms at C-9 and C-14 are in α configuration.
(3)   The configuration at C-20 is R.

All these configurations are implied in the root (*cholest*) of the systematic name for cholesterol and are usually omitted in structural formulae of cholesterol unless there is a specific reason for denoting them. Many less informative modifications of (**1.29**) are in common use, particularly (**1.30**). In some cases the configuration of the 3-hydroxyl group is not denoted, the bond being drawn as a line of normal thickness.

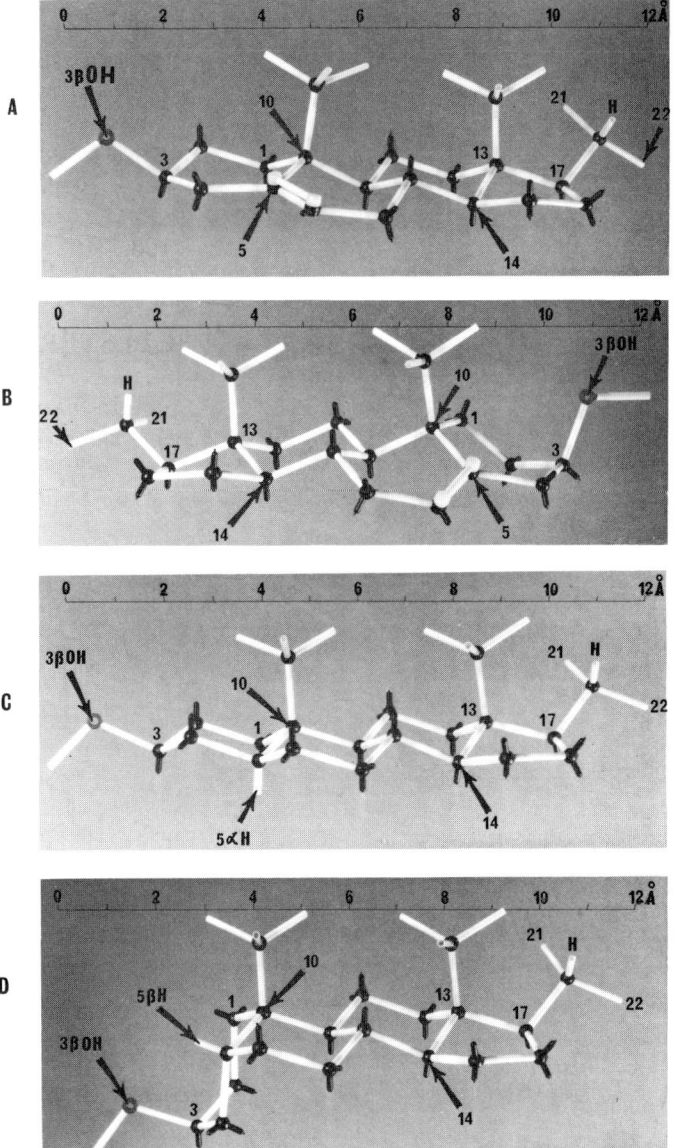

Figure 1.4
Models of cholesterol and of closely related sterols to show the flattening effect of the Δ^5 double bond and the 5α-configuration.

A, cholesterol. B, the enantiomer of cholesterol ('Cholesterol Through the Looking-Glass'). The configuration at each of the eight asymmetric centres in B is the opposite of that in A. B could not be superimposed on A but either could be superimposed on the mirror image of the other. C, 5α-cholestan-3β-ol. D, 5β-cholestan-3β-ol.

The fragment of side-chain attached to C-22 is omitted in each model. The models were made with the Orbit Molecular Building System. Note the scale in Å units.

In the unconstrained state, the ring system of cholesterol is flatter than that of 5α-cholestane (Fig. 1.2), owing to the presence of the double bond in ring B. Fig. 1.4 shows models of cholesterol and of 5α- and 5β-cholestanol illustrating the flattening effect of the Δ^5 double bond.

6 HISTORY OF THE ELUCIDATION OF STEROID STRUCTURE AND CONFIGURATION

6.1 Early history

Although cholesterol was recognized as a distinct chemical substance in 1816, little progress towards elucidating its structure had been made by the end of the nineteenth century. The observation that cholesterol is capable of forming esters (Berthelot, 1859) and a dibromide (Wislicenus and Moldenhauer, 1868) showed that it is an alcohol with one double bond. The empirical formula ($C_{27}H_{46}O$) established by Reinitzer (1888) excluded a straight-chain compound with one double bond, since this would not have had enough hydrogen atoms to satisfy the carbon valency of four, but was consistent with a structure containing four rings with two shared carbon atoms at each ring junction (four fused rings). Two other lines of investigation made before the turn of the century were to become important in the subsequent development of ideas about the structure of steroids. First, establishment of the empirical formula of cholic acid by Strecker (1848) and of deoxycholic acid by Mylius (1886) showed that the ratio of C to H in bile acids (1.67) is similar to that in cholesterol (1.70). This, together with the association of bile acids with cholesterol in bile, suggested that bile acids and cholesterol have structural features in common. The second investigation of historical importance made during this period was the demonstration that a substance isolated from human faeces by Flint (1862), and later called coprosterol (Gr. *kopros*, dung), was formed by the saturation of cholesterol by bacteria in the intestine (Bondzyński and Humnicki, 1896). According to present-day nomenclature, coprosterol (or coprostanol; see Table 2) is 5β-cholestan-3β-ol. Structural studies of this compound played an important role in the elucidation of the configuration of sterols. References to most of this early work are given in Fieser and Fieser (1959).

6.2 Background to later history

During the early years of the present century several of the most gifted organic chemists of their day devoted the greater part of their working, lives to the problem of steroid structure. By 1932 the structure of cholesterol and the commoner bile acids had been established and some features of their stereochemistry had been elucidated, largely owing to the work of Diels (1876–1954), Windaus (1876–1959), Wieland (1877–1957) and their collaborators. The approach used initially was to deduce structural features of cholesterol by identifying the products obtained by attacking the molecule at its two reactive sites (the OH group and the double bond). Once Windaus and Neukirchen (1919) had proved that the carbon skeleton of bile acids is identical with that of the greater part of the cholesterol molecule, information obtained from structural studies of bile acids could be applied directly to the study of cholesterol. The advantage of this approach was that the presence of the OH group in ring C of cholic and deoxycholic acids enabled Wieland and his collaborators to penetrate further into the steroid ring system than was possible with cholesterol.

To appreciate fully the achievement of these early workers it must be remembered that modern physical techniques for structural analysis of steroids were not available to them and that an analysis of a complex mixture which can now be completed in a few hours could then have taken months. A detailed historical account of the work of this period will be found in Fieser and Fieser (1959) and a more condensed account has been given by Kritchevsky (1958). In this chapter, only a brief outline is given, with a few illustrative examples. In order to simplify the narrative, chemical reactions from which structural features were first deduced are described in terms of present-day knowledge of steroid chemistry, a knowledge that was not, of course, available at the time. Finally, stereochemical studies, culminating in the establishment of the absolute configuration at all centres of asymmetry, are dealt with separately although some of the relative configurations at asymmetric centres in cholesterol and bile acids had been deduced correctly from chemical evidence by 1932.

6.3 The functional groups and the side-chain

In 1904 Diels and Abderhalden showed that the hydroxyl group of cholesterol is attached to a ring carbon atom. At about the same time, Windaus and coworkers showed that the double bond of cholesterol is in a ring adjacent to the one containing the hydroxyl group and they suggested correctly that the double bond and the OH group are related according to the sequence

However, *proof* that the hydroxyl group is at C-3 was not obtained until many years later (Farmer and Kon, 1937). The structure of the side-chain of cholesterol was elucidated by Windaus and Resau (1913), who identified methyl isohexyl ketone (**1.31**) as a product of the oxidation of cholesterol by chromic acid, the keto group being at the site of cleavage of the side-chain from the steroid nucleus.

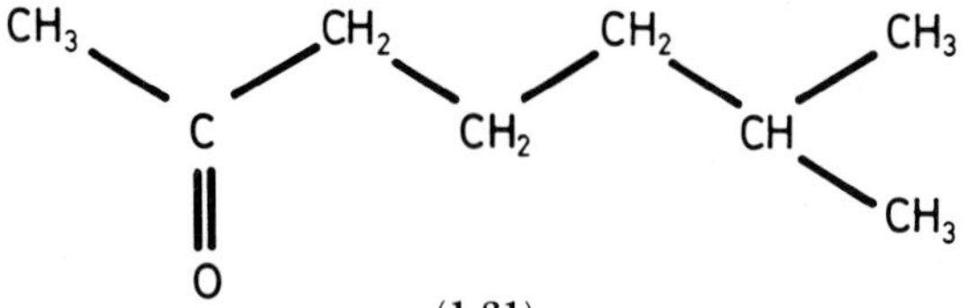

(1.31)

The position of the steroid side-chain was established by Wieland and Dane (1933), who showed that compound (**1.32**) is formed by cyclization of the side-chain of a 12-keto bile acid, C-23 becoming linked to C-12 to form a new six-membered ring with loss of CO_2.

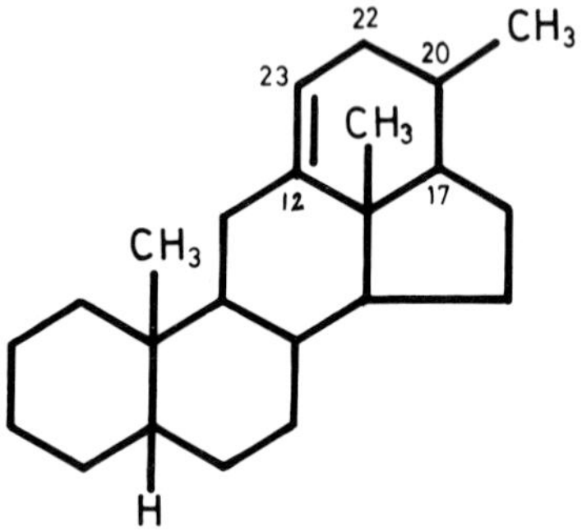

(1.32)

6.4 The four steroid rings

The approach used initially for investigation of steroid ring structure was to open the rings successively by oxidative cleavage and then to deduce the number of carbon atoms in each ring by applying the Blanc rule (see Kritchevsky, 1958). Using this approach, Windaus and Dalmer (1919) proved that ring A of cholesterol is six-membered. Further progress became possible when Windaus and Neukirchen (1919) prepared cholanoic acid by removing the terminal three carbon atoms of the side-chain of 5β-cholestane. This showed that cholesterol and cholic acid have the same ring skeleton, since 5β-cholestane had already been synthesized from cholesterol. Thus, bile acids could now be used for studies of the ring system of sterols.

Wieland and his collaborators investigated the ring system of deoxycholic acid by successive oxidation of rings A, C (then defined

Chemistry 37

as the ring containing the hydroxyl group) and B, followed by application of the Blanc rule. They concluded, correctly, that rings A and B are six-membered but, incorrectly, that ring C is five-membered. Wieland *et al.* (1926) later succeeded in opening ring D after stepwise removal of the carbon atoms of the side-chain of methyl cholanoate. Application of Blanc's rule showed that this ring was five-membered.

In 1928 Wieland, reviewing current knowledge of the chemistry of steroids, suggested formula (**1.33**) for bile acids. According to Wieland's working hypothesis, rings A, B and C of the steroid nucleus met at a common point. Wieland also assumed that ring C, as well as ring D, was five-membered and that there was only one angular methyl group. The two missing carbon atoms were tentatively accommodated by proposing that a C_2H_4 group was attached to the ring system. The double bond of cholesterol was correctly placed in relation to the hydroxyl group, but the hydroxyl group was placed at C-4. In 1932 Bernal showed, by X-ray crystallography of ergosterol, that the steroid molecule is longer and flatter than Wieland's proposed structure. This, together with an earlier observation of Diels and Gädke (1927) that selenium dehydrogenation of cholesterol gives rise to chrysene (**1.34**), led Rosenheim and King (1932a) to suggest a modified structural formula for deoxycholic acid with four six-membered rings and one angular methyl group (**1.35**). Later in the same year Wieland and Dane (1932) and Rosenheim and King (1932b) proposed a new structure for deoxycholic acid (**1.36**), now known to be correct, in which rings C and B of the earlier Rosenheim–King formula were transposed, ring D was changed to the five-membered structure originally deduced by Wieland and an additional methyl group was placed at C-10.

6.5 Configuration

The study of the stereochemistry of steroids grew out of attempts made at the beginning of this century to understand the chemical relationship between cholesterol and coprostanol. In the following brief account of some of this early work, modern terminology is used to describe reactions studied before the introduction of the α/β system for denoting the configuration of substituents in the steroid ring system.

In 1904 Diels and Abderhalden prepared an isomer of coprostanol, now known to be cholestanol (5α-cholestan-3β-ol) (**1.38**), by reduction of cholestenone (cholest-4-en-3-one) (**1.37**)

Dorée and Gardner (1908) then showed that coprostanone (**1.40**), prepared by oxidizing coprostanol (**1.39**), was different from cholestanone (**1.42**) (previously prepared by oxidizing cholestanol (**1.38**)). They also showed that coprostanol could be isomerized to a substance which, on oxidation, yielded a ketone identical with coprostanone. The product of isomerization (epicoprostanol (**1.41**)) was therefore identical with coprostanol except for the configuration of the hydroxyl group.

A few years later, Windaus and Uibrig (1914) showed that cholestanol could also be converted into an isomer which, on oxidation, gave cholestanone. The isomer (epicholestanol (**1.43**)) therefore differed from cholestanol only in the configuration of the hydroxyl group:

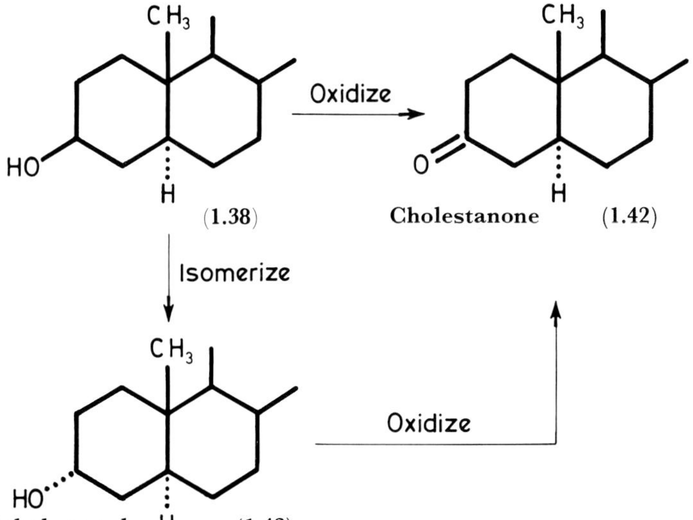

In the following year Windaus and Uibrig (1915) showed that coprostane, the saturated hydrocarbon formed by dehydration and reduction of coprostanol, is an isomer of cholestane, the parent hydrocarbon of cholestanol. It was later recognized that the isomerism between the cholestane and coprostane series, i.e. between the α- and β-cholestane series, is due to a difference in the configuration at the junction between rings A and B.

For historical reasons, the configuration of the hydroxyl group of cholesterol and cholestanol was designated β in the early literature. All configurations at other asymmetric centres in the steroid nucleus were subsequently related to the configuration at C-3 of cholesterol. Thus, if the configuration of a substituent was shown to be the same as that of the C-3 hydroxyl group of cholesterol it was designated β; if the opposite, it was designated α. By 1953, the configuration at all asymmetric centres of cholesterol, relative to that at C-3, had been established. When the absolute configurations at C-7 of 5α-cholestan-7α-ol (Prelog, 1953) and C-20 of 5α-cholest-14-en-3β-ol (Cornforth *et al.*, 1954; Riniker *et al.*, 1954) were established, it became possible to deduce the absolute configuration of the whole cholesterol molecule.

40   The Biology of Cholesterol and Related Steroids

The configuration at the asymmetric centres of steroids has been established largely by chemical methods of the kind described above, but other methods, including X-ray crystallography, ultra-violet and infra-red spectroscopy, polarimetry and nuclear magnetic resonance spectroscopy, have provided independent or confirmatory evidence. This section may be ended appropriately with a description of the proof of the absolute configuration at C-20 of cholesterol.

The absolute configuration about an asymmetric carbon atom in a molecule containing more than one asymmetric centre may be established by isolating a fragment of the molecule containing the carbon atom in question as the sole asymmetric centre and then comparing the optical activity of the fragment (or of a derivative thereof) with that of a reference compound of known absolute configuration. This method was used by Cornforth et al. (1954) and by Riniker et al. (1954) to determine the absolute configuration at C-20 of the cholesterol side-chain. Cornforth et al. (1954) prepared a C_{11} unsaturated aldehyde (**1.44**) from 5α-cholest-14-en-3β-ol containing a portion of ring D and the whole of the side-chain. The C_{11} aldehyde, which contained C-20 of cholesterol as the sole asymmetric centre, gave a laevorotatory semicarbazone which was identical with this semicarbazone prepared from (+)-citronellal (**1.45**). Since the absolute configuration of (+)-citronellal was known from its relationship to D-glyceraldehyde to be that shown in (**1.45**), the absolute configuration at C-20 of cholesterol is that shown in (**1.45**).

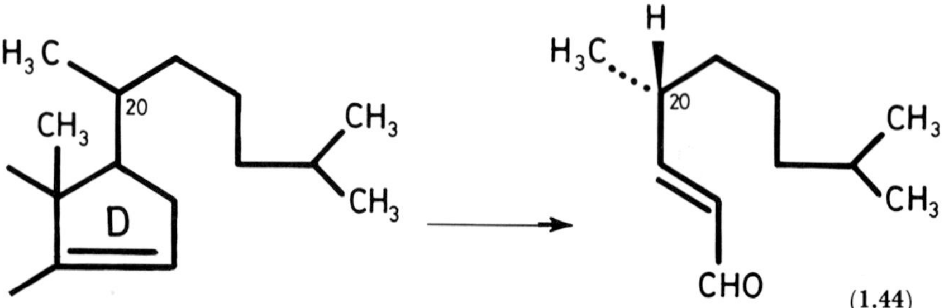

5α-Cholest-14-en-3β-ol

(1.44)

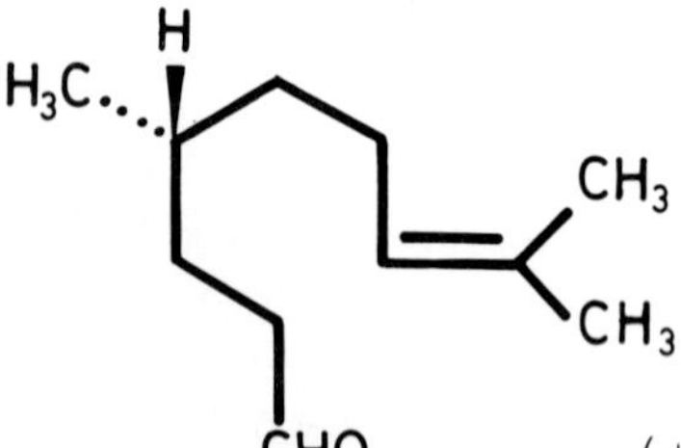

(1.45)

(+)-Citronellal

7 SOME PHYSICAL AND CHEMICAL PROPERTIES

7.1 Physical constants

When crystallized from anhydrous solvents, cholesterol forms colourless triclinic needles; m.p., 149–151 °C*; [α]D, −39 (in chloroform). The molecular weight is 387 (386.7, based on ^{12}C = 12.000). Cholesterol is insoluble in water (180 µg/100 ml at 20 °C (Haberland and Reynolds, 1973)) but is soluble in many organic solvents (Table 1.4). As deduced from a Dreiding model, the cholesterol ring system is about 10 Å long and 5 Å wide and the sidechain is about 10 Å long when extended. The general shape of the cholesterol ring system has already been considered (see Fig. 1.4). A more detailed discussion of bond lengths and bond angles in various steroids, calculated from data obtained by X-ray diffraction analysis, will be found in the review by Romers et al. (1974). The melting points, specific rotations and other physical constants of many steroids related to cholesterol are tabulated in Cook (1958). Some of these are included in Table 1.5. Other physical properties of cholesterol are dealt with in Chapter 2.

Table 1.4
Solubility of cholesterol in some organic solvents (g/100 g of solvent)

Solvent	Solubility
Methyl alcohol (0 °C)	0.34
Methyl alcohol (50 °C)	2.94
Ethyl alcohol (0 °C)	0.68
Ethyl alcohol (50 °C)	5.25
Chloroform (20 °C)	22.2
Benzene (0 °C)	14.24
Hexane (0 °C)	1.92
Pyridine (20 °C)	67.7
Diethylether (20 °C)	38.7

Compiled from Rosin (1923), Gemant (1962) and other sources.

---

* The m.p. reported by Chevreul (1816) was 137 °C.

42   The Biology of Cholesterol and Related Steroids

Table 1.5
Melting points of some sterols related to cholesterol and of some cholesteryl esters

Compound	Melting point (°C)
Cholestanol	142
Coprostanol	101
7-Dehydrocholesterol	143–147
Epicholestanol	182
Epicoprostanol	117
7α-Hydroxycholesterol	188
Desmosterol	121
Cholesteryl benzoate	147 (181)
Cholesteryl linoleate	41–48
Cholesteryl linolenate	36–49
Cholesteryl oleate	35–51
Cholesteryl palmitate	75
Cholesteryl palmitoleate	52

From Cook (1958) and Small (1970). Where reported values differ widely, a range is given. For systematic names, see Table 1.2. Note that although cholesteryl esters are usually capable of forming one or more liquid-crystalline (mesomorphic) phases, most cholesteryl esters of long-chain fatty acids melt directly to isotropic liquids when the crystals are heated, the mesomorphic phases forming only when the melt is cooled slowly (Small, 1970). Cholesteryl benzoate forms a mesophase when crystals are heated, and on raising the temperature further the melt clears to an isotropic liquid (m.p. given in parentheses). Note also that cholesteryl esters which, when pure, have m.p. above body temperature could exist in a liquid or liquid-crystalline state in the presence of other lipids (including other cholesteryl esters) in living tissues (see Small, 1970).

7.2   Liquid crystal formation

Cholesterol and its esters tend to form liquid crystals, in which the molecules have some degree of order but are not in the completely ordered state characteristic of true crystals (see Chapter 7). Under certain conditions, liquid crystals are *doubly refracting* or *birefringent*. Birefringence is often exhibited by cholesterol and its esters, and by other substances, in biological materials *in situ*.

Note: A doubly refracting crystal splits an incident ray of light (other than one parallel to its axis) into two divergent plane-polarized rays whose directions of polarization are perpendicular to each other. Double refraction may be detected by viewing the specimen between the crossed Nicol prisms of a polarizing microscope. If a ray of polarized light from the lower prism passes through a liquid crystal of cholesterol whose axis is not parallel to the ray of light, double refraction will take place, permitting the upper prism to transmit light from the crystal. Hence, the doubly refracting material appears luminous against a dark background. The term *anisotropy* (Gr. *anisos*, unlike; *tropos*, turning) is often used incorrectly as a synonym for double refraction. A substance is said to be anisotropic if its physical properties are not the same in all directions. Double refraction is one of several manifestations of the anisotropy exhibited by many substances in which there is a degree of order in the arrangement of their molecules. One of the characteristics of double refraction, its dependence on direction, is shared by other properties of anisotropic substances.

7.3 Some chemical reactions of cholesterol

The information built up by steroid chemists has played an essential part in the study of the biology of cholesterol. In particular, the biosynthetic pathways for cholesterol could not have been elucidated unless it had been possible to synthesize chemically a large number of labelled potential intermediates. Nor would it have been possible to assign particular atoms of a non-steroid precursor to particular positions in the steroid molecule without the knowledge required for the isolation of specific fragments of labelled steroids (see Chapter 4). Many of the chemical reactions undergone by cholesterol and related steroids are described in Fieser and Fieser (1959) and Shoppee (1964), and the chapter by Bladon in Cook (1958) contains a remarkable amount of information summarized in the form of charts. More recent information on the chemistry of steroids may also be found in *Terpenoids and Steroids* and in other review articles listed at the end of this chapter. Here we shall consider only a few chemical reactions of cholesterol, all of which have a direct bearing on methods of preparation, purification and assay.

7.3.1 Formation of digitonides

While investigating the inhibitory effect of cholesterol on the haemolytic action of saponins,* Windaus (1909) discovered that digitonin forms an alcohol-insoluble complex with cholesterol containing equimolar amounts of the two components. This complex, though dissociable by certain organic solvents, is known as *cholesterol digitonide*. Insoluble sterol-saponin complexes are formed with sterols other than cholesterol and with saponins other than digitonin, though the complexes with lowest solubility are usually those formed with digitonin.

Windaus noted a high degree of stereospecificity in digitonide formation, a precipitate being formed with 5α-cholestan-3β-ol (cholestanol) but not with 5α-cholestan-3α-ol (epicholestanol). He also noted that cholesteryl esters do not form digitonides. The structural conditions required for digitonide formation have since

---

* Saponins are glycosides in which a chain of one or more sugar residues is attached by a glycosidic bond to C-3 of a sapogenin. A sapogenin is a C_{27} steroid with a heterocyclic C_8 side-chain and, almost invariably, a 3β hydroxyl group.

been investigated in considerable detail (Fernholz, 1935; Fieser and Fieser, 1949; Haslam and Klyne, 1953). Although there is no infallible way of predicting whether or not a given steroid will form an insoluble digitonide, the following rules hold in most cases:

(1) Steroids based on a wide variety of parent hydrocarbons, including androstane, pregnane, cholane, cholestane, ergostane and stigmastane, may form insoluble digitonides.

(2) Almost all steroids which form insoluble digitonides have an unprotected 3β-hydroxyl group and either a 5α-hydrogen or a Δ^5 double bond. Examples are: ergosterol, cholesterol, cholestanol, dehydroepiandrosterone (3β-hydroxyandrost-5-en-17-one) and 5α-pregnan-3β-ol.

(3) The introduction of keto groups or of additional double bonds or hydroxyl groups into the ring system usually has little effect on the ability of a steroid to form an insoluble digitonide. For example, 3β-hydroxy-5α-cholestan-6(or 7)-one, cholesta-5,7-dien-3β-ol, 5α-cholest-7-en-3β-ol and cholest-5-ene-3β,4β-diol all form insoluble complexes with digitonin.

(4) Steroids in which there is no 3β-hydroxyl group, or in which a 3β-hydroxyl group is present but is esterified, almost invariably fail to form insoluble digitonides.

In general, the structural features most favourable for precipitation with digitonin seem to be a hydroxyl group at C-3 in equatorial conformation with respect to ring A and a flat ring system (see Fig. 1.2). Thus, cholestanol (A/B *trans* and 3-hydroxyl group equatorial) gives a more insoluble digitonide than coprostanol (A/B *cis* and 3-hydroxyl group axial), and epicholestanol (A/B *trans* and 3-hydroxyl group axial) is not digitonin-precipitable.

Digitonin precipitation has been used extensively for the gravimetric assay of cholesterol and for the separate assay of free and esterified cholesterol in mixtures of the two (see Methods of assay). Precipitation as the digitonide is also used as a final step in the purification of cholesterol extracted from biological materials. The method is convenient, owing to the ease of crystallization of digitonides, but has the disadvantage that digitonide formation is non-specific. In biological samples in which almost all the sterol is cholesterol, such as human plasma, it may be justifiable to assume that all digitonin-precipitable material in the non-saponifiable fraction is cholesterol. But this assumption is not justified in tissues, such as animal skin, which contain significant amounts of sterol other than cholesterol. Digitonin precipitation may also be used as a preliminary step in the purification of mixtures of sterols. For example, the sterols of plant tissues may be precipitated with digitonin and the sterols may then be regenerated from a pyridine solution of the digitonide after precipitating the digitonin with ether.

When radioactive precursors of sterols are used in investigations of cholesterol biosynthesis in animal tissues, it is common practice to express the results in terms of the amount of radioactivity incorporated into the digitonin-precipitable fraction ('digitonin-precipitable sterols'). Under certain conditions (see p. 342) this probably gives a good indication of the sterol-synthesizing activity of the tissue. However, the digitonin-precipitable fraction may contain all the radioactive intermediates in the biosynthetic pathway from lanosterol to cholesterol and the specific radioactivity of some of these intermediates may be very different from that of the cholesterol. Hence, the specific radioactivity of the cholesterol cannot be deduced from the mass of cholesterol and the total radioactivity in the digitonin-precipitable sterols.

7.3.2 Formation of a dibromide

When bromine is added to a solution of cholesterol in ether, the ether-insoluble dibromide ($5\alpha,6\beta$-dibromocholestan-3β-ol) is formed. This reaction is the basis of a standard method for separating cholesterol from 5α-cholestanol, lathosterol (5α-cholest-7-en-3β-ol), 7-dehydrocholesterol (cholesta-5,7-dien-3β-ol) and other sterols present as contaminants in most crude preparations of cholesterol. After bromination, the dibromide is separated from the mother liquor and the cholesterol regenerated by treatment with zinc and acetic acid (Fieser, 1953). This method of purification is useful for removing radioactive contaminants from cholesterol formed biosynthetically from radioactive precursors and for purifying commercial preparations of labelled cholesterol.

7.3.3 Oxidation by molecular oxygen

Cholesterol in the form of an aqueous emulsion undergoes oxidation when the emulsion is aerated. The products formed include 7-ketocholesterol, 7α-hydroxycholesterol, 7β-hydroxycholesterol, cholestane-$3\beta,5\alpha,6\beta$-triol and 25-hydroxycholesterol. Aerial oxidation is enhanced by the presence of cupric ions and is diminished by the presence of EDTA or of glutathione or other SH-containing compounds. Under the most favourable conditions, more than 40% of an emulsion of cholesterol may be oxidized by molecular oxygen within a few hours (Bergström and Wintersteiner, 1941). Cholesterol stored as crystals without exclusion of air undergoes slow oxidation (Bergström, 1943), with the formation of substances that give a positive Lifschütz reaction (see Section 7.3.4). Samples that have been stored in this way for months or years should therefore be purified before use. Crystals of [^{14}C]cholesterol form detectable amounts of radioactive oxidation products when stored for many months if air is not excluded (Dauben and Payot, 1956). When spread as a thin film on glass or paper, cholesterol is oxidized rapidly in the presence of air and this effect is enhanced by exposure to daylight (Hais and Myant, 1965).

Non-enzymic oxidation of cholesterol by molecular oxygen should always be borne in mind as a possible cause of the presence of oxidized sterols in biological material. 7α-Hydroxycholesterol and other Lifschütz-positive substances have been identified in the sterols obtained from animal tissues. Some of this material may have been present in the fresh tissue as a result of enzymic or non-enzymic oxidation *in vivo*, but some or all of it may have been formed by aerial oxidation during the extraction, analysis and storage of the sample. A particularly difficult problem arises with incubations of tissue preparations *in vitro* when non-enzymic aerial oxidation of cholesterol gives rise to the same compounds as those formed enzymically. For example, radioactive 7α-hydroxycholesterol is formed during the incubation of [^{14}C]cholesterol with suspensions of liver microsomes. Some of this is formed enzymically by a microsomal hydroxylating system, but some is also formed non-enzymically. The contribution from non-enzymic sources can only be found by measuring the formation of radioactive 7α-hydroxycholesterol in boiled preparations of the tissue incubated under identical conditions.

In order to minimize aerial oxidation of cholesterol in biological experiments the extraction and analysis should be carried out as rapidly as possible, exposure to air should be avoided as far as possible, direct sunlight should be excluded and samples should always be stored in the dark, preferably under nitrogen. Radioactive cholesterol should be stored as solutions in non-polar solvents such as benzene. The use of certain anti-oxidants in incubation mixtures may help to reduce aerial oxidation, though it cannot eliminate it entirely.

7.3.4 Colour reactions of sterols

Many steroids form highly coloured products when treated with strong acids under dehydrating conditions. This property is the basis of several qualitative tests for detecting steroids possessing more or less specific structural features. It is also the basis of almost all colorimetric methods for assaying cholesterol.

7.3.4.1 The Liebermann-Burchard reaction.
Salkowski (1872) showed that a sequence of colours develops in a chloroform solution of cholesterol shaken with concentrated sulphuric acid. Liebermann (1885) then showed that when concentrated sulphuric acid is added to a solution of cholesterol in cold acetic anhydride the mixture turns red, the colour changing gradually to blue-green. Burchard (1890)

found that a similar colour reaction occurs when a mixture of concentrated sulphuric acid and acetic anhydride is added to a solution of cholesterol in chloroform. The term 'Liebermann-Burchard reaction' is now commonly used for any colour reaction of a steroid in which the colour reagent is a mixture of sulphuric acid and acetic anhydride or glacial acetic acid. In general, the reaction is positive for any steroid containing either two double bonds in the same ring, or a double bond adjacent to a ring containing a double bond or a hydroxyl group. However, there are exceptions to this general rule. Coprostanol, for example, gives a delayed Liebermann-Burchard reaction. Cholesteryl esters give a more intense colour than free cholesterol.

The speed, intensity and duration of the colour reaction with cholesterol depend on several factors, including the concentration of sulphuric acid, the nature of the solvent for cholesterol and the temperature at which the reaction is carried out (Kabara, 1962). With non-polar solvents (e.g. toluene) the colour develops more quickly and is less stable than with polar solvents (e.g. acetic acid). As the ratio of sulphuric acid to acetic anhydride in the colour reagent is decreased progressively, the colour develops more slowly, the maximum intensity decreases and the stability increases. As the temperature of the reaction is increased, the rate of development of the colour increases and its stability decreases.

The rate of colour development under given conditions is characteristic for certain classes of steroids. Fast-reacting steroids (maximum colour within 2 minutes at 25 °C) include sterols with a Δ^7 double bond or a hydroxyl group at C-7. Slow-reacting steroids (maximum colour at 30–35 minutes at 25 °C) include cholesterol and other C_{27}, C_{28} and C_{29} sterols with a Δ^5 double bond but no Δ^7 double bond.

7.3.4.2 The Lifschütz reaction. Lifschütz (1908) showed that when cholesterol dissolved in acetic acid is heated with benzoyl peroxide, an oxidation product is formed which gives an intense blue or blue-green colour on addition of sulphuric acid to the cooled mixture. Lifschütz called the oxidation product 'oxycholesterol', but oxycholesterol is now known to be a mixture of several substances, not all of which give a colour in the Lifschütz reaction with sulphuric acid. Lifschütz also used a modification of this procedure for the detection and assay of certain steroids. The steroid to be tested is dissolved in chloroform. When a mixture of acetic acid, sulphuric acid and a drop of 5% $FeCl_3$ in acetic acid is added to the solution, a blue-green colour develops immediately. Under these conditions, a positive Lifschütz reaction is given by most steroids with two conjugated double bonds (two double bonds separated by a single bond) or with a double bond separated from a hydroxyl group by a single bond. In the latter case, conjugated double bonds can be formed by removal of water from the ring system. Typical Lifschütz-positive steroids are 7α-hydroxycholesterol and 7β-hydroxycholesterol (the chromogenic components of oxycholesterol), cholest-4-en-3β-ol and cholest-5-ene-3β,6β-diol. Cholesterol and 7-ketocholesterol are Lifschütz-negative.

Note the use of the term 'Lifschütz reaction' in two different senses is apt to be confusing. If the oxidation step with benzoyl peroxide is included, a positive colour reaction is given by many steroids with one or more double bonds in the ring system which do not give a colour with the modified procedure described above.

7.3.4.3 Other colour reactions.

In the reaction described by Rosenheim (1929), the steroid is dissolved in chloroform. On addition of a few drops of aqueous trichloroacetic acid, a red colour develops immediately, the colour changing gradually to a clear blue. Cholesterol does not give a colour in the cold, but ergosterol and cholest-4-en-3β-ol are both Rosenheim-positive. Rosenheim concluded that the structural feature required for a positive colour reaction was a Δ^4 double bond, either already present in the steroid molecule or capable of being formed by dehydration or double-bond migration. It is likely, however, that the structural requirements for a positive Rosenheim reaction are the same as those for a positive Lifschütz reaction. In the Tschugaeff (1900) reaction, zinc chloride in acetyl chloride is added to a solution of the steroid in glacial acetic acid. A red colour develops when the mixture is boiled.

A histochemical test for cholesterol developed by Schultz and Lahr has been modified by Zlatkis *et al.* (1953) for use as a method for assaying cholesterol. A purple colour develops when a mixture of sulphuric acid and glacial acetic acid containing $FeCl_3$ is added to a solution of cholesterol in acetic acid.

7.3.4.4 Mechanism of colour reactions.

The mechanism of these colour reactions, and of many others listed by Kritchevsky (1958), is not fully understood. Kritchevsky (1958) suggests that in colour reactions with sterols in which sulphuric acid is a component of the colour reagent, the following sequence of events occurs: the sterol is dehydrated to a colourless cholestadiene with conjugated double bonds (e.g., cholesta-3,5-diene); two molecules of the cholestadiene combine to form a dimer which is then sulphated to give a blue or purple product; the sulphated dimer undergoes further polymerization to brown or yellow compounds as the initial colour fades.

REFERENCES

In addition to the references listed below, the following general articles may be consulted:

Brooks, C. J. W. Steroids: sterols and bile acids. Chapter in: *Rodd's Chemistry of Carbon Compounds*, 2nd Edition, Vol. II, Part D (Steroids). Ed. S. Coffey. Elsevier, Amsterdam, pp. 1–196, 1970.

Florkin, M. From proto-biochemistry to biochemistry. In: *Comprehensive Biochemistry*, Vol. 30, Part II. Ed. M. Florkin and E. H. Stotz. Elsevier, Amsterdam, pp. 107–127, 1972.

Florkin, M. Early studies on biosynthesis. In: *Comprehensive Biochemistry*, Vol. 32, Part IV. Ed. M. Florkin and E. H. Stotz. Elsevier, Amsterdam, 1972.

Goodwin, T. W. (1973). Prochirality in biochemistry. *Essays in Biochemistry*, **9**, 103–160

Terpenoids and Steroids. In: *Specialist Periodical Reports*. Published annually by The Chemical Society, Burlington House, London.

Arigoni, D. and Eliel, E. L. Chirality due to the presence of hydrogen isotopes at noncyclic positions. In: *Topics in Stereochemistry*, Vol. 4. Ed. E. L. Eliel and N. L. Allinger. Wiley-Interscience, New York, pp. 127–243, 1969.

Ayrton, M. In: *Labrys-3, Michael Ayrton Issue*. Published from Labrys, 91 Wimborne Avenue, Hayes, Middlesex, 1978.

Bergström, S. (1943). On the oxidation of cholesterol and other unsaturated sterols in colloidal aqueous solution by molecular oxygen. *Arkiv för Kemi, Mineralogi och Geologi*, **16A**, 1–72.

Bergström, S. and Wintersteiner, O. (1941). Autoxidation of sterols in colloidal aqueous solution. The nature of the products formed from cholesterol. *Journal of Biological Chemistry*, **141**, 597–610.

Bernal, J. D. (1932). Carbon skeleton of the sterols. *Chemistry and Industry*, **51**, 466.

Berthelot, M. (1859). Sur plusiers alcools nouveaux. Combinaisons des acides avec la cholestérine, l'éthal, le camphre de Bornéo et la méconine. *Annales de Chimie et de Physique*, **56**, 51–98.

Bondziński, S. and Humnicki, V. (1896). Ueber das Schicksal des Cholesterins im thierischen Organismus. *Zeitschrift für physiologische Chemie*, **22**, 396–410.

Burchard, H. (1890). Beiträge zur Kenntnis des Cholesterins. *Chemisches Zentralblatt*, **61**, 25–27.

Cahn, R. S. (1964). An introduction to the sequence rule. A system for the specification of absolute configuration. *Journal of Chemical Education*, **41**, 116–125.

Cahn, R. S., Ingold, C. and Prelog, V. (1966). The specification of molecular chirality. *Angewandte Chemie, International Edition*, **5**, 385–415.

Chambers, V. M. A., Evans, E. A., Elvidge, J. A. and Jones, J. R. Tritium nuclear magnetic resonance (tnmr) spectroscopy. Review 19, *The Radiochemical Centre*, Amersham, U.K., 1978.

Chevreul, M. E. (1816). Examen des graisses d'homme, de mouton, de boeuf, de jaguar et d'oie. *Annales de Chimie et de Physique*, **2**, 339–372.

Cook, R. P. *Cholesterol. Chemistry, Biochemistry and Pathology*. Academic Press, New York, 1958.

Cornforth, J. W., Youhotsky, I. and Popják, G. (1954). Absolute configuration of cholesterol. *Nature*, London, **173**, 536.

Cross, C. Clerics doubt Christ's divinity. *The Observer Newspaper*, June 26th, 1977.

Dauben, W. G. and Payot, P. H. (1956). Radiation induced oxidation of cholesterol. *Journal of the American Chemical Society*, **78**, 5657–5660.

Diels, O. and Abderhalden, E. (1904). *Zur Kenntniss des Cholesterins. Chemische Berichte*, **37**, 3092–3103.

Diels, O. and Gadke, W. (1927). Über die Bildung von Chrysen bei der Dehydrierung des Cholesterins. *Chemische Berichte*, **60**, 140–147.
Dorée, C. and Gardner, J. A. (1908). Coprosterol. Part I. *Journal of the Chemical Society* (London), **93**, 1625–1633.
Farmer, S. N. and Kon, G. A. R. (1937). Sapogenins. Part II. Sarsasapogenin and smilagenin. *Journal of the Chemical Society* (London) (1), 414–420.
Fernholz, E. (1935). Notiz über das Verhalten von Sterniabkömmlingen gegenüber Digitonin. *Zeitschrift fur physiologische Chemie*, **232**, 97–100.
Fieser, L. F. (1953). Cholesterol and companions. VII Steroid dibromides. *Journal of the American Chemical Society*, **75**, 5421–5422.
Fieser, L. F. and Fieser, M. *Natural Products Related to Phenanthrene*, 3rd Edition, Reinhold, New York, 1949.
Fieser, L. F. and Fieser, M. *Steroids*. Reinhold, New York, 1959.
Flint, A. (1862). Experimental researches into a new excretory function of the liver; consisting in the removal of cholesterine from the blood, and its discharge from the body in the form of stercorine. *American Journal of Medical Sciences*, **44**, 305–365.
Gemant, A. (1962). Solubilization of cholesterol. *Life Sciences*, **1**, 233–238.
Gibbons, G. F., Mitropoulos, K. A. and Myant, N. B. *The Biochemistry of Cholesterol*. Elsevier, Amsterdam, 1982.
Haberland, M. E. and Reynolds, J. A. (1973). Self-association of cholesterol in aqueous solutions. *Proceedings of the National Academy of Sciences of the U.S.A.*, **70**, 2313–2316.
Hais, I. M. and Myant, N. B. (1965). Photolysis of cholesterol during biological experiments. *Biochemical Journal*, **94**, 85–90.
Hanson, K. R. (1966). Applications of the sequence rule. I. Naming the paired ligands g,g at a tetrahedral atom Xggij. II. Naming the two faces of a trigonal atom Yghi. *Journal of the American Chemical Society*, **88**, 2731–2742.
Hart, H. Isomerism. In: *Encyclopaedia Britannica*, 15th Edition, **9**, 1032–1043, 1975.
Haslam, R. M. and Klyne, W. (1953). The precipitation of 3β-hydroxysteroids by digitonin. *Biochemical Journal*, **55**, 340–346.
IUPAC (1977). Nomenclature of isotopically labelled organic compounds. In: *Provisional Nomenclature Appendix No. 62* (July 1977) to IUPAC Information Bulletin, Section H.
IUPAC-IUB (1971). IUPAC-IUB 1971 *Definitive Rules for Steroid Nomenclature*. Obtainable from IUPAC Secretariat, Bank Court Chambers, 2–3 Pound Way, Cowley Centre, Oxford OX4 3YF, U.K.
Kabara, J. J. (1962). Determination and microscopic localization of cholesterol. *Methods of Biochemical Analysis*, **10**, 263–318.
Kritchevsky, D. *Cholesterol*. John Wiley & Sons, New York, 1958.
Liebermann, C. (1885). Ueber das Oxychinoterpen. *Chemische Berichte*, **18**, 1803–1809.
Liftschütz, J. (1908). Eine Farbenreaktion auf Cholesterin durch Oxydation. *Chemische Berichte*, **41**, 252–255.
Mylius, F. (1886). Ueber die Cholsäure. *Chemische Berichte*, **19**, 369–379.
Newman, H. H. *Twins and Super-twins: A Study of Twins, Triplets, Quadruplets and Quintuplets*. Hutchinson's Scientific and Technical Publications, London, 1942.
Popják, G. and Cornforth, J. W. (1966). Substrate stereochemistry in squalene biosynthesis. *Biochemical Journal*, **101**, 553–568.
Prelog, V. (1953). Untersuchungen über asymmetrische Synthesen I. Über den sterischen Verlauf der Reaktion von α-Ketosäure-estern optisch activer Alkohole mit Grignardschen Verbindungen. *Helvetica Chimica Acta*, **36**, 308–319.
Prelog, V. (1976). Chirality in chemistry. *Science*, **193**, 17–24.

Reinitzer, F. (1888). Beiträge zur Kenntniss des Cholesterins. *Sitzber. Akad. Wiss. Wien*, **97**, 167–187.
Riniker, B., Arigoni, D. and Jeger, O. (1954). Über die direkte Konfigurative Verknüpfung der Steroide mit dem Citronellal, ein Beitrag zur Bestimmung der absoluten Konfiguration der Steroide. *Helvetica Chimica Acta*, **37**, 546–552.
Romers, C., Altona, C., Jacobs, H. J. C. and De Graaff, R. A. G. Steroid conformation from X-ray analysis data. In: *Terpenoids and Steroids, Vol. 4*. Ed. K. H. Overton. Published by The Chemical Society, Burlington House, London, pp. 531–583, 1974.
Rosenheim, O. (1929). A specific colour reaction for ergosterol. *Biochemical Journal*. **23**, 47–53.
Rosenheim, O. and King, H. (1932a). The ring-system of sterols and bile acids. *Chemistry and Industry*, **51**, 464–466.
Rosenheim, O. and King, H. (1932b). The ring system of sterols and bile acids. *Nature*, **130**, 315.
Rosin, A. (1923). Über die Lösung von Gallensteinen. *Zeitschrift fur physiologische Chemie*, **124**, 282–286.
Salkowski, E. (1872). Kleinere Mittheilungen physiologisch-chemischen Inhalt (II). *Pflügers Archiv für die gesamte Physiologie*, **6**, 207–222.
Shoppee, C. W. *Chemistry of the Steroids*, 2nd Edition. Butterworths, London, 1964.
Small, D. M. The physical state of lipids of biological importance: cholesteryl esters, cholesterol, triglyceride. In: *Surface Chemistry of Biological Systems*. Ed. M. Blank, Plenum Press, New York, pp. 55–83, 1970.
Strecker, A. (1848). Untersuchung der Ochsangalle. *Annalen der Chemie*, **65**, 1–37.
Tanret, C. (1889). Sur un nouveau principe immédiat de l'ergot de seigle, l'ergostérine. *Comptes Rendus*, **108**, 98–100.
Tschugaeff, L. (1900). Report of a meeting of the Russian Society for Physical Chemistry (May, 1900). *Zeitschrift fur Angewandte Chemie*, **14**, 618.
Wieland, H. and Dane, E. (1932). Untersuchungen über die Konstitution der Gallensäuren. 39. Mitteilung. Zur Kenntnis der 12-Oxy-cholansäure. *Zeitschrift fur physiologische Chemie*, **210**, 268–281.
Wieland, H. and Dane, E. (1933). Über die Haftstelle der Seitenkette. *Zeitschrift fur physiologische Chemie*, **219**, 240–244.
Wieland, H., Schlichting, O. and Jacobi, R. (1926). Über die Natur der Seitenkette und des vierten Ringes. *Zeitschrift fur Physiologie*, **161**, 80–115.
Windaus, A. (1909). Über die Entgiftung der Saponine durch Cholesterin. *Chemische Berichte*, **42**, 238–246.
Windaus, A. and Dalmer, O. (1919). Zur Kentnis der Ring-Systeme in Cholesterin. *Chemische Berichte*, **52**, 162–169.
Windaus, A. and Hauth, A. (1906). Ueber Stigmasterin, ein neues Phytosterin aus Calabar-Bohnen. *Chemische Berichte*, **39**, 4378–4384.
Windaus, A. and Neukirchen, K. (1919). Die Umwandlung des Cholesterins in Cholansäure. *Chemische Berichte*, **52**, 1915–1919.
Windaus, A. and Resau, C. (1913). Methyl-isohexyl-keton, ein Abbauprodukt des Cholesterins. *Chemische Berichte*, **46**, 1246–1248.
Windaus, A. and Uibrig, C. (1914). Über β-Cholestanol. *Chemische Berichte*, **47**, 2384–2388.
Windaus, A. and Uibrig, C. (1915). Über Koprosterin. *Chemische Berichte*, **48**, 857–863.
Wislicenus, J. and Moldenhauer, W. (1868). Ueber das Cholesterindibromür. *Annalen der Chemie*, **146**, 175–180.
Zlatkis, A., Zak, B. and Boyle, A. J. (1953). A new method for the direct determination of serum cholesterol. *Journal of Laboratory and Clinical Medicine*, **41**, 486–492.

Chapter 2

Analysis of Sterols and Related Steroids

1	INTRODUCTION	55
2	EXTRACTION	56
2.1	Saponification	56
2.2	Mechanical homogenization	56
2.3	Lipid extraction	57
3	SEPARATION	58
3.1	General principles	58
3.2	Column chromatography	58
3.3	Thin-layer chromatography	59
3.3.1	General principles	59
3.3.2	Methods of detection	60
3.3.3	Relation between structure and mobility	61
3.3.3.1	R_f of sterols	61
3.3.3.2	R_f of bile acids	63
3.4	Gas-liquid chromatography	64
3.4.1	General principles	64
3.4.2	Methods of detection	65
3.4.3	Solid supports and liquid phases	66
3.4.4	Formation of derivatives	66
3.4.5	Relation between structure and retention time	68
3.4.5.1	General remarks	68
3.4.5.2	Influence of the liquid phase	69
3.4.5.3	The effect of derivative formation	70
3.4.5.4	R_T of sterols	70
3.4.5.5	R_T of bile acids	72
3.4.6	Quantitative gas-liquid chromatography	74
3.4.7	Radioassay combined with GLC	76
4	IDENTIFICATION	77
4.1	General principles	77
4.2	Preliminary steps	78
4.3	Gas-liquid chromatography	79
4.4	Other methods of identification	79
4.4.1	General remarks	79

4.4.2	UV spectroscopy	81
4.4.3	IR spectroscopy	82
4.4.4	Nuclear magnetic resonance spectroscopy	84
4.4.5	Electron spin resonance	87
4.4.6	Mass spectrometry	87
4.4.7	Optical rotatory disperson and circular dichroism	88
5	THREE ILLUSTRATIVE EXAMPLES	90
5.1	Determination of the structure of presqualene pyrophosphate	90
5.2	The use of GC-MS in the identification of bile alcohols	97
5.3	Peak shifts in the identification of bile acids	98
6	ASSAY	99
6.1	Assay of plasma cholesterol	99
6.1.1	Importance of the plasma cholesterol concentration	99
6.1.2	Reliability and quality control	100
6.1.3	Cholesterol standards	101
6.1.4	Colorimetric methods	101
6.1.4.1	Liebermann-Burchard methods	102
6.1.4.2	Kiliani-Zak and other colorimetric methods	103
6.1.5	Gas-liquid chromatographic methods	103
6.1.6	Enzymic methods	104
6.1.7	Esterified cholesterol	106
6.1.8	Automation	106
6.2	Other aspects of the assay of sterols	107
6.3	Assay of bile acids	108
6.3.1	Relevance to cholesterol metabolism	108
6.3.2	Bile acids in duodenal bile	109
6.3.3	Measurement of sterol balance	111
6.3.4	Serum bile acids	113
6.3.5	Sulphated bile acids	114

Analysis of Sterols and Related Steroids

1 INTRODUCTION

Qualitative analysis of steroids in biological material is concerned with the identification and isolation of known steroids and the elucidation of the structure of new ones. Identification of all the steroids present in a plant or animal tissue may be of considerable interest, even if the amounts of each compound identified are not measured. For example, identification of the sterols and methyl sterols in skin has provided important clues to the sequence of intermediates through which cholesterol is biosynthesized (Clayton *et al.*, 1963).

Quantitative analysis of steroids is concerned with the measurement of the amount of a particular steroid or group of steroids in a biological sample. In most cases one wishes to assay individual compounds, as in the measurement of tissue cholesterol concentration. However, for some purposes it is sufficient to assay the total amount of steroid present in a given class, as in investigations of sterol balance in the whole animal. Since few methods for assaying steroids are specific, some degree of purification or separation is usually necessary if a single steroid is to be assayed in material containing a mixture of several steroids. In some instances, particularly when the steroid in question is a minor constituent in a mixture of steroids, it may be necessary to isolate and purify the compound before it can be assayed. If, on the other hand, the compound is the major steroid in the biological sample, it may be possible to assay it with a non-specific method without preliminary separation. This is done, for example, in the measurement of total cholesterol in normal human plasma by the Liebermann-Burchard reaction. Even when this is possible, extraction of the total lipids from the sample is almost always necessary. In work with radioactive compounds one may wish to know the total amount of radioactivity present in a particular steroid or group of steroids, as in the measurement of incorporation of radioactivity from a labelled precursor into cholesterol or into total sterols. On the other hand, in the study of biosynthetic pathways it may be necessary to know the specific radioactivity of an intermediate. In this case, recovery of total radioactivity in the intermediate is not required, but it is essential to obtain a pure specimen of the labelled substance for assay of the mass and radioactivity.

Thus, depending upon the purpose to be achieved, the analysis of sterols and related steroids may require various combinations of four procedures—extraction, separation, identification and assay. These four procedures are considered in this chapter.

2 EXTRACTION

The steroids of tissues or biological fluids are first extracted by organic solvents under conditions in which all the lipids are removed. The subsequent treatment of the total lipid extract will depend upon the information required. In order to achieve complete extraction, the intracellular lipids must be made accessible to the solvent and the lipids must be disrupted from water-soluble complexes with proteins (lipoproteins) so that they become soluble in the lipid solvent.

2.1 Saponification

A preliminary saponification by heating the material in alcoholic KOH digests animal cells and disrupts lipoproteins, but treatment with strong acids is usually required for digestion of plant cells. Saponification before extraction is the most convenient method for many purposes, but is ruled out if cholesteryl esters or other unsaponified lipids are required for further study. Methods for saponifying lipids in animal tissues have been described by Entenman (1957), Cook and Rattray (1958) and Radin (1969).

Hydrolysis of the peptide bond of conjugated bile acids requires more rigorous conditions than those suitable for ester-bond hydrolysis. Conjugated bile acids may be hydrolysed by heating at 110° in aqueous NaOH in Teflon or siliconized glass tubes for 3–5 hours. Alkaline hydrolysis under these conditions may cause considerable loss of bile acid, particularly of lithocholic acid. For this reason, some workers advocate the use of bacterial enzymes for hydrolysing conjugated bile acids (Section 6.3).

2.2 Mechanical homogenization

If alkaline digestion is ruled out, the tissue must be homogenized by a mechanical method capable of bringing about complete disruption of all cells. This can be achieved by several methods (for details, see Entenman, 1957). The best method for small pieces of soft tissue is to homogenize a weighed portion in a glass homogenizer with solvent and then to transfer the homogenate, with washings, to the vessel in which the extraction is to be carried out. For larger pieces of tissue (more than 1 g), the material should be divided into small fragments with a steel mincer or, if this is not possible, with scissors. The tissue fragments may then be homogenized with 3 volumes of ethanol in a blendor. Alternatively, the tissue may be frozen in liquid air, transferred to a steel block cooled in solid CO_2 and acetone, and then crushed to a fine powder. Skin is particularly difficult to homogenize. A blendor is unsatisfactory because the skin sticks to the blades of the instrument and no fragmentation occurs. Small pieces of skin may be homogenized in a glass homogenizer, provided that the tissue has been cut into very small pieces (1 mm^3) with fine scissors. For larger pieces, a Polytron homogenizer (Kinematica, Lucerne, Switzerland) may be used. Homogenization of skin is facilitated by preliminary digestion of collagen fibres by incubation with trypsin for 2 hours at 37 °C.

2.3 Lipid extraction

The extraction of lipids from the lipoproteins present in all tissues may be accomplished either by drying the tissue before extraction, or by using mixtures of polar and non-polar solvents. The tissue may be dried from the frozen state *in vacuo* or by repeated extraction with acetone, the acetone extracts being added to the total lipid extract. Solvent mixtures commonly used are acetone-ethanol (1:1, v/v), ether-ethanol (1:3, v/v) and chloroform-methanol (1:1, or 2:1, v/v). The extraction may be carried out in the cold by vigorous shaking in a stoppered vessel, by boiling under a reflux condenser or by prolonged extraction in a Soxhlet apparatus. Chloroform-methanol (2:1) was introduced by Folch *et al.* (1957) for the removal of lipids from brain, but is now generally regarded as a suitable solvent for extracting lipids from most tissues or body fluids. The paper by Folch *et al.* (1957) should be consulted for details of this method. Folch's method includes a step in which the lipid extract is washed with physiological saline equilibrated with the solvent. This is useful for removing water-soluble radioactive compounds from lipid extracts of tissues or incubation mixtures in which the biosynthesis of steroids from precursors of low molecular weight is under investigation.

For analysis of the bile acids of bile, an extraction step is not required. After removal of proteins by precipitation with ethanol the mixture is taken to dryness and dissolved in a suitable solvent for analysis by chromatography. Since all the biliary bile acids are conjugated, rigorous hydrolysis before or after preliminary separation of the conjugated acids must be carried out if the individual bile acids are to be analysed. Methods for extracting bile acids from blood and liver have been described by Eneroth and Sjövall (1969, 1971).

3 SEPARATION

3.1 General principles

Many well-tried methods are available for the separation and purification of lipids from the lipid extract. If the tissue or lipid extract has been saponified, it is usual to remove the unsaponifiable lipid, including the sterols, by extracting the alkaline hydrolysate with a non-polar solvent such as diethylether or petroleum ether. The hydrolysate is then acidified with strong acid and the saponifiable lipids, including fatty acids and bile acids, are removed with a suitable solvent. The steroids in an unsaponified extract, or in the neutral and acidic fractions obtained after saponification, may be separated by column chromatography, TLC or GLC. Paper chromatography has been largely replaced by TLC for the routine separation of lipids, but is still favoured by some workers for the separation of plant sterols and conjugated bile acids. The two most versatile methods for separation of steroids are undoubtedly TLC and GLC, either separately or in combination. Directions for carrying out separations by these two methods will be found in the review articles listed below, but a few general comments on chromatography in relation to sterols and bile acids may be helpful.

3.2 Column chromatography

In conventional column chromatography the most commonly used solid phases for work with steroids are silicic acid and alumina, the solid phase acting either as adsorbant in adsorption chromatography or as support for the stationary liquid phase in reversed-phase partition chromatography. Ion-exchange columns have been used for separation of bile acids but have found little application in the separation of sterols. Conventional column chromatography was for many years a popular method for the small-scale separation of steroids. It was used for much of the classical work on the identification of intermediates in the biosynthesis of sterols (Frantz and Schroepfer, 1967) and still has a place in the preliminary separation of lipid extracts and of mixtures of steroids into classes before their final separation by GLC. It has also been used successfully with silver-nitrate-impregnated solid phases for the resolution of unsaturated sterols differing only in the positions of their double bonds (see, for example, Lutsky et al., 1971). However, for work of this kind long columns are required if high resolution is to be achieved. Hence, the rate of elution is slow, the separation of a complex mixture of sterols sometimes taking many hours. For this reason, most workers ceased to use column chromatography when TLC was introduced. However, recent technical developments have brought column chromatography back into favour (Vestergaard, 1973; Knox, 1978). A combination of high resolution with high speed may be achieved by using very fine solid-phase particles (less than 40 µ in diameter) of uniform size, long columns and very high elution pressures instead of the conventional gravity flow. With modern high-pressure liquid chromatography the solutes in the eluate are monitored continuously by a non-destructive method, such as UV absorption or change in refractive index.

High-pressure column chromatography is now used increasingly in the separation of sterols and related compounds. For the separation of certain compounds of this class it has several advantages over GLC. In particular, the fact that it does not subject the solutes to a high temperature makes it the method of choice for separation of unusually heat-labile steroids such as the moulting hormones of insects (Schooley and Nakanishi, 1973) and the dihydroxy metabolites of vitamin D (Matthews *et al.*, 1974), although the methods of detection that can be used in conjunction with high-pressure liquid column chromatography are relatively insensitive. The use of reversed-phase high-pressure column chromatography for the separation of closely similar sterols has been described by Rees *et al.* (1976) and by Hansbury and Scallen (1978).

3.3 Thin-layer chromatography

3.3.1 General principles

The separation of compounds by thin-layer adsorption chromatography is due largely to differential adsorption to the solid supporting medium, the more polar compounds in the mixture being more strongly adsorbed and therefore remaining closer to the origin. In reversed-phase partition chromatography the supporting medium is impregnated with a non-polar solvent which acts as the stationary phase. Separation of compounds in the mixture is due in this case to differences in their relative solubilities in the stationary and moving phases, the most polar compounds moving furthest from the origin. Reversed-phase partition TLC may have advantages over adsorption TLC for certain separations, particularly for the separation of non-polar steroids. TLC methods for the separation of sterols have been described by Lisboa (1969) and those suitable for the separation of bile salts have been described by Eneroth and Sjövall (1971).

It is possible to use TLC for small-scale preparation of steroids (mg amounts on 20-cm plates), although the need to use layers of supporting medium 1–2 mm thick diminishes the resolving power of the method. Silica gel is the most generally useful supporting medium, but alumina, Florisil, Anasil and other adsorbents have advantages over silica gel for certain separations. When TLC is used for separation of the lipids in a total lipid extract, it is useful to separate polar from non-polar lipids by a preliminary step with a solvent system which leaves the more strongly adsorbed polar lipids at the origin. The lipid bands may then be eluted from the supporting medium and submitted to further TLC with different solvent systems. Improved separation of closely related compounds may often be achieved by the formation of derivatives. Examples are the formation of methyl esters for improving the separation of $5\alpha/5\beta$ isomers of bile acids (see p. 63) and the formation of epoxides for separating Δ^5 sterols from their saturated 5α analogues, e.g. cholesterol from cholestanol. However, it should be noted that some TLC separations are decreased by the formation of derivatives. For example, differences in the mobility of the 3α and 3β epimeric cholestanols on adsorption chromatography are considerably reduced if the effect of the hydroxyl group is masked by acetylation. Steroids differing only in the number of double bonds cannot be separated by TLC with silica gel as the supporting medium. However, if the silica gel is impregnated with silver nitrate ('argentation chromatography'), unsaturated sterols form complexes with the silver nitrate, thus permitting the separation of analogues with different numbers of double bonds.

3.3.2 Methods of detection

When the chromatographic separation has been completed, the positions of the individual compounds must be located. If the steroid is to be eluted and used for further study, a non-destructive method of detection must be used. One such method is to stand the plate in a glass tank containing a few crystals of iodine. The steroid spots will absorb iodine and appear as yellow areas against a white background. On removal from the tank, the iodine may be evaporated from the plate under a stream of air. Alternatively, if the supporting medium is impregnated with a fluorescent substance, such as Rhodamine B, the steroids show up as non-fluorescent areas against a fluorescent background when the plate is viewed under UV. Both these methods are applicable to all steroids. A non-destructive method that can be used to detect some steroids containing one or more double bonds is to spray the plate with a fluorescence indicator and then to view the plate under UV. The spots will appear as fluorescent areas against a non-fluorescent background. If the steroid is radioactive, its position may be located by autoradiography. With all non-destructive methods, the area occupied by the steroid is demarcated while it is visible by pricking with a needle.

A large number of destructive methods for the detection of steroids on TLC plates has been described by Lisboa (1969). Two of the best general methods are spraying with sulphuric acid or a perchloric-acid-ammonium molybdate mixture (Witter and Stone, 1957), followed by heating. Many colour reactions, including those described in Chapter 1, may be used for detecting steroids. Some of these give colours characteristic for specific classes of steroids and are capable of revealing less than 0.01 µg of steroids. Provided that a non-destructive method has been used for detection, the steroids may be eluted from the adsorbent after scraping off the area containing the steroid spot. There is usually no difficulty in recovering the less polar steroids from TLC adsorbents, but large volumes of polar solvents (e.g. chloroform-methanol 2:1 or diethyl ether-alcohol 1:1) may be required for complete recovery of the more polar steroids such as free bile acids.

3.3.3 Relation between structure and mobility

The mobility of a compound on TLC is expressed as an R_f value (the distance run by the compound, divided by the distance run by the solvent). Since the mobility of a compound chromatographed on a given supporting medium and with a given solvent system varies from one laboratory to another, and even with different batches of supporting medium, absolute R_f values are of little use for characterizing the chromatographic behaviour of steroids. R_f values should therefore be expressed in relation to the R_f of a pure, readily available, standard steroid run on the same TLC plate (relative R_f). Relative R_f values are reproducible, provided that the supporting medium, the solvent system, the distance run by the solvent and other conditions are specified.

The polarity of a steroid, as exhibited during TLC, is influenced by the nature, position, configuration and number of its nuclear substituents, by the configuration of the A/B ring junction and by the number and position of nuclear double bonds; the length and the degree of saturation of an alkyl side-chain usually have little effect on the polarity of a steroid in adsorption TLC. A knowledge of the effect of these structural features on polarity is helpful in predicting the R_f of a given steroid relative to that of other steroids on TLC under specified conditions. It may also enable one to select conditions, such as the formation of derivatives or the use of argentation chromatography, for improving the separation of closely related compounds. However, although there is, in general, a close relation between structure and polarity, the behaviour of many steroids on TLC is anomalous, so that few rules for predicting relative R_f values are absolute.

3.3.3.1 R_f of sterols. Some general rules applicable to sterols are illustrated in the following examples, most of which are taken from the reviews by Tschesche (1964), Lisboa (1969) and Eneroth and Sjövall (1969).

Saturated sterols with 5α configuration are usually more polar than their 5β isomers, an equatorial OH group (e) at C-3 usually contributes more polarity to the sterol molecule than an axial one (a) and a Δ^5 double bond has the same effect on polarity as the 5α configuration. Thus, the polarities of cholesterol and three isomeric cholestanols decrease in the order: $3\beta, 5\alpha(e) = 3\beta, \Delta^5(e) > 3\alpha, 5\beta(e) > 3\alpha, 5\alpha(a)$. (Sterols are here designated by the configurations at C-3 and C-5).

Sterols differing only in the structure of a saturated side-chain show little difference in polarity. For example, cholesterol (C_{27}, Δ^5), campesterol (C_{28}, Δ^5) and β-sitosterol (C_{29}, Δ^5) cannot be separated by adsorption TLC, though some separation may be achieved on reversed-phase partition TLC if the dominating effect of the OH group is masked by acetylation.

Unsaturated sterols differing in the number and positions of their double bonds tend to exhibit only small differences in polarity on TLC. For example, the following pairs of C_{27} sterols cannot be separated effectively by standard TLC:

$$\Delta^5/\Delta^{5,24}; \quad \Delta^5/\Delta^7; \quad \Delta^{8,24}/\Delta^{5,24}; \quad \Delta^{5,7}/\Delta^0, 5\alpha.$$

Separation of unsaturated sterols with different numbers of double bonds can usually be achieved by reversed-phase partition or argentation TLC and is often improved if the effects of small differences in polarity due to differences in the double bonds are accentuated by acetylation of the hydroxyl group. Some sterols differing only in the

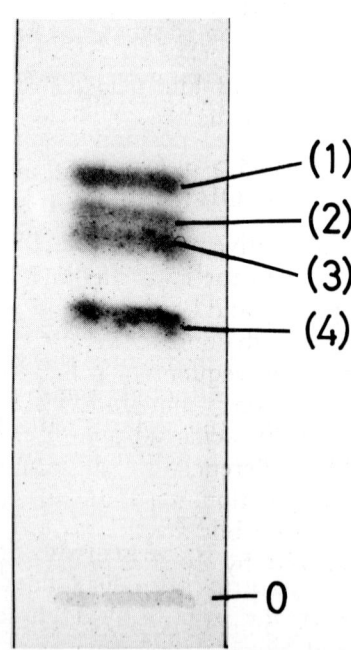

Figure 2.1
The separation of four closely related sterols by thin-layer chromatography with alumina impregnated with $AgNO_3$ as supporting medium. The compounds shown are the acetates of (1), 4,4-dimethylcholest-8(14)-enol; (2), 4,4-dimethylcholest-8(9)-enol; (3), 4,4-dimethylcholest-7-enol; (4), cholesterol. O = line of application of the mixture. The alumina-silver-nitrate plate was prepared as described by Gibbons et al. (1973) and the chromatogram was developed with hexane-toluene (3:1, v/v) at 4 °C. The developed plate was sprayed with 50% sulphuric acid and charred at 110 °C for 10 min.

I am indebted to G. F. Gibbons for preparing this chromatogram for me.

position of a single double bond may be separated by TLC with alumina impregnated with silver nitrate as the supporting medium (Gibbons et al., 1973) (see Fig. 2.1). A combination of argentation and reversed-phase partition TLC has been used successfully for the separation of a mixture of cholesterol, lathosterol and isomeric cholestanols (Truswell and Mitchell, 1965).

The presence of a methyl group at C-4 decreases the polarity of a sterol owing to hindrance of the 3β hydroxyl group. The presence of two methyl groups at C-4 has a greater effect than a single methyl group. The effect of 4-methyl groups on polarity may be used to separate mixtures of steroids into sterols, 4α-methyl sterols and 4,4-dimethyl sterols by adsorption TLC on a preparative scale (Goad and Goodwin, 1966). (On standard adsorption TLC the presence or absence of a 14α-methyl group makes little difference to the mobility of a sterol.)

3.3.3.2 R_f of bile acids.
Detailed information about the behaviour of bile acids on TLC will be found in the reviews by Hofmann (1964) and Eneroth and Sjövall (1969). Only a few of the more useful rules need be mentioned here.

In the normal (5β) mono-substituted bile acids an equatorial OH group at a given position confers greater polarity than an axial one and the effect of the substituent depends upon its position, the polarity decreasing in the order:

$$3\alpha OH(e) > 3\beta OH(a) > 7\beta OH(e) > 12\beta OH(e) > 7\alpha OH(a)$$
$$\geqslant 12\alpha OH(a) > 3\text{-keto} > 7\text{-keto} > 12\text{-keto}.$$

For normal bile acids with one or more substituents, polarity decreases in the order:

tri-OH > di-OH > mono-OH;   triketo > diketo > monoketo;
mono-OH > monoketo;   di-OH > diketo;   tri-OH > triketo.

The relative polarities of hydroxyketo bile acids are difficult to predict owing to the combined influence of the position and number of the hydroxy and keto groups. The separation of mixtures of bile acids into mono-, di- and tri-substituted classes is usually possible with single runs or sequential runs using different solvent systems and the separation is sometimes improved by formation of the methyl esters.

5α-Bile acids are usually more polar on TLC than their 5β isomers. This difference, due probably to the flattening effect of the trans A/B ring junction, may be exploited in the separation of normal (5β) from allo (5α) bile acids, particularly if the effect of the carboxyl group is masked by esterification (Table 2.1). There are exceptions to the general rule that 5α bile acids are more polar than their 5β isomers. For example, the presence of a 3αOH group (which is equatorial in

Table 2.1
Separation of 5β from 5α isomers of bile acids by adsorption TLC

Bile acid	Configuration at C-5	Relative R_f (5β = 100)	Solvent system	Adsorbent
(1) Propyl cholanoate	β	100	I	Anasil B
	α	79		
(2) 3αOH	β	100	II	Anasil B
(Me ester)	α	116		
(3) 3αOH,12αOH	β	100	III	Anasil B
(Me ester)	α	126		
(4) 3αOH,12αOH	β	100	IV	Silica gel G
(acid)	α	129		
(5) 3αOH,7αOH	β	100	IV	Silica gel G
(Me ester)	α	79		
(6) 3αOH,7αOH,12αOH	β	100	V	Silica gel G
(Me ester)	α	72		
(7) 3αOH,7αOH,12αOH	β	100	VI	Silica gel G
(acid)	α	86		

(Adapted from Eneroth and Sjövall, 1969)
Bile acids are designated by their hydroxyl groups (e.g., 3αOH = lithocholic acid). Me ester = methyl ester. For key to solvent systems see Eneroth and Sjövall (1969).

Note that a 3αOH group (2, 3 and 4) reverses polarity compared with that of the parent bile acid (1), unless a 7αOH group is present (5, 6 and 7). Note also that formation of the Me ester increases the separation between the 5α and 5β isomers of the 3αOH, 7αOH, 12αOH acid but has no significant effect on the separation of isomers of the 3αOH, 12αOH acid.

the 5β series) outweighs the effect of the 5α configuration. Thus, in most solvent systems lithocholic acid (3αOH, 5β) is more polar than allolithocholic acid (3αOH, 5α). Finally, it should be noted that a conjugated bile acid is always more polar than the corresponding free acid and that within a given class of mono-, di- and tri-hydroxy acid, taurine conjugates are more polar than glycine conjugates.

3.4 Gas-liquid chromatography
3.4.1 General principles
GLC is now the most rapid and versatile method for separating steroids on a micro scale and it can also be used for their assay, provided that appropriate conditions are chosen. The probable identity of a steroid can often be inferred by comparing its behaviour on GLC with that of a standard of known structure (see p. 98). By combining GLC with other methods of analysis, such as mass spectrometry, it may also be possible to elucidate the structure of a new steroid available only in microgram amounts in biological material. GLC equipment available in the laboratory is not suitable for preparative work, other than on the micro scale. However, GLC columns can be adapted for measurement of radioactivity combined

with mass assay and may therefore be used to measure the specific radioactivity of radioactive steroids (see pp. 76–7).

In GLC, the compounds to be analysed are vaporized at high temperature and are then carried by a stream of inert gas through a heated column of solid supporting medium whose particles are coated with a liquid (the 'liquid phase') in which the compounds are soluble. Separation depends on differential distribution between the liquid and gas phases.

Instructions for the preparation and operation of GLC columns will be found in the Handbook prepared by the Varian Instruments Company (McNair and Bonelli, 1969). The application of GLC to the qualitative and quantitative analysis of steroids is described in reviews by Vandenheuvel and Horning (1964), Kuksis (1966), Wotiz and Clark (1969), Eneroth and Sjövall (1969) and Heftmann (1975). The last three of these reviews include Tables of relative retention times (R_T) of a large number of the derivatives of sterols and bile acids submitted to GLC with different liquid phases.

3.4.2 Methods of detection

The vaporized compounds in the effluent gas may be detected by various methods, of which the most suitable for work with steroids are the flame-ionization detector and the electron-capture detector.

In the flame-ionization detector the gas leaving the column passes through a hydrogen flame between two electrodes. Some of the molecules of the eluted sample are ionized by the hydrogen flame as they pass through the electrode gap, allowing a current to flow. The current due to the ionization of impurities in the carrier gas and of volatile components of the liquid phase is adjusted to zero, so that the recorder traces the current due to the ionization of the components of the sample eluted from the column. Since the current is proportional to the concentration of ions in the gas between the electrodes, the elution of a pure compound should be recorded as a single symmetrical peak. The flame-ionization detector responds to all organic compounds and is capable of detecting less than 10 ng (0.01 µg) of sample under appropriate conditions.

In the electron-capture detector the carrier gas is ionized by a source of radiation (usually tritium or ^{63}Ni). The ions migrate to the anode of an electrode gap, producing a steady current. If an electron-absorbing compound is eluted from the column, the current is decreased while the electron-absorbing molecules pass through the detector. Electron-capture detectors are capable of detecting less than 0.1 ng of sample.

Flame-ionization detectors are preferable to electron-capture detectors for most steroid work. The electron-capture detector is more sensitive and has the additional advantage that it does not destroy the sample, but it is less stable, it has a narrower range over which the response is proportional to the mass of the sample and it can be used only for compounds that are electron absorbers or that can be converted into electron-absorbing derivatives.

3.4.3 Solid supports and liquid phases

Most solid supports used for GLC are prepared from diatomaceous earths and are of graded particle size. Liquid phases suitable for the separation of sterols and bile acids by GLC must be stable as thin films at high temperatures (200–300 °C) and should have negligible vapour pressure at these temperatures. Many synthetic polar and non-polar liquid phases are available commercially and their number and range is continually being added to. A useful non-polar liquid phase for separating steroids is SE-30, a straight-chain polymer of methyl siloxane:

$$H_3C-\underset{\underset{CH_3}{|}}{\overset{\overset{CH_3}{|}}{Si}}-O{\left[\underset{\underset{CH_3}{|}}{\overset{\overset{CH_3}{|}}{Si}}-O\right]}_x\underset{\underset{CH_3}{|}}{\overset{\overset{CH_3}{|}}{Si}}-CH_3 \quad ; \quad x = 15{,}000-35{,}000$$

Non-polar phases (sometimes referred to as 'non-selective') separate steroids largely on the basis of differences in molecular size and shape, interaction between a non-polar liquid phase and the functional groups of a steroid having little selective effect on its retention time. Non-polar liquid phases are therefore unsatisfactory for separating steroids differing only in the position or configuration of functional groups, unless the difference leads to a difference in molecular shape.

Two of the most useful polar liquid phases are QF-1, a polysiloxane containing fluoroalkyl groups:

$$(CH_3)_3Si{\left[O-\underset{\underset{CH_3}{|}}{\overset{\overset{\overset{\overset{CF_3}{|}}{(CH_2)_2}}{|}}{Si}}\right]}_x{\left[O-\underset{\underset{CH_3}{|}}{\overset{\overset{CH_3}{|}}{Si}}\right]}_y O-Si(CH_3)_3$$

and the polymerized ester NGS (neopentylglycol succinate):

$$\left[-\text{O}-\text{CH}_2-\underset{\underset{\text{CH}_3}{|}}{\overset{\overset{\text{CH}_3}{|}}{\text{C}}}-\text{CH}_2-\text{O}-\overset{\overset{\text{O}}{\|}}{\text{C}}-\text{CH}_2-\text{CH}_2-\overset{\overset{\text{O}}{\|}}{\text{C}}-\text{O} \right]_x$$

With polar liquid phases, the separation of steroids is due largely to differences in the nature, number and position of their functional groups. However, the effect of a given functional group is not the same for all polar phases. For example, QF-1 separates isomers of hydroxylated steroids with great efficiency but has little ability to separate on the basis of double bonds, whereas the polyester phases show selective retention of unsaturated steroids. It is sometimes possible to combine the selective properties of two liquid phases by forming co-polymers, e.g. by the addition of a siloxane monomer to ethylene glycol succinate during its polymerization.

3.4.4 Formation of derivatives

Although many steroids, including cholesterol itself, can be chromatographed successfully on GLC columns without modification, the formation of derivatives has several advantages, including increased volatility, increased thermal stability and decreased adsorption to the solid support, resulting in narrower peaks with less tailing. The separation of some steroids may also be improved by derivative formation. With SE-30, for example, cholesterol and epicholesterol cannot be separated as the free sterols but can be separated if they are converted into their trimethylsilyl (TMS) ethers, presumably because the presence of the bulky substituent at C-3 accentuates the difference in molecular shape of the two epimers. Separation of steroids differing in the degree of saturation of the ring system, or in the configuration of the A/B ring junction, may also be improved if the influence of OH groups is masked by the formation of esters or ethers, e.g. the separation of cholesterol from 5α-cholestanol on QF-1 is improved by formation of the trifluoroacetates (Kuksis, 1966). The formation of derivatives also helps in the identification of steroids by the 'peak shift' method (see p. 98) and is necessary for the quantitative analysis of some steroids. The derivatives most commonly used for GLC of steroids are methyl esters, trifluoroacetates and TMS ethers. Other chemical modifications useful for improving the separation of closely related steroids or for producing peak shifts, include oxidation of steroid alcohols, the formation of hydroborides from unsaturated steroids and the formation of epoxides. Epoxide formation is particularly useful in the separation of Δ^5-sterols from their saturated analogues. For example, the separation of cholesterol from 5α-cholestanol is facilitated by conversion of the cholesterol into the much more polar 5,6-epoxide by p-nitroperbenzoic acid.

Steroids containing a carboxyl group should be esterified before they are submitted to GLC. The best method of esterification is to form the methyl ester by treating the compound with a freshly prepared solution of diazomethane in dry ether. The ether is evaporated and the methylated sample is dissolved in a suitable solvent for further treatment or for application to the GLC column.

For the formation of a trifluoroacetate, the steroid is dissolved in pyridine or hexane and allowed to react with trifluoroacetic anhydride. When the reaction is complete the solvent is evaporated under nitrogen. Trifluoroacetates decompose in the presence of moisture and should not be stored for more than a few hours before GLC.

Many silylating reagents are available commercially, but the most widely used for steroids is Tri-Sil (Pierce Chemical Company), a mixture of hexamethyldisilazane (HMDS) and trimethylchlorosilane (TMCS) dissolved in pyridine. With this reagent, the formation of TMS ethers proceeds as follows:

$$3\text{R-OH} + \text{HN}\begin{matrix}\text{Si}\equiv(\text{CH}_3)_3 \\ \text{Si}\equiv(\text{CH}_3)_3\end{matrix} + \text{Cl-Si}\equiv(\text{CH}_3)_3$$

(Hydroxy-steroid)   (HMDS)   (TMCS)

$$\rightarrow 3\text{R-O-Si}\equiv(\text{CH}_3)_3 + \text{NH}_4\text{Cl}$$

The NH_4Cl is precipitated during the reaction and does not interfere with the chromatography. With Tri-Sil, most hydroxylated steroids are completely silylated within 30 min at room temperature, but hindered hydroxyl groups (e.g., 11β and 17α) may not be completely silylated unless more rigorous conditions are used. Keto groups are not usually silylated, but a 3-keto group may form a TMS ether, presumably after enolization, if pyridine is used as solvent. By modifying the conditions or by using different reagents it is possible to achieve selective silylation of the hydroxyl groups. For example, in the 5β series of bile acids, 6α, 7β and 12β hydroxyl groups may be silylated without silylation of 6β, 7α and 12αOH groups (Eneroth and Sjövall, 1969). Halogenated silanes may be used for forming steroid derivatives with high-electron-absorbing capacity for use with an electron-capture detector.

3.4.5 Relation between structure and retention time

3.4.5.1 General remarks.
The behaviour of steroids on GLC is usually more difficult to predict than their behaviour on TLC.

Attempts to formulate precise rules for predicting the R_T of steroids from a knowledge of their structure, and for deducing their structure from their GLC behaviour, have not been entirely successful. The retention time of a steroid, relative to that of a standard reference compound, is usually influenced markedly by the nature of the liquid phase and may also be affected by the operating conditions, including the temperature of the column and the gas flow. However, provided that different classes of liquid phase are considered separately, it is possible to make limited generalizations of use in the selection of suitable conditions for separating known compounds and in the preliminary steps in identification of unknown compounds. These empirical rules are based on measurements of the R_T of large numbers of steroids examined under specified conditions (see, for example, Clayton, 1962; Vandenheuvel and Horning, 1962; Brooks, 1964). Although it is often possible to explain the GLC behaviour of a steroid in terms of molecular size, molecular shape and polarity of its substituents, many steroids have anomalous R_T values for which no convincing explanation can be offered. The influence of certain double bonds on R_T in polar and non-polar liquid phases is a case in point (see examples listed below).

3.4.5.2 Influence of the liquid phase. With *non-polar liquid phases* such as SE-30, differences in the R_T of steroids can usually be explained by differences in molecular size or in the shape of the ring system. In general, R_T increases with increasing molecular size and increasing flatness of the ring system. Exceptions to the rule relating R_T to molecular size can often be explained by steric hindrance of substituents which interact non-selectively with the liquid phase, e.g. the anomalously low R_T of lanosterol and its analogues is probably due to hindrance of the 3β-OH by the 4,4-dimethyl group, the steric effect outweighing the effect on molecular size. Differences in the configuration of nuclear substituents have little effect on retention time with non-polar liquid phases. Hence, epimers cannot be separated on these phases. R_T may be influenced by the number and positions of double bonds in the nucleus and side-chain, but these effects are usually due to modification of the shape of the ring system rather than to specific interactions with the liquid phase, such as occur between carbon–carbon double bonds and some of the more polar liquid phases, as described below.

With *polar liquid phases*, in addition to effects due to differences in molecular size and shape, retention time is influenced by the polarity and position of substituents. For example, with a moderately polar liquid phase such as QF-1 it is possible to separate hydroxy steroids from their corresponding ketones and to separate methyl esters of bile acids differing only in the positions of hydroxyl groups. It may also be possible to separate isomers differing in the configuration of substituents, an equatorial substituent conferring longer R_T than the corresponding axial substituent. Other polar liquid phases, particularly the polyester resins, are capable of separating steroids on the basis of differences in the number and positions of carbon–carbon double bonds. This property seems to be due mainly to specific interaction of the liquid phase with the double bonds. However, in the case of nuclear double bonds it is not always possible to distinguish between a direct interaction with the liquid phase and an effect mediated by an influence on the geometry of the A/B and B/C ring junctions.

3.4.5.3 The effect of derivative formation.
The formation of derivatives to achieve better separation of closely related steroids has already been discussed (p. 67). The blocking of substituents by the formation of esters or ethers usually increases R_T with non-polar liquid phases but may markedly shorten R_T with polar phases.

3.4.5.4 R_T of sterols.
The following examples illustrate some of the more useful rules for predicting the R_T of sterols.

The effect of *molecular size* is shown by the increase in R_T of Δ^5 sterols with increasing number of carbon atoms in the side-chain:

$$\text{cholesterol} < \text{campesterol} < \beta\text{-sitosterol}.$$

Differences in the *configuration* of the A/B ring junction usually permit separation on most liquid phases. Thus, $5\alpha/5\beta$ isomers of sterols and their keto analogues can be separated on SE-30, the 5α isomer having a longer R_T than the 5β isomer. For example, 5α-cholestanol can be separated from 5β-cholestanol and the separation is improved if the effect of the 3β-OH groups is blocked by TMS-ether formation. Sterols differing only in the configuration of a nuclear hydroxyl group have similar R_T on non-polar phases but can often be separated on a polar phase, the epimer with the equatorial OH having the longer R_T, e.g. 5α-cholestan-3β-ol (equatorial OH) has a longer R_T than 5α-cholestan-3α-ol (axial OH). Increasing the size of the C-3 substituent by TMS-ether formation improves the separation. Sterols differing only in the configuration of an alkyl substituent at C-24 cannot be separated effectively by GLC. For example, stigmasterol (24 S) and its 24 R isomer (poriferasterol) have the same R_T on all liquid phases tested. However, pairs of sterols isomeric at a $\Delta^{24\,(28)}$ double bond may be separated on some phases (Knights, 1973).

Differences in the nature and position of *substituents* in a sterol molecule usually affect its R_T on polar phases. For example, a keto group usually confers longer R_T than a hydroxyl group at a given position. With monoketo derivatives, R_T may be affected by the position of the keto group, so that some pairs of positional isomers can

Analysis of Sterols and Related Steroids   71

be separated. In general, the effects of more than one substituent are additive provided that the substituents are not close enough to interact. For example, for compounds differing only in their substituents, R_T increases in the order:

monohydroxy < monoketo < monohydroxy, monoketo < diketo.

With non-polar liquid phases the effect of *double bonds* is usually negligible unless the double bond influences molecular shape. Thus, with SE-30, cholesterol cannot be separated from 5α-cholestanol but can be separated from C_{27} sterols containing a Δ^7 or Δ^{24} double bond, such as lathosterol and desmosterol.

Many polar liquid phases interact selectively with C—C double bonds in a sterol, the effect on R_T depending upon the number and positions of the double bonds. When two or more non-conjugated double bonds are present, their effect on R_T is usually additive. An interesting exception to this is the effect of a Δ^{22} double bond which, in some series of sterols, decreases the R_T, presumably by influencing the rigidity of the side-chain. These effects of double bonds are illustrated by the retention times of sterols of the ergostanol series (24 β-methylcholestanols) analysed as their methyl ethers on diethyleneglycol succinate polymer (Clayton, 1962). For this series, R_T increases in the order:

$\Delta^{5,22} < \Delta^{8}(^{14}) < \Delta^{5} < \Delta^{7,22} < \Delta^{7,9,22} < \Delta^{7} < \Delta^{5,24}(28) < \Delta^{5,7,22} < \Delta^{5,7}$.

Thus, the Δ^{22} double bond decreases R_T in the presence of Δ^5, Δ^7 or $\Delta^{5,7}$. A similar effect of Δ^{22} is seen in the 24α-ethylcholestanol series, stigmasteryl methyl ether ($\Delta^{5,22}$) having a shorter R_T than β-sitosteryl methyl ether (Δ^5).

The gas-liquid chromatogram of 6 sterols shown in Fig. 2.2

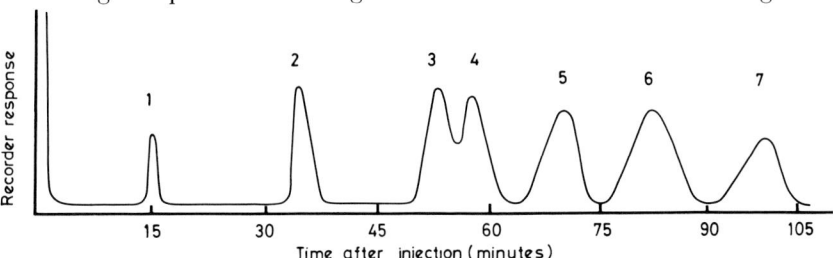

Figure 2.2
Gas-liquid chromatogram of a mixture of the methyl ethers of six sterols. *Peak 1*, 5α-cholestane; *peak 2*, 5β-cholestan-3β-ol (coprostanol); *peak 3*, 5α-cholestan-3β-ol; *peak 4*, cholesterol; *peak 5*, 5α-cholest-7-en-3β-ol; *peak 6*, cholest-5,7-dien-3β-ol; *peak 7*, ergosterol.

GLC was carried out with a 6 ft × 4 mm stainless steel column and with an ionization detector. The liquid phase was 5% diethyleneglycol succinate polymer supported on acid-washed chromosorb W; column temperature was 195 °C; detector temperature was 212 °C. (Drawn from Clayton, 1962, with the permission of R. B. Clayton.)

illustrates some of the effects of sterol structure on R_T. With the polar liquid phase used for this analysis of a mixture of known sterol methyl ethers: 5α-cholestanol has a longer R_T than 5β-cholestanol (coprostanol); cholesterol is not separated from 5α-cholestanol; three sterols differing only in their nuclear double bonds (Δ^5, Δ^7 and $\Delta^{5,7}$) are well separated; ergosterol has the longest R_T, owing to a combination of the $\Delta^{5,7}$ double-bond system and the 24β-methyl group. Note, however, that cholesterol and 5α-cholestanol can be separated as their TMS ethers on QF-1 columns (Fig. 2.3), presumably because the effect of the 3β-OH group is masked.

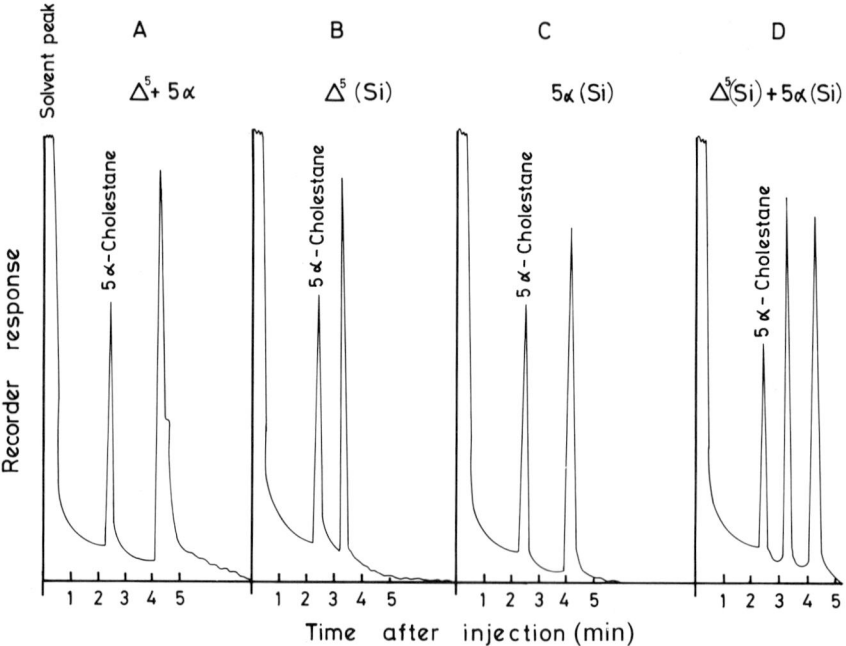

Figure 2.3
The effect of trimethylsilylation on the separation of cholesterol and 5α-cholestanol on GLC columns with QF-1 as liquid phase. A mixture of unsilylated cholesterol (Δ^5) and 5α-cholestanol (5α) gave a single peak (A). Formation of the TMS ether (Δ^5(Si)) and (5α(Si)) decreased the retention time of both sterols relative to that of a 5α-cholestane marker (B, C), but permitted separation of the two sterols (D).

GLC was carried out with a Pye-Unicam Chromatograph (Series 204), with a 6-foot glass column and a hydrogen-flame ionization detector. Column conditions were: 1% QF-1 on 80–100 mesh Varaport; column temp., 220 °C; detector temp., 255 °C; the carrier gas was N_2 (35 ml/min). (Analysis by S. Niththyananthan).

3.4.5.5 R_T of bile acids. A full discussion of the GLC behaviour of bile acids will be found in two reviews by Eneroth and Sjövall (1969, 1971), so that only the more important aspects need be mentioned here. Owing to their high polarity, bile acids must be esterified, preferably by methylation, before GLC. All the following remarks refer to the behaviour of the methyl esters of bile acids and their derivatives.

With non-polar phases, separation is due mainly to differences in the number of hydroxyl or keto groups, R_T increasing with the total number of substituents. Positional effects do, however, occur. For example, chenodeoxycholic acid (3α, 7α) has a longer R_T than deoxycholic acid (3α, 12α) on some non-polar phases owing to hindrance of the 12α-OH group by the side-chain.

With polar phases, a keto group confers longer R_T than a hydroxyl group and the effect of two or more substituents is usually additive. Thus, for most bile-acid methyl esters analysed on QF-1, R_T increases in the order:

mono-OH < monoketo < di-OH < mono-OH, monoketo < tri-OH
    < diketo < di-OH, monoketo < mono-OH, diketo < triketo.

Exceptions to this are noted by Eneroth and Sjövall (1969). With polar liquid phases many positional and configurational isomers of bile acids can be separated (see Fig. 2.4). For hydroxyl groups, the

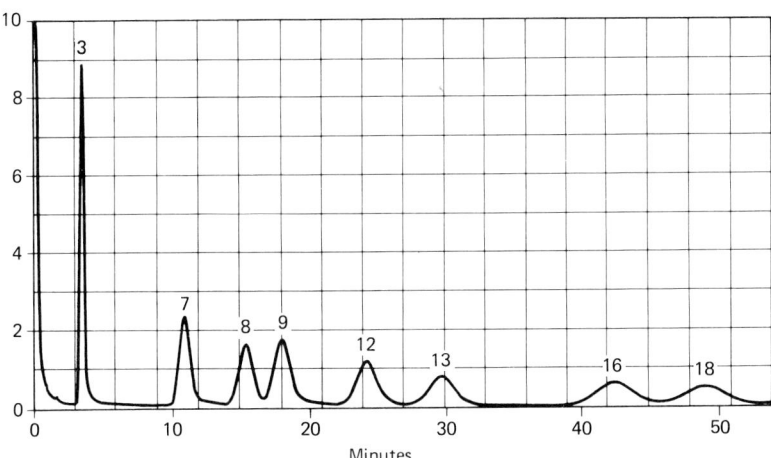

Figure 2.4
Gas-liquid chromatography of a mixture of eight bile acids separated as the trifluoroacetates of their methyl esters. The bile acids shown are cholanoic acid (3) and the following derivatives of cholanoic acid: 3α-hydroxy (7); 3β,12α-dihydroxy (8); 3α-12α-dihydroxy (9); 3α,7α-dihydroxy (12); 3α,6α-dihydroxy (13); 3α,7α,12α-trihydroxy (16); 3α-hydroxy,7-keto (18). Column conditions were: 1% QF-1 on 100–120 mesh Gas-Chrom P (5 ft × $\frac{1}{8}$ in); column temp., 205 °C; gas, N_2 at a flow rate of 100 ml/min. (Reproduced from Kuksis (1966), with the permission of the author and of John Wiley and Sons.)

less hindered 3 position confers longer R_T than the 6, 7 and 12 positions, and an equatorial group confers longer R_T than an axial one in the same position. For example, on QF-1 the R_T of the methyl esters of 5β-monohydroxy bile acids increases in the order:

$$12\alpha(a) < 12\beta(e) < 7\alpha(a) < 7\beta(e) < 6\alpha(a) < 3\beta(a) < 3\alpha(e).$$

As with sterols, a 5α (allo) bile acid usually has a longer R_T than its 5β isomer. However, the presence of an equatorial 3-OH group diminishes, and may even outweigh, the effect of 5α configuration and this anomalous effect is enhanced if the bulk of the C-3 substituent is increased by derivative formation. For example, on QF-1 the TMS ether of methyl cholanoate (5β with equatorial 3α-OH) has a longer R_T than the TMS ether of methyl allocholanoate (5α with axial 3α-OH).

Figure 2.4 illustrates the power of GLC to separate bile acids. On this chromatogram, four isomeric dihydroxy bile acids are well separated and the elution sequence of the hydroxy acids is that to be expected from the additive effects of the individual hydroxyl groups. Note that for the trifluoroacetates of the methyl esters of bile acids, monohydroxy monoketo acids have *longer* R_T than the trihydroxy acids on QF-1.

3.4.6 Quantitative gas-liquid chromatography

GLC may be used for the assay of steroids and is, indeed, the method of choice in many cases. Compared with most other methods it has the advantage of speed, specificity and sensitivity, and is particularly well suited to the simultaneous assay of several closely related steroids in a mixture. For this purpose, the liquid phase and column conditions must be such that there is little or no overlap between successive peaks. If this cannot be achieved, the steroids must be separated (for example, by TLC) before GLC. For some purposes, however, the steroids in a mixture need only be assayed as a class. In this case, separation of individual steroids on the column is not necessary, provided that the detector response per unit mass is the same for all the steroids in the mixture. An example of this will be found on p. 112.

Although quantitative GLC is simple in principle, several conditions must be satisfied before it can be applied to the assay of any steroid.

The steroid must be shown to pass through the column without appreciable degradation or reversible adsorption. Recovery of the steroid from the column may be determined either by injecting a radioactive sample on to the column and measuring radioactivity in the effluent gas or by mixing the steroid with a known amount of a closely related inert steroid hydrocarbon and then measuring the relative areas of the peaks due to the two compounds. For example, recovery of cholesterol from a column could be determined from the relative areas of the two peaks obtained by injecting a mixture of equal amounts of cholesterol and 5α-cholestane. If there were no loss of cholesterol on the column, the peak areas should be equal. It is permissible to correct for small constant losses of a steroid during GLC, but recoveries of less than 80% should not be accepted. Adsorption to the solid support may be minimized by careful attention to the preparation and packing of the column. In particular, losses on the column may be diminished by acid-washing and silylation of the supporting medium and by increasing the percentage of liquid phase. Recovery of steroids with polar substituents is often improved by conversion to derivatives with greater thermal stability.

The response of the detector must be linear with respect to the quantity of sample injected over the range to be assayed. Standard curves should be constructed by measuring the response to increasing amounts of the steroid injected in a constant volume of solvent. Under favourable conditions linearity may be achieved over the range 0.1 to 5.0 µg for sterols and bile acids. Automatic injectors are now available commercially and give more reproducible results than manual injection.

The method used for injecting known volumes of sample on to the column must be accurate. Alternatively, injection errors can be eliminated by using an internal standard. A known amount of a standard steroid is added to the solvent containing the steroid to be assayed and a sample (whose volume need not be known accurately) is injected on to the column. The relative areas of the peaks due to the unknown and the standard are then determined. The standard must have GLC properties similar to those of the unknown and it must produce a peak completely separate from the peaks produced by all other compounds in the sample. If the peak area/mass ratios are not the same for the standard and unknown, an appropriate correction factor must be used. The 'internal standard ratio' method may be used to assay several steroids in a mixture with a single internal standard provided that the peak area/mass ratios are the same for all unknowns and the standard, or that appropriate factors to correct for differences in peak area/mass ratio have been determined. Correction factors cannot, of course, be determined for peaks due to unidentified steroids in a mixture.

A simple example will illustrate the use of an internal standard for the assay of a single sterol. A solution containing 1 mg of 5α-cholestane is added to a tissue extract containing an unknown amount of cholesterol and a sample of the mixture is submitted to GLC under conditions in which the 5α-cholestane and cholesterol peaks are separate and the peak area/mass ratios are the same for the two compounds. The area of the peak due to cholesterol is found to be twice that of the 5α-cholestane peak. Therefore the extract contains 2 mg of cholesterol.

The method for estimating the areas of the peaks must be accurate. If the peaks are sharp and are superimposed on a flat base-line, relative peak areas may be determined from relative peak heights. For direct measurement of peak areas a simple and accurate method (error less than 2%) is to make a photocopy of the chart and to cut out and weigh the peaks on the photocopy. A more accurate and less time-consuming method is to use an electronic digital integrator capable of measuring areas of peaks superimposed on a flat or falling base-line.

For specific examples of the use of GLC for assaying steroids, see Sections 6.1 and 6.3.

3.4.7 Radioassay combined with GLC

It is often desirable to measure the radioactivity in steroids separated by GLC. For example, in studies of sterol biosynthesis one may wish to know the specific radioactivity of each of the labelled steroid intermediates formed during the incubation of a tissue with a radioactive precursor. Provided that the specific radioactivity of the intermediates is high enough for measurement of radioactivity in microgram amounts, this may be achieved by simultaneous GLC and radioassay.

If a non-destructive mass detector is used, the whole of the effluent gas can be conducted from the detector into the radiation counting system. If a destructive detector system is used, a stream-splitter must be inserted between the column and the detector so that a known proportion of the effluent can be diverted into the counting system. Since most radioactive compounds encountered in steroid work are labelled with ^{14}C or ^{3}H, the counting system must be capable of detecting low-energy beta radiations. The steroids eluted from the column may be assayed for radioactivity without modification, or they may be burnt to CO_2 and water before radioassay, the water being reduced to hydrogen if ^{3}H is to be assayed. Conversion into gases eliminates contamination of the counting system by local condensation of steroids.

The radiation detectors that have been used successfully in combination with GLC of steroids are Geiger–Müller tubes with very thin end-windows (not suitable for ^{3}H), proportional counters and scintillation systems with liquid or solid scintillators. If the radioactive compounds in the effluent accumulate in the counting system, as in the liquid-scintillation system described by Popják et al. (1959), an integrated response is obtained, the radioactivity recorder showing the total counts/min accumulated at any time during the chromatography of the sample. With other counting systems a continuous record of counting rate is obtained, each radioactive steroid that emerges from the column producing a separate peak of radioactivity superimposed on a flat baseline. A simple manual method for combining GLC with radioassay is to collect serial fractions from the column, using a stream-splitter if necessary, by condensing the vaporized steroids in capillary tubes during timed intervals. The contents of the capillary tubes are then transferred to vials for scintillation counting. The disadvantage of this method is that it cannot provide a continuous record of radioactivity. Hence its power to resolve adjacent peaks of radioactivity is limited.

4 IDENTIFICATION

4.1 General principles

There are two rather different aspects to the problem of identifying a steroid. On the one hand, the compound may be one whose structure is already established and for which a reference compound is available. Examples that come to mind are the detection of 5α-cholestanol in the lesions of cerebrotendinous xanthomatosis, of allo bile acids in human faeces and of desmosterol in the plasma of triparanol-treated animals. On the other hand, one may be faced with the more difficult problem of identifying a previously unknown steroid. In the latter case it is usually necessary to synthesize reference compounds with which to compare the unknown.

For the complete identification of a steroid in a biological sample it is necessary to establish the structure of the whole carbon skeleton, the nature, position and configuration of all substituents and the positions of any double bonds present. When double bonds are present in the side-chain it may also be necessary to determine their configuration. Although it is always desirable to achieve complete identification, partial identification (identification of some but not all structural features of the compound) may be very useful, for example in confirming or disproving the participation of a postulated intermediate in a biosynthetic sequence. In some cases the steroid in question can be obtained in quantities sufficient for conventional chemical and physical analysis. Frequently, however, it can only be obtained in microgram quantities, or in trace amounts detectable only by the presence of radioactivity. In the latter case, the problem of complete identification may test to the limit the ingenuity, technical skill and deductive powers of the investigator. An impressive example of this is the identification, by Gautschi and Bloch, of a new radioactive intermediate formed in trace amounts during the biosynthesis of cholesterol from [^{14}C]acetate in rat liver. From a consideration of its biological origin and behaviour, and of its radiochemical properties when mixed with lanosterol, Gautschi and Bloch (1957) deduced that the new compound was a sterol with a *gem*-dimethyl substituent at C-4, a Δ^{24} double bond and a nuclear double bond close to the B/C ring junction. Identification was established by correlation of the radioactive intermediate with chemically synthesized 14-desmethyl-lanosterol (4,4-dimethyl-5α-cholesta-8,24-dien-3β-ol) (Gautschi and Bloch, 1958).

For final proof of a proposed structure, the behaviour of the unknown compound must be shown to be identical with that of a reference compound whose complete structure is known. If no reference compound is available, decisive information may sometimes be obtained by comparison with a model compound possessing structural features presumed to be present in the unknown, as in the elucidation of the structure of presqualene pyrophosphate described below (Section 5.1).

4.2 Preliminary steps

The first step in the identification of any steroid should always be the extraction of all the lipids present in the sample. This may be followed by saponification and successive extraction of the hydrolysate before and after acidification. Non-saponifiable lipid will be extracted from the alkaline hydrolysate, acidic lipids remaining behind. The sterols in the non-saponifiable fraction may be partially purified by precipitation with digitonin and subsequently recovered from their digitonides for further study (see Goad and Goodwin, 1967). This procedure removes quinones, squalene, polyisoprenoid alcohols and other non-sterols from the mixture, but does not precipitate lanosterol and other trimethyl sterols completely.

The total non-saponifiable fraction, or the sterols recovered from the digitonin precipitate, may be separated into classes by column chromatography or preparative TLC, using non-destructive methods of detection so that the fraction containing the compound to be identified can be recovered at each step. For example, with columns or TLC plates of alumina it is possible to separate a complex mixture of sterols into 4,4-dimethyl sterols (with or without a 14α-methyl group), sterols with one methyl group at C-4 and sterols, such as cholesterol, with no methyl group at C-4 (4-di-desmethyl sterols). This method has been used successfully in the preliminary stages in the separation of complex mixtures of sterols obtained from animals (Clayton *et al.*, 1963) or plants (Goad and Goodwin, 1967). Sterols with different numbers of double bonds in each class may then be separated by TLC or column chromatography with $AgNO_3$-impregnated solid phases. Argentation chromatography may also be used to separate closely similar sterols differing in the positions of their double bonds. Lutsky *et al.* (1971), for example, have separated 5α-cholesta-8,14-dien-3β-ol from the $\Delta^{7,14}$ diene by column chromatography on Silica Gel G-Super-Gel-silver nitrate. Separation of sterols by argentation TLC on the basis of differences in the positions of double bonds may be much improved if the effect of the 3βOH group is masked by acetylation (Gibbons *et al.*, 1973).

A similar approach, using column or thin-layer chromatography with more polar solvents, may be used to separate acidic steroids into classes. For example, bile acids may be separated into free and conjugated acids, and some degree of separation within each class may be achieved on the basis of the number and nature of substituents (see pp. 63–64).

The information obtained at this stage will usually point to the general structure of the steroid, the presence of substituents, and the number, and possibly the positions, of double bonds. This may be sufficient to suggest a tentative identification or at least to narrow the search to a small number of possible compounds. Comparison between the TLC behaviour of the compound and that of reference compounds, before and after derivative formation and in different solvent systems, may lead to exclusion of some of these possible structures.

4.3 Gas-liquid chromatography

Additional evidence may be obtained from the behaviour of the compound on GLC with polar and non-polar liquid phases. Measurement of the changes in R_T (peak shifts) brought about by the formation of derivatives will also provide valuable information. The peak-shift method has been found especially useful for the identification of bile acids, particularly in the hands of Eneroth and Sjövall (1969). (For an example of the peak-shift method see Section 5.3).

4.4 Other methods of identification

4.4.1 General remarks

For some purposes, identification by a combination of TLC and GLC may be sufficient, as in cases where the presence of a particular sterol in the biological material under investigation is already well established. But for complete identification of unknown steroids additional methods must be used. At some stage in the identification of a steroid it is necessary to obtain it in a pure state. In this connection, it should be noted that the demonstration that a steroid gives a single peak on GLC does not prove that it is pure. The sample may contain impurities that do not chromatograph because they are non-volatile or heat-labile, or it may contain a mixture of compounds that are not separated under the GLC conditions used. A mixture of cholesterol and 5α-cholestanol, for example, would give a single peak on SE-30 or QF-1. If the sample still gives a single peak when tested after derivative formation and on several different liquid phases, the probability that it is pure is increased. However, as noted above, sterols differing only in the configuration of an alkyl group at C-24 cannot be distinguished by GLC. Hence, complete identification of a C-24 alkylated sterol cannot be achieved by GLC.

If the steroid to be identified is radioactive, it may be mixed with a non-radioactive reference compound and the specific radioactivity determined after successive recrystallization before and after derivative formation. If the specific radioactivity falls, the unknown steroid differs from the reference compound. If the specific radioactivity remains unchanged, identity is probable, but not certain since steroids with different structures may co-crystallize even after derivative formation.

In addition to measurement of the melting-point and the optical rotation, other methods applicable to the identification of steroids include UV and IR spectroscopy, magnetic-resonance spectroscopy, mass spectrometry and measurement of chiroptical properties (see Section 4.4.7). These methods are discussed briefly in this section in relation to steroid chemistry. More detailed explanations will be found in the introductory chapters of any advanced textbook of organic chemistry. Each method has its own advantages and disadvantages in the solution of a structural problem in steroid work and it is often necessary to use a combination of several methods if a complete elucidation is to be achieved (see Section 5). At present, the most widely used methods in steroid analysis are IR spectroscopy and mass spectrometry, usually after preliminary investigation by TLC and GLC, but it is probable that some of the other methods, particularly magnetic resonance spectroscopy and chiroptical techniques, will be used much more widely in the future if the necessary instrumentation is improved. The crucial role of X-ray crystallography in the final stages of the elucidation of the structure of cholesterol has already been mentioned in Chapter 1. A discussion of other contributions of X-ray crystallography in the steroid field will be found in the review by Karle (1973). It should also be noted that the determination of the *absolute* configuration of virtually all steroids must be traced back ultimately to the determination of the absolute configuration of a chiral reference compound by differential X-ray analysis. Determination of the absolute configuration of cholesterol by isolation of a fragment containing C-20 as the single chiral centre is a case in point (see p. 40). The use of X-ray crystallography and fluorescence depolarization in the investigation of the physical state of sterols in membranes is discussed in Chapter 7. For a critical discussion of methods now available for the analysis of steroids, see Gibbons *et al.* (1982).

4.4.2 UV spectroscopy

Absorption of radiations in the UV region (≃185–400 mµ) is due mainly to changes in the energy of electrons involved in the formation of valency bonds. UV absorption spectra are therefore of value in revealing the presence of double bonds and, in particular, of conjugated double-bond systems. Certain structural features have characteristic effects on the wave-length and intensity of absorption peaks in the UV spectrum. For example, the intensity of the absorption peak due to a single double bond at about 210 µm increases with the degree of substitution of the $\diagdown_/\diagup$ C=C $\diagup^\diagdown$ group. Thus, the absorption at 210 mµ for mono-unsaturated steroids increases in the order: Δ^2 (di-substituted) $< \Delta^4 = \Delta^5$ (tri-substituted) $< \Delta^{8(9)} = \Delta^{8(14)}$ (tetra-substituted). This property may provide evidence about the position of a nuclear double bond (Bladon, Henbest and Wood, 1952).

Conjugated double-bond systems in steroids also give characteristic UV spectra, as shown in Fig. 2.5. If the two conjugated double bonds are present in the steroid nucleus it is often possible to tell whether they are in the same or different rings. The $\Delta^{5,7}$ conjugated double bond system present in provitamins D gives a characteristic UV absorption spectrum, with peaks at 271, 282 and 293.5 mµ. This

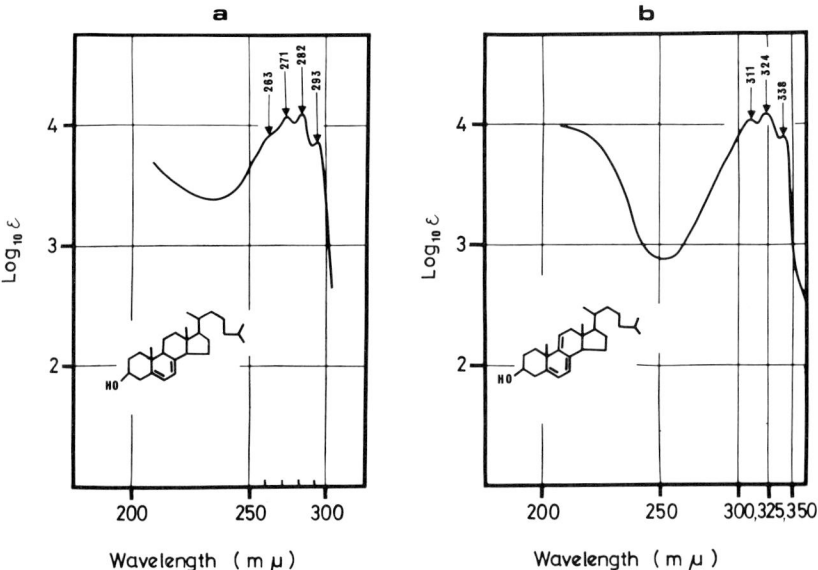

Figure 2.5
Ultraviolet spectra of two sterols, both containing nuclear double bonds. (a), Cholesta-5,7-dien-3β-ol; (b), cholesta-5,7,9(11)-trien-3β-ol. Note in (a) the peaks at 271, 282 and 293 characteristic of the ergosterol nucleus.

82   The Biology of Cholesterol and Related Steroids

property was exploited in the early work on the formation of vitamin D from provitamin D, since the transformation can be followed by observing the disappearance of the absorption peaks at these wavelengths.

4.4.3   IR spectroscopy

The IR absorption spectrum is a highly characteristic property of a compound and is now widely used in the identification of steroids (See Fig. 2.6). The wavelength of IR radiation is usually expressed in terms of wave-number, defined as the reciprocal of the wavelength in

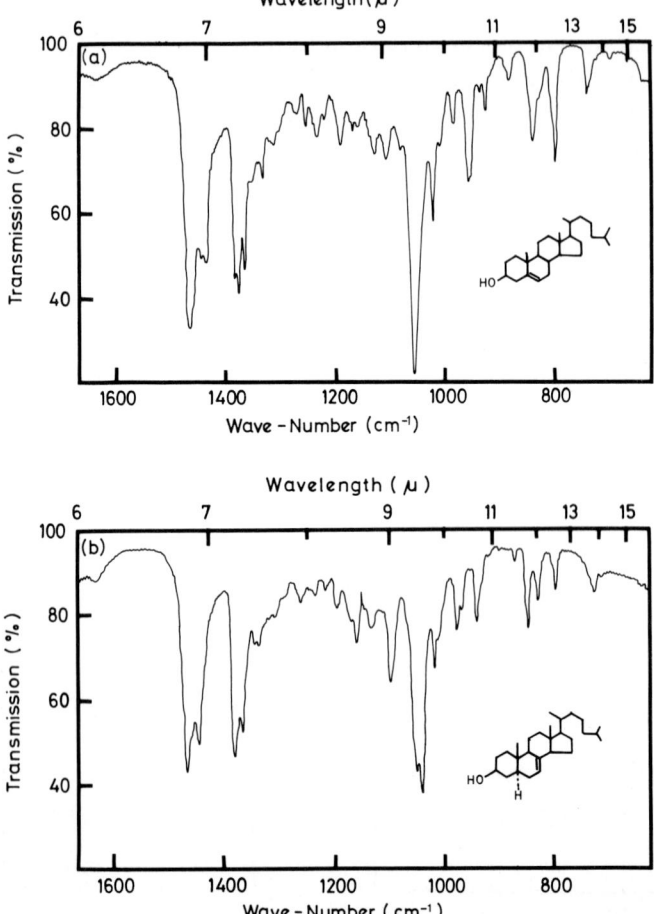

Figure 2.6
IR spectra of four closely related sterols: (a), cholest-5-en-3β-ol (cholesterol); (b), 5α-cholest-7-en-3β-ol (lathosterol); *overleaf*; (c), 5α-cholestan-3α-ol (epicholestanol); (d), 5β-cholestan-3α-ol (epicoprostanol). Note the marked differences between the four spectra in the region between 800 and 1200 cm^{-1}. Comparison

centimeter units. Since $f = c/\lambda$, where f is the frequency of vibration, c is the velocity of propagation of electromagnetic waves and λ is the wavelength, wave-number is directly proportional to frequency. The IR region usually scanned in absorption spectroscopy ranges between about 4000 and 625 cm^{-1} (2.5 to 16 μ).

When a beam of IR radiation passes through a molecule, radiations of certain frequencies are selectively absorbed, so that a series of peaks or bands appears in the spectrum of transmitted radiations. The frequencies of the absorbed radiations correspond to the frequencies of stretching and bending vibrations of the various bonds

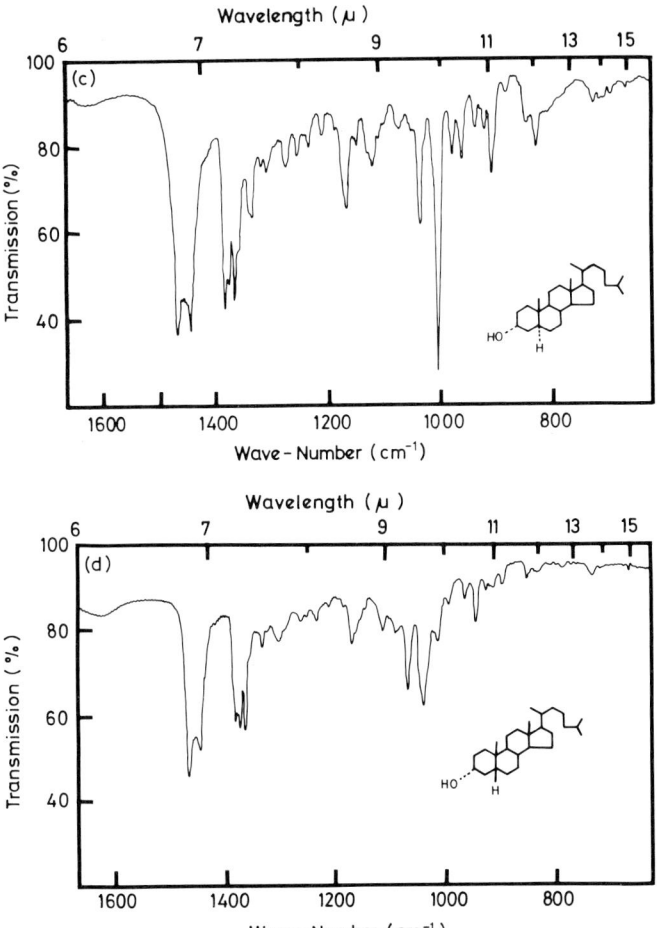

between (a) and (b) shows the effect of a difference in the position of a single nuclear double bond. Comparison between (c) and (d) shows the effect of a difference in the configuration of the C-5 hydrogen atom. (I am indebted to G. F. Gibbons and C. Pullinger for these spectra.)

linking the atoms in the molecule. Certain structural features of the molecule give rise to absorption peaks which always appear within the same general region of the spectrum, irrespective of the structure of the molecule as a whole. Hence, the IR absorption spectrum provides evidence for the presence or absence of certain groups, such as the $\diagdown\mathrm{C}{=}\mathrm{O}\diagup$ group in a ketone (stretch frequency in the region 1705–1725 cm^{-1}) or the $\diagdown\mathrm{C}{=}\mathrm{C}\diagup$ group (stretch frequency in the region 1620–1680 cm^{-1}). These *group frequencies* have been used extensively for deducing structural features of steroids (Bellamy, 1968), but they are of limited value because of overlap between the frequencies of different bonds. However, in the region between about 650 and 1600 cm^{-1} the pattern of absorption bands is very characteristic of the molecule as a whole. This region of the IR spectrum is therefore known as the *fingerprint region*. By comparing the IR fingerprint of an unknown steroid with that of a reference compound, a positive identification can often be made or alternative possibilities can be excluded. IR spectroscopy in the fingerprint region is particularly valuable for distinguishing between isomers differing in the configuration of a single nuclear substituent, but often fails to reflect differences in the configuration of a side-chain substituent. IR absorption spectra of many steroids have been recorded and are available in atlas form (Neudert and Röpke, 1965). The fingerprint of an unknown steroid may now be compared with the fingerprints of several hundred reference compounds by means of the Infrared Information Search (IRIS) computer programme (Noone, 1973).

The examples shown in Fig. 2.6 illustrate the effect, on the IR spectrum, of a difference in the position of a nuclear double bond and in the configuration of the A/B ring junction of a sterol.

4.4.4 Nuclear magnetic resonance spectroscopy

The nucleus of a hydrogen atom (a proton) possesses an intrinsic spin and therefore behaves like a bar magnet, tending to align itself in a direction parallel to an applied magnetic field, with the N pole of the nuclear magnet nearest the S pole of the external magnet. When a substance containing hydrogen atoms is placed in a strong magnetic field, their nuclei will absorb radiofrequency radiations of discrete wavelength, the absorption of energy resulting in a brief realignment to the less stable, antiparallel, position (the N pole nearest the N pole of the external magnet). On returning to the more stable alignment, the nuclei emit a radiation signal. This phenomenon is known as *nuclear magnetic resonance* (NMR) and the frequency of the radiation absorbed by a nucleus in a magnetic field of given strength is known as its *resonance frequency*. The relation between the resonance frequency (v) of a nucleus and the strength of the magnetic field in which it is immersed (H) is given by $v = \gamma H/2\pi$, where γ is constant for each type of nucleus (^{1}H, ^{13}C, etc.). Thus, for a given type of nucleus the resonance frequency is directly proportional to the strength of the magnetic field at the nucleus. Other atomic nuclei, including ^{3}H, ^{13}C and ^{31}P, act as magnetic dipoles and are therefore capable of emitting NMR signals under appropriate conditions.

Since the electrons near a nucleus exert a shielding effect, the effective strength of the magnetic field at any magnetic nucleus of a molecule placed in an applied magnetic field will differ from that of the applied field to an extent which varies according to the intramolecular environment of the nucleus. Hence, in an applied field, nuclei of the same type but in different positions within the molecule may have different resonance frequencies. For example, the hydrogen nuclei of the OH, CH$_2$ and CH$_3$ groups of ethanol have different resonance frequencies and therefore give rise to three absorption bands in the NMR spectrum of ethanol. These shifts in the resonance frequencies of nuclei of the same type due to differences in their chemical environment are known as *chemical shifts*. (Since $v = \gamma H/2\pi$, chemical shifts may also be thought of as shifts in the strength of the applied magnetic field required to cause nuclear absorption of radiation of a given frequency.)

The chemical shift value of a particular nucleus or group of equivalent nuclei is expressed in terms of the position of the NMR absorption band relative to that of an internal reference compound which gives a single band in a convenient region of the spectrum. The usual internal standard for proton NMR spectroscopy of substances studied in organic solvents is tetramethylsilane.

Examination of the high-resolution NMR spectrum of ethanol shows that the proton absorption bands due to the CH$_2$ and CH$_3$ groups are split into sets of equidistant spikes; the CH$_2$ signal has four spikes (a quartet) and the CH$_3$ signal has three (a triplet). The formation of 'multiplets' in NMR absorption bands is due to an influence of the spin characteristics of a proton (or group of equivalent protons) upon the magnetic field at the protons on nearby carbon atoms. This mutual interaction of nearby protons is known as *spin-spin* splitting. Spin-spin interaction is transmitted by valency bonds and its magnitude depends on the spatial relation between the interacting protons and on the number and nature (whether single, double or triple) of the intervening valency bonds. For example, for the hydrogen protons at opposite ends of an olefinic double bond, spin-spin interaction is greater for *cis* than for *trans* configuration, and in a system with no double bonds interaction occurs with hydrogen protons separated by two carbon atoms (H—C—C—H) but is negligible when the protons are separated by three carbon atoms.

An atom of a paramagnetic metal linked to a molecule may alter the resonance frequency and NMR splitting pattern of neighbouring protons. Since the effects of a paramagnetic atom on the resonance frequency of a proton are generally dependent on distance and also on the orientation of the proton with respect to the metal atom, these effects may lead to information about the conformation of a molecule. Of special value in work of this kind with steroids are certain metal complexes containing rare-earth elements. These reagents are known as *Lanthanide shift reagents* (lanthanum is a rare earth). Examples of the use of these reagents in the study of steroid structure will be found in the review by Hinckley (1973).

Since chemical shift values are more or less typical for certain proton-containing groups, NMR spectroscopy may be used to confirm or exclude the presence of particular groups in a molecule. However, in steroid work this technique is not as useful in the identification of compounds as are, for example, GLC, IR spectroscopy and mass spectrometry. The great value of NMR spectroscopy in this field lies, rather, in the fact that one can obtain information about the configuration and conformation of structural features already known to be present, by exact measurement of chemical shift values attributable to protons in known parts of the molecule and by detailed examination of the fine-structure of the resonance signals. One of the fields in which NMR spectroscopy is likely to be most rewarding is the study of the conformation of steroid molecules as they exist in biological systems. In this work the use of lanthanide shift reagents will undoubtedly play an increasingly important role.

NMR spectroscopy of steroids has in the past been confined almost entirely to the study of the hydrogen protons (^{1}H-NMR). However, NMR spectra of ^{13}C nuclei may also give useful information about steroid structure, although they are difficult to obtain owing to the low natural abundance of ^{13}C (1.1%). Improvement in the sensitivity of NMR spectrometers will lessen this difficulty. ^{13}C-NMR may also be used to determine the distribution, within a steroid molecule, of specific carbon atoms derived from a biological precursor. Thus, Popják et al. (1977) have used NMR spectroscopy to confirm the positions of the carbon atoms in cholesterol originating biosynthetically from C-3′ of [3′-^{13}C]mevalonic acid. Both ^{13}C-NMR and ^{31}P-NMR have already provided valuable information about the physical state of the molecules in cholesterol-phospholipid bilayers (see Chapter 7). An example of the use of ^{1}H-NMR in the determination of the structure of an unknown sterol precursor will be found in Section 5.1.

4.4.5 Electron spin resonance

Molecules containing unpaired electrons, or molecules in which unpaired electrons have been produced by ion-formation, absorb electro-magnetic radiations when placed in a strong magnetic field. This phenomenon is known as electron spin resonance (ESR) or electron para-magnetic resonance and is similar in principle to NMR, except that ESR absorption spectra lie within a much higher range of frequencies than the radio-frequencies used in NMR spectroscopy. ESR may provide information about the structure of a steroid complementary to that provided by NMR. The use of spin-labelled compounds in the study of the fluidity of sterol-phospholipid membranes is mentioned in Chapter 7.

4.4.6 Mass spectrometry

In the mass spectrometer, as used for the study of organic molecules, the sample is converted into positively charged molecular ions by bombardment in a high vacuum with a stream of electrons from a hot filament. The ions are then accelerated electrically towards a negatively charged collecting electrode. As they move towards the electrode they are deflected by a magnet, the amount of deflection being proportional to the mass/charge (m/e) ratio. At appropriate energies of bombardment, the ionized molecules are split into ionized fragments of different mass, the nature of the fragments being influenced by the structure of the compound. Hence, the mass spectrum shows a series of peaks corresponding to fragments of different mass. The pattern of peaks given by a particular compound is known as its *cracking pattern*. With modern instruments a mass spectrum may be obtained with sub-microgram quantities of a steroid.

The mass spectrometer may be used for the accurate determination of the molecular weight of a steroid, the peak with highest m/e in the spectrum usually corresponding to the ion of the unfragmented parent ion, of mass M. Comparison of the cracking pattern of an unknown steroid with that of a reference compound provides useful, and sometimes decisive, information as to the identity of the unknown. This procedure for identifying unknown steroids may be refined by converting the unknown steroid into derivatives and observing the effect of derivative formation on the cracking pattern. Although the cracking pattern is not unique for every steroid, some stereoisomers (e.g. some $5\alpha/5\beta$ isomers) may be distinguished from each other by their mass spectra. If a reference compound is not available, structural features of an unknown steroid may sometimes be deduced from the pattern of fragments produced in the mass spectrometer, using empirical rules for predicting points of cleavage derived from the study of the fragmentation patterns of large numbers of known steroids (Budzikiewicz et al., 1967).

The sensitivity and speed of response of modern mass spectrometers are such that steroids can now be analysed in microgram quantities by a combination of mass spectrometry with GLC (Ryhage, 1964; McCloskey, 1969). A variable proportion of the effluent from the GLC column is freed from carrier gas and introduced into the mass spectrometer. By this means, the fragmentation pattern of the steroids in successive peaks obtained from a gas chromatogram can be examined. This combined technique (GC-MS) is now considered by many workers to be the most powerful method available for steroid analysis. A good example of the use of this method is the identification of a large number of bile acids in normal human faeces by Eneroth et al. (1966). By comparing the R_T values and MS fragmentation patterns of derivatives of bile acids in faecal extracts with the corresponding properties of reference compounds, Eneroth and his coworkers were able to assign probable structures to at least 23 mono-, di- and tri-substituted cholanoic acids, many of which were present in amounts too small for conventional chemical analysis. This paper also provides an example of the chain of reasoning by which the structure of a steroid may be deduced from its GC-MS behaviour and from the effects of known chemical modifications upon its R_T. Other examples of the use of mass spectrometry in the elucidation of structure are given in Section 5. Fig. 2.7 shows the cracking patterns of 5α-cholestane and the TMS ether of cholesterol.

4.4.7 Optical rotatory dispersion and circular dichroism

The rotation of a beam of polarized light by a compound with one or more chiral centres varies with the wavelength of the light. This is known as optical rotatory dispersion (ORD) and the curve obtained by plotting absorption of polarized light against wavelength is known as an ORD curve; for many compounds with chiral centres the ORD curve is sinusoidal (the 'Cotton effect'). The form of the ORD curve is often influenced predictably by the configuration at chiral centres near a specific group (e.g. a carbonyl or a carboxyl group) at a known position in the molecule. For example, the ORD curve of a 3-keto steroid is markedly influenced by the configuration of the H atom at C-5 and may therefore give decisive information as to the configuration of the A/B ring junction. Other examples in the steroid field will be found in the review by Scopes (1975). ORD analysis may also be used to determine the *absolute* configuration of a compound provided that a reference compound of closely similar structure and known absolute configuration is available for comparison. In the simplest case, the ORD curve of the unknown substance is compared with that of a reference compound with identical relative configuration. If the

Analysis of Sterols and Related Steroids   89

(a) 5α-Cholestane

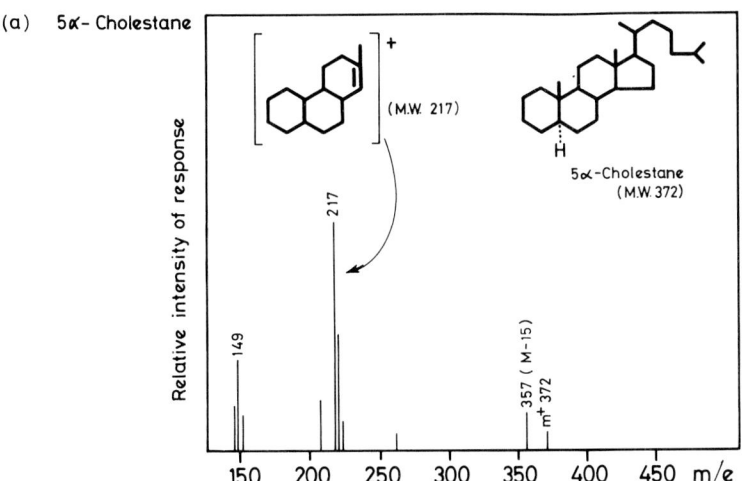

(b) TMS ether of cholesterol

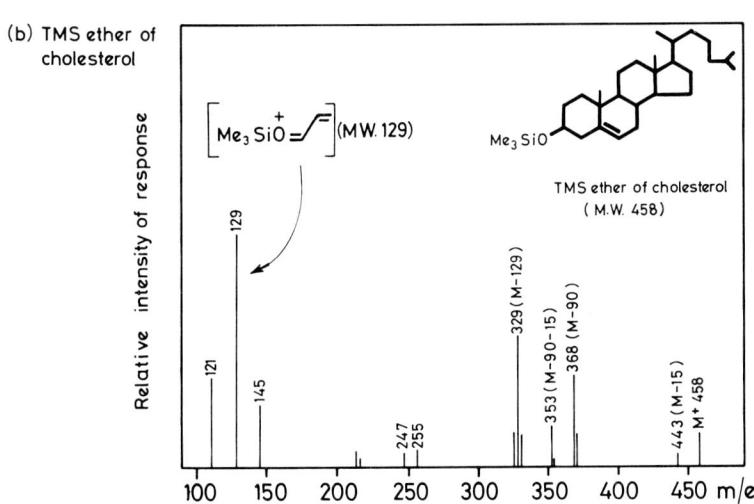

Figure 2.7
Mass spectrum of 5α-cholestane (a) and of the trimethylsily (TMS) ether of cholesterol (b) to show the fragmentation patterns. Each spectrum shows a parent ion (M^+) with the mass of the unfragmented sterol (5α-cholestane = 372; TMS ether of cholesterol = 458). 5α-Cholestane gives a fragment at m/e 357 (M-15), due to loss of one CH_3 radicle, and another intense peak at m/e 217 resulting from loss of the side-chain together with C-15, C-16 and C-17. Cholesterol TMS ether gives fragments at M-15, M-90 (loss of the TMS residue) and M-105 (loss of m/e 90 and m/e 15). This spectrum also shows a prominent peak at m/e 129, with the complementary fragment at M-129. The fragment at m/e 129 is indicative of a 3-trimethylsilyloxy-Δ^5 structure in the parent ion and its formation is due to the presence of the Δ^5 double bond in cholesterol. Note that the peaks with m/e greater than 300 have been amplified fivefold.

I am indebted to T. A. Baillie for determining the mass spectra of these two sterols and for interpreting the fragmentation patterns. The figures were redrawn from the original records.

curves are identical the unknown compound and the reference have the same absolute configuration; if the curves are mirror images of one another, the unknown and reference are enantiomers.

An effect related to ORD is known as circular dichroism (CD). If a substance absorbs right-handed (clockwise) and left-handed circularly polarized light of a given wavelength to different extents it is said to exhibit CD. A CD curve is obtained by plotting the difference in the absorption of right and left circularly polarized light against wavelength. The curve so obtained has a single maximum within the UV range. The CD curve gives stereochemical information similar to that obtainable from ORD, but the CD curve often gives the more unequivocal information because it is less influenced than is the ORD curve by interactions between different regions within a molecule.

A discussion of the unique value of ORD and CD (together known as *chiroptical* effects) in the determination of absolute configuration will be found in the review by Klyne and Scopes (1969). An example of the way in which the absolute configuration of a substance can be deduced by comparing its chiroptical properties with those of a valid reference compound is given in Section 5.1 of this Chapter.

5 THREE ILLUSTRATIVE EXAMPLES

Three examples will help the reader to appreciate how the methods described in the preceding sections may be used in combination to answer a difficult structural problem in steroid chemistry. The first illustrates, among other things, the way in which isotopic labelling, used in conjunction with mass spectrometry and the study of the enzymic steps leading to the formation of the substance in question, may provide important clues during the progress of the investigation. The second example shows how much structural information can be obtained by a combination of GLC and MS when a great deal of information about the GLC and MS behaviour of analogues of the unknown steroid is already available. The third example illustrates the use of the peak-shift method as a means of enhancing the value of GLC.

5.1 Determination of the structure of presqualene pyrophosphate

The discovery and structural analysis of presqualene pyrophosphate, an intermediate in the conversion of farnesyl pyrophosphate (FPP) into squalene, illustrate the use of modern methods of analysis in the study of a compound available initially only in microgram quantities. The events leading ultimately to the correct assignment of its absolute configuration are worth describing in some detail because they show

how information derived from widely different sources may lead to the complete identification of a newly-discovered compound.

In 1961 Popják et al. showed that during the condensation of two molecules of FPP to form squalene (a symmetrical molecule) one of the four H atoms on the two C-1 carbons of the condensing pair is lost and replaced by H from NADPH. In order to explain this, Popják et al. (1961) suggested that the immediate product of the condensation of the two farnesyl residues is an asymmetrical molecule, which is then converted into squalene. One of the structures they proposed for this intermediate was a compound containing a cyclopropane ring:

$$\begin{array}{c} \text{①} \\ \text{CH}_2 \\ \text{H}_3\text{C} \diagdown \diagup \diagdown \diagup \text{OPP} \\ \text{C}=\text{CH}-\text{CH}\text{CH}-\text{C}-\text{CH}_2\text{R} \\ \text{RH}_2\text{C} \diagup \text{③}\text{②} \diagdown \text{CH}_3 \end{array}$$

$$\text{R}=\text{H}_3\text{C}-\overset{\overset{\text{CH}_3}{|}}{\text{C}}=\text{CH}-\text{CH}_2-\text{CH}_2-\overset{\overset{\text{CH}_3}{|}}{\text{C}}=\text{CH}-\text{CH}_2$$

(Geranyl)
(2.1)

Rilling (1966) later isolated a radioactive intermediate in the biosynthesis of squalene from incubations of [^{14}C, ^{32}P]FPP in the absence of NADPH and showed that this compound (Compound X, later termed *presqualene pyrophosphate*) could be converted into squalene by a yeast enzyme system containing NADPH. Although this intermediate was not obtained in amounts sufficient for structural analysis at this stage, certain features of its structure could be deduced from its radioactive composition and GLC behaviour. The ^{32}P:^{14}C and ^{3}H:^{14}C ratios in the specimens synthesized, respectively, from [^{14}C, ^{32}P]FPP and [^{14}C, 1-^{3}H$_2$]FPP showed that the compound contained one less PP group than the two FPP molecules and that the loss of one H atom from C-1 of FPP (Popják et al., 1961) took place during the formation of the intermediate. Treatment with LiAlH$_4$ (known to cleave phosphate esters) led to the formation of an alcohol (*presqualene alcohol*) and a mixture of hydrocarbons. The latter, on catalytic reduction, gave a saturated hydrocarbon whose R$_T$ on GLC was only slightly less than that of squalene. Rilling concluded that the intermediate was the pyrophosphate ester of a C$_{30}$ alcohol with a carbon skeleton different from that of squalene and with only three of the four hydrogen atoms on C-1 of the two farnesyl residues. He suggested structure (2.1) to account for his observations.

However, Corey and Ortiz de Montellano (1968) showed that this structure could not be correct. They synthesized the diastereomers of the *cis* and *trans* isomers of the alcohol of (2.1) (i.e. of the isomers in which the two side-chains are on the same and opposite faces, respectively, of the cyclopropane ring) and showed, by implication, that the TLC behaviour of all the eight stereoisomers was different from that of the labelled alcohol obtained from the biosynthetically labelled intermediate. Moreover, when radioactive specimens of the chemically synthesized compounds were pyrophosphorylated and incubated with a yeast enzyme system containing NADPH, no radioactive squalene was formed.

In an attempt to obtain more definite information about the structure of presqualene PP, Popják et al. (1969) prepared the compound enzymically from FPP in amounts sufficient for examination of some of its physical properties. They showed that it was optically active and must therefore contain at least one asymmetric centre. The NMR and mass spectra of presqualene PP and the mass spectrum of the products of its acid hydrolysis led them to conclude that presqualene PP did not contain a cyclopropane ring and that it was probably a cyclic pyrophosphoryl ester of squalene-10,11-glycol.

Epstein and Rilling (1970) then prepared up to 50 mg of radioactive or deuterium-labelled presqualene PP enzymically from [1-^{3}H$_2$]FPP and [1-^{2}H$_2$]FPP. With these quantities at their disposal they were able to study the structure of the intermediate by a combination of conventional chemical methods with NMR and mass spectrometry. A sample of the labelled material was converted into presqualene alcohol and a mixture of hydrocarbons by treatment with LiAlH$_4$. The alcohol was purified by column chromatography and its purity checked by TLC and GLC under a variety of conditions. Since the alcohol, after chemical pyrophosphorylation, was efficiently converted into squalene by a yeast enzyme system, it could be assumed that no rearrangement of the carbon skeleton of presqualene PP had occurred during its conversion into the alcohol.

Examination of the alcohol in the mass spectrometer revealed a molecular ion at m/e 426, giving C$_{30}$H$_{50}$O($\equiv$C$_{30}$H$_{49}$OH) as the empirical formula and thus confirming the earlier evidence of Rilling (1966) that one of the 50 carbon-bound H atoms of the condensing farnesyl pair is lost in the formation of presqualene PP. The fragmentation pattern included a peak at m/e 395 (M-31), indicating loss of a CH$_2$OH group, and a peak at M-137, indicating loss of a C$_{10}$H$_{17}$ fragment. The fragmentation pattern of the alcohol obtained from presqualene PP biosynthesized from [1-^{2}H$_2$]FPP included a molecular ion at m/e 429 (not 430), providing additional evidence that only three of the four C-1 hydrogen atoms of the two farnesyl residues are present in the intermediate. The fragmentation pattern of the deuterated alcohol included a peak at m/e 396 (M-33), indicating loss of a CD$_2$OH group and thus showing that the carbon of the CH$_2$OH group of presqualene PP is derived from C-1 of FPP.

The hydrocarbons formed from presqualene PP by LiAlH$_4$ treatment were examined by MS before and after catalytic hydrogenation. The fragmentation patterns were consistent with the presence of a cyclopropane ring at the position shown in Structure (**2.2**). In particular, the fragmentation pattern of the fully saturated hydrocarbon was consistent with its formation by opening of the cyclopropane ring of (**2.2**) between positions (1) and (3), with subsequent fragmentation around position (2).

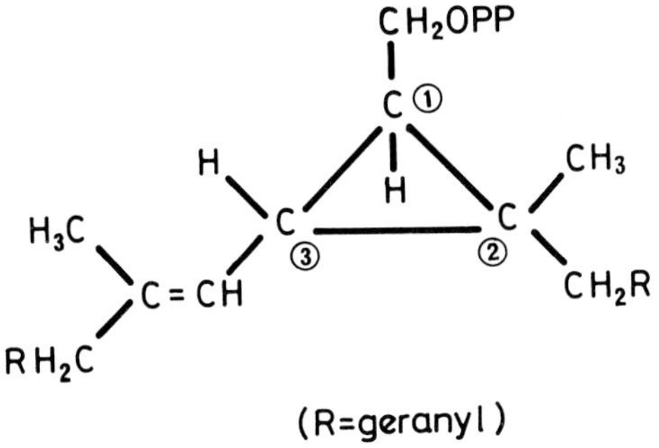

(R=geranyl)
(**2.2**)

Epstein and Rilling (1970) obtained more direct evidence for the presence of a substituted cyclopropane ring in presqualene PP by comparing the NMR spectrum of presqualene PP with that of chrysanthemyl PP, and of presqualene alcohol with that of chrysanthemyl alcohol (**2.3**).

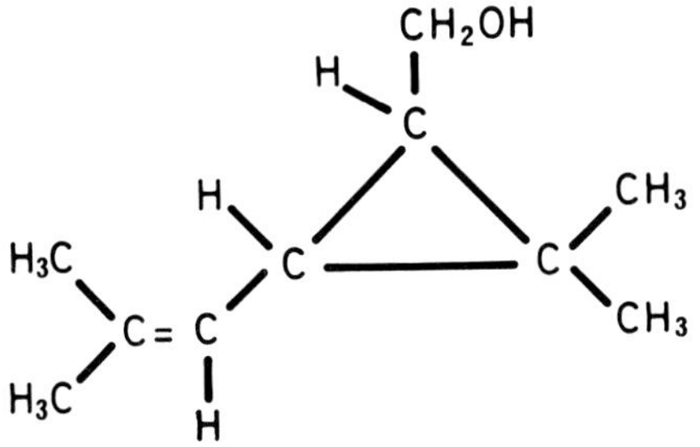

(**2.3**)

Chemical shifts could be assigned to a CH$_2$O group and to cyclopropyl hydrogens and a cyclopropyl methyl in presqualene PP and presqualene alcohol.

From a consideration of the known geometry of chrysanthemyl alcohol and of the probable mechanism of synthesis of presqualene PP, Epstein and Rilling suggested that the relative configurations at the three carbon atoms of the cyclopropane ring of presqualene PP are those shown in (**2.2**).

94 The Biology of Cholesterol and Related Steroids

Edmond et al. (1971) confirmed and extended the observations of Epstein and Rilling (1970), using presqualene alcohol prepared enzymically from labelled FPP under conditions in which the presqualene PP formed during the incubation was hydrolyzed to the alcohol by a microsomal phosphatase. The MS fragmentation pattern of this material, including that of the tri-deuterated alcohol biosynthesized from [1-^{2}H$_2$]FPP, was similar to that of the preparations used by Epstein and Rilling and fully supported structure (**2.2**) for presqualene PP. In the course of this work, Edmond et al. reconsidered their earlier suggestion (Popják et al., 1969) that presqualene PP is a cyclic ester of squalene-10,11-glycol. They concluded that the formation of squalene-10,11-glycol from presqualene PP by acid hydrolysis, an important part of the evidence for their proposed structure, must have involved rearrangement of the carbon skeleton, with loss of the cyclopropane ring.

Their examination of the NMR spectrum of presqualene alcohol gave conclusive evidence as to the geometry of the substituents on the cyclopropane ring, providing an excellent example of the power of this technique in the elucidation of three-dimensional structure. Comparison of the spectrum of presqualene alcohol with the spectra of *cis*- and *trans*-chrysanthemyl alcohols enabled them to assign absorption lines to the following structural features shown in the structural formula (**2.4**) and designated by letters in brackets:

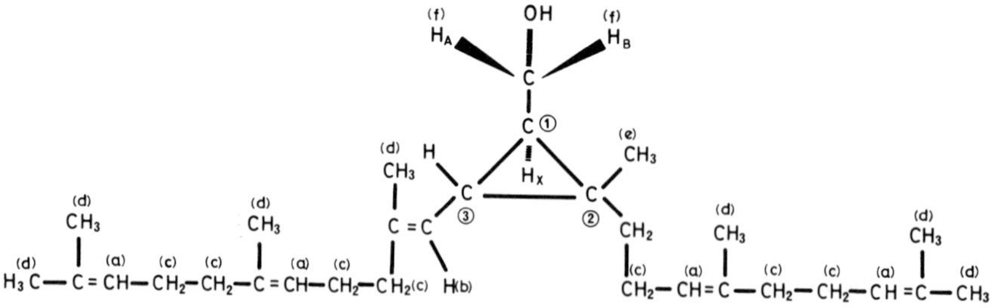

(Presqualene alcohol)

(**2.4**)

(a), 4 olefinic protons (=CH—); (b), 1 isolated proton; (c), 14 allylic methylene protons (=C—CH$_2$—); (d), 21 allylic methyl

$$\overset{\mid}{\underset{\mid}{CH_3}}$$

protons (=C—); (e), 1 isolated methyl group; (f), 2 carbinyl protons; (g), an ABX-system (**2.5**), giving an octet in the spectrum and represented by the structural element shown in (**2.4**) and also present in chrysanthemyl alcohol (**2.3**). The H$_x$ of the ABX-system was shown to be a methine proton (≡C—).

Analysis of Sterols and Related Steroids 95

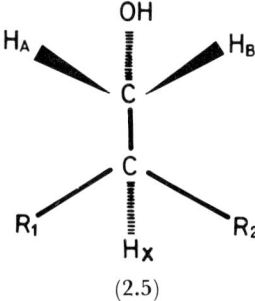

(2.5)

Comparison with the spectra of *cis*- and *trans*-chrysanthemyl alcohols proved that the vinyl group attached to C ③ of the ring was *trans* to the carbinol (—CH$_2$OH) and that the methyl group attached to C ② was *cis* to the carbinol. Thus, interpretation of the NMR spectrum of presqualene alcohol provided decisive evidence for the presence of a substituted cyclopropane structure and for the geometry of its substituents as shown in (2.7).

Further evidence for the configurations around the 3 carbon atoms of the cyclopropane ring of presqualene alcohol was obtained by reductive ozonolysis of a 50-mg specimen of the biosynthetically labelled alcohol, followed by acetylation of the products. A triacetate was isolated from the acetylated products by preparative GLC and assigned structure (2.6) by GLC, GC-MS, NMR spectroscopy and IR spectroscopy.

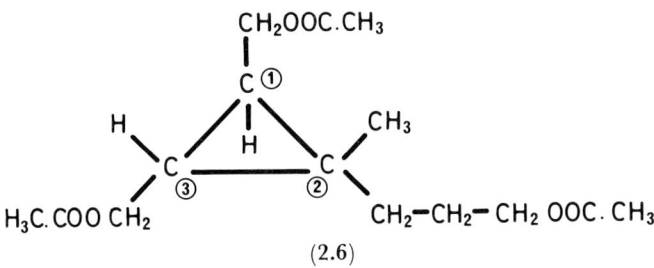

(2.6)

This compound has two asymmetric centres (at positions 1 and 3). Hence, if the configuration at these two positions are as shown in (2.6) (i.e., either 1R, 3R or 1S, 3S) the compound should be optically active. If, on the other hand, the substituents at positions 1 and 3 are in *cis* relationship, the configurations would be either 1S, 3R or 1R, 3S and the compound would be optically inactive, since the two halves of the molecule would be mirror images of each other. Edmond *et al.* (1971) showed that the triacetate was dextrorotatory and they therefore concluded that the relative configurations at positions 1 and 2 were as shown in (2.6). Since it could be assumed that the configurations at these positions in the parent presqualene alcohol had not been inverted, this must also hold for the cyclopropane ring of presqualene PP. Since the NMR studies had shown that the methyl group at position 2 is *cis* to the substituent at position 1, Edmond *et al.* concluded that the absolute configuration must be either 1R, 2R, 3R or its enantiomer (1S, 2S, 3S), thus excluding six of the eight possible stereoisomers.

Shortly after this report, Altman *et al.* (1971) described the chemical synthesis of the racemate of presqualene alcohol (**2.7**) by the addition of an allylic diazo compound to *trans-trans*-farnesol.

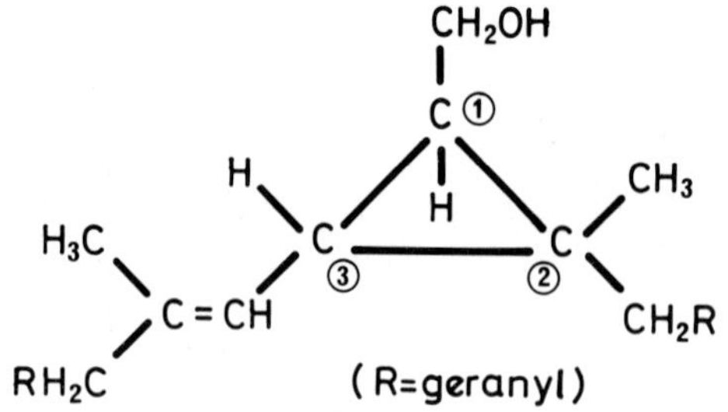

(2.7)

They then prepared the pyrophosphate of tritiated (**2.7**) and showed that it was convertible enzymically into squalene with a yield of 34%, equivalent to a yield of 68% for the natural radioactive enantiomer. Structure (**2.7**) for presqualene alcohol was confirmed independently by stereoselective chemical synthesis in two other laboratories (Coates and Robinson, 1971; Campbell *et al.*, 1971).

Although the evidence from structural analysis of biosynthesized presqualene PP and from stereoselective chemical synthesis proved conclusively that the relative configurations at positions 1, 2 and 3 were those shown in (**2.2**) (CH$_2$OH *syn* to the CH$_3$ at position 2 and *anti* to the vinyl group at position 3) none of the methods used was capable of distinguishing between the two enantiomers of this structure. Hence, it remained to be shown whether the absolute configuration was that depicted in (**2.8**) or its mirror image. The solution to this problem was achieved by Popják *et al.* (1973), who showed that the CD spectra of the benzoates of presqualene alcohol and *trans*-chrysanthemyl alcohol, and of their ozonolysis products, were

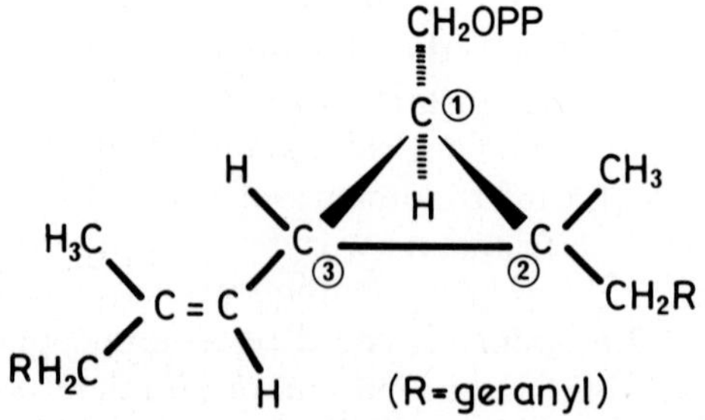

(2.8)

similar. Since it was known that the configuration of the two asymmetric centres in *trans*-chrysanthemyl alcohol is 1R, 3R, this observation showed that the carbons at positions 1 and 3 of presqualene alcohol must also have R configuration, and since all three asymmetric carbons of presqualene alcohol had been shown to have the same configuration, it followed that the absolute configuration of presqualene alcohol (and of presqualene PP) must be R, R, R, as shown in (2.8). In this stereochemical formula, the plane of the ring is considered to be at right angles to the plane of the paper with C(1) to the rear.

Thus, even with the help of almost every technique available for modern structural investigation, 12 years elapsed between the recognition that the biosynthesis of squalene from FPP must involve the formation of an intermediate and the complete elucidation of the three-dimensional structure of this intermediate.

5.2 The use of GC-MS in the identification of bile alcohols

The identification of two unusual bile alcohols in the faeces of patients with cerebrotendinous xanthomatosis (Setoguchi *et al.*, 1974) illustrates the power and limitations of GC-MS. The non-saponifiable fraction of a lipid extract of faeces from a patient was separated into sterols and bile alcohols by column chromatography with reversed-phase partition, and the bile alcohol fraction was separated into several components by adsorption TLC. One of the less polar of these components was submitted to GC-MS after conversion into its TMS ether. The mass spectrum showed the presence of a molecular ion with m/e 724, indicating a bile alcohol with four OH groups, each of which was silylated (mass of TMS group = 90). The mass spectrum also included a prominent peak at m/e 131. This would be expected if the side-chain contained a silylated OH group at C-25, resulting in the formation of a fragment containing the isopropyl unit of the side-chain with one TMS group (mass, 131) by rupture of the 24–25 bond. A likely structure was therefore 5β-cholestane-3α,7α,12α,25-tetrol. This structure was established by the demonstration that the melting point, IR spectrum, fragmentation pattern in the mass spectrum and GLC behaviour of the faecal bile alcohol were all identical with those of a chemically synthesized reference compound.

Another, more polar TLC fraction gave a molecular ion with m/e 452 (M) and a peak at m/e 253 (M − 199) when submitted to GC-MS without derivative formation. This suggested the presence of a C_{27} bile alcohol with three nuclear and two side-chain hydroxyl groups, giving rise to a fragment formed by removal of the three nuclear OH groups as water (mass 3 × 18) and of a complete side-chain containing the two OH groups (mass, 146 minus one H atom). GC-MS of the

TMS ether of the unknown bile alcohol gave a peak at m/e 131, indicating the presence of one OH group at C-25.

This fraction was subsequently separated into two subfractions, one shown to contain 5β-cholestane-3α,7α,12α,23ξ,25-pentol and the other to contain the corresponding 3α,7α,12α,24ξ,25-pentol (Shefer et al., 1975). Since no reference compound was available for comparison with the 23-hydroxy pentol, the configuration at C-23 could not be determined. However, Shefer et al. (1975) showed that the 24-hydroxy pentol had the same melting point, mass spectrum, IR spectrum and TLC and GLC properties as a chemically synthesized reference compound to which the structure 5β-cholestane-3α,7α,12α,24α,25-pentol (the 24R hydroxy epimer) had been assigned. They therefore concluded that the 24-hydroxy pentol present in the bile of patients with cerebrotendinous xanthomatosis has the 24R configuration.

5.3 Peak shifts in the identification of bile acids

A useful procedure for deducing the probable structure of a bile acid by the GLC peak-shift method has been outlined by Eneroth and Sjövall (1969) and may be illustrated by a consideration of Table 2.2. Suppose that the methyl ester of an unknown trihydroxy bile acid isolated from human faeces by TLC was found to have an R_T value of 2.17 when chromatographed on QF-1. Comparison with the R_T values of the methyl esters of the reference compounds 1–6 would exclude structures 3, 4, 5 and 6, but not structures 1 and 2. Hence, the unknown could be either cholic acid (1) or the 7β isomer

Table 2.2

Retention times of the derivatives of some trihydroxy bile acids on GLC with 3% QF-1 as liquid phase

Compound	Derivative		
	OH	TFA	TMSE
1. (5β) 3α,7α,12α	2.14	1.29	1.23
2. (5β) 3α, 7β,12α	2.17	1.18	0.74
3. (5β) 3β,7α,12α	1.81	0.95	1.13
4. (5β) 3β,7β,12α	1.93	1.00	0.65
5. (5α) 3α,7α,12α	2.37	1.37	—
6. (5α) 3β,7α,12α	2.50	—	—

OH, methyl ester with unprotected OH groups; TFA, trifluoroacetate; TMSE, trimethylsilyl ether. Abbreviated formulae denote configurations of the three OH groups and the hydrogen at C-5. All values are relative to the retention time of methyl deoxycholate. Values for reference compounds taken from Eneroth and Sjövall (1969).

of cholic acid (2). If conversion into the TFA and TMS ethers showed that the shift in the R_T of the GLC peaks was similar to that of compound 2 and different from that of 1, cholic acid could be excluded and the unknown could be identified tentatively as 3α,7β,12α-trihydroxy-5β-cholanoic acid (2). In the absence of other suitable reference compounds (e.g. the 12β isomer of compound 2), this identification would remain uncertain.

This example shows how TLC followed by GLC analysis, including the use of the peak-shift method, may lead to a tentative identification of the structure of a bile acid and may be used to exclude possible alternatives, provided that appropriate reference compounds are available. If enough reference compounds are available, identification may be made with a high degree of probability. Moreover, it is often possible to make positive inferences about the structure of the unknown compound by observing the effect of known structural changes on the GLC behaviour of closely related compounds. However, it is easier to exclude possible structures than to deduce a particular structure unequivocally by GLC alone, since some pairs of isomers cannot be separated by GLC. In the present example, the structure inferred from GLC analysis would need confirmation by IR spectroscopy and mass spectrometry. The latter technique is of special value in the elucidation of bile-acid structure.

6 ASSAY

In this section we shall be concerned mainly with the principles underlying methods for assaying sterols and bile acids and with the relative merits of those in current use. Practical details are given in the relevant articles listed at the end of this Chapter. For the reasons given below, measurement of the plasma cholesterol concentration is discussed separately and at some length.

6.1 Assay of plasma cholesterol

6.1.1 Importance of the plasma cholesterol concentration

The belief that plasma lipids play a causal role in the development of ischaemic heart disease has led to extensive investigations of the plasma cholesterol concentration in large numbers of human subjects. These investigations include measurements in different populations and in the same population over long intervals of time. In epidemiological studies of human plasma cholesterol there is also an increasing tendency to combine results obtained from different research centres, sometimes in different countries, in order to obtain enough observations for statistical significance. In view of the enormous effort and expense involved in carrying out these investigations, and of the importance of the social decisions that may flow from them, it is clearly essential that the methods used for assaying cholesterol should be as reliable as possible. However carefully the investigation is designed, its value will be nullified if the laboratory measurements are erroneous. Yet experience during the past two or three decades has shown that it is surprisingly difficult to achieve and maintain an acceptable degree of reliability in the measurement of plasma cholesterol concentration, a problem that is reflected in the number of published methods; Tonks (1967) mentions more than sixty colorimetric methods for assaying plasma cholesterol and many others have been published since his review.

6.1.2 Reliability and quality control

The term 'reliability' usually refers to two aspects of an assay method: first, the degree to which it gives reproducible results when tested against samples taken from a standard pool (precision); second, the degree to which it gives results close to the true value (accuracy). Several surveys have shown that unless a high standard of laboratory work is maintained, plasma cholesterol assays will inevitably lack both precision and accuracy. In a survey by Tonks (1963), for example, values reported by 170 Canadian laboratories for samples of serum from a single pool containing 86 mg of cholesterol/100 ml ranged from 84 to > 158 mg/100 ml, the great majority being considerably higher than the true value. There is also a tendency, well-known in every routine lipid laboratory, for the values given by the standard serum sample to drift, usually towards higher values, from day to day.

Much thought has been given to ways of overcoming these deficiencies, so that valid conclusions can be drawn from data obtained from multi-centre studies continued for many years, e.g. from large-scale trials of the effects of modifying plasma cholesterol concentration on the incidence of heart disease. This has led to the setting up of organizations for promoting the standardization of assay methods for cholesterol. The first of these was the *National and International Cooperative Cholesterol Standardization Program*, organized by the National Institutes of Health (NIH) of the U.S. Public Health Service. The object of this organization, which includes a *Lipid Standardization Laboratory*, is to provide facilities for evaluating cholesterol assay methods and for the continuous testing of the performance of laboratories in which cholesterol is assayed routinely. An outcome of this is the system developed by the NIH for their *Lipid Research Clinics Program*. Procedures for the automated assay of plasma cholesterol by laboratories participating in this program are described in U.S. DHEW (1974) (and see Section 6.1.8, p. 107). The essential features of the NIH system are as follows:

The procedures for obtaining blood plasma, for the preparation of reagents and for the operation of the autoanalyser are standardized, and the standard solution of pure cholesterol is supplied by the *Lipid Standardization Laboratory*. Control samples, taken from a pool of frozen serum containing cholesterol at a concentration known to the operator, are analysed with each batch of unknown samples. If the variation of the control values exceeds a pre-selected limit, the results are rejected and the procedure, including the reagents, is checked for faults (internal quality control). In addition to internal quality control, each laboratory tests its performance at regular intervals by analysing samples of serum containing cholesterol at concentrations known to the *Lipid Standardization Laboratory* but not to the operator (external quality control).

6.1.3 Cholesterol standards

The need to use pure standards for cholesterol assay is obvious, yet it is not always realized that most 'pure' commercial samples of cholesterol contain impurities and that cholesterol undergoes autoxidation during storage unless precautions are taken to prevent this. The major contaminants in commercial preparations of cholesterol are 5α-cholestanol, lathosterol and 7-dehydrocholesterol. These are not removed by recrystallization from ethanol, but can be removed by bromination to give the insoluble 5α,6β-dibromide of cholesterol, followed by regeneration of cholesterol from the dibromide. Cholesterol for use as a standard should therefore be purified *via* the dibromide. Moreover, since cholesterol crystallizes from moist solvents as the monohydrate, it should also be dried at 80 °C for 2 hours before the sample is weighed. Radin and Gramza (1963) examined samples of cholesterol obtained from several different commercial sources and found considerable variation in the melting point determined in evacuated capillary tubes. After purification *via* the dibromide each sample melted at a higher temperature and over a narrower temperature range than before purification. In 14 commercial samples of cholesterol examined by TLC and quantitative GLC, Williams *et al.* (1965) found 4–5% of impurities—a source of error that would be within the limits of detection of most colorimetric methods for assaying cholesterol. It should also be noted that sterols containing a Δ^7 double bond give a stronger colour with some reagents than cholesterol itself.

6.1.4 Colorimetric methods

Most of the colorimetric methods for cholesterol assay that have stood the test of time are based either on the Liebermann-Burchard (L-B) reaction (colour formation with reagents containing concentrated H_2SO_4 and acetic anhydride) or on the Kiliani-Zak (K-Z) reaction (colour formation with a ferric salt-H_2SO_4 reagent). Other colorimetric or fluorimetric methods still favoured by some workers are those based on the Tschugaeff colour reaction (Hanel and Dam, 1955), on the colour formed in the presence of *p*-toluenesulphonic acid (*p*-TSA) (Pearson *et al.*, 1953) and on the fluorescence produced by reacting a solution of cholesterol in trichloroethane with acetic anhydride-H_2SO_4 (Carpenter *et al.*, 1957).

6.1.4.1 Liebermann-Burchard methods. The intensity and time-course of the L-B reaction are influenced by many variables, including the temperature, the presence of moisture in the cholesterol solvent and colour reagent, the nature of the solvent for cholesterol, the presence of light during the reaction and the presence of substances, such as bilirubin, that give a positive L-B reaction. With most solvents, the intensity of the colour is influenced by the proportion of esterified to free cholesterol in the sample, esterified cholesterol giving a stronger L-B reaction than free cholesterol. These variables have been discussed in considerable detail by Cook and Rattray (1958) and Kabara (1962).

In the most successful adaptations of the L-B reaction the cholesterol is extracted from plasma with an organic solvent, either before saponification (Schoenheimer and Sperry, 1934) or after saponification (Abell *et al.*, 1952) of the plasma lipids. In the Schoenheimer-Sperry procedure, digitonin is added to the acetone-ethanol extract before saponification to precipitate free cholesterol, or after saponification to precipitate total cholesterol. The digitonides are then dissolved in acetic acid and the cholesterol is assayed by the L-B reaction. In the Abell procedure the dried extract containing total cholesterol is dissoved in acetic acid and assayed by the L-B reaction. Interference by L-B-positive substances in plasma is minimized by the lipid extraction in the Abell procedure and is eliminated by the digitonin precipitation in the Schoenheimer-Sperry procedure. Both methods have the additional advantage that free cholesterol is measured in the L-B reaction, so that no correction need be made for the difference in reactivities of free and esterified cholesterol.

Despite the fact that all methods based on the L-B reaction suffer from the disadvantages that the development of the colour is temperature-dependent and that the final colour is unstable, the procedure of Abell *et al.* gives very reproducible results and is generally regarded as the best reference method for evaluating other methods for assaying total cholesterol (Tonks, 1967; U.S. DHEW, 1974). The Abell procedure and its subsequent modifications cannot be used for assay of plasma esterified cholesterol (see Section 6.1.7). Several colorimetric and fluorimetric methods are considerably more sensitive than the Abell method (Kabara, 1962), but lack of sensitivity is seldom a disadvantage in a method for assaying total cholesterol in the plasma of adults. With all L-B methods a colour reaction is given by sterols other than cholesterol (Cook and Rattray, 1958, Table II). However, L-B positive sterols other than cholesterol are present in normal plasma only in traces, so that high specificity towards sterols is not required (but see Section 6.2 for exceptions to this).

Attempts to develop direct methods, in which the L-B reagent is added to untreated plasma, are open to serious objection. These methods give erroneously high values, owing partly to their failure to eliminate interfering substances and partly to the absence of a step for hydrolysing esterified cholesterol.

6.1.4.2 Kiliani-Zak and other colorimetric methods.

Many variations on the original, direct, method of Zlatkis *et al.* (1953) have been proposed. These include: an initial extraction of lipid with organic solvent, which need not be evaporated since the colour reaction is uninfluenced by organic solvents; precipitation of plasma proteins before addition of the full colour reagent; stabilization of the reagent by citric acid.

Methods based on the K-Z reaction and on the colour developed with *p*-TSA have several advantages over those based on the L-B reaction. They are capable of greater sensitivity (some K-Z methods can be modified for microassay); the colour developed is relatively stable and is not affected by light; they give equal colour intensities with free and esterified cholesterol and can therefore be used for assay of total plasma cholesterol without a saponification step. An additional advantage is that they can be used for assay of esterified cholesterol by measuring cholesterol in the supernatant after digitonin precipitation, since the colour reactions are not affected by the presence of digitonin.

Despite these advantages, K-Z and *p*-TSA methods tend to be less accurate than L-B methods, usually giving higher values than those obtained with the method of Abell *et al.* (1952). This seems to be due largely to the fact that the L-B reaction is less sensitive to substances other than sterols in the plasma and in the reagents; acetic acid, even of Analar grade, may contain traces of glyoxylic acid, which gives an intense colour with plasma proteins in the unmodified Zlatkis procedure. Other substances that may cause erroneously high values with K-Z and *p*-TSA methods are bilirubin, haemoglobin, salicylates, thiouracil, bromide and iodide.

6.1.5 Gas-liquid chromatographic methods

The plasma cholesterol is well suited to assay by quantitative GLC. Procedures based on GLC have the advantages of sensitivity, specificity and precision. A high degree of accuracy can also be achieved, provided that the precautions outlined in Section 3.4.6 are observed. In principle, 5α-cholestane is added to the serum as an internal standard, the sample is saponified and the saponified lipids are extracted into an organic solvent for injection on to the column. The amount of cholesterol in the sample is estimated from the ratio of the heights or areas of the cholesterol and 5α-cholestane peaks (peak-height or peak-area ratios). In the micro-method of Ishikawa *et al.* (1974) the peak-height ratio given by the unknown sample is compared with the peak-height ratio given by a reference sample of serum containing a known amount of cholesterol (previously determined by a ferric chloride method) together with 5α-cholestane as internal standard. Ishikawa *et al.* used OV-17 as liquid phase, but equally satisfactory results can be obtained with SE-30 or QF-1.

GLC may be used for the assay of cholesterol in the presence of desmosterol and the plant sterols, all of which can be separated from cholesterol on several liquid phases. The GLC assay of 5α-cholestanol in the presence of cholesterol is difficult with most liquid phases (Klause and Subbiah, 1975) and is best carried out after separation of the two sterols by argentation chromatography. The GLC steps of the assay can be automated by means of an automatic injector, making it possible to inject one saponified and extracted sample on to the column every 15 minutes. Many workers regard GLC as the method of choice for assaying cholesterol in the research laboratory, particularly for measurement at the microgram level. GLC methods have been used extensively in the investigation of cholesterol concentration in cord-blood plasma and the plasma of newborn infants. Kuksis *et al.* (1975) have described a method for the GLC assay of free and esterified cholesterol in plasma without preliminary separation and saponification of the esterified cholesterol.

6.1.6 Enzymic methods

Several strains of soil bacteria form cholesterol oxidase (EC 1.1.3.6), an enzyme catalyzing the oxidation of cholesterol to cholest-4-en-3-one in the presence of molecular oxygen, with the formation of hydrogen peroxide:

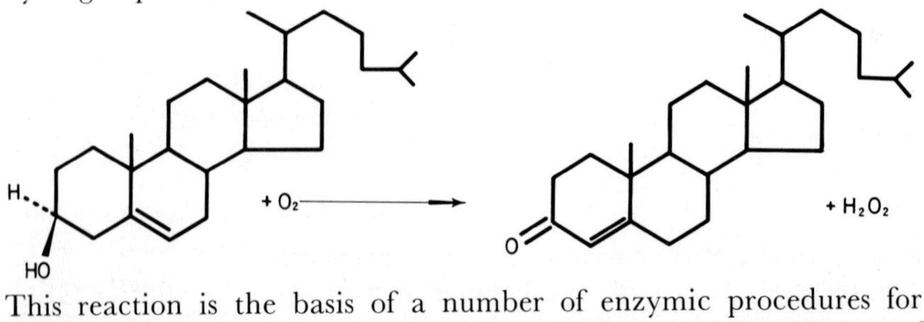

This reaction is the basis of a number of enzymic procedures for assaying cholesterol in plasma. Enzymic methods based on the use of cholesterol oxidase consist essentially of three steps: the hydrolysis of esterified cholesterol, the oxidation of cholesterol and, finally, the measurement of the amount of cholest-4-en-3-one or H_2O_2 formed.

Numerous variants of this basic combination have been proposed and several have been tested rigorously by comparing them with other methods. Hydrolysis of cholesteryl esters by saponification is generally considered to be unsatisfactory, owing to the formation of reducing substances, and has been superseded by enzymic hydrolysis. In the procedure of Allain *et al.* (1974), esterified cholesterol is hydrolyzed with cholesteryl ester hydrolase (EC 3.1.1.13), cholesterol is oxidized by a partially purified oxidase from *Nocardia* sp. and the H_2O_2 produced is measured by a colour reaction in which horse-radish peroxidase (EC 1.11.1.7) is used to effect the oxidative coupling of 4-aminoantipyrine with phenol, resulting in the formation of a coloured compound absorbing at 500 nm. Other methods of measuring the products of the oxidation of cholesterol are discussed in a review by Smith and Brooks (1976). The enzymic method may also be adapted for fluourimetric assay of the product of the peroxidase reaction, with much increased sensitivity (Heider and Boyett, 1978). Since cholesteryl esters do not act as substrate for the bacterial oxidase, cholesterol oxidase methods can be adapted for measurement of esterified cholesterol by carrying out the oxidation step before and after hydrolysis.

A major advantage of the enzymic method for assaying cholesterol in plasma is its specificity. The specificity of the oxidase is such that it can only use sterols with a 3β-hydroxyl group as substrate and is virtually inactive against steroid hormones (see Smith and Brooks (1976), Table 2.2, for substrate specificity of the oxidase from *N. erythropolis*). Furthermore, non-sterol plasma constituents that give so much trouble with colorimetric methods have little or no influence on any of the steps in the enzymic method. Another considerable advantage of the enzymic method is the absence of saponification and solvent extraction. This makes it particularly suitable for automation. Moreover, since the three enzymes used in the Allain procedure are stable, the method lends itself to use in the form of commercially prepared 'kits'; kits based on colorimetric methods, it may be noted, have not been very successful (Tonks, 1967).

Witte *et al.* (1974) have compared the results obtained with an automated modification of the Allain procedure with those obtained by three other methods: a manual Abell method, the automated Auto Analyzer method used in the *Lipid Research Clinics Program* and an automated direct colorimetric method (i.e., no saponification and no solvent extraction). With the enzymic method, precision was comparable with that of the *Lipid Research Clinics* method and the values estimated in serum samples containing cholesterol ranging from < 100 to 430 mg/100 ml were lower than those estimated by the other three methods. The lower values obtained with the enzymic method reflect the absence of interference from non-sterol plasma constituents and the lower reactivity of cholesterol oxidase with traces of sterol other than cholesterol in human plasma. In conclusion, the automated enzymic method is rapid, sensitive and relatively specific. If it were not for the high cost per assay, the procedure might justifiably be regarded as the method of choice for the assay of plasma cholesterol in the routine clinical laboratory.

An additional use of cholesterol oxidase may be noted in passing. The properties of the enzyme have been exploited for the formation of 3-ketosteroids from 3β-hydroxysterols in analytical work (e.g. in the GLC separation of a mixture of cholesterol and 5α-cholestanol by enzymic conversion into the Δ^4- and 5α-3-ketosteroid) and in the preparation of intermediates in the chemical synthesis of steroids (Smith and Brooks, 1976).

6.1.7 Esterified cholesterol

Although more than half the cholesterol of normal human plasma is esterified, for routine purposes it is usually sufficient to measure total plasma cholesterol concentration. However, in the investigation of certain abnormal clinical states it may be desirable to measure separately the concentrations of free and esterified cholesterol in plasma.

The reference method for measurement of plasma esterified cholesterol is the Schoenheimer-Sperry procedure or one of its modifications, but these are time-consuming and are not sensitive enough for some purposes. In the procedure favoured by most workers, total lipids are extracted from plasma by the Folch method, free and esterified cholesterol are separated by column chromatography (Hirsch and Ahrens, 1958) or TLC, the eluted esterified cholesterol is hydrolysed to free cholesterol and the cholesterol assayed by an appropriate method (usually GLC if high sensitivity is required, or a colorimetric method if the quantities of cholesterol are adequate). As mentioned in Section 6.1.6, the cholesterol oxidase method can be adapted for assay of esterified cholesterol in plasma, so that automation for routine measurement is theoretically possible. Quantitative GLC may also be used for the assay of cholesteryl esters without a preliminary hydrolysis (Kuksis *et al.*, 1975).

6.1.8 Automation

In view of the increasing numbers of plasma cholesterol assays that have to be performed daily in routine clinical work and in epidemiological surveys, an important factor in the choice of a suitable procedure is the ease with which it can be fully automated. Apart from their greater speed and lower running cost, automated methods also give greater reproducibility than manual methods since pipetting errors are largely eliminated. In general, automation is facilitated by minimizing the number of separate steps, avoiding the use of corrosive or unstable reagents and eliminating the need for saponification.

Nevertheless, several well-tried automated methods requiring solvent extraction and the use of the K-Z or L-B colour reagent are in current use.

In the fully automated method of van der Honing *et al.* (1968), the serum is saponified, the saponified lipids are extracted into carbon tetrachloride and the cholesterol in the unevaporated solvent is assayed with the L-B colour reagent (which is miscible with carbon tetrachloride). Horse serum containing cholesterol at known concentrations is used as standard. Serum esterified cholesterol may be determined by carrying out the procedure with and without saponification.

In the automated AutoAnalyzer methods I and II for the simultaneous assay of cholesterol and triglycerides in the same sample, adopted by the NIH for their *Lipid Research Clinics Program*, the plasma lipids are extracted into isopropanol, phospholipids and certain substances that interfere with the subsequent colour reactions are removed by adsorption with Zeolite, and the cholesterol in the isopropanol extract is assayed with the K-Z (method I) or L-B (method II) colour reagent without prior saponification or evaporation of the solvent. The standard is a solution of pure unesterified cholesterol. The use of free cholesterol as standard for the assay of a mixture of free and unesterified cholesterol in plasma is no disadvantage in method I since free and esterified cholesterol react equally with the K-Z reagent. However, values obtained with method II are higher than those obtained with the reference method (manual Abell, with saponification), owing to the greater reactivity of esterified than of free cholesterol with the L-B reagent. A correction factor for this error is calculated by assaying a 'calibration' sample of serum whose total cholesterol concentration has been determined previously by the reference method.

The full automation of the cholesterol oxidase method and the partial automation of GLC methods for assay of plasma cholesterol have been referred to in Sections 6.1.6 and 6.1.7 of this chapter.

6.2 Other aspects of the assay of sterols

In the routine assay of human serum cholesterol, speed, simplicity, low cost and comparability between laboratories are of prime importance. In other circumstances, however, the need for sensitivity or for a high degree of specificity towards particular sterols may determine the method of choice. For example, the assay of cholesterol in needle biopsies taken from human subjects or in small pieces of tissue obtained from experimental animals may require measurement of submicrogram quantities. In this case, quantitative GLC is usually the most appropriate method. Specificity with respect to sterols is essential if one wishes to assay the sterols other than cholesterol present in serum or tissues. As we shall see in Chapter 3, cholesterol in the animal body is always accompanied by other sterols, including 5α-cholestanol, lathosterol, 7-dehydrocholesterol and desmosterol. In normal serum these are present only in traces, but in certain tissues, such as the skin of some animals, developing brain and intestinal wall, one or other of these 'companions' of cholesterol may account for a significant proportion of the total sterols. Colorimetric methods capable of discriminating between Δ^5 sterols (slow-acting sterols) and Δ^7 and $\Delta^{5,7}$ sterols (fast-acting sterols) have been superseded by quantitative GLC. Desmosterol, lathosterol and 7-dehydrocholesterol can be separated from cholesterol and from each other by GLC with a polar liquid phase, and the separation on most phases is improved by derivative formation. 5α-Cholestanol cannot readily be assayed by GLC in the presence of cholesterol. However, these two sterols can be separated by TLC with $AgNO_3$-treated silicic acid, eluted from the silicic acid and assayed separately on GLC columns (but see Fig. 2.3).

Colorimetric and enzymic methods cannot be used to assay cholesterol in foods containing vegetable matter or shell-fish, since the sterols of plants and the desmosterol present in shell-fish give a positive reaction with both types of method. The cholesterol content of foods is considered in Chapter 3. Since plant sterols react with the colour reagents used for assaying cholesterol, the plant sterols present in the tissues of omnivorous and herbivorous animals cannot be assayed colorimetrically without prior separation. GLC is now the method of choice for assaying plant sterols in animal tissues. The assay of faecal neutral sterols in the sterol balance prodecure is discussed in Section 6.3.3.

6.3 Assay of bile acids

6.3.1 Relevance to cholesterol metabolism

In this section, the assay of bile acids is considered primarily in so far as it is called for in the study of cholesterol metabolism. Since a substantial fraction of the exchangeable cholesterol in the animal body is converted into bile acids, an important aspect of the quantitative investigation of cholesterol metabolism is the measurement of the rate of production of total bile acids *in vivo*. This can be achieved by measurement of the rate of turnover of the primary bile acids (cholic acid and chenodeoxycholic acid in most mammals, including man), or of the rate of excretion of total bile acids in the faeces. The assay of bile acids in serum and gall-bladder bile may also be required in the study of abnormal clinical states affecting cholesterol metabolism. Details of the methods available for assay of bile acids for different purposes will be found in the references given in the reviews by Eneroth and Sjövall (1971), Danielsson and Sjövall (1975) and Hofmann (1976).

6.3.2 Bile acids in duodenal bile

The absolute rate of turnover of cholic or chenodeoxycholic acid may be measured by a radioisotopic method introduced by Lindstedt (1957) and subsequently modified after the development of improved methods for assaying bile acids (see Hofmann and Hoffman, 1974). The bile acid, labelled with ^{14}C or ^{3}H, is injected intravenously into the subject and the rate of decline of the specific radioactivity of the injected bile acid in serial samples of duodenal fluid is measured over a period long enough for estimation of the pool size and half life of the labelled acid.

When used for measurement of the turnover of cholic acid alone, the method is simple in principle; the only complicating factor is the presence, in duodenal fluid, of radioactive deoxycholic acid formed in the intestinal lumen by 7α-dehydroxylation of cholic acid. The conjugated bile acids in the duodenal sample are separated by TLC or column chromatography, preferably after hydrolysis to the free acids, into cholic acid and a dihydroxy fraction containing chenodeoxycholic and deoxycholic acids. The cholic acid, now separated from radioactive deoxycholate, is assayed for radioactivity and its mass determined either by GLC of the TFA derivative of the methyl ester, or by enzymic oxidation with *3-hydroxysteroid dehydrogenase* (EC 1.1.1.50 (or 51)). This enzyme, prepared from the soil bacterium *Pseudomonas testosteroni*, catalyzes the NAD-linked oxidation of the 3α- or 3β-hydroxyl group of a 5α or 5β steroid to a 3-keto group, as in the oxidation of cholic acid:

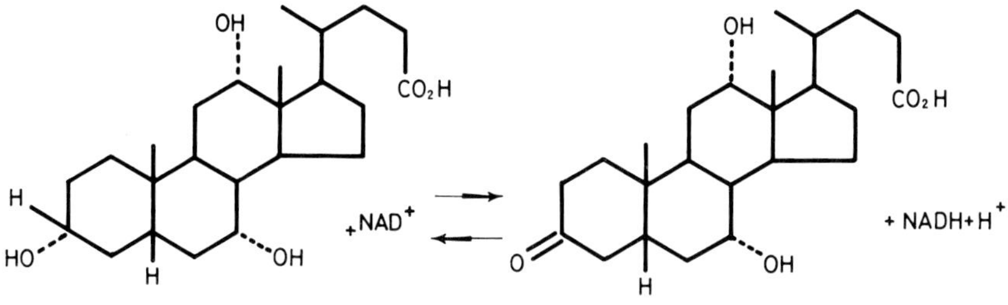

The reaction, adapted for use in the microassay of free or conjugated normal or allo bile acids containing a 3-hydroxyl group, is measured by spectrophotometric determination of NADH (Iwata and Yamasaki, 1964). The nomenclature of this enzyme is rather unsatisfactory. Many commercial preparations, including that used by Iwata and Yamasaki (1964), use 3α- or 3β-hydroxysteroids as substrate, though Iwata and Yamasaki referred to their enzyme as β-hydroxysteroid dehydrogenase (EC 1.1.1.51). However, enzyme preparations with such broad specificity appear to consist of a mixture of two distinct enzymes, one with specificity for 3α-hydroxysteroids (EC 1.1.1.50) and the other specific for 3β-hydroxysteroids (EC 1.1.1.51).

The Enzyme Commission nomenclature of these enzymes is 3α- (or 3β)hydroxysteroid:NAD(P)oxidoreductase (EC 1.1.1.50 (or 51)) (Bergmeyer, 1974). If one wishes to assay 3α- and 3β-hydroxy bile acids by the enzymic method, it is necessary to use an enzyme preparation containing both enzymes. A method based on the use of a 3-hydroxysteroid dehydrogenase could not be used for assaying bile acids with a sulphate group at C-3.

The simultaneous measurement of the rates of turnover of cholic acid and chenodeoxycholic acid in the same subject is complicated by the fact that when both radioactive primary bile acids are administered, duodenal bile contains radioactivity in the two dihydroxy acids (chenodeoxycholic and deoxycholic), as well as in cholic acid. Hence, if the injected cholic and chenodeoxycholic acids are labelled with ^{14}C, the dihydroxy fraction obtained by chromatography will contain [^{14}C] chenodeoxycholic acid and [^{14}C] deoxycholic acid. It will therefore be impossible to measure ^{14}C in the chenodeoxycholic acid without first separating it from deoxycholic acid. This is difficult to achieve by thin-layer or column chromatography. An alternative method is to inject a mixture containing [4-^{14}C] cholic acid and chenodeoxycholic acid labelled with ^{3}H at C-2, C-4, C-11 or C-12 (positions in which the tritium atoms are stable). The ^{3}H in chenodeoxycholic acid can then be assayed in the presence of [^{14}C] deoxycholic acid by liquid scintillation spectrometry. The mass of chenodeoxycholic acid in the dihydroxy fraction may be assayed by GLC or with a bacterial NAD-7α-hydroxysteroid dehydrogenase for which chenodeoxycholic acid (the 3α,7α-dihydroxy acid), but not deoxycholic acid (the 3α,12α-dihydroxy acid), acts as substrate (Haslewood et al., 1973). The enzyme is prepared from a strain of *E. coli* and uses as substrate either free or conjugated bile acids containing a 7α-hydroxyl group. The reaction is analogous to that catalyzed by 3α-hydroxysteroid dehydrogenase, resulting in the formation of NADH and a 7-keto bile acid. With the combined use of the 3-hydroxysteroid and 7α-hydroxysteroid dehydrogenases it is possible to assay deoxycholic and chenodeoxycholic acids in a mixture of the two.

The enzymic method is the most convenient for measurement of the total bile acids in hepatic or gall-bladder bile as, for example, in the investigation of cholesterol stones in the gall bladder. Although all the bile acids in bile are conjugated, saponification is not necessary because 3-hydroxysteroid dehydrogenase reacts equally with conjugated and free bile acids. Measurement of the individual bile acids in human bile requires, in principle, a preliminary separation of the bile-acid mixture into mono-, di- and tri-hydroxy bile acids, together with a method for assaying deoxycholic acid and chenodeoxycholic acid in a mixture of the two steroids.

6.3.3 Measurement of sterol balance

In the sterol balance method for measuring cholesterol synthesis *in vivo*, the rate of production of exchangeable cholesterol by the whole body is estimated as the difference between the intake of dietary cholesterol and the output of cholesterol and its metabolites in the faeces (for the assumptions on which the method is based, see Chapter 10). Thus, it is only necessary to measure *total* faecal bile acids and *total* faecal cholesterol plus its neutral derivatives; separate assay of each of the numerous bile acids and neutral steroids excreted in the faeces is not required.

Enzymic assay of total faecal bile acids with 3α-hydroxysteroid dehydrogenase is not feasible, owing to the presence of faecal bile acids with no 3-hydroxyl group and of substances in the acidic steroid fraction that interfere with the enzymic reaction.

The most widely accepted method is the GLC procedure developed by Grundy *et al.* (1965) and Miettinen *et al.* (1965) for the assay of total bile acids and neutral steroids in a single sample of human or animal faeces. The method for bile acids was later modified (Grundy and Metzger, 1972) by the additional use of a keto bile acid, not normally present in faeces, as internal standard. The critical features of the complete procedure are the use of GLC conditions under which the area of the GLC peak given by each bile acid or neutral steroid is directly proportional to its mass, and the separation of dietary plant sterols from cholesterol and its neutral derivatives by a combination of TLC and GLC.

For the assay of bile acids in a sample of faeces, the bile acid extract, containing 5α-cholestane as GLC marker and 3α,7α-dihydroxy-12-keto-5β-cholanoic acid as internal standard, is methylated and the methyl esters are converted into their TMS ethers. The mixture of silylated bile acids is analysed by GLC with SE-30 or QF-1 as liquid phase and with a hydrogen-flame ionization detector. Under critical conditions of column temperature, gas flow and detector temperature (which must be established for each column and should be checked periodically), the area under the peak given by a bile acid or neutral steroid is proportional to the mass of the unsilylated, unmethylated, parent compound. All the bile acids normally present in faeces, when analysed by this procedure, are eluted after 5α-cholestane and before the dihydroxy 12-keto acid used as internal standard. Moreover, all the acidic contaminants present in the faecal bile acid fraction are eluted before 5α-cholestane. Hence, the total mass of bile acid in the faecal sample may be estimated from the ratio:

$$\frac{\text{total area under all the peaks between the 5α-cholestane and internal standard peaks}}{\text{area under the peak due to the internal standard}}$$

112   The Biology of Cholesterol and Related Steroids

This analysis is illustrated in Fig. 2.8.

For the assay of cholesterol and its neutral derivatives in the faecal sample, preliminary separation of the neutral steroid fraction by TLC must be carried out before silylation and subsequent analysis by GLC. This step is necessary because some of the 5β-saturated plant sterols present in faeces cannot be completely separated from cholesterol or 5β-cholestan-3-one (coprostanone) by GLC. The neutral steroid fraction is separated by TLC into three subfractions, each of which is

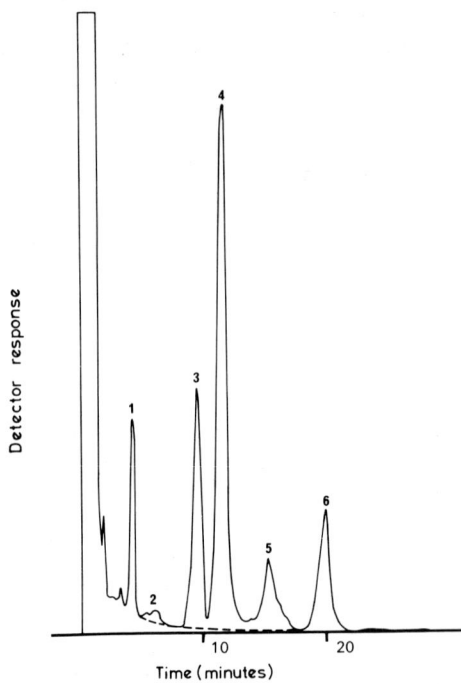

Figure 2.8
Gas-liquid chromatogram of the TMS ethers of the methyl esters of total bile acids extracted from a homogenate of normal human faeces. Before extraction, exactly 2 mg of 3α,7α-dihydroxy-12-keto-5β-cholanoic acid was added to the faecal sample as internal standard. 5α-Cholestane was added to the methylated bile acid mixture before silylation. The mass of bile acids in the sample was calculated from the ratio of the area under the peaks between peaks 1 and 6 (shown as the total area above the broken line) to the area under peak 6. Peak 1, 5α-cholestane; peak 2, unidentified; peak 3, lithocholic acid; peak 4, deoxycholic acid; peak 5, cholic acid and other minor components; peak 6, internal standard (dihydroxy-12-keto acid).

GLC was carried out on a Varian Aerograph, model 2740, with a 6 ft × 4 mm glass column and with a hydrogen flame detector (H_2 flow, 30 ml/min; air flow 300 ml/min). The liquid phase was 1.5% SE-30 supported on Varaport; the carrier gas was N_2 (30 ml/min); column temperature was 240 °C; detector temperature was 255 °C. Note that samples from some human subjects give one or more peaks with longer retention time than the dihydroxy-12-keto acid. Unequivocal identification of the compounds responsible for these peaks would require the use of GLC-mass spectrometry. (This analysis was carried out by A. V. Jadhav.)

eluted separately, silylated and analysed by GLC with 5α-cholestane as internal standard. By this means it is possible to measure the amounts of cholesterol, coprostanone, 5α-cholestanol and 5β-cholestanol in faeces in the presence of plant sterols and the products of their metabolism in the intestine.

6.3.4 Serum bile acids

Methods for measuring serum bile acids are needed for investigations of the enterohepatic circulation of bile salts in normal conditions and in various diseases affecting the hepato-biliary system or the gastrointestinal tract. In obstructive jaundice, when the serum from peripheral blood may contain more than 200 µg of bile acid/ml, there is no difficulty in assaying serum bile acids by the enzyme/spectrophotometry method of Iwata and Yamasaki. In normal human subjects, however, total serum bile acid concentration may be less than 1 µg/ml (<2.5 µmol/l) in the fasting state. The unmodified enzymic method is not nearly sensitive enough for measurement at this level.

The first successful method, suitable for assaying both total and individual bile acids in normal serum, was developed by Sandberg *et al.* (1965). In this method, the bile acids are extracted by anion-exchange column chromatography, saponified, methylated and assayed as their TFA derivatives by GLC with QF-1 or CNSi as liquid phase. The method may be adapted for measurement of the very small amounts of unconjugated bile acids present in normal serum by omitting the saponification. Enzymic hydrolysis of the conjugated bile acids with an enzyme from *Clostridium perfringens* may also be used as an alternative to saponification. The Sandberg procedure is a sensitive and accurate method for assaying individual bile acids in serum, but the initial extraction step makes the method too time-consuming for routine use. Bile acids may be rapidly and efficiently extracted from serum by shaking with Amberlite XAD-7, a non-ionic resin (van Berge Henegouwen *et al.*, 1976). This alternative to column chromatography greatly simplifies the assay of serum bile acids by GLC and may be used for handling large batches of samples. In the method of Panveliwalla *et al.* (1970), free and conjugated serum bile acids are separated by TLC, eluted from the plates and assayed by measurement of fluorescence in the presence of concentrated H_2SO_4.

The enzymic method for assay of total serum bile acids has been modified by Murphy *et al.* (1970), who determined NADH spectrofluorimetrically. This method is much more sensitive than the original spectrophotometric method of Iwata and Yamasaki and has been improved by combining it with XAD-extraction procedures (Schwartz *et al.*, 1974).

The most sensitive method for measuring serum bile acids, and potentially the easiest to adapt for routine use, is the radioimmunoassay developed by Simmonds et al. (1973). In the method for assaying conjugated cholic acid, antiserum to glycocholic acid coupled to serum albumin by amide linkage is raised in rabbits. Conjugated cholic acid in less than 0.1 ml of normal serum may be assayed by measuring the displacement of glyco[^{3}H]cholic acid from the antibody. The antibody binds glycocholate and taurocholate equally, but shows only limited cross-reactivity with conjugated chenodeoxycholic and deoxycholic acids. It is possible to extend this method to the assay of conjugated bile acids other than cholic acid (Murphy et al., 1976).

6.3.5 Sulphated bile acids

The recognition that sulphate esters account for a substantial proportion of the total bile acids in the bile and urine of patients with biliary obstruction has led to increasing interest in the problem of assaying bile-acid sulphates in biological materials. This concern has been reinforced by the need to measure sulphated bile acids in the bile and faeces, as an investigative procedure, in the growing number of gallstone patients treated with chenodeoxycholic acid or ursodeoxycholic acid (Chapter 18), both of which are metabolized extensively to bile-acid sulphates. The methodology in this field is developing very rapidly and it is likely that procedures now in use will be superseded or greatly modified within the next few years. A detailed discussion of current methods for assaying bile-acid sulphates would therefore be premature. However, a few general points are worth making.

First, there is the question as to how far conventional methods for assaying total bile acids or the total amount of a given bile acid, in bile or other materials, are valid in circumstances in which an appreciable proportion of the total bile-acid mixture is present as sulphate esters. If, for example, a significant fraction of the bile acids in human faeces is sulphated and if, as the observations of Palmer and Bolt (1971) suggest, sulphated bile acids are partially degraded during rigorous alkaline hydrolysis, then the total bile acid content of faeces would be underestimated by the method of Grundy et al. (1965) (see Section 6.3.3), since this method includes a rigorous saponification without a preliminary step to remove the sulphate group from sulphated bile acids that may be present in the faeces. Any sulphated bile acids in the original sample would also fail to contribute to the gas-liquid chromatogram unless the sulphate group was removed at some stage in the procedure. Thus, it would seem desirable to check this method for completeness of recovery of the bile acids of sulphate esters at the final stage of gas-liquid chromatographic assay of the TMS ethers of the methyl esters of free bile acids.

The second problem concerns the assay of the bile-acid sulphates themselves, particularly in bile, urine and faeces. Although the predominant bile-acid sulphate in human bile is the 3α-sulphate ester of lithocholic acid conjugated with glycine or taurine, sulphation can also occur at the 7α and 12α positions in the di- and trihydroxy conjugated bile acids, as well as in the unconjugated acids. Hence, the total number of possible sulphated bile acids is considerable. There are at present no simple methods for assaying all sulphated bile acids in a complex mixture, though Almé et al. (1977) have described a procedure applicable to the assay of bile acids in human urine. In this procedure the total bile acid mixture is extracted from acidified urine with an XAD column. Group separation into unconjugated and glyco- or tauro-conjugated sulphated and non-sulphated bile acids is then achieved by column chromatography with Sephadex LH-20, a lipophilic anion exchanger. The bile acids in each fraction eluted from the column are assayed by GLC, either directly or after removal of the sulphate group by solvolysis followed by deconjugation by alkaline hydrolysis.

In practice, such detailed analysis is seldom required. More commonly one merely wishes to know how much of a particular bile acid is present in sulphated form. For example, the extent to which lithocholic acid (a potentially toxic agent) is sulphated in gallstone patients treated with large doses of chenodeoxycholic acid has an obvious bearing on the possible hazards from this treatment. For purposes such as this a 'difference' method is the most suitable. Thus Danzinger et al. (1973) measured the total amount of sulphated lithocholic acid (unconjugated plus glyco- and tauro-conjugated) in bile as the difference between the amount assayed by GLC with and without a preliminary acid solvolysis to remove the sulphate group before deconjugation by alkaline hydrolysis. Stiehl et al. (1975) have extended this method to the group assay of conjugated and unconjugated sulphated and non-sulphated bile acids in human urine. Essentially, their method involves the GLC assay of individual bile acids in samples of urine that have been submitted to enzymic deconjugation (Nair et al., 1967), or acid solvolysis or a combination of both, or that have not been treated by either procedure. In the last case the assay will, of course, provide an estimate of the amount of each bile acid that is neither conjugated nor sulphated.

In conclusion, it should be noted that the removal of the sulphate group from a bile-acid sulphate ester by non-hydrolytic solvolysis takes place when the sulphate ester is left in solution at room temperature in an organic solvent such as ethanol, acetone or ether at acid pH. Hence, in any procedure in which the bile acids are extracted from an acidified aqueous phase into an organic solvent such as ether, any sulphated bile acids taken into the organic solvent will undergo solvolysis in a matter of hours at room temperature (van Berge Henegouwen et al., 1977). Therefore if sulphate esters of bile acids are to be assayed, the organic solvent should be evaporated promptly.

REFERENCES

Abell, L. L., Levy, B. B., Brodie, B. B. and Kendall, F. E. (1952). A simplified method for the estimation of total cholesterol in serum and demonstration of its specificity. *Journal of Biological Chemistry*, **195**, 357–366.

Allain, C. C., Poon, L. S., Chan, C. S. G., Richmond, W. and Fu, P. C. (1974). Enzymatic determination of total serum cholesterol. *Clinical Chemistry*, **20**, 470–475.

Almé, B., Bremmelgaard, A., Sjövall, J. and Thomassen, P. (1977). Analysis of metabolic profiles of bile acids in urine using a lipophilic anion exchanger and computerized gas-liquid chromatography-mass spectrometry. *Journal of Lipid Research*, **18**, 339–362.

Altman, L. J., Kowerski, R. C. and Rilling, H. C. (1971). Synthesis and conversion of presqualene alcohol to squalene. *Journal of the American Chemical Society*, **93**, 1782–1783.

Bellamy, L. J. *Advances in Infrared Group Frequencies*. Methuen, London, 1968.

Bergmeyer, H. U. Reagents for enzymatic analysis. In: *Methods of Enzymatic Analysis*, Vol. 1. Ed. H. U. Bergmeyer. Academic Press, New York, pp. 476–477, 1974.

Bladon, P., Henbest, H. B. and Wood, G. W. (1952). Studies in the sterol group. LV. Ultra-violet absorption spectra of ethylenic centres. *Journal of the Chemical Society*, 2737–2744.

Brooks, C. J. W. Gas-chromatographic examination of sterols. In: *The Determination of Sterols*. Six Papers originally presented at a Meeting of the Society held on 2nd May, 1962, Monograph No. 2, pp. 18–29. The Society for Analytical Chemistry, London, 1964.

Budzikiewicz, H., Djerassi, C. and Williams, D. H. *Mass Spectrometry of Organic Compounds*. Holden-Day, San Francisco, 1967.

Campbell, R. V. M., Crombie, L. and Pattenden, G. (1971). Synthesis of presqualene alcohol. *Chemical Communications*, 218–219.

Carpenter, K. J., Gotsis, A. and Hegsted, D. M. (1957). Estimation of total cholesterol in serum by a micro method. *Clinical Chemistry*, **3**, 233–238.

Clayton, R. B. (1962). Gas-liquid chromatography of sterol methyl ethers and some correlations between molecular structure and retention data. *Biochemistry*, **1**, 357–366.

Clayton, R. B., Nelson, A. N. and Frantz, I. D. (1963). The skin sterols of normal and triparanol-treated rats. *Journal of Lipid Research*, **4**, 166–178.

Coates, R. M. and Robinson, W. H. (1971). Stereoselective total synthesis of ($\pm$)-presqualene alcohol. *Journal of the American Chemical Society*, **93**, 1785/1786.

Cook, R. P. and Rattray, J. B. M. Methods of isolation and estimation of sterols. In: *Cholesterol*. Ed. R. P. Cook. Academic Press, New York, pp. 117–143, 1958.

Corey, E. J. and Ortiz de Montellano, P. R. (1968). A simple synthetic route to a proposed intermediate in the biosynthesis of squalene from farnesyl pyrophosphate. *Tetrahedron Letters*, No. 49, 5113–5115.

Danielsson, H. and Sjövall, J. (1975). Bile acid metabolism. *Annual Review of Biochemistry*, **44**, 233–253.

Danzinger, R. G., Hofmann, A. F., Thistle, J. L. and Schoenfield, L. J. (1973). Effect of oral chenodeoxycholic acid on bile acid kinetics and biliary lipid composition in women with cholelithiasis. *Journal of Clinical Investigation*, **52**, 2809–2821.

Edmond, J., Popják, G., Wong, S. M. and Williams, V. P. (1971). Presqualene alcohol. Further evidence on the structure of a C_{30} precursor of squalene. *Journal of Biological Chemistry*, **246**, 6254–6271.

Eneroth, P., Gordon, B., Ryhage, R. and Sjövall, J. (1966). Identification of mono-

and dihydroxy bile acids in human feces by gas-liquid chromatography and mass spectrometry. *Journal of Lipid Research*, **7**, 511–523.

Eneroth, P. and Sjövall, J. Methods of analysis in the biochemistry of bile acids. In: *Methods in Enzymology*, **XV**. Ed. R. B. Clayton. Academic Press, New York, pp. 237–280, 1969.

Eneroth, P. and Sjövall, J. Extraction, purification, and chromatographic analysis of bile acids in biological materials. In: *The Bile Acids. Chemistry, Physiology, and Metabolism*, Vol. 1. Chemistry, Ed. P. P. Nair and D. Kritchevsky. Plenum Press, New York, pp. 121–171, 1971.

Entenman, C. General procedures for separating lipid components of tissue. In: *Methods in Enzymology*, **III**. Ed. S. P. Colowick and N. O. Kaplan. Academic Press, New York, pp. 299–317, 1957.

Epstein, W. W. and Rilling, H. C. (1970). Studies on the mechanism of squalene biosynthesis. The structure of presqualene pyrophosphate. *Journal of Biological Chemistry*, **245**, 4597–4605.

Folch, J., Lees, M. and Sloane Stanley, G. H. (1957). A simple method for the isolation and purification of total lipids from animal tissues. *Journal of Biological Chemistry*, **226**, 497–509.

Frantz, I. D. and Schroepfer, G. J. (1967). Sterol biosynthesis. *Annual Review of Biochemistry*, **36**, 691–726.

Gautschi, F. and Bloch, K. (1957). On the structure of an intermediate in the biological demethylation of lanosterol. *Journal of the American Chemical Society*, **79**, 684–689.

Gautschi, F. and Bloch, K. (1958). Synthesis of isomeric 4,4-dimethylcholestenols and identification of a lanosterol metabolite. *Journal of Biological Chemistry*, **233**, 1343–1347.

Gibbons, G. F., Mitropoulos, K. A. and Myant, N. B. *The Biochemistry of Cholesterol*. Elsevier, Amsterdam, 1982.

Gibbons, G. F., Mitropoulos, K. A. and Ramananda, K. (1973). A method for the rapid qualitative and quantitative analysis of 4,4-dimethyl sterols. *Journal of Lipid Research*, **14**, 589–592.

Goad, L. J. and Goodwin, T. W. (1966). The biosynthesis of sterols in higher plants. *Biochemical Journal*, **99**, 735–746.

Goad, L. J. and Goodwin, T. W. (1967). Studies on phytosterol biosynthesis: the sterols of *Latrix decidua* leaves. *European Journal of Biochemistry*, **1**, 357–362.

Grundy, S. M., Ahrens, E. H. Jr. and Miettinen, T. A. (1965). Quantitative isolation and gas-liquid chromatographic analysis of total fecal bile acids. *Journal of Lipid Research*, **6**, 397–410.

Grundy, S. M. and Metzger, A. L. (1972). A physiological method for estimation of hepatic secretion of biliary lipids in man. *Gastroenterology*, **62**, 1200–1217.

Hanel, H. K. and Dam, H. (1955). Determination of small amounts of total cholesterol by the Tschugaeff reaction with a note on the determination of lathosterol. *Acta Chemica Scandinavica*, **9**, 677–682.

Hansbury, E. and Scallen, T. J. (1978). Resolution of desmosterol, cholesterol, and other sterol intermediates by reverse-phase high-pressure liquid chromatography. *Journal of Lipid Research*, **19**, 742–746.

Haslewood, G. A. D., Murphy, G. M. and Richardson, J. M. (1973). A direct enzymic assay for 7α-hydroxy bile acids and their conjugates. *Clinical Science*, **44**, 95–98.

Heider, J. G. and Boyett, R. L. (1978). The picomole determination of free and total cholesterol in cells in culture. *Journal of Lipid Research*, **19**, 514–518.

Heftmann, E. Chromatography of steroids. In: *Chromatography*. Ed. E. Heftmann. Van Nostrand Reinhold Co., New York, pp. 610–636, 1975.

Henegouwen, van Berge, G. P. See van Berge Henegouwen, G. P.

Hinckley, C. C. Applications of lanthanide shift reagents. In: *Modern Methods of Steroid Analysis*. Ed. E. Heftmann. Academic Press, New York, pp. 265–279, 1973.

Hirsch, J. and Ahrens, E. H. Jr. (1958). The separation of complex lipid mixtures by the use of silicic acid chromatography. *Journal of Biological Chemistry*, **233**, 311–320.

Hofmann, A. F. Thin-layer chromatography of bile acids and their derivatives. In: *New Biochemical Separations*. Ed. A. T. James and L. J. Morris. Van Nostrand, London, pp. 261–282, 1964.

Hofmann, A. F. (1976). The enterohepatic circulation of bile acids in man. *Advances in Internal Medicine*, **21**, 501–534.

Hofmann, A. F. and Hoffman, N. E. (1974). Measurement of bile acid kinetics by isotope dilution in man. *Gastroenterology*, **67**, 314–323.

Ishikawa, T. T., MacGee, J., Morrison, J. A. and Glueck, C. J. (1974). Quantitative analysis of cholesterol in 5–20 μl of plasma. *Journal of Lipid Research*, **15**, 286–291.

Iwata, T. and Yamasaki, K. (1964). Enzymatic determination and thin-layer chromatography of bile acids in blood. *Journal of Biochemistry* (Tokyo), **56**, 424–431.

Kabara, J. J. (1962). Determination and microscopic localization of cholesterol. *Methods of Biochemical Analysis*, **10**, 263–318.

Karle, J. Application of direct methods of x-ray structure analysis to steroids. In: *Modern Methods of Steroid Analysis*. Ed. E. Heftmann. Academic Press, New York, pp. 293–319, 1973.

Klause, K. A. and Subbiah, M. T. R. (1975). Improved resolution of cholestanol and cholesterol by gas-liquid chromatography. Application to testicular sterols. *Journal of Chromatography*, **103**, 170–172.

Klyne, W. and Scopes, P. M. (1969). Stereochemical correlations. *Progress in Stereochemistry*, **4**, 97–166.

Knights, B. A. Qualitative and quantitative analysis of plant sterols by gas-liquid chromatography. In: *Modern Methods of Steroid Analysis*. Ed. E. Heftmann. Academic Press, New York, pp. 103–138, 1973.

Knox, J. H. *High-performance liquid chromatography*. Ed. J. H. Knox. Edinburgh University Press, Edinburgh, 1978.

Kuksis, A. (1966). Newer developments in determination of bile acids and steroids by gas chromatography. *Methods of Biochemical Analysis*, **14**, 325–454.

Kuksis, A., Myher, J. J., Marai, L. and Geher, K. (1975). Determination of plasma lipid profiles by automated gas chromatography and computerized data analysis. *Journal of Chromatography*, **13**, 423–430.

Lindstedt, S. (1957). The turnover of cholic acid in man. Bile acids and steroids. 51. *Acta Physiologica Scandinavica*, **40**, 1–9.

Lisboa, B. P. Thin-layer chromatography of steroids, sterols and related compounds. In: *Methods in Enzymology*, **XV**. Ed. R. B. Clayton. Academic Press, New York, pp. 3–158, 1969.

Lutsky, B. N., Martin, J. A. and Schroepfer, G. J. Jr. (1971). Studies of the metabolism of 5α-cholesta-8,14-dien-3β-ol and 5α-cholesta-7,14-dien-3β-ol in rat liver homogenate preparations. *Journal of Biological Chemistry*, **246**, 6737–6744.

McCloskey, J. A. Mass spectrometry of lipids and steroids. In: *Methods in Enzymology*, **XIV**. Ed. J. M. Lowenstein. Academic Press, New York, pp. 382–450, 1969.

McNair, H. M. and Bonelli, E. J. *Basic Gas Chromatography*, 5th edition. Varian Aerograph, Walnut Creek, California, 1969.

Matthews, E. W., Byfield, P. G. H., Colston, K. W., Evans, I. M. A., Galan, T. E. L. S. and MacIntyre, I. (1974). Separation of hydroxylated derivatives of vitamin D_3 by high speed liquid chromatography (HSLC). *FEBS Letters*, **48**, 122–125.

Miettinen, T. A., Ahrens, E. H. Jr. and Grundy, S. M. (1965). Quantitative isolation and gas-liquid chromatographic analysis of total dietary and fecal neutral steroids. *Journal of Lipid Research*, **6**, 411–424.

Murphy, G. M., Billing, B. H. and Baron, D. N. (1970). A fluorimetric and enzymatic method for the estimation of serum total bile acids. *Journal of Clinical Pathology*, **23**, 594–598.

Murphy, G. M., Sampson, D. G., Cross, L. M. and Catty, D. (1976). The methodology of bile acid radioimmunoassay. *Clinical Science and Molecular Medicine*, **50**, 25P.

Nair, P. P., Gordon, M. and Reback. T. (1967). The enzymatic cleavage of the carbon-nitrogen bond in 3α,7α,12α-trihydroxy-5β-cholan-24-oylglycine. *Journal of Biological Chemistry*, **242**, 7–11.

Neudert, W. and Röpke, H. *Atlas of Steroid Spectra*. Sadler Research Laboratories. Springer-Verlag, Heidelberg, 1965.

Noone, M. A computerized method for rapid comparison and retrieval of infrared spectral data. In: *Modern Methods of Steroid Analysis*. Ed. E. Heftmann. Academic Press, New York, pp. 221–230, 1973.

Palmer, R. H. and Bolt, M. G. (1971). Bile acid sulfates. 1. Synthesis of lithocholic acid sulfates and their identification in human bile. *Journal of Lipid Research*, **12**, 671–679.

Panveliwalla, D., Tabaqchali, S., Lewis, B. and Wootton, I. D. P. (1970). Determination of individual bile acids in biological fluids by thin-layer chromatography and fluorimetry. *Journal of Clinical Pathology*, **23**, 309–314.

Pearson, S., Stern, S. and McGavack, T. H. (1953). A rapid, accurate method for the determination of total cholesterol in serum. *Analytical Chemistry*, **25**, 813–814.

Popják, G., Edmond, J., Anet, F. A. L. and Easton, N. R. Jr. (1977). Carbon-13 NMR studies on cholesterol biosynthesized from [^{13}C]mevalonates. *Journal of the American Chemical Society*, **99**, 931–935.

Popják, G., Edmond, J., Clifford, K. and Williams, V. (1969). Biosynthesis and structure of a new intermediate between farnesyl pyrophosphate and squalene. *Journal of Biological Chemistry*, **244**, 1897–1918.

Popják, G., Edmond, J. and Wong, S.-M. (1973). Absolute configuration of presqualene alcohol. *Journal of the American Chemical Society*, **95**, 2713–2714.

Popják, G., Goodman, D. S., Cornforth, J. W., Cornforth, R. H. and Ryhage, R. (1961). Studies on the biosynthesis of cholesterol. XV. Mechanism of squalene biosynthesis from farnesyl pyrophosphate and from mevalonate. *Journal of Biological Chemistry*, **236**, 1934–1947.

Popják, G., Lowe, A. E., Moore, D., Brown, L. and Smith, F. A. (1959). Scintillation counter for the measurement of radioactivity of vapors in conjunction with gas-liquid chromatography. *Journal of Lipid Research*, **1**, 29–39.

Radin, N. S. Preparation of lipid extracts. In: *Methods in Enzymology*, **XIV**. Ed. J. M. Lowenstein. Academic Press, New York, pp. 245–254, 1969.

Radin, N. and Gramza, A. L. (1963). Standard of purity for cholesterol. *Clinical Chemistry*, **9**, 121–134.

Rees, H. H., Donnahey, P. J. and Goodwin, T. W. (1976). Separation of C_{27}, C_{28} and C_{29} sterols by reversed-phase high-performance liquid chromatography on small particles. *Journal of Chromatography*, **116**, 281–291.

Rilling, H. C. (1966). A new intermediate in the biosynthesis of squalene. *Journal of Biological Chemistry*, **241**, 3233–3236.

Ryhage, R. (1964). Use of mass spectrometer as a detector and analyser for effluents emerging from high temperature gas liquid chromatography columns. *Analytical Chemistry*, **36**, 759–764.

Sandberg, D. H., Sjövall, J., Sjövall, K. and Turner, D. A. (1965). Measurement of human serum bile acids by gas-liquid chromatography. *Journal of Lipid Research*, **6**, 182–192.

Schoenheimer, R. and Sperry, W. M. (1934). A micromethod for the determination of free and combined cholesterol. *Journal of Biological Chemistry*, **106**, 745–760.

Schooley, D. A. and Nakanishi, K. Application of high-pressure liquid chromatography to the separation of insect molting hormones. In: *Modern Methods of Steroid Analysis*. Ed. E. Heftmann. Academic Press, New York, pp. 37–54, 1973.

Schwartz, H. P., Bergmann, K. v. and Paumgartner, G. (1974). A simple method for the estimation of bile acids in serum. *Clinica Chimica Acta*, **50**, 197–206.

Scopes, P. M. Applications of the chiroptical techniques to the study of natural products. In: *Progress in the Chemistry of Organic Natural Products*, Vol. 32. Ed. W. Herz, H. Grisebach and G. W. Kirby. Springer-Verlag, New York, pp. 167–265, 1975.

Setoguchi, T., Salen, G., Tint, S. and Mosbach, E. H. (1974). A biochemical abnormality in cerebrotendinous xanthomatosis. Impairment of bile acid synthesis associated with incomplete degradation of the cholesterol side-chain. *Journal of Clinical Investigation*, **53**, 1393–1401.

Shefer, S., Dayal, B., Tint, G. S , Salen, G. and Mosbach, E. H. (1975). Identification of pentahydroxy bile alcohols in cerebrotendinous xanthomatosis: characterization of 5β-cholestane-3α,7α,12α,24ξ,25-pentol and 5β-cholestane-3α,7α,23ξ,25-pentol. *Journal of Lipid Research*, **16**, 280–286.

Simmonds, W. J., Korman, M. G., Go, V. L. W. and Hofmann, A. F. (1973). Radioimmunoassay of conjugated cholyl bile acids in serum. *Gastroenterology*, **65**, 705–711.

Smith, A. G. and Brooks, C. J. W. (1976). Cholesterol oxidases: properties and applications. *Journal of Steroid Biochemistry*, **7**, 705–713.

Stiehl, A., Earnest, D. L. and Admirand, W. H. (1975). Sulfation and renal excretion of bile salts in patients with cirrhosis of the liver. *Gastroenterology*, **68**, 534–544.

Tonks, D. B. (1963). A study of the accuracy and precision of clinical chemistry determinations in 170 Canadian laboratories. *Clinical Chemistry*, **9**, 217–233.

Tonks, D. B. (1967). The estimation of cholesterol in serum: a classification and critical review of methods. *Clinical Biochemistry* **1**, 12–29.

Truswell, A. S. and Mitchell, W. D. (1965). Separation of cholesterol from its companions, cholestanol and Δ^7-cholestenol, by thin-layer chromatography. *Journal of Lipid Research*, **6**, 438–441.

Tschesche, R. Thin-layer chromatography of steroids. In: *New Biochemical Separations*. Ed. A. T. James and L. J. Morris. D. Van Nostrand, London, pp. 197–245, 1964.

U.S. DHEW. Manual of Laboratory Operations, Lipid Research Clinics Program, Vol. 1, Lipid and Lipoprotein Analysis, National Heart and Lung Institute, National Institutes of Health, Bethesda, pp. 1–81, 1974. *DHEW Publication No. (NIH)* 75–628.

van Berge Henegouwen, G. P., Allan, R. N., Hofmann, A. F. and Yu, P. Y. S. (1977). A facile hydrolysis-solvolysis procedure for conjugated bile acid sulfates. *Journal of Lipid Research*, **18**, 118–122.

van Berge Henegouwen, G. P., Hofmann, A. F. and Ruben, A. T. (1976). A simple batch adsorption procedure for the isolation of sulfated and non-sulfated bile acids from serum. *Clinica Chimica Acta*, **73**, 469–474.

Vandenheuvel, W. J. A. and Horning, E. C. (1962). A study of retention-time relationships in gas chromatography in terms of the structure of steroids. *Biochimica et Biophysica Acta*, **64**, 416–429.

Vandenheuvel, W. J. A. and Horning, E. C. In: *Biomedical Application of Gas Chromatography*. Ed. H. Szymanski. Plenum Press, New York, p. 89, 1964.

van der Honing, J., Saarloos, C. C. & Styp, J. (1968). Method for fully automated determination of total cholesterol in blood serum, including saponification and extraction. *Clinical Chemistry*, **14**, 960–966.

Vestergaard, P. Liquid column chromatography of hormonal steroids. In: *Modern Methods of Steroid Analysis*. Ed. E. Heftmann. Academic Press, New York, pp. 1–35, 1973.
Williams, J. H., Kuchmak, M. and Witter, R. F. (1965). Purity of cholesterol to be used as a primary standard. *Journal of Lipid Research*, **6**, 461–465.
Witte, D. L., Barrett, D. A. and Wycoff, D. A. (1974). Evaluation of an enzymatic procedure for determination of serum cholesterol with the Abbott ABA-100. *Clinical Chemistry*, **20**, 1282–1286.
Witter, R. F. and Stone, S. (1957). Spot test for 3-hydroxy delta^{-5} steroids. *Analytical Chemistry*, **29**, 156–157.
Wotiz, H. H. and Clark, S. J. Gas-liquid chromatographic methods for the analysis of steroids and sterols. In: *Methods in Enzymology*, **XV**. Ed. R. B. Clayton. Academic Press, New York, pp. 158–200, 1969.
Zlatkis, A., Zak, B. and Boyle, A. J. (1953). A new method for the direct determination of serum cholesterol. *Journal of Laboratory and Clinical Medicine*, **41**, 486–492.

Chapter 3

The Distribution of Sterols and Related Steroids in Nature

1	INTRODUCTION	125
2	VERTEBRATES	126
2.1	General	126
2.2	Liver and bile	127
2.3	Skin	130
2.3.1	Whole skin	130
2.3.2	Sebum	131
2.4	Nervous tissue	132
2.5	Fat, muscle, connective tissue and artery	133
2.6	Intestine and faeces	136
2.7	Glands	137
2.8	Milk	138
2.9	Subcellular distribution	139
2.10	Dietary cholesterol	141
2.11	Squalene	142
2.12	Steroidal toad poisons	143
3	INVERTEBRATES	144
3.1	General	144
3.2	Insects	145
3.3	Echinoderms	146
3.4	Porifera	148
3.5	Other invertebrates	149
4	PLANTS AND FUNGI	149
4.1	General	149
4.2	Higher plants	150
4.2.1	Types of sterol found	150
4.2.2	Other plant steroids	150
4.2.3	Possible functions of steroids in higher plants	155
4.3	Algae	155
4.4	Fungi and lichens	156

The Distribution of Sterols and Related Steroids in Nature

1 INTRODUCTION

Sterols are found in almost all living organisms. They are present in vertebrates, invertebrates, green plants, fungi and yeasts and they have been identified in very small amounts in some bacteria. They are also present in the most primitive of the algae, the Cyanophyta or 'blue-green algae', and in some animal viruses cholesterol accounts for up to 10% of the weight of the virus (Blough and Tiffany, 1973). Sterols are present in many species of protozoa. Some protozoans synthesize their own sterol but others have an absolute requirement for sterol in the medium. In some protozoan species that parasitize vertebrates, cholesterol obtained ready-made from the host is the major sterol present.

Sterols may be unconjugated, or they may be present as their fatty acid or sulphate esters (e.g. 3.1) or as glycosides. In addition to sterols themselves, numerous steroids and terpenoids related metabolically to sterols are found in animals, plants and fungi. Many of these are precursors of sterols or are derived from such precursors; others are products of the metabolism of sterols. The distribution of sterols and of

(3.1) Cholesteryl sulphate

some of the more interesting of these related compounds is considered in this chapter. The two groups of metabolites of cholesterol of major biological importance in vertebrates—bile acids and steroid hormones—are considered separately in Chapter 5.

2 VERTEBRATES

2.1 General

Cholesterol is by far the most abundant sterol in vertebrates. Most of the cholesterol in the whole body is present in free (unesterified) form in the plasma membranes and subcellular membranes of cells and in the myelin of nervous tissue. However, in certain specialized tissues, and under some pathological conditions, substantial quantities of cholesterol are esterified with long-chain fatty acids. In the plasma of all mammals, for example, the bulk of the cholesterol is esterified. The presence of cholesteryl sulphate and of other steryl sulphates has been demonstrated in several mammalian tissues and body fluids, including the adrenal cortex, brain, kidney, liver, plasma, bile and urine; meconium and faeces from newborn infants also contain cholesteryl sulphates and the disulphate esters of several hydroxylated derivatives of cholesterol. (For references to steryl sulphates, see Drayer and Lieberman, 1967; Gustafsson and Eneroth, 1972; Iwamori *et al.*, 1976.)

The probable *functions* of cholesterol in higher animals are: (a) to serve as an essential stabilizing constituent of cell membranes, plasma lipoproteins and myelin, and (b) to act as a precursor of bile acids and steroid hormones and, in the unusual case of toads, as a precursor of poisonous substances. One of the functions of esterified cholesterol is to act as a store of cholesterol for steroid-hormone synthesis; another may be to act as a reservoir of surplus cholesterol in a form in which it cannot interact with membranes.

In addition to cholesterol and its esters, other sterols and related steroids are present in measurable amounts in many animal tissues. These occur either as intermediates in the biosynthesis of cholesterol or as products of its enzymic or non-enzymic modification. Strictly speaking, all the steroidal precursors of cholesterol should be present at finite concentrations in all tissues in which cholesterol is synthesized. However, the concentrations of many intermediates is such that their presence in the tissues can only be demonstrated by special techniques involving the use of radioactive tracers. Although plant sterols are poorly absorbed from the diet, many tissues of omnivorous and herbivorous animals contain detectable amounts of β-sitosterol and other phytosterols.

In much of the work done before the 1950's on the sterol composition of animal tissues, the methods used for extraction, separation and assay of sterols are open to criticism. This applies particularly to estimations of 'non-cholesterol' sterols and methyl sterols present in the unsaponifiable lipids; in many cases, the assay methods were not sufficiently specific to permit a distinction between closely related stenols such as lathosterol and 7-dehydrocholesterol. D'Hollander and Chevallier (1969) have analysed the digitonin-precipitable sterols of most of the tissues of adult rats, using quantitative GLC (Table 3.1). No comparable values are available for human tissues as a whole, though some information is available on the sterols of human skin (Nikkari et al., 1974). Analyses of various tissues from rabbits, guinea pigs and other species suggest that the sterol composition of the tissues of rats is representative, with some interesting exceptions, of that of mammals in general.

In rat tissues, the concentration of total (digitonin-precipitable) sterol varies widely from less than 100 mg/100 g in plasma, bone and adipose tissue, to very high values in brain, nerve, adrenal glands and hair. In most rat tissues, less than 10% of the total sterol is esterified and in some tissues, including brain, nerve and red blood cells, virtually all the sterol is free. However, in liver, skin, hair, adrenals and plasma, a substantial proportion of the total sterol is esterified. In all rat tissues, with the partial exception of hair, almost all the *free* sterol is cholesterol but the *esterified* fraction in several tissues contains non-cholesterol sterols in amounts ranging from 10% to over 60% of the total.

The whole body of an adult rat contains about 450 mg of cholesterol (free plus esterified). More than a fifth of this is present in the brain and nervous system, but other organs, including skeletal muscle, skin, hair, liver and adipose tissue make substantial contributions to the total, largely by virtue of their mass.

In the tissues of most mammals, including man, the predominant fatty acids in the steryl ester fraction are oleate and palmitate. Exceptions to this general rule are the plasma and the adrenal glands, in which the esterified sterols contain high proportions of fatty acids with two or more double bonds (see pages 509 and 138, and the review by Goodman (1965)).

In this section, the sterols of certain animal tissues of special interest are considered in more detail.

2.2 Liver and bile

Cholesterol is the major sterol of liver in mammals, though lanosterol, zymosterol, 7-dehydrocholesterol, lathosterol and 5α-cholestanol are detectable in the non-saponifiable fraction of liver lipids. Normal

128 The Biology of Cholesterol and Related Steroids

Table 3.1

Free and esterified sterols of organs and tissues of adult rats
(Values compiled from D'Hollander and Chevallier (1969))

Organ or tissue	*Total sterols (mg/100 g fresh weight) F	E	E/F+E (%)	Composition of sterols (%) F Cholesterol	E Cholesterol	†Other sterols	Cholesterol in whole organ or tissue (mg) F	E
Plasma	19	61	76	98	98	<1	1.7	5.2
Stomach	234	7	3	97	75	20	3.2	0.1
Small intestine	186	9	5	99	94	4	17.4	0.8
Colon + caecum	190	3	2	98	84	13	3.6	0.1
Liver	159	87	35	98	98	2	27.0	14.8
Spleen	379	6	2	99	89	5	2.3	0
Kidneys	332	4	1	99	96	2	10.5	0.1
Testes	156	9	5	99	94	<1	4.5	0.1
Adrenals	855	2590	75	95	95	3	0.2	0.5
Lungs	391	18	4	99	98	<1	5.6	0.3
Skin	94	102	52	94	25	64	53.0	15.3
Hair	375	750	67	88	18	68	32.9	13.5
Adipose	54	5	8	99	96	2	15.0	1.3
Aorta	127	7	5	99	94	2	—	—
Heart	111	2	2	99	92	<1	1.3	0.1
Muscle	63	2	3	98	83	15	74.2	1.5
Tendons	152	11	7	96	68	22	—	—
Bone marrow	264	10	4	98	94	2	21.4	0.8
Brain	1653	2	<1	99	91	3	30.0	0
Spinal cord	4120	2	<1	98	88	5	26.6	0
Nerve	3720	10	<1	98	81	11	36.4	0.1
Bone	28	6	18	96	86	12	10.7	2.1
Red blood cells	145	0	<1	99	<1	<1	10.1	0
Total:							387.6	444.2

mammalian liver, including human liver, contains 200–400 mg of sterol/100 g of fresh tissue. In animals given a normal diet 20–30% of the total liver sterol is esterified with fatty acids, oleic acid being the major fatty acid of the hepatic cholesteryl esters in most mammalian species. However, the feeding of cholesterol-rich diets produces marked increases in the cholesterol content of the liver, due mainly to an increase in the concentration of cholesteryl oleate, which may in extreme cases account for more than 80% of the total liver sterol. The fatty acid composition of liver cholesteryl esters can be altered to some extent by changing the fatty acid composition of the dietary triglycerides. There is no correlation between plasma and liver cholesterol concentration in adult human subjects (Insull *et al.*, 1967).

The liver of the newly-hatched chick is remarkably rich in cholesterol, containing up to 1 g of total cholesterol/100 g of fresh tissue, most of which is esterified. As the bird matures, the liver cholesterol concentration decreases to values similar to those observed in mammalian liver. The liver of the fattened goose, used for making paté de foie gras, contains up to 2 g of total cholesterol/100 g of fresh tissue. There are wide species differences in the sterol content of fish liver. The livers of some bony fish (e.g. the cod) and of some cartilagenous fish are rich in lipid and may contain up to 600 mg of cholesterol/100 g of fresh tissue. The livers of many cartilagenous fish (sharks, dogfish, skates and rays) contain large amounts of squalene. Though squalene is not a steroid, it is worth mentioning here because of its importance in the biosynthesis of sterols (see Chapter 4). The biological function of squalene in the liver is probably to impart buoyancy to the fish and thus to reduce the work needed to keep its body at a given depth; the specific gravity of squalene (0.85 g/ml at 20 °C) is much less than that of the whole body. Cartilagenous fish lack the swim bladder which is present in most bony fish and which provides them with a mechanism for controlling their buoyancy.

Cholesterol is present in the bile of all mammals, though the concentration varies widely from one species to another. In both hepatic and gall-bladder bile essentially all the cholesterol is unesteri-

---

Values are averaged from several analyses. The mean body weight of the rats used for estimation of total cholesterol in whole organs or tissues was 341 g. F, free; E, esterified; —, not recorded.

* *Total sterols* included all free and esterified sterols precipitable with digitonin after alkaline hydrolysis. The mixture of digitonin-precipitable sterols was analyzed by GLC of the free sterols with 1% QF-1 as liquid phase. Under the GLC conditions used, cholesterol was separated from lathosterol, 7-dehydrocholesterol and methyl sterols, but lathosterol and 7-dehydrocholesterol were probably not separated from each other; any traces of 5α-cholestanol present in the tissues would have been included in the cholesterol peak.

† *Other sterols* include all sterols with the R_T of lathosterol, 7-dehydrocholesterol or methostenol (peaks 4 and 5 of D'Hollander and Chevallier (1969)) but do not include dimethyl- or trimethyl sterols.

fied. The cholesterol concentration and the cholesterol:bile salt:phospholipid ratio in the bile vary widely between species and in some species may be modified by dietary and other factors (Portman, Osuga and Tanaka, 1975). Values reported for the cholesterol concentration in human bile draining from a bile-duct fistula after cholecystectomy have ranged from 30–300 mg/100 ml; in the five patients studied by Nilsson and Scherstén (1969) the mean concentration was 197 mg/100 ml (range, 127–297). This variability may be due in part to the fact that the composition of hepatic bile is influenced by the rate of flow of bile. In healthy human subjects the concentration of cholesterol in gall-bladder bile is two to four times that in hepatic bile (reported range for gall-bladder bile: 170–800 mg/100 ml). There is no correlation between the plasma and biliary cholesterol concentrations in man. However, in some species of animals, including non-human primates, hypercholesterolaemia induced by dietary means may be associated with an increase in the biliary cholesterol concentration (Portman *et al.*, 1975). Human cholesterol gallstones contain small amounts of cholesteryl sulphate (Drayer and Lieberman, 1965). Further discussion of the cholesterol in bile will be found in Chapter 18.

2.3 Skin

From the point of view of sterol biochemistry, skin is of considerable interest because in many mammals it contains relatively large quantities of sterols that are present in other tissues only in trace amounts. Many of these sterols, including lanosterol (a major component of wool fat) and several of the sterols found in normal rat skin (see Table 3.2), are intermediates in sterol biosynthesis. Their accumulation in skin is due, presumably, to low activity of the enzymes catalyzing some of the steps in the biosynthetic sequence between lanosterol and cholesterol. The identification of these sterols has played a significant part in the elucidation of the final stages of cholesterol biosynthesis.

Mammalian skin has two layers—a superficial epidermis and an underlying dermis which, in most areas of the body surface, contains hair follicles and sebaceous glands. Skin containing sebaceous glands is covered with a layer of lipid (sebum) secreted by these glands. Since the two structural layers and the surface layer of sebum contain different amounts of sterol, and since the relative amounts of these layers differ in different areas of the body, it is difficult to generalize about the sterol content of whole skin. Furthermore, there are marked species differences in the composition of skin sterols.

2.3.1 Whole skin

Whole skin from the human thigh, taken without removing surface lipid, contains 200–300 mg of total sterol/100 g of fresh tissue, of which at least 95% is cholesterol. Between 50 and 60% of the total cholesterol is esterified, the proportion of esterified to free cholesterol being higher in surface lipids than in epidermal lipids, suggesting that esterified cholesterol is secreted by the sebaceous glands. Human whole skin contains sterols other than cholesterol, including lathosterol and 7-dehydrocholesterol, but in smaller relative amounts than in most other mammalian species in which skin sterols have been studied.

In the whole skin of rats, cholesterol accounts for less than half the total sterols. Clayton et al. (1963) have identified a large number of other sterols in the non-saponifiable fraction of rat-skin lipids. The more abundant of these are listed in Table 3.2. Note that if all these sterols are indeed precursors of cholesterol synthesized in rat skin, they cannot all lie on the same pathway. Thus, the presence of sterols 2, 3 and 8 shows that reduction of the Δ^{24} double bond can take place before or after loss of the 4,4-dimethyl groups of lanosterol. Desmosterol is of historical interest because it was at first thought to be an obligatory intermediate in the biosynthesis of cholesterol. It was first reported by Stokes et al. (1956) as a constituent of the tissues of chick embryos and was shown by these workers to be converted into cholesterol *in vivo*; hence it was given the name desmosterol (Gr. *desmos*, a link).

2.3.2 Sebum

Cholesterol is present in the sebum of all mammals, but other sterols

Table 3.2
Sterols present in the non-saponifiable fraction of the lipids of the whole skin of rats

Sterol	% of total sterols recovered
1. Lanosterol	1
2. 4,4-Dimethylcholest-7-en-3β-ol	3
3. 4,4-Dimethylcholest-8-en-3β-ol	10
4. 4,4-Dimethylcholesta-8,24-dien-3β-ol	3
5. 4α-Methylcholest-7-en-3β-ol	7
6. 4α-Methylcholest-8-en-3β-ol	7
7. Cholesterol	32
8. Desmosterol	4
9. Lathosterol	21
10. 7-Dehydrocholesterol	0.5–1.0

Sterols were separated by silicic acid column chromatography and gas-liquid chromatography. All sterols other than those with a Δ^5 double bond are 5α. Systematic names of the sterols given trivial names will be found in Chapter 1, Table 2.
(Modified from Clayton et al., 1963.)

are also present, often in surprisingly large amounts. In wool fat, the sebum secreted by the sheep's skin, lanosterol and agnosterol account for as much as 10% of the total sterol. The lipids of human sebum contain up to 17% of squalene (Nicolaides et al., 1968), as well as small amounts of lathosterol and 7-dehydrocholesterol. In the surface lipids of the human forehead, cholesterol accounts for more than 90% of the total sterol (Nikkari et al., 1974). The sterols of human preputial sebum (smegma) contain a high proportion of 5α-cholestanol, mainly in esterified form. Squalene is present only in traces in the sebum of most species other than man (Nicolaides et al., 1968). Squalene is present in the human sebaceous secretions of ear wax, hair fat and vernix caseosa (see Goodman, 1964).

2.4 Nervous tissue

In adult mammals 20–25% of the cholesterol in the whole body is present in the nervous system, including the brain, spinal cord and peripheral nerves. Most of the cholesterol in the nervous system is present in unesterified form as a major constituent of myelin, but small quantities of esterified cholesterol and related sterols are found in other cellular constituents of brain. Several sterols other than cholesterol have been identified in brain. These include lanosterol, 14α-desmethyllanosterol, 5α-cholestanol, lathosterol, desmosterol, 26-hydroxycholesterol and 24β-hydroxycholesterol. Desmosterol is present in considerable amounts in the brains of immature birds and mammals and may be an intermediate in the main pathway for cholesterol biosynthesis in brain tissue during the early stages of myelination. Table 3.3 shows the percentages of cholesterol and other sterols in the total sterol fraction of immature rat brain. In mature rat brain, desmosterol is present only in traces, possibly because of its conversion into cholesterol during maturation.

Owing to the high cholesterol content of myelin, there are marked regional differences in the sterol composition of brain. Furthermore, since myelination of the central nervous system continues after birth

Table 3.3
Sterols of developing rat brain (% total free sterols)

Sterol	%
Cholesterol	91.4
Desmosterol	8.3
14α-Desmethyllanosterol	0.19
Lanosterol	0.12

(From Ramsey and Nicholas (1972)).

in all mammals, and in some is confined almost entirely to the postnatal period, the cholesterol content of whole brain, and of specific anatomical regions of brain, changes markedly during maturation (see Chapter 6, Section 2.3).

2.5 Fat, muscle, connective tissue and artery

Mammalian white fat consists mainly of triglyceride-rich adipocytes, but it also contains variable amounts of blood-vessel, nerve and connective tissue. The sterol content of whole adipose tissue is usually between 1 and 2 mg/g fresh weight, but wide variations may occur in relation to age, diet and other factors. In particular, the cholesterol content of whole fat (mg/g fresh weight or total protein) increases with age. More than 95% of the total sterol of adipose tissue is cholesterol, with lanosterol and other sterols present only in trace amounts. It should be noted that in much of the earlier work considerably higher values for the sterol content of adipose tissue were reported, probably owing to inadequacy of the methods used for assaying sterols. The total mass of fat in the whole body is such that an adult rat may store as much as 50 mg of cholesterol in its 'adipose organ' (more than the cholesterol content of the whole liver and about half that of the whole mass of skeletal muscle); in an obese human subject with 25 kg of body fat, about 50 g of cholesterol would be stored in adipose tissue.

Recognition that adipose tissue may store large quantities of exchangeable cholesterol in obese human subjects has focused attention on the cholesterol content of the isolated adipocyte in man and experimental animals. The proportion of the total cholesterol in adipose tissue that is present in the adipocytes increases with age and body weight, rising from 65% in young rats to 90% in old rats. This increase may be explained by changes in the lipid composition of adipocytes as a function of cell size and maturity of the animal (Björntorp and Sjöström, 1972; Farkas et al., 1973). In adipocytes of different sizes obtained from the same specimen of subcutaneous human fat, the amount of cholesterol in a given cell is roughly proportional to cell volume and the bulk of the cholesterol is present as free cholesterol in the lipid droplets. This suggests that most of the cholesterol in adipocytes, other than that in membranes, is dissolved in unesterified form in the triglycerides of the lipid droplets and that as the adipocyte increases in size by enlargement of its lipid droplets, the amount of cholesterol in the cell increases. This would help to explain the rise in cholesterol content of adipose tissue with age, since fat cells are known to increase in size as the animal ages. However, the amount of triglyceride stored in the adipocytes cannot be the only factor that determines their cholesterol content because the cholesterol/triglyceride ratio in isolated adipocytes increases with age. The amount of cholesterol/adipocyte in human subjects is not significantly correlated with the plasma cholesterol concentration (Schreibman and Dell, 1975).

Mammalian skeletal muscle contains 300–500 mg of total cholesterol per 100 g dry weight, the bulk of the cholesterol being in unesterified form. In man, there is little or no change in the cholesterol content of skeletal muscle (mg/100 g dry weight) with increasing age.

The cholesterol content of human connective tissue, expressed in terms of dry weight, increases with age and is positively correlated with the plasma cholesterol concentration. Crouse *et al.* (1972) measured the cholesterol content of the connective tissue of men and women who died suddenly at ages ranging from 23–78 years and found a three- to sevenfold increase in the cholesterol content of dura mater and biceps tendon between the ages of 30 and 70. The increase was due almost entirely to an increase in esterified cholesterol.

The cholesterol content of the arterial wall has received a great deal of attention because free and esterified cholesterol are the major lipid components of atheromatous lesions in large and medium-sized arteries. The cholesterol content of atheromatous lesions is considered in Chapter 13. In this section we shall consider the normal arterial wall, including the changes that occur in the lipid composition of histologically normal regions of the artery. Since 'fatty streaks' (localized aggregations of fat-filled smooth-muscle cells in the intima) are present in the arteries of healthy children, these may also be considered normal. Most analyses of arterial lipids have been carried out on the aorta, usually after removal of the outer layer of connective tissue (adventitia). A few measurements of the lipids of veins and pulmonary arteries obtained *post mortem* suggest that their total sterol content is lower than that of the aorta in human adults (see Cook, 1958).

In newborn animals and human beings there is very little lipid in the aortic intima and the small amount of cholesterol that is present is unesterified. In lesion-free human aortic intima, the concentrations of free cholesterol, phospholipid and triglyceride increase progressively with age, the increase being due mainly to accumulation of perifibrous (extracellular) lipid droplets. Cholesteryl esters accumulate slowly at first, but from the age of about 20 years their concentration increases rapidly (at about 0.6 mg/100 mg of defatted dried tissue/decade (Smith, 1974)), so that after age 40 the major lipid component of normal human aortic intima is esterified cholesterol. In addition to the accumulation of extracellular cholesterol in the intima, there is also accumulation in the lipid droplets of the smooth-muscle cells of fatty streaks. The proportion of esterified to total

Table 3.4
Total and esterified cholesterol in lesion-free areas of aorta from monkeys and human subjects

Tissue	Total cholesterol	% of cholesterol esterified	% of total cholesteryl ester fatty acids 18:1	% of total cholesteryl ester fatty acids 18:2
Adult human intima (perifibrous)	6.0 mg/100 mg dry weight	76.5	28.0	38.6
Adult human intima (fatty streak)	30.1 mg/100 mg dry weight	87.4	50.1	14.0
Rhesus intima (near term foetus)	120 mg/100 g fresh weight	5	—	—
Rhesus intima (adult)	185 mg/100 g fresh weight	15	—	—
Adult human intima (whole)	658 mg/100 g fresh weight	64	—	—
Adult human media	480 mg/100 g fresh weight	40	—	—
Adult human (fatty streak)	960–2190 mg/100 g fresh weight	—	—	—

Values are derived from Smith (1974), Portman (1970) and Insull and Bartsch (1966).

cholesterol is higher in the intracellular than in the extracellular cholesterol of normal adult intima and there are differences in the fatty acid composition of the cholesteryl esters in these two regions. In the intracellular cholesteryl esters the predominant fatty acid is oleate (18:1), whereas linoleate (18:2) predominates in the extracellular cholesteryl esters. These differences almost certainly reflect a difference in the origin of the intracellular and extracellular cholesteryl esters that accumulate in the ageing human aortic intima. Despite the age-related increase in total cholesterol concentration and in the ratio of esterified to free cholesterol in the aortic intima, the ratio of free cholesterol to total phospholipid concentration remains more or less constant, the relative concentrations corresponding to a molar ratio of about 1:1. Since this is the molar ratio of free cholesterol to phospholipid in the plasma membranes of many cells, it is possible that the increase in free cholesterol in the intima reflects an increase in the amount of plasma membrane of smooth-muscle cells. Some of these regional and age-related differences in intimal cholesterol are shown in Table 3.4.

The feeding of cholesterol-rich diets to experimental animals leads to accumulation of free and esterified cholesterol in the intima plus inner media in areas of the aorta other than those in which localized atheromatous plaques may develop.

7-Ketocholesterol and 26-hydroxycholesterol have been demonstrated in human atheromatous lesions (Brooks *et al.*, 1966).

2.6 Intestine and faeces

The concentration of cholesterol in the intestinal wall of mammals usually lies between 100 and 200 mg/100 g fresh weight and is higher in the upper than in the lower intestine. In rats, the concentration of total sterol in the intestinal mucosa is higher than that in the submucosal layers. In the rat's small intestine only 5–10% of the total cholesterol is esterified. During the absorption of dietary cholesterol, when there is a considerable flux of cholesterol through the intestinal wall, there is an increase in the concentration of total cholesterol and in the ratio of esterified to free cholesterol in the small intestine (Swell *et al.*, 1958).

Although cholesterol is the major sterol in the intestinal mucosal cells of mammals, other sterols, including phytosterols, lathosterol and 7-dehydrocholesterol, are also present in the intestinal mucosa of guinea pigs, rats and other animals. The phytosterols arise from the diet and are taken up into the mucosal cells, with little transfer into intestinal lymph. Mucosal lathosterol and 7-dehydrocholesterol, both intermediates in the biosynthesis of cholesterol, probably arise mainly by synthesis *in situ*. However, lathosterol is also present in the lumen of the rat's stomach and intestine, probably as a result of ingestion of skin lipids after licking the fur. In addition to sterols derived from the diet, from the bile, from skin-grooming and from mucosal cells extruded into the lumen of the small intestine, coprostanol and other faecal steroids formed by bacterial action in the large intestine may be present in the upper intestine of coprophagous animals.

The unsaponifiable fraction of the faecal lipids contains cholesterol and its metabolites formed by bacteria in the large intestine. The faeces of herbivorous and omnivorous animals also contain phytosterols and a series of their metabolites analogous to those formed from cholesterol by intestinal bacteria. The amounts and proportions of these faecal steroids are extremely variable, depending upon the composition of the diet and the micro-organisms present in the intestinal lumen. There are wide variations from one species to another and even in a given animal or human subject at different times. In the faeces of a normal human subject eating a mixed diet, the major sterols and their bacterial metabolites are cholesterol, coprostanol, coprostanone, β-sitosterol, stigmasterol and campesterol, together with the 5β-saturated and 3-keto derivatives of the three plant sterols. 5α-Cholestanol and the 5α-saturated derivatives of plant sterols may also be present in smaller amounts. The faeces of rats and guinea pigs, but not of adult human beings, contain lathosterol, some of which may be derived from fur-licking. The faeces of germ-free animals fed a mixed diet contain cholesterol, lathosterol and plant sterols, but no 5β-saturated sterols or 3-keto derivatives of sterols (Kellog, 1971).

The faeces of adult humans contain appreciable amounts of cholesteryl sulphate (15–85 mg/day), probably derived from the bile (Gustafsson *et al.*, 1968). Meconium and the faeces of newborn infants also contain cholesteryl sulphate and the disulphate esters of (22R)-22-hydroxycholesterol, (20S)-20,22ξ-dihydroxycholesterol and cholesterol hydroxylated in the 23 or 24 positions (Gustafsson and Eneroth, 1972). The sterol moiety of some of these disulphate esters may be derived from the hypertrophied adrenal cortex of the fetus and newborn infant (see Chapter 6). Coprostanol does not appear in the faeces of infants until the age of 5–12 months, but 5α-cholestanol is present in meconium.

The neutral steroids of dried faeces appear to be very stable, as is shown by the observation of Lin *et al.* (1978) that the GLC pattern of cholesterol and plant sterols, and of their intestinal metabolites, was indistinguishable from the normal in specimens of human coprolites more than 2000 years old.

2.7 Glands

The glandular tissue of mammals is usually rich in cholesterol. For example, the human thymus contains 400–500 mg of total cholesterol/100 g fresh weight and the cholesterol content of the human pancreas is even higher.

In many mammalian species the adrenal glands and the gonads contain very large amounts of cholesterol. In the rat and guinea pig and in man, cholesterol may comprise 5% of the wet weight of the adrenals. In these steroid-hormone-forming tissues 80–90% of the cholesterol is esterified and in the adrenals, corpus luteum and placenta this esterified cholesterol is present in large cytoplasmic droplets up to 1.5 μ in diameter. These lipid droplets are thought to be enclosed by membranes and may be isolated from tissue homogenates by centrifugal flotation. Under conditions in which steroid-hormone synthesis is stimulated, the lipid droplets decrease in size and the tissue content of cholesteryl ester decreases. Thus, when luteinizing hormone is injected into a rat after the ovary has been luteinized by gonadotrophin treatment, the cholesteryl ester content of the ovary decreases markedly within 3 to 5 hours of the injection (Herbst, 1967). Similarly, acute stress leads to rapid loss of lipid droplets and a fall in the cholesteryl ester content of the zona fasciculata of the rat's adrenal cortex.

The cholesteryl esters of the adrenal cortex of several species contain unusual long-chain fatty acids, including a C_{22} acid with four double bonds in the ω6, 9, 12 and 15 positions. This acid presumably arises by addition of a C_2 unit to the carboxyl end of arachidonic acid (Goodman, 1965). Small amounts of cholesteryl sulphate (1–2 mg/kg fresh weight) are present in bovine adrenal cortex (Drayer et al., 1964).

2.8 Milk

The cholesterol content of milk shows wide species differences, the concentration of total cholesterol tending to vary in parallel with the triglyceride concentration in different species. The cholesterol content of colostrum is several times that of the milk secreted a few days after parturition. Representative values for total cholesterol in milk secreted during fully established lactation are shown for seven species in Table 3.5. At least 90% of the cholesterol in milk is unesterified. The bulk of this free cholesterol is associated with phospholipid in the formation of surface membrane covering the fat droplets and may be derived from the plasma membrane of the secreting cells of the mammary gland. Up to 20% of the total cholesterol in whole milk is present in skim milk (milk from which the fat has been removed by centrifugation) in the form of plasma membrane fragments, microvilli and other membranous material derived from the mammary gland.

In some species, the concentration of cholesterol in the milk can be increased by feeding cholesterol-rich diets. In lactating women,

Table 3.5
Concentration of total cholesterol in whole milk from seven species

Species	Cholesterol concentration (mg/100 ml)
Cow	10–15
Goat	10–15
Guinea-pig	30–50
Horse	10–15
Man	15–25
Rabbit	50–100
Rat	60–70

Values are taken from various sources. Within a given species there is considerable individual variation and in a given individual the value may vary during lactation and according to the number of milkings/day.

however, the cholesterol content of the milk is unaffected by changes in cholesterol intake or fatty acid composition of dietary triglycerides, despite changes in the plasma cholesterol concentration resulting from these dietary modifications (Potter and Nestel, 1976).

In addition to cholesterol, lanosterol and plant sterols have been identified in the milk of ruminants.

2.9 Subcellular distribution

Knowledge of the subcellular distribution of cholesterol is essential if we are to understand fully the physiology of cholesterol at the level of the cell. For example, within the hepatocyte cholesterol is synthesized, esterified, metabolized to bile acids, transported into the bile, incorporated into lipoproteins for secretion into the plasma, or used in the formation of subcellular membranes. As a first step towards understanding the dynamics of these intracellular events we need to know how free and esterified cholesterol is distributed between the various components of the liver cell. However, despite intensive study it remains difficult to draw any firm conclusions about the subcellular distribution of cholesterol in many tissues.

The problem is largely a question of the methods used for separating broken-cell preparations into the various components that can be recognized in the intact cell. The method most commonly used is to disrupt the cells of a tissue by some carefully standardized procedure and then to separate the fragments by sequential centrifugation into particles with different sedimentation properties. The particulate fractions are then identified with structural elements of the intact cell by their physical appearance and other properties. Contamination of one fraction by elements from another is usually assessed by the presence of marker enzymes assumed to be restricted to specific subcellular components of the intact cell.

In most of the work that has been done on the subcellular distribution of cholesterol, broken cells have been separated into a heavy fraction containing nuclei and plasma membrane, a mitochondrial fraction sedimenting at 10 000 to 20 000 × g (S_{10}), a fraction sedimenting at about 100 000 × g (S_{100}) and a 'soluble supernatant' fraction containing all components that do not sediment at 100 000 × g. The S_{100} particles are referred to, operationally, as 'microsomes' and are usually considered to consist predominantly of fragments derived from the endoplasmic reticulum, including the ribosomes; the soluble supernatant is assumed to contain all the components present in solution in the cytosol of the intact cell. However, the development of improved methods for separating subcellular particles, especially the technique of centrifugation to equilibrium in density gradients, has shown that these interpretations are too simple. It is now recognized, for example, that the S_{100} particles from liver cells contain (in addition to elements of the endoplasmic reticulum) small fragments of plasma membrane, various secretory vesicles, pieces of the outer walls of mitochondria and fragments of the Golgi apparatus. Furthermore, free cholesterol may shift from membrane components into the soluble fraction or from one type of particle to another during the fractionation procedure (Rouser *et al.* 1972). Hence, although it is legitimate to speak of microsomal cholesterol, it must not be assumed that all the cholesterol in the S_{100} fraction is present in the endoplasmic reticulum of the intact cell. Much of the earlier work on the subcellular distribution of cholesterol may have to be re-appraised in the light of future work with newer methods of separation. The following brief summary should be read with this proviso in mind.

The lipid composition differs from one subcellular fraction to another and in a given subcellular fraction from one organ to another. However, the differences between organs is less than the difference between particles. Thus, in cells of most organs the bulk of the cholesterol is in the microsomal fraction and the proportion of esterified to total cholesterol is highest in the microsomes. Table 3.6 shows some representative values for the distribution of cholesterol in subcellular fractions of liver from normal rats. In cholesterol-fed rats, cholesterol accumulates in the liver, mainly as cholesteryl esters in the microsomes and soluble supernatant. It should be noted that analysis of homogenates of liver cells by density-gradient centrifugation has shown that much of the cholesterol in the microsomal fraction (as defined above) is present in fragments of plasma membrane and of the Golgi apparatus (Beaufay *et al.*, 1974), though there is now no doubt that some of the microsomal cholesterol of liver cells is contributed by elements of the endoplasmic reticulum (Mitropoulos *et al.*, 1978).

The Distribution of Sterols and Related Steroids in Nature 141

Table 3.6
Representative values for the subcellular distribution of total cholesterol in microsomes, mitochondria and supernatant of normal rat liver

Subcellular fraction	Cholesterol content (μg/mg of protein)	% of total*
Microsomes	20–30	55
Mitochondria	5–10	20
Supernatant	10–15	25

* Very approximate values, not corrected for recoveries within each fraction, or for the cholesterol in the heavy fraction containing unbroken cells, nuclei and plasma membranes.

Certain specialized cells with an unusually high content of cholesterol have already been mentioned. These include: myelinated nerve cells, in which the bulk of the cholesterol in myelin is free; adipocytes, which contain large amounts of free cholesterol dissolved in the triglyceride droplets; the hormone-producing cells of the adrenal cortex and other tissues, in which high concentrations of esterified cholesterol are present in lipid droplets. The cholesterol content of the plasma membranes of different types of cell is dealt with in Chapter 7.

2.10 Dietary cholesterol

The sources of cholesterol in the diets normally eaten by Europeans and North Americans are meat (including organ meats), poultry, fish, milk and its products, eggs and, to a very variable extent, shellfish. Cholesterol is present in green plants but only in amounts too small to contribute significantly to the total dietary intake.

Knowledge of the cholesterol content of foods is needed by dietitians for the compilation of low-cholesterol menus, by individuals wishing to limit their intake of dietary cholesterol and by epidemiologists carrying out dietary surveys. Tables showing the amount of cholesterol per unit of cooked or uncooked weight in many foods have been published in numerous books and journals. However, much of this information is of limited use as a basis for calculating the amount of cholesterol present in standard quantities of foods. Values quoted in the older literature, and reproduced in some current articles, are usually based on assay by digitonin precipitation or the Liebermann-Burchard reaction, neither of which is specific for cholesterol. Although in most foods of animal origin virtually all the sterol is cholesterol, this is not always so. In some shellfish, for example, cholesterol accounts for less than half the total sterol. Another source of error is variability in the cholesterol content of a given food item according to the species, breed, age, sex and diet of the animal and, in the case of meats, the part of the carcass from which the cut is taken. Examples of this variability will be found in the comprehensive Table of 'Cholesterol content of foods' compiled and critically reviewed by Feeley et al. (1972). The values listed in this Table show that the cholesterol content of fresh meat ranges from 60–70 mg/100 g in lamb, beef, port and veal, while that of fresh whole fish ranges from 35 (sockeye salmon) to 95 mg/100 g (mackerel). Other points of interest in this Table are (1) the very high cholesterol content of brain, egg yolk (egg white contains no cholesterol), liver, kidney, sweetbread (thymus) and fish roe and, contrary to popular belief, (2) the absence of cholesterol from chocolate and peanut butter. It is also of interest to note that the cholesterol content of fresh visible fat is not very different from that of fresh meat trimmed of fat; hence, removal of visible fat from a cut of fresh meat does not change the amount of cholesterol per 100 g portion.

While the information given in Table 3.1 of Feeley et al. (1972) should enable the dietitian to calculate cholesterol intakes from mixed diets with an accuracy sufficient for general purposes, no food Tables, however carefully compiled, can provide the information required for accurate estimation of cholesterol intake, e.g., in the investigation of sterol balance in human subjects. In work of this kind, the cholesterol content of a mixed diet must be measured directly, preferably by digitonin precipitation of the total sterols extracted from duplicate portions of the diet, followed by quantitative GLC of the digitonin-precipitable sterols.

2.11 Squalene

The presence of substantial amounts of squalene in shark liver and human sebaceous secretions has already been mentioned (Sections 2.2 and 2.3). Squalene is also present in human and rat plasma, predominantly in the very-low density lipoprotein fraction (Goodman, 1964) and has been detected in rat liver (Langdon and Bloch, 1953). A systematic analysis of the distribution of squalene in animal tissues has not been reported, but Liu et al. (1976) have measured the concentration of squalene in human plasma and in a large number of human tissues, as well as in some of the commoner foods. Some of their results, illustrating the wide range of values obtained for squalene concentration and squalene:cholesterol ratio in different tissues, are shown in Table 3.7.

In human tissues, the highest concentrations of squalene are found in skin and adipose tissue, while the squalene concentration is comparatively low in liver and small intestine, the two tissues in which cholesterol synthesis is most active. There is also a very wide

The Distribution of Sterols and Related Steroids in Nature 143

Table 3.7
Squalene content of human plasma and tissues, and of some foods

Tissue	µg/g dry weight	µg/mg cholesterol
Subcutaneous fat	390	97
Skin	478	65
Artery wall (intima)	134	5
Adrenals	65	0.4
Liver	75	6
Small intestine	42	4
Kidney	101	6
Plasma (µg/100 ml)	26	0.1

Food	µg/g fresh weight
Olive oil	up to 6855
Safflower oil	37
Beef	20
Liver	18
Poultry	16–36
Egg yolk	47
Fish	30–97
Milk	2.4
Typical U.S. diet	24–38 mg/2000 calories

Squalene was assayed by GLC with squalane as standard. (Assembled from Liu et al., 1976.)

range of values in foods, from about 2 µg/g in milk to nearly 7 mg/g in olive oil. Liu and coworkers estimate that the daily intake of squalene in the United States is about 30 mg/person.

2.12 Steroidal toad poisons

The skin secretions of toads (Bufonidae) contain a mixture of poisonous substances, including cardiotonic steroids known as *bufogenins* e.g. (**3.2**). Several structurally related bufogenins have been isolated from the poisons secreted by toads of different species. All of them resemble the aglycones* of the cardiotonic principles of plants in that the C/D ring fusion is *cis* and the side-chain consists of a six-membered δ-lactone ring. Bufogenins may be unconjugated or they may be esterified with suberylarginine at C-3 of the steroid ring system to form *bufotoxins*. Both the unconjugated and esterified forms are highly toxic to mammals when taken by mouth, but are not toxic to toads. Presumably the function of these poisons is to teach predators not to eat toads. Even if the toad is killed by the predator and therefore fails

* An aglycone is the non-sugar residue of a glycoside.

(3.2)

Gamabufogenin (≡gamabufotalin); isolated from the skin of the Japanese *gama* toad (*Bufo formosus*).

to benefit from its poison, the genes for converting cholesterol into cardiotoxins could still have evolved, on Darwinian principles, by what is known as kinship selection (see Wilson, 1975 for examples).

3 INVERTEBRATES

3.1 General

Although cholesterol is the major sterol of most insects and crustacea and of some molluscs, in many invertebrates it is not detectable, or is present only in traces. In some invertebrate phyla, notably the Echinodermata and the Porifera, the sterols present in free and conjugated form are extremely diverse. In one species of starfish, for instance, more than 20 sterols have been identified. It is difficult to assign a definite biological function to many of the invertebrate sterols. Some may play a structural role, analogous to that of free cholesterol in higher animals, but there is no clear evidence for this in invertebrates other than insects. Other sterols of invertebrates may act as precursors of complex molecules with specific functions, such as the asterosaponins formed by certain starfish. Cholesterol itself may participate in membrane formation in those invertebrates in which it is present, but it also serves as a precursor of moulting hormones in insects. The steryl sulphates found in the tissues of echinoderms may act as precursors of asterosaponins or they may be inactivated sterol products in a form suitable for excretion.

Bergmann (1958) has suggested that the diversity of invertebrate sterols, many of which appeared to him to perform closely related functions, represents a stage in the evolution of the biosynthesis of cholesterol, the 'fittest' sterol and almost the sole sterol of vertebrates. However, it seems equally probable that most of the unusual sterols of marine invertebrates are of dietary origin, arising ultimately from the phytoplankton of the sea, and that they then undergo a limited number of enzymic modifications in the body of the animal. This explanation would fit in better with the fact that echinoderms cannot synthesize sterols with a side-chain other than that of cholestane.

3.2 Insects

Cholesterol is the major sterol in most insects and is present in all their tissues, with the greatest concentrations in mid-gut, Malpighian tubules and nerve. Omnivorous and phytophagous (plant-eating) insects contain phytosterols. Ergosterol is also present in the tissues of some insects, probably originating from micro-organisms in the gut. 7-Dehydrocholesterol, a precursor of moulting hormones, is a major sterol of the prothoracic gland of insects at certain stages of development. Several steroidal hormones, among which are α-ecdysone (**3.3**),

(3.3) α-Ecdysone (ecdysone) ((22R)-2β,3β,14α,22,25-pentahydroxy-5β-cholest-7-en-6-one)

(20R)-20-hydroxyecdysone and (20R)-20,26-dihydroxyecdysone, have been isolated from insects and are found in highest concentration in the prothoracic gland. All the moulting and pupating hormones that have been isolated from insects are steroids with a Δ^7 double bond and a 6-keto group. Note that systematic names of ecdysones are based on the cholestane skeleton. Trivial names are based on ecdysone (formula (**3.3**)).

Fatty-acid esters of cholesterol (mainly 16:1 and 18:1) are present in all insect tissues, with the highest ratios of esterified to total cholesterol in nerve and fat body. Sulphate esters and glucosides of cholesterol, phytosterols and ecdysones are present in the faeces of insects.

146 The Biology of Cholesterol and Related Steroids

Cholesterol is probably an essential structural constituent of insect tissues, though feeding experiments with 'sparing' sterols suggest that the requirement for structural sterol in insects can be partially satisfied by analogues of cholesterol. Cholesterol also serves as a precursor of ecdysones. The fatty-acid esters of cholesterol probably act as stores of free cholesterol needed for structural components during rapid growth or for the synthesis of ecdysones at certain stages in the life-cycle of the insect. The water-soluble sulphate esters and glucosides of sterols and ecdysones are presumably formed as excretory products. The ecdysones are moulting or pupating hormones, causing the insect to shed its cuticle or to pupate at specific stages in the growth of the larva. Steroids with the α,β-unsaturated keto system in ring B, and with the biological properties of ecdysone, are widely distributed in plants. Some plant-eating insects may therefore obtain preformed moulting hormones from their diet (see Section 4.2).

3.3 Echinoderms

The echinoderms (Gr. *echinos*, a hedgehog; *dermatos*, skin) are a group of marine invertebrates that includes the starfish (Asteroidea), sea cucumbers (Holothuroidea) and sea urchins (Echinoidea). Echinoderms contain very complex mixtures of C_{26}, C_{27}, C_{28}, C_{29} and C_{30} sterols, differing mainly in the number and position of double bonds in the nucleus and side-chain and in the position, nature and stereochemistry of side-chain substituents. These sterols may be free or they may be present as sulphate or fatty-acid esters. In starfish and sea cucumbers the predominant free sterols have a 5α-Δ^7 ring system as in *asterosterol* (**3.4**), whereas those of the sea urchins are mainly Δ^5

(3.4) **Asterosterol**

sterols (including cholesterol). In one species of starfish alone (*Asterias rubens*), 18 sterols have been identified in the unesterified fraction (Goad *et al.*, 1972). *Acansterol* (**3.5**), an unusual sterol with a cyclopropane ring in the side-chain, is found in the tissues of the 'crown-of-thorns' starfish (*Acanthaster planci*) and is probably formed

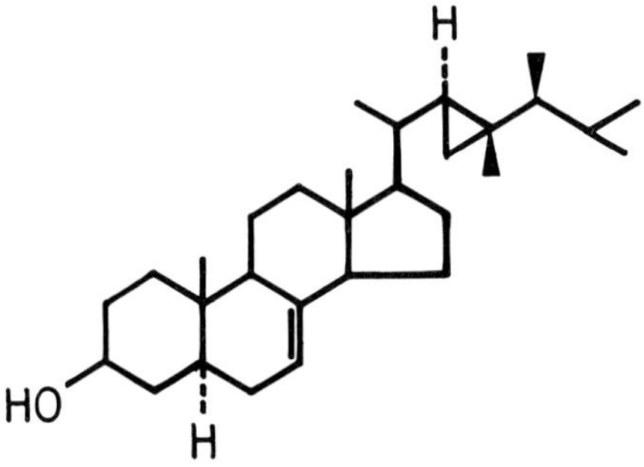

(3.5) Acansterol

from *gorgosterol* (a sterol present in the corals eaten by this starfish) by isomerization of the Δ^5 double bond to the Δ^7 position.

The striking variety of sterols in the echinoderms must be a reflection of species differences in the sterol composition of the diet and in the capacity to synthesize specific sterols *de novo* or to modify those absorbed from the food.

Sterols also occur in starfish as the aglycones of asterosaponins, an interesting group of steroidal glycosides present in the reproductive tissues. Asterosaponins are sulphate esters of glycosides which, on hydrolysis, give sulphuric acid, a mixture of monosaccharides and a steroid with 3β- and 6α-OH groups and, in most cases, a $\Delta^{9(11)}$ double bond, as in *asterosaponin A* (**3.6**) (Sheikh *et al.*, 1972). In other

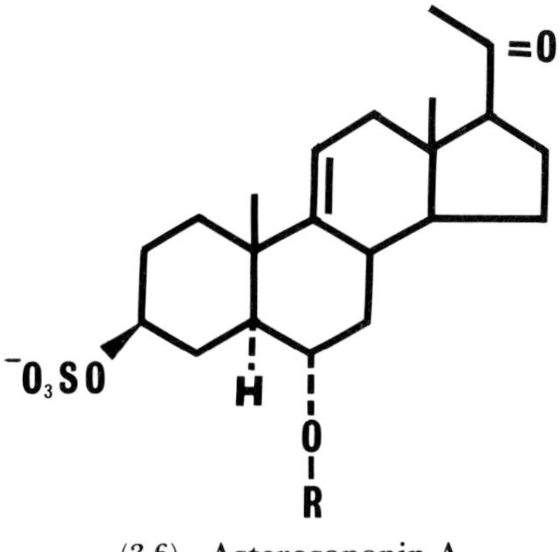

(3.6) Asterosaponin A

asterosaponins isolated from *A. rubens* the aglycone has a cholestane carbon skeleton with a substituted side-chain. Asterosaponins are spawning inhibitors and are thought to play a specific role in the reproductive cycle of the starfish. In these animals, reproduction involves the congregation of both sexes during the breeding season

148 The Biology of Cholesterol and Related Steroids

and the regulation of spawning times, males shedding their spawn before females. Other steroidal saponins, known as *holothurins*, are produced by sea cucumbers. In some holothurins the aglycone is based upon the lanostane skeleton.

3.4 Porifera

The Porifera (sponges) are said to contain the greatest variety of sterols found in any invertebrate phylum. In most sponges the predominant sterols have a $\Delta^{5,7}$ or Δ^5 ring system and include cholesterol. In a few species the major components of the sterol mixture have a saturated 5α ring system. Many of the sterols encountered in sponges have a conventional ring system with a normal C_8 side-chain alkylated at C-24, but some very unusual features have been described in the sterols of some species. These unusual sterols include one with a five-membered ring A from which C-3 has been removed and another with a side-chain lacking one of the carbon atoms between C-20 and C-25. The formulae of two of the commoner sterols found in sponges are shown in (**3.7**) and (**3.8**). A detailed account of the sterols of sponges will be found in Bergmann (1962), Minale and Sodano (1977) and Nes and McKean (1977).

(**3.7**) **Poriferasterol** (from *Cliona celata*)

(**3.8**) **Placosterol** (from *Tethya aurantia*)

3.5 Other invertebrates

All the Coelenterata (jelly-fish, sea anemones, corals, etc.) contain complex mixtures of Δ^5 sterols, with cholesterol as the major sterol in many species. Sterols with a Δ^5 ring system, including cholesterol, are also the predominant sterols in the higher molluscs, including bivalves, gastropods, squids and octopuses, but in most primitive molluscs the major sterol is 5α-cholest-7-en-3β-ol. Desmosterol is present in substantial amounts in the sterols of barnacles and of some bivalves, probably arising by the formation of a Δ^{24} double bond in cholesterol rather than as an intermediate in the biosynthesis of cholesterol.

Cholesterol is the major sterol of Crustacea (crabs, shrimps, etc.) and is present in earthworms, in some flatworms and in many protozoa living as parasites in the bodies of vertebrates. 20-Hydroxyecdysone has been isolated from a marine crayfish (*Jasus lalandei*) and for this reason is sometimes called crustecdysone. For references to invertebrate sterols in general, see Brooks (1970) and Nes and McKean (1977).

4 PLANTS AND FUNGI

4.1 General

Cholesterol is present in green plants and in a few species of fungi, and in some red algae it is the major sterol present. However, the numerous sterols found in higher plants, fungi and algae are, in the main, characterized by the presence of an alkyl group at C-24. The substituent at C-24 may be a methyl, an ethyl, a methylene or an ethylidene group. The methyl and ethyl groups may be in α or β configuration and the ethylidene group may exist in two different configurations (E and Z). Since there may also be a Δ^{22} *trans* double bond, and since there may be one or more double bonds at different positions in the ring system, the number of possible analogues of these sterols is extremely large. Many have already been identified in plants and fungi; others are certain to be discovered as the search for new sterols is extended to a wider range of species.

Most of the sterols of photosynthetic organisms and of fungi are known by trivial names based on the genus or species from which the sterol was first isolated. A few of these sterols are referred to in the remaining sections of this chapter. More complete lists will be found in Table 19 of the article by Brooks (1970), in the comprehensive review by Goad and Goodwin (1972) and in Tables 10.9 and 10.10 of the book by Nes and McKean (1977).

In the following sections we shall consider some of the sterols of higher plants (the Bryophyta and Tracheophyta), algae, fungi and lichens.

4.2 Higher plants

4.2.1 Types of sterol found

The major sterols of higher plants possess a B ring with a Δ^5 or Δ^7 double bond. Examples are β-sitosterol, stigmasterol (named after Physostigma), campesterol (named after Brassica campestris) and spinasterol. Table 3.8 shows the trivial names, partial formulae, and systematic names of these and other phytosterols found in leaves, oils, seeds, nuts and fruits. Other phytosterols of interest are Δ^7-avenasterol (the Δ^7 analogue of isofucosterol), found in sunflower seeds, and chalinasterol (24-methylenecholesterol), a constituent of many plant pollens.

In the higher plants, β-sitosterol is usually the most abundant sterol. However, in the tissues of a few species the amount of stigmasterol exceeds that of any other sterol present. The principal sterols are usually those of the Δ^5 series with an alkyl group at C-24 in α configuration, 24-ethyl sterols usually predominating over 24-methyl sterols. However, some families or genera have a characteristic sterol pattern that differs from this. Examples are plants of the genus *Vernonia*, in which the major sterols have a 24-ethylidene group, and some of the *Verbenaceae*, in which the major sterol is clerosterol, a sterol with an ethyl group in the 24β position and a Δ^{25} double bond (see Table 3.8). Another exception to the general rule that Δ^5 sterols predominate in the higher plants is the relative abundance of spinasterol (see Table 3.8) and other Δ^7 sterols in the *Cucurbitaceae*.

4.2.2 Other plant steroids

As well as the true phytosterols, in which the carbon skeleton is that of cholestane with or without an additional alkyl group at C-24, closely related steroids with methyl groups at C-4 or C-14 are widely distributed in plants; several are considered in Chapter 4 in relation to the biosynthesis of phytosterols from cycloartenol. The formulae and sources of some of these ring-methylated sterols are shown in (**3.9**) to (**3.13**). Other plant terpenoids of interest from the point of view of the mechanism of sterol biosynthesis are referred to in Chapter 4 (see index for references to farnesol, squalene, euphol and dammarenediol).

(**3.9**)   **Cycloartenol** (many plants)

The Distribution of Sterols and Related Steroids in Nature 151

(3.10) **Cycloeucalenol** (Eucalyptus)

(3.11) **Lophenol≡Methostenol** (Cactus, *Lophocereus schottii*)

(3.12) **Parkeol** (from *Butyrospermum parkii*)

(3.13) **Macdougallin** (Cactus, *Peniocereus macdougalli*)

Table 3.8
Structural formulae of some typical sterols found in higher plants

Trivial name	Formula	Systematic name	Source
1. Campesterol		24α-Methylcholest-5-en-3β-ol (24R)	Brassica campestris
2. Dihydrobrassicasterol		24β-Methylcholest-5-en-3β-ol (24S)	Ferns
3. β-Sitosterol		24α-Ethylcholest-5-en-3β-ol (24R)	Widely distributed
4. Clerosterol		24β-Ethylcholesta-5,25-dien-3β-ol (24S)	Verbenaceae
5. Brassicasterol		24β-Methylcholesta-5,22-dien-3β-ol (24R)	Rapeseed oil

The Distribution of Sterols and Related Steroids in Nature

6. Stigmasterol	(structure with R₁)	24α-Ethylcholesta-5,22-dien-3β-ol (24S)	Calabar bean and soybean oil
7. α-Spinasterol	(structure with R₂)	24α-Ethylcholesta-7,22-dien-3β-ol (24S)	Spinach, cucumber family
8. 24-Methylene cholesterol (Chalinasterol)	(structure with R₁)	Ergosta-5,24(28)-dien-3β-ol	Pollen of many plants
9. 28-Isofucosterol (Δ⁵-Avenasterol; L. *avena*, wild oats)	(structure with R₁)	Stigmasta-5,Z-24(28)-dien-3β-ol	Oats (also in some green algae)

R₁ = (steroid nucleus with HO- and H) ; R₂ = (steroid nucleus with HO- and H)

Notes:
1. The α/β system is used to denote the configuration of the 24 alkyl group in this Table; the *R/S* configuration is included at the end of each systematic name.
2. The presence of the Δ²² double bond may alter the *R/S* assignment (compare (3) with (6)). See Cahn *et al.* (1966).
3. In β-sitosterol, the 'β' prefix is not a stereochemical designation and is now often omitted.
4. Systematic names of sterols with a 24α methyl or 24-methylene group may be based on the ergostane carbocycle; those of sterols with a 24α ethyl or 24-ethylidene group may be based on the stigmastane carbocycle (as in (9)).
5. Source usually refers to the plant from which the sterol was first isolated. Most of the sterols are present in more than one genus.
6. This list illustrates the fact that in most sterols of higher plants ((1), (3) and (6)) the 24 alkyl group has the α configuration.
7. In higher plants with an ethylidene group at C-24 the configuration is always Z (as in (9)). Brown algae contain sterols with a C-24 ethylidene group with E configuration (as in *fucosterol*, the E-24(28) isomer of 28-isofucosterol).

α-Ecdysone and at least 30 analogues of ecdysone, all possessing the characteristic Δ^7, 6-keto system, have been isolated from many species of green plants. Among these analogues are 20-hydroxyecdysone and ponasterone A (Thompson et al., 1973).

Steroids are also found in higher plants as the aglycones of cardiotonic glycosides (e.g. digoxin, which is the glycoside of digoxigenin) and of saponins, and also as azasteroids (steroidal alkaloids containing one or more nitrogen atoms in the molecule). Saponins are detergent glycosides (hence their name) found in plants of the genus Digitalis and in several other genera. The aglycones of saponins, the *sapogenins*, are C_{27} sterols with the stereochemistry of 5α-cholestane and with two additional oxygen-containing rings in the side-chain joined at C-22. Most of the sapogenins have a 3β-OH group, to which the sugar residues are attached in the parent saponin, and additional OH groups at other positions in the ring system. Digitogenin (**3.14**), the aglycone of digitonin (from *D. purpurea*), is a typical sapogenin. Formula (**3.15**) shows digitoxigenin, the aglycone of digitoxin (never to be confused with digitonin) and formula (**3.16**) shows solasodine, an azasteroid obtained from *Solanum sodomaeum*, the Dead Sea apple. For more detailed information, the reviews by Marshall (1970) and Elks (1971) should be consulted.

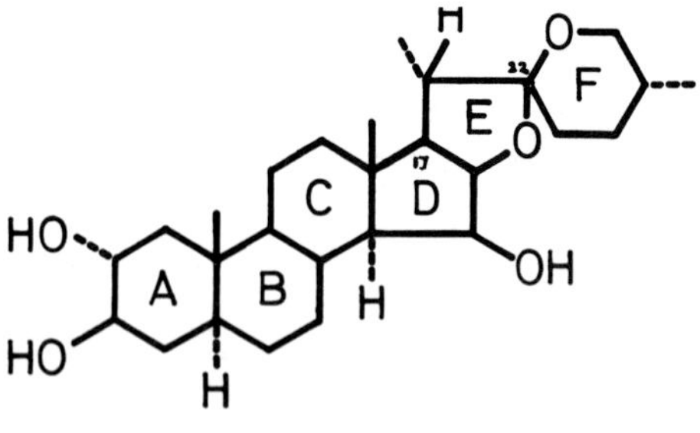

(**3.14**) Digitogenin

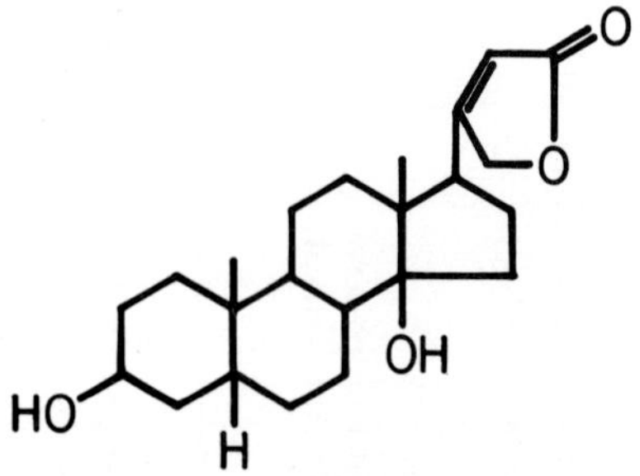

(**3.15**) Digitoxigenin

(3.16) Solasodine

4.2.3 Possible functions of steroids in higher plants

Much of the free sterol of plants is associated with plasma membrane and intracellular particles, suggesting that plant sterols participate in the formation of membranes. In keeping with this, free phytosterols are capable of entering the membranes of red cells and liposomes, though the presence of an alkyl group or a Δ^{22} double bond in the side-chain reduces the ability of a sterol to form a liquid-crystalline bilayer with phospholipid. Cholesterol may also take part in membrane formation in plants. However, a more important function of cholesterol in higher plants seems to be to act as a precursor of ecdysones and of the steroid residues of cardiotonic glycosides, saponins and azasteroids.

It is not known why ecdysones are so widely distributed among the higher plants. They may be required as essential hormones by plant-eating insects, but this does not explain the biological advantage of ecdysones to the plants that synthesize them, unless the insects are of advantage to the plant. Cardiotonic glycosides, saponins and azasteroid glycosides are found in a restricted number of plant species, particularly in the *Scrophulariaceae* (e.g. foxglove, potato, tomato and deadly nightshade) and in some *Strophanthus* sp. Some of these complex glycosides inhibit the growth of micro-organisms, including fungi. It is possible, therefore, that their synthesis gives the plant some resistance to pathogens. The cardiotonic glycosides have certain physiological properties which are unlikely to be of value to the plant in which they are synthesized, but which have been exploited by man for medicinal purposes and as arrow poisons. It should be noted that the cardiac stimulants used in medicine are the *glycosides*; the steroidal aglycones are convulsive poisons.

4.3 Algae

In the blue-green algae, a group of primitive organisms lacking a nuclear membrane, a variety of sterols has been identified. Those

156 The Biology of Cholesterol and Related Steroids

most frequently found in this phylum have an ethyl group at C-24 and a ring system with Δ^5, Δ^7 or $\Delta^{5,7}$ double bonds. Cholesterol has been demonstrated in various species of blue-green algae. In some of the eukaryotic algae (those possessing a true nucleus), cholesterol is the most abundant sterol. Other sterols in higher algae include desmosteral and 5α-cholestanol, present in some red algae, fucosterol (the E-24(28) isomer of isofucosterol, shown in Table 3.8), isolated from a marine species of brown alga (*Fucus vesiculosus*) and several 24β-alkylated sterols with Δ^5 or Δ^7 double bonds.

4.4 Fungi and lichens

Sterols have been found in almost all species of fungus that have been examined (Weete, 1976). The predominant sterols in fungi usually have a 24-alkyl substituent in β configuration and a $\Delta^{5,7}$ ring system, as in ergosterol, the most widespread and abundant fungal sterol. Other fungal sterols include fungisterol (**3.17**), a major sterol in the bracket fungus (*Fomes applanatus*), and zymosterol (**3.18**), present in some yeasts as an intermediate in the biosynthesis of sterols. Cholesterol has been isolated from a few species, e.g. *Penicillium funiculosum*. In addition to conventional sterols, unusual steroidal compounds have been identified in some fungi. Among the more interesting of these are fusidic acid, a protosterol present in

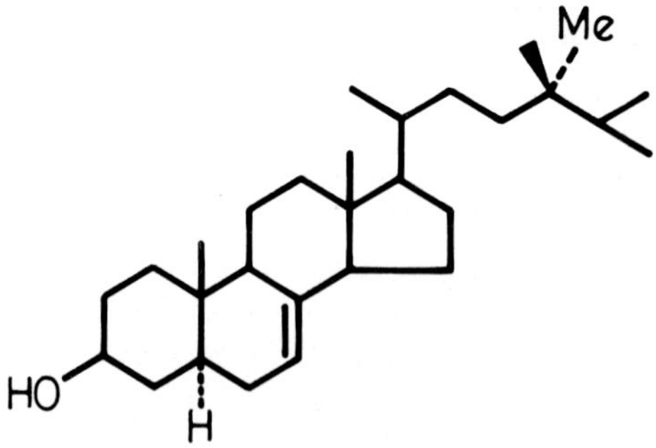

(3.17) **Fungisterol**

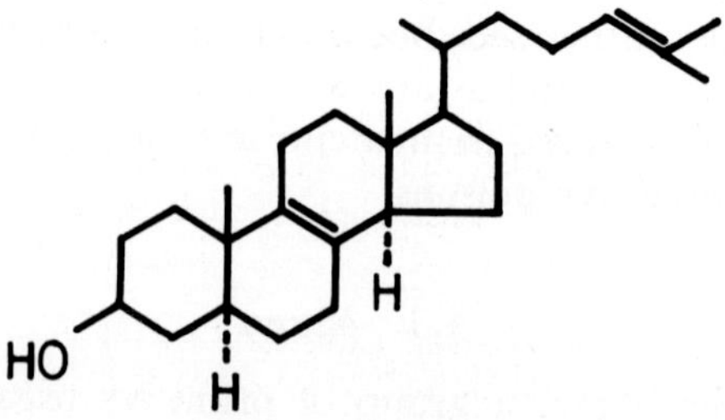

(3.18) **Zymosterol**

Fusidium coccineum (see Fig. 4.10 and Chapter 4, Section 7.5.3) and antheridiol, an oxygenated sterol with a five-membered ring in the side-chain. Antheridiol acts as a fungal sex hormone, inducing the formation of the male sex organs in the fungus in which it is synthesized. Lichens are symbiotic aggregations of an alga and a fungus and they therefore possess sterols characteristic both of algae and of fungi. Among the sterols identified in lichens are ergosterol, brassicasterol and cholesterol.

REFERENCES

Beaufay, H., Amar-Costesec, A., Thinès-Sempoux, D., Wibo, M., Robbi, M. and Berthet, J. (1974). Subfractionation of the microsomal fraction by isopycnic and differential centrifugation in density gradients. *Journal of Cell Biology*, **61**, 213–231.

Bergmann, W. Evolutionary aspects of the sterols. In: *Cholesterol*. Ed. R. P. Cook. Academic Press, New York, pp. 435–444, 1958.

Bergmann, W. Sterols: their structure and distribution. In: *Comparative Biochemistry. A Comprehensive Treatise, Vol. III, Constituents of Life, Part A*. Ed. M. Florkin and H. S. Mason, Academic Press, New York, pp. 103–162, 1962.

Björntorp, P. and Sjöström, L. (1972). The composition and metabolism *in vitro* of adipose tissue fat cells of different sizes. *European Journal of Clinical Investigation*, **2**, 78–84.

Blough, H. A. and Tiffany, J. M. (1973). Lipids in viruses. *Advances in Lipid Research*, **11**, 267–339.

Brooks, C. J. W. Steroids: sterols and bile acids. In: *Rodd's Chemistry of Carbon Compounds*, 2nd edition, Vol. II, Part D. Steroids. Ed. S. Coffey. Elsevier, Amsterdam, 1970.

Brooks, C. J. W., Harland, W. A. and Steel, G. (1966). Squalene, 26-hydroxycholesterol and 7-ketocholesterol in human atheromatous plaques. *Biochimica et Biophysica Acta*, **125**, 620–622.

Clayton, R. B., Nelson, A. N. and Frantz, I. D. (1963). The skin sterols of normal and triparanol-treated rats. *Journal of Lipid Research*, **4**, 166–178.

Cook, R. P. *Cholesterol. Chemistry, Biochemistry and Pathology*. Ed. R. P. Cook. Academic Press, New York, 1958.

Crouse, J. R., Grundy, S. M. and Ahrens, E. H. Jr. (1972). Cholesterol distribution in the bulk tissues of man: variation with age. *Journal of Clinical Investigation*, **51**, 1292–1296.

Drayer, N. M. and Lieberman, S. (1965). Isolation of cholesterol sulfate from human blood and gallstones. *Biochemical and Biophysical Research Communications*, **18**, 126–130.

Drayer, N. M. and Lieberman, S. (1967). Isolation of cholesterol sulfate from human aortas and adrenal tumours. *Journal of Chemical Education*, **27**, 136–139.

Drayer, N. M., Roberts, K. D., Bandi, L. and Lieberman, S. (1964). The isolation of cholesterol sulfate from bovine adrenals. *Journal of Biological Chemistry*, **239**, 3112–3114.

Elks, J. Steroid saponins and sapogenins. In: *Rodd's Chemistry of Carbon Compounds*, 2nd edition, Vol. II, Part E, Steroids. Ed. S. Coffey. Elsevier, Amsterdam, pp. 1–53, 1971.

Farkas, J., Angel, A. and Avigan, M. I. (1973). Studies on the compartmentation of lipid in adipose cells. II. Cholesterol accumulation and distribution in adipose tissue components. *Journal of Lipid Research*, **14**, 344–356.

Feeley, R. M., Criner, P. E. and Watt, B. K. (1972). Cholesterol content of foods. *Journal of the American Dietetic Association*, **61**, 134–148.

Goad, L. J. and Goodwin, T. W. (1972). The biosynthesis of plant sterols. *Progress in Phytochemistry*, **3**, 113–198.

Goad, L. J., Rubinstein, I. and Smith, A. G. (1972). The sterols of echinoderms. *Proceedings of the Royal Society of London (B)*, **180**, 223–246.

Goodman, De W. S. (1964). Squalene in human and rat blood plasma. *Journal of Clinical Investigation*, **43**, 1480–1485.

Goodman, De W. S. (1965). Cholesterol ester metabolism. *Physiological Reviews*, **45**, 747–839.

Gustafsson, B. E., Gustafsson, J-Å. and Sjövall, J. (1968). Steroids in germfree and conventional rats. 3. Solvolyzable sterol conjugates in germfree and conventional rat faeces. *European Journal of Biochemistry*, **4**, 574–577.

Gustafsson, J-Å. and Eneroth, P. (1972). Steroids in meconium and faeces from newborn infants. *Proceedings of the Royal Society of London (B)*, **180**, 179–186.

Herbst, A. L. (1967). Response of rat ovarian cholesterol to gonadotropins and anterior pituitary hormones. *Endocrinology*, **81**, 54–60.

D'Hollander, F. and Chevallier, F. (1969). Estimation, qualitative et quantitative des stérols libres et estérifiés du rat in toto et de 23 de ses tissus ou organes. *Biochimica et Biophysica Acta*, **176**, 146–162.

Insull, W. Jr. and Bartsch, G. E. (1966). Cholesterol, triglyceride, and phospholipid content of intima, media, and atherosclerotic fatty streak in human thoracic aorta. *Journal of Clinical Investigation*, **45**, 513–523.

Insull, W. Jr., Yoshimura, S. and Yamamoto, T. (1967). Comparison of cholesterol concentration in serum and liver of Japanese and American men. *Circulation*, **36** (Supplement II), 19.

Iwamori, M., Moser, H. W. and Kishimoto, Y. (1976). Cholesterol sulfate in rat tissues. Tissue distribution, developmental change and brain subcellular localization. *Biochimica et Biophysica Acta*, **441**, 268–279.

Kellogg, T. F. (1971). Microbiological aspects of enterohepatic neutral sterol and bile acid metabolism. *Federation Proceedings*, **30**, 1808–1814.

Langdon, R. G. and Bloch, K. (1953). The biosynthesis of squalene. *Journal of Biological Chemistry*, **200**, 129–134.

Lin, D. S., Connor, W. E., Napton, L. K. and Heizer, R. F. (1978). The steroids of 2000-year-old human coprolites. *Journal of Lipid Research*, **19**, 215–221.

Liu, G. C. K., Ahrens, E. H. Jr., Schreibman, P. H. and Crouse, J. R. (1976). Measurement of squalene in human tissues and plasma: validation and application. *Journal of Lipid Research*, **17**, 38–45.

Marshall, P. G. Steroids: cardiotonic glycosides and aglycons; toad poisons. In: *Rodd's Chemistry of Carbon Compounds*, 2nd edition, Vol. II, Part D. Ed. S. Coffey. Elsevier, Amsterdam, pp. 360–421, 1970.

McNamara, D. J., Quackenbush, F. W. and Rodwell, V. W. (1972). Regulation of hepatic 3-hydroxy-3-methylglutaryl Coenzyme A reductase. *Journal of Biological Chemistry*, **247**, 5805–5810.

Minale, L. and Sodano, G. (1977). Non-conventional sterols of marine origin. In: *Marine Natural Products Chemistry. NATO Special Program Panel on Marine Science*, Jersey, 1976. Ed. D. J. Faulkner and W. H. Fenical. Plenum Press, New York and London, pp. 87–109.

Mitropoulos, K. A., Venkatesan, S., Balasubramaniam, S. and Peters, T. J. (1978). The submicrosomal localization of 3-hydroxy-3-methylglutaryl-coenzyme-A reductase, cholesterol 7α-hydroxylase and cholesterol in rat liver. *European Journal of Biochemistry*, **82**, 419–429.

Nes, W. R. and McKean, M. L. *Biochemistry of Steroids and Other Isopentenoids.* University Park Press, Baltimore, 1977.

Nicolaides, N., Fu, H. C. and Rice, G. R. (1968). The skin surface lipids of man compared with those of eighteen species of animals. *Journal of Investigative Dermatology*, **51**, 83–89.

Nikkari, T., Schreibman, P. H. and Ahrens, E. H. Jr. (1974). In vivo studies of sterol and squalene secretion by human skin. *Journal of Lipid Research*, **15**, 563–573.

Nilsson, S. and Scherstén, T. (1969). Importance of bile acids for phospholipid secretion into human hepatic bile. *Gastroenterology*, **57**, 525–532.

Portman, O. W. (1970). Arterial composition and metabolism: esterified fatty acids and cholesterol. *Advances in Lipid Research*, **8**, 41–114.

Portman, O. W., Osuga, T. and Tanaka, N. (1975). Biliary lipids and cholesterol gallstone formation. *Advances in Lipid Research*, **13**, 135–194.

Potter, J. M. and Nestel, P. J. (1976). The effects of dietary fatty acids and cholesterol on the milk lipids of lactating women and the plasma cholesterol of breast-fed infants. *American Journal of Clinical Nutrition*, **29**, 54–60.

Ramsey, R. B. and Nicholas, H. J. (1972). Brain lipids. *Advances in Lipid Research*, **10**, 143–232.

Rouser, G., Kritchevsky, G., Yamamoto, A. and Baxter, C. F. (1972). Lipids in the nervous system of different species as a function of age: brain, spinal cord, peripheral nerve, purified whole cell preparations, and subcellular particulates: regulatory mechanisms and membrane structure. *Advances in Lipid Research*, **10**, 261–360.

Schreibman, P. H. and Dell, R. B. (1975). Human adipocyte cholesterol. Concentration, localization, synthesis, and turnover. *Journal of Clinical Investigation*, **55**, 986–993.

Sheikh, Y. M., Tursch, B. and Djerassi, C. (1972). 5α-Cholesta-9(11),17(20),24-triene-3β,6α-diol, a minor genin from the star fish *Acanthaster planci*. *Tetrahedron Letters*, **35**, 3721–3724.

Smith, E. B. (1974). The relationship between plasma and tissue lipids in human atherosclerosis. *Advances in Lipid Research*, **12**, 1–49.

Stokes, W. M., Fish, W. A. and Hickey, F. C. (1956). Metabolism of cholesterol in the chick embryo. II. Isolation and chemical nature of two companion sterols. *Journal of Biological Chemistry*, **220**, 415–430.

Swell, L., Trout, E. C., Hopper, J. R., Field, H. and Treadwell, C. R. (1958). Mechanism of cholesterol absorption. II. Changes in free and esterified cholesterol pools of mucosa after feeding cholesterol-4-C^{14}. *Journal of Biological Chemistry*, **233**, 49–53.

Thompson, M. J., Kaplanis, J. N., Robbins, W. E. and Svoboda, J. A. (1973). Metabolism of steroids in insects. *Advances in Lipid Research*, **11**, 219–265.

Weete, J. D. Algae and fungal waxes. In: *Chemistry and Biochemistry of Natural Waxes.* Ed. P. E. Kolattukudy. Elsevier, Amsterdam, pp. 349–418, 1976.

Wilson, E. O. *Sociobiology.* Harvard University Press, 1975.

Chapter 4

The Biosynthesis of Sterols

1	INTRODUCTION	163
1.1	The extent of existing knowledge	163
1.2	Intermediates in the biosynthetic sequence	163
2	REACTION MECHANISMS	164
2.1	Some definitions	164
2.2	Stereochemical aspects	165
2.2.1	Saturation of an olefinic double bond	165
2.2.2	Nucleophilic substitution at a saturated carbon centre	166
2.2.3	Intramolecular rearrangements	166
3	ISOPRENOID UNITS AND THE ISOPRENE RULE	167
4	THE SOURCES OF EVIDENCE	168
4.1	Evidence from natural substances	169
4.2	Evidence from experiments with labelled compounds	170
4.3	The use of enzyme inhibitors	172
5	PREPARATION OF LABELLED INTERMEDIATES	173
6	HISTORICAL BACKGROUND	174
6.1	The squalene hypothesis	174
6.2	The importance of acetyl units	175
6.3	The distribution of acetate carbons in isoprenoid units	176
6.4	Location of the acetate carbons in cholesterol and squalene	176
6.5	The search for the isoprenoid unit	179
6.6	The cyclization of squalene and its conversion into cholesterol	183
7	THE BIOSYNTHETIC PATHWAY TO STEROLS	184
7.1	The formation of mevalonic acid from acetyl units	185
7.1.1	The reactions	185
7.1.2	The sources of acetyl-CoA	185
7.1.3	Enzymes and reaction mechanisms	185
7.2	The conversion of mevalonic acid into isopentenyl pyrophosphate	188
7.2.1	The reactions	188
7.2.2	Enzymes and reaction mechanisms	188

162 The Biology of Cholesterol and Related Steroids

7.3	Other pathways for the synthesis and metabolism of mevalonic acid	190
7.4	The conversion of isopentenyl pyrophosphate into squalene	191
7.4.1	The reactions	191
7.4.2	Enzymes and reaction mechanisms	192
7.4.2.1	Enzymes	192
7.4.2.2	Stereochemistry	193
7.5	The oxidative cyclization of squalene to lanosterol	198
7.5.1	Squalene epoxidase	198
7.5.2	The mechanism of the cyclization of squalene	199
7.5.3	Evidence for the Ružička hypothesis	202
7.5.4	The cyclase	205
7.6	The conversion of lanosterol into cholesterol	207
7.6.1	The probable sequence of reactions	207
7.6.2	Demethylation at C-14	207
7.6.3	Demethylations at C-4	209
7.6.4	Reduction of Δ^{24}	211
7.6.5	Rearrangement of the Δ^8 double bond	211
7.7	Summary of the origins of the carbon and hydrogen atoms of lanosterol and cholesterol biosynthesized from mevalonic acid	212
7.8	Sterol carrier proteins	213
7.9	Polyprenols	214
8	COMPARATIVE ASPECTS OF STEROL SYNTHESIS	215
8.1	Plants	215
8.1.1	The formation of cycloartenol	215
8.1.2	Conversion of cycloartenol into phytosterols	216
8.1.3	Other plant steroids	216
8.1.4	Biosynthesis of carotenes	217
8.2	Sterols of fungi (mycosterols)	218
8.3	Insects and other invertebrate animals	218
8.3.1	Insects	218
8.3.2	Other invertebrates	220
8.3.3	Bacteria	220

The Biosynthesis of Sterols

1 INTRODUCTION

1.1 The extent of existing knowledge

To the biochemist, the existence of sterols in nature poses the question as to how a living cell is able to assemble simple starting materials into molecules of a particular sterol whose three-dimensional structure is one of many possible stereoisomers. For a complete answer to this, we should need to know all the intermediates from the simplest precursor to the final product, the mechanism and stereochemistry of all the reactions in the biosynthetic sequence, and the properties and distribution of each of the enzymes catalyzing these steps. Most of the intermediates in the biosynthesis of plant and animal sterols have been identified and we have a fair understanding of many of the reaction mechanisms involved, including those that are stereospecific. However, with a few notable exceptions, our knowledge of the enzymes participating in these reactions is decidedly sketchy. Few have been obtained in a pure state and some exist only on paper—those, for example, that have been postulated in order to explain the formation of the ring system of steroids with atypical stereochemistry.

1.2 Intermediates in the biosynthetic sequence

A word or two about the meaning of the term *intermediate* in relation to sterol synthesis may be helpful at this point. The biosynthetic route to sterols may be envisaged as a single pathway along which all the carbon contributing to the skeleton of the sterol molecule must flow. Thus, if one could follow the fate of any carbon atom destined for cholesterol it would be found to appear successively in a series of compounds and the *primary intermediate* would be the first in the sequence from which all the carbon of cholesterol is derived. On a strict interpretation of this definition, β-hydroxy-β-methylglutaryl-CoA (HMG-CoA) is the primary intermediate in sterol biosynthesis (see Fig. 4.1). However, it is more usual to regard the acetyl unit (acetate or acetyl-CoA) as the starting-point for the biosynthetic sequence, since it is the final common pathway through which most of the carbon contributing to sterols is channelled. Note that in this discussion the alkyl residue of the phytosterol side-chain is not considered to be part of the sterol skeleton. More generally, the above definition of a primary intermediate is not applicable in cases where a molecule is synthesized *via* two or more separate pathways, each contributing to a specific portion of the final product; for example, the alkyl residue at C-24 of plant sterols is derived from methionine.

As shown in Fig. 4.1, the acetyl unit lies at the junction of several metabolic pathways. Moreover, several minor tributaries add to the carbon flow between acetate and mevalonic acid. Hence many substances that are sterol precursors, in the sense that they supply carbon for sterol synthesis, are not intermediates in this pathway in any useful sense of the term. The relevance of these metabolic interconnections to the design and interpretation of experiments with isotopically labelled compounds is considered in Section 1.2.

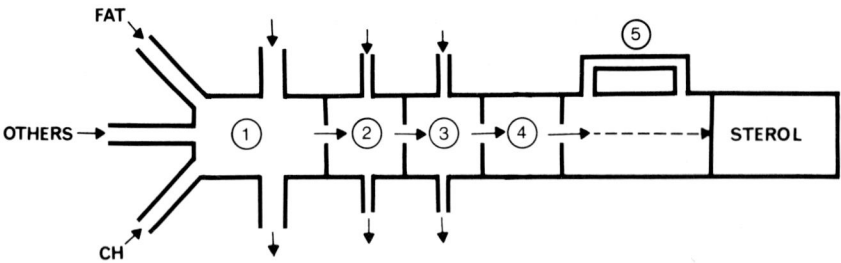

Figure 4.1
Diagram to show the sources of carbon in the critical steps in the biosynthesis of sterols. Arrows show the direction of flow of carbon. CH, carbohydrate; OTHERS, sources of carbon other than carbohydrate and fat; (1) acetate or acetyl-CoA; (2) acetoacetyl-CoA; (3) HMG-CoA; (4) mevalonic acid; (5) indicates the existence of alternative pathways in the later stages of sterol biosynthesis. No carbon enters the pathway after mevalonic acid, other than that used for alkylating the side-chain of a phytosterol. Routes from mevalonate to non-sterol polyisoprenoids are omitted.

2 REACTION MECHANISMS

2.1 Some definitions

Although most, if not all, of the chemical reactions in sterol biosynthesis are catalyzed by enzymes, it is safe to assume that the mechanisms of these reactions conform to the well-established laws

The Biosynthesis of Sterols 165

governing non-enzymic reactions. The reactions leading to the biosynthesis of a sterol are *additions, substitutions, eliminations and rearrangements*. Some of the terms used in discussion of these reactions in relation to sterol biochemistry are mentioned briefly in this section. A more detailed account, in terms of valence theory, will be found in any general textbook of organic chemistry.

In certain additions and substitutions, the *attacking group* or reagent (defined as the smaller of the two reactants) is either *nucleophilic* or *electrophilic*. A nucleophilic reagent is electron-rich and therefore seeks an atomic nucleus. An electrophilic reagent is electron-deficient and therefore seeks to combine with unpaired electrons. Examples of nucleophilic reagents or sites within a molecule are OH^- and $\diagdown C = C \diagup$; examples of electrophilic reagents or sites are H^+, OH^+, carbonium ions ($-C^+$) and $-C-OH$. A nucleophilic reaction is defined as one in which the attacking group is nucleophilic and the substrate is electrophilic, and *vice versa*. In a *concerted* or *non-stop* reaction a sequence of two or more chemical changes occurs more or less instantaneously without the formation of any stable intermediates.

2.2 Stereochemical aspects

Certain stereochemical aspects of reaction mechanisms are especially relevant to the biosynthesis of sterols.

2.2.1 Saturation of an olefinic double bond

The usual reaction by which a C=C double bond is saturated is thought to consist of two stages. First, an electrophilic agent (X^+) attacks the nucleophilic double-bond system to produce an unstable bridged cation (b). The cation may than be stabilized by loss of a proton from another part of the molecule (as in the isomerization of isopentenyl pyrophosphate), or by addition of a nucleophilic agent to the opposite, unhindered, face of the cation. This type of addition, in which an electrophile and a nucleophile are added in sequence to opposite sides of the double bond, is known as *antiplanar* or *antiparallel*.

(a)   (b)   (c)

In (a) the four substituents and the two carbon atoms are in the same plane at right angles to the plane of the paper. In (c), X and Y are in the plane of the paper at the moment when Y is added. If Y is provided by another double bond within the same molecule, the reaction leads to cyclization. In this case, the C—C bond will not be free to rotate and X and Y will remain on opposite sides of the ring. The significance of this *trans* relationship will be seen when we consider the stereochemistry of the cyclization of 2,3-oxidosqualene.

2.2.2 Nucleophilic substitution at a saturated carbon centre

In a *bimolecular nucleophilic substitution* (abbreviated to S_N2) the attacking nucleophile (N^-) replaces a group X attached to a saturated carbon centre. The nucleophile approaches the carbon centre from the side opposite to that occupied by X, forming a transitional ion in which N, the carbon centre and X lie along the same straight line. X is then expelled, producing a carbon centre in which the configuration has become inverted. Why this inversion must occur should be clear from the following three-dimensional equation showing an S_N2 reaction involving a deuterated pyrophosphate:

$$\underset{R}{\underset{D}{\overset{H}{|}}}C-OPP \xrightarrow{N^-} \left[\underset{D\quad R}{\overset{H}{N\cdots C\cdots OPP}} \right]^- \longrightarrow \underset{R}{\underset{D}{\overset{H}{|}}}N-C + OPP^-$$

When viewed from the OPP side of the substrate, H, D and R are clockwise; when viewed from the N side of the product, H, D and R are anti-clockwise. The change in bond angles of H, D and R may be likened to an umbrella turning inside out.

2.2.3 Intramolecular rearrangements

In steroid biochemistry the most important rearrangement is the *1,2 shift*, in which a unit (C⟨ or H—) migrates from one carbon atom to an adjacent electron-deficient carbon atom. The usual reaction mechanism includes the formation of a symmetrical bridged cation, the migrating unit never leaving the molecule during the rearrangement, as in the following example of a rearranged carbonium ion:

$$\underset{X}{-C-C-} \longrightarrow \underset{X}{-C\cdots C-} \longrightarrow \underset{X}{-C-C-}$$

(Carbonium ion)   (Bridged cation)   (Rearranged carbonium ion)

The configuration of the migrating unit is retained but that of the two adjacent C atoms is inverted. The position originally filled by the migrating unit may subsequently be filled by a nucleophilic group approaching from the opposite (unhindered) side ot the C—C system. All these stereochemical aspects of the 1,2 shift are seen in the rearrangement of the product of cyclization of 2,3-oxidosqualene.

3 ISOPRENOID UNITS AND THE ISOPRENE RULE

An *isoprenoid unit* (or isoprene unit) is a five-carbon-atom structure with the isopentane carbon skeleton of isoprene, a product of the distillation of natural rubber:

$$CH_2{=}C(CH_3){-}CH{=}CH_2$$ Isoprene (2-methyl-1,3-butadiene)

In the biological isoprenoid unit, the branched end is known as the 'tail' and the other end is known as the 'head'. The terms *prenyl*, e.g. 'a prenyl alcohol', and *polyisoprenoid* are both in common use.

Terpenes are usually defined as compounds whose carbon skeleton can be dissected into isoprenoid units joined to each other by head-to-tail (regular) condensation or in irregular linkage, e.g. the 1,1 linkage in the central C—C bond of squalene or the 4-2,3 linkage in the cyclopropane ring of presqualene PP (see p. 196). Terpenes may be acyclic or cyclic and are usually classified according to the number of C_{10} units in the carbon skeleton:

Monoterpenes (C_{10}), e.g. geraniol (acyclic);
Sesquiterpenes (C_{15}) (L. *Sesqui*, one and a half), e.g. farnesol (acyclic);
Diterpenes (C_{20}), e.g. vitamin A (cyclic);
Triterpenes (C_{30}), e.g. squalene (acyclic), lanosterol (tetracyclic);
Polyterpenes, e.g. natural rubber (acyclic).

Note that cholesterol (C_{27}) is not a triterpene and that lanosterol, although classified as a triterpene, cannot be dissected completely into isoprenoid units (but see the Biogenetic Isoprene Rule below).

By the beginning of this century it was clearly recognized that many cyclic and acyclic monoterpenes possess a carbon skeleton consisting of two isoprenoid units. The subsequent elucidation of the structure of farnesol and of several cyclic sesquiterpenes showed that these also possess a polyisoprenoid carbon skeleton. This, together with other structural studies of higher terpenes, led to the working hypothesis (the *isoprene rule*) that all terpenes found in nature are formed by the polymerization of isoprenoid units to acyclic terpenes which may then undergo cyclization. An account of the ideas leading up to the formulation of the isoprene rule, and of its value in providing clues in analytical work on terpene structure, will be found in the autobiographical memoir of Ružička (1973). A modification of the classical isoprene rule was suggested by Ružička *et al.* (1953) when it became clear that part of the carbon skeleton of lanosterol, a C_{30} triterpene whose structure had been elucidated by Voser *et al.* in 1952, could not be dissected into isoprenoid units:

(4.1)   (4.2)

In lanosterol, the carbon skeleton (**4.1**) contains a central C_5 unit (■■■■) that is not isoprenoid. In the incorrect structure (**4.2**), proposed by Barnes *et al.* (1951) in accordance with the classical isoprene rule, the side-chain is attached to C-15 and the whole carbon skeleton can be dissected into 6 isoprenoid units. Ružička's revised *biogenetic isoprene rule* was essentially an extension of the proposal of Woodward and Bloch (1953) that the carbon skeleton of lanosterol is formed from squalene by cyclization, followed by two 1,2 methyl shifts. According to the biogenetic isoprene rule, 'terpenes are compounds formed by combination of isoprene units to aliphatic substances such as geraniol, farnesol, geranyl-geraniol, squalene, and others of a similar kind, and can be derived from these aliphatic precursors by accepted cyclization and, in certain cases, by rearrangement mechanisms' (Ružička, 1959). The revised isoprene rule provides the basis for a rational definition of terpenes in which lanosterol and other 'steroidal triterpenes' containing the steroid ring system may be included, even though they are not polyisoprenoids in a structural sense.

4 THE SOURCES OF EVIDENCE

Much of the evidence relating to sterol biosynthesis has come from experiments initiated by imaginative speculation, based usually on analogies with non-enzymic reactions familiar to organic chemists. However, some of the biosynthetic reactions by which one sterol

The Biosynthesis of Sterols 169

intermediate is converted into another have turned out to be contrary to expectation, for example, the reaction leading to the formation of C—C bonds in the polymerization of isoprenoid units. This is hardly surprising, since living organisms, being products of their evolutionary history and having to function at relatively low temperatures, seldom achieve their biosynthetic ends by the most obvious route. An organic chemist wishing to synthesize cholesterol from acetate would be unlikely to choose the 30 or more steps used by a liver cell.

4.1 Evidence from natural substances

The occurrence in nature of a substance whose structure suggests that it might be an intermediate in the biosynthesis of sterols has often provided significant clues. Examples are the presence of lanosterol in wool fat, of squalene in shark liver and human skin, and of geraniol and farnesol in certain plants. All of these exist as, or are closely related to, stable intermediates in the biosynthesis of cholesterol in animal tissues. The accumulation of a potential intermediate in a specific tissue or organism is due presumably to the absence or deficiency of an enzyme system that would normally catalyze its further metabolism along the pathway to a sterol. The wide distribution of these compounds in yeasts, plants and animals is, of course, a reflection of the universality of the main features of the mode of synthesis of sterols in nature.

The structure of a natural product may not only suggest a biosynthetic pathway, which may then be examined experimentally; it may also be used as evidence for the formation of a hypothetical transient intermediate. An example of this approach is the study of fusidic acid, isolated from the fungus *Fusidium coccineum*. This substance has a carbon skeleton identical, except for the absence of a single methyl group, with that of the carbonium ion thought to arise by the cyclization of 2,3-oxidosqualene during the biosynthesis of sterols. In animals and plants the hypothetical carbonium ion must rearrange immediately to lanosterol or cycloartenol, but in *F. coccineum* it appears to be stabilized without rearrangement by the formation of a $\Delta^{17(20)}$ double bond (Mulheirn and Caspi, 1971). The occurrence of fusidic acid and of other unusual triterpenoids in nature provides the only direct evidence for the ionic mechanism proposed by Ružička *et al.* (1953) for the cyclization of squalene in the formation of lanosterol (see p. 199). Evidence of the kind discussed in this section is in some ways analogous to evidence about other metabolic pathways derived from the study of inborn errors of metabolism. In fact, inborn errors of sterol metabolism in man have, as yet, provided little or no information about the intermediates concerned in sterol synthesis.

4.2 Evidence from experiments with labelled compounds

The most fruitful source of evidence for the biosynthetic pathway to sterols is the study of the incorporation of isotopically labelled precursors. In principle, a labelled specimen of a hypothetical precursor is introduced into an intact organism, a perfused organ or a cellular or cell-free preparation, and the label is then looked for in the sterol and in possible intermediates. The results of such an experiment may be unambiguous. For instance, the observation from which it was deduced that more than 80% of the ^{14}C from the natural enantiomer of [2-^{14}C]mevalonic acid is incorporated into cholesterol by liver preparations left little doubt that mevalonic acid lies on the biosynthetic pathway to sterols or is directly convertible into a true intermediate. More often, interpretation of the results is less straightforward than this.

In general, if B is an intermediate in the synthesis of a sterol *via* a series of steps A → B → C, etc., label should appear in B and C when labelled A is added to the system and in C when labelled B is added. Since steady-state concentrations of intermediates are usually very low, detection of the label in B may be facilitated by adding an excess of unlabelled B with A (the 'cold trap'). Alternatively, if A and B are labelled with two different isotopes, the label of A should be detectable in B and both labels should be detectable in C (the 'hot trap'). Additional information may sometimes be obtained by measuring specific radioactivities after addition of a radioactive precursor to the system. For example, when radioactive A is added to a system synthesizing a sterol through an A, B, C sequence, specific radioactivities would be expected to decrease in the order A > B > C and the specific radioactivity of C should be diminished by addition of non-radioactive B with A. Such experiments are seldom carried out because it is usually difficult to measure the mass of an intermediate in a biosynthetic pathway. In any case, evidence from isotopic experiments almost always needs to be confirmed by evidence derived from other approaches; e.g., proof of the presence of the requisite enzyme system and of the proposed intermediate in the tissue in question.

Figure 4.2 illustrates some of the difficulties that may be encountered in the interpretation of isotopic experiments on sterol biosynthesis. A more complex problem is discussed on p. 90.

(1) A remote precursor (X) supplies carbon for acetyl-CoA or acetoacetyl-CoA but is not a true intermediate. Some of the confusion in the early stages of the search for the active isoprenoid unit in sterol biosynthesis was due to failure to recognize this possibility.

(2) A true intermediate, B, when added to the system may fail to reach the intracellular site at which B is generated from A or is

The Biosynthesis of Sterols   171

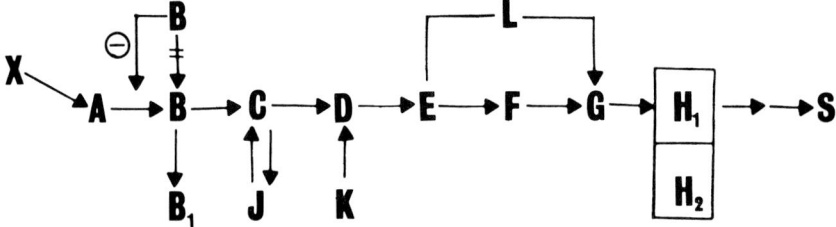

Figure 4.2
Steps in a hypothetical biosynthetic sequence from a precursor A to a sterol S. X, a remote precursor supplying carbon for acetyl-CoA; B, an intermediate derived from A and converted into C or B_1 (not an intermediate). Exogenous B may fail to reach the site of metabolism of endogenous B and, in excess, may inhibit the enzyme converting A into B; C, an intermediate in reversible equilibrium with J; K, a substance, not an intermediate, convertible into D; E, an intermediate converted into G *via* F or L; H_1 and H_2, a compound, H, present in two compartments. H_1 is an intermediate but H_2 is not.

metabolized to C. Hence, addition of labelled B to the system, or of unlabelled B in a trapping experiment, may give false-negative results. This problem arises with many of the water-insoluble intermediates near the end of the biosynthetic pathway to cholesterol. An excess of B, or a detergent used to solubilize it, might also inhibit the enzyme converting A into B, thus giving a false-negative result in a trapping experiment. Note, also, that mevalonic acid is not incorporated efficiently into cholesterol by intact mucosal cells of the intestine, though this tissue synthesizes cholesterol actively.

(3) An intermediate (B) is degraded to a substance (B_1) that is not on the sterol pathway. B_1 would become labelled if labelled A were added to the system and thus a false-positive result would be obtained.

(4) An intermediate (C) is inconvertible with a substance (J) that is not on the sterol pathway. False-positive results would be obtained from experiments in which label was measured in S after adding labelled J or in which J was trapped after adding labelled A or B.

(5) A substance (K) is converted directly into a true intermediate (D). Addition of labelled K would give labelling in S which might be as intense as that from labelled D (false-positive result).

(6) An intermediate (E) may be converted into another intermediate (G) by more than one route. This is a frequent occurrence in the later stages of the pathway to cholesterol and is a necessary consequence of the incomplete substrate-specificity of some of the enzymes catalyzing the metabolism of complex molecules. For example, the Δ^{24} double bond in the side-chain of a sterol precursor may be saturated either before or after the modification of some of the nuclear double bonds (see p. 211).

(7) A substance (H) may be present in more than one intracellular

172   The Biology of Cholesterol and Related Steroids

compartment (H_1 and H_2) and may act as an intermediate only when present in one of the compartments. If H_1 and H_2 cannot be isolated separately, the specific radioactivity in H could be lower than that in the intermediates formed from H when a labelled precursor is added to the system (false-negative result). Compartmentation almost certainly occurs with hepatic squalene and lanosterol and has been demonstrated for cholesterol in liver microsomes.

Some of these problems can be resolved by additional experiments. For example, label in B_1 would not be incorporated into S and label in C would not be incorporated into K. However, in some cases it may be difficult to reach a decision from isotopic evidence alone, particularly when there is a possibility of multiple pathways between two intermediates. A distinction between a true intermediate and a compound that acts merely by generating acetyl carbon may sometimes be made by determining the distribution of isotopic carbon atoms incorporated into sterol from the compound labelled in specific positions. For example, the distribution of ^{14}C in cholesterol synthesized from [2-^{14}C]mevalonate excludes the possibility that mevalonic acid is incorporated into sterol *via* acetate. The problem of determining the relative contributions of different endogenous or exogenous substrates to the total amount of carbon incorporated into sterol in biological system is discussed in Chapter 8.

4.3   The use of enzyme inhibitors

Inhibitors of enzymes catalyzing steps in sterol biosynthesis may be used to cause the accumulation of normal intermediates in quantities sufficient for their identification by conventional methods. An example of this approach is the inhibition of the reduction of the Δ^7 double bond of cholesterol precursors by the drug AY-9944, leading to the accumulation of cholesta-5,7-dien-3β-ol in whole animals or tissue preparations. In conjunction with other evidence, this suggests that the $\Delta^{5,7}$ sterol with a saturated side-chain is the last intermediate in the pathway to cholesterol. Another example is the inhibition of isopentenyl pyrophosphate (IPP) isomerase by iodoacetamide to enhance the accumulation of IPP. However, evidence of this kind should be viewed with caution because inhibition of a specific reaction in the biosynthesis of sterols may lead to the accumulation of metabolites which do not lie on the normal pathway. A case in point is the accumulation of desmosterol in the plasma and tissues of animals treated with triparanol, an inhibitor of the reduction of the Δ^{24} sterol double bond. Desmosterol is probably not on the major pathway to cholesterol biosynthesis in the tissue of mature animals (see p. 207 for discussion of this point).

An approach analogous to the use of enzyme inhibitors is the

The Biosynthesis of Sterols   173

omission of a cofactor required for a specific reaction in sterol biosynthesis. For example, the omission of NADPH from yeast systems has been used to enhance the accumulation of radioactive farnesyl pyrophosphate in the presence of [^{14}C]mevalonate (Lynen, 1967) and of radioactive presqualene pyrophosphate in the presence of radioactive farnesyl pyrophosphate (Rilling, 1970).

5 PREPARATION OF LABELLED INTERMEDIATES

Large numbers of labelled compounds are needed in the investigation of sterol biosynthesis. In many cases, as in the identification of intermediates or the measurement of rates of synthesis of sterols, the label need not be in any specific position, or even in any known position, as long as it is in a part of the molecule that is retained in the product. For purposes such as these, labelled compounds can usually be prepared by established chemical routes developed for non-isotopic synthesis or, when tritium-labelled compounds are required, by the Wilsbach procedure (Evans, 1974). Labelling by a biosynthesis from simple labelled precursors such as acetate and mevalonic acid is also useful, though high specific radioactivities or enrichments are seldom achieved by this method.

When more detailed information is required, as in the study of the mechanism by which intermediates are converted into their products, it may be necessary to use compounds labelled with isotopic carbon at specific positions or labelled stereospecifically with isotopic hydrogen attached to a specific carbon atom. Methods for the preparation of specifically labelled compounds used in the study of sterol biosynthesis have been described by Cornforth and Popják (1969). The synthesis of specifically labelled mevalonic acid has attracted a good deal of attention owing to the importance of mevalonate as a precursor of the isoprenoid unit. It is now possible to prepare mevalonic acid labelled with isotopic carbon at any of the six carbon positions or labelled stereospecifically with tritium or deuterium at any of the six prochiral hydrogen positions (Cornforth and Cornforth, 1970; Cornforth and Ross, 1970). Some of the methods used for preparing these compounds are highly ingenious and are based on combinations of partially stereo-selective chemical synthesis with enzyme-catalyzed modification. A noteworthy example is the synthesis of the natural enantiomer (3R) of mevalonic acid in which the *pro-R* and *pro-S* hydrogen positions at C-2 and C-4 are specifically labelled with deuterium or tritium. In brief, the procedure for preparing the deuterated compounds is as follows:

A mixture of (3S,4R)-[4-^{2}H$_1$] and (3R,4S)-[4-^{2}H$_1$]mevalonic acids is prepared by a stereoselective chemical synthesis, including a

174   The Biology of Cholesterol and Related Steroids

reduction with lithium borodeuteride. The 3R compound is separated from the mixture by enzymic conversion into the pyrophosphate by the action of mevalonic kinase, an enzyme that cannot use the 3S enantiomer as substrate, and is regenerated by hydrolysis. The 3S compound is then converted into $(2S,3R)$-[2-^{2}H$_1$]mevalonic acid by converting the COOH group into CH$_2$OH and the CH$_2$OH group into COOH through a three-step chemical procedure (Fig. 4.3).

(3R)Mevalonic acid labelled with deuterium in the 2R and 4R positions is prepared by an analogous procedure, starting with a mixture of the 3S, 4S and 3R, 4R compounds.

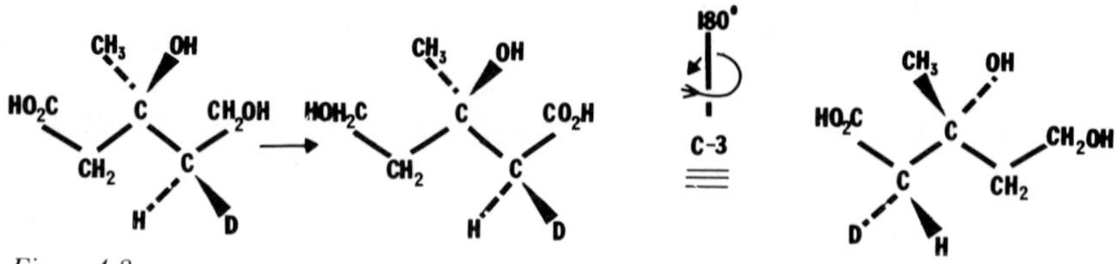

Figure 4.3
The chemical conversion of $(3S,4R)$-[4-^{2}H$_1$]mevalonic acid into $(2S,3R)$-[2-^{2}H$_1$]mevalonic acid by reversing the positions of the COOH and CH$_2$OH groups. The relation between the two specimens of mevalonic acid can be appreciated by imagining the 3R acid swivelled through 180° about an axis passing through C-3 in the plane of the paper.

6   HISTORICAL BACKGROUND

6.1   The squalene hypothesis

The first rational attempt to explain the biosynthesis of cholesterol was the suggestion (Heilbron *et al.*, 1926; Channon, 1926) that it was formed from squalene, a substance isolated from the livers of certain sharks by Tsujimoto in 1916 and since shown to be widely distributed in plants and animals. Squalene (C$_{30}$H$_{50}$) was shown by Heilbron and his co-workers to be an aliphatic triterpene with the structure shown in (**4.3**), each stroke representing a methyl group:

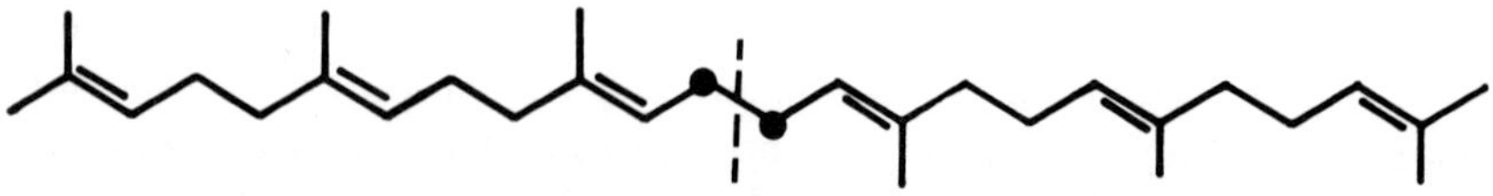

(4.3)

In isoprenoid language, the squalene molecule consists of two regular tri-isoprenoid or sequiterpenoid chains joined symmetrically by head-to-head union at the two central carbon atoms (●). Thus, the possibility that isoprenoid units participate in the biosynthesis of cholesterol was always implicit in the squalene hypothesis.

When the structure of cholesterol was established, Robinson (1934) suggested that the carbon skeleton was formed from squalene by the folding shown in (**4.4**), followed by cyclization and loss of three methyl groups (—O).

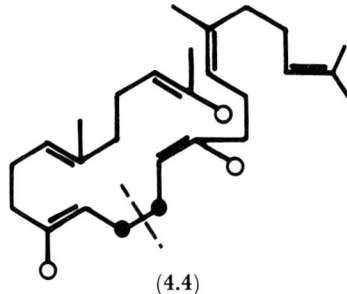

(4.4)

An attractive feature of Robinson's scheme was the absence of any rearrangement of the carbon skeleton.

Proof that squalene is, in fact, an intermediate in the biosynthesis of cholesterol was to come much later from experiments showing that [^{14}C]squalene can be 'trapped' in the livers of squalene-fed rats (Langdon and Bloch, 1953a) and is incorporated efficiently into cholesterol in mice (Langdon and Bloch, 1953b), and from the detailed studies of Bloch and co-workers on the enzymes catalyzing the conversion of squalene into lanosterol.

6.2 The importance of acetyl units

The first clue to the primary intermediate in cholesterol biosynthesis was the discovery of Bloch and his co-workers (see Bloch, 1952) that label from acetate labelled with D or ^{13}C is incorporated into cholesterol by intact animals or tissue slices. Investigation of other potential intermediates showed that most of those capable of providing carbon for cholesterol synthesis are first degraded to smaller units.

Two additional points of great significance were established by Bloch and coworkers at this stage. First, they showed that both carbon atoms of acetate contribute to the cholesterol molecule and that acetate contributes carbon to both the ring system and the side-chain. Secondly, they showed that when rats fed acetate labelled with ^{14}C in the methyl group and with ^{13}C in the carboxyl group (^{14}C:^{13}C ratio = 1:1), the ratio of ^{14}C to ^{13}C in the cholesterol synthesized in the animals was about 5:4. If it is assumed that all the carbon of cholesterol is derived from acetyl units, this result would suggest that 15 of its 27 carbon atoms are derived from the methyl group and that 12 are derived from the carboxyl group of acetate. In the light of the hypothesis that cholesterol is synthesized from isoprenoid units, the location of the methyl and carboxyl carbon atoms of acetate within the cholesterol molecule, and within certain of its precursors, played

176   The Biology of Cholesterol and Related Steroids

an important part in the next stage of the study of sterol biosynthesis. Meanwhile, however, evidence from a different direction had already suggested how the isoprenoid unit might be synthesized.

6.3   The distribution of acetate carbons in isoprenoid units

A detailed investigation of the biosynthesis of rubber, long known to be a polyisoprenoid, led Bonner and Arreguin (1949) to suggest that the isoprenoid unit is formed from three acetate units with loss of one carboxyl group, resulting in the formation β,β-dimethylacrylic acid $((CH_3)_2C=CH.CO_2H)$. According to this scheme, the methyl (m) and carboxyl (c) carbons of acetate would be incorporated into the isoprenoid unit in the following manner:

$$2(m-c) \longrightarrow m-c-m-c \xrightarrow{-CO_2} m-\overset{m}{\underset{|}{c}}$$

$$m-\overset{m}{\underset{|}{c}} + m-c \longrightarrow m-\overset{m}{\underset{|}{c}}-m-c \quad (\text{isoprenoid})$$

Hence, in a polyisoprenoid chain the distribution of the methyl and carboxyl carbons of acetate would be:

$$\left[-c-m-\overset{m}{\underset{|}{c}}-m-c-m-\overset{m}{\underset{|}{c}}-m-\right]^n$$

(4.5)

6.4   Location of the acetate carbons in cholesterol and squalene

If cholesterol is formed biosynthetically from squalene and if the distribution of acetate carbons in the isoprenoid unit is that suggested by Bonner and Arreguin, the distribution in cholesterol should be predictable for a given mode of folding of the squalene chain. Moreover, the distribution in squalene should be that shown in (**4.10**). Determination of the distribution of acetate carbons in cholesterol and squalene was carried out mainly by Bloch and his co-workers and by Popják and Cornforth. In principle, their approach was to measure or infer the radioactivity incorporated into specific positions of the molecule in specimens biosynthesized *in vitro* from [1-^{14}C]- or [2-^{14}C]acetate. Details of the methods used for isolating specific carbon atoms or groups of atoms in cholesterol and squalene will be found in the monograph by Popják (1955).

Wüersch *et al.* (1952), by isolating the individual carbon atoms of the side-chain of cholesterol biosynthesized from carboxy-labelled and methyl-labelled acetate, showed that the distribution of methyl and carboxyl carbons was indeed that predicted for a regular di-isoprenoid unit:

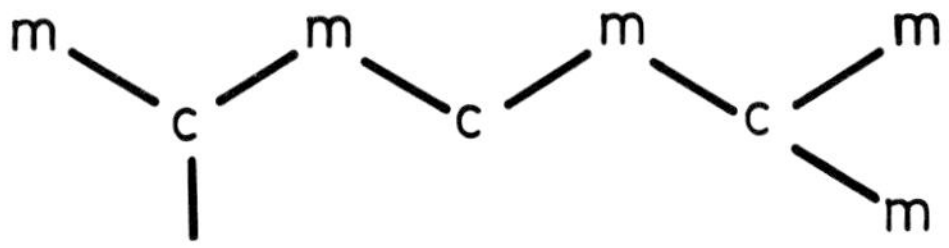

Cornforth *et al.* (1953) then showed that carbons 1, 3, 5 and 19 were derived from the methyl carbon of acetate and that carbons 2, 4, 6 and 10 were derived from the carboxyl carbon.

All these assignments were consistent with Robinson's scheme for the folding of squalene which, if squalene is derived as in (**4.5**), should give the pattern of methyl (m) and carboxyl (c) carbons of acetate shown in (**4.6**).

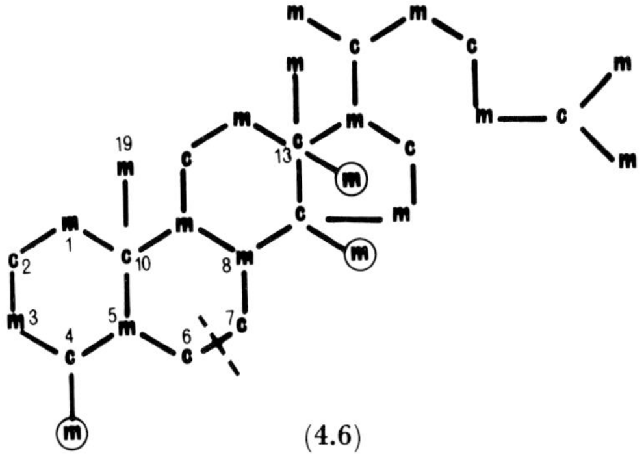

(**4.6**)

However, in 1953 Woodward and Bloch reported an experiment from which they deduced that C-13 is derived from the methyl group of acetate and not, as would be predicted from Robinson's scheme, from the carboxyl group. They therefore proposed a new scheme in which squalene folds as shown in (**4.7**)

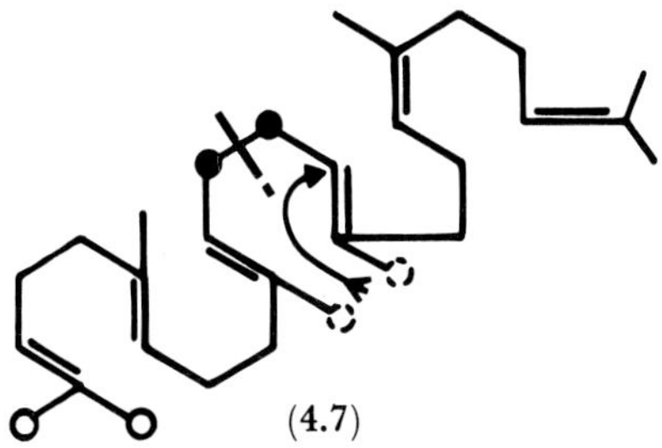

(**4.7**)

178 The Biology of Cholesterol and Related Steroids

and then cyclizes with, at some stage, one or more methyl migrations from C-8 or C-14 to give the angular methyl group at C-13 of the sterol skeleton. According to this scheme, the distribution of the methyl and carboxyl carbons of acetate in the product of cyclization and rearrangement would be that shown in (**4.8**).

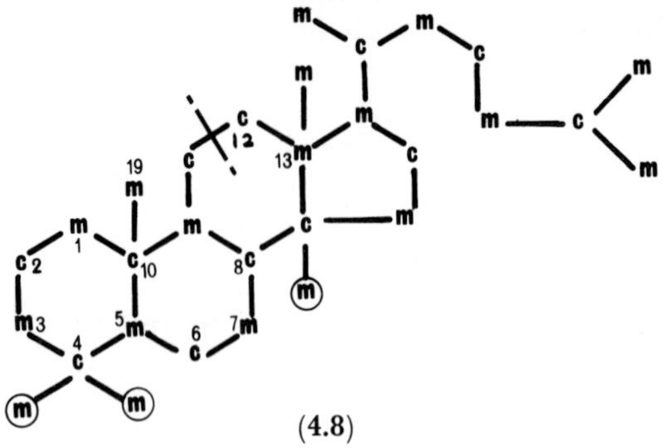

(4.8)

The new scheme was firmly established when Bloch (1953) showed that C-7 is a 'methyl' carbon and Cornforth, Gore and Popják (1957) showed that C-8 and C-12 are both 'carboxyl' carbons (compare **4.8** with **4.6**). Thus, the origin of all four crucial carbon atoms (C-7, -8, -12 and -13) is decisively in favour of the Woodward and Bloch proposal. In his Nobel lecture, Bloch (1965) records the background to this proposal. When Voser *et al.* (1952) established the structure of lanosterol, Robinson's scheme for the folding of squalene became suspect since it did not account for the origin of the *gem*-dimethyl groups at C-4. Woodward therefore suggested a new type of squalene folding which rationalized the structure of lanosterol. Bloch then examined the origin of C-13 of cholesterol and showed that, as predicted by the new scheme, it was a 'methyl' carbon.

In putting forward their scheme, Woodward and Bloch pointed out that it provided a reasonable explanation for the biosynthesis of lanosterol (**4.9**) and that it placed lanosterol on the pathway from squalene to cholesterol.

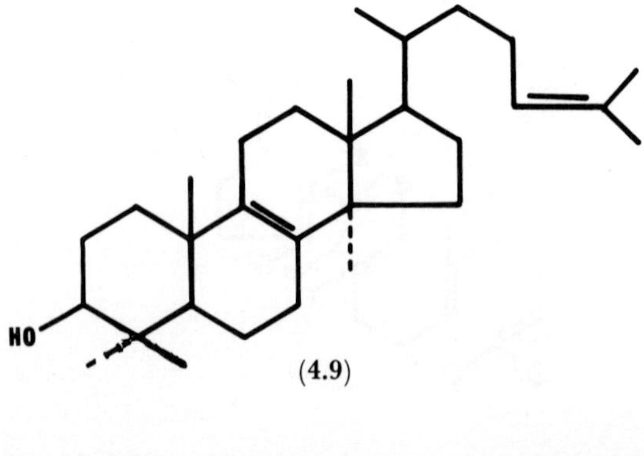

(4.9)

The Biosynthesis of Sterols 179

The formation of lanosterol by the folding of squalene shown in (**4.7**) followed by methyl migrations, explains why the carbon skeleton of lanosterol is not fully isoprenoid (see **4.1**). That lanosterol is, in fact, an intermediate in cholesterol biosynthesis was shown later by Tchen and Bloch (1955) and by Clayton and Bloch (1956). Further confirmation of the squalene hypothesis was provided by the demonstration (Cornforth and Popják, 1954) that the distribution of methyl and carboxyl carbons of acetate in squalene (**4.10**) is that predicted from the scheme proposed by Bonner and Arreguin for the biosynthesis of a polyisoprenoid and assumed by Woodword and Bloch in their scheme for the folding of squalene:

$$m-\overset{m}{\underset{|}{c}}-m-\overset{m}{\underset{|}{c}}-m-\overset{m}{\underset{|}{c}}-m-c-m-\overset{m}{\underset{|}{c}}-m-c\overset{|}{\underset{|}{}}\overset{m}{\underset{|}{c}}-m-\overset{m}{\underset{|}{c}}-m-c-m-\overset{m}{\underset{|}{c}}-m-c-m-\overset{m}{\underset{|}{c}}-m$$

(4.10)

6.5 The search for the isoprenoid unit

When it became clear that cholesterol is biosynthesized from acetate *via* isoprenoid units, a search began for possible intermediates in the formation of the isoprenoid unit and its conversion into polyisoprenoids. The approach used at this stage was to test compounds for their ability to provide carbon for sterol biosynthesis other than by conversion into acetate. Brady and Gurin (1951) showed that the carbon skeleton of acetoacetate is incorporated into sterol *in vitro* without breakdown to a C_2 unit. This finding, which must have depended upon the conversion of some acetoacetate into acetoacetyl-CoA in the liver slices used by Brady & Gurin, was not compatible with the scheme of Bonner and Arreguin, in which CO_2 is lost from a C_4 unit:

$$C_2 + C_2 \longrightarrow C_4$$

$$C_4 \xrightarrow{-CO_2} C_3$$

$$C_3 + C_2 \longrightarrow C_5 \longrightarrow \text{polyisoprenoid}$$

However, if the methyl group of an acetyl unit condenses with the keto group of acetoacetate, and if this is followed by loss of CO_2 from the third acetyl unit:

$$C_2 + C_2 \longrightarrow C_4$$

$$C_4 + C_2 \longrightarrow C_6$$

$$C_6 \xrightarrow{-CO_2} C_5 \longrightarrow \text{polyisoprenoid}$$

the m—c—m—c distribution of methyl and carboxyl carbons would
$$\overset{m}{|}$$
be retained in the C_5 unit and all the arguments based on the assumption that this is the pattern in the isoprenoid unit would still be valid. It is worth noting that Bloch pointed out in 1952 that the formation of β-hydroxy-β-methylglutarate (HMG) by the addition of an acetyl unit to acetoacetate, followed by loss of CO_2, would explain the incorporation of ^{14}C from carboxy-labelled acetoacetate into sterol. At that time it was not known that the reductive step, implicit in the formation of an isoprenoid from acetyl units, precedes the decarboxylation of the C_6 unit. Nor was it then recognized that acetoacetate and the C_6 unit arising from it participate in sterol biosynthesis only as their CoA esters.

Early work with branched-chain C_5 and C_6 acids labelled with ^{14}C gave conflicting results (summarized by Bloch, 1957). HMG was a much less efficient sterol precursor than acetate *in vivo* and *in vitro*, but two of the acids tested—isovalerate and β,β-dimethylacrylate (see Fig. 4.4)—were considerably more efficient than acetate as sterol precursors in intact rats. However, experiments with these acids labelled in specific positions showed that the methyl portion was incorporated into cholesterol with much greater efficiency than the carboxyl portion, suggesting that the carbon skeleton was broken into smaller units before being incorporated into sterol. Meanwhile, work in the laboratories of Rudney and Lynen had shown that HMG-CoA is biosynthesized by the condensation of acetyl-CoA with acetoacetyl-

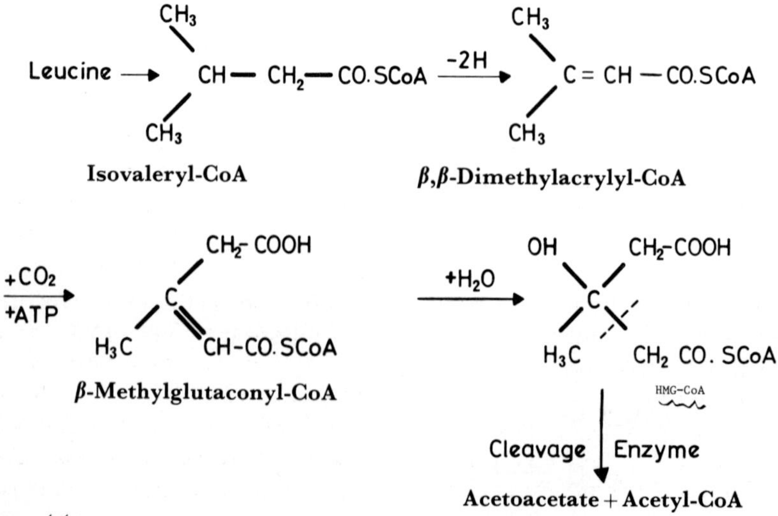

Figure 4.4
The steps by which leucine may be converted into acetoacetate *via* HMG-CoA.

CoA, a reaction catalyzed by the HMG-CoA condensing enzyme, HMG-CoA synthase (EC 4.1.3.5). Coon had also shown that HMG-CoA is split by a widely-distributed enzyme, the 'HMG-CoA cleavage enzyme' (HMG-CoA lyase) (EC 4.1.3.4) to acetyl-CoA and acetoacetate, and Lynen had shown that HMG-CoA can be synthesized from leucine by a pathway involving a biotin-dependent carboxylation (Fig. 4.4).

More recent work has shown that whereas the HMG-CoA cleavage enzyme is confined to the mitochondria, the HMG-CoA condensing enzyme is present both in the mitochondria and in the microsomes or cytosol (see p. 186).

The systematic search for branched-chain precursors of the isoprenoid unit ended abruptly in 1956, a vintage year in this story, when Folkers and his group (Wright et al., 1956) identified the lactone of the asymmetric compound, mevalonic acid (3,5-dihydroxy-3-methylpentanoic acid) (4.11), in dried 'distillers' solubles' and showed that it was an extremely efficient precursor of cholesterol.

The importance of this discovery in relation to the whole field of polyisoprenoid biochemistry is such that some aspects of its historical background are worth mentioning. Folkers (1959) has described how he and his co-workers were attempting to identify a factor in distillers' solubles that was capable of replacing acetate in the culture medium of *Lactobacillus acidophilus*, a micro-organism requiring acetate as a growth factor. When the structure of the growth factor was elucidated, its resemblance to HMG, long considered to be a possible intermediate in sterol biosynthesis, was noted by a group working on cholesterol biosynthesis 'only a few doors away'. This group (Tavormina et al., 1956) then showed that 43.4% of the ^{14}C in the racemate of [2-^{14}C]mevalonate was incorporated into cholesterol by a cell-free system of rat liver, whereas none of the ^{14}C of [1-^{14}C]mevalonate was incorporated. This suggested that mevalonic acid was decarboxylated to give the biologically active isoprenoid unit, a suggestion that has been fully substantiated by subsequent work.

Although these observations arose from an interest in *L. acidophilus*,

182 The Biology of Cholesterol and Related Steroids

several years were to elapse before the role of mevalonic acid in the metabolism of bacteria was elucidated (see p. 220). Thus, from the point of view of steroid biochemistry the discovery of mevalonic acid is a perfect example of serendipity.*

Overwhelming evidence that mevalonic acid is an obligatory intermediate on the biosynthetic pathway from acetate to sterols was provided by the demonstration that HMG-CoA is reduced to mevalonic acid by an enzyme system in yeast (Lynen, 1959; Rudney, 1959) and animal tissues (Bucher *et al.*, 1960) and by the identification (mainly in the laboratories of Bloch and Lynen, and of Popják and Cornforth) of a series of phosphorylated intermediates between mevalonic acid and squalene. That mevalonic acid does indeed provide the carbon skeleton for the elusive C_5 isoprenoid unit was proved conclusively by Cornforth, Popják and their co-workers (1957, 1958), who showed that squalene and cholesterol biosynthesized from [2-^{14}C]mevalonate are labelled in the expected positions (Fig. 4.5).

In the light of subsequent knowledge of the role of HMG-CoA in sterol biosynthesis it is now possible to suggest explanations for some of the results obtained in the early 1950's with labelled C_5 and C_6 branched-chain acids. The poor utilization of some of these acids when tested *in vitro* may have been due to absence of the requisite enzyme system for activation by esterification with CoA or to failure of the acid to enter cells. For example, the low efficiency of incorporation of HMG into cholesterol by liver slices is probably due to the virtual absence of an HMG-activating enzyme system in liver (Burch *et al.*, 1964). The very efficient incorporation of the methyl groups of β,β-dimethylacrylic and isovaleric acids, compared with the incorporation of acetate carbon, suggests that both acids are activated and that a part of the molecule containing the methyl groups then enters the pathway to sterol without passing through intracellular pools of acetyl-CoA.

Thus, selective incorporation of the methyl groups of isovaleryl-CoA into sterol could occur through the formation of HMG-CoA (Fig. 4.4), followed by the cleavage and resynthesis of HMG-CoA from acetoacetate (see Section 7.1).

Isovaleryl-CoA → → HMG → Acetoacetate + Acetyl-CoA
↓ Acetyl-CoA
HMG-CoA → Sterol

* *Serendipity*: *Serendib* is the old Arabic name for Sri Lanka, formerly Ceylon. The word 'serendipity' was coined by Horace Walpole (1717–1797), the putative son of Sir Robert Walpole (Prime Minister of George I and George II), and was suggested to him by the Persian fairy story 'The Three Princes of Serendip', in which the heroes were always making important discoveries by accident. The identification of mevalonic acid, one of the most significant events in the history of steroid biochemistry, was an unpredictable by-product of fundamental research in an entirely unrelated field—a point worth noting by those responsible for science policy.

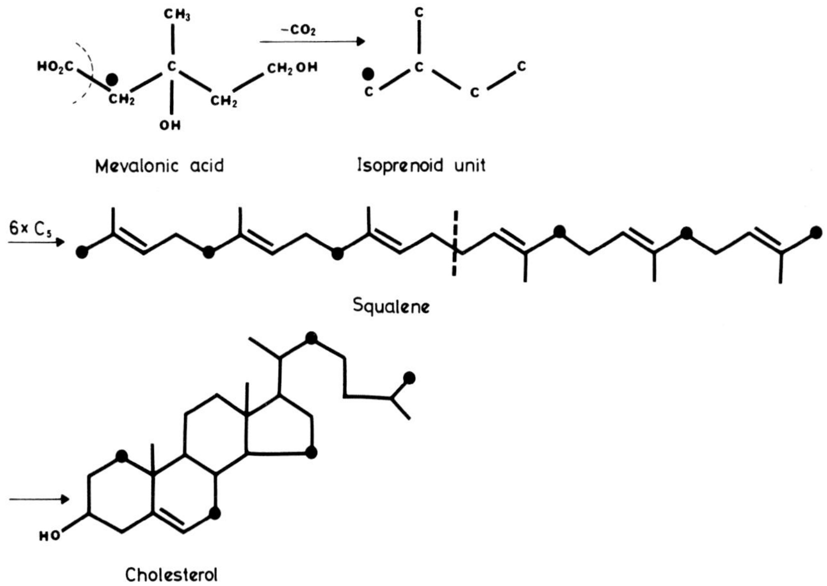

Figure 4.5
The distribution of labelled carbon atoms in squalene and cholesterol biosynthesized from [2-¹⁴C]mevalonate, showing that the isoprenoid portion of the carbon skeleton of mevalonic acid is incorporated as an intact unit and not *via* acetate. Note that only five positions in cholesterol are labelled because one carbon derived from C-2 of mevalonate is lost during the 4α-demethylation of lanosterol. (From Cornforth *et al.*, 1957, 1958*a*.)

The methyl carbons of isovalerate would be retained in the HMG-CoA after its cleavage and resynthesis, but the carboxyl carbon of isovalerate transferred to acetyl-CoA formed by the cleavage of HMG-CoA would be incorporated into sterol only after considerable dilution with endogenous acetyl-CoA.

A scheme such as this explains how ^{14}C in a specific position in a labelled compound could be incorporated into sterol with much greater efficiency than [^{14}C]acetate, even though the total amount of carbon provided by the compound for sterol synthesis is very small. Hence, the efficient incorporation of methyl-labelled isovalerate into cholesterol cannot be taken as evidence that leucine, or the C₅ acids arising from its metabolism, make a significant contribution to sterol synthesis.

6.6 The cyclization of squalene and its conversion into cholesterol

In 1953, Ružička suggested that all cyclic triterpenes are derived biosynthetically from squalene by cyclization of the squalene back-

184 The Biology of Cholesterol and Related Steroids

bone followed by various intramolecular rearrangements. Ružička and his Swiss co-workers (Eschenmoser et al., 1955) later put forward more detailed proposals for the biogenesis of lanosterol and other cyclic triterpenes, based on the assumptions that the cyclization of squalene and the subsequent rearrangements are concerted and that the rearrangements take place by 1,2 shifts. These proposals have, in the main, been substantiated by experimental observations, though it is now recognized that in the biosynthesis of steroidal triterpenes containing an oxygen function at C-3 the substrate for cyclization is not squalene but 2,3-oxidosqualene (Corey et al., 1966).

The first step in the conversion of lanosterol into cholesterol was shown by Gautschi and Bloch (1958) to be the removal of the 14α-methyl group. Olson et al. (1957) measured the $^{14}CO_2$ evolved from lanosterol, labelled biosynthetically with [2-^{14}C]acetate, during its enzymic conversion into cholesterol. They concluded that all of the three methyl groups removed (4,4-dimethyl and 14α-methyl) were oxidized to CO_2. More recent work, discussed below, has indicated that the 14α-methyl group is removed as formaldehyde. The order in which the remaining changes occur has not been established with certainty, but it is likely that the Δ^{24} double bond is saturated before the rearrangement of the Δ^8 to the Δ^5 position (see Frantz and Schroepfer, 1967 and Goad, 1970).

7 THE BIOSYNTHETIC PATHWAY TO STEROLS

In this section, the steps leading to the biogenesis of cholesterol from acetate will be described with, as far as possible, an account of the enzyme concerned and the mechanism and stereochemistry of the reaction at each step.

The whole sequence of reactions, beginning with acetate, may be divided for convenience into five stages: the formation of mevalonic acid from three acetyl units, the conversion of mevalonic acid into the biological isoprenoid unit, the formation of squalene from six isoprenoid units, the cyclization of squalene (as the 2,3-epoxide) to form lanosterol and the conversion of lanosterol into cholesterol. The enzymes required for all these reactions are present in the extra-mitochondrial components of the cell so that, as first demonstrated by Bucher and McGarrahan (1956), cholesterol can be synthesized from acetate in cell-free preparations from which the mitochondria have been removed. In the intact cell, however, free acetate is probably not a significant source of sterol carbon, the acetyl units used for cholesterol synthesis being derived largely from acetyl-CoA resulting indirectly from the breakdown of fatty acids and carbohydrate.

7.1 The formation of mevalonic acid from acetyl units

7.1.1 The reactions

Acetate is converted into mevalonic acid by the following sequence of reactions:

Acetate + ATP + CoA → Acetyl-CoA + AMP + PP (*1*)
2 Acetyl-CoA ⇌ Acetoacetyl-CoA + CoA (*2*)
Acetoacetyl-CoA + Acetyl-CoA + H_2O ⇌ HMG-CoA + CoA (*3*)
HMG-CoA + 2 NADPH + $2H^+$ → Mevalonate + 2 $NADP^+$ + CoA (*4*)

7.1.2 The sources of acetyl-CoA

Most of the acetyl-CoA used for sterol synthesis is not derived from reaction (*1*) but from a sequence of reactions in which citrate acts as an intermediate. The acetyl-CoA generated within the mitochondria by the β-oxidation of fatty acids or the oxidative decarboxylation of pyruvate is converted into citrate by intramitochondrial citrate synthase:

Acetyl-CoA + oxaloacetate + H_2O $\xrightarrow{\text{citrate synthase}}$ citrate + CoA (*5*)

The citrate formed within the mitochondria diffuses into the cytosol and is hydrolysed to acetyl-CoA and oxaloacetate by citrate-ATP lyase (citrate cleavage enzyme)

Citrate + ATP + CoA $\xrightarrow{\text{citrate lyase}}$ Acetyl-CoA + oxaloacetate + ADP + P + H_2O (*6*)

The citrate participating in these reactions may be regarded as a carrier for transporting acetyl carbon across a mitochondrial membrane impermeable to acetyl-CoA. In this way, fatty acids and carbohydrates provide the acetyl units needed for sterol synthesis outside the mitochondria. The importance of this source of acetyl-CoA in experiments on the incorporation of ^{14}C-acetate into sterol in intact cells is considered below.

7.1.3 Enzymes and reaction mechanisms

Reaction (*1*) is catalyzed by extramitochondrial acetyl-CoA synthase (acetate:CoA ligase (AMP)) (EC 6.2.1.1). Reaction (*2*) is catalyzed by β-ketoacyl thiolase (acetyl-CoA acyltransferase) (EC 2.3.1.9). The thiolase participating in sterol biosynthesis in liver is present in the cytosol or microsomes and is probably an isoenzymic form of the intramitochondrial thiolase catalyzing the last step in the β-oxidation of fatty acids (Clinkenbeard *et al.*, 1973). The cytosolic thiolase from chicken liver has been purified and appears to consist of a tetramer (M.W. 169 000) of four identical subunits (M.W. 41 000). The

186 The Biology of Cholesterol and Related Steroids

equilibrium constant, K, of reaction (2), defined by the equation

$$K = \frac{[\text{Acetoacetyl-CoA}][\text{CoA}]}{[\text{Acetyl-CoA}]^2}$$

is 6.0×10^{-5} at pH 8.5 and 30 °C, i.e. the equilibrium lies very far in the direction of thiolytic cleavage of acetoacetyl-CoA. However, when the reaction is coupled to the condensation of acetoacetyl-CoA with acetyl-CoA (reaction 3), the equilibrium constant of the overall reaction

$$3 \text{ Acetyl-CoA} + \text{H}_2\text{O} \rightleftharpoons \text{HMG-CoA} + 2 \text{ CoA}$$

at pH 8.0 and 30 °C is 1.33, i.e. the equilibrium lies in the direction of HMG-CoA synthesis.

Reaction (3), an essentially irreversible condensation, is catalyzed by extramitochondrial HMG-CoA synthase (the HMG-CoA condensing enzyme) (EC 4.1.3.5). In the liver, there are two isoenzymic forms of this enzyme, a cytosolic or microsomal form concerned in sterol synthesis and a mitochondrial form concerned in the formation of ketone bodies by the synthesis of HMG-CoA followed by the cleavage of HMG-CoA to acetyl-CoA and acetoacetate. The latter reaction is catalyzed by HMG-CoA lyase. The extramitochondrial HMG-CoA synthase of chicken liver is a dimer (M.W. 100 000) of two similar subunits (M.W. 55 000). Rudney *et al.* (1966) have shown that in the condensation of acetyl-CoA with acetoacetyl-CoA, CoA is lost from acetyl-CoA and the CoA of acetoacetyl-CoA (4.12) is retained in the product. The condensation takes place in three stages:

(1) The formation of an acetyl-Enzyme complex
    $\text{CH}_3.\text{CO}.\text{SCoA} + \text{Enzyme (E)} \rightarrow \text{CH}_3.\text{CO}-\text{E} + \text{HSCoA}$;
(2) The coupling of acetoacetyl-CoA with the acetyl unit on the enzyme surface;
(3) The hydrolysis of the HMG-CoA-Enzyme complex.

Note that the configuration of the asymmetric carbon (C-3) of the natural enantiomer of HMG-CoA is *S*. With the liver enzyme, the K_m for acetoacetyl-CoA is less than 2.5 µM and the K_m for acetyl-

CoA is 300 µM. The presence of acetoacetyl-CoA synthase and HMG-CoA synthase outside the mitochondria, and the restriction of HMG-CoA lyase to the mitochondria, permit the independent regulation of sterol synthesis and ketogenesis in the liver.

Reaction (**4**) (Section 7.1) is catalyzed by HMG-CoA reductase (mevalonate:NADP oxidoreductase (acylating CoA)) (EC 1.1.1.34), an enzyme first identified in yeast and later shown to be present in bacteria and in all animal and plant cells capable of synthesizing sterols. In most animal tissues the enzyme is confined largely to the microsomes, but it has also been detected in the mitochondria of intestinal mucosal cells. The purified yeast enzyme has a molecular weight of about 150 000 and is inhibited by thiol-binding reagents. The partially purified liver enzyme has a molecular weight of about 200 000 (Kawachi and Rudney, 1970); the subunit molecular weight of the enzyme purified by affinity chromatography is 52 000 (Edwards *et al.*, 1980). During the reaction, which is essentially irreversible, CoA is lost and the esterified carboxyl group of HMG-CoA is reduced to a primary alcohol, with NADPH as hydrogen donor. The overall reaction presumably proceeds with the intermediate formation of an aldehyde. However, the free aldehyde, known trivially as mevaldic acid (**4.13**), is not formed during the enzymic conversion of HMG-CoA into mevalonic acid (Ferguson *et al.*, 1959).

$$CH_2 . CHO$$
$$|$$
$$CH_3 . COH . CH_2 . COOH \qquad (4.13)$$

The most probable sequence is the reduction of HMG-CoA to the hemithioacetal of mevaldate with CoA (**4.14**), followed by the reduction of (**4.14**) to mevalonic acid, with displacement of CoA (Retey *et al.*, 1970). Both reactions are catalyzed by a single enzyme, HMG-CoA reductase. Both the hydrogen atoms incorporated into C-5 of mevalonate are derived from the 4R position of NADPH ('A side'), the first hydrogen atom becoming the 5*pro*-R (H_E) and the second becoming the 5*pro*-S (H_F) of mevalonic acid:

(3S)-HMG-CoA   (3R)-Mevalonic acid
(**4.14**)   (**4.15**)

The net reaction is

$$CH_3.COH.CH_2CO.SCoA + 2\ NADPH + 2\ H^+ \rightarrow$$
$$\begin{array}{c} CH_2.COOH \\ | \end{array}$$
(at top of left side)

$$\begin{array}{c} CH_2.COOH \\ | \\ CH_3.COH.CH_2.CH_2OH + 2\ NADP^+ + HSCoA \end{array}$$

Note that the enzyme is stereospecific, converting the S enantiomer of HMG-CoA into $(3R)$-mevalonic acid. The change from S to R is merely a consequence of the change in the order of priority at C-5 according to the R/S system of nomenclature and does not signify a change in the configuration around C-3. With the rat-liver enzyme, the K_m for $(3S)$-HMG-CoA is 6 µM.

Animal tissues and yeasts have been shown to contain enzymes catalyzing the reduction of free mevaldic acid to mevalonic acid with NADH or NADPH as hydrogen donor (mevaldate reductase; EC 1.1.1.32 and EC 1.1.1.33). Mevaldate reductase from mammalian liver catalyzes the stereospecific introduction of the 'A side' $(4R)$ hydrogen of NADPH or NADH into the $5R$ position of mevalonic acid, using either $(3R)$- or $(3S)$-mevaldic acid as substrate. Thus, this unusual enzyme shows no stereospecificity towards its substrate. Although mevaldate reductase has no known physiological role, its catalytic properties have been exploited in the synthesis of mevalonic acid labelled stereospecifically with tritium or deuterium in the $5R$ position (Popják, 1969).

7.2 The conversion of mevalonic acid into isopentenyl pyrophosphate

7.2.1 The reactions

The conversion of mevalonic acid into the C_5 isoprenoid unit, elucidated in the laboratories of Bloch, Lynen and Popják and Cornforth, takes place according to the following sequence:

Mevalonate + ATP → 5-phosphomevalonate (**4.16**) + ADP (*7*)
5-Phosphomevalonate + ATP → 5-pyrophosphomevalonate
  (**4.17**) + ADP (*8*)
5-Pyrophosphomevalonate + ATP → isopentenyl pyrophosphate
  (PP)(**4.18**) + CO_2 + P + ADP (*9*)

7.2.2 Enzymes and reaction mechanisms

Each of the enzymes catalyzing these reactions has been obtained free from the others.

Reaction (*7*) is catalyzed by mevalonate kinase (EC 2.7.1.36), an enzyme using only the R enantiomer of mevalonate as substrate. Reaction (*8*) is catalyzed by phosphomevalonate kinase (EC 2.7.4.2).

The Biosynthesis of Sterols   189

[Structures 4.16 and 4.17 with +ATP arrows]

Reaction (**9**) is catalyzed by pyrophosphomevalonate decarboxylase (EC 4.1.1.33). This enzyme has been demonstrated in yeast, plants and animal tissues but has proved difficult to purify owing to its instability. The overall reaction consists in the formation of isopentenyl PP (**4.18**) by the concerted elimination, from mevalonic acid, of C-1 as CO_2 and of the tertiary hydroxyl group. The need for ATP in the reaction suggests that 5-pyrophospho-3-phosphomevalonate (**4.19**) is formed as a transitory intermediate, though this compound has not been identified.

[Structures 4.17, 4.19, 4.18 with $+CO_2$ and $+H_3PO_4$]

(Note change in numbering of C atoms)

Reaction (**9**), it should be noted, leads to the formation of an isoprenoid unit with a nucleophilic methylene ($=CH_2$) and an electrophilic pyrophosphoryl group. Popják and Cornforth (1966) have shown that the elimination of the carboxyl and C-3 hydroxyl groups of mevalonic acid is *trans*, i.e. the conformation of pyrophosphomevalonate while attached to the enzyme surface is such that the carboxyl and hydroxyl groups are in *trans* relationship. Proof of this was obtained by showing that $(2R, 3R)$-[2-$^2H_1$]mevalonic acid (**4.20**), when decarboxylated enzymically, gives deuterated isopentenyl PP in which the D atom is *trans* to the methyl group (**4.21**)

[Structures 4.20 and 4.21]

(**Shown in trans conformation with the COOH and OH groups in the plane of the paper**).

190 The Biology of Cholesterol and Related Steroids

Inspection of an atomic model of (**4.20**) will show that if the elimination took place with the COOH and OH groups in *cis* relationship, the deuterated isopentenyl PP formed enzymically would be the *cis* isomer of (**4.21**).

7.3 Other pathways for the synthesis and metabolism of mevalonic acid

The observation that carbon from malonyl-CoA is incorporated into HMG-CoA by liver preparations led Brodie *et al.* (1964) to postulate an alternative pathway for the biosynthesis of sterols. This hypothetical pathway begins with the biotin-dependent carboxylation of acetyl-CoA to malonyl-CoA. Enzyme-bound forms of malonate, acetoacetate and HMG are then formed sequentially, followed by release of the enzyme-bound HMG as HMG-CoA and conversion of the HMG-CoA into mevalonate. However, it now seems unlikely that a pathway involving malonyl-CoA can supply significant amounts of carbon for sterol biosynthesis, since incorporation of acetate into sterol by yeast or liver systems is unaffected by avidin, an inhibitor of biotin-requiring reactions. Moreover, Higgins and Kekwick (1973) have shown that the pattern of carbon labelling in HMG-CoA and ergosterol biosynthesized from specifically labelled malonyl-CoA is consistent only with decarboxylation of malonyl-CoA to acetyl-CoA, followed by incorporation of acetyl-CoA into HMG-CoA *via* the pathway described in Section 7.1.

Popják and co-workers (Popják, 1977) have shown that all but C-1 of the carbon skeleton of mevalonic acid is incorporated into fatty acids and ketone bodies in certain tissues of the rat. Investigation of the intermediates concerned in this pathway has revealed the existence of a shunt (the '*trans*-methylglutaconate shunt') (Fig. 4.6) by which mevalonic acid is converted into HMG-CoA by a series of enzyme-catalyzed steps, the HMG-CoA so produced being cleaved to acetyl-CoA and acetoacetyl-CoA by a specific lyase. The labelling pattern of the fatty acids synthesized from mevalonate labelled in

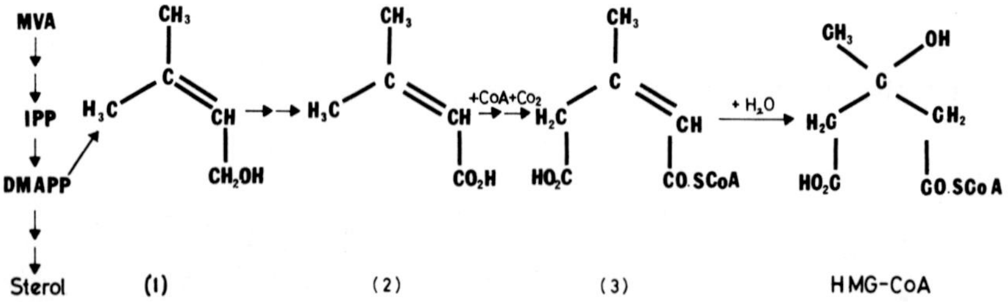

Figure 4.6
The *trans*-methylglutaconate shunt. MVA, mevalonic acid; IPP, isopentenyl PP; DMAPP, dimethylallyl PP; (1), dimethylallyl alcohol; (2), dimethylacrylic acid; (3), *trans*-methylglutaconyl-CoA.

known positions is consistent with the conclusion that incorporation takes place *via* acetyl-CoA or acetoacetate. The existence of the shunt has been established in man (Fogelman *et al.*, 1975), as well as in the rat. Since this shunt may divert up to 20% of mevalonate from the pathway of sterols, it could play a significant role in the regulation of cholesterol biosynthesis in the whole animal. The role of the kidney in the operation of the shunt pathway is considered in Chapter 8.

7.4 The conversion of isopentenyl pyrophosphate into squalene

7.4.1 The reactions

The reactions by which isopentenyl PP is converted into squalene, the first three of which were elucidated in Lynen's laboratory, are:

$$H_2C{=}\underset{\underset{\text{Isopentenyl PP }(\mathbf{4.22})}{|}}{\overset{CH_3}{C}}.CH_2.CH_2OPP \rightleftharpoons H_3C{-}\underset{\underset{\text{Dimethylallyl PP }(\mathbf{4.23})}{|}}{\overset{CH_3}{C}}{=}CH.CH_2OPP \qquad (10)$$

$$H_3C{-}\underset{\underset{(\mathbf{4.23})}{|}}{\overset{CH_3}{C}}{=}CH.CH_2OPP + H_2C{=}\underset{\underset{(\mathbf{4.22})}{|}}{\overset{CH_3}{C}}.CH_2.CH_2OPP \rightarrow$$

$$H_3C{-}\underset{|}{\overset{CH_3}{C}}{=}CH.CH_2.CH_2.\underset{|}{\overset{CH_3}{C}}{=}CH.CH_2OPP + PP$$
$$\text{Geranyl PP }(\mathbf{4.24}) \qquad (11)$$

$$\underset{(\mathbf{4.24})}{R.OPP} + \underset{(\mathbf{4.22})}{H_2C{=}\underset{|}{\overset{CH_3}{C}}.CH_2.CH_2OPP} \rightarrow \underset{\text{Farnesyl PP }(\mathbf{4.25})}{R.CH_2.\underset{|}{\overset{CH_3}{C}}{=}CH.CH_2OPP} + PP \qquad (12)$$

$$2\ \underset{(\mathbf{4.25})}{R.CH_2.\underset{|}{\overset{CH_3}{C}}{=}CH.CH_2OPP} \rightarrow$$

$$\underset{\text{Presqualene PP }(\mathbf{4.26})}{R.CH_2.\underset{|}{\overset{CH_3}{C}}{=}CH{-}CH{-}\overset{CH_2OPP}{\overset{|}{C}}{-}CH_2.R} + PP + H \qquad (13)$$

$$(R = \text{geranyl} = H_3C{-}\underset{|}{\overset{CH_3}{C}}{=}CH.CH_2:CH_2.\underset{|}{\overset{CH_3}{C}}{=}CH.CH_2{-})$$

192 The Biology of Cholesterol and Related Steroids

$$\text{R.CH}_2.\overset{\overset{\displaystyle CH_3}{|}}{C}=CH-\overset{\overset{\displaystyle CH_2OPP}{|}}{CH}-\overset{\overset{\displaystyle CH\ CH_3}{\diagup\diagdown}}{C}-CH_2.R + NADPH \rightarrow$$
(**4.26**)

$$\text{R.CH}_2.\overset{\overset{\displaystyle CH_3}{|}}{C}=CH.CH_2.CH_2.CH_2.\overset{\overset{\displaystyle CH_3}{|}}{C}.CH_2.R + NADP + PP$$

Squalene (**14**)

$$(R = \text{geranyl} = H_3C-\overset{\overset{\displaystyle CH_3}{|}}{C}=CH.CH_2.CH_2.\overset{\overset{\displaystyle CH_3}{|}}{C}=CH.CH_2-)$$

In its simplest essentials this reaction sequence consists in the formation of dimethylallyl PP, which acts as a primer for the condensation of three isoprenoid units to give the C_{15} compound farnesyl PP, followed by the head-to-head condensation of two molecules of farnesyl PP to give squalene.

7.4.2 Enzymes and reaction mechanisms

7.4.2.1 Enzymes. Reaction (**10**) is catalyzed by isopentenyl pyrophosphate isomerase (EC 5.3.3.2). The isomerization is reversible, but at equilibrium more than 90% of the product is dimethylallyl PP. The enzyme is markedly inhibited by iodoacetamide, a property utilized by Lynen and co-workers in their identification of isopentenyl PP as the product of the decarboxylation of pyrophosphomevalonate. From the point of view of sterol biosynthesis the significance of this reaction is that it results in the formation of an isoprenoid unit with a potentially electrophilic group (the allylic pyrophosphate, $\overset{\diagdown}{\underset{\diagup}{C}}=\overset{|}{C}-\overset{|}{C}-OPP$) well suited to attacking the nucleophilic methylene group of isopentenyl PP.

Reactions (**11**) and (**12**) are similar as regards their mechanism and stereochemistry, both involving the formation of a C—C bond between an allylic carbon atom at the head of one prenyl unit and a methylene carbon atom at the tail of another. The two reactions are probably catalyzed by a single enzyme, geranyl transferase ('prenyl transferase') (EC 2.5.1.1), first demonstrated by Lynen *et al.* (1959) in yeast. Reaction (**13**) is catalyzed by an enzyme present in yeast microsomes. The enzyme system catalyzing reaction (**14**) has been demonstrated in yeast and rat-liver microsomes. The products of all these four reactions are all-*trans*.

The conversion of farnesyl PP into presqualene PP and the conversion of presqualene PP into squalene are probably catalyzed by a single particulate enzyme complex with two distinguishable sites (*trans*-farnesyl pyrophosphate-squalene synthetase or 'squalene synthetase') (Agnew and Popják, 1978). The enzyme has been purified from liver microsomes and yeast particles. The yeast enzyme has a molecular weight of 426 000–450 000.

7.4.2.2 Stereochemistry. The steric course of the reactions leading from isopentenyl PP to squalene has been worked out by Cornforth and Popják, using substrates in which the hydrogen atoms at various positions were replaced stereospecifically by tritium or deuterium. The apparently simple question 'To which side of the Δ^3 double bond of isopentenyl PP is the hydrogen atom added during the isomerization to dimethylallyl PP?' was the most difficult to answer and the last to be solved (Cornforth *et al.*, 1972).

For the solution to this problem, (3*R*)-mevalonic acid labelled stereospecifically with tritium either in the 2*pro-R* or the 2*pro-S* position was converted enzymically into farnesyl PP *via* isopentenyl PP in the presence of D_2O. During the isomerization of the isopentenyl PP formed from mevalonic acid, a deuterium atom from water was added stereospecifically to the methylene carbon (C-4 of isopentenyl PP, originally C-2 of mevalonic acid) to produce a chiral methyl group:

$$D \sim \overset{T}{\underset{H}{C}}-R, \text{ where R is the } -C(CH_3)=CH.CH_2OPP$$

residue of dimethylallyl PP. The chiral methyl group, which eventually became the terminal methyl group of farnesyl PP (see Fig. 4.7), was isolated as acetic acid and its absolute configuration determined. With each of the two labelled specimens of (3*R*)-mevalonic acid, the configuration was such that the D atom must have been added to that side of the double bond of isopentenyl PP from which $CH_2.CH_2.OPP$; CH_3; H_B and H_A appear in anti-clockwise order (the 3*re*, 4*re* face of the double bond). In other words, when the isopentenyl PP molecule is oriented as in Fig. 4.7, the hydrogen atom H_G approaches from above the plane of the paper. To appreciate the imaginative power behind this experiment the reader should study the paper by Cornforth *et al.* (1972).

Other stereochemical features of the reactions leading to squalene have been reviewed by Popják and Cornforth (1966) and are shown in Fig. 4.7 and Fig. 4.8.

During the isomerization of isopentenyl PP to dimethylallyl PP the

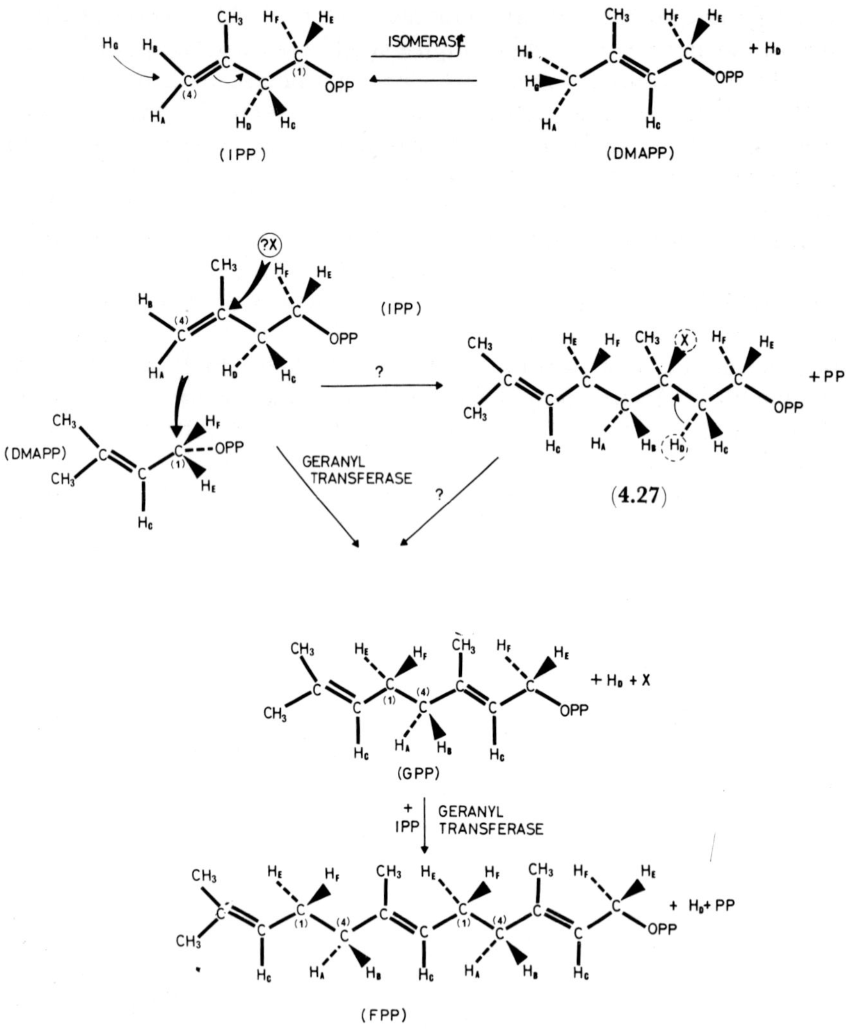

194 The Biology of Cholesterol and Related Steroids

Figure 4.7
Stereochemistry of the isomerization of isopentenyl PP (IPP) to dimethylallyl PP (DMAPP), the condensation of IPP with DMAPP to give geranyl PP (GPP) and of GPP with IPP to give farnesyl PP (FPP). The hydrogen atoms are labelled, according to their original position in *mevalonic acid*, as follows: H_A is the 2*pro-R*, H_B the 2*pro-S*, H_C the 4*pro-R*, H_D the 4*pro-S*, H_E the 5*pro-R* and H_F the 5*pro-S*. Note that the numbering of the carbon atoms in mevalonic acid is not the same as in IPP (for example, the 4*pro-S* hydrogen of mevalonic acid is the 2*pro-R* (H_D) of IPP). The numbers in brackets show the carbon atoms originating from C-1 (1) and C-4 (4) of IPP. Note the inversion of the hydrogen atoms at C(1) of GPP and FPP (H_E and H_F) and the loss of H_D at each condensation.

The Biosynthesis of Sterols 195

addition of the hydrogen atom to the *re, re* face of the double bond is accompanied by the concerted elimination of H_D (the 2*pro-R* hydrogen of isopentenyl PP), the new methyl group being *trans* to the —CH_2OPP group of dimethylallyl PP.

During the head-to-tail condensation of dimethylallyl PP with isopentenyl PP: (1) the C-1 of dimethylallyl PP is added to that side of the double bond of isopentenyl PP from which $CH_2.CH_2.OPP$, CH_3, H_B and H_A (Fig. 4.7) appear in clockwise order (the 3*si*, 4*si* face of the double bond, or the face seen from beneath the plane of the paper); (2) the configuration at C-1 of dimethylallyl PP is inverted and (3) H_D is eliminated to form the Δ^2 double bond of geranyl PP. In the condensation reaction between IPP and DMAPP shown in Fig. 4.7, the arrangement of the two molecules at the moment when the C—C bond is formed should be visualized with C-1 of dimethylallyl PP in the plane of the paper, the methylene carbon of isopentenyl PP directly above C-1 and the pyrophosphate group of dimethylallyl PP directly below C-1. This linear arrangement would be required for an S_N2 reaction (see p. 166), the $H_2C=$ group of isopentenyl PP acting as the attacking nucleophilic agent and the displacement of the pyrophosphate group resulting in inversion of the configuration at C-1.

R = GERANYL

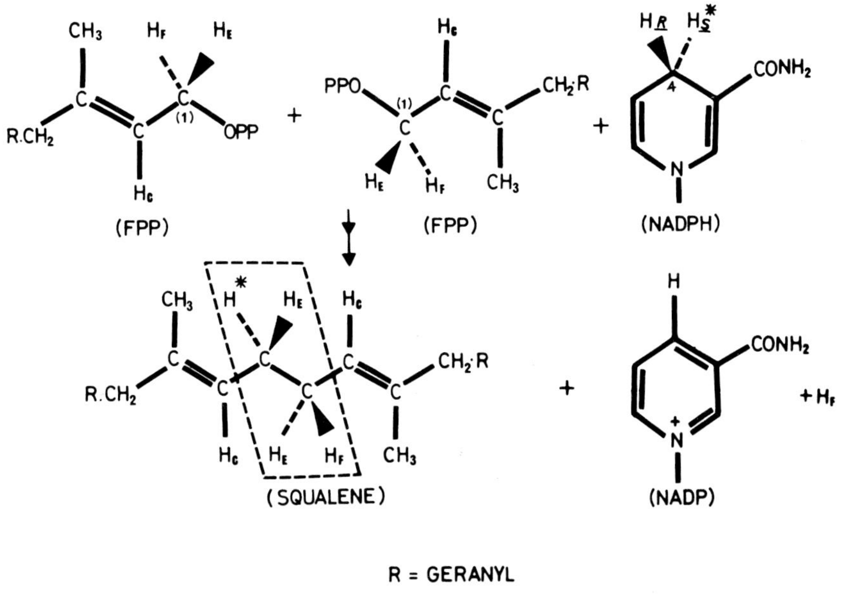

Figure 4.8
Stereochemistry of the formation of squalene from two molecules of farnesyl PP (FPP). The lettering of the hydrogen atoms is explained in Fig. 4.7. The four central hydrogen atoms of squalene are enclosed by the broken lines. Note the replacement of H_F on C-1 of one FPP molecule (left side) by a 4*pro-S* hydrogen of NADPH and the inversion of H_E and H_F on C-1 of the other FPP molecule (right side).

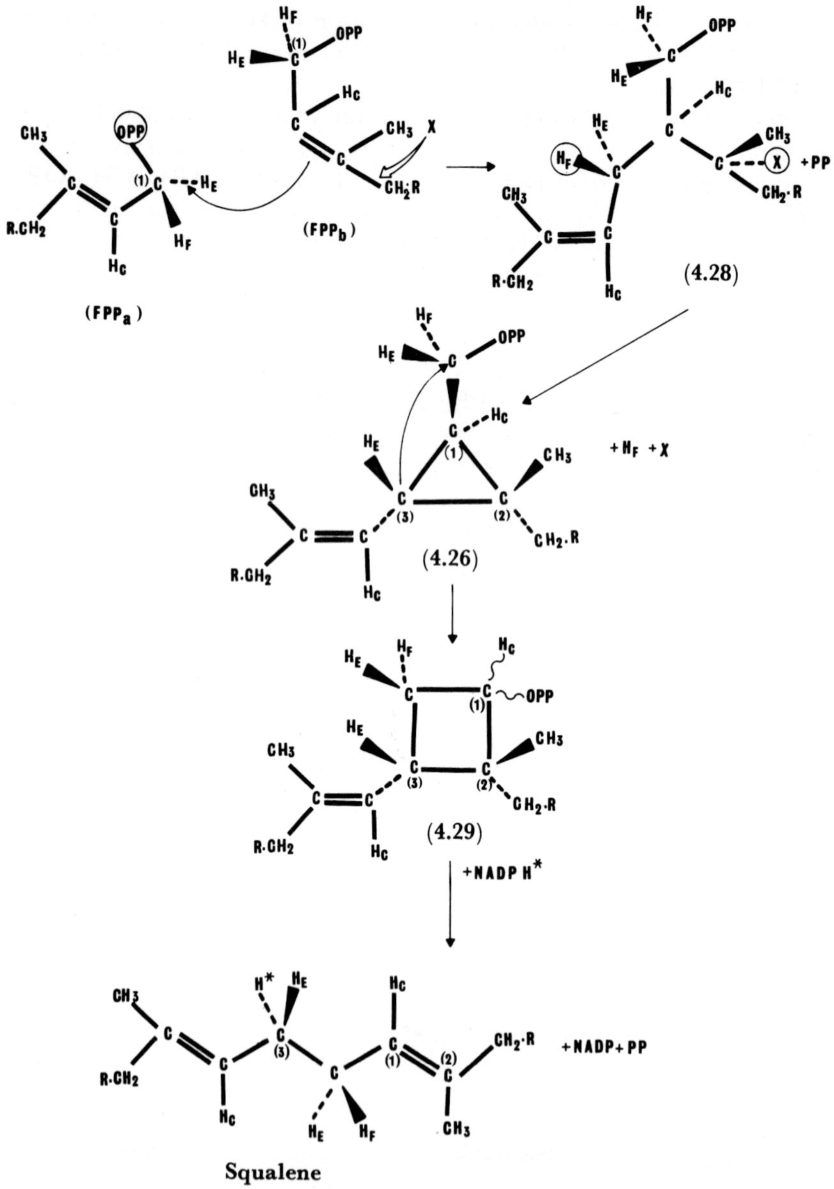

196   The Biology of Cholesterol and Related Steroids

Figure 4.9
Hypothetical scheme for the formation of squalene from farnesyl PP (FPP). The nucleophilic group X approaches FPP$_b$ from below the plane of the paper. The rings in (**4.26**) and (**4.29**) should be visualized as lying in the plane of the paper. Inversion of the configuration at C-1 of FPP$_b$ occurs when the C—C bond is formed between C-3 of (**4.26**) and the pyrophosphate-bearing carbon atom to give (**4.29**).

The Biosynthesis of Sterols   197

In order to account for the elimination of the 2*pro-R* hydrogen of isopentenyl PP (H_D), rather than the 2*pro-S* hydrogen, during the condensation of isopentenyl PP with dimethylallyl PP, Popják and Cornforth (1966) have suggested that reaction (*11*) takes place in two stages: addition of a group X (possibly a group in the enzyme) to C-3 of isopentenyl PP in *trans* relationship to H_D of Fig. 4.7 simultaneously with the formation of the new C—C bond to give the intermediate (**4.27**), followed by *trans* elimination of X and H_D to form the new *trans* double bond. The stereochemistry and mechanism of the formation of farnesyl PP by the condensation of isopentenyl PP with geranyl PP are identical with those of reaction (*11*).

In the biosynthesis of rubber, an all-*cis* polyisoprenoid, the 2*pro-S* hydrogen of isopentyl PP is lost during the condensation of the isopentenyl PP with dimethylallyl PP. Popják and Cornforth (1966) suggest that the mechanism of the condensation is the same as that shown in Fig. 4.7, except that the conformation of the —CH_2.CH_2.OPP group of the isopentenyl PP molecule bound to the enzyme surface is such that *trans* elimination of X and the H atom results in the formation of a *cis* double bond.

During the conversion of farnesyl PP into squalene the *pro-S* hydrogen atom at C-1 of one farnesyl residue is replaced by a 4*pro-S* hydrogen atom from NADPH ('B side') and the configuration at C-1 of the other farnesyl residue is inverted (Fig. 4.8). In order to reconcile these stereochemical events with the known geometry of presqualene PP (see Chapter 2), Edmond *et al.* (1971) have suggested the sequence shown in Fig. 4.9 for the formation of (1*R*, 2*R*, 3*R*)-presqualene PP (**4.26**) and its reduction to squalene. They propose that the reaction is initiated by addition of a nucleophilic group (X) in the enzyme to C-3 of one farnesyl PP molecule (FPP_b), resulting in the formation of a C—C bond between C-2 of FPP_b and C-1 of the other farnesyl PP (FPP_a) and the expulsion of PP from FPP_a. The C_{30} acyclic intermediate (**4.28**) cyclizes to presqualene PP by elimination of X and of the hydrogen atom that was in the 1*pro-S* position of FPP_a. A cyclobutyl intermediate (**4.29**) is then formed by expansion of the cyclopropane ring. Reduction of (**4.29**) by NADPH leads to ring cleavage, with addition of a hydrogen atom at C-3, loss of PP and the formation of a double bond between C-1 and C-2.

Other possible mechanisms for the formation of squalene from presqualene PP have been considered by Rees and Goodwin (1975).

Schechter and Bloch (1971) have noted that squalene is formed twice as rapidly from farnesyl PP as from presqualene PP in the presence of yeast squalene synthetase, a surprising finding if presqualene PP is a free intermediate in the biosynthesis of squalene. Schechter and Bloch suggest that presqualene PP formed from farnesyl PP enzymically is converted into squalene without leaving the

198   The Biology of Cholesterol and Related Steroids

enzyme surface. If so, presqualene PP may be a more efficient precursor of squalene if it is generated enzymically than if it is added to an incubation mixture containing squalene synthetase. A possible alternative route from farnesyl PP to squalene, not involving presqualene PP, has been discussed by Cornforth (1973). However, this possibility seems very remote (Popják et al., 1975).

7.5 The oxidative cyclization of squalene to lanosterol

7.5.1 Squalene epoxidase

As already mentioned, the conversion of squalene into lanosterol takes place in two separate stages. In the first stage, squalene is oxidized stereospecifically to (3S)-2,3-oxidosqualene (**4.30**) by squalene epoxidase (squalene monooxygenase (2,3-epoxidizing)) (EC 1.14.99.7), a mixed-function oxidase present in liver microsomes, yeasts and green plants. The enzyme requires NADPH, FAD and O_2, one atom of oxygen from O_2 becoming incorporated into the substrate:

Squalene

Squalene oxidase   + NADPH + H$^+$ + O–O*

2,3-Oxidosqualene   (**4.30**)   + NADP$^+$ + H$_2$O

Unlike many mixed-function oxidases, squalene epoxidase does not require cytochrome P450 (Ono and Bloch, 1975). For full activity, the squalene epoxidase of rat liver requires a cytosolic heat-stable factor, probably a phospholipid, and a cytosolic protein (M.W. 44 000) distinct from the two sterol-carrier proteins reported by Scallen et al. (1971) and Ritter and Dempsey (1971) in rat-liver supernatant fractions (Tai and Bloch, 1972). The enzyme can accept 10,11-dihydrosqualene as substrate, but the product of epoxidation of this squalene analogue is not cyclized (Corey and Russey, 1966). 10,11-Dihydrosqualene may therefore be used as a convenient substrate in the assay of squalene epoxidase. When squalene, labelled with ^{3}H at one of the two central C atoms by a biosynthesis from farnesyl PP and [^{3}H]NADPH (see Fig. 4.8), is converted enzymically into cholesterol, the ^{3}H becomes equally distributed between C-11 and C-12 of the cholesterol so produced (Samuelsson and Goodman, 1964). This proves that the symmetrical squalene molecule has an equal chance of being epoxidized at either end and excludes the possibility that squalene synthesized from FPP remains stereospecifically attached to the enzyme surface until epoxidation has occurred.

In animal tissues and fungi, 2,3-oxidosqualene undergoes enzymically catalyzed cyclization to lanosterol. In considering this process, possibly 'the most complex chemical reaction yet known' (Cornforth, 1959), it will be convenient to deal separately with the mechanism postulated by Ružička and the Swiss school (already mentioned briefly) and the enzyme system catalyzing the cyclization.

7.5.2 The mechanism of the cyclization of squalene

The theoretical work of Ružička and his co-workers (Eschenmoser, Ružička, Jeger and Arigoni) was done before it was recognized that 2,3-oxidosqualene, rather than squalene itself, is the substrate for oxidative cyclization. However, the only effect of this is to substitute H^+ for OH^+ as the initiating electrophile in Ružička's scheme.

The Ružička hypothesis, modified to take account of the initial formation of 2,3-oxidosqualene, is depicted in Fig. 4.10. Oxidosqualene, folded in a specific conformation, is attacked by an electron-deficient species (H^+), with the formation of a C-3 hydroxyl group and an electron deficiency at C-4 (steroid numbering) (3). This leads to the formation of a C—C bond by nucleophilic attack from the adjacent double bond, the electron deficiency moving to C-10 (4). In this manner, the electron deficiency moves through four double bonds to form a carbonium ion with a positive charge at C-20 or, more probably, a bridged cation (7). This positively charged 'protosterol' is then converted into lanosterol by a sequence of 1,2 shifts, beginning with the migration of the C-17 hydrogen atom to C-20 (8) and ending with stabilization by expulsion of H^+ from the 9β position to form the Δ^8 double bond of the uncharged molecule, lanosterol (10). According to Ružička's hypothesis the whole process, including the 'zip-fastener' effect of the electron shift along the folded squalene chain and the rearrangements of the hydrogen atoms and methyl groups, is a concerted reaction. That is, no stable intermediates are formed by neutralization of the positive charge and, hence, no hydrogen from the medium can enter the molecule during the cyclization and rearrangements.

When putting forward their proposal for the formation of lanosterol from squalene, Eschenmoser *et al.* (1955) made the assumption that the generation of the new C—C bonds in the cyclization of squalene follows the normal rule of antiplanar addition to olefinic double bonds, the nucleophilic agent (see Section 2.2.1) being supplied by another double bond in the squalene chain. They also assumed that the rearrangements of the positively charged protosterol take place by stereospecific 1,2 shifts. They pointed out that if these assumptions are correct, the stereochemistry of the ring system of the tetracyclic

200 The Biology of Cholesterol and Related Steroids

triterpene produced by the cyclization of all-*trans* squalene must be determined by the conformation of the carbon chain of squalene during its cyclization. The configuration at C-20 is presumably determined by enzymically directed stereospecificity of the hydrogen migration from C-17 to C-20.

The effect of the conformation of the squalene backbone on the geometry of the ring junctions formed by antiplanar additions has been discussed by Arigoni (1959). If the carbon atoms are in chair conformation the new bonds will be in *trans* relation; if in boat conformation, they will be *cis*. The protosterol (Fig. 4.10 (7)) that would form lanosterol by the requisite 1,2 shifts has the following configuration: 5α, 10β, 9β, 8α, 14β, 13α, 17β. Inspection of a

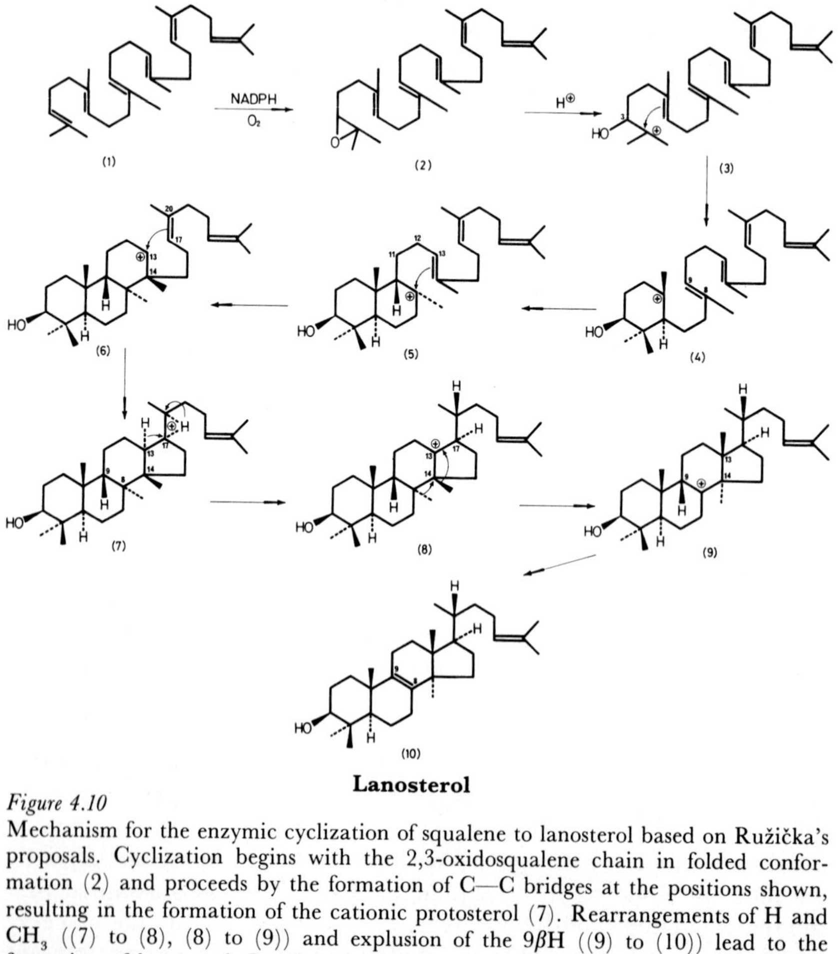

Lanosterol

Figure 4.10
Mechanism for the enzymic cyclization of squalene to lanosterol based on Ružička's proposals. Cyclization begins with the 2,3-oxidosqualene chain in folded conformation (2) and proceeds by the formation of C—C bridges at the positions shown, resulting in the formation of the cationic protosterol (7). Rearrangements of H and CH$_3$ ((7) to (8), (8) to (9)) and explusion of the 9βH ((9) to (10)) lead to the formation of lanosterol. R$_1$, R$_2$, R$_3$, R$_4$ are the uncyclized residues of the folded chain.

molecular model will show that for this geometry to result from antiplanar addition to double bonds, the conformation of the four potential rings, A—B—C—D, must be chair-boat-chair-boat.

An important feature of the Ružička hypothesis is the fact that it provides a mechanistic explanation for the stereochemistry, not only of lanosterol, but of all known natural cyclic triterpenes and the compounds derived from them. Thus, by various combinations of: (a) different modes of folding of an all-*trans* squalene chain, (b) stabilization at different stages in the rearrangement of the protosterol; (c) cyclization from both ends of the chain, and (d) initiation of cyclization by an attack by H$^+$ without the intermediate formation of 2,3-oxidosqualene, it is possible to explain the formation of all known cyclic triterpenes from squalene and to predict the existence in nature of others not yet identified. The special case of cycloartenol is considered below. Other examples are:

(a) Euphol (**4.32**), a diastereomer of lanosterol, may be supposed to arise by cyclization of 2,3-oxidosqualene in chair-chair-chair-boat conformation to produce the cationic protosterol (**4.31**), which would stabilize by expulsion of H$^+$ from the 9α position after a series of 1,2 shifts giving a 17α side-chain and methyl groups in the 13α and 14β positions.

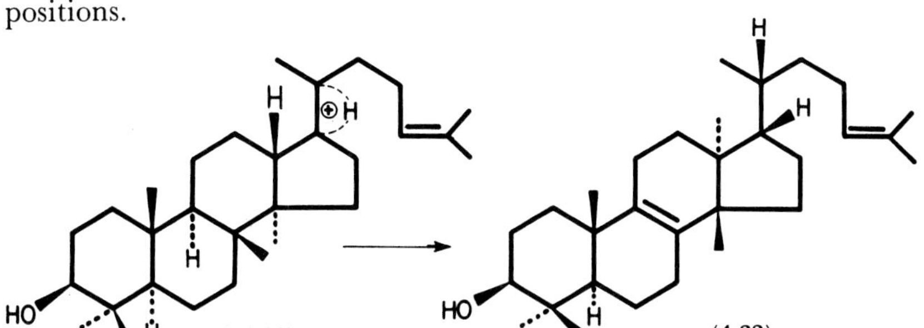

(4.31) (4.32)

(b) Dammarenediol (**4.33**) would arise by cyclization of 2,3-oxidosqualene in chair-chair-chair-boat conformation to give the cationic protosterol (**4.31**), which would then stabilize by addition of OH$^-$ at C-20 in *R* or *S* configuration without further rearrangement.

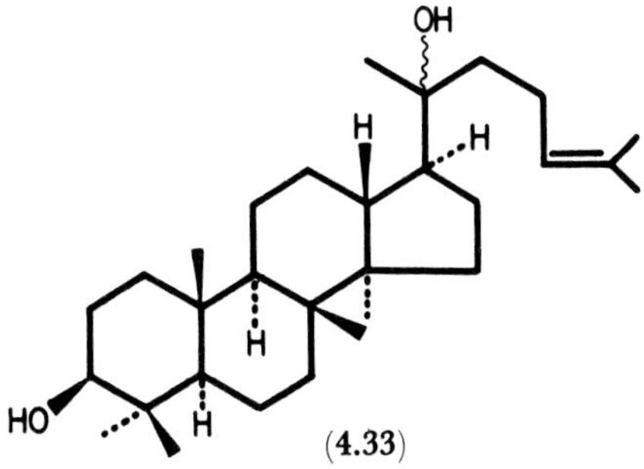

(4.33)

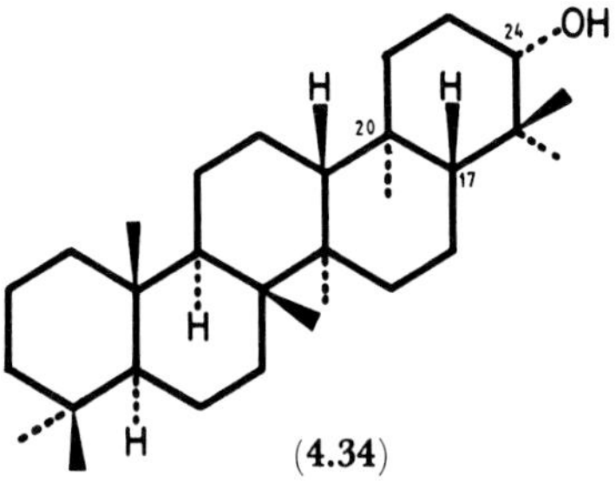

(4.34)
(Steroid numbering)

(c) Tetrahymanol (**4.34**), a pentacyclic triterpene isolated from the protozoan *Tetrahymena pyriformis*, would be formed by nonoxidative cyclization of squalene (not oxidosqualene) in chair-chair-chair-chair conformation, with electrophilic attack at one end by H$^+$ to produce a cationic protosterol stabilized by nucleophilic addition of OH$^-$ at C-24 (Caspi *et al.*, 1968).

7.5.3 Evidence for the Ružička hypothesis

In support of Ružička's proposal that the cyclization of the squalene carbon chain and the subsequent rearrangements are part of a single concerted reaction, Tchen and Bloch (1957) have shown that no stably bound hydrogen from the medium enters the product during the biogenesis of lanosterol from squalene. Proof that the postulated 1,2 methyl shifts occur during the biogenesis of lanosterol has been obtained by ingenious experiments carried out independently in the laboratories of Bloch and of Cornforth and Popják.

Maudgal *et al.* (1958) synthesized chemically a mixture of four species of squalene doubly labelled with ^{13}C in the following positions (11 and 12 = steroid numbering):

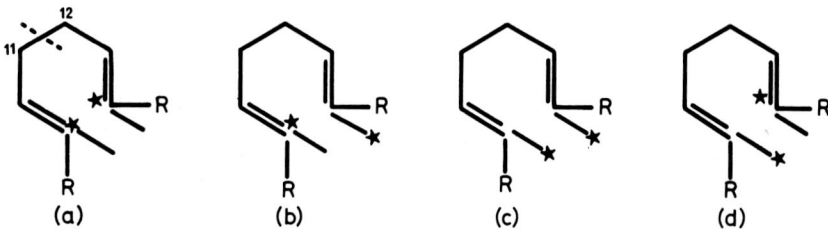

The mixture was converted enzymically into lanosterol and all the C—CH$_3$ units of the lanosterol were isolated as ethylene. If the methyl group at C-13 of lanosterol arises by a 1,3 shift from the C-8 position, no molecules of ethylene would have ^{13}C in both carbon positions. If, however, the C-13 methyl arises from two 1,2 shifts, species (d) would yield doubly-labelled molecules:

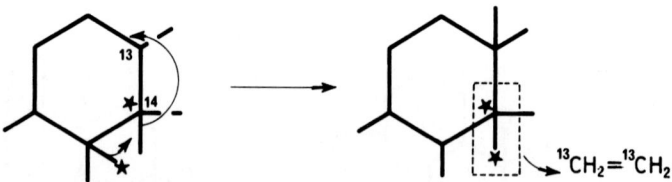

Examination of the ethylene in the mass spectrometer revealed the presence of doubly-labelled molecules with an abundance consistent only with a shift of the C-8 methyl group to C-14.

Cornforth *et al.* (1958*b*), using a different approach, biosynthesized cholesterol from mevalonic acid labelled with ^{13}C in the 3′ and 4 positions. The squalene from which the cholesterol was formed must have been labelled in 12 positions, including those shown in Fig. 4.11 (11 and 12 = steroid numbering). If the C-13 methyl group of

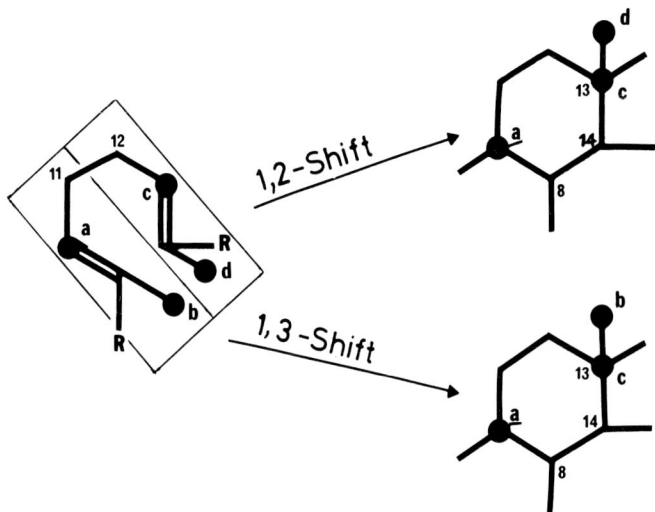

Figure 4.11
Experiment proving that the methyl group at C-13 of cholesterol arises by a 1,2-shift from C-14. Left, the central portion of the squalene molecule biosynthesized from [3′,4-$^{13}C_2$]mevalonic acid, showing the distribution of ^{13}C atoms (●) in the adjacent isoprenoid units. Right, the origin of the C-13 methyl groups arising either by a 1,2- or a 1,3-shift. With a 1,2-shift, the C-13 and C-18 carbon atoms arise from the same isoprenoid unit.

cholesterol arises by a 1,2 shift from C-14, every C-14 methyl group that migrates within a doubly-labelled isoprenoid unit will pair with another ^{13}C atom (*d* pairing with *c*) and will give rise to doubly-labelled acetic acid molecules (mass, 62) when the C—CH$_3$ groups of cholesterol are isolated by oxidative degradation. Since the probability that two labelled mevalonate residues will become adjacent during the biosynthesis of squalene is small, a 1,3 shift (*b* pairing with *c*) would give rise to a much smaller number of doubly-labelled C—CH$_3$ groups. The abundance of acetic acid molecules of mass 62 obtained from the biosynthesized cholesterol in this experiment was consistent only with a 1,2 shift.

The two experiments of Maudgal *et al.* (1958) and of Cornforth *et al.* (1958*b*) are complementary in that, together, they confirm the occurrence of both the methyl shifts postulated by Ružička.

The occurrence of the two 1,2 shifts of hydrogen atoms may be deduced from two independent lines of evidence, as follows:

When a sterol is biosynthesized from $(3R, 4R)$-[2-^{14}C,4-T_1] meva-

204 The Biology of Cholesterol and Related Steroids

Ionic acid (T = ³H), the T/¹⁴C ratio in squalene, lanosterol and cholesterol, and the distribution of T in cholesterol (Cornforth et al., 1965; Mulheirn and Caspi, 1971), are consistent with the cyclization and the rearrangements of hydrogen atoms postulated by Ružička. All the T atoms from six mevalonate units are retained in squalene (T/¹⁴C ratio, 6:6), one T atom is lost during the conversion of squalene into lanosterol (ratio, 5:6) and two T atoms and one ¹⁴C atom are lost during the conversion of lanosterol into cholesterol (ratio, 3:5). The cholesterol contains one T atom in the 17α position, one at C-20 and one at C-24. This change in the pattern of labelling (Fig. 4.12) shows that the H atom at C-20 of cholesterol originates by

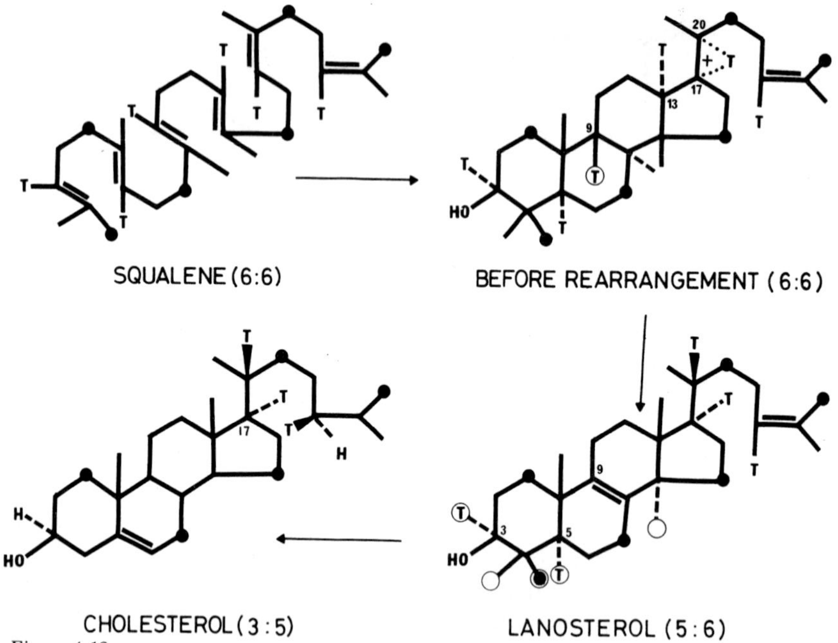

SQUALENE (6:6)   BEFORE REARRANGEMENT (6:6)

CHOLESTEROL (3:5)   LANOSTEROL (5:6)

Figure 4.12
The pattern of labelling with tritium and ¹⁴C in squalene, in the protosterol formed by the cyclization of 2,3-oxidosqualene, and in lanosterol and cholesterol under conditions in which sterol is synthesized from mevalonic acid labelled with ¹⁴C at C-2 and with T in the 4pro-R position (3R,4R)-[2-¹⁴C,4-T]mevalonic acid. Each molecule of squalene has six atoms of ¹⁴C and six of T in the positions shown. All these atoms are retained in the protosterol (T:¹⁴C = 6:6). During the rearrangements to form lanosterol, the 9β tritium atom is lost (T:¹⁴C = 5:6). The conversion of lanosterol to cholesterol results in loss of one ¹⁴C atom (the 4β methyl) and of two more tritium atoms (7α and 5α) (T:¹⁴C = 3:5). The pattern of labelling in cholesterol, compared with that in squalene, shows that the hydrogen at C-20 must originate either from the C-13 or the C-17 position. Atoms or groups that are removed during conversion to the next intermediate are circled.

●, ¹⁴C originating from C-2 of mevalonate.
T, tritium originating from the 4pro-R position of mevalonate.

intramolecular rearrangement, although it does not show whether it originates from C-17 (1,2 shift) or C-13 (1,3 shift). Direct evidence for the migration of a hydrogen atom from C-13 to C-17 during the biosynthesis of lanosterol from squalene has been obtained by Barton *et al.* (1971).

Further evidence for the formation of the cyclic cation postulated in the biosynthesis of lanosterol (Fig. 4.10 (**7**)) has come from the study of natural triterpenoids that are thought to arise by stabilization of the hypothetical cation without rearrangement. Perhaps the most interesting of these is the triterpenoid fusidic acid (**4.35**).

(4.35)

The stereochemistry at C-8, 9, 13 and 14 suggests that this compound arises by stabilization of the cationic protosterol by elimination of a proton from C-17 without the rearrangements that would lead to lanosterol. In agreement with this, Mulheirn and Caspi (1971) have shown that tritium is retained in the 9β and 13α positions of fusidic acid biosynthesized from $(3R, 4R)$-[2-^{14}C, 4-T$_1$]mevalonic acid.

Using a different approach to the problem, Corey and his group have shown that rat liver will convert certain analogues of 2,3-oxidosqualene into stable protosterols with the same stereochemistry as that of the hypothetical cyclic cation shown in Fig. 4.10 (**7**). Presumably, these abnormal protosterols cannot undergo the rearrangement that would convert them into analogues of lanosterol.

7.5.4 The cyclase

The enzyme system catalyzing the cyclization of 2,3-oxidosqualene to lanosterol (2,3-oxidosqualene:lanosterol-cyclase) (EC 5.4.99.7) is present in liver microsomes and yeast soluble fractions. The solubilized enzyme from hog-liver microsomes has a molecular weight of about 90 000 and requires high concentrations of organic salts for full activity (Dean, 1969). The enzyme is strongly inhibited by the imino analogue of squalene. In the absence of high salt concentrations the solubilized enzyme undergoes reversible aggregation to an inactive form. The steric requirements of the cyclase system have been examined in some detail. The enzyme is relatively insensitive to changes in the oxygen-free end of the substrate, though the products of cyclization of analogues of 2,3-oxidosqualene do not necessarily rearrange to analogues of lanosterol. An essential function of the enzyme is undoubtedly to hold the squalene backbone in the conformation required for cyclization to the correct protosterol, but it is not clear whether the same enzyme, or a different one, catalyzes the subsequent methyl and hydrogen shifts or, indeed, whether the stereospecific rearrangements leading to lanosterol take place without the cooperation of any enzyme.

The observation that the protolanosterol (**4.36**) rearranges in the presence of acid to give the lanosterol analogue dihydroparkeol (5α-lanost-9(11)-en-3β-ol) (van Tamelen and Anderson, 1972) might suggest that the formation of lanosterol follows automatically once the protosterol has been formed enzymically from 2,3-oxidosqualene.

(**4.36**)

However, this leaves unexplained the natural occurrence of steroidal triterpenes in which the rearrangement has not proceeded as far as the formation of the Δ^8 double bond to produce lanosterol, or has followed a different course, as in the formation of cycloartenol. Possibly, specific enzymes are required to produce stabilization at earlier stages, e.g., for formation of the $\Delta^{17(20)}$ double bond of fusidic acid. It should be noted that non-enzymic, acid-catalyzed, cyclization of 2,3-oxidosqualene always produces the natural A/B *trans* fusion, but it also produces a 5-membered C ring, indicating an absolute requirement for enzymic assistance in the biogenesis of lanosterol from 2,3-oxidosqualene. In any case, non-enzymic cyclization could never give rise to 100% of the single enantiomer formed in the living cell. For references to non-enzymic cyclization of analogues of 2,3-oxidosqualene, see Connolly (1972); for an illuminating discussion of the various cyclases catalyzing the biosynthesis of sterols and cyclic triterpenes, see Dean (1971).

7.6 The conversion of lanosterol into cholesterol

7.6.1 The probable sequence of reactions

During the formation of cholesterol from lanosterol the three 'extra' methyl groups at C-4 and C-14 are removed, the Δ^8 double bond is isomerized to the Δ^5 position, the Δ^{24} double bond is saturated and certain changes take place in the origin and configuration of carbon-bound hydrogen atoms. All these modifications are catalyzed by microsomal enzymes, some of which have been partially purified. A good deal is known about the reactions responsible for these changes, but there is some doubt as to the order in which they occur. There is probably a *preferred* pathway from lanosterol through which most cholesterol is synthesized in a given tissue, and this must be determined by the substrate specificities and relative activities of the relevant enzymes. However, it is likely that minor pathways are also followed, owing to incomplete specificity of some of these enzymes. This would explain the large number of potential intermediates between lanosterol and cholesterol that have been demonstrated in animal tissues and that are enzymically convertible into cholesterol. Inspection of the structure of these compounds (Frantz and Schroepfer, 1967) shows that they cannot all lie on the same pathway to cholesterol. For example, the presence in animal tissues of 24:25-dihydrolanosterol, zymosterol, cholest-7-en-3β-ol and desmosterol suggests that saturation of the Δ^{24} double bond can occur before removal of the first methyl group from lanosterol, or as the final step in the formation of cholesterol or at intermediate stages.

It may be possible to get some idea of the relative importance of different pathways from time-course experiments with labelled precursors and from studies of the kinetics of enzymes catalyzing specific reactions in the conversion of lanosterol into cholesterol, but an unequivocal interpretation of such experiments is not always possible. Figure 4.13 shows, in broad outline, a pathway that is consistent with what is known about the biosynthesis of cholesterol in animal tissues. In this pathway, the first step is the removal of the 14α-methyl group and the last step is the formation of the Δ^5 double bond, the saturation of the Δ^{24} double bond occurring after removal of the three methyl groups and before transposition of the nuclear double bond.

7.6.2 Demethylation at C-14

Gautschi and Bloch (1957, 1958) identified radioactive 14α-desmethyllanosterol (**4.37**) in the livers of rats killed shortly after injection of ^{14}C-acetate and showed that it was converted into cholesterol by rat-liver homogenates. They concluded that removal of the 14α methyl group was the first step in the pathway from lanosterol to cholesterol. Subsequently, it was shown that the product of

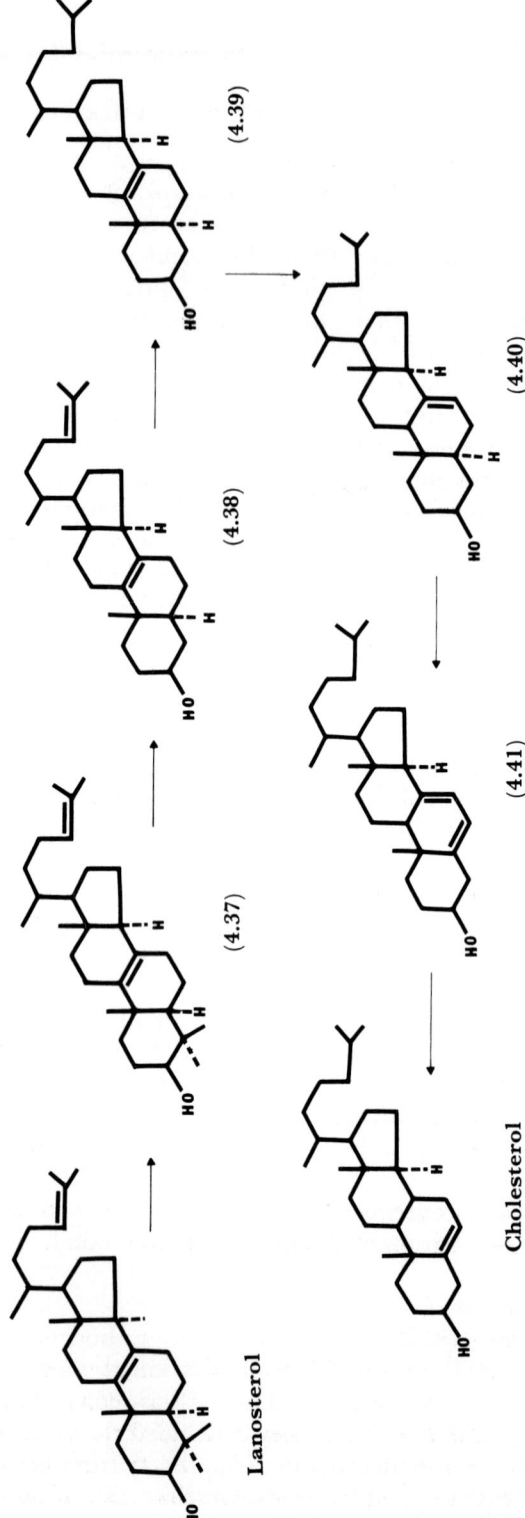

Figure 4.13
Probable steps in the conversion of lanosterol into cholesterol.

(**4.37**), 4,4-Dimethyl-5α-cholesta-8,24-dien-3β-ol (14α-desmethyllanosterol); (**4.38**), 5α-cholesta-8,24-dien-3β-ol (zymosterol); (**4.39**), 5α-cholest-8-en-3β-ol; (**4.40**), 5α-cholest-7-en-3β-ol (lathosterol); (**4.41**), cholesta-5,7-dien-3β-ol (7-dehydrocholesterol).

(4.37)

cleavage at the 14α position is formic acid (Alexander et al., 1972) and that cleavage is accompanied by loss of the 15α hydrogen atom (Gibbons et al., 1968; Canonica et al., 1968) and the formation of a Δ^{14} double bond (Akhtar et al., 1969), trans reduction of the double bond taking place by addition of a hydrogen atom from NADPH to the 14α position and of a proton from the medium to the 15β position. Loss of the 15α hydrogen could be explained by hydroxylation at C-15 at an early stage in the demethylation, the OH group facilitating the removal of a partially oxidized 14α methyl group. Gibbons and Mitopoulos (1973) have shown that CO inhibits the synthesis of cholesterol from [^{14}C]mevalonate in rat-liver homogenates and leads to the accumulation of radioactive lanosterol. This suggests that the first step in the removal of the 14α methyl group is a hydroxylation catalyzed by a mixed-function oxidase requiring cytochrome P450.

It is not known whether the hydroxylation at C-15 precedes or follows that at C-32 (the 14α methyl carbon). The available evidence (see Akhtar et al. (1978) and Gibbons et al. (1979)) suggests an initial hydroxylation at C-32, with the formation of 5α-lanosta-8,24-diene-3β,32-diol (Fig. 4.14 (**4.42**)), but other pathways to 14α-demethylation cannot be excluded. Fig. 4.14 shows a possible sequence in which the first step is a cytochrome P450-dependent hydroxylation of the 14α methyl group, with subsequent removal of C-32 as formic acid (but see Akhtar et al. (1978) for an alternative mechanism). Saturation of the Δ^{14} double bond, resulting in the inversion of the configuration of the 15β hydrogen atom of lanosterol, probably occurs before the demethylations at C-4 (Gibbons and Mitropoulos, 1975).

7.6.3 Demethylations at C-4

The gem-dimethyl groups at C-4 of lanosterol are removed as CO_2 during the formation of cholesterol in animal tissues, both demethylations requiring O_2, NADPH, NAD and at least three microsomal enzymes. The sequence of reactions (Fig. 4.15), elucidated mainly in Gaylor's laboratory (Gaylor, 1972), begins with the oxidation of the

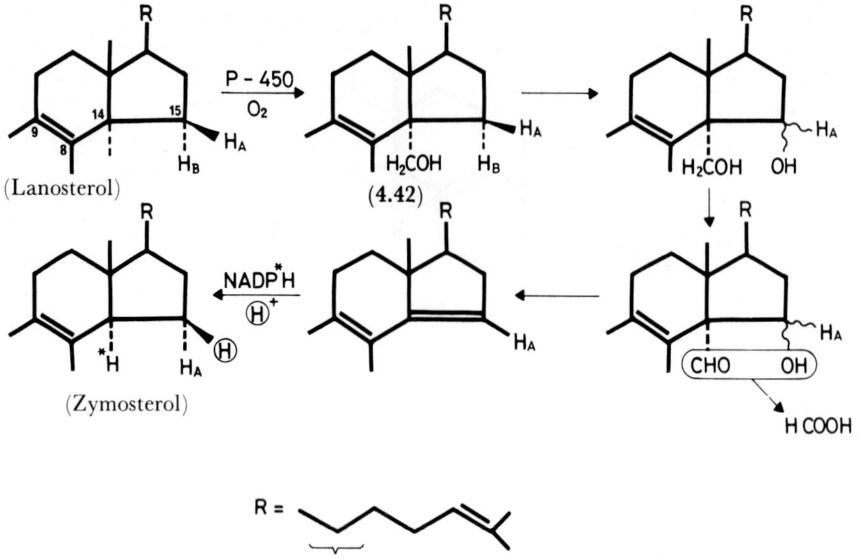

210   The Biology of Cholesterol and Related Steroids

Figure 4.14
A possible sequence of steps by which the 14α methyl group of lanosterol is removed during the biosynthesis of cholesterol. The 14α methyl is hydroxylated, C-32 eventually leaving as formic acid with the formation of a Δ^{14} double bond. The 15α hydrogen atom is replaced by a hydroxyl group. There is no direct evidence as to the stage at which the 15 hydroxylation occurs, but the stereochemistry of the reduction of the Δ^{14} double bond has been established (see text). Note that the 15β hydrogen of lanosterol becomes the 15α hydrogen of cholesterol after the formation and reduction of the Δ^{14} double bond. Compound (**4.42**) is 5α-lanosta-8,24-diene-3β, 32-diol.

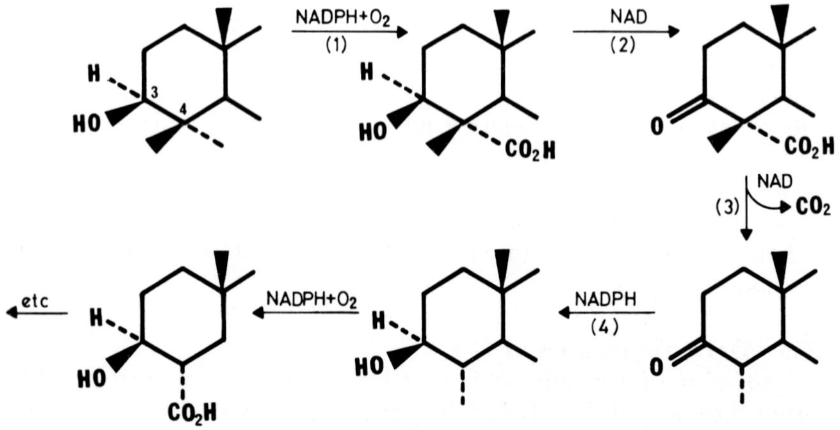

Figure 4.15
Steps in the sequential removal of the 4α and 4β methyl groups of lanosterol during the biosynthesis of cholesterol.

4α-methyl group to COOH. The 3β-OH is then oxidized to a keto group before, or simultaneously with, loss of the 4α carboxyl group as CO_2. The 3-keto group is then reduced to 3β-OH and the same sequence of reactions is repeated, leading to removal of the second 4-methyl group and, finally, reduction of the 3-keto group to 3β-OH.

Step (1) is catalyzed by a mixed-function oxidase in which cytochrome P450 is not involved (Gaylor and Mason, 1968). This enzyme (methyl sterol oxidase) acts first on the 4α-methyl group. The 4β-methyl group epimerizes to the 4α position during reaction (3) and is then oxidized by the same oxidase after the 3-keto group has been reduced. Both decarboxylations are catalyzed by the same NAD-requiring 4α-carboxylic acid decarboxylase and both reductions (step (4) and the final reduction after removal of the second methyl group) are catalyzed by a microsomal NADPH-requiring 3-ketosteroid reductase.

7.6.4 Reduction of Δ^{24}

The Δ^{24} double bond is saturated by addition of a proton from water ⓗ⁺ at the 24pro-S position, with cis addition of a hydrogen atom from NADPH at C-25:

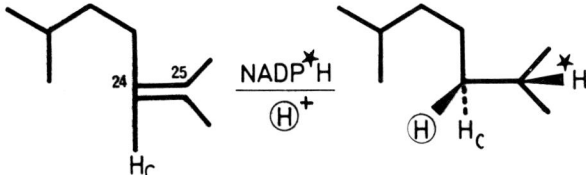

The reduction is catalyzed by a microsomal enzyme. Liver microsomes catalyze the reduction of the Δ^{24} double bond of lanosterol and of desmosterol and other Δ^{24} sterols. Since all these reductions are selectively inhibited by the same drugs, it is likely that they are catalyzed by a single Δ^{24}-reductase. If so, this enzyme must have low specificity with respect to the number and positions of nuclear double bonds and methyl groups.

7.6.5 Rearrangement of the Δ^8 double bond

Work done mainly in the laboratories of Dempsey, Schroepfer and Akhtar has shown that the rearrangement of the Δ^8 double bond to Δ^5 during the biosynthesis of cholesterol in animal tissues takes place via the sequence $\Delta^8 \rightarrow \Delta^7 \rightarrow \Delta^{5,7} \rightarrow \Delta^5$. The isomerization of Δ^8 to Δ^7 involves the addition of a proton from the medium to the 9α position and the elimination of the 7β hydrogen atom. Introduction of the Δ^5 double bond into 5α-cholest-7-en-3β-ol requires the presence of O_2 and is effected by cis elimination of the 5α and 6α hydrogen atoms. Saturation of the Δ^7 double bond of the $\Delta^{5,7}$ dienol requires NADPH

212   The Biology of Cholesterol and Related Steroids

and involves the *trans* addition of a proton from the medium to the 8β position and of a hydrogen atom from NADPH to the 7α position. The net effect of these changes (Fig. 4.16) is an inversion of the configuration of the hydrogen originally present in the 7α position of lanosterol.

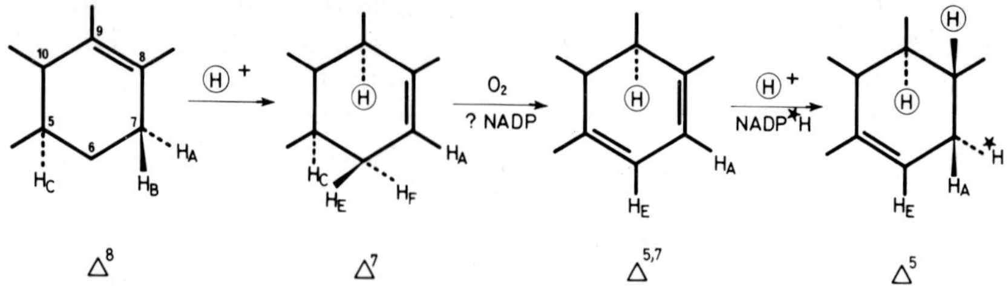

Figure 4.16
Steps in the isomerization of the Δ^8 double bond to Δ^5 in the final stage of the biosynthesis of cholesterol. Ring B is shown. Ⓗ⁺, hydrogen ion from the medium; H*, hydrogen from NADPH. H_A, H_B, H_C, H_E and H_F are as in Fig. 4.17.

The Δ^8 isomerase and the enzyme catalyzing the formation of the Δ^5 double bond in rat liver are microsomal; the reduction of the Δ^7 double bond is catalyzed by a microsomal enzyme that is inhibited by the drug AY-9944.

7.7   Summary of the origins of the carbon and hydrogen atoms of lanosterol and cholesterol biosynthesized from mevalonic acid

Figure 4.17 shows the origin of the C and H in lanosterol and cholesterol derived from mevalonic acid. The origin of the carbon atoms of lanosterol, as determined from the pattern of labelling with ^{14}C incorporated from specifically labelled [^{14}C]mevalonate, is shown in (1). In (2) and (3); H_A, H_B, H_C, H_D, H_E and H_F were originally the 2*pro-R*, 2*pro-S*, 4*pro-R*, 4*pro-S*, 5*pro-R* and 5*pro-S* hydrogen atoms of mevalonic acid, respectively.

*H atoms are derived from NADPH (or NADH); Ⓗ atoms are derived from the medium. Owing to the asymmetry in the origin of two of the central H atoms of squalene and to the fact that cyclization can begin with equal probability at either end of the molecule, the origin of the H atoms at C-11 and C-12 in half the cholesterol molecules synthesized will be that shown in Fig. 4.17 and will be the converse in the other half. In a biological system in which the reductive H of NADPH and NADH is derived ultimately from the medium, twelve of the H atoms of cholesterol synthesized from mevalonic acid should be derived from water.

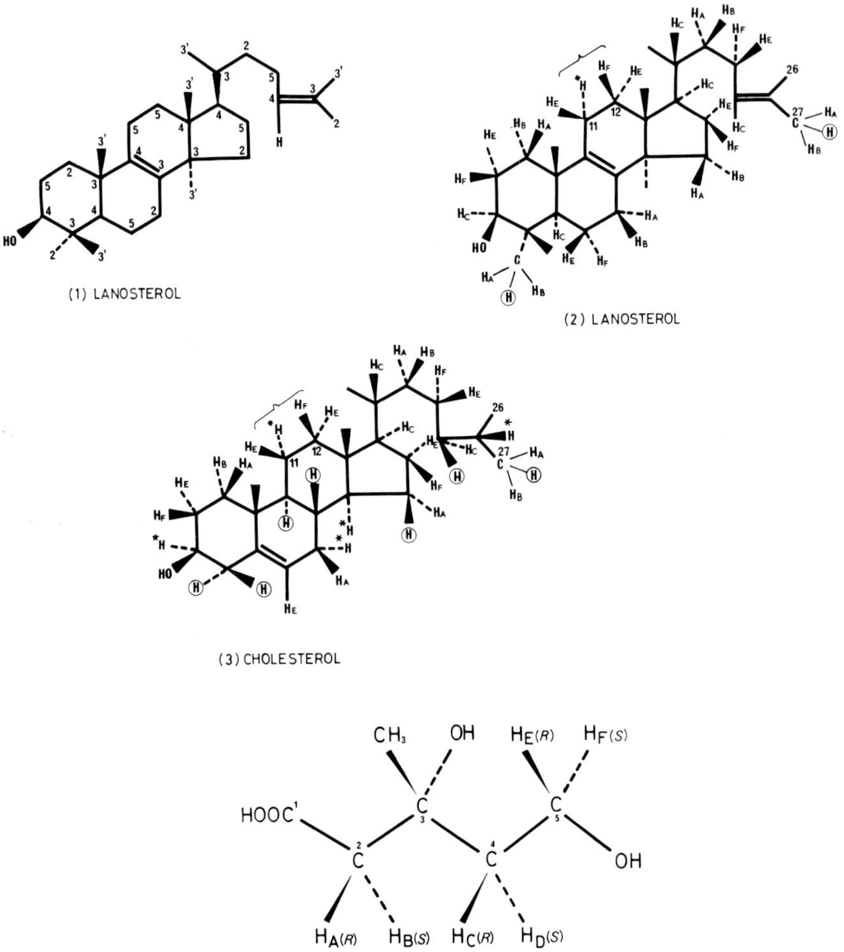

Figure 4.17
The origin of the carbon and hydrogen atoms in lanosterol and cholesterol synthesized from mevalonate. In (1) the numbers show the positions in the mevalonic acid molecule from which each carbon atom arises. In (2) and (3) the hydrogen atoms are labelled in accordance with their origin from NADPH or NADH (*H), from the medium Ⓗ and from C-2, C-4 and C-5 of mevalonic acid (see formula of mevalonic acid in text).

7.8 Sterol carrier proteins

Dempsey (1974) has shown that the cytosol of liver contains a heat-stable non-catalytic protein (squalene and sterol carrier protein, SCP) that stimulates the synthesis of cholesterol from its water-insoluble precursors by washed microsomes. SCP from rat liver has been purified (M.W. of the protomer, 16 000) and has been shown to have a high affinity for all the intermediates in the biosynthetic pathway from squalene to cholesterol, and also for other lipids. Proteins with the properties of SCP have been found in animal tissues other than liver and in protozoa. Another protein that stimulates the conversion of squalene into cholesterol by liver microsomes *in vitro* has been described by Scallen *et al.* (1971), but this protein is heat-labile and appears to be confined to the liver. Unfortunately, it is also referred to as SCP. Other proteins with SCP-like activity include the apoprotein of low-density lipoprotein (apoLDL), apoA-II, apoA-I and a heat-stable protein present in adrenal mitochondria that stimulates the enzymic conversion of cholesterol into pregnenolone.

Dempsey suggests that SCP acts by forming water-soluble complexes with water-insoluble sterol precursors, thus facilitating their transport from one membrane-bound enzyme to the next in the biosynthetic sequence. This seems a very reasonable interpretation of the effects of SCP and other proteins on the synthesis of sterols from exogenous precursors added to suspensions of microsomes. However, a similar role for SCP in the intact living cell has yet to be demonstrated conclusively.

7.9 Polyprenols

Acyclic polyisoprenoid alcohols containing up to 23 isoprenoid units, the *polyprenols*, are widely distributed in nature, occurring in bacteria (see Section 8.3.3), fungi, plants and animal tissues. Among the most carefully studied are the *dolichols*, which are polyprenols containing both *trans* and *cis* double bonds. Their general formula is

$$R - \left[CH_2 . \underset{cis}{C} = CH . CH_2 \right]_{n-4} - CH_2 . \underset{\alpha}{CH} . CH_2 . CH_2OH$$

where R = farnesyl (with 3 *trans* double bonds) and n = 17 to 22. Note that the terminal isoprenol (α) is saturated. Dolichols are present in many animal tissues and have also been isolated from plants and yeast.

Though they are not sterols, their biosynthesis is close enough to that of the acyclic precursors of sterols to warrant a brief mention in this section (see Hemming, 1970 for a review). Observations on the incorporation of stereospecifically labelled mevalonic acid into dolichols in rat liver have shown that the first stage in the biosynthetic sequence is the formation of all-*trans* farnesyl PP by the pathway described in Section 7.4, with loss of the 2*pro-R* hydrogen of isopentenyl PP both during its isomerization to dimethylallyl PP and during the sequential addition of two isopentenyl units to form

The Biosynthesis of Sterols 215

farnesyl PP with 3 *trans* double bonds. In the further elongation of the polyisoprenoid chain the addition of isopentenyl units is accompanied by loss of the 2*pro-S* hydrogen, resulting in the formation of *cis* double bonds, as in the formation of rubber (see Section 7.4.2). The final product of chain elongation is probably a dolichyl monophosphate, which then acts as a carrier for transferring oligosaccharide units to nascent proteins to form N-glycosidic glycoproteins, the free dolichol being formed as a by-product by hydrolysis of dolichyl monophosphate (Hemming, 1977).

8 COMPARATIVE ASPECTS OF STEROL SYNTHESIS

8.1 Plants

8.1.1 The formation of cycloartenol

Green plants and most algae synthesize sterols from mevalonic acid *via* 2,3-oxidosqualene, but the product of cyclization is cycloartenol (**4.43**), not lanosterol. In cycloartenol biosynthesized from (4*R*)-[2-^{14}C, 4-^{3}H$_1$]mevalonic acid the T:^{14}C ratio (T = ^{3}H) is 6:6 (not 5:6 as in lanosterol; see p. 204), one of the six tritium atoms occupying the 8β position (Rees *et al.*, 1968). This may be explained by cyclization of 2,3-oxidosqualene in chair-boat-chair-boat conformation to give the cationic protosterol formed in animal tissues (Fig. 4.10 (**7**)), followed by a backward rearrangement terminated by migration of a hydrogen atom from 9β to 8β and expulsion of a proton from C-19 to give the cyclopropane ring (Fig. 4.18). The cyclase (2,3-oxidosqualene:cycloartenol-cyclase) (EC 5.4.99.8) has been obtained in soluble form from the alga *Ochromonas malhamensis*.

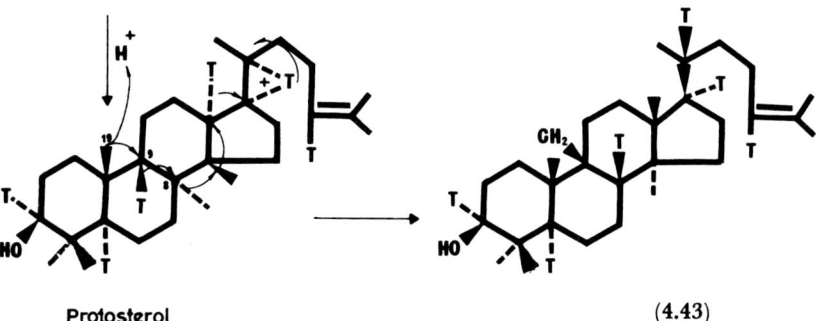

Figure 4.18
The formation of cycloartenol (**4.43**) from the cationic sterol formed by the cyclization of 2,3-oxidosqualene in plant tissues. The 9β hydrogen atom of the cationic protosterol migrates to the 8β position and a bond is formed between C-19 and C-9 with loss of a proton from C-19.

8.1.2 Conversion of cycloartenol into phytosterols

The formation of a phytosterol from cycloartenol requires opening of the cyclopropane ring, removal of the C-4 and C-14 methyl groups, alkylation at C-24, the formation of a nuclear double bond and, in some cases, the formation of a *trans* Δ^{22} double bond.

The structures of many naturally occurring potential precursors of plant sterols suggest that there are multiple pathways from cycloartenol to phytosterols. A possible metabolic route to β-sitosterol, with a branch point to campesterol, is shown in Fig. 4.19. All the inter-

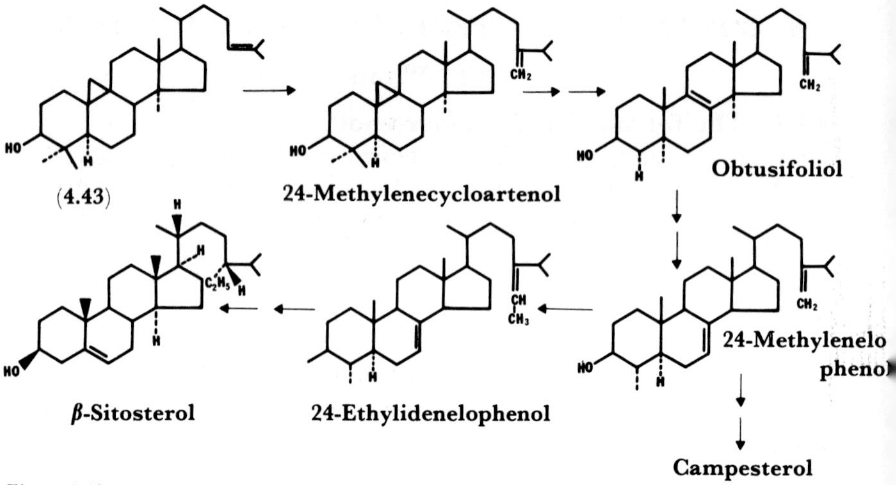

Figure 4.19
Probable steps in the conversion of cycloartenol (**4.43**) into β-sitosterol.

mediates shown in this scheme, and many other likely ones not included, have been identified in plants. Evidence in support of some of the steps postulated has also been obtained from experiments with labelled compounds. The C-24 alkyl group arises by transmethylation from methionine, a second methylation being required for the formation of 24-ethylidene or 24-ethyl sterols.

Since lanosterol is not found in green plants (other than those of the genus *Euphorbia*), it is likely that the cholesterol present in many green plants is usually formed from cycloartenol by a pathway in which alkylation at C-24 is omitted.

8.1.3 Other plant steroids

Sapogenins, the C_{27} steroid components of saponins (see Chapter 3), are synthesized in certain plants from mevalonic acid *via* cycloartenol and cholesterol without cleavage of the cholesterol side-chain. Cardenolides, the C_{23} steroidal aglycones of cardiotonic glycosides such as digoxin, are synthesized from sterol (probably cholesterol) in the leaves of *Digitalis sp.* and other plants. Cleavage of the cholesterol side-chain gives pregnenolone (C_{21}) and then progesterone (**4.44**). Progesterone is converted into a cardenolide, e.g. (**4.45**), by addition to the side-chain of two carbon atoms, not derived from mevalonic acid, and various other modifications. The *cis* A/B ring junction is probably formed by saturation of the Δ^4 double bond of progesterone with the formation of the 5β steroid. The mechanism of the formation of the unusual *cis* C/D ring junction by 14β-hydroxylation is not understood.

(**4.44**)   Digoxigenin   (**4.45**)

8.1.4 Biosynthesis of carotenes

Though carotenoids are not sterols, their formation in plants is worth mentioning here because the early intermediates in sterol biosynthesis also lie on the pathway to carotenoids. In the biosynthesis of carotenoids, an additional isopentenyl PP unit is added to farnesyl PP, giving geranylgeranyl PP (C_{20}). Two units of geranylgeranyl PP then form phytoene (**4.46**) by head-to-head condensation. Phytoene is

(**4.46**)

converted into carotenes by stepwise desaturation, followed by cyclization at one or both ends of the carbon chain in the formation of cyclic carotenoids. The mechanism of the condensation of the two units of geranylgeranyl PP is different from that of farnesyl PP in the formation of squalene. The former does not require NADPH and leads to the formation of a central double bond.

8.2 Sterols of fungi (mycosterols)

Yeasts and other fungi synthesize their sterols from mevalonic acid *via* lanosterol. The metabolic pathway to lanosterol is identical with that followed in animal tissues. The conversion of lanosterol into ergosterol (**4.47**) requires the removal of the C-4 and C-14 methyl groups, addition of a methyl group at C-24, saturation of Δ^8 and the formation of Δ^5, Δ^7 and Δ^{22} double bonds. The structures of naturally occurring potential intermediates in ergosterol biosynthesis indicate that, as in plants, there are multiple pathways in the final stages of sterol synthesis in fungi. The presence of zymosterol (**4.48**) in yeast suggests that methylation of the side-chain does not occur until the three nuclear demethylations have taken place. However, the presence of 24-methylenelanosterol in some fungi, together with the results of experiments with labelled intermediates (Barton *et al.*, 1973), suggests that transmethylation at C-24 can also occur before demethylation of lanosterol.

(4.48) $\longrightarrow$? $\longrightarrow$ (4.47)

8.3 Insects and other invertebrate animals

8.3.1 Insects

Insects cannot synthesize sterols, the metabolic block occurring between farnesyl PP and squalene. Nevertheless, they have an absolute requirement for cholesterol as a structural constituent of their cells and as a precursor for the formation of hormones and other steroid metabolites such as 'defence substances'. Most insects cannot grow or undergo metamorphosis unless cholesterol, or a sterol precursor of cholesterol, is present in the diet. The only exceptions are insects that obtain their sterol from symbiotic micro-organisms. Carnivorous insects obtain their cholesterol ready-made from their diet. However, many plant-eating and omnivorous insects can convert phytosterols into cholesterol by removal of the alkyl group at C-24 and, in some cases, saturation at Δ^{22}. The tobacco hornworm (*Manduca sexta*), a very versatile insect int this respect, converts phytosterols with at least seven different types of side-chain into cholesterol. Some omnivorous insects, including the house-fly, cannot use phytosterols as substitutes for cholesterol and therefore have an absolute dietary requirement for cholesterol. Dealkylation of phytosterols by insects probably involves the intermediate formation of fucosterol or isofucosterol, followed by formation of the 24,28-epoxide before removal of the C-28,29 unit.

One of the functions of cholesterol in insects is to act as a precursor of ecdysone (**3.3**) and its hydroxylated derivatives. The enzymes required for the formation of ecdysone are known to be present in the prothoracic glands of insects, but the metabolic pathway has not been fully elucidated. The conversion of cholesterol into 7-dehydrocholesterol, and of 7-dehydrocholesterol into ecdysone, has been demonstrated in several insect species, suggesting that the introduction of a Δ^7 double bond into cholesterol is the first step in the formation of moulting hormones in most insects. However, insects of at least two species lack a sterol 7-desaturase; these insects have an absolute requirement for dietary Δ^7 or $\Delta^{5,7}$ sterols. Studies of the incorporation of potential labelled intermediates into ecdysones suggest that the nuclear substituents are introduced before the side-chain is hydroxylated.

Certain beetles are able to convert sterols into C_{21} and C_{19} steroids, including deoxycorticosterone and testosterone. These substances are secreted by the insect as a means of defence against predators. Defence substances have marked pharmacological effects on the predator. In some cases, for instance, the prey is vomited out immediately after being eaten.

It is worth noting that although insects are unable to synthesize sterols, many of them can synthesize isoprenoids from acetate or mevalonic acid. An example is the group of substances known as juvenile hormones, so called because they maintain the larva in an immature state after moulting. The carbon skeleton of a juvenile hormone is essentially that of an alkylated farnesane (C_{15}) built from three isoprenoid units.

Pheromones, a fascinating group of substances secreted as trail-laying or assembling signals by social insects, or as sex attractants, are usually isoprenoids. Some of these have been shown to be synthesized in the insect from mevalonate, but some are present in plants. They may therefore be obtained by plant-eating insects from the diet and stored until their secretion is called for.

More detailed information about the origin and metabolism of sterols and other polyisoprenoids in insects will be found in Clayton (1964), Thompson *et al.* (1973), Nes and McKean (1977) and *Terpenoids and Steroids*. (See Chapter 1 for reference.)

Other arthropods, including spiders, shrimps and crabs are also incapable of synthesizing sterols *de novo*, though some crustaceans can dealkylate the side-chain of C_{28} and C_{29} dietary sterols to form cholesterol.

8.3.2 Other invertebrates

Many invertebrates, including molluscs, echinoderms and annelids have been shown to synthesize sterols from mevalonic acid. In some of the echinoderms that have been most carefully investigated, the major sterols synthesized are cholesterol and 5α-cholest-7-en-3β-ol. Some echinoderms are also capable of introducing a $\Delta^{9(11)}$ double bond into the sterol ring, but the numerous sterols with modified side-chains found in many marine invertebrates presumably arise from the diet, with or without minor modification of the ring system after ingestion by the animal. None of the sponges so far investigated has been shown unequivocally to synthesize sterols *de novo*, though at least one species seems to be capable of synthesizing squalene from mevalonate.

8.3.3 Bacteria

Almost all bacteria that have been examined contain little or no sterol and none has been shown to synthesize sterol from simple precursors. However, many bacteria possess the enzymic machinery for synthesizing isoprenoid units and for building these into acyclic polyprenyl pyrophosphates with up to eleven isoprenoid units (C_{55}). These polyprenols are thought to play an essential role as carriers of the carbohydrate components of the cell walls of all bacteria.

REFERENCES

Agnew, W. S. and Popják, G. (1978). Squalene synthetase. Solubilization from yeast microsomes of a phospholipid-requiring enzyme. *Journal of Biological Chemistry*, **253**, 4574–4583.

Akhtar, M., Alexander, K., Boar, R. B., McGhie, J. F. and Barton, D. H. R. (1978). Chemical and enzymic studies on the characterization of intermediates during the removal of the 14α-methyl group in cholesterol biosynthesis. *Biochemical Journal*, **169**, 449–463.

Akhtar, M., Watkinson, I. A., Rahim-Tulla, A. D., Wilton, D. C. and Munday, K. A. (1969). The role of a cholesta-8,14-dien-3β-ol system in cholesterol biosynthesis. *Biochemical Journal*, **111**, 757–761.

Alexander, K., Akhtar, M., Boar, R. B., McGhie, J. F. and Barton, D. H. R. (1972). The removal of the 32-carbon atom as formic acid in cholesterol biosynthesis. *Journal of the Chemical Society Chemical Communications*, 383–385.

Arigoni, D. Steric aspects of the biosynthesis of terpenes and steroids. In: *Steric Aspects of the Chemistry and Biochemistry of Natural Products*, Biochemical Society Symposium No. 19. Ed. J. K. Grant and W. Klyne, pp. 32–45, 30 June 1959.

Barnes, C. S., Barton, D. H. R., Fawcett, J. S., Knight, S. K., McGhie, J. F., Pradham, M. K. and Thomas, B. R. (1951). The nature of the lanosterol side chain. *Chemistry and Industry*, 1067–1068.

Barton, D. H. R., Corries, J. E. T., Mrs. Marshall, P. J. and Widdowson, D. A. (1973). Biosynthesis of terpenes and steroids. VII. Unified scheme for the

biosynthesis of ergosterol in Saccharomyces cerevisiae. *Bioorganic Chemistry*, **2**, 363–373.
Barton, D. ·H. R., Mellows, G., Widdowson, D. A. and Wright, J. J. (1971). Biosynthesis of terpenes and steroids. Part IV. Specific hydride shifts in the biosynthesis of lanosterol and β-amyrin. *Journal of the Chemical Society* (C), 1142–1148.
Bloch, K. (1952). Biological synthesis of cholesterol. *Harvey Lectures*, **48**, 68–88.
Bloch, K. (1953). The origin of carbon atom 7 in cholesterol. A contribution to the knowledge of the biosynthesis of steroids. *Helvetica Chimica Acta*, **36**, 1611–1614.
Bloch, K. (1957). The biological synthesis of cholesterol. *Vitamins and Hormones*, **XV**, 119–150.
Bloch, K. (1965). The biological synthesis of cholesterol. *Science*, **150**, 19–28.
Bonner, J. and Arreguin, B. (1949). The biochemistry of rubber formation in the Guayule. I. Rubber formation in seedlings. *Archives of Biochemistry*, **21**, 109–124.
Brady, R. O. and Gurin, S. (1951). The synthesis of radioactive cholesterol and fatty acids *in vitro*. *Journal of Biological Chemistry*, **189**, 371–377.
Brodie, J. D., Wasson, G. and Porter, J. W. (1964). Enzyme-bound intermediates in the biosynthesis of mevalonic and palmitic acids. *Journal of Biological Chemistry*, **239**, 1346–1356.
Bucher, N. L. R. and McGarrahan, K. (1956). The biosynthesis of cholesterol from acetate-1-C^{14} by cellular fractions of rat liver. *Journal of Biological Chemistry*, **222**, 1–15.
Bucher, N. L. R., Overath, P. and Lynen, F. (1960). β-hydroxy-β-methylglutaryl coenzyme A reductase, cleavage and condensing enzymes in relation to cholesterol formation in rat liver. *Biochimica et Biophysica Acta*, **40**, 491–501.
Burch, R. E., Rudney, H. and Irias, J. J. (1964). The activation and metabolism of β-hydroxy-β-methylglutaric acid. *Journal of Biological Chemistry*, **239**, 4111–4116.
Canonica, L., Ficchi, A., Kienle, M. G., Scala, A., Galli, G., Paoletti, E. G. and Paoletti, R. (1968). The fate of the 15β hydrogen of lanosterol in cholesterol biosynthesis. *Journal of the American Chemical Society*, **90**, 3597–3598.
Caspi, E., Greig, J. B. and Zander, J. M. (1968). The biosynthesis of tetrahymanol *in vitro*. *Biochemical Journal*, **109**, 931–932.
Channon, H. J. (1926). The biological significance of the unsaponifiable matter of oils. I. Experiments with the unsaturated hydrocarbon, squalene (spinacene). *Biochemical Journal*, **20**, 400–408.
Clayton, R. B. (1964). The ultilization of sterols by insects. *Journal of Lipid Research*, **5**, 3–19.
Clayton, R. B. and Bloch, K. (1956). The biological conversion of lanosterol to cholesterol. *Journal of Biological Chemistry*, **218**, 319–325.
Clinkenbeard, K. D., Sugiyama, T., Moss, J., Reed, W. D. and Lane, M. D. (1973). Molecular and catalytic properties of cytosolic acetoacetyl coenzyme A thiolase from avian liver. *Journal of Biological Chemistry*, **248**, 2275–2284.
Connolly, J. D. Triterpenoids. In: *Terpenoids and Steroids, Specialist Periodical Reports of the Chemical Society*, Vol. 2. Burlington House, London, pp. 155–179, 1972.
Corey, E. J. and Russey, W. E. (1966). Metabolic fate of 10,11-dihydrosqualene in sterol-producing rat liver homogenate. *Journal of the American Chemical Society*, **88**, 4751–4752.
Corey, E. J., Russey, W. E. and Ortiz de Montellano, P. R. (1966). 2,3-Oxidosqualene, an intermediate in the biological synthesis of sterols from squalene. *Journal of the American Chemical Society*, **88**, 4750–4751.
Cornforth, J. W. (1959). Biosynthesis of fatty acids and cholesterol considered as chemical processes. *Journal of Lipid Research*, **1**, 3–28.
Cornforth, J. W. (1973). The logic of working with enzymes. *Chemical Society Reviews*, **2**, 1–20.

Cornforth, J. W., Clifford, K., Mallaby, R. and Phillips, G. T. (1972). Stereochemistry of isopentenyl pyrophosphate isomerase. *Proceedings of the Royal Society of London, B*, **182**, 277–295.

Cornforth, J. W. and Cornforth, R. H. Chemistry of mevalonic acid. In: *Natural substances formed biologically from mevalonic acid*, Biochemical Society Symposium, Vol. 29. Ed. T. W. Goodwin, pp. 5–15, 1970.

Cornforth, J. W., Cornforth, R. H., Donninger, C., Popják, G., Shimizu, Y., Ichii, S., Forchielli, E. and Caspi, E. (1965). The migration and elimination of hydrogen during biosynthesis of cholesterol from squalene. *Journal of the American Chemical Society*, **87**, 3224–3228.

Cornforth, J. W., Cornforth, R. H., Pelter, A., Horning, M. G. and Popják, G. (1958*b*). Rearrangement of methyl groups in the enzymic cyclization of squalene to lanosterol. *Proceedings of the Chemical Society*, 112–113.

Cornforth, J. W., Cornforth, R. H., Popják, G. and Youhotsky-Gore, I. (1957). Biosynthesis of squalene and cholesterol from DL-β-hydroxy-β-methyl-δ-[2-^{14}C]valerolactone. *Biochemical Journal*, **66**, 10P.

Cornforth, J. W., Cornforth, R. H., Popják, G. and Gore, I. Y. (1958*a*). Studies on the biosynthesis of cholesterol. 5. Biosynthesis of squalene from DL-3-hydroxy-3-methyl-[2-^{14}C]pentano-5-lactone. *Biochemical Journal*, **69**, 146–155.

Cornforth, J. W., Gore, I. Y. and Popják, G. (1957). Studies on the biosynthesis of cholesterol. 4. Degradation of rings C and D. *Biochemical Journal*, **65**, 94–109.

Cornforth, J. W., Hunter, G. D. and Popják, G. (1953). Studies of cholesterol biosynthesis. 2. Distribution of acetate carbon in the ring structure. *Biochemical Journal*, **54**, 597–601.

Cornforth, J. W. and Popják, G. (1954). Studies on the biosynthesis of cholesterol. 3. Distribution of ^{14}C in squalene biosynthesized from [*Me*-^{14}C]acetate. *Biochemical Journal*, **58**, 403–407.

Cornforth, J. W. and Popják, G. Chemical syntheses of substrates of sterol biosynthesis. In: *Methods of Enzymology*, Vol. 15. Ed. R. B. Clayton. Academic Press, New York, pp. 357–390, 1969.

Cornforth, J. W. and Ross, F. P. (1970). Synthesis of 5*S*-5-[^{3}H$_1$]mevalonic acid. *Chemical Communications*, 1395–1396.

Dean, P. D. G. Enzymatic cyclization of squalene 2,3-oxide. In: *Methods in Enzymology, Vol. 15*. Ed. R. B. Clayton. Academic Press, New York, pp. 495–501, 1969.

Dean, P. D. G. (1971). The cyclases of triterpene and sterol biosynthesis. *Steroidologia*, **2**, 143–157.

Dempsey, M. E. (1974). Regulation of steroid biosynthesis. *Annual Review of Biochemistry*, **43**, 967–990.

Edmond, J., Popják, G., Wong, S.-M. and Williams, V. P. (1971). Presqualene alcohol. Further evidence on the structure of a C_{30} precursor of squalene. *Journal of Biological Chemistry*, **246**, 6254–6271.

Edwards, P. A., Lemongello, D., Kane, J., Schechter, I. and Fogelman, A. M. (1980). Properties of purified rat hepatic 3-hydroxy-3-methylglutaryl coenzyme A reductase and regulation of enzyme activity. *Journal of Biological Chemistry*, **255**, 3715–3725.

Eschenmoser, A., Ružička, L., Jeger, O. and Arigoni, D. (1955). Zur Kenntnis der Triterpene. Eine stereochemische Interpretation der biogenetischen Isoprenregel bei den Triterpenen. *Helvetica Chimica Acta*, **38**, 1890–1904.

Evans, E. A. Tritium and Its Compounds. 2nd Edition. Butterworths, London, 1974.

Ferguson, J. J., Durr, I. F., and Rudney, H. (1959). The biosynthesis of mevalonic acid. *Proceedings of the National Academy of Sciences of the USA*, **45**, 499–504.

Fogelman, A. M., Edmond, J. and Popják, G. (1975). Metabolism of mevalonate in rats and man not leading to sterols. *Journal of Biological Chemistry*, **250**, 1771–1775.

Folkers, K., Shunk, C. H., Linn, B. O., Robinson, F. M., Wittreich, P. E., Huff, J. W., Gilfillan, J. L. and Skeggs, H. R. Discovery and elucidation of mevalonic acid. In: *Biosynthesis of Terpenes and Sterols*, Ciba Foundation Symposium. Ed. G. E. W. Wolstenholme and C. M. O'Connor, pp. 20–43, 1959.

Frantz, I. D. and Schroepfer, G. J. (1967). Sterol biosynthesis. *Annual Review of Biochemistry*, **36**, 691–726.

Gautschi, F. and Bloch, K. (1957). On the structure of an intermediate in the biological demethylation of lanosterol. *Journal of the American Chemistry Society*, **79**, 684–689.

Gautschi, F. and Bloch, K. (1958). Synthesis of isomeric 4,4-dimethylcholestenols and identification of a lanosterol metabolite. *Journal of Biological Chemistry*, **233**, 1343–1347.

Gaylor, J. L. (1972). Microsomal enzymes of sterol biosynthesis. *Advances in Lipid Research*, **10**, 89–141.

Gaylor, J. L. and Mason, H. S. (1968). Investigation of the component reactions of oxidative sterol demethylation. Evidence against participation of cytochrome P-450. *Journal of Biological Chemistry*, **243**, 4966–4972.

Gibbons, G. F., Goad, L. J. and Goodwin, T. W. (1968). The sterochemistry of hydrogen elimination from C-15 during cholesterol biosynthesis. *Chemical Communications*, 1458–1460.

Gibbons, G. F. and Mitropoulos, K. A. (1973). The rôle of cytochrome P-450 in cholesterol biosynthesis. *European Journal of Biochemistry*, **40**, 267–273.

Gibbons, G. F. and Mitropoulos, K. A. (1975). Effect of trans-1,4-bis (2-chlorobenzyl-aminomethyl) cyclohexane dihydrochloride and carbon monoxide on hepatic cholesterol biosynthesis from 4,4-dimethyl sterols *in vitro*. *Biochimica et Biophysica Acta*, **380**, 270–281.

Gibbons, G. F., Pullinger, C. R. and Mitropoulos, K. A. (1979). Studies on the mechanism of 14α-demethylation. A requirement for two distinct types of mixed-function oxidase systems. *Biochemical Journal*, **183**, 309–315.

Goad, J. L. Sterol biosynthesis. In: *Natural Substances Formed Biologically From Mevalonic Acid, Biochemical Society Symposia, No. 29*. Ed. T. W. Goodwin, pp. 45–77, 1970.

Heilbron, I. M., Hilditch, T. P. and Kamm, E. D. (1926). The unsaponifiable matter from the oils of elasmobranch fish. Part II. The hydrogenation of squalene in the presence of nickel. *Journal of the Chemical Society*, 3131–3136.

Hemming, F. W. Polyprenols. In: *Natural Substances Formed Biologically From Mevalonic Acid, Biochemical Society Symposia, No. 29*. Ed. T. W. Goodwin, pp. 105–117, 1970.

Hemming, F. W. (1977). The rôle of polyprenol-linked sugars in eukaryotic macro-molecular synthesis. *Biochemical Society Transactions*, **5**, 1682–1687.

Higgins, M. J. P. and Kekwick, R. G. O. (1973). An investigation into the role of malonyl-coenzyme A in isoprenoid biosynthesis. *Biochemical Journal*, **134**, 295–310.

Kawachi, T. and Rudney, H. (1970). Solubilization and purification of β-hydroxy-β-methylglutaryl Coenzyme A reductase from rat liver. *Biochemistry*, **9**, 1700–1705.

Langdon, R. G. and Bloch, K. (1953a). The biosynthesis of squalene. *Journal of Biological Chemistry*, **200**, 129–134.

Langdon, R. G. and Bloch, K. (1953b). The utilization of squalene in the biosynthesis of cholesterol. *Journal of Biological Chemistry*, **200**, 135–144.

Lynen, F. (1967). Biosynthetic pathways from acetate to natural products. *Pure and Applied Chemistry*, **14**, 137–167.

Lynen, F., Knappe, J., Eggerer, H., Henning, U. and Agranoff, B. W. (1959). Biosynthesis of terpenes. *Federation Proceedings*, **18**, 278.

Maudgal, R. K., Tchen, T. T. and Bloch, K. (1958). 1,2-Methyl shifts in the cyclization of squalene to lanosterol. *Journal of the American Chemical Society*, **80**, 2589–2590.

Mulheirn, L. J. and Caspi, E. (1971). Mechanism of squalene cyclization. Biosynthesis of fusidic acid. *Journal of Biological Chemistry*, **246**, 2494–2501.
Nes, W. R. and McKean, M. L. *Biochemistry of Steroids and Other Isopentenoids*. University Park Press, Baltimore, 1977.
Olson, J. A., Lindberg, M. and Bloch, K. (1957). On the demethylation of lanosterol to cholesterol. *Journal of Biological Chemistry*, **226**, 941–956.
Ono, T. and Bloch, K. (1975). Solubilization and partial characterization of rat liver squalene epoxidase. *Journal of Biological Chemistry*, **250**, 1571–1579.
Popják, G. Chemistry, biochemistry and isotopic tracer technique. *Royal Institute of Chemistry Lectures, Monographs and Reports*, No. 2, 59 pp, 1955.
Popják, G. Enzymes of sterol biosynthesis in liver and intermediates of sterol biosynthesis. In: *Methods in Enzymology*, Vol. 15. Ed. R. B. Clayton. Academic Press, New York, pp. 393–454, 1969.
Popják, G. (1977). As I remember it. Research on biosynthesis of fatty acids, triglycerides, squalene, and cholesterol. *Journal of the American Oil Chemists*, **54**, 647A–655A.
Popják, G. and Cornforth, J. W. (1966) Substrate stereochemistry in squalene biosynthesis. *Biochemical Journal*, **101**, 553–568.
Popják, G., Edmond, J., Anet, F. A. L. and Easton, N. R. Jr. (1977). Carbon-13 NMR studies on cholesterol biosynthesized from [^{13}C]mevalonates. *Journal of the American Chemical Society*, **99**, 931–935.
Popják, G., Ngan, H.-L. and Agnew, W. (1975). Stereochemistry of the biosynthesis of presqualene alcohol. *Bioorganic Chemistry*, **4**, 279–289.
Rees, H. H., Goad, L. J. and Goodwin, T. W. (1968). Studies in phytosterol biosynthesis. Mechanism of biosynthesis of cycloartenol. *Biochemical Journal*, **107** 417–426.
Rees, H. H. and Goodwin, T. W. Biosynthesis of triterpenes, steroids and carotenoids. *Special Periodical Reports of the Chemical Society, Biosynthesis*,Vol. 3, pp. 14–88, 1975.
Retey, J., von Stetten, E., Coy, U. and Lynen, F. (1970). A probable intermediate in the enzymic reduction of 3-hydroxy-3 methylglutaryl Coenzyme A. *European Journal of Biochemistry*, **15**, 72–76.
Rilling, H. C. (1970). Biosynthesis of presqualene pyrophosphate by liver microsomes. *Journal of Lipid Research*, **11**, 480–485.
Ritter, M. C. and Dempsey, M. E. (1971). Specificity and role in cholesterol biosynthesis of a squalene and sterol carrier protein. *Journal of Biological Chemistry*, **246**, 1536–1539.
Robinson, R. (1934). Structure of cholesterol. *Chemistry and Industry*, **53**, 1062–1063.
Rudney, H. The biosynthesis of β-hydroxy-β-methyl-glutaryl coenzyme A and its conversion to mevalonic acid. In: *Biosynthesis of Terpenes and Sterols, Ciba Foundation Symposium*. Ed. G. E. W. Wolstenholme and M. O'Connor, pp. 75–90, 1959.
Rudney, H., Stewart, P. R., Majerus, P. W. and Vagelos, P. R. (1966). The biosynthesis of β-hydroxy-β-methylglutaryl Coenzyme A in yeast. V. The role of acyl carrier protein. *Journal of Biological Chemistry*, **241**, 1226–1228.
Ružička, L. (1959). History of the isoprene rule. *Proceedings of the Chemical Society*, 341–360.
Ružička, L. (1973). In the borderland between bioorganic chemistry and biochemistry. *Annual Review of Biochemistry*, **42**, 1–20.
Ružička, L., Eschenmoser, A. and Heusser, H. (1953). The isoprene rule and the biogenesis of terpenic compounds. *Experienta*, **9**, 357–367.
Samuelsson, B. and Goodman, D. S. (1964). Stereochemistry at the center of squalene during its biosynthesis from farnesyl pyrophosphate and subsequent conversion to cholesterol. *Journal of Biological Chemistry*, **239**, 98–101.

Scallen, T. J., Schuster, M. W. and Dhar, A. K. (1971). Evidence for a noncatalytic carrier protein in cholesterol biosynthesis. *Journal of Biological Chemistry*, **246**, 224–230.
Schechter, I. and Bloch, K. (1971). Solubilization and purification of *trans*-farnesyl pyrophosphate-squalene synthetase. *Journal of Biological Chemistry*, **246**, 7690–7696.
Tai, H.-H. and Bloch, K. (1972). Squalene epoxidase of rat liver. *Journal of Biological Chemistry*, **247**, 3767–3773.
Tavormina, P. A., Gibbs, M. H. and Huff, J. W. (1956). The utilization of β-hydroxy-β-methyl-δ valerolactone in cholesterol biosynthesis. *Journal of the American Chemical Society*, **78**, 4498–4499.
Tchen, T. T. and Bloch, K. (1955). *In vitro* conversion of squalene to lanosterol and cholesterol. *Journal of the American Society*, **77**, 6085–6086.
Tchen, T. T. and Bloch, K. (1957). On the mechanism of enzymatic cyclization of squalene. *Journal of Biological Chemistry*, **226**, 931–939.
Thompson, M. J., Kaplanis, J. N., Robbins, W. E. and Svoboda, J. A. (1973). Metabolism of steroids in insects. *Advances in Lipid Research*, **11**, 219–265.
van Tamelen, E. E. and Anderson, R. J. (1972). Biogenetic-type total synthesis. 24,25-Dihydrolanosterol, 24,25-dihydro-$\Delta^{13(17)}$-protosterol, isoeuphenol, (—)-isotirucallol, and parkeol. *Journal of the American Chemical Society*, **94**, 8225–8228.
Voser, W., Mijović, M. V., Heusser, H., Jeger, P. and Ružička, L. (1952). Steroids and sex hormones. CLXXXVI. The constitution of lanostadienol (lanosterol) and its relationship to the steroids. *Helvetica Chimica Acta*, **35**, 2414–2430.
Woodward, R. B. and Bloch, K. (1953). The cyclization of squalene in cholesterol synthesis. *Journal of the American Chemical Society*, **75**, 2023–2024.
Wright, L. D., Cresson, E. L., Skeggs, H. R., MacRae, G. D. E., Hoffman, C. H., Wolf, D. E. and Folkers, K. (1956). Isolation of a new acetate-replacing factor. *Journal of the American Chemical Society*, **78**, 5273–5275.
Wüersch, J., Huang, R. L. and Bloch, K. (1952). The origin of the isoctyl side chain of cholesterol. *Journal of Biological Chemistry*, **195**, 439–446.

Chapter 5

The Metabolism of Cholesterol

1	BILE ACIDS	229
1.1	Introduction	229
1.2	Biosynthesis	230
1.2.1	Historical background	230
1.2.2	The metabolic pathways	230
1.2.3	The formation of secondary bile acids	235
1.2.4	Enzymes and reaction mechanisms.	235
1.2.4.1	Cholesterol 7α-hydroxylase.	235
1.2.4.2	Other enzymes catalyzing changes in the nucleus	236
1.2.4.3	Side-chain cleavage enzymes	237
1.2.5	Allo bile acids	241
1.2.5.1	Distribution	241
1.2.5.2	Derivation	241
1.2.6	Sulphate esters and glucuronides	242
1.3	The enterohepatic circulation of bile salts	243
1.3.1	Secretion and reabsorption	243
1.3.2	Pool size and rates of synthesis and secretion	245
1.3.3	The effect of interrupting the EHC	249
1.4	The regulation of bile-acid synthesis	252
1.4.1	Feedback inhibition by bile salts	252
1.4.2	Effects of diet.	253
1.4.3	Effects of hormones	253
1.4.4	Effects of drugs	254
1.4.4.1	Anionic exchange resins	254
1.4.4.2	Phenobarbital	255
1.4.4.3	Antimicrobial agents	256
1.4.5	Cholesterol 7α-hydroxylase	256
1.4.5.1	The 7α-hydroxylation of cholesterol as a rate-limiting step	256
1.4.5.2	The regulation of cholesterol 7α-hydroxylase activity	257
2	STEROID HORMONES	259
2.1	Introduction	259
2.1.1	Comparative aspects	259
2.1.2	Quantitative aspects	260
2.2	Biosynthesis	261
2.2.1	Adrenocortical hormones	261

2.2.1.1	The biologically active hormones	261
2.2.1.2	The metabolic pathways	261
2.2.2	Steroid hormones of the gonads and placenta.	263
2.2.2.1	Biologically active hormones	263
2.2.2.2	The metabolic pathways	263
2.2.3	Enzymes and reaction mechanisms.	267
2.2.3.1	The formation of adrenocorticoids	267
2.2.3.2	The formation of androgens and oestrogens	268
2.2.3.3	Consequences of the subcellular distribution of enzymes	268
2.2.4	Regulation of the production of steroid hormones	269
3	FORMATION OF FATTY ACYL ESTERS OF CHOLESTEROL.	273
3.1	Introduction	273
3.2	ACAT	273
3.3	Cholesteryl ester hydrolase	275
3.4	LCAT	276
3.4.1	The LCAT reaction	276
3.4.2	Distribution	277
3.4.3	Properties	277
3.4.4	Substrate specificity	278
3.4.5	Assay	279
3.4.6	Physiological function	280
4	HYDROLYSIS OF FATTY ACYL ESTERS OF CHOLESTEROL.	281
4.1	Introduction	281
4.2	Pancreas	281
4.3	Liver.	282
4.4	Artery	283
4.5	Steroid-hormone-forming tissues	284
4.6	Other tissues	284
5	5α-CHOLESTANOL	287
6	STERYL SULPHATES	287
7	VITAMIN D	288
7.1	Sterol precursors of vitamin D	288
7.2	Metabolism of vitamin D	290
7.3	Biologically active analogues of vitamin D.	291

The Metabolism of Cholesterol

Cholesterol is metabolized in animals mainly by conversion into bile acids and steroid hormones and by esterification with long-chain fatty acids. Other pathways of minor quantitative significance are the formation of cholesteryl sulphate and of various C_{27} metabolites, including 5α-cholestanol, 5β-cholestanol and 5β-cholestan-3-one. The formation of vitamin D from sterols closely related to cholesterol may also be conveniently considered in this chapter. Some of the modifications undergone by cholesterol in insects and plants have been mentioned in Chapter 4.

1 BILE ACIDS

1.1 Introduction

In rats and human beings the formation of bile acids in the liver is the major metabolic outlet for cholesterol of endogenous and exogenous origin, accounting for 80–90% of the turnover of the total exchangeable cholesterol in rats and for about half the total turnover of that in normal man. Under conditions in which bile-acid synthesis in human subjects is stimulated, up to 80% of the total exchangeable cholesterol removed from the body may be excreted as bile acids. In addition to the potential importance of bile-acid formation as a means of preventing the accumulation of excessive amounts of cholesterol in the body, cholesterol metabolism and bile-acid metabolism interact mutually. Thus, bile acids are essential for the absorption of cholesterol from the intestine and they influence the rate of synthesis of cholesterol in the liver and the intestine; conversely, in rats and animals of most other species, synthesis of bile acids is influenced by the amount of cholesterol absorbed from the diet.

In this section, the biochemistry and physiology of the bile acids are considered in relation to the metabolism of cholesterol. The role of bile acids in cholesterol absorption and in maintaining the biliary cholesterol in solution is dealt with elsewhere in this book (Chapters 10 and 18). More detailed information on bile acids will be found in several reviews (Danielsson and Einarsson, 1969; Hofmann, 1977) and monographs (Van Belle, 1965; Haslewood, 1978) and in a three-volume treatise dealing comprehensively with the chemistry, physiology and metabolism of bile acids (Nair and Kritchevsky, 1971, 1973, 1976). The comparative and evolutionary aspects of bile acids are dealt with in Haslewood's monograph (1978).

1.2 Biosynthesis

1.2.1 Historical background

The biosynthetic origin of bile acids from cholesterol was suggested by several workers in the 1920's and 1930's as it became increasingly clear that bile acids are closely related structurally to the sterols. Proof that cholesterol is, in fact, the precursor of bile acids was obtained by Bloch *et al.* (1943), who isolated deuterium-labelled cholic acid from a dog given an intravenous injection of deuterium-labelled cholesterol. The isotopic enrichment in the cholic acid approached the value to be expected if cholesterol was the sole source of cholic acid in the animal's body. Since this observation was made, the sequence of steps by which cholesterol is converted into cholic and chenodeoxycholic acids, the two primary bile acids synthesized in the livers of most mammals, has been elucidated mainly by experiments on the incorporation of radioactive hypothetical intermediates into bile acids *in vivo* and by identification of these labelled intermediates in cell-free preparations of liver incubated in the presence of radioactive cholesterol. Corroborative evidence has also been obtained by the isolation of certain intermediates in small quantities from normal bile.

1.2.2 The metabolic pathways

Inspection of the structures of cholesterol, cholic acid and chenodeoxycholic acid (Fig. 5.1) shows that the formation of a primary bile acid from cholesterol requires the oxidative cleavage of the side-chain between C-24 and C-25 to give a C_5 side-chain, the formation of a 5β saturated ring system, epimerization of the 3β-hydroxyl group and the introduction of 7α- and 12α-hydroxyl groups to give cholic acid, or of a 7α-hydroxyl group to give chenodeoxycholic acid.

The probable reactions by which the cholesterol nucleus and side-chain are modified to give cholic acid (Schemes 1 and 2) have been deduced largely from work on rats and mice. In these species, the initial step is the introduction of a 7α-hydroxyl group into the

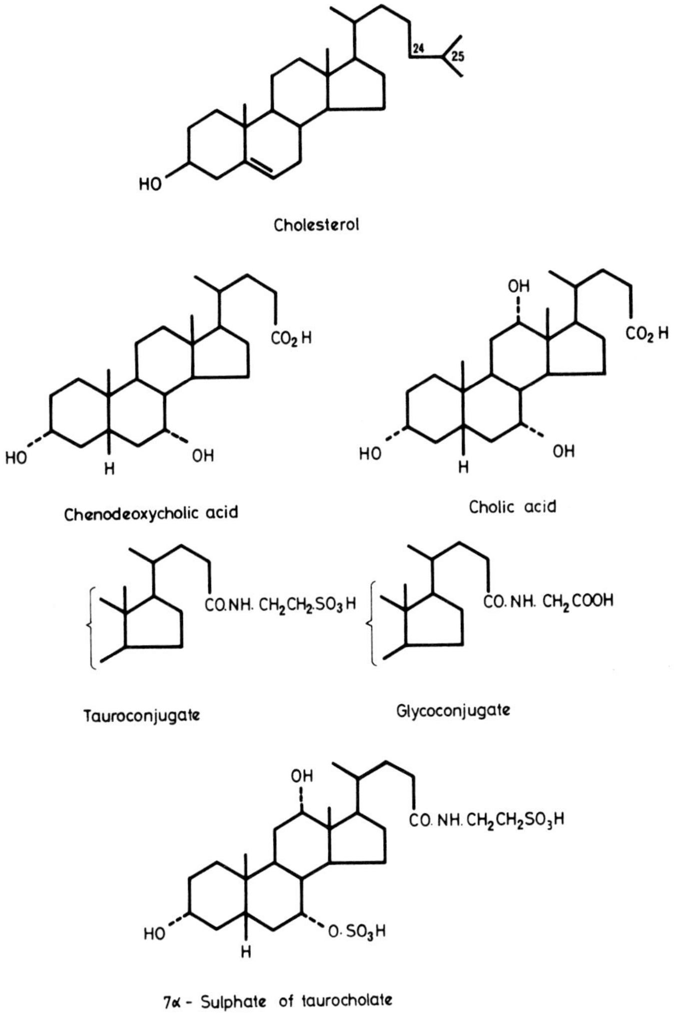

Figure 5.1
Structural formulae of cholesterol and of the primary bile acids and their conjugates. The bottom formula shows the 7α-sulphate of taurocholic acid.

cholesterol nucleus to give cholest-5-ene-3α,7α-diol (7α-hydroxycholesterol) (**5.1**). This is followed by oxidation of the 3β-OH group to a keto group and the isomerization of the Δ^5 double bond to the Δ^4 position to give 7α-hydroxycholest-4-en-3-one (**5.2**). The 3-keto steroid (**5.2**) is hydroxylated at the 12α position to give 7α,12α-dihydroxycholest-4-en-3-one (**5.3**), which is then converted into 5β-cholestane-3α,7α,12α-triol (**5.4**) by saturation of the Δ^4 double bond and reduction of the 3-keto group.

The oxidative cleavage of the side-chain (Scheme 2) is initiated by

Formula	Enzyme	Subcellular fraction	Cofactors
Cholesterol 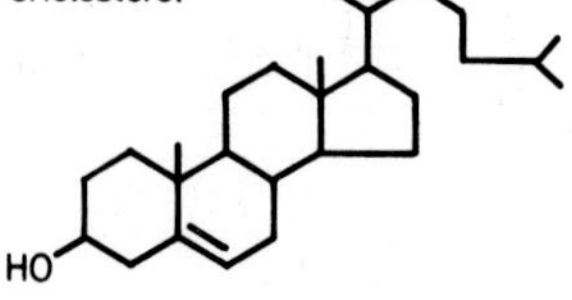			
	Cholesterol 7α-hydroxylase	Microsomal	NADPH; cytochrome P450
(5.1)	Δ⁵-3β-Hydroxy(C₂₇) steroid oxidoreductase	Microsomal	NAD or NADP
	Δ⁵-3-Ketosteroid isomerase	Microsomal	
(5.2)	12α-Hydroxylase	Microsomal	NADPH; ? cytochrome P450
(5.3)	Δ⁴-3-Ketosteroid-5β-reductase	Soluble	NADPH
	3α-Hydroxy(C₂₇)steroid ketoreductase	Soluble	NADH or NADPH
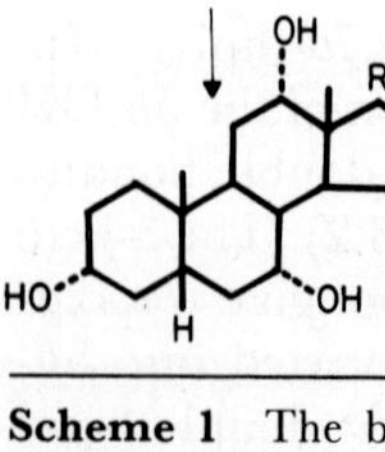 (5.4)	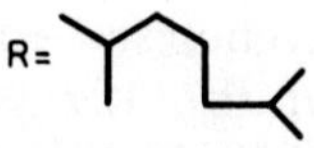 R =		

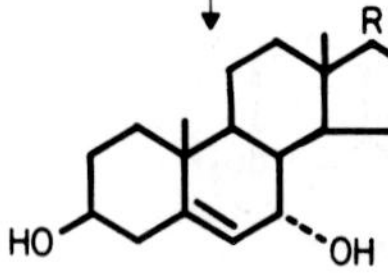

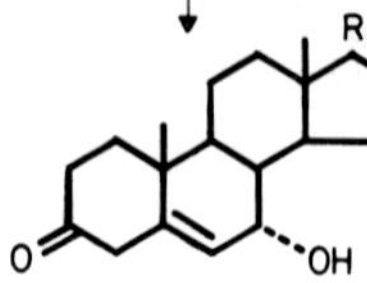

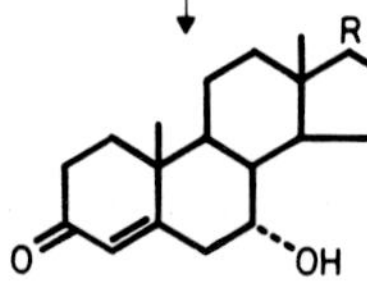

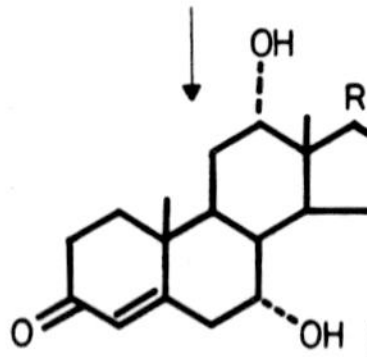

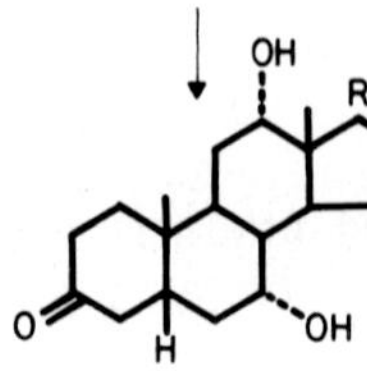

Scheme 1 The biosynthesis of bile acids; the conversion of cholesterol into 5β-cholestane-3α,7α,12α-triol.

(**5.1**), 7α-Hydroxycholesterol (cholest-5-ene-3β,7α-diol); (**5.2**), 7α-hydroxycholest-4-en-3-one; (**5.3**), 7α,12α-dihydroxycholest-4-en-3-one; (**5.4**), 5β-cholestane-3α,7α,12α-

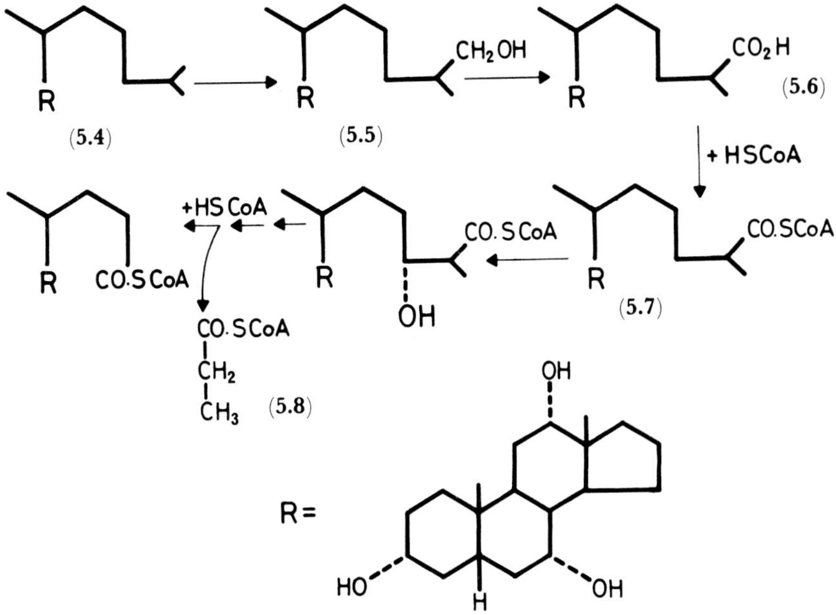

Scheme 2 The biosynthesis of bile acids; the oxidative cleavage of the side-chain of 5β-cholestane-3α,7α,12α-triol (**5.4**) to give the CoA ester of cholic acid.

(**5.5**), 5β-Cholestane-3α,7α,12α,26-tetrol; (**5.6**), 3α,7α,12α-trihydroxy-5β-cholestanoic acid; (**5.7**). cholyl-CoA; (**5.8**), propionyl-CoA.

hydroxylation of the triol (**5.4**) at C-26 to give the 3α,7α,12α,26-tetrol (**5.5**), followed by a further oxidation to give 3α,7α,12α-trihydroxy-5β-cholestanoic acid (**5.6**). The subsequent steps in the cleavage of the side-chain are thought to be those shown in Scheme 2. According to this Scheme, the trihydroxy acid (**5.6**) is esterified with CoA and the CoA ester is oxidized by a β-oxidation, ending with a thiolytic cleavage to give cholyl-CoA (**5.7**) and propionyl-CoA (**5.8**). The cholyl-CoA released by the cleavage reaction is conjugated with glycine or taurine by the formation of a peptide bond between the carboxyl carbon of cholic acid and the amino group of the amino acid.

The major pathway for the formation of chenodeoxycholic acid is similar to that shown in Schemes 1 and 2, with the exception that no 12α-hydroxylation occurs, the modification to the ring system resulting in the formation of 5β-cholestane-3α,7α-diol rather than compound (**5.4**). The side-chain of the diol is then cleaved, as in Scheme 2, to give chenodeoxycholyl-CoA. Chenodeoxycholic acid may also be formed by other minor pathways, differing from each other in the stage at which side-chain cleavage begins. In the extreme case, 26-hydroxylation occurs before the introduction of the 7α-hydroxyl group, giving cholest-5-ene-3β,26-diol (26-hydroxycholesterol). Cleavage of the side-chain may occur before further modification to the ring system, giving rise to the formation of 3β-hydroxycholest-5-enoic acid. The monohydroxy acid may then be converted into chenodeoxycholic acid by modification of the ring system (Mitropoulos and Myant, 1967) or, as in obstructive human liver disease, it may appear in the serum and urine without further modification (Makino et al., 1971). The absence of these alternative pathways for the formation of cholic acid is probably due to substrate specificity of the 12α-hydroxylase. In rats, this enzyme appears to be unable to catalyze the introduction of a 12α-hydroxyl group into substrates lacking an intact cholestane side-chain, so that once the first step in side-chain oxidation has taken place the pathway to cholic acid is closed. In some species, chenodeoxycholic acid is converted into α- and β-muricholic acids (3α,6β,7α- and 3α,6β,7β-trihydroxy-5β-cholanoic acid). Since these conversions take place in the liver, the muricholic acids may be regarded as primary bile acids.

Observations on cell-free preparations of human liver (Björkhem et al., 1968) indicate that the pathway for the conversion of cholesterol into (**5.4**) in man is broadly similar to that in rats. The presence of small amounts of 3α,7α,12α-trihydroxy-5β-cholestanoic acid in human bile (Carey and Haslewood, 1963) suggests that the major pathway for the oxidation of the side-chain in man also resembles that in rats, at least in so far as the process is initiated by an oxidation at C-26 in both species. In keeping with this, Carey (1964) has isolated radioactive 3α,7α,12α-trihydroxy-5β-cholestanoic acid from the bile of a human subject given [^{14}C]cholesterol and has shown that this acid is converted into cholic acid in man. Observations on the conversion of labelled precursors into bile acids in patients with bile fistulas suggest that, in man, small amounts of cholic and chenodeoxycholic acid are formed by alternative pathways when bile-acid synthesis is stimulated. These pathways include routes to cholic acid in which the formation of 7α-hydroxycholesterol is bypassed or the 12α-hydroxyl group is introduced after 26-hydroxylation of the side-chain, and a route to chenodeoxycholic acid involving the 26-hydroxylation of (**5.2**). (For references, see Swell et al., 1980).

Human liver homogenates also catalyze the introduction of a 25-hydroxyl group into (**5.4**). This may be the initial step in an alternative pathway for the formation of cholic acid in human liver, oxidative cleavage at C-24 giving acetone and the bile acid. In favour of the existence of this pathway for cholic-acid synthesis in man, Mosbach and his co-workers (1977) have isolated considerable amounts of the two bile alcohols, 5β-cholestane-3α,7α,12α,25-tetrol and the corresponding 3α,7α,12α,24α,25-pentol, from the bile and faeces of patients suffering from cerebrotendinous xanthomatosis.

They have also shown that the tetrol is converted into cholic acid in man. For reasons discussed in Chapter 17, the pathway to bile acids initiated by 25-hydroxylation is probably no more than a minor route uncovered only when the normal pathway via 26-hydroxylation is blocked.

1.2.3 The formation of secondary bile acids

After their secretion into the intestinal lumen, the conjugated primary bile acids are modified by the action of bacteria in the lower ileum and large intestine. These modifications include hydrolysis of the peptide bond of tauro- and glyco-conjugated bile acids and the removal of the 7α-hydroxyl group, resulting in the formation of deoxycholate from cholic acid, of lithocholate from chenodeoxycholic acid and of allodeoxycholate from allocholic acid. Other enzymic modifications brought about by intestinal bacteria include inversion of α-hydroxyl groups, oxidation of the 3α, 7α or 12α-hydroxyl group to the corresponding keto group and the inversion of the 5β hydrogen to give the 5α (allo) bile acid. As a result of these reactions, which must require the presence of several distinct bacterial enzymes, normal human faeces may contain more than twenty different bile acids, and human bile contains reabsorbed deoxycholic, lithocholic and ursodeoxycholic (3α,7β-dihydroxy) acids as well as the two primary bile acids.

1.2.4 Enzymes and reaction mechanisms

1.2.4.1 Cholesterol 7α-Hydroxylase.
The 7α-hydroxylation of cholesterol is catalyzed by cholesterol 7α-monooxygenase (cholesterol 7α-hydroxylase) (EC 1.14.13.17), a microsomal enzyme system requiring molecular oxygen, NADPH, cytochrome P450 and a flavoprotein (NADPH-cytochrome c reductase, sometimes referred to as NADPH-cytochrome P450 reductase) (see Myant and Mitropoulos (1977) for review). The overall reaction is typical of many enzyme-catalyzed 'mixed-function' hydroxylations in which one atom of a molecule of O_2 is reduced to water by NADPH and the other oxygen atom is introduced into the substrate, cytochrome P450 functioning as oxygen activator. The general reaction may be written:

$$RH + NADPH + O_2 + H^+ \rightarrow ROH + NADP^+ + H_2O$$

where RH is the substrate.

The study of cytochrome P450-requiring hydroxylases obtained from bacteria and animal tissues suggests that these hydroxylations involve the following sequence of reactions: first, the substrate combines with oxidized (Fe^{3+}) cytochrome P450 to form a complex which is then reduced to the Fe^{2+} form by the transfer of one electron from NADPH *via* NADPH-cytochrome c reductase. Next, molecular O_2 combines with the complex to form a reduced cytochrome-substrate-O_2 complex. A second electron is then transferred to the ternary complex and the complex undergoes a molecular rearrangement in which one atom of oxygen is introduced into the substrate and the cytochrome P450 is oxidized. The reaction is completed by the expulsion of water from the complex, with the release of hydroxylated substrate and cytochrome P450 in the Fe^{3+} form. (See Fig. 5.6 for an example of a cytochrome P450-requiring hydroxylation).

Cytochrome P450 acts as activator for O_2 and the substrate in a considerable number of hydroxylations catalyzed by liver microsomes. The multiplicity of these hydroxylations is not due to the presence of a single cytochrome P450-containing enzyme system with broad specificity but, rather, to the presence of a number of distinct hydroxylating systems differing from each other with regard to the preferred substrate or to the position in the molecule at which the OH group is inserted. It seems clear, for example, that cholesterol 7α-hydroxylase is distinct from the enzyme system catalyzing the 7α-hydroxylation of deoxycholate and that both differ from the microsomal 26-hydroxylase, though in all three systems the known elements are the same, i.e. cytochrome P450, NADPH and a mechanism for transferring electrons from NADPH to the cytochrome. What, then, determines the substrate specificity and the nature of the hydroxylation in each case? There is increasing evidence to suggest that 'microsomal cytochrome P450' is really a mixture of several forms of the cytochrome. It is possible, therefore, that each hydroxylating system contains a specific cytochrome P450. In keeping with this, Haugen *et al.* (1975) have isolated several different cytochromes P450 from liver microsomes.

Although liver microsomes contain esterified as well as free cholesterol, the substrate for cholesterol 7α-hydroxylase is probably free cholesterol. Observations on the conversion of [^{14}C]cholesterol into 7α-hydroxycholesterol by liver microsomes *in vitro* show that only a portion of the total endogenous microsomal cholesterol acts as substrate for the enzyme. This fraction has been termed the 'substrate pool' of microsomal cholesterol (Balasubramaniam *et al.*, 1973).

1.2.4.2 Other enzymes catalyzing changes in the nucleus. The enzymes catalyzing the nuclear changes required for the conversion of 7α-hydroxycholesterol into bile acids, together with their subcellular localization in the liver and cofactor requiremens, are shown in Scheme 1.

The oxidation of the 3β-hydroxyl group and the migration of the Δ^5 double bond to the Δ^4 position are catalyzed by microsomal enzymes:

an NAD-linked 3β-hydroxysteroid oxidoreductase and a Δ⁵-3-ketosteroid isomerase. The isomerization of the double bond involves a partial transfer of the hydrogen from the 4β to the 6β position. The 12α-hydroxylation of (5.2) is catalyzed by a microsomal NADPH-linked microsomal enzyme that requires molecular O_2 but does not have an absolute requirement for cytochrome P450. The enzyme shows some activity towards 7α-hydroxycholesterol and 5β-cholestane-3α,7α-diol. However, the preferred substrate is (5.2); hence the pathway to 5β-cholestane-3α,7α,12α-triol (5.4) shown in Scheme 1.

The two enzymes required for saturation of the Δ⁴ double bond and reduction of the 3-keto group of (5.3) are present in the cytosol. The reduction of the Δ⁴ double bond is catalyzed by an NADPH-linked Δ⁴-3-ketosteroid-5β-reductase. The reaction consists in the transfer of one hydrogen atom from the A side of NADPH to the 5β position of the steroid and the introduction of another H from the medium into the 4α position. The enzyme catalyzing this reaction in the synthesis of bile acids differs from the hepatic Δ⁴-3-ketosteroid reductases concerned in the metabolism of steroid hormones containing a 3-keto group and a Δ⁴ double bond. The reduction of the 3-keto group to a 3α-hydroxyl group is catalyzed by an NAD- or NADPH-linked 3α-hydroxysteroid ketoreductase. In this reaction, a hydrogen atom is transferred from the A side of NADPH to the 3β position, a proton entering from the medium to form the 3α-hydroxyl group. The 3α-hydroxysteroid dehydrogenase concerned in bile acid synthesis shows considerable activity towards C_{19}, C_{21} and C_{24} steroids possessing a 3-keto group, even after the enzyme has been purified more than 200-fold.

1.2.4.3 Side-chain cleavage enzymes. Rat-liver mitochondria are capable of bringing about the 26-hydroxylation of cholesterol in the presence of NAD. This hydroxylation is stereospecific, resulting in the introduction of a hydroxyl group into the C-25 methyl carbon that was originally C-3' of mevalonic acid (see Chapter 4, p. 213) (Berséus, 1965; Mitropoulos and Myant, 1965). This methyl carbon is in the 25*pro*-S position (see Fig. 5.2); addition of an oxygen atom to this carbon gives rise to the (25R) compound. Rat-liver microsomes contain an enzyme system that catalyzes the 26-hydroxylation of 5β-cholestane-3α,7α,12α-triol (5.4) but is inactive towards cholesterol. The microsomal enzyme requires NADPH, molecular O_2 and cytochrome P450, and is possibly the enzyme responsible for initiating the oxidative cleavage of the side-chain in the pathway from cholesterol to cholic acid in rats.

The 26-hydroxylation of (5.4), and the subsequent carboxylation of the terminal methyl group, must also be stereospecific, since

3α,7α,12α-trihydroxy-5β-cholestanoic acid (**5.6**) usually occurs predominantly as only one of the two C-25 isomers (the 25*R* and the 25*S* acids) in a given species. However, there is some uncertainty as to the configuration at C-25 of the (**5.6**) formed by the liver in different species or by different hepatic enzymes within a species. Haslewood (1952) and Carey and Haslewood (1963) isolated the same hydroxy acid (**5.6**) from the bile of *Alligator mississippiensis* and from human bile. Shah *et al.* (1968) concluded that this was the D isomer (m.p. 180°–182°), whereas the major constituent of the bile of two species of caiman crocodiles studied by them was the L isomer (m.p. 194°–196°) (Shah *et al.*, 1968). Batta *et al.* (1979) have examined the X-ray crystallographic properties of the two trihydroxy acids (**5.6**) isomeric at C-25 and have concluded that the configuration of the L isomer is 25*S* and that that of the D isomer is 25*R*. If these identifications are correct, it follows that in the enzymic formation of (**5.6**) in human liver the initial hydroxylation of the side-chain occurs at the 25*pro-S* methyl group. If so, the stereospecificity of the enzyme catalyzing this hydroxylation is the same as that of the mitochondrial cholesterol 26-hydroxylase in rat liver. Oxidation of the steroid side-chain in the formation of chenodeoxycholic acid from 5β-cholestane-3α,7α-diol in man also appears to be catalyzed by a mitochondrial hydroxylase which hydroxylates the 25*pro-S* methyl group, giving the 25*R* triol (Shefer *et al.*, 1978). On the other hand, Gustafsson and Sjöstedt (1978) have shown that rat-liver microsomal 26-hydroxylase oxidizes the 25*pro-R* methyl carbon of (**5.4**). This would lead to the formation of the 25*S* trihydroxy acid (**5.6**), which would therefore be the C-25 isomer of the (**5.6**) apparently isolated from human bile by Carey and Haslewood (1963).

If the mitochondrial and microsomal 26-hydroxylases do indeed have opposite stereospecificities, it should be possible to determine the relative contributions of the mitochondrial and microsomal 26-hydroxylation pathways to bile acids in the intact animal or human subject by analysing the distribution of labelled carbon atoms in the propionic acid formed *in vivo* from stereospecifically labelled cholesterol (as in the *in vitro* experiment of Mitropoulos and Myant (1965)).

Human liver microsomes also exhibit some 26-hydroxylating activity towards (**5.4**), but the major product formed during an incubation of human liver microsomes with (**5.4**) is 5β-cholestane 3α,7α,12α,25-tetrol (Björkhem *et al.*, 1975). The probable pathway for side-chain cleavage in the formation of bile acids in man is discussed in more detail in Chapter 17, Section 6.5.1.

Partial separation of the rat-liver microsomal enzymes catalyzing the 7α-hydroxylation of cholesterol, the 12α-hydroxylation of (**5.2**) and the 26-hydroxylation of (**5.4**) has been achieved by Cottman *et al.* (1977).

The Metabolism of Cholesterol 239

A note on nomenclature of 26-hydroxycholesterol. According to the IUPAC rules for steroid nomenclature (IUPAC, 1972), if one of the two terminal methyl groups of the sterol side-chain is substituted, that methyl carbon is designated C-26, as in *26-hydroxycholesterol*. Thus, according to this rule the mammalian enzyme catalyzing the first step in the oxidative cleavage of the side-chain in the pathway to bile acids is a 26-hydroxylase, and this is how it has always been designated. However, the IUPAC rule raises a difficulty in that C-25 is a prochiral carbon, stereospecific substitution at C-26 or C-27 giving rise to one or other of two diastereomers. As mentioned above, the terminal methyl that is hydroxylated by rat-liver mitochondria is the one derived from C-3' of mevalonic acid. Hence, to be consistent with the current IUPAC ruling we should designate this methyl carbon C-26 and the terminal methyl derived from C-2 of mevalonic acid should be C-27. A more direct system of nomenclature would be to number the terminal methyls on the basis of their stereochemistry. Kienle *et al.* (1973) have deduced, from the stereochemistry of the reduction of the Δ^{24} double bond during the biosynthesis of cholesterol, that the 25*pro-R* methyl carbon is derived from C-2 and that the 25*pro-S* is derived from C-3' of mevalonate (Fig. 5.2). Hence, it would be consistent with the IUPAC rule to define C-26 as the *pro-S* and C-27 as the *pro-R* carbon atom. A major advantage of this nomenclature would be that 26-hydroxycholesterol would remain the correct name for the diol formed by hepatic 26-hydroxylation in human liver, though the cholesterol 26-hydroxylase of Mycobacterium smegmatis, which hydroxylates the 25*pro-R* methyl of cholesterol (Kienle *et al.*,

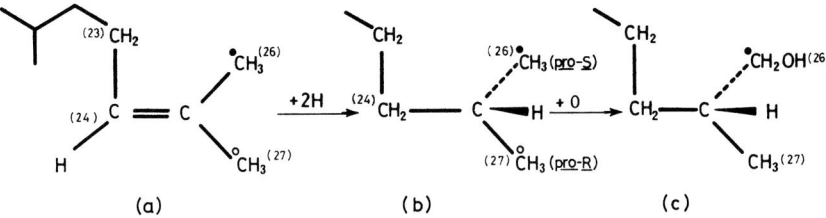

Figure 5.2
Stereochemistry of the enzymic reduction of the Δ^{24} double bond of the sterol side-chain and of the 26-hydroxylation of the saturated side-chain by mammalian liver enzyme. C̊, derived from C-3' of mevalonate: Ċ, derived from C-2 of mevalonate. If the side-chain is drawn with the conformation shown and with C-26 above C-27, the reduction of Δ^{24} gives the configuration and numbering shown in (b) (ĊH₃ becoming the *pro-S* methyl group). 26-Hydroxylation then introduces the OH group into the *pro-S* methyl to give the (25*R*)-26-hydroxylated product. Note that if the side-chain is drawn in extended conformation (⋎⋀⋀⋋), ĊH₃ would be drawn below C̊H₃ and would be numbered 27 in (a) if the convention of numbering the upper methyl 26 was followed. The stereochemistry shown in (a) (ĊH₃ *trans* to the H at C-24) was demonstrated by Popják and Cornforth (1966); the stereochemistry shown in (b) is deducible from Kienle *et al.* (1973).

1973), and the 26-hydroxylase of rat-liver microsomes, which must also hydroxylate the 25*pro-R* methyl group, should be called 27-hydroxylases. In the absence of a definitive rule, it would seem best to refer to the terminal methyl carbon atom derived from C-3 of mevalonate as C-26 (but see Popják *et al.*, 1977). When the configuration at C-25 of a C-26- or C-27-substituted side-chain is known, the compound is denoted (25*R*) or (25*S*).

The oxidation of the 26-hydroxylated side-chain to the 26-carboxy acid (Scheme 2, (**5.4**)–(**5.8**)) is catalyzed by NAD-linked enzymes in the cytosol of liver cells. The oxidation probably occurs in two steps, with the aldehyde as intermediate, each step being catalyzed by a separate enzyme.

The nature and subcellular distribution of the enzymes catalyzing the further oxidation of the carboxylated side-chain is controversial. Suld *et al.* (1962) showed that preparations containing the mitochondria and cytosol of liver cells catalyze the conversion of (**5.4**) into cholyl-CoA and propionyl-CoA, with the intermediate formation of the CoA ester of the 26-carboxy acid (3α,7α,12α-trihydroxy-5β-cholestanoyl-CoA). On the basis of this observation they suggested that cleavage of the side-chain of the 26-carboxy acid takes place by β-oxidation of the CoA ester, a process analogous to the β-oxidation of long-chain fatty acids. Such a pathway would require the presence of a dehydrogenase to give the 24-enoyl CoA, a hydratase to give the 24-hydroxylated derivative, a second dehydrogenase to give the 24-keto derivative and a 24-keto thiolase to cleave the 24-25 bond.

Although this scheme seems reasonable, there is little direct evidence in support of it. The introduction of a 24-hydroxyl group, probably in α configuration, into 3α,7α,12α-trihydroxy-5β-cholestanoic acid is catalyzed by rat-liver mitochondria plus cytosol (but not by the cytosol alone) (Masui and Staple, 1966) and by rat-liver microsomes (Gustafsson, 1975). Most of the published work on the formation of cholic and chenodeoxycholic acids from cholesterol by subcellular preparations of rat liver is consistent with the generally held view that liver mitochondria are needed for the complete sequence of changes involved in the modification of the sterol side-chain, though the nature of the reactions catalyzed by mitochondrial enzymes is far from clear. It should also be noted that Mendelsohn and Mendelsohn (1968) have reported the formation of cholic and chenodeoxycholic acids from cholesterol in rat-liver preparations from which the mitochondria have been removed. In human liver, the only 26-hydroxylase with significant activity towards C_{27} substrates is confined to the mitochondria, whereas the enzyme system catalyzing the 25-hydroxylation of (**5.4**) is confined to the microsomes (Björkhem *et al.*, 1975).

The Metabolism of Cholesterol 241

The question of the subcellular localization of the enzymes needed for cleavage of the C_8 side-chain in the formation of the primary bile acids is likely to remain in doubt until more work has been done with subcellular fractions of liver prepared by methods which minimize contamination of one fraction with enzymes derived from another. If intramitochondrial enzymes do play an essential part in bile acid synthesis this would raise the further problem as to how the relevant intermediates are transported into and out of the mitochondrion.

1.2.5 Allo bile acids

1.2.5.1 Distribution. Although the predominant bile acids in the bile of most mammals and of many lower vertebrates have the 5β (normal) configuration, allo (5α) bile acids have been found, if only in traces, in all mammalian species in which their presence has been sought and have also been identified in the bile of many lower vertebrates. Allocholic acid is present in significant amounts in the bile of the leopard seal (*Hydrurga leptonyx*), possibly originating from the penguins and fish eaten by these animals, and is a constituent of the bile of several species of birds, reptiles and fish. It has also been isolated from human faeces. In certain reptiles, allocholic acid is the major bile acid secreted in the bile. Allodeoxycholic acid is a normal constituent of rabbit faeces and accounts for about 5% of the total biliary bile acid in this species. In rabbits fed a diet containing 5α-cholestanol, the glycine conjugate of allodeoxycholic acid may comprise more than 25% of the total bile acids in the bile. Allodeoxycholic acid arises by bacterial 7α-dehydroxylation of allocholic acid in the intestinal lumen and undergoes reabsorption and 7α-hydroxylation in the liver, as in the enterohepatic circulation of deoxycholic acid (see Section 2).

1.2.5.2 Derivation. Allo bile acids are derived from three sources:— from 5α-cholestanol, from cholesterol by a modification of the pathway to normal bile acids, and from 5β bile acids.

5α-Cholestanol is converted into allocholic and allochenodeoxycholic acids in rats, and into allodeoxycholic acid (*via* allocholic acid) in rabbits. The first step in the pathway from 5α-cholestanol to allo bile acids is almost certainly the introduction of the 7α-hydroxyl group, since 5α-cholestanol is an efficient substrate for cholesterol 7α-hydroxylase. The later steps must include the inversion of the 3β hydroxyl group without the introduction of a Δ^4 double bond, since loss of the 5α hydrogen would presumably lead to the formation of a 5β bile acid by the pathway shown in Scheme 1. In so far as cholesterol is converted into 5α-cholestanol in animal tissues, the pathway from 5α-cholestanol to allo bile acids must constitute a minor route for the metabolism of cholesterol.

Hoshita et al. (1968) have shown that liver microsomes from the green iguana, a species in which the major biliary bile acid is the taurine conjugate of allocholic acid, convert 7α,12α-dihydroxycholest-4-en-3-one (5.3) into 5α-cholestane-3α,7α-12α-triol in the presence of NADPH. This suggests the presence of an alternative pathway to allo bile acids in which cholesterol is the primary precursor and in which saturation of the Δ^4 double bond of (5.3) is catalyzed by a microsomal 5α-reductase and not, as in rat liver, by a soluble 5β-reductase. A microsomal NADPH-linked 5α-reductase using 7α-hydroxycholest-4-en-3-one as substrate has also been demonstrated in rat liver by Björkhem (1969). The stereochemistry of the reaction catalyzed by this enzyme is the opposite of that catalyzed by the soluble 5β-reductase participating in the biosynthesis of normal bile acids. During the reduction of the Δ^4 double bond by the 5α-reductase, a hydrogen atom is transferred to the 5α position from the B side of NADPH and a hydrogen from the medium is transferred to the 4α position, i.e. saturation involves a *cis* addition. The existence of a Δ^4-3-ketosteroid 5α-reductase in liver suggests that 5α-cholestanol is not required for the formation of allo bile acids in the liver. In keeping with this, 5α-cholestanol does not form an unusually large proportion of the total liver sterols in those species in which allo bile acids are the major bile acids synthesized in the liver.

Bile acids of the 5β series are converted into allo acids by microorganisms in the lumen of the large intestine. The pathway from normal to allo bile acids involves the intermediate formation of a Δ^4-3-keto acid, followed by saturation of the double bond by a 5α-reductase and reduction of the 3-keto group by a 3α-hydroxysteroid dehydrogenase (Kallner, 1967). Allo bile acids may be re-converted into normal bile acids, presumably through the Δ^4-3-keto intermediate, but with saturation of the Δ^4 double bond by a 5β-reductase.

1.2.6 Sulphate esters and glucuronides

The sulphate esters of conjugated bile salts are detectable in normal human serum and urine in trace amounts and a considerable proportion of the lithocholic acid in normal human bile is present as the 3-sulphate ester of the glyco- or tauro-conjugated bile salt. In patients taking large doses of chenodeoxycholic acid for treatment of gall stones, the excretion of lithocholic and ursodeoxycholic acids increases markedly in the bile and, to a smaller extent, in the urine. This increase is accompanied by a rise in the proportion of sulphated to non-sulphated bile acid. After prolonged treatment with chenodeoxycholic acid, more than 75% of the biliary lithocholic acid may be sulphated (Stiehl et al., 1975). Conversion to the sulphate ester reduces the toxicity and facilitates the excretion of this poorly soluble bile acid (Gr. *lithos*, a stone).

In biliary obstruction, up to 100 mg of conjugated bile salts may be excreted daily in the urine of an adult human subject, the urinary bile salts containing a high proportion of mono- and di-sulphated esters. The sulphated bile acids include cholic, chenodeoxycholic and lithocholic acids, together with 3β-hydroxychol-5-enoic acid, a monohydroxy bile acid not normally present in the bile or urine of adults. Sulphation of bile salts probably takes place mainly in the liver but may also occur in the kidneys (Barnes *et al.*, 1976; Czygan *et al.*, 1976). The sulphotransferase catalyzing the transfer of a sulphate group from adenosine 3-phosphate 5'-sulphatophosphate to the bile salt is present in both liver and kidney of rats (Chen *et al.*, 1975). The cytosol of hamster liver, intestine and adrenals has also been shown to contain a sulphotransferase that catalyzes the sulphation of glycochenodeoxycholate in the 7α-position (Barnes *et al.*, 1979). Some bacterial hydrolysis of bile-acid sulphate esters may occur in the intestinal lumen, but this process must be very incomplete since substantial quantities of sulphated bile salts may be excreted in the faeces (see Chapter 2, Section 6.3 for further discussion of bile-acid sulphates).

The glucuronides of conjugated cholic, chenodeoxycholic, deoxycholic and lithocholic acids have been detected in the urine of patients with obstructive liver disease.

1.3 The enterohepatic circulation of bile salts

The bile salts undergo an enterohepatic circulation (EHC) which enables the body to conserve at least 95% of the bile acids secreted into the lumen of the intestine. The EHC of the bile salts also plays an essential role in the absorption of cholesterol from the intestine and in the regulation of cholesterol metabolism in the liver. Figure 5.3 shows the main features of the EHC of bile salts in diagrammatic form.

1.3.1 Secretion and reabsorption

The bile salts secreted by the liver into the biliary tree enter the intestine *via* the common bile duct; in animals with a gall bladder the flow of bile into the duodenum is intermittent, most of the bile secreted in the fasting state passing into the gall bladder for storage until food is eaten, when the contents of the gall bladder are discharged into the duodenum. After participating in the digestion and absorption of lipids in the upper part of the small intestine, the bile salts are almost completely reabsorbed. The small quantity that escapes reabsorption is excreted in the faeces, almost entirely in unconjugated form. The reabsorbed bile salts, which include conjugated and unconjugated primary and secondary bile acids, enter the portal bloodstream and are bound reversibly to the plasma

244   The Biology of Cholesterol and Related Steroids

albumin. On reaching the liver, the bile salts are largely removed from the plasma during a single passage, very little bile salt passing through the liver into the systemic circulation under normal conditions. Within the hepatocytes, unconjugated bile acids are reconjugated, deoxycholate is 7α-hydroxylated to cholic acid (completely in some species, but only partially in others) and some of the reabsorbed lithocholate is sulphated. The re-absorbed bile salts, together with a small amount of conjugated, newly-synthesized primary bile acid, is secreted into the biliary tree to begin a new cycle of the EHC.

Absorption of bile salts from the intestine takes place by two mechanisms: active transport and passive nonionic diffusion. Active transport is confined to the distal part of the ileum and is probably the major absorptive mechanism for bile salts as a whole in normal human subjects. Nonionic diffusion, which may occur along the whole length of the small intestine and colon, plays little part in the

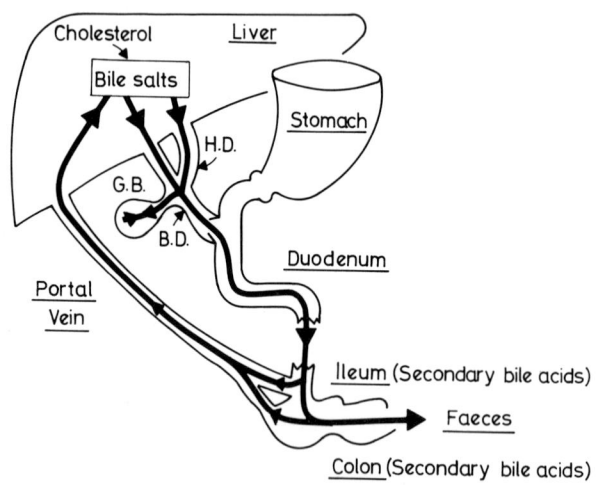

Figure 5.3
Diagrammatic representation of the main features of the enterohepatic circulation of the bile salts. The organs are not drawn to scale. Bile salts are secreted *via* the hepatic ducts (HD) into the common bile duct (BD) and thence into the second part of the duodenum, the flow of bile into the duodenum being regulated by the sphincter of Oddi. During fasting most of the bile salt secreted into the hepatic ducts is diverted into the gall bladder (GB), where it is stored until the gall bladder contracts in response to a meal. Bile salts are reabsorbed from the ileum and, to a small extent, from the colon after conversion into unconjugated secondary bile acids. Absorption occurs *via* the portal vein. The small proportion of the bile salts that are not reabsorbed are excreted in the faeces. The bile salts are cleared from the portal blood by a single passage through the liver and resecreted, after conjugation, together with bile salts formed in the liver from cholesterol derived from the plasma or synthesized *in situ*. In the steady state, the amount of bile salt synthesized in the liver is equal to the amount of unabsorbed bile salts lost in the faeces. For quantitative aspects see Fig. 5.4.

absorption of conjugated bile salts because most tauro- and glyco-conjugated bile acids have pK values lower than the pH of the intestinal lumen and are therefore present in the intestine largely in ionized form. Unconjugated bile acids, on the other hand, have relatively high pK values and are therefore more readily absorbed by nonionic diffusion. This mechanism probably accounts for the reabsorption of free bile acids from the colon under normal conditions, and for the reabsorption of free bile acids from the jejunum in the blind-loop syndrome, a condition in which the lumen of the upper small intestine becomes heavily contaminated with deconjugating micro-organisms.

1.3.2 Pool size and rates of synthesis and secretion

The pool of a given bile acid may be defined as the total amount present in the liver, biliary system and portal circulation and in the walls and lumen of the intestine above the level below which no reabsorption occurs; in the presence of a normal EHC, the small amount present in the systemic circulation may be ignored. The pool of a bile acid may also be defined operationally as the total exchangeable mass measured by isotope dilution, but this definition is not valid unless the rate of mixing of the isotopically labelled bile acid with the endogenous pool is rapid compared with the fractional rate of turnover of the pool. This condition is probably satisfied in normal human subjects but does not hold when the reabsorption of bile acids is defective, as in certain clinical abnormalities of the intestinal tract, when the pool of bile acid may be grossly overestimated by the isotope-dilution technique.

The sum of the absolute rates of turnover of the two primary bile acids (estimated from the pool size and fractional rate of turnover of each acid) gives the rate at which newly-synthesized bile acid is added to the pool and, under steady-state conditions, should also give the rate at which bile acid is lost from the pool by faecal excretion. Table 5.1 shows values for the pool size and turnover of the primary and secondary bile acids estimated by isotope dilution in normal man.

The total bile acid pool is between 1.3 and 2.3 g. The pools of cholic and chenodeoxycholic acids are roughly equal, but the fractional rate of turnover of chenodeoxycholic acid is lower than that of cholic acid, so that the rate of synthesis of chenodeoxycholic acid is only about half that of cholic acid. The fractional rate of turnover of lithocholate is much higher than that of the other bile acids, probably because of the low rate of intestinal absorption of the sulphate ester, the form in which a large proportion of the lithocholate taken up by the liver is secreted into the intestine. The sum of the rates of synthesis of cholic and chenodeoxycholic acids, estimated by isotope dilution, varies from 400 to 500 mg per day in most normal human subjects.

Table 5.1.
Pool size and turnover of bile acids in normal man

Bile acid	Pool (mg)	Pool (μmoles kg^{-1})	FRT (day^{-1})	ART (mg day^{-1})	ART (μmoles kg^{-1} day^{-1})
Cholic	600–1000	12.0–14.2	0.32	192–320	3.8–4.6
Chenodeoxycholic	500–800	10.0–11.4	0.20	100–160	2.0–2.3
				Total 292–480	5.8–6.9
Deoxycholic	200–400	4.0–5.7	0.20	40–80	0.8–1.1
Lithocholic	40–80	0.8–1.1	1.0	40–80	0.8–1.1
Total	1340–2280	26.8–32.4			

FRT, fractional rate of turnover; ART, absolute rate of turnover (equivalent to rate of synthesis of primary bile acids from cholesterol and to rate of formation of secondary bile acids from primary bile acids). (Values collected by Hofmann (1977) from published work of many authors.)

Table 5.2.

The enterohepatic circulation of bile salts in rhesus monkeys and rats

	Pool		Synthesis		Secretion	
	mg	µmoles kg^{-1}	mg day^{-1}	µmoles kg^{-1} day^{-1}	g day^{-1}	mmoles kg^{-1} day^{-1}
Monkey	500	200	50	20	5.0	2.0
Rat	16	130	5.0	40	0.5	2.5

(1) *Monkeys*. Values are taken from Dowling et al. (1970). Pool size was estimated from the amount of bile salt drained from the pool immediately after cannulating the bile duct (wash-out method); synthesis was estimated as the rate of loss of bile salt from the enterohepatic circulation in the steady state; secretion was measured directly from the amount passing through the external measuring system in the steady state. All values are rounded.

(2) *Rats*. Values for pool size and synthesis are taken from Strand (1963) and were estimated by isotope dilution of labelled cholic and chenodeoxycholic acids. Other workers (Shefer et al., 1969; Mitropoulos et al., 1973) using the wash-out method have obtained higher values for pool size in rats than those reported by Strand. Values for secretion rate have been estimated from the values obtained by Shefer et al. (1969) for taurocholate, on the assumption that rat bile contains cholate and chenodeoxycholate in the ratio 4:1. The weight of a rat is assumed to be 250 g. All values are rounded.

Note: The molecular weight of a bile salt is taken to be 500.

This is considerably higher than the rate of excretion of total bile acids in the faeces (200–400 mg/day) reported by most workers who have used the GLC method for analyzing faecal bile acids. A possible reason for this discrepancy is overestimation of the cholic and chenodeoxycholic acid pools by the isotope-dilution method. Another is the use of residue-free formula diets in much of the work on the faecal excretion of bile acids in human subjects; this would tend to give low values for bile-acid excretion because bile-acid synthesis may be decreased by the feeding of diets containing no indigestible residue (see Chapter 10). It is also possible that some methods for determining total faecal bile acids give erroneously low values because sulphated bile acids are not included in the assay (see Chapter 2, Section 6.3).

The rate of secretion of bile salts (the total mass of bile salt entering the duodenum per day) may be estimated in man by a technique which involves measurement of the degree of dilution of a marker infused at a constant rate into the proximal duodenum and assayed at a point just below the opening of the common bile duct (Go et al., 1970; Grundy and Metzger, 1972). In the presence of a normal EHC, 12–24 g of bile salt are secreted daily. During the fasting state, when much of the bile is diverted into the gall bladder, the secretion rate falls to a low level, rising rapidly when a test meal is infused into the stomach. The *cycling frequency*, or the virtual number of circulations of the pool of bile salts through the EHC in a given time, is defined as the secretion rate divided by the pool size. Thus, if the pool size is assumed to be 2 g, the pool of bile salts would be said to circulate between 6 and 12 times per day in a healthy man. The cycling frequency has been much discussed in relation to the possible causes of the lithogenic bile secreted in patients with cholesterol stones in the gall bladder.

The fractional rate of deconjugation of glycocholate or taurocholate can be estimated from the relative rates of decline of the specific activities of the amino acid and steroid residues in each bile salt after administration of [^{14}C]glyco-[^{3}H]cholate or [^{35}S]tauro-[^{3}H]cholate. Hepner et al. (1973) have shown that about 18% of the glycocholate pool and about 7% of the taurocholate pool is deconjugated during each cycle of the EHC in man. For a comprehensive discussion of the quantitative aspects of bile-salt turnover, see Hofmann (1977).

The methods developed for studying the pool size and rate of synthesis of bile salts in man have also been used for the study of bile acid metabolism in animals. Pool sizes and rate of synthesis have been measured in intact animals by isotope-dilution techniques and Dowling et al. (1970) have developed a method for measuring the secretion rate of bile salts in monkeys by diverting the bile through a bile-duct cannula into an external measuring system and then returning it to the duodenum. Representative values for rats and monkeys with an intact EHC are shown in Table 5.2.

1.3.3 The effect of interrupting the EHC

In the presence of a normal intestine and hepato-biliary system, 95–98% of the bile salt passing down the intestine is reabsorbed. After uptake by the liver the reabsorbed bile salts partially repress the synthesis of bile acids by a mechanism discussed in the next section. The net result of the homeostatic regulation of bile-acid synthesis is that the size of the bile-salt pool remains more of less constant from day to day, the amount of newly-synthesized bile salt balancing the amount lost by faecal excretion. If the bile salts are diverted from the EHC so that the amount returning to the liver is diminished, the rate of synthesis of bile acids increases. This situation can arise if the bile is drained through a bile fistula or if the reabsorption of bile salts is diminished by an abnormality of the terminal ileum such as chronic inflammation, surgical resection or bypass. It can also be brought about by the oral administration of a non-absorbable resin that binds bile acids in the lumen of the intestine. If the interruption to the EHC is only partial, the increase in bile-acid synthesis may be sufficient to maintain a normal rate of secretion of bile salts into the intestine. In this case the size of the bile-salt pool remains unchanged, though its rate of turnover increases. If, however, the rate of loss of bile salts *via* the faeces exceeds the maximal capacity of the liver for making bile acids (2–3 g/day in man), the bile-salt pool decreases and a new steady-state is achieved in which the rate of secretion of bile salts is subnormal. These changes in the EHC have been discussed by Hofmann (1967) in relation to the effects of ileal resection and are shown diagrammatically in Fig. 5.4. The stimulatory effect of interruption of the EHC on bile-acid synthesis is sometimes exploited deliberately in the treatment of primary hypercholesterolaemia. Interference with the reabsorption of bile salts by an operation for ileal bypass or by the oral administration of cholestyramine (see Section 1.4.4) may lower the plasma cholesterol concentration by stimulating the catabolism of cholesterol to bile acids.

The effect of total diversion of the EHC by cannulating the bile duct of a rat is shown in Fig. 5.5. The rat was kept under conditions of regulated lighting and feeding such that the rate of synthesis of bile acids varied rhythmically, with a maximum at night and a minimum during the day. When the cannula was inserted into the common bile duct, bile salts were secreted through the cannula initially at a rapid rate while the pool was emptying. After 5–10 hours, when emptying was complete, the secretion rate fell to a low level corresponding to the basal rate of synthesis before cannulation. The mean rate then

250   The Biology of Cholesterol and Related Steroids

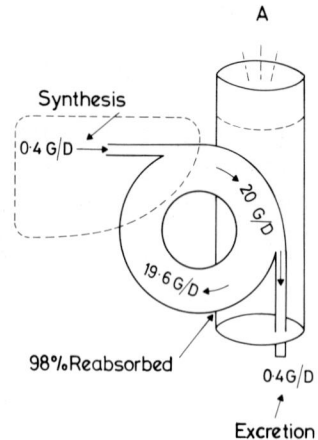

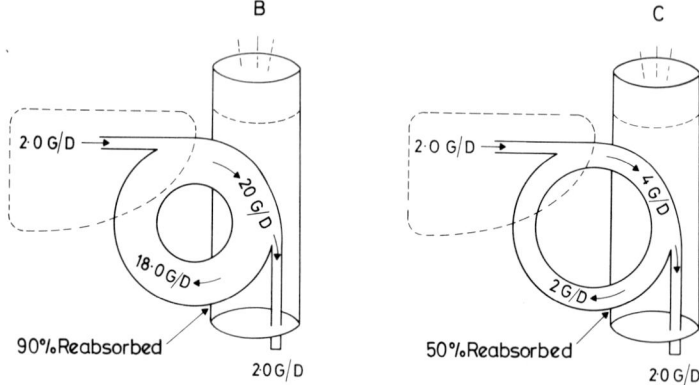

Figure 5.4
The effect of interruption of the enterohepatic circulation of the bile salts on bile-acid synthesis.

A. Normal enterohepatic circulation. 98% of secreted bile salt is reabsorbed. Secretion rate is 20 g/day, of which 0.4 g is lost by faecal excretion and *19.6 g* are reabsorbed. Excretion is balanced by synthesis of 0.4 g of bile salt per day.

B. Resection of less than 100 cm of ileum, causing reabsorption to fall to 90%. Secretion rate is 20 g/day, of which 2 g are lost by faecal excretion and *18 g* are reabsorbed. Increased excretion is balanced by increasing synthesis to 2 g/day. Secretion rate and pool size are normal, but note that a slight decrease in % reabsorbed requires a large proportional increase in synthesis to maintain the *status quo*.

C. Resection of more than 100 cm of ileum, causing reabsorption to fall to 50%. Secretion is 4 g/day, of which 2 g are lost by faecal excretion and 2 g are reabsorbed. Increased excretion is balanced by increasing synthesis to 2 g/day (the maximum possible in this hypothetical situation) but pool size and secretion rate are greatly diminished.

This Figure is taken, with slight modification, from Hofmann (1967).

The Metabolism of Cholesterol 251

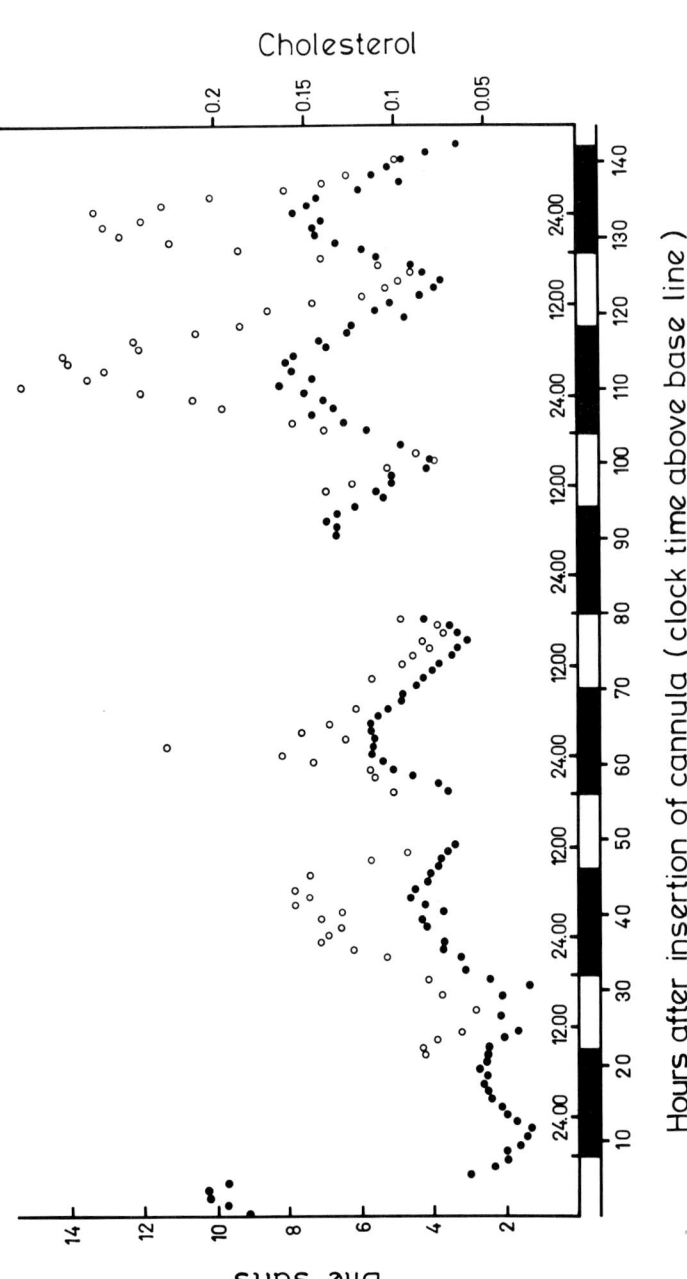

Figure 5.5
The effect of bile-duct cannulation on the secretion of bile salts (●) and cholesterol (○) in a rat. The rat was kept under conditions of regulated lighting and feeding, with food allowed only at night. Dark periods are shown in black, light periods in white. The cannula was inserted into the common bile duct at zero time and total bile acids were assayed enzymically in serial samples of bile collected from the cannula. After about 10 hours, no bile salts remain in the pool and the rate of secretion through the cannula becomes equal to the rate of synthesis in the liver. All values are expressed in μmoles of cholesterol or bile acid excreted per hour. (Mitropoulos, Balasubramaniam and Myant, unpublished.)

rose progressively over the next four or five days as bile-acid synthesis in the liver was released from its normal repression by reabsorbed bile salts. Note that the diurnal rhythm in bile-acid synthesis was maintained after complete interruption of the EHC, an increase occurring in both the maximum and minimum rates.

In the monkey preparation devised by Dowling *et al.* (1970), bile-acid synthesis increases roughly in proportion to the fraction of the bile diverted from the EHC, until about a fifth of the bile is diverted. At this point, bile-acid synthesis reaches a maximum value of about 400 μmoles/kg/day, any further increase in the fraction diverted having no additional effect on the rate of synthesis.

1.4 The regulation of bile-acid synthesis

In this section we shall consider various factors that modify bile-acid metabolism. In some cases, as in the feedback inhibition of bile-acid synthesis by bile acids, the modification clearly plays a regulatory role, in the sense that it enables the animal to alter its bile-acid metabolism in response to a biological need. In other cases, as in the effects of thyroid hormone, a true regulatory role is not so obvious. The effects of diet and drugs are included here simply for convenience. Changes in bile-acid metabolism that occur in disorders of lipoprotein metabolism are considered in Chapter 15.

1.4.1 Feedback inhibition by bile salts

The increase in the rate of synthesis of bile acids that occurs in response to diversion of bile salts from the EHC has been referred to in the preceding section. This effect was first observed by Thompson and Vars (1953) in rats and has since been demonstrated in other species, including man, the rhesus monkey and the rabbit. The subsequent demonstration that hepatic synthesis of bile acids in bile-fistula rats can be restored to the normal by infusing taurochenodeoxycholate (Bergström and Danielsson, 1958) or taurocholate (Shefer *et al.*, 1969) into the duodenum indicated that bile salts themselves are responsible for the normal feedback inhibition of bile-acid synthesis in the intact animal.

The biological function of this homeostatic mechanism must be to ensure an optimal supply of bile salts for the digestion and absorption of lipid, any change in the amount of bile salt returning from the intestine *via* the portal blood acting as a signal to the liver to adjust its rate of synthesis of bile acids. The immediate need for bile salts in the upper intestine when a meal is eaten can, of course, be satisfied by the contraction of a full gall bladder, but in the longer term bile-acid synthesis must be regulated to compensate for the continual leak from the EHC due to faecal excretion of bile acid. The diurnal rhythm in bile-acid synthesis in rats must also be related functionally to the need for bile salts during digestion. In the wild state, rats sleep by day and eat at night. Since the rat has no gall bladder and therefore cannot store bile salts for intermittent secretion, a diurnal rhythm in synthetic rate, with a maximum at night, must clearly be advantageous.

1.4.2 Effects of diet

In several species, bile-acid synthesis increases when cholesterol is added to the diet. This may be looked upon as a regulatory mechanism which enables the animal to compensate for increased absorption of dietary cholesterol by increasing the rate of catabolism of cholesterol, but at the small price of making more than the optimal amount of bile acid. Bile-acid synthesis is also influenced by the amount of fibre in the diet, increasing when certain types of fibre are added to the food and decreasing when the animal is fed a fibre-free diet. These effects of fibre, discussed more fully in Chapter 10 in relation to cholesterol metabolism, may be mediated by effects on the reabsorption of bile salts from the intestine. The effects of dietary fat and fibre on bile acid synthesis are considered in Chapter 10. A discussion of other clinical aspects of the influence of diet on bile-acid synthesis in man will be found in the review by Miettinen (1973).

1.4.3 Effects of hormones

Several hormones have been shown to influence the metabolism of bile acids in experimental animals. However, with the possible exception of the effects of corticosteroids on the diurnal rhythm in bile-acid synthesis in rats (discussed below in relation to cholesterol 7α-hydroxylase), there is little to suggest that these effects play any part in the regulation of bile-acid synthesis under physiological conditions. Sex differences in the side-chain cleaving activity of liver mitochondria incubated with cholesterol have been reported (Kritchevsky *et al.*, 1963), but there is no evidence to suggest that these differences are causally related to the well-established sex differences in human plasma cholesterol concentration.

The hypercholesterolaemia that occurs in myxoedematous human subjects is accompanied by a diminished rate of synthesis of cholesterol. This suggests that in the absence of a normal supply of thyroid hormone the rate of catabolism of cholesterol is diminished—a possibility that has led several workers to examine the effects of changes in thyroid function upon the synthesis of bile acids. Taken as a whole, the results obtained from experimental animals and from human subjects suffering from disorders of thyroid function have not provided any clear evidence in favour of this suggestion.

Bile-acid synthesis is essentially normal in intact hypothyroid rats. However, thyroid hormone given to intact rats in non-calorigenic doses leads to a slight increase in the synthesis of total bile acids and a marked change in the ratio of chenodeoxycholic to cholic acid in the bile. Whereas a normal rat synthesizes about four times as much cholic as chenodeoxycholic acid, the synthesis of chenodeoxycholic acid may equal or exceed that of cholic acid in the hyperthyroid rat. These changes are accompanied by a decrease in the rate of 12α-hydroxylation of 7α-hydroxycholest-4-en-3-one by liver microsomes, an increase in the activity of cholesterol 7α-hydroxylase and an increase in the side-chain-cleaving activity of liver mitochondria and in the 26-hydroxylation of 5β-cholestane-3α,7α,12α-triol. The combination of increased 7α-hydroxylation of cholesterol with increased side-chain cleavage and decreased 12α-hydroxylation would be expected to stimulate bile-acid synthesis and to increase the ratio of chenodeoxycholic to cholic acid.

The effects of altered thyroid function on bile-acid metabolism in man are less obvious than in rats. In many hyperthyroid and myxoedamatous patients the faecal excretion of total bile acids is within the normal range, though excretion per kg of body weight tends to be high in thyrotoxicosis and to be low in myxoedema (Miettinen, 1973). The absolute rate of turnover of cholic acid, estimated by isotope dilution, has also been shown to be lower in hypothyroid than in thyrotoxic patients (Hellström and Lindstedt, 1964). These small differences from the normal may be due indirectly to changes in gastrointestinal function rather than to any direct effect of thyroid hormone on bile-acid synthesis in the human liver. It is possible, for example, that in the hyperthyroid state increased intestinal motility reduces the reabsorption of bile salts from the ileum, thus releasing hepatic synthesis of bile acids from feedback inhibition. The ratio of chenodeoxycholic to cholic acid in the bile is not consistently altered in thyrotoxic patients.

1.4.4 Effects of drugs

1.4.4.1 Anionic exchange resins. The use of cholestyramine in the treatment of primary hypercholesterolaemia was mentioned in the preceding section. The events leading to the development of this drug are of interest because they illustrate the way in which an advance in the treatment of a disease may result from a consideration of physiological principles and not, as is so often the case, from empirical observation. Some years ago, Siperstein *et al.* (1952) showed that bile salts are necessary for the absorption of cholesterol from the intestine; this suggested that it might be possible to prevent the absorption of exogenous and endogenous cholesterol by precipitating the bile salts within the lumen of the intestine. Siperstein *et al.* (1953) then showed that ferric chloride, a precipitating agent for bile salts, lowers the plasma cholesterol concentration in cholesterol-fed cockerels when given in the drinking water.

Ferric chloride cannot be given to patients because it is too toxic. However, the approach initiated by Siperstein and co-workers has led to the development of non-absorbable resins that bind bile salts by anionic exchange and can be given safely to human subjects. The most effective and widely used of these resins is cholestyramine, a polymer containing quaternary ammonium groups. When cholestyramine is given by mouth in the chloride form, bile salts are bound by the resin in exchange for chloride so that their reabsorption from the ileum is diminished, leading to increased formation of bile acids from cholesterol in the liver. The effect of large doses (20–30 g/day) given to patients is to increase bile-acid synthesis to 2 or more g/day and to bring about a substantial fall in plasma cholesterol concentration. Cholestyramine may also diminish the absorption of cholesterol from the small intestine, but since this effect is small and inconstant, it is probable that the fall in plasma cholesterol concentration is, in fact, due largely to increased cholesterol catabolism in the liver rather than to decreased absorption of cholesterol. As shown in Fig. 5.3, the response of the liver to interruption of the EHC is such that a relatively small decrease in the reabsorption of bile salts causes a large increase in bile-acid synthesis. Thus, it may be that a therapeutically effective dose of cholestyramine binds enough bile salt to stimulate the catabolism of cholesterol but not enough to affect cholesterol absorption significantly.

Other anionic exchangers that bind bile salts in the intestine are diethylaminoethyl (DEAE)-Sephadex (a modified dextran), DEAE-cellulose and colestipol. DEAE-Sephadex and colestipol have been shown to be effective in the treatment of primary hypercholesterolaemia.

1.4.4.2 Phenobarbital. Barbiturates are inducers of many hepatic microsomal enzymes, including those catalyzing drug hydroxylations. Hence, barbiturates might be expected to stimulate bile-acid synthesis, since several of the enzymes required for this process are present in liver microsomes. In view of the tendency shown by gallstone patients to secrete a bile with a low bile-salt:cholesterol ratio, any drug that stimulates bile-acid synthesis has potential value for the treatment of gall stones.

Large does of phenobarbital (85 mg/kg/day) given to bile-fistula rats increase bile flow without a corresponding fall in bile-salt concentration (Siegfried and Elliott, 1972). The net result is an increase in the daily output of bile acids. The effect of the drug on bile-acid output and bile flow may be due to the increase in liver weight that occurs after treatment with a barbiturate and does not necessarily indicate a specific influence on bile-acid synthesis. Much smaller doses of phenobarbital (5 mg/kg/day) increase the rates of synthesis and secretion of bile salts in rhesus monkeys with intact or totally interrupted EHC's (Redinger and Small, 1973). Since the increased rate of synthesis in a phenobarbital-treated monkey with an intact EHC is maintained despite a considerable increase in the rate of return of reabsorbed bile salts to the liver, phenobarbital must in some way modify the feedback inhibition of bile-acid synthesis by bile salts. An increase in bile-acid synthesis, determined from the daily output of faecal bile acids, may occur in some human subjects given phenobarbital (Miller and Nestel, 1973).

1.4.4.3 Antimicrobial agents. In animals whose intestinal contents have been sterilized by the feeding of chemotherapeutic agents (Lindstedt and Norman, 1956) or in animals born and reared under germ-free* conditions (Gustafsson et al., 1957), deconjugation of bile salts does not occur and no secondary bile acids are formed. Under these conditions the fractional rate of turnover and the rate of synthesis of bile acids are both considerably diminished. For example, the time required for the faecal excretion of half the ^{14}C in a dose of [^{14}C]cholic acid is 11 days in germ-free rats but is only 2 days in conventional rats (i.e. those with a normal intestinal microflora); likewise, germ-free rats synthesize only about half as much cholic acid per day as conventional animals. The decreased rate of synthesis of bile acids in rats with sterile intestinal contents is due to increased reabsorption of bile salts from the intestine, resulting in increased feedback inhibition of bile-acid synthesis in the liver (Kellog, 1971). The increased reabsorption of bile salts is not due to the absence of deconjugation, since the faecal excretion of bile salts by germ-free rats is not significantly increased when their intestinal contents are infected with a· strain of *Clostridium perfringens* capable of splitting the peptide bond of taurocholate *in vitro* and *in vivo*. It is possible, however, that the dehydroxylated bile acids formed in the intestines of conventional animals are less efficiently absorbed than are primary bile acids, possibly because dehydroxy bile acids tend to be adsorbed to bacteria and to dietary fibre in the intestine.

1.4.5 Cholesterol 7α-hydroxylase
1.4.5.1 The 7α-hydroxylation of cholesterol as a rate-limiting step. The step that determines the rate of synthesis of bile acids under most conditions is thought to be the 7α-hydroxylation of cholesterol. This view is based on two lines of evidence (see Myant and Mitropoulos, 1977). First, observations on the incorporation of radioactive precursors into bile acids in conditions in which bile-acid

* For definitions of the terms 'germ-free' and 'gnotobiotic', see Kellog (1971).

synthesis is stimulated or depressed show that there are essentially no rate-limiting steps in the biosynthetic sequence beyond 7α-hydroxycholesterol. Second, changes in the rate of bile-acid synthesis, whether brought about physiologically or experimentally, are almost always accompanied by parallel changes in the activity of cholesterol 7α-hydroxylase (Table 5.3). For example, the activity of this enzyme in rat liver rises and falls in parallel with the diurnal rise and fall in bile-acid synthesis (see Fig. 5.5) and the increase in bile-acid synthesis brought about by interruption of the EHC, by cholesterol feeding and by treatment with thyroid hormone is in each case accompanied by an increase in enzyme activity.

Although it has not been possible to measure the capacities of the enzymes catalyzing all the steps in the biosynthetic pathway to bile acids, or to measure steady-state concentrations of intermediates under conditions in which the rate of synthesis is varied, this evidence is at least consistent with the conclusion that the 7α-hydroxylation of cholesterol is the control point for bile-acid synthesis. However, in several conditions in which cholesterol 7α-hydroxylase activity is altered there is also a parallel change in the activity of HMG-CoA reductase, the enzyme whose activity determines the rate of synthesis of cholesterol in liver microsomes. Since Balasubramaniam *et al.* (1973) have shown that the substrate pool of cholesterol is usually insufficient to saturate cholesterol 7α-hydroxylase and that newly-synthesized cholesterol is the preferred substrate for the enzyme, this raises the possibility that the rate of production of 7α-hydroxycholesterol may in some conditions be determined by the rate of synthesis of cholesterol in the microsomes. When an increase in the activity of HMG-CoA reductase precedes an increase in that of cholesterol 7α-hydroxylase, as in glucose feeding after a fast (Takeuchi *et al.*, 1974), it is reasonable to suppose that the initial increase in cholesterol 7α-hydroxylase activity is due to an increase in the supply of its preferred substrate. After thyroxine treatment, on the other hand, the rise in cholesterol 7α-hydroxylase activity occurs several hours before the rise in HMG-CoA reductase activity (Balasubramaniam *et al.*, 1975). In this case, it seems more likely that the primary event is increased 7α-hydroxylation of microsomal cholesterol, and that this leads to induction of HMG-CoA reductase owing to removal of cholesterol from the microsomes. When the two enzymes are induced or repressed more or less simultaneously, as in the diurnal changes observed in the activities of the enzymes in rat liver, it is likely that they are both responding to a common signal.

1.4.5.2 The regulation of cholesterol 7α-hydroxylase activity. The important question of the mechanism by which cholesterol 7α-hydroxylase is regulated has proved difficult to answer.

Table 5.3.

The effect of various agents on the components of the cholesterol 7α-hydroxylase enzyme system and on HMG-CoA reductase activity in rat-liver microsomes

Modifying agent	Cholesterol 7α-hydroxylase activity	Cytochrome P450 (total concentration)	NADPH-cytochrome c reductase activity	HMG-CoA reductase activity
Bile fistula or cholestyramine	↑	↑	↑	↑
Portacaval anastomosis	↑	→	→	↑
Diurnal rhythm (peak)	↑	↑	↑	↑
Thyroid hormone	↑	→	←	↑
Phenobarbital[a]	→ or ↑ or ↓	←	?	?
Cholesterol feeding	↑	↑	?	→
β-Sitosterol[b]	↑	↑	?	←

Enzyme activities and cytochrome P450 concentration are per mg of microsomal protein.

(a) There is disagreement as to the effect of phenobarbital on the activity of cholesterol 7α-hydroxylase per mg of microsomal protein. The increased bile-acid synthesis reported in phenobarbital-treated rats may be due to increased liver mass.

(b) β-Sitosterol induces HMG-CoA reductase by interfering with the intestinal absorption of endogenous and exogenous cholesterol.

(For references, see Myant and Mitropoulos, 1977).

This is due partly to the fact that it is impossible to achieve assay conditions in which the enzyme is saturated with its substrate, but also to the difficulty of separating and recombining the components of the enzyme complex without loss of activity. Observations on the size of the substrate pool and on the effects of inhibitors of protein synthesis suggest that in some conditions, such as cholesterol feeding in rats, the increase in enzyme activity is due to an increase in the supply of microsomal substrate, but that in other conditions, as in bile-fistula animals, it is due to induction of the synthesis of enzyme protein. A rhythmic change in the rate of enzyme synthesis also seems to be responsible for the diurnal rise and fall in enzyme activity observed in rats kept under conditions of controlled lighting and feeding. The well-known diurnal rhythm in plasma corticosterone concentration in rats is partly responsible for the alternating cycle of induction and repression of cholesterol 7α-hydroxylase. However, this cannot be the sole factor, since a diurnal rhythm in enzyme activity may still be observed after removal of both adrenals, though the amplitude of the rhythm is greatly reduced.

The activity of cholesterol 7α-hydroxylase is not correlated with the concentration of total cytochrome P450 or with NADPH-cytochrome c reductase activity in liver microsomes in a variety of states in which the activity of the hydroxylase is altered. Several examples of this lack of correlation are shown in Table 5.3. Perhaps the most striking is seen in the bile-fistula rat, in which cholesterol 7α-hydroxylase activity rises severalfold without detectable change in the two known components of the enzyme system. This raises the question as to what it is that is induced when cholesterol 7α-hydroxylase activity increases after interruption of the EHC or during the night in rats kept under regulated conditions. As discussed earlier in this section, it is possible that the total cytochrome P450 in liver microsomes is a mixture of several cytochrome pigments, all giving the same difference spectrum under the conditions in which cytochrome P450 is routinely assayed. If so, it may be that only one of these is involved in the 7α-hydroxylation of cholesterol, and that only this one is induced after interruption of the EHC and during the peak of activity in the diurnal cycle.

2 STEROID HORMONES

2.1 Introduction

2.1.1. Comparative aspects

In mammals, steroid hormones are synthesized in the adrenal cortex, the gonads and the placenta. Steroids structurally identical with mammalian adrenocortical and gonadal hormones are synthesized by almost all vertebrates, including the most primitive (the cyclostomes), and have been isolated from the gonads and other tissues of many invertebrates; progesterone, testosterone and oestrone are also present in some higher plants. Comparative studies indicate that in plants and animals all these C_{18}, C_{19} and C_{21} steroids are formed by a common pathway in which cholesterol is converted into pregnenolone by cleavage of the side-chain (see Scheme 3). It thus seems clear that the ability to convert cholesterol into 'steroid hormones' appeared at an early stage in the evolution of living organisms, and that the nature and mode of biosynthesis of these steroids have undergone little or no change during the subsequent course of evolution. What has evolved is the response of specific tissues to steroids and the complexity of the mechanisms by which their synthesis and secretion are regulated. Progesterone and other vertebrate steroid hormones do not necessarily act as hormones in those plants in which they are found. Progesterone is an intermediate in the biosynthesis of cardenolides and of other plant steroids (Burstein and Gut, 1971), and this may be one reason for its presence in the leaves of many plants. In some invertebrates, the male and female gonads produce steroids similar to the corresponding sex hormones produced in the gonads of mammals. This suggests, but is far from proving, that steroids had already acquired a hormonal role before the appearance of vertebrates.

Numerous observations on fish, amphibia, reptiles and birds (see Idler and Truscott, 1972) suggest that in all nonmammalian vertebrates the corticosteroids and the gonadal hormones have actions broadly similar to their actions in mammals, and that the synthesis and secretion of these hormones is regulated by pituitary hormones analogous to those secreted by the mammalian pituitary. This is particularly clear in the case of the gonadal steroids, which seem to be responsible for the development of secondary sexual characters throughout the vertebrate phylum. Corticosteroids also participate in the regulation of electrolyte balance in vertebrates of all classes and are known to have effects on muscle metabolism in fish and amphibia similar to the effects of cortisol in mammals. However, the more or less complete functional separation between mineralocorticoids and glucocorticoids that is characteristic of mammals is not apparent in all nonmammalian vertebrates. In some bony fish, for example, cortisol (the major glucocorticoid in many mammals) has marked effects on salt metabolism. A discussion of the evolution of the function of adrenocortical hormones will be found in Bellamy and Chester Jones (1965) and Barrington (1979).

2.1.2 Quantitative aspects
In man, the daily amount of cholesterol converted into steroid

hormones is much less than that converted into bile acids. Nevertheless, the metabolic pathway from cholesterol to steroid hormones is by no means negligible. For example, a normal man may excrete 50 mg of total adrenocortical and gonadal hormones per 24 hours, and a normal woman may excrete considerably more than this quantity per 24 hours during the luteal phase of the sexual cycle. Since steroid hormones and their metabolites are excreted almost entirely in the urine, this route for the removal of cholesterol from the body may be a source of error in the estimation of sterol balance based on measurement of the dietary intake of cholesterol and the faecal excretion of total steroids derived from cholesterol.

2.2 Biosynthesis

2.2.1 Adrenocortical hormones

2.2.1.1 The biologically active hormones.
The major biologically active hormones secreted by the adrenal cortex are the two glucocorticoids, corticosterone (**5.15**) and cortisol (**5.18**) and the mineralocorticoid, aldosterone (**5.17**). Other C_{21} and C_{19} steroids are also secreted by the adrenals. Some of these C_{21} steroids, such as progesterone (**5.12**) and pregnenolone (**5.10**), are known intermediates in the biosynthesis of the three biologically active adrenocorticoids, their appearance in adrenal-vein blood being due to escape from the metabolic pathway. The C_{19} steroids are presumably formed by cleavage of the C_2 side-chain of the C_{21} steroids. In man and in many other species, including cattle, sheep, dogs and guinea-pigs, cortisol is the major glucocorticoid. However, in rats, mice and rabbits, and also in many non-mammalian species, little or no cortisol is formed owing to lack of the adrenocortical 17α-hydroxylase (see Scheme 3); in these species corticosterone is the predominant, if not the sole, glucocorticoid.

2.2.1.2 The metabolic pathways.
Cholesterol is an obligatory precursor of the adrenocortical hormones, although early radioisotopic evidence suggested the contrary. Scheme 3 shows the major pathway for the conversion of cholesterol into corticosterone, cortisol and aldosterone. The initial event consists in the splitting of the cholesterol side-chain between C-20 and C-22 to give pregnenolone (**5.10**) and isocaproaldehyde (**5.11**). The steps leading to the cleavage reaction probably include the formation of (20*R*, 22*R*)-20,22-dihydroxycholesterol (**5.9**). However, notwithstanding the usual textbook description of this sequence of reactions, it is not known whether the first hydroxylation is at C-20 to give (20*S*)-20-hydroxycholesterol (see legend to Scheme 3 concerning nomenclature) or at C-22 to give (22*R*)-22-hydroxycholesterol, or whether the two hydroxylations

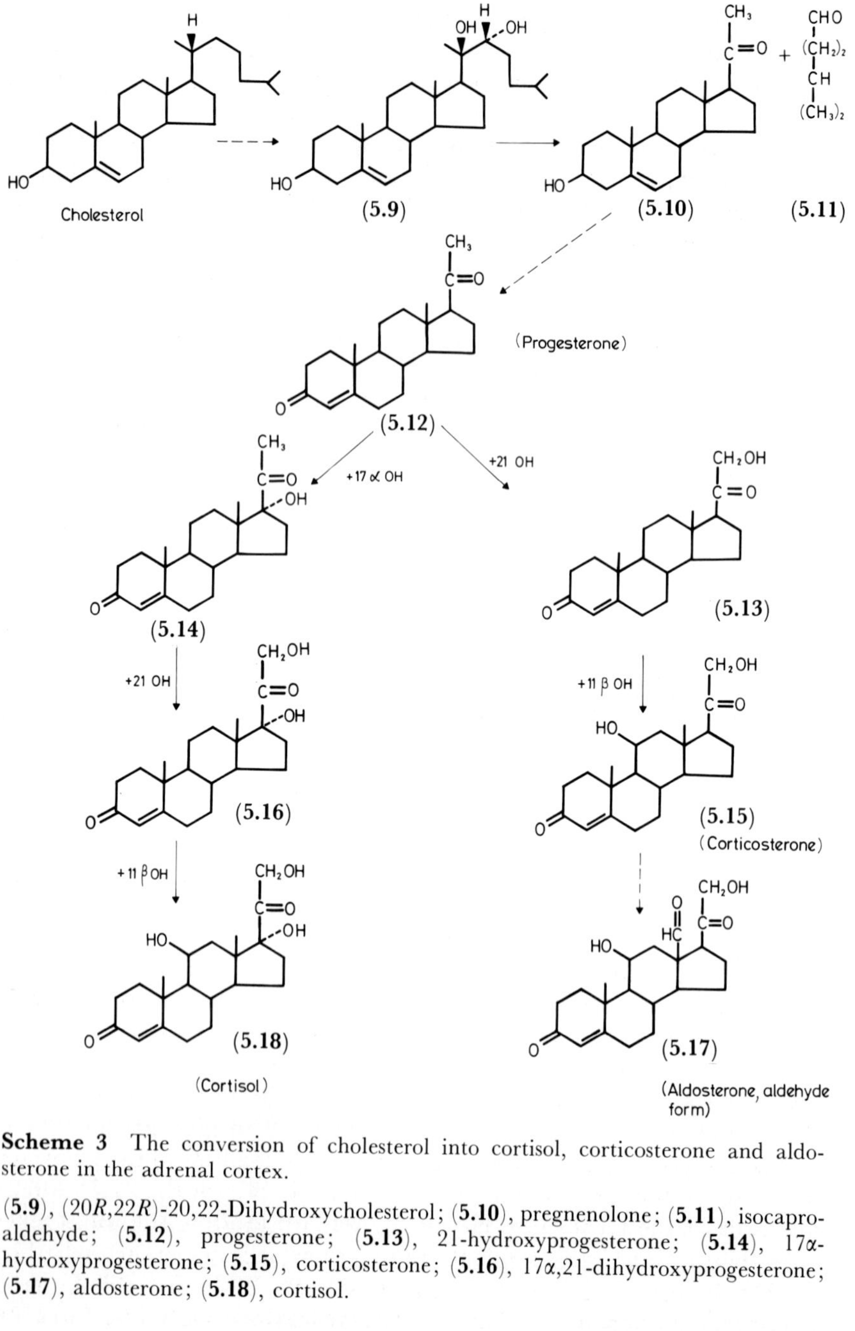

Scheme 3 The conversion of cholesterol into cortisol, corticosterone and aldosterone in the adrenal cortex.

(**5.9**), (20R,22R)-20,22-Dihydroxycholesterol; (**5.10**), pregnenolone; (**5.11**), isocaproaldehyde; (**5.12**), progesterone; (**5.13**), 21-hydroxyprogesterone; (**5.14**), 17α-hydroxyprogesterone; (**5.15**), corticosterone; (**5.16**), 17α,21-dihydroxyprogesterone; (**5.17**), aldosterone; (**5.18**), cortisol.

occur together by a concerted attack by O_2. The pregnenolone formed by loss of the C_6 unit from cholesterol is converted into progesterone (**5.12**), which is then converted into corticosterone by sequential hydroxylations in the 21 and 11β positions, or into cortisol by sequential hydroxylations in the 17α, 21 and 11β positions. Aldosterone is formed from corticosterone by oxidation of the C-18 methyl group to an aldehyde, probably *via* the alcohol (—CH_2OH).

In Scheme 3, progesterone is an intermediate in the formation of corticosterone and cortisol. The pathway through progesterone probably accounts for most of the corticosteroid and aldosterone formed in rat adrenal cortex, but in other species the introduction of the 17α and 21 hydroxyl groups may occur at earlier stages than those shown in Scheme 3. In the sheep, progesterone is bypassed by the 21-hydroxylation of pregnenolone to give 21-hydroxypregnenolone, which is then converted into deoxycorticosterone (**5.13**) by modification of the nucleus. In man, cortisol is formed by the 17α-hydroxylation of pregnenolone, followed by the conversion of 17α-hydroxypregnenolone into (**5.14**). Other minor variants of Scheme 3 have been described, presumably reflecting incomplete specificity of the hydroxylases. The possibility that cholesteryl sulphate is the primary precursor in the biosynthetic pathway to steroid hormones in the adrenal cortex is considered briefly on p. 287.

2.2.2 Steroid hormones of the gonads and placenta

2.2.2.1 Biologically active hormones. The major androgenic hormones secreted by the interstitial cells of the mammalian testis are testosterone (**5.22**), androstenedione (**5.20**) and dehydroepiandrosterone (**5.21**). C_{21} intermediates in the biosynthesis of the androgenic hormones are also secreted by the testis. The major oestrogenic hormones secreted by the ovary are oestrone (**5.23**) and oestradiol-17β (**5.24**); the progestational hormone produced by the ovary is progesterone (**5.12**). 17α-Hydroxyprogesterone (**5.14**), androstenedione (**5.20**) and other intermediates in the biosynthesis of oestrogens are also released by the ovary in small amounts. The placenta is the predominant source of the progesterone and oestrogens secreted during pregnancy, oestriol (**5.25**) being the major oestrogen synthesized by the primate placenta.

2.2.2.2 The metabolic pathways. Scheme 4 shows the major metabolic routes to the androgenic steroids. Pregnenolone (**5.10**) is formed from cholesterol by cleavage of the side-chain. Dehydroepiandrosterone (**5.21**) is formed from pregnenolone by 17α-hydroxylation to give (**5.19**), followed by removal of the C_2 side-chain. Androstenedione (**5.20**) is formed from progesterone (**5.12**) by 17α-hydroxylation to give (**5.14**), followed by loss of the side-chain.

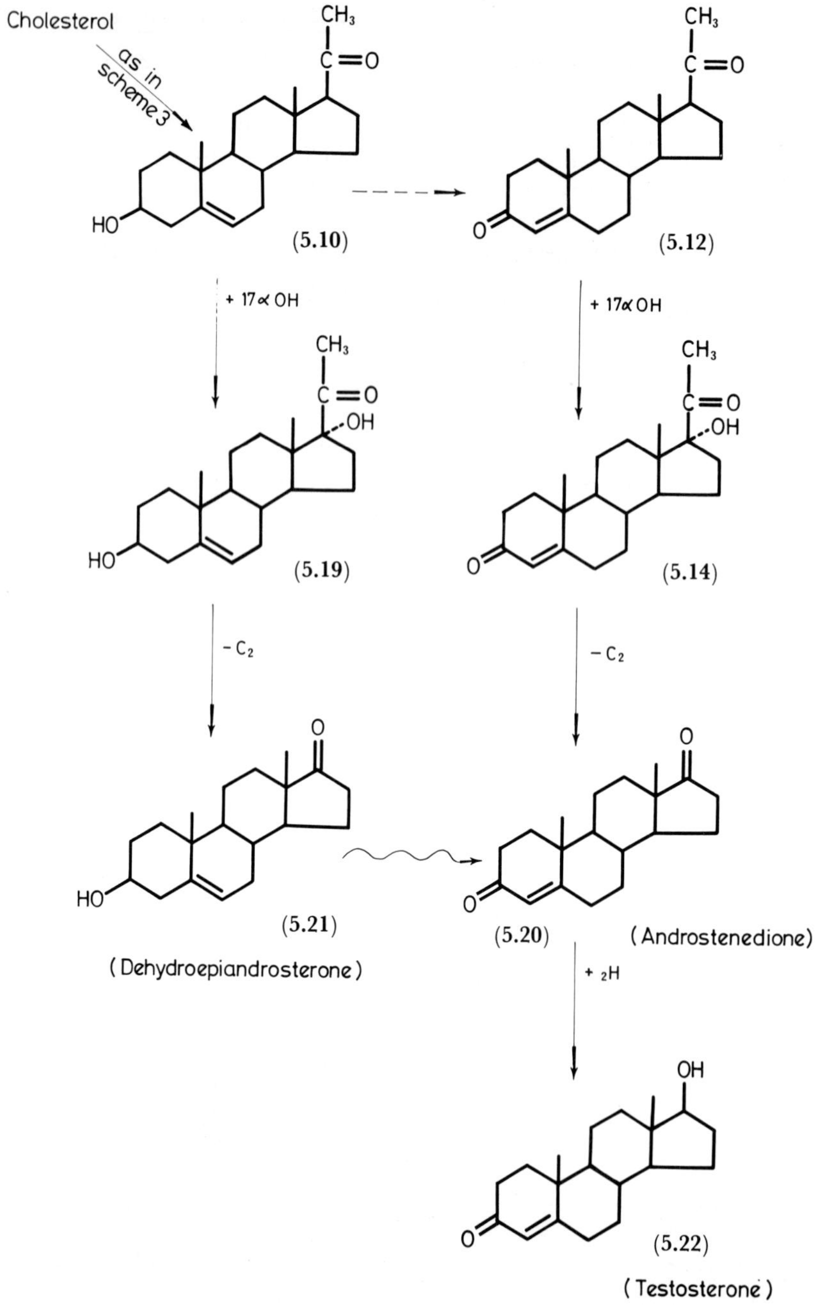

Scheme 4 The conversion of cholesterol into dehydroepiandrosterone and testosterone in the testis.

(**5.10**), Pregnenolone; (**5.12**), progesterone; (**5.14**), 17α-hydroxyprogesterone; (**5.19**), 17α-hydroxypregnenolone; (**5.20**), androstenedione; (**5.21**), dehydroepiandrosterone; (**5.22**), testosterone.

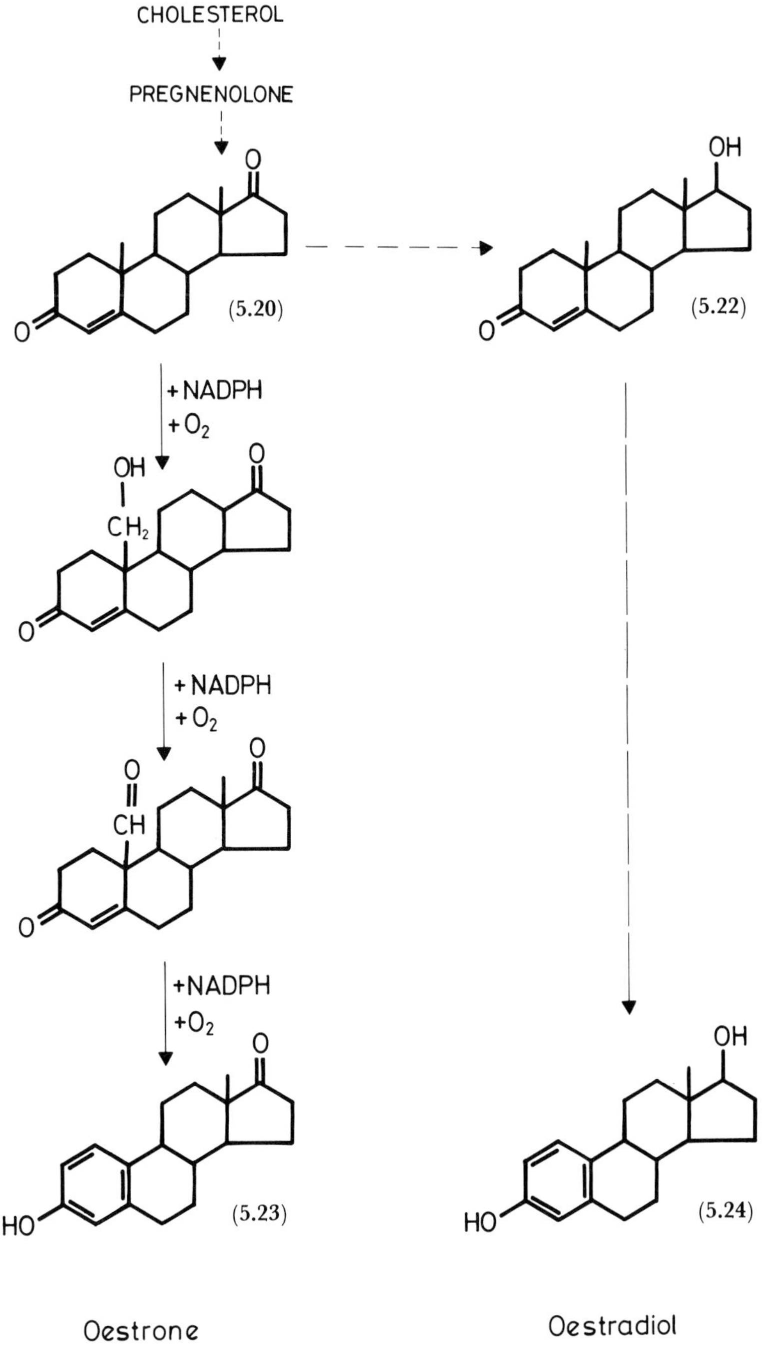

The Metabolism of Cholesterol 265

Oestrone   Oestradiol

Scheme 5 The conversion of cholesterol into oestrone and oestradiol in the ovary. (**5.20**), Androstenedione; (**5.22**) testosterone; (**5.23**), oestrone; (**5.24**), oestradiol.

266 The Biology of Cholesterol and Related Steroids

Testosterone (**5.22**) is formed from androstenedione by reduction of the 17-keto group to give the 17β-hydroxysteroid. In some species, testosterone may also be formed by an alternative route in which (**5.21**) is converted into (**5.20**).

In the ovaries, oestrogens are formed from cholesterol *via* androstenedione (**5.20**) and testosterone (**5.22**), the two androgenic hormones arising by the pathway shown in Scheme 4. Oestrone (**5.23**) and oestradiol-17β (**5.24**) are formed from androstenedione and testosterone, respectively, by removal of the C-19 methyl group and conversion of ring A into the aromatic form ('aromatization'). Scheme 5 shows the probable sequence of reactions involved in the aromatization of androgens to form oestrone and oestradiol-17β.

The human placenta forms progesterone from cholesterol by the pregnenolone pathway (Scheme 3) but lacks the enzymes required for conversion of C_{21} steroids into C_{19} or C_{18} steroids. However, 16α-hydroxydehydroepiandrosterone (**5.26**), formed in the fetal adrenal cortex from cholesterol and pregnenolone and transported thence to

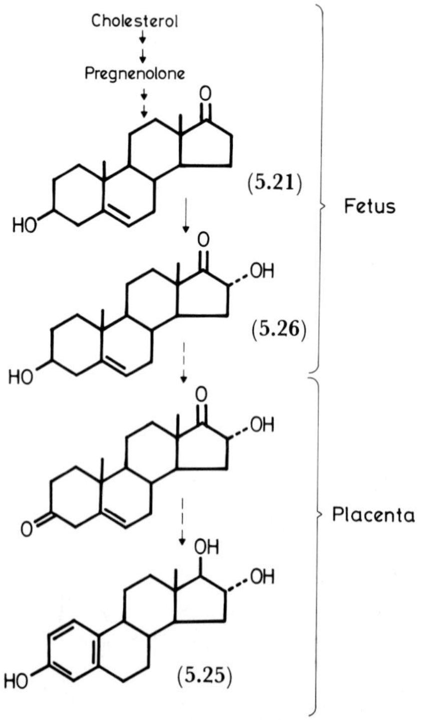

Scheme 6 The conversion of cholesterol into oestriol by the combined action of the fetus and placenta.

(**5.21**), Dehydroepiandrosterone; (**5.25**), oestriol; (**5.26**), 16α-hydroxydehydroepiandrosterone.

the placenta *via* the umbilical artery, is readily converted into oestriol (**5.25**) by enzymes in the placenta (Scheme 6) (for details see Chapter 6, Section 2.2).

2.2.3 Enzymes and reaction mechanisms

2.2.3.1 The formation of adrenocorticoids.

The overall reaction resulting in the oxidative cleavage of the cholesterol side chain between C-20 and C-22 (the cleavage reaction) and the introduction of 11β and 18 hydroxyl groups into the substrates shown in Scheme 3 are catalyzed by mixed-function oxidases in the inner membranes of adrenal cortex mitochondria. The 20-22 lyase and the 11β- and 18-hydroxylases require NADPH, molecular O_2, a flavoprotein, cytochrome P450 and a non-haem iron-containing electron carrier (adrenodoxin) not present in liver microsomes. The probable sequence of the reactions concerned in these mixed-function oxidations is shown in simplified form in Fig. 5.6.

As in the 7α-hydroxylation of cholesterol catalyzed by liver microsomes, the substrate is thought to combine with cytochrome P450 in the Fe^{3+} form, the Fe^{3+} cytochrome-substrate complex then being reduced to the Fe^{2+} form before formation of the cytochrome-substrate-O_2 complex (not shown in Fig. 5.6). In adrenal cortex mitochondria, however, the electron donor for the Fe^{3+} cytochrome-substrate complex is reduced adrenodoxin and not, as in hepatic microsomal hydroxylations, reduced flavoprotein. Adrenal cortex mitochondria contain two forms of cytochrome P450 which have been partially separated from one another (Jefcoate *et al.*, 1970). One form is associated with side-chain cleavage activity (P450$_{scc}$) and gives a characteristic difference spectrum in the presence of (20S)-20-hydroxycholesterol; the other (P450$_{11\beta}$) has 11β-hydroxylase activity, with little or no side-chain cleavage activity, and gives a characteristic difference spectrum in the presence of deoxycorticosterone

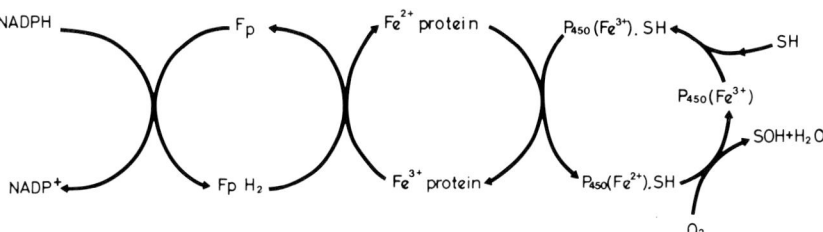

Figure 5.6
Mechanism of the hydroxylations in steroid hormone biosynthesis (much simplified). Fp, flavoprotein (adrenodoxin reductase); Fe protein, non-haem iron protein (adrenodoxin); P450, cytochrome P450 in oxidized (Fe^{3+}) or reduced (Fe^{2+}) form; SH, substrate for hydroxylation (cholesterol for cytochrome P450$_{scc}$ and deoxycorticosterone for cytochrome P450$_{11\beta}$).

(5.13). Furthermore, the ESR spectrum of the cytochrome P450 of the 20-22 lyase changes from a 'low-spin' to a 'high-spin' form on combination of the free Fe^{3+} cytochrome with cholesterol (see Fig. 5.6). This change in the ESR spectrum can be detected in isolated intact mitochondria or in the mitochondria of whole adrenal cortex. Although the cleavage reaction is known to require cytochrome P450, it is not known whether the two oxidative attacks (at C-20 and C-22) and the final cleavage are catalyzed by different cytochrome P450-requiring enzymes or by a single enzyme complex.

The 21- and 17α-hydroxylations involved in the formation of adrenocorticocoids are catalyzed by microsomal cytochrome P450-requiring hydroxylases which probably do not use adrenodoxin as electron carrier. The oxidation of the 3β-hydroxyl group and the $\Delta^5 \rightarrow \Delta^4$ isomerization (see Scheme 3) are catalyzed by an NAD-dependent 3β-hydroxysteroid oxidoreductase and a Δ^5-3-ketosteroid isomerase. Both enzymes are confined largely to microsomes, but their presence has been reported in adrenal cortex mitochondria. Note that the 3β-hydroxysteroid oxidoreductase concerned in the formation of adrenocorticoids is different from the microsomal enzyme responsible for the oxidation of the 3β-hydroxyl group of 7α-hydroxycholesterol in the formation of bile acids (see Scheme 1).

2.2.3.2 The formation of androgens and oestrogens. The enzyme system catalyzing the conversion of cholesterol into pregnenolone in the ovary, placenta and interstitial cells of the testis is confined to the mitochondria and resembles the 20-22 lyase of adrenal cortex mitochondria in requiring O_2, NADPH, cytochrome P450 and adrenodoxin. All the enzymes required for the conversion of pregnenolone into the gonadal hormones formed in the ovary and testis are present predominantly in the microsomal fraction. The 17α-hydroxylase and the 17-20 lyase catalyzing the conversion of C_{21} into C_{19} steroids are microsomal mixed-function oxidases requiring NADPH, O_2 and cytochrome P450 but not, apparently, adrenodoxin. The reduction of the 17-keto group of androstenedione to a 17β-hydroxy group is catalyzed by a microsomal NADH- or NADPH-dependent 17β-hydroxysteroid oxidoreductase. The enzymic mechanism responsible for the formation of oestrogens by aromatization of C_{19} androgens is not fully understood, but there is some evidence to suggest that the final steps shown in Scheme 6 are catalyzed by a cytochrome P450-requiring mixed-function oxidase that is unusual in being insensitive to inhibition by CO (Thompson and Siiteri, 1973).

2.2.3.3 Consequences of the subcellular distribution of enzymes. The first step in the formation of all the steroid hormones from cholesterol is the cleavage of the side chain by an enzyme system embedded in the inner membrane of the mitochondria. Since the cholesterol used for steroid-hormone formation must ultimately come from outside the mitochondria, the formation of pregnenolone requires the translocation of cholesterol across the outer and inner membranes of the mitochondria, a step that could be potentially rate-limiting for pregnenolone synthesis. Furthermore, since the steps leading to the conversion of pregnenolone into deoxycorticosterone (**5.13**) and cortisol (**5.18**) in the adrenal cortex are microsomal, pregnenolone must leave the mitochondria before undergoing these changes. In so far as the 11β-hydroxylation required for corticosteroid formation takes place at the stage shown in Scheme 3, the steroid molecule must re-enter the mitochondrion in order to gain access to the intramitochondrial 11β-hydroxylase. The formation of aldosterone must also involve the re-entry into the mitochondrion of steroids formed by microsomal enzymes from pregnenolone. Each of these translocations may be expected to require the participation of a carrier whose supply might be rate-limiting for the biochemical transformation in question.

2.2.4 Regulation of the production of steroid hormones

The output of steroid hormones varies widely in different physiological conditions, usually in response to changes in the rate of secretion of pituitary hormones, ACTH controlling the production of glucocorticoids and the gonadotrophic hormones (LH and FSH) controlling the production of gonadal steroid hormones. (Aldosterone production is controlled primarily by the renin-angiotensin system but is also influenced to a minor extent by ACTH). The output of glucocorticoids by the adrenal cortex varies diurnally in many species, including man, and may exhibit a sustained increase in response to chronic stress. An increase in glucocorticoid output also occurs after acute stress, the increase being accompanied by a marked loss of cholesteryl ester from the lipid droplets of the zona fasciculata of the adrenal cortex. Increased output of aldosterone, probably from the cells of the zona glomerulosa of the adrenal cortex, occurs in response to the need to conserve salt. Phasic changes in the output of gonadal hormones also occur in relation to the reproductive cycle. The interstitial cells of the testis and the oestrogen-forming cells of the ovary do not contain lipid droplets comparable with those of the adrenal cortex, but the cells of the mature corpus luteum contain large droplets filled with cholesteryl ester; in rats, the lipid droplets in the corpus luteum become depleted when progesterone output is stimulated by LH. All these changes in steroid hormone output are accompanied by parallel changes in the rate of conversion of cholesterol into the hormone. In this chapter we shall consider only those aspects of the regulation of steroid hormone production that have a bearing on the metabolism of cholesterol in the endocrine glands in which these hormones are formed.

Work carried out many years ago on the effect of ACTH on the incorporation of labelled precursors into corticosteroids in perfused adrenals (Stone and Hechter, 1954) suggested that there are no rate-limiting steps in the biosynthesis of corticosterone beyond the formation of progesterone. Subsequent work has shown that the main effect of ACTH on the biosynthetic pathway to steroid hormones in the adrenal cortex is to stimulate the conversion of cholesterol into pregnenolone in the mitochondria. This effect occurs within a few minutes of an intravenous injection of ACTH and is associated with the rapid hydrolysis of esterified cholesterol in the lipid droplets, due to activation of a cytosolic cholesteryl ester hydrolase. Activation of this enzyme is thought to be caused by stimulation of adenyl cyclase by ACTH, leading to increased formation of cyclic AMP which, in turn, activates a protein kinase catalyzing the phosphorylation of an inactive form of the hydrolase to the active form (Boyd *et al.*, 1975).

There have been several attempts to explain all the effects of ACTH on steroid hormone synthesis in terms of a single primary action (Schulster, 1974). Perhaps the most plausible is the suggestion that the production of glucocorticoids is regulated by a single rate-limiting step—the conversion of intramitochondrial cholesterol into pregnenolone—and that the rate of this reaction is determined by the supply of cholesterol available to the 20-22 lyase. On this view, the increase in pregnenolone formation that occurs almost immediately in response to ACTH is a consequence of an increased flow, into the mitochondria, of free cholesterol released from the lipid droplets. In keeping with this explanation, Brownie *et al.* (1973) have shown that acute stress or an injection of ACTH increases the proportion of substrate-bound cytochrome $P450_{scc}$ in adrenal cortex mitochondria ($P450(Fe^{3+})$.SH in the scheme shown in Fig. 5.6) and decreases the proportion of free cytochrome $P450_{scc}$. This shows that ACTH stimulates a step in the cleavage reaction earlier than the reduction of the cytochrome P450-cholesterol complex and, hence, that neither the supply of reductive hydrogen nor the addition of O_2 to the reduced cytochrome-substrate complex is rate-limiting for pregnenolone formation.

However, it is difficult to explain the effect of ACTH on pregnenolone production solely in terms of increased hydrolysis of extramitochondrial cholesteryl ester, since pregnenolone synthesis is increased in isolated mitochondria from the adrenal cortex of ACTH-treated rats, even though the cholesterol content of the mitochondria is normal. ACTH must therefore have an additional effect on the mitochondria themselves, mediated perhaps by the cyclic AMP that is indirectly responsible for activation of cholesteryl ester hydrolase. For reasons discussed by Boyd and Trzeciak (1973), the intramitochondrial effect of ACTH may involve the translocation of cholesterol within the mitochondrion to a pool of cholesterol accessible to the 20-22 lyase. The effect of ACTH on pregnenolone formation in the mitochondria (but not the activation of cholesteryl ester hydrolase) is inhibited by pre-treatment with cycloheximide, suggesting that the effect requires the synthesis of a labile protein.

Thus, as with other hormones, the effect of ACTH is not confined to a single control point in a metabolic sequence. Rather, ACTH has many effects, all of which are co-ordinated so as to enable the organism to respond with maximum efficiency to a biological need—in this case, the need for a rapid increase in the production of glucocorticoid from cholesterol. In fact, the regulation of cholesterol metabolism in relation to glucocorticoid production is much more complex than that revealed by the influence of ACTH on the isolated adrenal cortex.

Although a sudden increase in the requirement for substrate for pregnenolone formation may be satisfied by increased breakdown of cytosolic cholesteryl esters, the store of cholesterol in the lipid droplets must, in the long term, be maintained by cholesterol supplied from the plasma or synthesized within the cells of the adrenal cortex. The source of this cholesterol seems to vary between different species. In guinea-pigs, about half the cholesterol used for corticosteroid synthesis in the adrenal glands in the resting state is derived directly from the plasma and about half is derived from synthesis of cholesterol *in situ*. In rats, dogs and man, on the other hand, almost all the glucocorticoid formed in the resting state is derived from cholesterol that enters the adrenal cortical cells from the plasma, possibly entering the pool of cholesteryl esters in the lipid droplets before being transported as free cholesterol into the mitochondria. If, however, the plasma lipoprotein concentration of a rat is reduced to a very low level, so that the supply of plasma cholesterol no longer suffices to maintain the store of esterified cholesterol in the lipid droplets, the cholesteryl ester content of the adrenal cortex falls and the activities of HMG-CoA reductase and HMG-CoA synthase increase markedly (Balasubramaniam *et al.*, 1977). The net effect of these changes is to substitute newly-synthesized cholesterol for plasma cholesterol as the substrate for pregnenolone formation in the mitochondria. A similar co-ordinated response occurs during the diurnal cycle in corticosterone production in rats, though the nocturnal rise in HMG-CoA reductase and HMG-CoA synthase activities is less than that seen in response to depletion of plasma lipoprotein. Further discussion of cholesteryl-ester metabolism in the adrenal cortex will be found in Section 3 of this chapter.

The scheme shown in Fig. 5.7 shows a working hypothesis which

272 The Biology of Cholesterol and Related Steroids

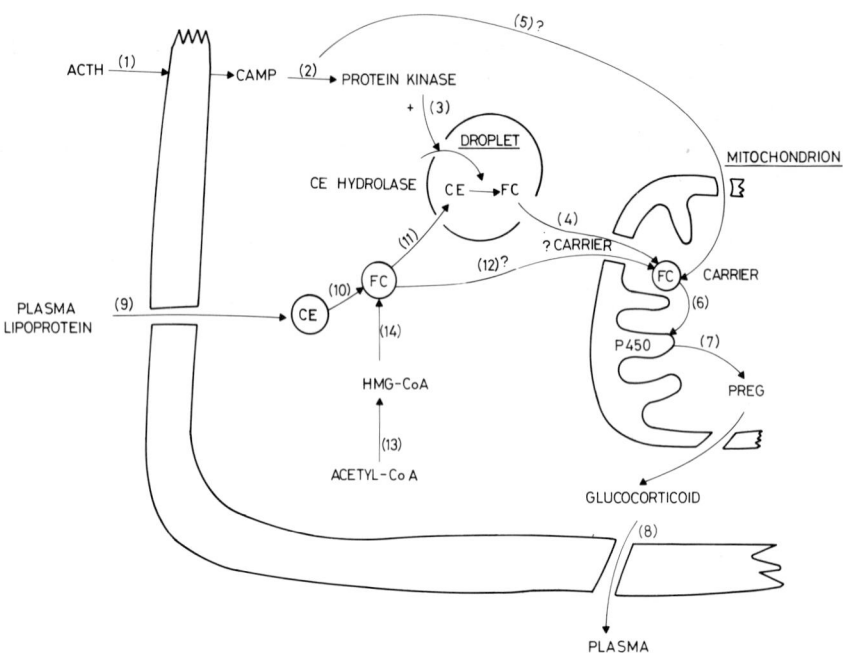

Figure 5.7
Diagram suggesting possible mechanisms by which glucocorticoid production is regulated in a cell of the zona fasciculata of the rat's adrenal cortex.

ACTH, adrenocorticotrophic hormone; CAMP, cyclic AMP; CE, cholesteryl ester; FC, free cholesterol; PREG, pregnenolone; P450, cytochrome $P450_{scc}$; carrier, a labile protein concerned in the transport of cholesterol.

1, Stimulation of CAMP synthesis by ACTH; 2, activation of a protein kinase by CAMP; 3, phosphorylation of cytosolic CE hydrolase; 4, entry of FC, released by the action of CE hydrolase, into the mitochondria (possibly mediated by a carrier protein); 5, induction of a protein carrier (possibly by CAMP) required for translocation of FC to cytochrome $P450_{scc}$ (6); 7, formation of pregnenolone and exit of prenenolone from mitochondrion for conversion into glucocorticoid; 8, secretion of glucocorticoid into plasma; 9, entry of plasma lipoprotein CE into the cell followed by 10, hydrolysis of lipoprotein CE to FC; 11, re-esterification of FC to form CE in lipid droplet; 12, possible direct entry of FC (derived by 10) into the mitochondrion; 13, 14, induction of HMG-CoA synthase and HMG-CoA reductase in response to depletion of droplet CE by decreased supply of plasma lipoprotein cholesterol or increased utilization of cholesterol for glucocorticoid synthesis. The relative contributions of the plasma cholesterol and cholesterol synthesized within the adrenal-cortical cell vary widely from species to species.

incorporates most of what is known about the relation between cholesterol metabolism and corticoid production in the adrenal cortex. Some of the steps shown have been clearly established experimentally; others have been inferred indirectly from experimental observations; others (marked '?') are possible but are not supported by any evidence. The possible role of lipoprotein receptors on adrenal cortical cells is discussed in Chapter 9.

The regulation of steroid-hormone formation in the gonads resembles that in the adrenal cortex, at least in so far as the conversion of cholesterol into pregnenolone is rate-limiting for hormone production. However, little is known about the relative importance of plasma cholesterol and cholesterol synthesized *in situ* as substrates for the cleavage reaction in gonadal mitochondria. The cells of the corpus luteum have a rich store of extramitochondrial cholesteryl ester and it is possible that regulation of progesterone synthesis in this tissue is mediated partly by control of the supply of free cholesterol to the mitochondria from the esterified cholesterol in the lipid droplets. Regulation of the synthesis of aldosterone raises an interesting question in that corticosterone is an obligatory intermediate in the biosynthesis of aldosterone. We do not know how independent regulation of the synthesis of these two corticoids is achieved. Information about the control of the 18-hydroxylation of corticosterone would undoubtedly help to throw light on this problem.

3 FORMATION OF FATTY ACYL ESTERS OF CHOLESTEROL

3.1 Introduction

As we have seen in Chapter 3, cholesteryl esters of long-chain fatty acids are widely distributed in animal tissues and are the predominant form in which cholesterol is carried in the plasma. Three reactions, each catalyzed by a distinct enzyme or class of enzymes, are responsible for the formation of cholesteryl esters in the animal body. Two of these, acyl-CoA:cholesterol O-acyltransferase (ACAT) (EC 2.3.1.26) and cholesteryl ester hydrolase (cholesterol esterase) (EC 3.1.1.13) are present in most, if not all, tissues; the third enzyme, lecithin:cholesterol acyltransferase (LCAT) (EC 2.3.1.43), is thought to be active only in the plasma and peripheral lymph.

3.2 ACAT

ACAT is a microsomal enzyme catalyzing the reaction:

Long-chain acyl-CoA + cholesterol → cholesteryl ester + CoA   (1)

The optimum pH for this reaction is near 7.4. The enzyme is inhibited by bile salts and sulphhydryl-blocking agents and in some tissues requires Mg^{2+} for maximum activity. ACAT exhibits marked specificity towards its fatty acid substrate. In the presence of CoA and ATP (required for the enzymic formation of acyl-CoA from fatty acids) oleate (18:1) is the preferred substrate; in rat liver the order of preference is oleate > palmitate > stearate > linoleate. Specificity with respect to the sterol substrate has not been examined in detail, but it is likely that the fatty acyl esters of the sterol analogues of cholesterol found in skin and other tissues are formed by the action of ACAT.

ACAT has been demonstrated in the microsomes of many tissues, including liver, intestinal mucosa, skin fibroblasts, arterial smooth muscle cells, adrenal cortex and kidney, and is probably responsible for the preponderance of 18:1 fatty acid in the intracellular cholesteryl esters of most tissues. The enzyme is usually assayed by measuring the incorporation of radioactive oleate into cholesteryl ester by microsomal suspensions in the presence of CoA and ATP. Assays in which radioactive cholesterol is used as substrate are less satisfactory, because in some microsomal preparations ACAT does not esterify exogenous cholesterol and also because of the unavoidable presence, in the incubation mixture, of endogenous cholesterol which may not equilibrate completely with the added substrate. Thus, ACAT is not detectable in human liver when labelled cholesterol is used as substrate (Stokke, 1972) but is readily demonstrable in human liver microsomal preparations with labelled oleate as the substrate (Balasubramaniam et al., 1979).

The ACAT present in at least two tissues is subject to regulation. When human skin fibroblasts or arterial smooth muscle cells are cultured in a lipoprotein-deficient medium, ACAT activity is maintained at a very low level. On addition of low-density lipoprotein (LDL) (but not of high-density lipoprotein) to the medium, ACAT is activated. The activation of ACAT observed under these conditions is mediated by the uptake of LDL from the medium by specific LDL receptors on the surfaces of the cells, followed by a sequence of events discussed in Chapter 9. ACAT activity is also increased in aortic tissue and in arterial smooth muscle cells of cholesterol-fed animals (St. Clair, 1976). The significance of this increase in relation to changes in cholesterol metabolism that take place in atherosclerotic lesions is discussed in Chapter 13. Hepatic ACAT activity is also increased by cholesterol feeding, but there is little or no diurnal variation in ACAT activity in the livers of rats maintained under conditions of controlled lighting and feeding (Balasubramaniam et al., 1978).

3.3 Cholesteryl ester hydrolase

Acetone powders and high-speed supernatant fractions from many tissues catalyze the formation of cholesteryl esters from cholesterol and un-ionized fatty acid in the absence of CoA and ATP. The pH optimum for this activity varies between 5 and 6, depending upon the source of the enzyme system, the pK of the fatty acid substrate and other factors. Although the mechanism of the reaction is not known it is usually assumed that the formation of cholesteryl esters by these preparations is due to a hydrolase catalyzing the reversible reaction:—

$$\text{Cholesteryl ester} + H_2O \rightleftharpoons \text{Cholesterol} + \text{fatty acid} \qquad (2)$$

Hence, the enzyme system presumed to be responsible for this activity is called 'cholesteryl ester hydrolase' or 'cholesterol esterase'. The names 'cholesterol esterifying enzyme' and 'cholesteryl ester synthetase' have also been suggested. Since lysosomes contain a cholesteryl ester hydrolase with a pH optimum between 5 and 6 it is possible that some or all of the cholesteryl-ester synthesizing activity of high-speed supernatant fractions is due to lysosomal enzyme released during the fractionation of the tissue. This is perhaps more likely than that the cytosol of intact cells contains an enzyme with a pH optimum below 6. However, it should be noted that no-one has yet shown that the hydrolysis and synthesis of cholesteryl esters that occur under conditions in which cholesteryl ester hydrolase activity is observed are due to one and the same enzyme. The problem of the nature of the extra-microsomal cholesterol-esterifying system will not be resolved until one or more of the relevant enzymes has been isolated and characterized. Only then will it be possible to introduce an unambiguous system of nomenclature for these enzymes

Cholesteryl ester hydrolase has been found in many tissues, including liver, artery, intestinal wall and adrenal cortex. During the absorption of cholesterol from the intestine, free cholesterol is esterified within the mucosal cells to cholesteryl esters containing a high proportion of oleate. Although the mucosal cells of the intestine contain microsomal ACAT, there is some evidence to suggest that much of the cholesterol-esterifying activity of intestinal mucosa is present in the cytosol, has a pH optimum of 6.1 for cholesteryl oleate, is stimulated by bile salts and does not require CoA or ATP when free fatty acids are used as substrate (Treadwell and Vahouny, 1968). This suggests that ACAT is not entirely responsible for the synthesis of intra-mucosal cholesteryl esters during cholesterol absorption. On the other hand, the soluble enzyme system investigated by Treadwell and Vahouny has a pH optimum different from that of the cholesteryl ester hydrolase in other tissues.

3.4 LCAT

3.4.1 The LCAT reaction

The presence in plasma of an enzyme system that catalyzes the esterification of plasma free cholesterol was demonstrated many years ago by Sperry (1935). Early work, showing that the esterification of cholesterol is accompanied by loss of plasma lecithin, led to the suggestion that the overall reaction consists in the transfer of a fatty acyl group from lecithin to cholesterol by the coupled actions of plasma lecithinase and a cholesterol esterase catalyzing reaction (2) in reverse. However, it is now known that the esterification takes place by the direct transfer of the β fatty acid of lecithin (i.e., the acyl group linked to the C-2 of the glycerol residue) to cholesterol (Glomset, 1968). The enzyme catalyzing the reaction is therefore called lecithin:cholesterol acyltransferase, in accordance with the EC rules for naming enzymes. During the esterification of cholesterol by the LCAT reaction, one mole of lecithin is converted into lysolecithin for each mole of cholesterol esterified (Fig. 5.8). On theoretical grounds

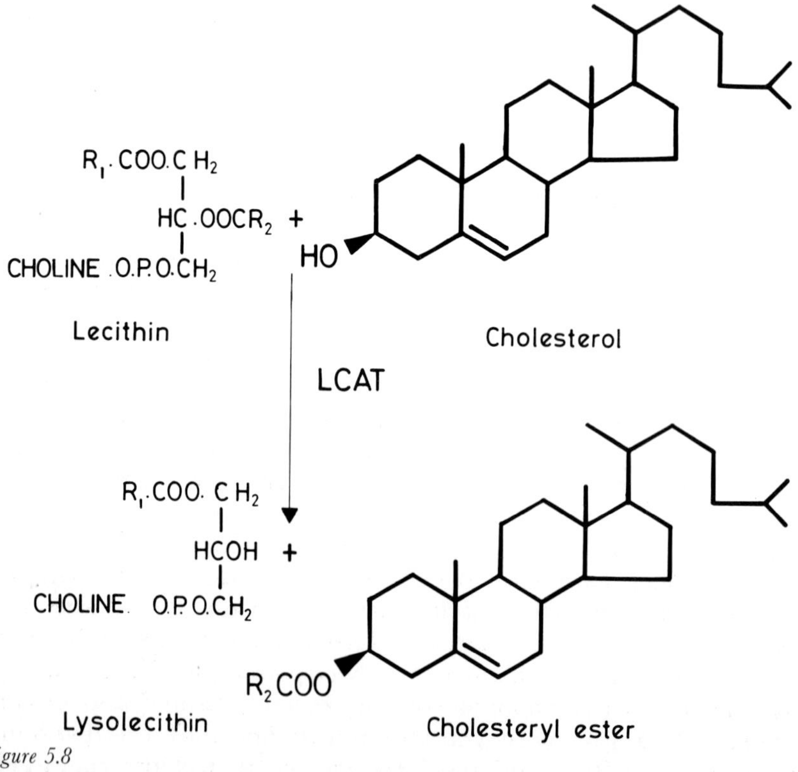

Figure 5.8
The LCAT reaction, showing the conversion of lecithin and cholesterol into lysolecithin and cholesteryl ester by the enzyme-catalyzed transfer of a fatty acyl residue (OOCR$_2$) from C-2 of lecithin to the 3β position of cholesterol.

LCAT should also catalyze the reverse reaction (the transacylation of lysolecithin to give lecithin), but under natural conditions in plasma the reaction would proceed exclusively in the direction shown in Fig. 5.8 owing to the continuous removal of lysolecithin and cholesteryl ester from the site of the reaction.

3.4.2 Distribution

LCAT has been demonstrated in the plasma of many species, including dogs, rats, rabbits, guinea-pigs, cattle, pigs, human beings and chickens. It is also present in the plasma of amphibians and reptiles (Gillett, 1978). The enzyme is synthesized in the liver and secreted into the circulation, probably in close association with the plasma lipoproteins. However, the enzyme in the liver is inactive in the LCAT reaction, possibly because catalytic activity requires the presence of cofactors in the plasma. LCAT has not been demonstrated unequivocally in any cellular tissue, but cholesterol-esterifying activity probably due to LCAT has been reported in peripheral lymph of human subjects and dogs. The presence of LCAT in the arterial wall has also been reported, but it is unlikely that LCAT plays any significant role in the esterification of cholesterol by normal or atherosclerotic arteries. LCAT activity is barely detectable in intestinal lymph (Bennett Clark and Norum, 1977).

3.4.3 Properties

The pH optimum for the LCAT reaction is about 7.5 when either native plasma lipoproteins or artificial cholesterol-lecithin dispersions are used as substrate. The enzyme is inhibited by SH-blocking agents and by polyvalent cations and is stimulated by polyvalent anions (sulphate, phosphate, citrate). LCAT from human plasma has been purified 12 000-fold to homogeneity by a combination of differential ultracentrifugation and column chromatography (Albers *et al.*, 1976). The enzyme tends to form reversible complexes with triglyceride-phospholipid emulsions, a property that has been exploited in its isolation from plasma. The human enzyme has a molecular weight of about 70 000 and is unstable in the absence of plasma lipoproteins. Highly purified preparations of LCAT are almost inactive with artificial lipid substrates unless apoA-I (the major apoprotein of HDL) is added to the incubation mixture and the stimulatory effect of apoA-I is inhibited by apoA-II (a minor apoprotein of HDL); apoC-I and apoD may also stimulate the LCAT reaction under some conditions. The role of apoprotein cofactors in the LCAT reaction is not understood. Possibly, apoA-I acts specifically by exerting a favourable influence on the physical state or spacing of the lipid molecules in the substrate (see below).

3.4.4 Substrate specificity

The LCAT reaction can only take place when the cholesterol and lecithin substrate molecules are oriented in a natural or artificial lipid layer, as described in Chapter 7. All the lipoproteins of normal plasma contain lecithin and free cholesterol present as a monolayer on the surface of the lipoprotein molecule. However, LCAT exhibits a high degree of specificity when different lipoproteins are used as substrate. Lipoprotein-free preparations of the enzyme show little ability to catalyze the formation of cholesteryl esters with VLDL or LDL as substrate, but are highly active with HDL. Furthermore, the HDL fraction with the highest density (HDL_3, d 1.12–1.21) is a better substrate than HDL_2 (d 1.063–1.12).

The reason for this preference for HDL as substrate has been sought by studying the reaction with artificial bilayers in which the lipid composition can be varied. With sonicated dispersions, lecithin is essentially the only phospholipid that can act as acyl donor and the rate of the reaction is influenced markedly by the relative amounts of lecithin and cholesterol incorporated into the bilayer, the rate of esterification decreasing when the lecithin:cholesterol molar ratio is decreased by increasing the proportion of cholesterol in the substrate mixture (Nichols and Gong, 1971). The reaction is also influenced by the nature of the fatty acid in the β position of lecithin, polyunsaturated or short-chain acyl groups being transferred to cholesterol more readily than long-chain saturated groups (Sgoutas (1972)). There are also species differences with respect to the preferred β fatty acid of lecithin. For rat LCAT the order of preference is $20:4 > 18:2 > 18:1$, but for human LCAT the order is $18:2 > 18:1 > 20:4$ (Portman and Sugano, 1964). In general, it appears that the specificity of the enzyme with respect to its lecithin substrate is determined partly by the position and partly by the nature of the fatty acids at the α and β positions. Thus, purified preparations of LCAT have some activity towards artificial lecithins with linoleate in the α position (Assmann et al., 1978).

These features of the LCAT reaction suggest that the effectiveness of HDL as a substrate for the enzyme is due to its high lecithin:cholesterol ratio (higher than that of any other plasma lipoprotein) and to the high proportion of polyunsaturated acyl groups on the β carbon of HDL lecithin. Nichols and Gong (1971) have suggested that the influence of the lecithin:cholesterol ratio on the rate of esterification is due to an effect on the lateral spacing of the substrate molecules such as to favour their combination with the active sites on the enzyme. However, it seems more likely that the effect of the lecithin:cholesterol ratio, and of the lecithin fatty acyl groups, on the LCAT reaction is due to an influence on the fluidity of the fatty acyl groups. Soutar et al. (1974) have shown that, as the temperature is raised, the rate of the LCAT reaction in a phospholipid bilayer increases abruptly at the transition temperature of the phospholipid, when the hydrocarbon chains change from a liquid-crystalline to a liquid state (see Chapter 7 for an explanation of these terms). Soutar *et al.* (1974) suggest that the fluidity of the acyl chains above the transition temperature facilitates penetration of the lipid layer by the enzyme and may also favour diffusion of the cholesteryl esters away from the active site.

3.4.5 Assay

There is no completely satisfactory method for measuring LCAT activity in plasma. The problems encountered in assaying the enzyme under conditions relevant to its activity *in vivo* have been discussed in a review by Norum (1974), which should be read by anyone intending to work on LCAT.

Assay methods based on the use of artificial substrates of standard composition and particle size are suitable for monitoring enzyme activity at successive stages in the purification of the enzyme from plasma, or for studies of the LCAT reaction. Enzyme preparations from which the plasma lipoproteins have been removed catalyze the formation of cholesteryl esters in lamellar dispersions of lecithin and cholesterol at a rate comparable with that observed when plasma lipoprotein is used as substrate. With highly purified preparations of the enzyme it is necessary to add HDL apoprotein, but apoA-I has been reported to have only a small stimulatory effect on partially purified enzyme preparations from which apoA-1 has been removed. If radioactive cholesterol is incorporated into the substrate mixture, the absolute rate of formation of the product may be calculated from the radioactivity recovered in cholesteryl esters and the specific radioactivity of the substrate cholesterol; under optimal conditions the reaction is linear for at least 60 min at 37 °C. It should be noted, however, that classical enzyme kinetics are not applicable to the LCAT reaction, whatever the method of assay used, since the total 'concentration' of membrane-bound substrate is not necessarily proportional to the amount of substrate accessible to the enzyme per unit volume of reaction mixture.

Several methods have been developed for measuring LCAT activity in whole plasma. In all these methods the substrate is the lipoprotein present in the plasma and in most of them the free cholesterol in the lipoproteins is labelled by equilibration with radioactive cholesterol, with subsequent measurement of the amount of radioactive cholesteryl ester formed during a standard incubation period. As an alternative to the use of labelled cholesterol, the decrease in free cholesterol may be measured by GLC. In order to ensure that the measured rate of the reaction is uninfluenced by depletion of substrate or accumulation of inhibitory end products, the reaction should always be followed only for the period during which it is linear. In the method of Glomset and Wright (1964), the substrate is a pool of normal plasma in which LCAT has been irreversibly inactivated by heating before equilibration of the endogenous unesterified cholesterol with radioactive cholesterol and the enzyme source is a relatively small volume of the unheated plasma in which LCAT is to be assayed. The main disadvantage of this method is the possibility that the lipoprotein acting as substrate for the enzyme is denatured by the heat inactivation. To obviate this, Stokke and Norum (1971) have devised a method in which the endogenous unesterified cholesterol in a sample of plasma is equilibrated with radioactive cholesterol for 4 hours while the LCAT in the plasma is reversibly inhibited by addition of an SH-blocking agent. After equilibration the LCAT is activated by addition of mercaptoethanolamine and the rate of formation of radioactive cholesteryl ester is measured. An advantage of this method is that the enzyme is assayed under near-physiological conditions. Hence, the initial rate of the reaction may be assumed to be close to the net rate of esterification of free cholesterol in the circulation *in vivo*. However, since enzyme and substrate are derived from the same plasma, it is not always possible to infer whether a difference in the rate of the reaction measured in two samples of plasma is due to a difference in enzyme capacity or in the 'efficiency' of the native substrate.

Methods for assaying plasma LCAT activity with radioactive cholesterol as substrate are valid only if the labelled cholesterol equilibrates completely with all the free cholesterol in the plasma sample before the reaction is started. If there is any free cholesterol in the plasma with specific radioactivity different from that of the HDL free cholesterol, estimates of the reaction rate based on the mean specific radioactivity of the free cholesterol in the whole sample would be in error. In normal plasma, complete equilibration is probably achieved with the Glomset and Wright method and with the Stokke and Norum method, but in abnormal plasmas, such as those containing large quantities of cholesterol-rich LpX, this may not be so (Kepkay *et al.*, 1973).

It is to be hoped that, in view of the difficulty of measuring the capacity of LCAT in plasma, it will eventually be possible to determine the mass of the enzyme by an immunochemical method. Progress in this direction has already been reported (Gustow *et al.*, 1978).

3.4.6 Physiological function
The distribution of LCAT in the animal body and the fact that HDL is the preferred substrate for the LCAT reaction suggest that the

enzyme is concerned mainly, perhaps exclusively, with the esterification of free cholesterol in the plasma and interstitial fluids. The significance of the LCAT reaction in relation to plasma and tissue free cholesterol is discussed in Chapter 11.

4 HYDROLYSIS OF FATTY ACYL ESTERS OF CHOLESTEROL

4.1 Introduction

Enzymes catalyzing the hydrolysis of cholesteryl esters are present in pancreatic juice and intestinal fluid and in many animal tissues. The pancreatic enzyme is well defined and has been studied in considerable detail, but there is still a good deal of uncertainty about the identity of the enzymes responsible for cholesteryl ester hydrolysis in the tissues. As already noted, it is not known whether the ability of high-speed supernatant fractions to catalyze the synthesis and hydrolysis of cholesteryl esters is due to the presence of at least two separate enzymes or to a single enzyme catalyzing the reversible reaction in both directions. Nor is it clear how far the presence of cholesterylester hydrolyzing activity observed in different subcellular fractions and under different assay conditions reflects the existence of several distinct cholesteryl ester hydrolases in animal tissues. Until these points have been settled, tissue enzyme systems catalyzing the hydrolysis of cholesteryl esters are best referred to in terms of the subcellular fraction in which the activity is observed, the nature and physical state of the cholesteryl ester substrate and the conditions under which activity is assayed. The question whether activity observed in different circumstances is due to multiple enzymes or to a single enzyme can then be left open. Many of the problems encountered in the study of the enzymic hydrolysis of long-chain fatty acid esters of sterols, especially in relation to the standardization of the substrate, have been discussed by Vahouny and Treadwell (1968).

4.2 Pancreas

Dietary cholesteryl esters are hydrolyzed in the lumen of the intestine before absorption. Pancreatic cholesteryl ester hydrolase, the enzyme responsible for this hydrolysis, is secreted in pancreatic juice and catalyzes the reversible reaction shown in equation (2). The pH optimum for the hydrolytic reaction is 6.5–7.0, a range over which most long-chain fatty acids are largely in the ionized form. (Below about pH 6 the reaction is catalyzed in the direction of steryl ester synthesis.) At equilibrium the ratio of steryl ester:free sterol is about

2:1. Bile salts are required for the reaction catalyzed in either direction. According to Treadwell and Vahouny (1968) pancreatic cholesteryl ester hydrolase has a specific requirement for cholic acid and this acid cannot be replaced by dihydroxy- or monohydroxy bile acids or by other detergents, suggesting that cholic acid does not act simply as an agent for maintaining the substrate in a suitable physical state in an aqueous medium. The fact that taurocholic acid also protects the enzyme against proteolytic inactivation suggests that the bile-salt activator combines with the enzyme and may therefore act as a true cofactor. The ability of dog plasma to hydrolyse cholesteryl esters in the presence of bile salts (Sperry and Stoyanoff, 1938) is due to the presence of pancreatic cholesteryl ester hydrolase in the dog's circulation.

The enzyme has been partially purified from acetone powders prepared from hog pancreas or rat pancreatic juice. These preparations exhibit substrate specificity with respect to the sterol moiety of the steryl ester. For steryl esters of oleic acid, the rate of the reaction measured in the direction of synthesis decreases in the order: cholesterol = 5α-cholestanol > β-sitosterol > stigmasterol > ergosterol. Sterols with a 3α-hydroxyl group or 5β configuration are very poorly esterified with oleic acid.

4.3 Liver

Homogenates of liver from animals of several species, including man, have been shown to catalyze the hydrolysis of long-chain fatty acid esters of cholesterol at pH 4.5–5.0. (At pH 4.0 the reaction is catalyzed in the direction of cholesteryl ester synthesis.) These preparations are active when tested with artificial emulsions of cholesteryl esters and with serum lipoproteins containing labelled cholesteryl esters synthesized by the LCAT reaction (Stokke, 1974). The hydrolytic activity exhibited at pH 4.5–5.0 is present in high-speed supernatant fractions of liver homogenates and in liver lysosomes.

A soluble enzyme catalyzing the hydrolysis of cholesteryl esters with a pH optimum in the range 6.5–7.5 has also been reported in rat liver (Deykin and Goodman, 1962). This enzyme has been purified 70-fold by ammonium sulphate precipitation and gel chromatography. The partially purified enzyme is inhibited by bile salts and shows some specificity with respect to the fatty acid moiety of the substrate. With substrates added as acetone solutions, hydrolytic activity decreases in the order: $18.2 \geqslant 18:1 > 16:0 \geqslant 18:0$.

No cofactors are required either by the preparations active at pH 4.5–5.0 or by those active in the range 6.5–7.5. Autoradiographic studies of the hydrolysis of tritium-labelled cholesteryl esters in chylomicrons suggest the presence of yet another hepatic cholesteryl ester hydrolase catalyzing the hydrolysis of chylomicron cholesteryl esters on the outer surface of the hepatocyte plasma membrane (Stein et al., 1969).

4.4 Artery

Cholesteryl ester hydrolase activity has been demonstrated in extracts or homogenates of aortic tissue and in isolated aortic smooth-muscle cells (Day, 1967; St. Clair, 1976). Cytoplasmic hydrolase activity has also been observed in arterial smooth-muscle cells (Stein et al., 1980). At least three different pH optima for the hydrolysis of cholesteryl esters by these preparations have been reported from different laboratories (pH 8.6, 6.6–7.5 and 4.0–4.5). The activity with a pH optimum between 4.0 and 4.5 is due to a lysosomal acid hydrolase in arterial smooth-muscle cells (Takano et al., 1974). Little is known about the enzymic basis of the hydrolytic activity observed at pH 8.6 and in the range 6.6–7.5. There may be more than one enzyme in the arterial wall with cholesteryl ester hydrolase activity. On the other hand, the pH optimum for the enzymic hydrolysis of cholesteryl ester is markedly influenced by the form in which the substrate is added to the assay system (St. Clair, 1976). It is possible, therefore, that some discrepancies in reports from different laboratories are due to differences in the method of adding the exogenous substrate, rather than to the presence of different cholesteryl-ester hydrolases. A comprehensive list of published reports of cholesteryl-ester hydrolyzing enzymes in arterial tissue from different species will be found in the review by Kritchevsky and Kothari (1978).

Stein et al. (1980) have investigated the hydrolysis of cytoplasmic (extralysosomal) cholesteryl esters in intact aortic smooth-muscle cells in culture. The cytoplasmic cholesteryl esters were labelled by incubating the cells in a medium containing radioactive free cholesterol at high concentration. Under these conditions free cholesterol in the medium crossed the plasma membrane to reach the interior of the cells, where it was esterified by ACAT and incorporated into the cytoplasmic pool of esterified cholesterol. When the cells were transferred to fresh medium containing an acceptor for cholesterol, the cytoplasmic cholesteryl esters were hydrolysed and the labelled free cholesterol so produced was excreted into the medium. Since hydrolysis of the labelled esters was not inhibited by chloroquine (an inhibitor of lysosomal enzymes) it may be assumed that the esters were hydrolysed by the cytosolic cholesteryl ester hydrolase active at neutral pH, rather than by a lysosomal hydrolase following their entry into lysosomes by autophagy (see Chapter 17, Section 2). In addition to throwing light on the mechanism by which smooth-muscle cells excrete cholesterol, these experiments confirm the presence of a physiological intracellular cholesteryl ester hydrolase other than the lysosomal acid-pH enzyme.

4.5 Steroid-hormone-forming tissues

Homogenates and acetone powders prepared from adrenal cortex of rats, pigs, dogs and other animals have been shown to catalyze the hydrolysis of long-chain fatty acid esters of cholesterol in the absence of added cofactors. There is disagreement about the subcellular distribution of this activity and about the optimum conditions of incubation. Cholesteryl-ester hydrolysing activity has been observed in high-speed supernatant fractions and in particulate fractions of adrenal cortex homogenates, and pH optima ranging from 6.6 to 7.4 have been reported from different laboratories. The soluble enzyme system prepared from rat adrenal cortex by Boyd *et al.* (1975) has a pH optimum at 7.4 when assayed with cholesteryl oleate as substrate and, as discussed on p. 270, is activated by the adenyl cyclase system. Enzymes catalyzing the hydrolysis of cholesteryl esters have also been reported in ovary, testis and human placenta. The human placental enzyme has been purified 350-fold, the partially purified enzyme having a pH optimum at 6.6 (Chen and Morin, 1971).

In view of the probable role of cholesteryl ester as a store of cholesterol for steroid-hormone synthesis, it is possible that the enzymic hydrolysis of cholesteryl esters in the tissues discussed in this section is functionally related to the production of steroid hormones. This certainly seems to be true for adrenal cortex. The mechanism by which the enzyme in its activated state gains access to its substrate in these tissues is not understood, but is clearly a question of much interest, especially in relation to those steroid-hormone-forming tissues in which cholesteryl esters are enclosed within lipid droplets.

4.6 Other tissues

Cholesteryl-ester hydrolysing activity has been reported in a wide variety of tissues, in addition to those considered in the previous sections. These tissues include intestinal wall, kidney, skeletal muscle, spleen, developing brain, adipose tissue, white blood cells, macrophages from various sources and cultured human fibroblasts. Not all these reports have been confirmed and there is disagreement as to the subcellular localization, substrate specificity and pH optimum of the hydrolytic activity in different cells. However, lysosomes from several cell types have been shown to contain an acid hydrolase capable of hydrolysing long-chain fatty acid esters of cholesterol. Hence it is possible that the ability to hydrolyse cholesteryl esters is an essential attribute of all metabolically active animal cells. The physiological function of the lysosomal hydrolase may be to convert intracellular cholesterol, originating by uptake of cholesterol-rich lipoproteins from the extracellular fluids, into unesterified cholesterol required for growth and maintenance of cell membranes. Lysosomal hydrolysis of cholesteryl esters may also be necessary for the removal of cholesterol from some types of cell. It is consistent with this possibility that cholesteryl esters accumulate in the cells of patients with Wolman's disease, a condition in which there is an inherited absence of a lysosomal ester hydrolase (see Chapter 17, Section 3.6 for discussion of this question).

On the other hand, lysosomal hydrolysis does not appear to be an essential step in the removal of esterified cholesterol from cytoplasmic pools in arterial smooth-muscle cells (see Section 4.4) or macrophages. In a study analogous to that of Stein et al. (1980), Brown et al. (1980) have shown that the cytoplasmic cholesteryl esters in mouse macrophages are hydrolysed by an extralysosomal esterase. In these experiments the cytoplasmic lipid droplets of macrophages in monolayer culture were loaded with cholesteryl ester by incubating them in a medium containing acetyl-LDL as an external source of cholesterol (see Chapter 9, Section 2.2.3). When the acetyl-LDL was removed and an acceptor for free cholesterol was added to the medium, the esterified cholesterol in the droplets underwent net hydrolysis and the free cholesterol so produced was excreted into the medium. As with arterial smooth-muscle cells, hydrolysis of cytoplasmic esterified cholesterol was not inhibited by inhibitors of lysosomal enzymes, showing that the hydrolytic enzyme is extralysosomal. Using doubly labelled cholesteryl ester, Brown and coworkers (1980) showed that the cholesteryl esters in the lipid droplets of macrophages undergo continual hydrolysis and re-esterification by ACAT, and that net hydrolysis is promoted, not by increased activity of the esterase, but by decreased re-esterification. These findings point to an essential role for extralysosomal hydrolysis of esterified cholesterol in the excretion of ingested cholesterol by macrophages *in vivo*.

In certain other tissues, cytoplasmic hydrolysis of esterified cholesterol serves other more specific functions. Examples are the controlled hydrolysis of cholesteryl esters in adrenal cortex during steroid-hormone formation and the cholesteryl-ester hydrolysing system in adipose tissue described by Pittman et al. (1975). The latter enzyme system appears to be the same as the hormone-sensitive lipase responsible for the hydrolysis of triglycerides in the lipid droplets of fat cells (Khoo et al., 1976). The importance of intracellular hydrolysis of cholesteryl esters in the turnover of esterified cholesterol in plasma lipoproteins is discussed in Chapters 9 and 11.

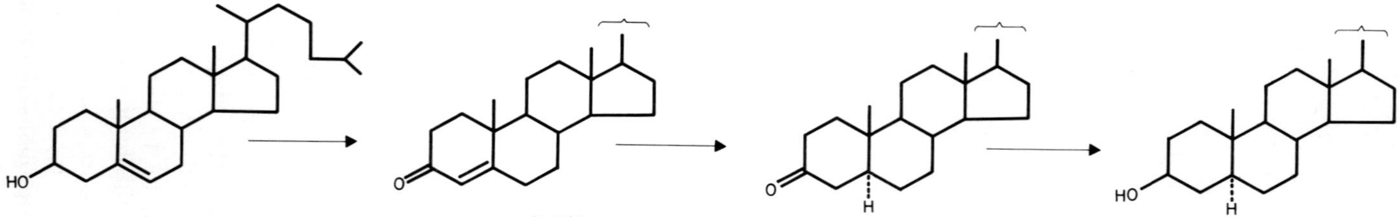

286 The Biology of Cholesterol and Related Steroids

Scheme 7 The conversion of cholesterol into 5α-cholestane-3β-ol (cholestanol). (**5.27**), Cholest-4-en-3-one; (**5.28**), 5α-cholestan-3-one; (**5.29**), 5α-cholestanol.

5 5α-CHOLESTANOL

5α-Cholestanol is formed from cholesterol in the intestinal lumen by the action of microbial enzymes. However, some of the 5α-cholestanol present in animal tissues must also be formed *in situ* by tissue enzymes, since [^{14}C]cholesterol is converted into 5α-cholestanol in germ-free animals. In the liver, 5α-cholestanol is derived from cholesterol by a sequence of steps requiring at least three separate enzymes. The first step (see Scheme 7) is the conversion of cholesterol into cholest-4-en-3-one (**5.27**) by a microsomal 3β-hydroxy-Δ^5-steroid oxidoreductase which requires NAD as H acceptor and is distinct from the steroid oxidoreductase concerned in the formation of bile acids from cholesterol (Björkhem and Karlmar, 1974). The second step is the reduction of the Δ^4 double bond of (**5.27**), to give 5α-cholestan-3-one (**5.28**) by a microsomal 5α-reductase which requires NADPH as H donor (Shefer *et al.*, 1966*a*). The final step consists in the reduction of the 3-keto group by a microsomal 3β-hydroxysteroid dehydrogenase, using NADPH as H donor, to give 5α-cholestanol (**5.29**). This enzyme differs from the hydroxysteroid dehydrogenase that uses C_{19} steroids as substrate (Shefer *et al.*, 1966*b*).

5α-Cholestanol is esterified with long-chain fatty acids in human plasma *in vivo* at a rate almost equal to the rate of esterification of the plasma free cholesterol (Salen and Grundy, 1973). As we have already seen (Section 1.2.5), 5α-cholestanol is a substrate for cholesterol 7α-hydroxylase and may thus enter the pathway to bile-acid formation.

6 STERYL SULPHATES

Cholesteryl sulphate is widely distributed in animal tissues and several sulphate esters of sterols closely related to cholesterol have been isolated from human faeces. The formation of 3β-monosulphate esters of sterols is catalyzed by a 3β-hydroxysteroid sulphotransferase (EC 2.8.2.2), the sulphotransferase catalyzing the transfer of the sulphate group from a donor of activated sulphate (adenosine 3'-phosphate 5'-sulphatophosphate) to the sterol acceptor. This enzyme is present in rat liver (Nose and Lipmann, 1958) and has been demonstrated in the high-speed supernatant from homogenates of human breast carcinoma (Adams and Wong, 1968).

The high polarity of sulphated sterols suggests that they are excretory products. However, Roberts *et al.* (1964) injected [7α-^{3}H]cholesteryl[^{35}S]sulphate into the artery supplying an adrenal tumour in a human subject and subsequently isolated radioactive monosulphate esters of C_{19} and C_{21} steroids from the patient's urine.

These steroids contained ³H and ³⁵S in the same ratio as that in the injected cholesteryl sulphate.

This finding suggests that cholesteryl sulphate can act as the immediate precursor in the biosynthetic sequence leading to the formation of steroid hormones in the adrenal cortex and that the enzymes catalyzing the cleavages between C-20 and C-22 and between C-17 and C-20 of the sterol side chain, as well as other modifications to the sterol molecule, can use sulphated intermediates as substrates.

7 VITAMIN D

7.1 Sterol precursors of vitamin D

Vitamin D$_2$ (5,6-*cis*-ergocalciferol) was the first vitamin with antirachitic properties to be isolated and identified. (Vitamin D$_1$ is the name given by Windaus to an antirachitic substance formed by ultraviolet irradiation of ergosterol and now known to be a mixture of vitamin D$_2$ and lumisterol, a biologically inactive isomer of the vitamin). Vitamin D$_2$ is formed from ergosterol by irradiation with ultraviolet light of wavelength 275–300 mμ; ergosterol is therefore the provitamin of D$_2$. The steps in the conversion of ergosterol into vitamin D$_2$ are probably those shown in Fig. 5.9. An unstable

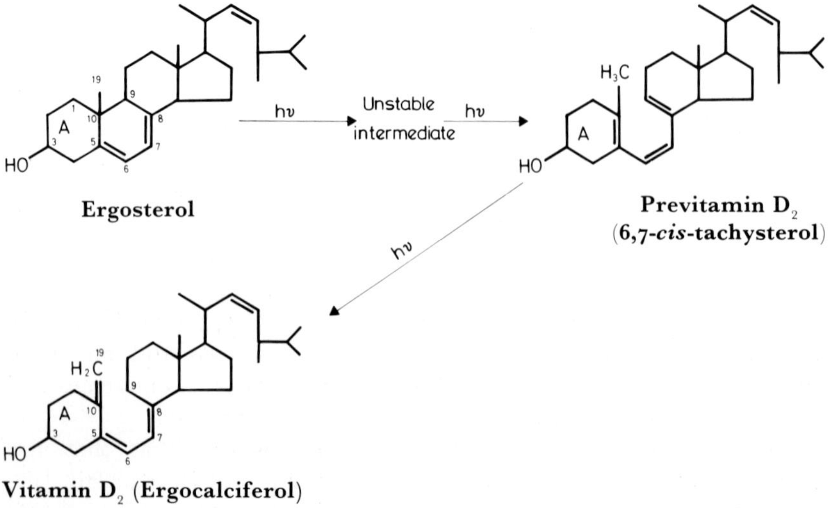

Figure 5.9
Probable steps in the conversion of ergosterol into vitamin D$_2$ *via* an unstable intermediate (X) and previtamin D$_2$.

intermediate is formed reversibly and is rapidly converted into previtamin D_2 by opening of ring B at the 9,10 bond and the formation of an additional double bond. Previtamin D_2 is then converted into vitamin D_2 by the transfer of a proton from C-19 to C-9 and the rearrangement of the three conjugated double bonds. X-ray analysis of a crystalline derivative of vitamin D_2 (the 4-iodo-5-nitrobenzoate) by Crowfoot and Dunitz (1948) has shown that the conformation of the vitamin D_2 molecule in the crystalline state is roughly that shown in Fig. 5.10. The molecule adopts an extended form with the 5,6 and 7,8 double bonds coplanar and more or less in line with one another. The 5,6 double bond is *cis*, in the sense that C-7 is *cis* to C-10.

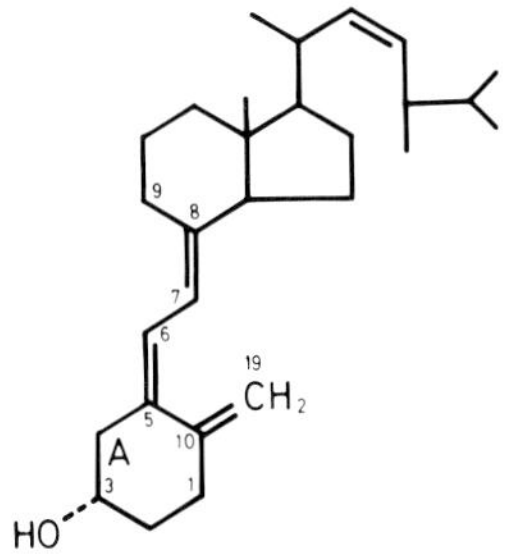

Vitamin D_2 (extended conformation)

Figure 5.10
The probable conformation of vitamin D_2 in the crystalline state. Note that the 3β-OH group projects below the plane of the paper when ring A is rotated into the extended conformation.

Vitamin D_3 (5,6-*cis*-cholecalciferol) is the antirachitic vitamin present in fish oils and mammalian skin. It is formed in the skin by the action of ultraviolet light on 7-dehydrocholesterol by a sequence analogous to that shown in Fig. 5.7. Hence, 7-dehydrocholesterol is the provitamin of D_3. The structure of vitamin D_3 differs from that of vitamin D_2 only in the nature of the side-chain, vitamin D_3 lacking the Δ^{22} double bond and the C-24 methyl group.

Other sterols with a $\Delta^{5,7}$-diene system (22-dihydroergosterol, for example) can be converted into compounds with antirachitic activity by ultraviolet irradiation, but sterols with a C_5 side-chain cannot act as precursors for vitamin D. The precursor of the vitamin D_3 present in fish liver oils is undoubtedly 7-dehydrocholesterol, but it is unlikely that conversion of the provitamin to the vitamin takes place in the body of the fish because the intensity of ultraviolet light beneath the surface of the sea would be too low for this to occur. A possible source of fish D_3 is the surface zooplankton on which young fish feed during the summer and which have been shown to have antirachitic activity in rats (Copping, 1934).

290 The Biology of Cholesterol and Related Steroids

7.2 Metabolism of vitamin D

Vitamin D is converted in the body into metabolites which have greater and more rapid biological effects than those of the unchanged vitamin. These biologically active metabolites are formed by the 25-hydroxylation of vitamin D in the liver, followed by 1α-hydroxylation in the kidneys to give 1α,25-dihydroxyvitamin D. The steps in the formation of the two active metabolites from vitamin D_3 are shown in Fig. 5.11. Metabolites of vitamin D with hydroxyl groups in the 21,

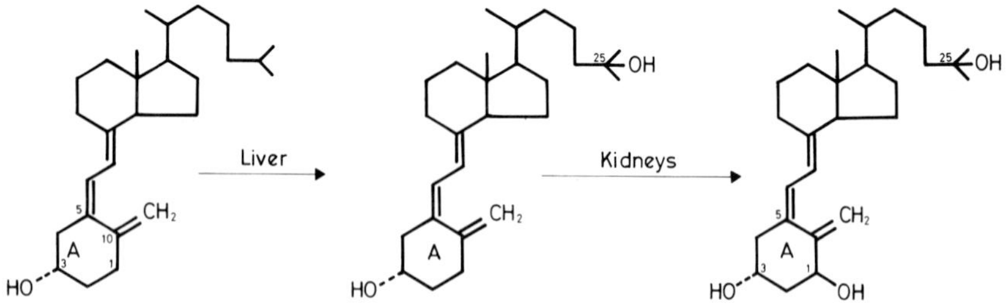

Vitamin D_3 25-Hydroxyvitamin D_3 1α,25-Dihydroxyvitamin D_3

Figure 5.11
The conversion of vitamin D_3 into biologically active metabolites. Note that the 1α-OH group is shown projecting above the plane of the paper owing to rotation of the A ring into the extended conformation.

24 and 26 positions have also been identified in plasma. Their physiological significance has not yet been fully established, but it seems likely that 24,25-dihydroxyvitamin D_3 is a normal biologically active metabolite in man (Kanis *et al.*, 1979). The enzyme catalyzing the 25-hydroxylation of vitamin D in the liver is microsomal and that catalyzing the 1α-hydroxylation of 25-hydroxyvitamin D in the kidneys is mitochondrial. Both enzyme systems require molecular O_2, NADPH and cytochrome P450.

25-Hydroxyvitamin D in very large doses stimulates the mobilization of calcium in cultures of embryonic bone and the transport of calcium in perfused intestines. However, the 1α,25-dihydroxylated compound must be regarded as the form in which the vitamin acts upon its target organs, since the mobilization of bone calcium and the intestinal transport of calcium are not stimulated by physiological doses of 25-hydroxyvitamin D_3 in nephrectomized animals, but are fully stimulated by physiological doses of 1α,25-dihydroxyvitamin D_3 in these animals (Holick *et al.*, 1972). The biological activity of the 25-hydroxyvitamin in intact animals is presumably due to its rapid 1α-hydroxylation in the kidneys.

The synthesis of 1α,25-dihydroxyvitamin D in the kidneys is regulated by a complex homeostatic mechanism tending to maintain a constant plasma calcium concentration. When an intact animal is given a diet low in calcium, the renal synthesis of 1α,25-dihydroxyvitamin D increases and this, in turn, leads to increased intestinal absorption of calcium and increased mobilization of bone calcium. This response to a low-calcium diet is mediated by increased secretion of parathyroid hormone and does not occur when the parathyroid glands have been removed. The effect of parathyroid hormone on the production of 1α,25-dihydroxyvitamin D appears to be due to stimulation of the 1α-hydroxylase in the renal tubules, possibly *via* the adenyl cyclase system (Rasmussen *et al.*, 1972). Increased 1α-hydroxylating activity in the kidneys also occurs as a direct response to a low plasma concentration of inorganic phosphorus without the participation of the parathyroid glands.

7.3 Biologically active analogues of vitamin D

Dihydrotachysterol and the 5,6-*trans* isomer of vitamin D_3, the two analogues of vitamin D shown in Fig. 5.12, have only about 1/500 the antirachitic activity of vitamin D_3 in intact animals. However, dose for dose these analogues are much more potent than vitamin D_3 in mobilizing bone calcium and stimulating intestinal transport of calcium in parathyroidectomized or nephrectomized animals. The biological effectiveness of dihydrotachysterol under these conditions seems to depend upon two factors. Inspection of the formula in Fig. 5.12 shows that the 3β-hydroxyl group of dihydrotachysterol is

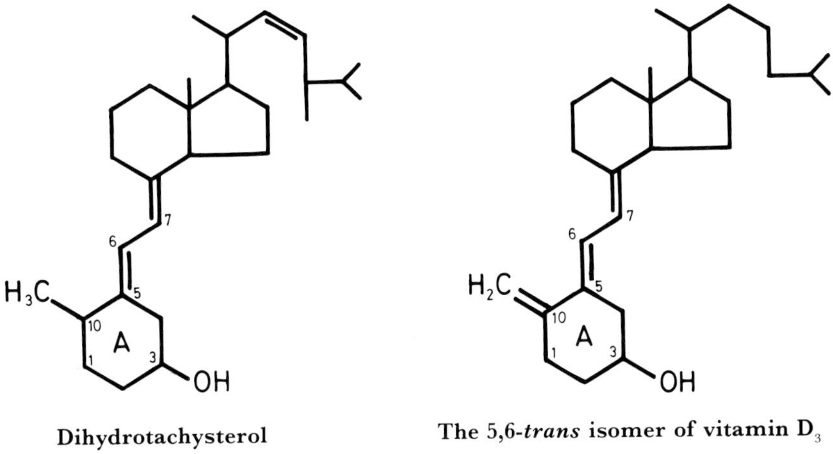

Dihydrotachysterol   **The 5,6-*trans* isomer of vitamin D_3**

Figure 5.12
Two biologically active analogues of vitamin D, dihydrotachysterol and the 5,6-*trans* isomer of vitamin D_3. Note the steric equivalence of the 3β-OH group of these analogues with the 1α-OH group of 1α,25-dihydroxyvitamin D, possibly helping to explain their biological activity.

stereochemically equivalent to the 1α-hydroxyl group of 1α,25-dihydroxyvitamin D (Fig. 5.11). Furthermore, dihydrotachysterol acts as an efficient substrate for the hepatic 25-hydroxylase. Thus it seems likely that dihydrotachysterol can be converted into a biologically active compound (25-hydroxydihydrotachysterol) without the need for the 1α-hydroxylation dependent upon the presence of intact kidneys and functioning parathyroid glands. The implications of this in relation to the treatment of bone disease in patients with disease of the parathyroid glands or the kidneys are obvious and have been discussed by Holick and De Luca (1974). The position with regard to the biological activity of the 5,6-*trans* isomer of vitamin D_3 is not so clear. Like dihydrotachysterol, this compound contains a hydroxyl group that is equivalent to the 1α-hydroxyl group present in the active metabolite of vitamin D_3. The 5,6-*trans* isomer mobilizes calcium from bone in nephrectomized rats. However, this activity is not increased by 25-hydroxylation. Possibly, the hydroxyl group in the pseudo 1α-position is sufficient to confer biological activity on this analogue of vitamin D_3.

For a full discussion of vitamin D in relation to calcium metabolism, the reader should consult the monograph by De Luca (1979).

REFERENCES

Adams, J. B. and Wong, M. S. F. (1968). Enzymic synthesis of steroid sulfates. VI. Formation of cholesteryl-3[35]S-sulfate on incubation of human breast carcinoma extracts with adenosine-3-phosphate-5'-phospho-^{35}S-sulfate. *Steroids*, **11**, 313–319.

Albers, J. J., Cabana, V. G. and Stahl, Y. D. B. (1976). Purification and characterization of human plasma lecithin:cholesterol acyltransferase. *Biochemistry*, **15**, 1084–1086

Assmann, G., Schmitz, G., Donath, N. and Lekin, D. (1978). Phosphatidyl choline substrate specificity of lecithin:cholesterol acyltransferase. *Scandinavian Journal of Clinical Laboratory Investigation*, **38**, Supplement 150, 16–20.

Balasubramaniam, S., Goldstein, J. L. and Brown, M. S. (1977). Regulation of cholesterol synthesis in rat adrenal gland through coordinate control of 3-hydroxy-3-methylglutaryl coenzyme A synthase and reductase activities. *Proceedings of the National Academy of Sciences of the USA*, **74**, 1421–1425.

Balasubramaniam, S., Mitropoulos, K. A. and Myant, N. B. (1973). Evidence for the compartmentation of cholesterol in rat-liver microsomes. *European Journal of Biochemistry*, **34**, 77–83.

Balasubramaniam, S., Mitropoulos, K. A. and Myant, N. B. Hormonal control of the activities of cholesterol-7α-hydroxylase and hydroxymethylglutaryl-CoA reductase in rats. In: *Advances in Bile Acid Research, Vol. 3, Bile Acid Meeting*, Freiburg. Ed. S. Matern, J. Hackenschmidt, P. Back and W. Gerok. F. K. Schattauer Verlag, Stuttgart, pp. 61–67, 1975.

Balasubramaniam, S., Mitropoulos, K. A., Myant, N. B., Mancini, M. and Postiglione, A. (1979). Acyl-coenzyme A-cholesterol acyltransferase activity in human liver. *Clinical Science*, **56**, 373–375.

Balasubramaniam, S., Mitropoulos, K. A. and Venkatesan, S. (1978). Rat-liver acyl-CoA:cholesterol acyltransferase. *European Journal of Biochemistry*, **90**, 377–383.
Barnes, S., Burhol, P. G., Zander, R., Haggstrom, G., Settine, R. L. and Hirschowitz, B. I. (1979). Enzymatic sulfation of glycochenodeoxycholic acid by tissue fractions from adult hamsters. *Journal of Lipid Research*, **20**, 952–959
Barnes, S., Summerfield, J. A., Gollan, J. L. and Billing, B. H. Renal mechanisms influencing the bile acid composition of cholestatic urine. In: *Bile Acid Metabolism in Health and Disease*. Ed. G. Paumgartner and A. Stiehl. MTP Press, London, pp. 89–92, 1976.
Barrington, E. J. W. *Hormones and Evolution*. Ed. E. J. W. Barrington, 2 Volumes, Academic Press, New York, 1979.
Batta, A. K., Salen, G., Blount, J. F. and Shefer, S. (1979). Configuration at C-25 in $3\alpha,7\alpha,12\alpha$-trihydroxy-5β-cholestan-26-oic acid by X-ray crystallography. *Journal of Lipid Research*, **20**, 935–940.
Bellamy, D. and Chester Jones, I. (1965). The evolution of adrenocortical hormones. *Excerpta Medica*, **83**, 153–157.
Van Belle, H. *Cholesterol, Bile Acids and Atherosclerosis*. North-Holland Publishing Company, Amsterdam, 1965.
Bennett Clark, S. and Norum, K. R. (1977). The lecithin-cholesterol acyl transferase activity of rat intestinal lymph. *Journal of Lipid Research*, **18**, 293–300.
Bergström, S. and Danielsson, H. (1958). On the regulation of bile acid formation in the rat liver. *Acta Physiologica Scandinavica*, **43**, 1–7.
Berséus, O. (1965). On the stereospecificity of 26-hydroxylation of cholesterol. Bile acids and steroids 155. *Acta Chemica Scandinavica*, **19**, 325–328.
Björkhem, I. (1969). On the mechanism of the enzymatic conversion of cholest-5-ene-$3\beta,7\alpha$-diol into 7α-hydroxycholest-4-en-3-one. *European Journal of Biochemistry*, **8**, 337–344.
Björkhem, I., Danielsson, H., Einarsson, K. and Johansson, G. (1968). Formation of bile acids in man: conversion of cholesterol into 5β-cholestane-$3\alpha,7\alpha,12\alpha$-triol in liver homogenates. *Journal of Clinical Investigation*, **47**, 1573–1582.
Björkhem, I., Danielsson, H. and Wikvall, K. (1976). Side-chain hydroxylations in biosynthesis of cholic acid. 25- and 26-hydroxylation of 5β-cholestane-$3\alpha,7\alpha,12\alpha$-triol by reconstituted systems from rat liver microsomes. *Journal of Biological Chemistry*, **251**, 3495–3499.
Björkhem, I., Gustafsson, J., Johansson, G. and Persson, B. (1975). Biosynthesis of bile acids in man. Hydroxylation of the C_{27}-steroid side chain. *Journal of Clinical Investigation*, **55**, 478–486.
Björkhem, I. and Karlmar, K.-E. (1974). Biosynthesis of cholestanol: conversion of cholesterol into 4-cholesten-3-one by rat liver microsomes. *Biochimica et Biophysica Acta*, **337**, 129–131.
Bloch, K., Berg, B. N. and Rittenberg, D. (1943). The biological conversion of cholesterol to cholic acid. *Journal of Biological Chemistry*, **149**, 511–517.
Boyd, G. S., Arthur, J. R., Beckett, G. J., Mason, J. I. and Trzeciak, W. H. (1975). The role of cholesterol and cytochrome P-450 in the cholesterol side chain cleavage reaction in adrenal cortex and corpora lutea. *Journal of Steroid Biochemistry*, **6**, 427–436.
Boyd, G. S. and Trzeciak, W. H. (1973). Cholesterol metabolism in the adrenal cortex: studies on the mode of action of ACTH. *Annals of the New York Academy of Sciences*, **212**, 361–377.
Brown, M. S., Ho, Y. K. and Goldstein, J. L. (1980). The cholesteryl ester cycle in macrophage foam cells. Continual hydrolysis and re-esterification of cytoplasmic cholesteryl esters. *Journal of Biological Chemistry*, **255**, 9344–9352.
Brownie, A. C., Alfano, J., Jefcoate, C. R., Orme-Johnson, W., Beinert, H. and

Simpson, E. R. (1973). Effect of ACTH on adrenal mitochondrial cytochrome P-450 in the rat. *Annals of the New York Academy of Sciences*, **212**, 344–360.
Burstein, S. and Gut, M. (1971). Biosynthesis of pregnane derivatives. *Advances in Lipid Research*, **9**, 291–333.
Carey, J. B. Jr. (1964). Conversion of cholesterol to trihydroxycoprostanic acid and cholic acid in man. *Journal of Clinical Investigation*, **43**, 1443–1448.
Carey, J. B. Jr. and Haslewood, G. A. D. (1963). Crystallization of trihydroxycoprostanic acid from human bile. *Journal of Biological Chemistry*, **238**, PC855–856.
Chen, L. J., Admirand, W. H. and Bolt, R. J. (1975). Cholyl sulfokinase enzymatic sulfation of bile salts. *Federation Proceedings*, **34**, 560.
Chen, L. & Morin, R. (1971). Purification of human placental cholesteryl ester hydrolase. *Biochimica et Biophysica Acta*, **231**, 194–197.
Copping, A. M. (1934). Origin of vitamin D in cod-liver oil: vitamin D content of zooplankton. *Biochemical Journal*, **28**, 1516–1520.
Cottman, J., Danielsson, H., Hansson, R. and Wikvall, K. Hydroxylations in biosynthesis and metabolism of bile acids catalyzed by reconstituted systems from rat liver microsomes. In: *Bile Acid Metabolism in Health and Disease*. Ed. G. Paumgartner and A. Stiehl. MTP Press, Lancaster, pp. 1–10, 1977.
Crowfoot, D. and Dunitz, J. D. (1948). Structure of calciferol. *Nature*, **162**, 608–609.
Czygan, P., Ast, E., Frohling, W., Stiehl, A. and Kommerell, B. Synthesis and excretion of bile acid sulfate esters in the isolated perfused rat kidney. In: *Bile Acid Metabolism in Health and Disease*. Ed. G. Paumgartner and A. Stiehl. MTP Press, Lancaster, pp. 83–87, 1976.
Danielsson, H. and Einarsson, K. Formation and metabolism of bile acids. In: *The Biological Basis of Medicine, Vol. 5*. Ed. E. E. Bittar and N. Bittar. Academic Press, London, pp. 279–315, 1969.
Day, A. J. (1967). Lipid metabolism by macrophages and its relationship to atherosclerosis. *Advances in Lipid Research*, **5**, 185–207.
De Luca, H. F. *Vitamin D: Metabolism and Function*. Springer Verlag, Berlin, 1979.
Deykin, D. and Goodman, DeW. S. (1962). The hydrolysis of long-chain fatty acid esters of cholesterol with rat liver enzymes. *Journal of Biological Chemistry*, **237**, 3649–3656.
Dowling, R. H., Mack, E. and Small, D. M. (1970). Effects of controlled interruption of the enterohepatic circulation of bile salts by biliary diversion and by ileal resection on bile salt secretion, synthesis, and pool size in the rhesus monkey. *Journal of Clinical Investigation*, **49**, 232–242.
Drayer, N. M., Roberts, K. D., Bandi, L. and Lieberman, S. (1964). The isolation of cholesterol sulfate from bovine adrenals. *Journal of Biological Chemistry*, **239**, PC3112–3114.
Gillett, M. P. T. (1978). Comparative studies of the lecithin:cholesterol acyltransferase reaction in the plasma of reptiles and amphibians. *Scandinavian Journal of Clinical Laboratory Investigation*, **38**, Supplement 150, 32–39.
Glomset, J. A. (1968). The plasma lecithin:cholesterol acyltransferase reaction. *Journal of Lipid Research*, **9**, 155–167.
Glomset, J. A. and Wright, J. L. (1964). Some properties of a cholesterol esterifying enzyme in human plasma. *Biochimica et Biophysica Acta*, **89**, 266–276.
Go, V. L. W., Hofmann, A. F. and Summerskill, W. H. J. (1970). Simultaneous measurements of pancreatic, biliary, and gastric outputs in man using a perfusion technique. *Gastroenterology*, **58**, 321–328.
Grundy, S. M. and Metzger, A. L. (1972). A physiological method for estimation of hepatic secretion of biliary lipids in man. *Gastroenterology*, **62**, 1200–1217.
Gustafsson, B. E., Bergström, S., Lindstedt, S. and Norman, A. (1957). Turnover and nature of fecal bile acids in germfree and infected rats fed cholic acid-24-^{14}C. Bile

acids and steroids 41. *Proceedings of the Society for Experimental Biology and Medicine*, **94**, 467–471.

Gustafsson, J. (1975). Biosynthesis of cholic acid in rat liver. 24-Hydroxylation of 3α,7α,12α-trihydroxy-5β-cholestanoic acid. *Journal of Biological Chemistry*, **250**, 8243–8247.

Gustafsson, J. and Sjöstedt, S. (1978). On the stereospecificity of microsomal "26"-hydroxylation in bile acid biosynthesis. *Journal of Biological Chemistry*, **253**, 199–201.

Gustow, E., Varma, K. G. and Soloff, L. A. (1978). Purification and characterization of lecithin:cholesterol acyltransferase. *Scandinavian Journal of Clinical and Laboratory Investigation*, **38**, *Supplement* 150, 1–5.

Haslewood, G. A. D. (1952). Comparative studies of 'bile salts'. 5. Bile salts of crocodylidae. *Biochemical Journal*, **52**, 583–587.

Haslewood, G. A. D. *The Biological Importance of Bile Salts*. Ed. A. Neuberger and E. L. Tatum. North-Holland Publishing Co., Amsterdam, 1978.

Haugen, D. A., van der Hoevan, T. A. and Coon, M. J. (1975). Purified liver microsomal cytochrome P-450. *Journal of Biological Chemistry*, **250**, 3567–3570.

Haussler, M. R. and McCain, T. A. (1977). Basic and clinical concepts related to vitamin D metabolism and action. *New England Journal of Medicine*, **297**, 974–983, 1041–1050.

Hellström, K. and Lindstedt, S. (1964). Cholic-acid turnover and biliary bile-acid composition in humans with abnormal thyroid function. Bile acids and steroids 139. *Journal of Laboratory and Clinical Medicine*, **63**, 666–679.

Hepner, G. W., Sturman, J. A., Hofmann, A. F. and Thomas, P. J. (1973). Metabolism of steroid and amino acid moieties of conjugated bile acids in man. III. Cholyltaurine. *Journal of Clinical Investigation*, **52**, 433–440.

Hofmann, A. F. (1967). The syndrome of ileal disease and the broken enterohepatic circulation: cholerheic enteropathy. *Gastroenterology*, **52**, 752–757.

Hofmann, A. F. (1977). The enterohepatic circulation of bile acids in man. *Clinics in Gastroenterology*, **6**, 3–24.

Holick, M. F. and DeLuca, H. F. (1974). Chemistry and biological activity of vitamin D, its metabolites and analogs. *Advances in Steroid Biochemistry and Pharmacology*, **4**, 111–155.

Holick, M. F., Garabedian, M. and DeLuca, H. F. (1972). 1,25-Dihydroxycholecalciferol: metabolite of vitamin D_3 active on bone in anephric rats. *Science*, **176**, 1146–1147.

Hoshita, T., Shefer, S. and Mosbach, E. H. (1968). Conversion of 7α,12α-dihydroxycholest-4-en-3-one to 5α-cholestane-3α,7α,12α-triol by iguana liver microsomes. *Journal of Lipid Research*, **9**, 237–243.

Idler, D. R. and Truscott, B. Corticosteroids in fish. In: *Steroids in Nonmammalian Vertebrates*. Ed. D. R. Idler. Academic Press, New York, pp. 126–252, 1972.

IUPAC (1972). Definitive rules for nomenclature of steroids. *Pure and Applied Chemistry*, **31**, 285–322.

Jefcoate, C. R., Hume, R. and Boyd, G. S. (1970). Separation of two forms of cytochrome P450 from adrenal cortex mitochondria. *FEBS Letters*, **9**, 41–44.

Kallner, A. (1967). On the biosynthesis and metabolism of allodeoxycholic acid in the rat. Bile acids and steroids 175. *Acta Chemica Scandinavica*, **21**, 315–321.

Kanis, J., Taylor, C. M., Heynen, G., Cundy, T., Andrade, A., Douglas, D. and Russell, R. G. G. What is the function of the renal metabolites of vitamin D in man? In: *Molecular Endocrinology*. Ed. I. MacIntyre and M. Szelke. Elsevier, Amsterdam, pp. 319–326, 1979.

Kellogg, T. F. (1971). Microbiological aspects of enterohepatic neutral sterol and bile acid metabolism. *Federation Proceedings*, **30**, 1808–1814.

Kepkay, D. L., Poon, R. and Simon, J. B. (1973). Lecithin-cholesterol acyltransferase and serum cholesterol esterification in obstructive jaundice. *Journal of Laboratory and Clinical Medicine*, **81**, 172–181.

Khoo, J. C., Steinberg, D., Huang, J. J. and Vagelos, P. R. (1976). Triglyceride, diglyceride, monoglyceride, and cholesterol ester hydrolases in chicken adipose tissue activated by adenosine 3′:5′-monophosphate-dependent protein kinase. Chromatographic resolution and immunochemical differentiation from lipoprotein lipase. *Journal of Biological Chemistry*, **251**, 2882–2890.

Kienle, M. G., Varma, R. K., Mulheirn, L. J., Yagen, B. and Caspi, E. (1973). The reduction of Δ^{24} of lanosterol in the biosynthesis of cholesterol by rat liver enzymes. II. Stereochemistry of addition of the C-25 proton. *Journal of the American Chemical Society*, **95**, 1996–2001.

Kritchevsky, D. and Kothari, H. V. (1978). Arterial enzymes of cholesteryl ester metabolism. *Advances in Lipid Research*, **16**, 221-266.

Kritchevsky, D., Tepper, S. A., Staple, E. and Whitehouse, M. W. (1963). Influence of sex and sex hormones on the oxidation of cholesterol-26-C[14] by rat liver mitochondria. *Journal of Lipid Research*, **4**, 188–192.

Lindstedt, S. and Norman, A. (1956). The excretion of bile acids in rats treated with chemotherapeutics. Bile acids and steroids 40. *Acta Physiologica Scandinavica*, **38**, 129–134.

Makino, I., Sjövall, J., Norman, A. and Strandvik, B. (1971). Excretion of 3β-hydroxy-5-cholenoic and 3α-hydroxy-5α-cholanoic acids in urine of infants with biliary atresia. *FEBS Letters*, **15**, 161–164.

Masui, T. and Staple, E. (1966). The formation of bile acids from cholesterol. The conversion of 5β-cholestane-3α,7α,12α-triol-26-oic acid to cholic acid via 5β-cholestane-3α,7α,12α,24ξ-tetraol-26-oic acid I by rat liver. *Journal of Biological Chemistry*, **241**, 3889–3893.

Mendelsohn, D. and Mendelsohn, L. (1968). The *in vitro* catabolism of cholesterol. A comparison of the formation of 26-hydroxycholesterol and chenodeoxycholic acid from cholesterol in rat liver. *Biochemistry*, **7**, 4167–4172.

Miettinen, T. A. Clinical implications of bile acid metabolism in man. In: *The Bile Acids, Chemistry, Physiology and Metabolism, Vol. 2, Physiology and Metabolism*. Ed. P. P. Nair and D. Kritchevsky. Plenum Press, New York, pp. 191–247, 1973.

Miller, N. E. and Nestel, P. J. (1973). Altered bile acid metabolism during treatment with phenobarbitone. *Clinical Science*, **45**, 257–262.

Mitropoulos, K. A., Balasubramaniam, S. and Myant, N. B. (1973). The effect of interruption of the enterohepatic circulation of bile acids and of cholesterol feeding on cholesterol 7α-hydroxylase in relation to the diurnal rhythm in its activity. *Biochimica et Biophysica Acta*, **326**, 428–438.

Mitropoulos, K. A. and Myant, N. B. (1965). Evidence that the oxidation of the side chain of cholesterol by liver mitochondria is stereospecific, and that the immediate product of cleavage is propionate. *Biochemical Journal*, **97**, 26C–28C.

Mitropoulos, K. A. and Myant, N. B. (1967). The formation of lithocholic acid, chenodeoxycholic acid and other bile acids from 3β-hydroxychol-5-enoic acid *in vitro* and *in vivo*. *Biochimica et Biophysica Acta*, **144**, 430–439.

Mosbach, E. H., Salen, G. and Shefer, S. Metabolism of 25-hydroxylated bile alcohols. In: *Bile Acid Metabolism in Health and Disease*. Ed. G. Paumgartner and A. Stiehl. MTP Press, Lancaster, pp. 11–15, 1977.

Myant, N. B. and Mitropoulos, K. A. (1977). Cholesterol 7α-hydroxylase. *Journal of Lipid Research*, **18**, 135–153.

Nair, P. P. and Kritchevsky, D. *The Bile Acids. Chemistry, Physiology and Metabolism, Vol. 1, Chemistry. Vol. 2, Physiology and Metabolism. Vol. 3, Pathophysiology.* Plenum Press, New York, 1971, 1973, 1976.

Nichols, A. V. and Gong, E. L. (1971). Use of sonicated dispersions of mixtures of cholesterol with lecithin as substrates for lecithin:cholesterol acyltransferase. *Biochimica et Biophysica Acta*, **231**, 175–184.

Norum, K. R. (1974). The enzymology of cholesterol esterification. *Scandinavian Journal of Clinical and Laboratory Investigation*, **33**, Supplement 137, 7–13.
Nose, Y. and Lipmann, F. (1958). Separation of steroid sulfokinases. *Journal of Biologica Chemistry*, **233**, 1348–1354.
Pittman, R. C., Khoo, J. C. and Steinberg, D. (1975). Cholesterol esterase in rat adipose tissue and its activation by cyclic adenosine 3′:5′-monophosphate-dependent protein kinase. *Journal of Biological Chemistry*, **250**, 4505–4511.
Popják, G., Edmond, J., Anet, F. A. L. and Easton, N. R. Jr. (1977). Carbon-13 NMR studies on cholesterol biosynthesized from [^{13}C]mevalonates. *Journal of the American Chemical Society*, **99**, 931–935.
Portman, O. W. and Sugano, M. (1964). Factors influencing the level and fatty acid specificity of the cholesterol esterification activity in human plasma. *Archives of Biochemistry and Biophysics*, **105**, 532–540.
Rasmussen, H., Wong, M., Bikle, D. and Goodman, D. B. P. (1972). Hormonal control of the renal conversion of 25-hydroxycholecalciferol to 1,25-dihydroxycholecalciferol. *Journal of Clinical Investigation*, **51**, 2502–2504.
Redinger, R. N. and Small, D. M. (1973). Primate biliary physiology VIII. The effect of phenobarbital upon bile salt synthesis and pool size, biliary lipid secretion, and bile composition. *Journal of Clinical Investigation*, **52**, 161–172.
Roberts, K. D., Bandi, L., Calvin, H. I., Drucker, W. D. and Lieberman, S. (1964). Evidence that steroid sulfates serve as biosynthetic intermediates. IV. Conversion of cholesterol sulfate *in vivo* to urinary C_{19} and C_{21} steroid sulfates. *Biochemistry*, **3**, 1983–1988.
St. Clair, R. W. (1976). Metabolism of the arterial wall and atherosclerosis. *Atherosclerosis Reviews*, **1**, 61–117.
Salen, G. and Grundy, S. M. (1973). The metabolism of cholestanol, cholesterol, and bile acids in cerebrotendinous xanthomatosis. *Journal of Clinical Investigation*, **52**, 2822–2835.
Schulster, D. (1974). Adrenocorticotrophic hormone and the control of adrenal corticosteroidogenesis. *Advances in Steroid Biochemistry and Pharmacology*, **4**, 233–245.
Severson, D. L. and Fletcher, T. (1978). Characterization of cholesterol ester hydrolase activities in rabbit and guinea pig aortas. *Atherosclerosis*, **31**, 21–32.
Sgoutas, D. S. (1972). Fatty acid specificity of plasma phosphatidylcholine: cholesterol acyltransferase. *Biochemistry*, **11**, 293–296.
Shah, P. P., Staple, E. and Rabinowitz, J. L. (1968). Trihydroxycoprostanic acid from Crocodilians. *Archives of Biochemistry and Biophysics*, **123**, 427–428.
Shefer, S., Cheng, F. W., Batta, A. K., Dayal, B., Tint, G. S. and Salen, G. (1978). Biosynthesis of chenodeoxycholic acid in man. Stereospecific side-chain hydroxylations of 5β-cholestane-3α,7α-diol. *Journal of Clinical Investigation*, **62**, 539–545.
Shefer, S., Hauser, S., Bekersky, I. and Mosbach, E. H. (1969). Feedback regulation of bile acid biosynthesis in the rat. *Journal of Lipid Research*, **10**, 646–655.
Shefer, S., Hauser, S. and Mosbach, E. H. (1966a). Biosynthesis of cholestanol:5α-cholestan-3-one reductase of rat liver. *Journal of Lipid Research*, **7**, 763–771.
Shefer, S., Hauser, S. and Mosbach, E. H. (1966b). Studies on the biosynthesis of 5α-cholestan-3β-ol. I. Cholestenone 5α-reductase of rat liver. *Journal of Biological Chemistry*, **241**, 946–952.
Siegfried, C. M. and Elliott, W. H. Effect of phenobarbital on the formation of bile acids from cholesterol-4-^{14}C in the bile fistula rat. In: *Pharmacological Control of Lipid Metabolism*. Ed. W. L. Holmes, R. Paoletti and D. Kritchevsky. Plenum Press, New York, p. 323, 1972.
Siperstein, M. D., Chaikoff, I. L. and Reinhardt, W. O. (1952). C^{14}-cholesterol. V. Obligatory function of bile in intestinal absorption of cholesterol. *Journal of Biological Chemistry*, **198**, 111–114.
Siperstein, M. D., Nichols, C. W. Jr. and Chaikoff, I. L. (1953). Effects of ferric

chloride and bile on plasma cholesterol and atherosclerosis in the cholesterol-fed bird. *Science*, **117**, 386–389.

Soutar, A. K., Pownall, H. J., Hu, A. S. and Smith, L. C. (1974). Phase transitions in bilamellar vesicles. Measurements by pyrene excimer fluorescence and effect on transacylation by lecithin:cholesterol acyltransferase. *Biochem.* **13**, 2828–2836.

Sperry, W. M. (1935). Cholesterol esterase in blood. *Journal of Biological Chemistry*, **111**, 467–478.

Sperry, W. M. and Stoyanoff, V. A. (1938). The enzymatic synthesis and hydrolysis of cholesterol esters in blood serum. *Journal of Biological Chemistry*, **126**, 77–89.

Stein, O., Coetzee, G. A. and Stein, Y. Deposition and hydrolysis of cytoplasmic triglyceride and cholesterol ester in aortic smooth muscle cells in culture. In: *Atherosclerosis V, Proceedings of the Fifth International Symposium*. Springer-Verlag, New York, 1980, pp. 796–799.

Stein, O., Stein, Y., Goodman, D. S. and Fidge, N. H. (1969). The metabolism of chylomicron cholesteryl ester in rat liver. A combined radioautographic-electron microscopic and biochemical study. *Journal of Cell Biology*, **43**, 410–431.

Stiehl, A., Czygan, P. and Raedsch, R. Sulphation of lithocholate in patients during chenodeoxycholate treatment. A protective mechanism. In: *Advances in Bile Acid Research. III. Bile Acid Meeting*, Freiburg. Ed. S. Matern, J. Hackenschmidt, P. Back and W. Gerok. F. K. Schattauer Verlag, Stuttgart, pp. 347–350, 1975.

Stokke, K. T. (1972). The existence of an acid cholesterol esterase in human liver. *Biochimica et Biophysica Acta*, **270**, 156–166.

Stokke, K. T. (1974). Cholesteryl ester metabolism in liver and blood plasma of various animal species. *Atherosclerosis*, **19**, 393–406.

Stokke, K. T. and Norum, K. R. (1971). Determination of lecithin:cholesterol acyltransferase in human blood plasma. *Scandinavian Journal of Clinical and Laboratory Investigation*, **27**, 21–27.

Stone, D. and Hechter, O. (1954). Studies on ACTH action in perfused bovine adrenals: The site of action of ACTH in corticosteroidogenesis. *Archives of Biochemistry and Biophysics*, **51**, 457–469.

Strand, O. (1963). Effects of D- and L-triiodothyronine and of propylthiouracil on the production of bile acids in the rat. *Journal of Lipid Research*, **4**, 305–311.

Suld, H. M., Staple, E. and Gurin, S. (1962). Mechanism of formation of bile acids from cholesterol: oxidation of 5β-cholestane-$3\alpha,7\alpha,12\alpha$-triol and formation of propionic acid from the side chain by rat liver mitochondria. *Journal of Biological Chemistry*, **237**, 338–344.

Swell, L., Gustafsson, J., Schwartz, C. C., Halloran, L. G., Danielsson, H. and Vlahcevic, Z. R. (1980). An *in vivo* evaluation of the quantitative significance of several potential pathways to cholic and chenodeoxycholic acids from cholesterol in man. *Journal of Lipid Research*, **21**, 455–466.

Takano, T., Black, W. J., Peters, T. J. and de Duve, C. (1974). Assay, kinetics and lysosomal localization of an acid cholesteryl esterase in rabbit aortic smooth muscle cells. *Journal of Biological Chemistry*, **249**, 6732–6737.

Takeuchi, N., Ito, M. and Yamamura, Y. (1974). Regulation of cholesterol 7α-hydroxylation by cholesterol synthesis in rat liver. *Atherosclerosis*, **20**, 481–494.

Thompson, E. A. and Siiteri, P. K. (1973). Studies on the aromatization of C-19 androgens. *Annals of the New York Academy of Sciences*, **212**, 378–388.

Thompson, J. C. and Vars, H. M. (1953). Biliary excretion of cholic acid and cholesterol in hyper-, hypo-, and euthyroid rats. *Proceedings of the Society for Experimental Biology and Medicine*, **83**, 246–248.

Treadwell, C. R. and Vahouny, G. V. Cholesterol absorption. In: *Handbook of Physiology*, Sec. 6, Vol. 3. Ed. C. F. Code. American Physiological Society, Washington, pp. 1407–1438, 1968.

Vahouny, G. V. and Treadwell, C. R. (1968). Enzymatic synthesis and hydrolysis of cholesterol esters. *Methods of Biochemical Analysis*, **16**, 219–272.

Chapter 6

Developmental Aspects of Cholesterol Metabolism

1	MATERNAL AND FETAL CONTRIBUTIONS TO THE FETUS	301
2	CHOLESTEROL METABOLISM IN FETAL AND NEONATAL TISSUES	303
2.1	General	303
2.2	The human feto-placental unit	304
2.3	The central nervous system	306
2.3.1	Deposition of cholesterol in the brain	306
2.3.2	Cholesterol synthesis in the developing brain	309
2.3.3	Turnover of cholesterol in developing brain	310

Developmental Aspects of Cholesterol Metabolism

The amount of cholesterol in the mammalian body increases throughout pre-natal and post-natal development. A major factor in this increase must be the continuous synthesis of membranes accompanying cell multiplication, but there is also a net accumulation of cholesterol in certain tissues at particular stages of development, as in the marked increase in the cholesterol content of the central nervous system during myelination in the white matter.

The total amount of free and esterified cholesterol in fetal plasma increases as the fetus grows, but in most species the plasma cholesterol concentration in the fetus is much lower than that in the mother. In man, for example, the fetal plasma cholesterol concentration is less than half the maternal concentration from the 18th week of gestation (Ross et al., 1973) until birth (see Chapter 16 for human cord-blood values). An interesting exception to this is the rabbit, in which the fetal concentration is higher than the maternal, particularly towards the end of gestation, when there is a marked fall in the maternal level associated with a decrease in the rate of synthesis of cholesterol in the maternal liver (Popják, 1954).

1 MATERNAL AND FETAL CONTRIBUTIONS TO THE FETUS

The cholesterol deposited in fetal tissues is derived partly from the mother and partly from synthesis within the fetus itself. The relative importance of these two sources differs from one species to another and, probably, at different stages of fetal development in a given species. Goldwater and Stetten (1947), who measured the deuterium content of the cholesterol of rat fetuses after the mother had been fed D_2O, concluded that only about 10% of the total fetal cholesterol is derived from the mother. Using a similar approach, with D_2O and [^{14}C]acetate as precursors, Popják and Beeckmans (1950) deduced that virtually all the cholesterol that accumulates in a rabbit fetus between the 16th and 28th day of gestation is synthesized within the fetus from small molecules, and that in the extrahepatic tissues of the fetus the rates of synthesis and net deposition of cholesterol are equal. More recent observations on the fate of radioactive cholesterol introduced into the maternal circulation indicate that the maternal contribution to the fetal cholesterol is greater than was suggested by the earlier D_2O experiments. Chevallier (1964) investigated cholesterol synthesis in rat fetuses by an extension of the isotopic equilibrium method used for determining the contribution of dietary cholesterol to the plasma in mature animals. Female rats were fed [^{14}C]cholesterol before and throughout pregnancy and the specific activity of the total fetal cholesterol was compared with that of the maternal plasma cholesterol at successive stages of gestation. Chevallier concluded that up to 70% of the fetal cholesterol accumulating during the first 13 days of gestation comes from the mother, but that the relative contribution from the fetus increases in the later stages so that by the end of gestation at least 80% of the total cholesterol in the fetus has been contributed by fetal synthesis. Connor and his co-workers (Connor and Lin, 1967; Pitkin et al., 1972), also using the isotopic equilibrium method, have shown that the relative importance of the mother and the fetus as sources of fetal cholesterol varies from one tissue to another. In guinea-pigs the mother's plasma contributes about 20% of the cholesterol in the fetal plasma and liver, but less than 5% of the fetal brain cholesterol. In rabbits the mother also makes a much smaller contribution to brain cholesterol than to plasma cholesterol in the fetus. In monkeys, the maternal contribution to the fetal cholesterol seems to be more important than in rabbits or guinea-pigs, more than 40% of the cholesterol in the plasma, liver and heart originating in the mother's plasma with, again, a very small contribution from the mother to the fetal brain.

There has been no systematic attempt to find out how cholesterol molecules cross the placenta from the maternal plasma into the umbilical venous blood. The concentration of cholesterol in the fetal plasma is very different from that in the maternal plasma and is uninfluenced by marked changes in the maternal plasma cholesterol concentration, such as those brought about by feeding the mother a cholesterol-rich diet (Connor and Lin, 1967). This indicates that the fetal plasma cholesterol concentration is determined by something a good deal more complex than equilibration between fetal and maternal plasma across a passive membrane. One important determinant of the fetal plasma cholesterol concentration may be the availability of apolipoproteins for the formation of cholesterol-carrying lipoproteins in the fetal circulation. But we know nothing about the physiology of fetal plasma apolipoproteins, nor do we know whether net transplacental transport of cholesterol involves the movement of intact lipoprotein molecules, or whether the maternal plasma lipoproteins can act as shuttles, depositing cholesterol in the placenta and then returning to the plasma in a manner analogous to that suggested for reverse cholesterol transport to the liver (Chapter 9, Section 6). If, as the observations of Ross *et al.* (1973) might suggest, there is a considerable uptake of cholesterol from the maternal plasma by the placenta in pregnant women, it would be of interest to know whether or not this is mediated by specific receptors for one or other of the maternal plasma lipoproteins.

2 CHOLESTEROL METABOLISM IN FETAL AND NEONATAL TISSUES

2.1 General

As we have already seen, the fetus is capable of synthesizing cholesterol from small molecules. This has been demonstrated in rats and rabbits *in vivo*, in the isolated perfused human fetus (Solomon *et al.*, 1967) and in preparations of fetal tissue *in vitro* in various species. The earliest stage at which the fetus begins to synthesize cholesterol is not known, nor do we know when, or in what order, the cholesterol-synthesizing enzymes first appear in particular tissues, but we do know that the whole human fetus incorporates acetate carbon into the cholesterol of liver and adrenal cortex as early as the 18th week of gestation (Solomon *et al.*, 1967). The developmental pattern of cholesterol synthesis in the liver has been studied in some detail in the rat (Carroll, 1964; Ballard and Hanson, 1967). Incorporation of the carbon of acetate and glucose into cholesterol is much higher in the late fetus than in the adult. At birth the rate of incorporation falls sharply, remains very low during suckling and then rises at weaning to a level higher than that in adults, eventually falling again to adult levels. McNamara *et al.* (1972) have shown that the activity of HMG-CoA reductase per mg of protein in the liver follows a closely similar pattern, suggesting that the reduction of HMG-CoA is the rate-limiting step in hepatic cholesterol synthesis in fetal and neonatal life as well as in the adult. McNamara *et al.* (1972) have demonstrated the presence of a heat-stable inhibitor of cholesterol synthesis in rat's milk. They suggest that this inhibitor, together with the significant amounts of cholesterol in milk, explains the complex developmental pattern of rat hepatic HMG-CoA reductase, suckling leading to inhibition of the enzyme, followed by a temporary rebound in enzyme activity when the inhibition is withdrawn. Hepatic HMG-CoA reductase appears to be subject to regulation at an early stage of post-natal development in rats, since a diurnal rhythm in enzyme activity (with a maximum during the *day*) is present at least as early as the 6th day of post-natal life. The developmental pattern of cholesterol synthesis in nervous tissue is considered in Section 2.3 below.

The presence of conjugated bile acids in the meconium of newborn human infants (Back and Ross, 1973) suggests that the fetal liver has all the enzymes required for the conversion of cholesterol into bile acids, and for conjugating bile acids with taurine and glycine. In agreement with this, Danielsson and Rutter (1968) have demonstrated the presence of enzymes catalyzing several steps in the formation and conjugation of bile acids in rat fetal liver, and DeBelle *et al.* (1973) have shown that cultures of 15-week-old human fetal liver are capable of converting cholesterol into conjugated bile acids. While there can be no doubt that some of the bile salts in meconium are synthesized and secreted by the fetus, it has been shown that cholic and chenodeoxycholic acids can cross the placenta from mother to fetus and from fetus to mother in pregnant dogs and monkeys (see Little *et al.*, 1975). The presence of deoxycholate and lithocholate in human meconium (Back and Ross, 1973) also shows that bile acids can cross from mother to fetus in pregnant women, since both these bile acids are derived exclusively from primary bile acids in the mother's intestine.

Human meconium contains considerable quantities of the sulphate ester of 3β-hydroxycholenoic acid (Back and Ross, 1973), a bile acid not normally present in the faeces of adult human subjects. Since it is not present in the plasma of pregnant women, Back and Ross suggest that the 3β-hydroxycholenoic acid in meconium is synthesized and sulphated in the fetal liver. Whereas bile acids are conjugated predominantly with glycine in the adult human, tauroconjugates predominate in meconium (Encrantz and Sjövall, 1959) and in the bile salts formed from cholesterol by cultured human liver (DeBelle *et al.*, 1973).

2.2 The human feto-placental unit

The participation of the fetus in the formation of steroid hormones by the human placenta has already been mentioned briefly in Chapter 5. In this section we shall consider the role of the human feto-placental unit in cholesterol metabolism in more detail. Our understanding of the remarkable sequence of events by which the human fetus and placenta co-operate to form steroid hormones is derived from three experimental approaches: (1) Measurement of the relative concentrations of hypothetical intermediates in plasma from the uterine and umbilical arteries and veins, (2) identification of the labelled steroids formed from radioactive acetate or cholesterol perfused into the isolated fetus or feto-placental unit, or into the feto-placental unit *in situ*, and (3) the study of the ability of slices or homogenates of placenta and fetal tissue to catalyze various steps in the overall pathway from acetate to steroid hormones (for references to methods and results, see Solomon *et al.*, 1967; Samuels and Eik-Nes, 1968; Diczfalusy and Mancuso, 1969; Gower and Fotherby, 1975).

The human placenta, though capable of forming squalene and lanosterol from acetate, cannot synthesize cholesterol. It does, however, form large quantities of pregnenolone and progesterone from cholesterol taken up from the maternal plasma. Contrary to earlier views, the human placenta can synthesize dehydroepiandrosterone (DHA) from cholesterol, though only in extremely small amounts. Thus, the placenta contains the enzyme system required for cleavage of the cholesterol side-chain at C-20 and, to a very limited extent, the C-17 lyase.

The fetal adrenal cortex can synthesize cholesterol from acetate and can also convert the cholesterol so formed *in situ* into various steroid hormones, including the glucocorticoids. However, the major substrates for side-chain cleavage of steroids in the fetal adrenal are cholesterol and pregnenolone transported to the fetus from the placenta *via* the umbilical veins. These compounds are converted mainly into the sulphate ester of DHA and of 16α-hydroxy DHA (a precursor of oestriol). DHA sulphate and 16α-hydroxy DHA sulphate are transported to the placenta *via* the umbilical artery. Within the placenta, the sulphated C_{19} steroids made in the fetal adrenal are hydrolysed to the free steroids by an active placental sulphatase and are then converted into 17β-oestradiol and oestriol by the enzyme systems considered in Chapter 5. The more important pathways in the formation of female sex hormones by the human feto-placental unit are shown in Fig. 6.1. These pathways are responsible for the enormous increase in the production of progesterone and oestrogens (mainly oestriol) that occurs in pregnant women.

Another aspect of cholesterol metabolism relevant to mammalian reproduction is the high rate of synthesis of cholesterol in the ovary of the pregnant rabbit. Shortly after mating, the production of progesterone by the rabbit's ovary increases in response to luteinizing hormone secreted by the pituitary. Kovanen *et al.* (1978) have shown that this increase is accompanied by a considerable rise in HMG-CoA reductase activity in the corpus luteum beginning before the 5th day after mating and persisting until the end of pregnancy, and that the rate of incorporation of acetate into cholesterol in the ovary increase in parallel with the rise in enzyme activity. The rise in HMG-CoA

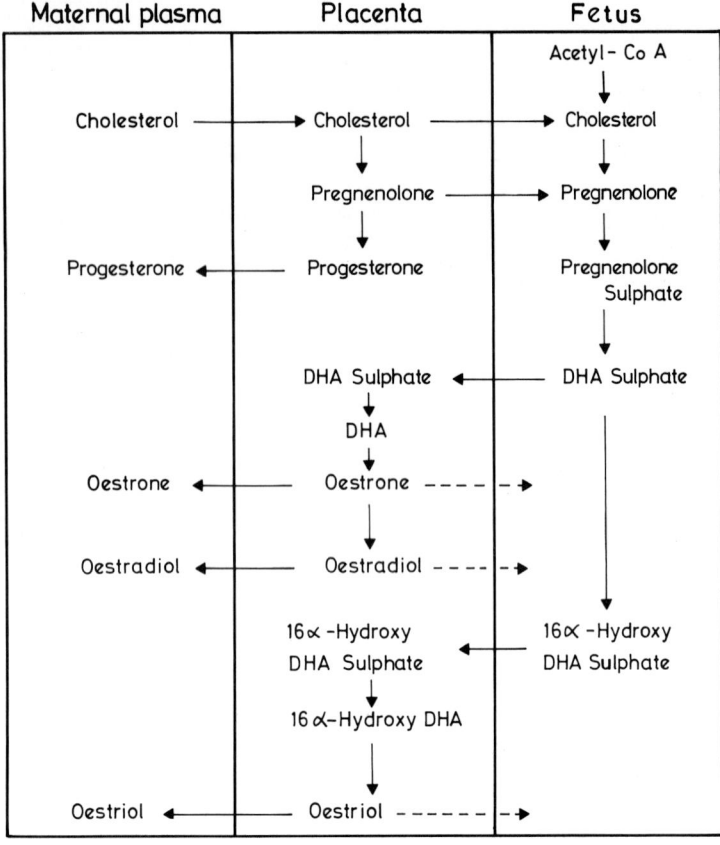

Figure 6.1
Probable major routes for the formation of progesterone and oestrogens by the human fetus and placenta.

DHA, Dehydroepiandrosterone.

Note. Each arrow may signify more than one biochemical step: oestrogens made in the placenta reach the fetus, where they are inactivated by hydroxylation and the formation of sulphates or glucuronides.

reductase activity in the cells of the corpus luteum is clearly an adaptive mechanism for supplying adequate substrate for increased progesterone production.

2.3 The central nervous system

2.3.1 Deposition of cholesterol in the brain

During the maturation of the mammalian central nervous system there is an increase in the total amount of cholesterol in the whole brain and in the amount of cholesterol per g of fresh or dry weight.

The observations of Cuzner and Davison (1968) on the deposition of cholesterol in the brains of rats throughout post-natal development provide a good example of these changes (Fig. 6.2). Between day 1 and day 100 there is a 40-fold increase in total brain cholesterol (from 0.93 to 38.2 mg/brain) and a 6-fold increase in brain cholesterol concentration (mg/g fresh weight). During the first 7 days the rate of deposition of cholesterol per whole brain is relatively slow, but there is a marked acceleration at day 7, followed by a somewhat slower rate beginning at about day 12 and continuing until day 50, after which there is little further increase in brain cholesterol content or concentration. A comparison of the three curves for brain weight, cholesterol content and cholesterol concentration shows that the initial slow increase in cholesterol content is due entirely to growth of the brain, but that the increase occurring after day 7 is due to a combination of brain growth and increased cholesterol concentration. Since myelination in the rat's central nervous system begins at about day 10 and is virtually complete by day 50, Cuzner and Davison (1968) suggest that the very rapid accumulation of cholesterol beginning at day 7 is

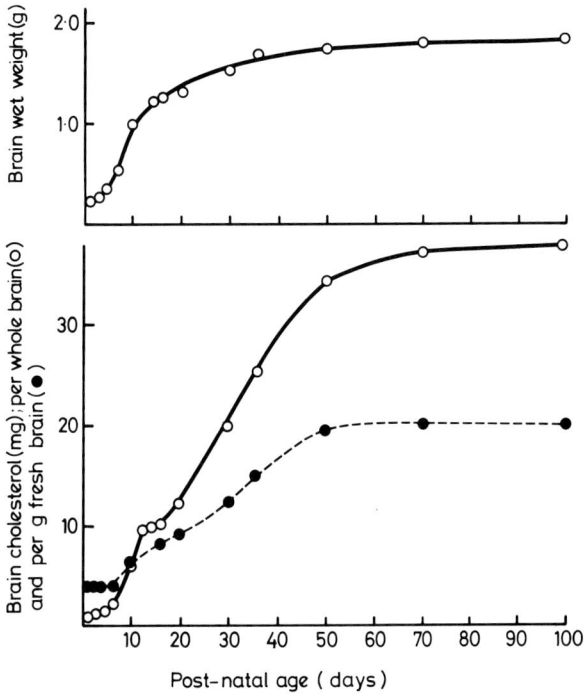

Figure 6.2
Changes in weight and cholesterol content of the brains of rats during the first 100 days after birth. Values taken from Cuzner and Davison (1968).

Table 6.1
The concentration of cholesterol in human whole brain, grey matter and white matter during pre-natal and post-natal development

	Age	Whole brain F	Whole brain D	Grey matter F	Grey matter D	White matter F	White matter D	Nerve F	Nerve D
Fetus	10 weeks	0.18	—	—	—	—	—		
	5 months	0.40	4.3	—	—	—	—		
	7 months	0.45	—	—	—	—	—		
	8 months	—	—	0.50	—	0.65	—		
	Full-term	—	—	0.60	—	0.76	—		
Post-natal	1 day	—	—	0.74	4.5	0.53	7.0		
	7 days	—	—	0.47	—	0.55	—		
	3 months	0.70	5.7	0.50	5.1	0.70	7.8		
	7 months	—	—	0.80	—	1.8	—		
	2 years	—	—	0.90	—	3.2	—		
	7 years	—	—	0.90	—	4.5	—		
	Adult	1.9	8.3	1.0	7.2	4.2	15.1	3.9	14.5

— = No values reported.
Values obtained from Brante (1949), Johnson et al. (1949), Cumings et al. (1958) and Davison (1970).
Values for peripheral nerve are shown for comparison. All values are expressed as g/100 g fresh weight (F) of dry weight (D).

due to the increase in cell mass accompanying the early spurt in brain growth (see Fig. 6.2, upper curve), and that the subsequent increase in brain cholesterol content is due to myelination.

A similar pattern of changes occurs during brain development in other species, though the time-course differs, depending upon the time at which myelination of the central nervous system begins in relation to birth. In rats, mice and rabbits myelin is not present in the brains of newborn animals. In man, on the other hand, some myelin is deposited in the basal areas of the brain during the last month of fetal life. Table 6.1 shows the cholesterol content of human brain at different stages of development, with values for peripheral nerve shown for comparison. In adult whole brain, cholesterol contributes about 2% of the fresh weight and about 8% of the dry weight. Owing to the abundance of myelinated nerves in white matter, the cholesterol content of adult white matter is similar to that of peripheral nerve and is considerably higher than that of grey matter. During development from the fetal to the fully mature state, the amount of cholesterol in the brain, expressed in terms of fresh or dry weight, increases markedly, the increase being greater in white matter than in grey matter.

During the development of the brain, significant changes occur in the lipid composition of myelin. In the brains of rats examined between day 15 and day 190 (Table 6.2), the proportion of cholesterol in myelin increases and that of phospholipid decreases, the net effect being a change in the cholesterol:phospholipid molar ratio from 0.97 at 15 days to 1.24 at 190 days after birth. During this period, desmosterol disappears almost completely from myelin.

Table 6.2
Lipid composition of rat-brain myelin

Age (days)	15	30	60	144	190
Cholesterol	25.1	25.7	25.9	27.8	27.9
Galactolipid	21.4	26.2	30.5	33.3	30.7
Phospholipid	50.4	48.0	44.0	43.7	43.5
Plasmalogen	14.1	13.7	14.4	13.9	13.7
Desmosterol	3.0	1.5	1.0	0.3	0.2

Values for desmosterol espressed as % of total sterol. All other values show % of total lipid; galactolipid includes cerebroside and cerebroside sulphates.
(Modified from Norton, 1971.)

2.3.2 Cholesterol synthesis in the developing brain

As we have seen, the bulk of the cholesterol deposited in the fetus is synthesized within the fetal tissues. Furthermore, the isotopic-equilibrium experiments on pregnant animals mentioned in Section 1 show that most of the cholesterol that accumulates in the fetal brain is synthesized *in situ* and is not brought to the brain from other organs in the fetus. In agreement with this, fetal brain has been shown to incorporate acetate into cholesterol *in vitro*. Synthesis of cholesterol within the brains of newborn animals was also demonstrated many years ago by Waelsch and co-workers (1940), who showed that when D_2O is fed to newborn rats, the deuterium enrichment of the cholesterol in brain is greater than that of the cholesterol in any other tissue. The incorporation of deuterium from D_2O into brain cholesterol is greatest when myelination is most active and falls to a low, though still detectable, level in the adult animal. Brain slices from newborn rats incorporate acetate into cholesterol very actively (Srere *et al.*, 1950); in line with the observations of Waelsch *et al. in vivo*, brain slices from adult rats synthesize cholesterol from acetate only at a very low rate.

The pathway for the biosynthesis of cholesterol in developing brain resembles that in the liver in broad outline, but there are some minor differences. Whereas the reduction of HMG-CoA is the rate-limiting step in the synthesis of cholesterol in the liver under almost all conditions, there seem to be two slow steps beyond mevalonic acid in the pathway to cholesterol in immature brain—one at the isomerization of the $\Delta^{8,9}$ double bond of zymosterol to the Δ^7 position and the other at the reduction of the Δ^{24} double bond. This, at any rate, is the most reasonable explanation for the presence of zymosterol and desmosterol in the brains of newborn animals, and for the accumulation of radioactive zymosterol and desmosterol in the brains of newborn rats and chick embryos injected with [^{14}C]acetate (see Davison, 1970). The observations of Kandutsch and Saucier (1969) on the activity of HMG-CoA reductase in the developing mouse brain also suggest that, in this species, during the first ten days of post-natal life the rate-limiting step in cholesterol synthesis is later than mevalonic acid. In the mature mammalian brain, the rate-limiting step in cholesterol synthesis is the reduction of HMG-CoA to mevalonic acid.

2.3.3 Turnover of cholesterol in developing brain

If radioactive cholesterol is injected into an immature animal or bird, a small proportion of the labelled cholesterol is incorporated into the lipids of the brain (Davison, 1970). The proportion of the injected dose deposited in the brain lipids is related directly to the rate of accumulation of brain lipid at the time of the injection. In rats, uptake reaches a peak at about 15 days after birth and then falls progressively to a low level in the mature animal.

The uptake of labelled exogenous cholesterol by the immature brain provides an opportunity to study the turnover of cholesterol in the central nervous system by observing the subsequent loss of label from the brain. Such observations have shown that the brain as a whole contains at least three pools of cholesterol, one with a half-life of about 80 min, another with slower turnover and a pool of metabolically stable cholesterol which turns over with a half-life measured in years. Since labelled cholesterol persists for much longer in white matter than in grey matter, the pool of very slowly-exchanging cholesterol is thought to be predominantly in myelin. In support of this, Cuzner *et al.* (1966) have shown that the turnover of cholesterol *in vivo* in myelin, isolated from brain homogenates by density-gradient centrifugation, is much slower than that in other subcellular fractions of brain.

Although cholesterol incorporated into the myelin of developing brain turns over exceedingly slowly, suggesting that once incorporated into the myelin sheath it ceases to be exchangeable, cholesterol and other myelin lipids in the myelin of the mature brain are exchangeable. Davison (1964) has suggested an explanation for this paradox in terms of the way in which myelin is laid down. The myelin sheath is formed by a glial cell wrapping itself many times around the axon of a nerve cell, so producing concentric rings of bilaminar membrane, with the oldest layer nearest the axon. In the developing brain, cholesterol molecules incorporated into the outer layer of the myelin sheath would soon be covered by layers of fresh myelin and would thus become non-exchangeable. In the adult brain, on the other hand, cholesterol and other lipids in the outer layers of myelin would remain available for exchange. An additional factor that would help to explain the prolonged persistence of cholesterol in brain myelin is the presence of a slowly-exchanging pool of brain cholesterol from which developing myelin is supplied (Spohn and Davison, 1972).

It should be noted that although significant amounts of radioactive cholesterol are incorporated into the brain lipids of immature animals, in terms of mass this represents a very small contribution to the total amount of cholesterol deposited in the brain during its maturation. Clarenburg *et al.* (1963) have estimated that only about 8% of the cholesterol laid down in the brains of rabbits between day 17 and day 33 is derived from sources other than synthesis *in situ*.

REFERENCES

Back, P. and Ross, K. (1973). Identification of 3β-hydroxy-5-cholenoic acid in human meconium. *Hoppe-Seyler's Zeitschrift für physiologische Chemie*, **354**, 83–89.

Ballard, F. J. and Hanson, R. W. (1967). Changes in lipid synthesis in rat liver during development. *Biochemical Journal*, **102**, 952–958.

Brante, G. (1949). Studies on lipids in the nervous system with special reference to quantitative chemical determination and topical distribution. *Acta Physiologica Scandinavica*, **18**, Supplement 63.

Carroll, K. K. (1964). Acetate incorporation into cholesterol and fatty acids by livers of fetal, suckling, and weaned rats. *Canadian Journal of Biochemistry*, **42**, 79–86.

Chevallier, F. (1964). Transferts et synthèse du cholestérol chez le rat au cours de sa croissance. *Biochimica et Biophysica Acta*, **84**, 316–339.

Clarenburg, R., Chaikoff, I. L. and Morris, M. D. (1963). Incorporation of injected cholesterol into the myelinating brain of the 17-day-old rabbit. *Journal of Neurochemistry*, **10**, 135–143.

Connor, W. E. and Lin, D. S. (1967). Placental transfer of cholesterol-4-^{14}C into rabbit and guinea pig fetus. *Journal of Lipid Research*, **8**, 558–564.

Cumings, J. N., Goodwin, H., Woodward, E. M. and Curzon, G. (1958). Lipids in the brains of infants and children. *Journal of Neurochemistry*, **2**, 289–294.

Cuzner, M. L. and Davison, A. N. (1968). The lipid composition of rat brain myelin and subcellular fractions during development. *Biochemical Journal*, **106**, 29–34.

Cuzner, M. L., Davison, A. N. and Gregson, N. A. (1966). Turnover of brain mitochondrial membrane lipids. *Biochemical Journal*, **101**, 618–626.

Danielsson, H. and Rutter, W. J. (1968). The metabolism of bile acids in the developing rat liver. *Biochemistry*, **7**, 346–352.

Davison, A. N. Myelin metabolism. In: *Metabolism and Physiological Significance of Lipids*. Ed. R. M. C. Dawson and D. N. Rhodes. John Wiley & Sons Ltd., London, pp. 527–537, 1964.

Davison, A. N. Cholesterol metabolism. In: *Handbook of Neurochemistry, Vol. III, Metabolic Reactions in the Nervous System*. Ed. A. Lajtha. Plenum Press, New York, pp. 547–560, 1970.

DeBelle, R., Brown, A., Blacklow, N. R., Donaldson, R. M. and Lester, R. (1973). Organ culture of fetal liver: a new model system. *Pediatric Research*, **7**, 292.

Diczfalusy, E. and Mancuso, S. Oestrogen metabolism in pregnancy. In: *Fetus and Placenta*. Ed. A. Klopper and E. Diczfalusy. Blackwell Scientific Publications, Oxford, pp. 191–248, 1969.

Encrantz, J.-C. and Sjövall, J. (1959). On the bile acids in duodenal contents of infants and children. *Clinica Chimica Acta*, **4**, 793–799.

Goldwater, W. H. and Stetten, De W. (1947). Studies in fetal metabolism. *Journal of Biological Chemistry*, **169**, 723–738.

Gower, D. B. and Fotherby, K. Biosynthesis of the androgens and oestrogens. In: *Biochemistry of Steroid Hormones*. Ed. H. L. J. Makin. Blackwell Scientific Publications, Oxford, pp. 77–104, 1975.

Johnson, A. C., McNabb, A. R. and Rossiter, R. J. (1949). Concentration of lipids in the brain of infants and adults. *Biochemical Journal*, **44**, 494–498.

Kandutsch, A. A. and Saucier, S. E. (1969). Regulation of sterol synthesis in developing brains of normal and jimpy mice. *Archives of Biochemistry and Biophysics*, **135**, 201–208.

Kovanen, P. T., Goldstein, J. L. and Brown, M. S. (1978). High levels of 3-hydroxy-3-methylglutaryl coenzyme A reductase activity and cholesterol synthesis in the ovary of the pregnant rabbit. *Journal of Biological Chemistry*, **254**, 5126–5132.

Little, J. M., Smallwood, R. A., Lester, R., Piasecki, G. J. and Jackson, B. T. (1975). Bile-salt metabolism in the primate fetus. *Gastroenterology*, **69**, 1315–1320.

McNamara, D. J., Quackenbush, F. W. and Rodwell, V. W. (1972). Regulation of hepatic 3-hydroxy-3-methylglutaryl coenzyme A reductase. *Journal of Biological Chemistry*, **247**, 5805–5810.

Norton, W. T. Recent developments in the investigation of purified myelin. In: *Advances in Experimental Medicine and Biology, Vol. 13, Chemistry and Brain Development*. Ed. R. Paoletti and A. N. Davison. Plenum, New York, pp. 327–337, 1971.

Pitkin, M., Connor, W. E. and Lin, D. S. (1972). Cholesterol metabolism and placental transfer in the pregnant rhesus monkey. *Journal of Clinical Investigation*, **51**, 2584–2592.

Popják, G. (1954). The origin of fetal lipids. *Cold Spring Harbor Symposia on Quantitative Biology*, **19**, 200–208.

Popják, G. and Beeckmans, M.-L. (1950). Synthesis of cholesterol and fatty acids in foetuses and in mammary glands of pregnant rabbits. *Biochemical Journal*, **46**, 547–561.

Ross, P. E., Coutts, J. R. T. and MacNaughton, M. C. (1973). Free cholesterol levels in plasma from the maternal, placental and fetal circulations during human pregnancy. *Clinica Chimica Acta*, **49**, 415–422.

Samuels, L. T. and Eik-Nes, K. B. Metabolism of steroid hormones. In: *Metabolic Pathways*, 3rd edition, Vol. II. Ed. D. M. Greenberg. Academic Press, New York, pp. 169–220, 1968.

Solomon, S., Bird, C. E., Ling, W., Iwamiya, M. and Young, P. C. M. (1967). Formation and metabolism of steroids in the fetus and placenta. *Recent Progress in Hormone Research*, **23**, 295–335.

Spohn, M. and Davison, A. N. (1972). Cholesterol metabolism in myelin and other subcellular fractions of rat brain. *Journal of Lipid Research*, **13**, 563–570.

Srere, P. A., Chaikoff, I. L., Treitman, S. S. and Burstein, L. S. (1950). The extrahepatic synthesis of cholesterol. *Journal of Biological Chemistry*, **182**, 629–634.

Waelsch, H., Sperry, W. M. and Stoyanoff, V. A. (1940). Lipid metabolism in brain during myelination. *Journal of Biological Chemistry*, **135**, 297–302.

Chapter 7

Sterols in Biological Membranes

1	LIPID COMPOSITION OF MEMBRANES	317
2	PHOSPHOLIPIDS AND MEMBRANE STRUCTURE	318
3	STEROL-PHOSPHOLIPID INTERACTIONS	320
3.1	Condensation in monolayers	320
3.2	Effect of sterols on phase changes	321
4	EFFECTS OF STEROLS ON MEMBRANE FUNCTION	326
4.1	Liposomes	327
4.2	Natural membranes	327
5	DISTRIBUTION AND MOBILITY OF MEMBRANE CHOLESTEROL	331
6	EVOLUTIONARY SIGNIFICANCE OF MEMBRANE STEROLS	333

Sterols in Biological Membranes

1 LIPID COMPOSITION OF MEMBRANES

Sterols are thought to play an essential role in determining the structure and physiological properties of biological membranes. Indeed, this may well be the most primitive, in an evolutionary sense, of all the functions of sterols, their other functions as precursors of essential metabolites probably arising only at a much later stage of the evolution of living systems. That sterols have a very long biological history is suggested by their presence in some modern prokaryotic organisms and by the identification of cyclic hydrocarbons with a cholestane skeleton, undoubtedly of organic origin, in shales known to be at least 3000 million years old (Calvin, 1969).

In the membranes of animal cells cholesterol is the major sterol, but other sterols including lathosterol, 7-dehydrocholesterol and 5α-cholesterol are found in small amounts in the membranes of human red cells and of other animal cells. In most plant-cell plasma membranes, stigmasterol and β-sitosterol are the predominant sterols. In myelin and in the plasma membranes of some animal cells the cholesterol:phospholipid molar ratio is close to 1:1. In the plasma membranes of normal human lymphocytes this ratio is less than 0.7 and is much reduced in the lymphocytes of patients with chronic lymphatic leukaemic (Gottfried, 1967). In the membranes of mammalian mitochondria, microsomes and nuclei the cholesterol:phospholipid molar ratio usually lies between 0.1 and 0.3 (Ashworth and Green, 1966); in intact liver mitochondria the cholesterol:phospholipid ratio is 3 to 4 times higher in the outer than in the inner membrane (Graham and Green, 1970). It has been claimed that the membranes of the endoplasmic reticulum, separated from fragments of plasma membrane and of other membranes by density gradient centrifugation, do not contain appreciable amounts of cholesterol (Amar-Costesec *et al.*, 1974). However, free cholesterol has been demonstrated in both rough and smooth endoplasmic reticulum of rat liver, though not necessarily in a form that is readily accessible to digitonin (Mitropoulos *et al.*, 1978).

The lipid composition of red-cell ghosts has been studied in considerable detail because they consist of plasma membrane almost entirely free from other cellular elements. In red-cell ghosts from a large number of different species, free cholesterol accounts for 25–30% of the total lipid, while phospholipid accounts for about 60%. However, the composition of the total phospholipid fraction varies widely from one species to another. For example, lecithin is the predominant phospholipid in human red cells but is barely detectable in the red cells of sheep, cows and goats (Rouser *et al.*, 1968). There are also marked differences between the lipid compositions of the inner and outer monolayers. In the human red cell, lecithin and sphingomyelin are largely confined to the outer layer, while the aminophosphatides occur mainly in the inner layer (Bretscher, 1973; Rothman and Lenard, 1977). Asymmetry in the distribution of cholesterol in the red-cell membrane is not nearly as marked as that of phospholipids, though Fisher (1976) has deduced, from analysis of the fragments of membrane produced by freeze-fracture, that there is more cholesterol in the outer leaflet than in the inner leaflet.

2 PHOSPHOLIPIDS AND MEMBRANE STRUCTURE

It is generally agreed that the structural feature common to all biological membranes is a double layer of phospholipid molecules with their long axes at right angles to the plane of the membrane and their polar head groups facing outwards into the water on either side of the membrane. Current ideas about the physical state of the molecules in the phospholipid bilayers of natural membranes have been developed from the study of phospholipid monolayers formed at an air/water interface and of bilayers formed by dispersions of phospholipid in water, and also from investigations of biological membranes examined in their natural state or after preparation by staining, partial dehydration or other procedures. These studies have been carried out with a variety of methods, including X-ray crystallography, IR spectroscopy, magnetic resonance spectrometry and the use of lipophilic fluorescent probes, all of which can provide information about the arrangement and mobility of the lipid molecules in lipid/water systems. Of particular interest are the bilaminar, or *lamellar*, structures formed by shaking phospholipids in aqueous media. These may be multilamellar, consisting of stacks of bilayers each separated by a layer of water (*myelin figures*, so called because of

Sterols in Biological Membranes 319

their similarity to the myelin sheath of nerve fibres), or they may consist of closed vesicles, each formed by multiple or single bilayers. Both types of structure may be formed by pure phospholipids of a single chemical form, by mixtures of different purified phospholipids or by mixtures of phospholipids with cholesterol or other lipids possessing both hydrophobic and hydrophilic groups (*amphiphiles*). They may also be formed by the lipid mixtures extracted from natural membranes.

Results obtained by X-ray crystallography and electron micrography agree in showing the presence of a bilaminar structure in aqueous dispersions of phospholipids and in various natural membranes (myelin sheath, red-cell plasma membrane, mitochondrial membranes and the membranes of chloroplasts). The electron-density profile of phospholipid bilayers, as revealed by the X-ray diffraction pattern, shows peaks of high density about 40 Å apart, separated by

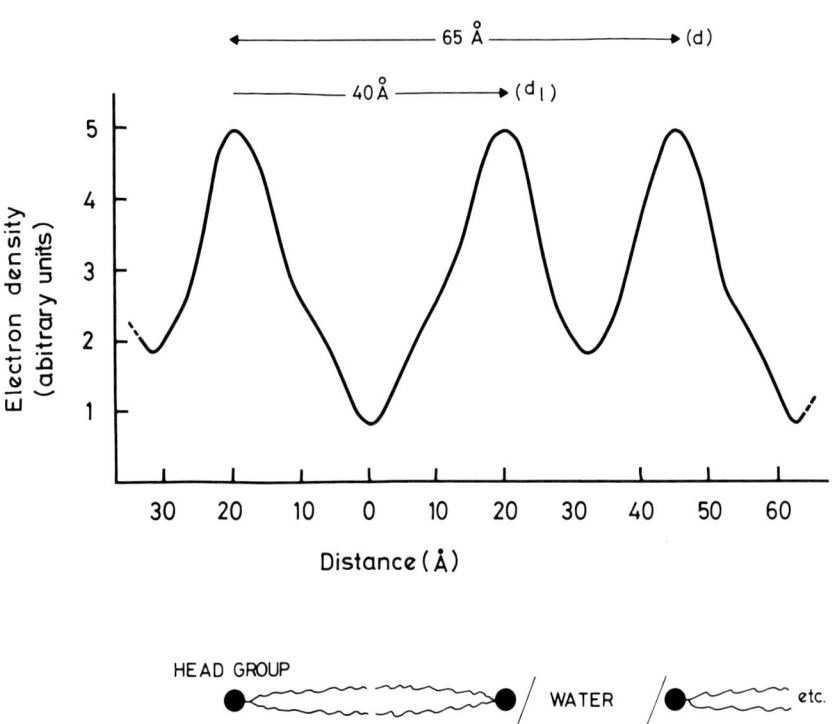

Figure 7.1
Idealized electron-density profile of a lecithin bilayer in a lecithin/water system. The arrangement of the phospholipid molecules, shown in cross-section, is shown below the profile. One layer of a second bilayer is shown to the right, with a layer of water between the two sheets of polar head groups (phosphoryl choline residues). d_l, thickness of one bilayer; d, repeat distance between bilayers.

troughs of low density. The peaks of high density are due to the polar head groups and the troughs are due to the electron-sparse hydrocarbon chains of the phospholipid molecules. The 40 Å distance between peaks is roughly twice the length of a phospholipid molecule (Fig. 7.1). In some natural membranes the electron-density profile is asymmetrical. This asymmetry has been attributed to a difference in the cholesterol:phospholipid ratio on the two sides of the bilayer. However, the evidence for significant asymmetry in the distribution of cholesterol in natural membranes is equivocal; but see Fisher (1976).

Observations on the effects of varying the cholesterol:phospholipid ratio in single-bilayer vesicles have suggested ways in which sterols may influence the permeability and physical state of natural membranes. However, it should be noted that although many of the properties of living membranes can be explained on the assumption that the basic structural element is a continuous bilayer of phospholipids, cholesterol and other amphiphilic lipids, the manner in which these lipids interact with each other and with membrane proteins is still far from clear. It is also worth noting that phospholipid-sterol mixtures are capable of forming various non-lamellar structures in water (Luzatti, 1968) and that some of these may participate in the formation of biological membranes. Indeed, it is possible that a living membrane is not a static structure but is capable of changing from one physical state to another under different physiological conditions. Such changes could affect different regions of the membrane at different times. (See Lucy (1968), Vandenheuval (1971) and Jain and White (1977) for contrasting views of membrane structure).

3 STEROL-PHOSPHOLIPID INTERACTIONS

3.1 Condensation in monolayers

The manner in which sterols influence the physical state of the phospholipid molecules in a monolayer has provided important clues to the significance of sterols in biological membranes (see Demel and de Kruyff, 1976). The minimum cross-sectional area (A) occupied by a phospholipid molecule in a monolayer formed at an air/water interface depends upon the nature of the polar head group and the length and degree of unsaturation of the hydrocarbon chains. For a given class of phospholipid, the longer the chains and the fewer the double bonds, the greater is the hydrophobic interaction between chains and the smaller is the area per molecule. For example, the limiting values for A are 41, 58 and 63 Å^2/molecule for lecithins with di-18:0, di-14:0 and 18:1, 18:0 hydrocarbon chains respectively.

When cholesterol is incorporated into a phospholipid monolayer, interaction between cholesterol molecules and the hydrocarbon chains may lead to a reduction in the mean area per phospholipid molecule. This effect is known as *condensation*. The condensing effect of cholesterol is most marked for phospholipids in which both chains are short (C_{14} or less) or in which one chain has up to 4 double bonds. If the phospholipids are already in a fully condensed state, as with di-18:0 chains, or if they are fully expanded, as when both chains are polyunsaturated, cholesterol has little or no condensing effect.

Many sterols other than cholesterol can bring about condensation of phospholipid monolayers composed of a single species of phospholipid, or of mixtures of the lipids extracted from biological membranes such as red-cell ghosts. The relative magnitudes of the condensing effect of various sterols and their analogues suggest that the structural features required for sterol-phospholipid interaction in monolayers (and, presumably, in the bilayers of membranes) are a planar ring system, a free 3β-OH group and an intact hydrophobic side-chain with or without an alkyl substituent at C-24. Thus, condensation occurs with 5α-saturated sterols, with sterols possessing a Δ^5 or Δ^7 double bond and with many plant sterols. 3α-Hydroxysterols and sterols in which the 3β-OH group is esterified with fatty acids do not interact with phospholipids and cannot participate in membrane formation, though there is some evidence to suggest that cholesteryl sulphate helps to stabilize human red-cell membranes (Bleau *et al.*, 1974).

The structural features of the sterol and hydrocarbon chains needed for condensation suggest that the effect is due to hydrophobic interaction between the hydrocarbon chains and a planar sterol ring system and side-chain. The need for a free 3β-OH group suggests that there may also be interaction between this group and the polar head group of the phospholipid. Against this, however, elimination of the oxygen linkages of a phospholipid does not influence its ability to interact with cholesterol in a monolayer, nor does cholesterol affect the ^{31}P-NMR spectrum of lecithin bilayers.

3.2 Effect of sterols on phase changes

The physical state of a phospholipid bilayer in an aqueous medium is influenced by the temperature and by the presence of sterols (see Chapman and Wallach, 1968). Below a critical temperature, known as the *phase transition temperature* (T_c), a bilayer of a single phospholipid species is in a quasi-crystalline state; the hydrocarbon chains are rigid and lateral diffusion in the plane of the bilayer is negligible, though rotation without lateral motion can occur. As the temperature is raised to a value approaching T_c, lateral diffusion increases and the hydrocarbon chains become mobile. When the transition temperature is reached there is an abrupt change of phase from a crystalline to a liquid-crystalline state, the hydrocarbon chains flexing and twisting so that their conformation becomes completely disordered, as in a solution of phospholipid in organic solvent. Although the hydrocarbon chains 'melt' and become fluid at the T_c, the polar head groups retain their two-dimensional order since they are anchored at the lipid/water interface. At the transition temperature the area per molecule of phospholipid increases and the thickness of the bilayer decreases. The phase transition is accompanied by various physical changes, all of which reflect the melting of the hydrocarbon chains. These changes include an increase in the short spacing of the X-ray diffraction pattern from 4.2 to 4.6 Å, an increase in the rate of heat uptake, a reduction in the line-width of the NMR signal due to the protons of the hydrocarbon chains (indicating increased freedom of motion of the chains) and a change in the ESR spectrum of bilayers in which the chains are spin-labelled, also indicating increased chain mobility. For a given class of phospholipid, T_c depends on the nature of the hydrocarbon chains. In general, phospholipids giving relatively condensed monolayers have high transition temperatures. Thus, the shorter and the more unsaturated the chains, the lower the transition temperature. For example, for lecithin bilayers with di-16:0, di-14:0 and di-18:1 chains, the values for T_c are 41 °C, 23 °C and −22 °C respectively.

When cholesterol is incorporated into a bilayer of a pure phospholipid, the phase transition is influenced in a complex manner (de Kruyff et al., 1974). As the proportion of cholesterol is increased, the transition becomes less sharply defined until, at cholesterol:phospholipid molar ratios approaching 1:1, it disappears altogether (Ladbrooke et al., 1968). This may be seen by observing the effect of cholesterol on the heat absorption at the phase transition in a bilayer of di-16:0 lecithin (Fig. 7.2). In the absence of cholesterol there is a sharp endothermic absorption peak at 41 °C due to melting of the hydrocarbon chains. When 12.5 moles % of cholesterol are incorporated into the bilayer the peak becomes broader and flatter; when the cholesterol concentration is raised to 50 moles % the peak can no longer be seen.

Changes in the liquid-crystalline state of the bilayer corresponding to these changes in thermal behaviour may be studied by examining the proton- and ^{13}C-NMR spectra given by the fatty acyl chains of the phospholipid molecules. Additional information may be obtained from the ESR spectrum given by spin-labelled molecules introduced into the phospholipid bilayer and from the behaviour of lipid-soluble fluorescent compounds, also incorporated into the bilayer. For a discussion of the use of these techniques in the study of membranes,

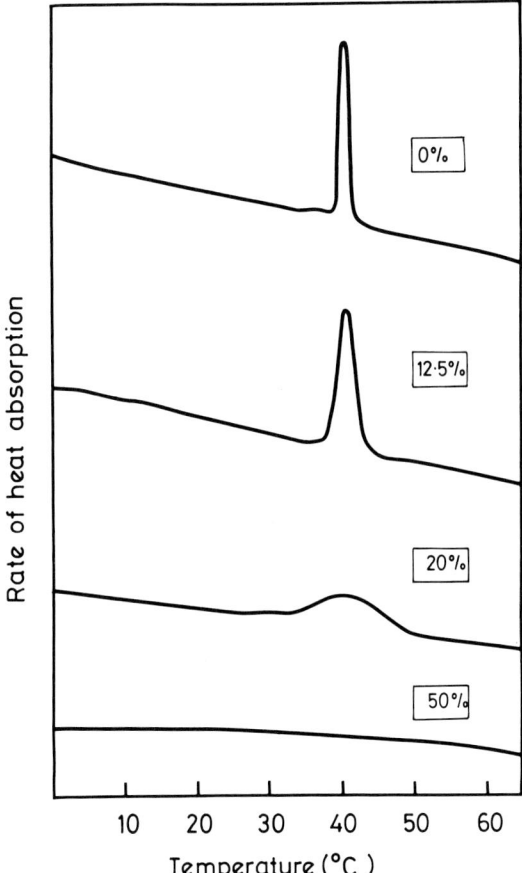

Figure 7.2
Effect of increasing concentrations of cholesterol on the rate of heat absorption at the phase transition temperature (41 °C) of an aqueous dispersion of di-16:0 lecithin, measured by differential scanning calorimetry. The molar concentration of cholesterol in the cholesterol-phospholipid mixture is shown beside each curve. Note the absence of any discernible absorption peak when the molar concentration is 50%. (Redrawn from Ladbrooke *et al.* (1968).)

see Chapman (1973). Observations obtained by these methods have shown that the effect of adding cholesterol to a phospholipid bilayer is to maintain the chains, over a relatively wide range of temperature, in a state intermediate between the crystalline and liquid-crystalline phases (the *intermediate gel phase*). The NMR spectrum of a bilayer of a 1:1 molar mixture of cholesterol and lecithin shows that over a 10–20 °C range of temperature on either side of the T_c for pure lecithin, the first 8 to 10 carbon atoms of the hydrocarbon chains are in a rigid state and the remaining terminal carbon atoms are freely mobile

(Rothman and Engelman, 1972) (Fig. 7.3). Molecular models show that if the hydroxyl group of cholesterol is close to the phosphate group of lecithin, the remainder of the sterol molecule would extend to about C-10 of the hydrocarbon chains. Thus, the net effect of cholesterol on a phospholipid bilayer is to increase the mean fluidity of the chains at temperatures below the T_c and to decrease their fluidity at temperatures above the T_c.

Of greater relevance to the properties of natural membranes are the effects of sterols on bilayers of pairs of phospholipids with different fatty-acid chains or head groups. If the two phospholipids have transition temperatures that are not very far apart, they will form mixed bilayers whose chains melt at a single well-defined T_c, as shown by the presence of a sharp endothermic peak at a temperature between the transition temperatures of the pure components. When cholesterol is incorporated into the mixture, the cholesterol molecules distribute themselves at random throughout the bilayer and the effect on the phase transition is the same as that in a bilayer of a single phospholipid. As the sterol concentration is increased, the heat-absorption peak becomes broader and flatter, finally disappearing; at this point all the fatty-acid chains may be assumed to be in the intermediate gel state over a wide range of temperature.

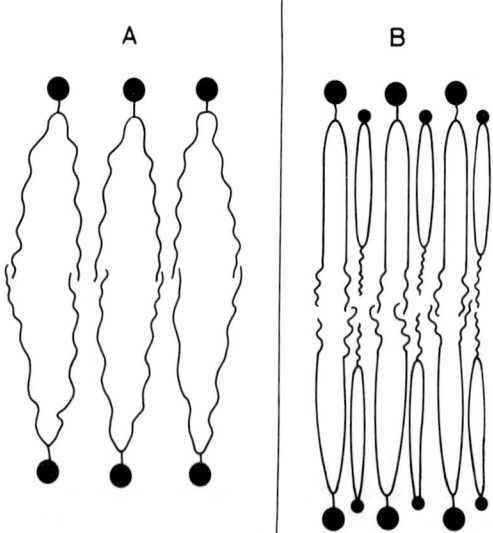

Figure 7.3
Effect of cholesterol on the physical state of a phospholipid bilayer at a temperature above the phase transition temperature. In the absence of cholesterol (A) the chains are fluid. In the presence of cholesterol (B) (50 moles %) the first eight to ten carbon atoms of the chains are rigid and the bilayer is condensed. The cholesterol molecules are shown with their hydroxyl groups (●) close to the head groups of the phospholipids (●).

If the two phospholipids have transition temperatures which differ by more than about 30 °C, e.g. a mixture of di-14:0 lecithin (T_c, 23 °C) and di-18;0 lecithin (T_c, 58 °C), each component of the bilayer will melt at a T_c close to that of the pure phospholipid and the heat-absorption curve will show two sharp peaks, indicating segregation of the mixture into regions containing only one species of phospholipid. When cholesterol is incorporated into the mixed bilayer at low concentrations (up to 20 moles %), the phase transition of the phospholipid with the lower T_c is modified or abolished without significant effect on that of the phospholipid with the higher T_c. When the cholesterol concentration reaches a value of about 35 moles % both phase transitions are abolished, as shown by the absence of peaks in the heat-absorption curve. These changes are due to the fact that cholesterol molecules interact preferentially with the phospholipid with the lower T_c. Hence, at low cholesterol:phospholipid molar ratios, when there is not enough cholesterol to interact with all the phospholipid molecules, over a wide range of temperatures below the T_c of the component with the higher transition temperature the bilayer contains regions of a cholesterol-phospholipid mixture in which the chains are fluid, or in the intermediate-gel state, and regions of pure phospholipid in which the chains are rigid. When there is enough cholesterol to interact with all the phospholipid molecules of both species, the whole bilayer assumes the intermediate-gel state.

Consideration of the possible ways in which the cholesterol and phospholipid molecules of a bilayer may pack suggests that two molecules of phospholipid can interact with each molecule of cholesterol (Phillips and Finer, 1974; Poznansky and Czekanski, 1979). If this is so, every molecule of phospholipid in a homogeneous bilayer should be adjacent to a cholesterol molecule when the cholesterol:phospholipid molar ratio is 1:2 and hence there should be one phase throughout the bilayer at a cholesterol concentration of 33.3 moles %. This may explain why there is little or no temperature-dependent phase change in a mixed phospholipid bilayer containing 35 moles % of cholesterol.

A further complication may arise when proteins are present in an artificial bilayer. Many proteins, including enzymes and structural proteins, are capable of interacting with cholesterol (Papahadjopoulos *et al.*, 1973, and see de Kruyff *et al.*, 1974). Hence, proteins in a cholesterol-phospholipid bilayer may reduce the number of cholesterol molecules available for interaction with phospholipid and may thus give rise to separation of the phospholipids into regions in which the hydrocarbon chains are in different states of fluidity, even though the cholesterol:phospholipid ratio exceeds 1:2.

Intrinsic membrane proteins may also influence the physical state of the phospholipids in the surrounding lipid bilayer, the effect of the protein depending upon such factors as the ratio of protein to membrane lipid, the temperature relative to the T_c of the phospholipids and the nature of the phospholipid acyl chains. Jost et al. (1973), using ESR spectroscopy and a spin-labelled probe, have examined the physical state of the lipids in the vicinity of cytochrome oxidase particles incorporated into phospholipid vesicles. They conclude that each enzyme particle in the vesicle is surrounded by a ring of immobilized phospholipid which they estimate to be one molecule thick. They point out that the effect of this segregation of lipid molecules must be to decrease the amount of phospholipid available for forming fluid bilayers in the membrane as a whole. Comparable experiments of Warren et al. (1975) and Hesketh et al. (1976) with complexes of dioleoyl lecithin and purified ATPase from sarcoplasmic reticulum also suggest that the ATPase in sarcoplasmic reticular membranes is surrounded by an annulus of rigid phospholipid molecules which, at physiological temperatures, prevents cholesterol in the membrane from coming into contact with the enzyme. If the phospholipid annulus is removed by a detergent and is then replaced by cholesterol, the enzyme is completely and reversibly inactivated. Warren et al. (1975) suggest that the presence of the phospholipid annulus around the enzyme enables it to maintain normal activity even when the cholesterol:phospholipid molar ratio in the bulk membrane lipids is 1:1. They speculate that other membrane-bound enzymes susceptible to inhibition by cholesterol maintain their activity by excluding cholesterol from their immediate environment.

It should be noted that the idea that many intrinsic membrane proteins are surroundeed by boundary layers of rigid phospholipid molecules has not gone unchallenged. Thus, Moore et al. (1978) have shown that the activity of sarcoplasmic-reticulum ATPase can be modified by changes in the lipid composition of the bulk lipids more readily than would be predicted if the enzyme is protected by an annulus of phospholipid whose molecules do not exchange with the lipid molecules of the surrounding membrane. Madden et al. (1979) have also described conditions under which the activity of ATPase in sarcoplasmic reticulum can be modified by changing the cholesterol:phospholipid ratio in the membrane. For a review of the evidence for and against the existence of immobile phospholipids surrounding membrane proteins, see Chapman et al. (1979).

4 EFFECTS OF STEROLS ON MEMBRANE FUNCTION

Information as to how sterols influence the physiological properties of natural membranes has been obtained mainly from two sources: (1) the study of single-bilayer or multilamellar vesicles (*liposomes*) in which different amounts of sterol have been incorporated into the bilayers and (2) the study of biological membranes in which the amount and structure of the sterol components vary naturally or have been altered experimentally.

4.1 Liposomes

Liposomes can be formed by sonicating phospholipids or phospholipid-sterol mixtures in an aqueous medium under suitable conditions. If the medium contains organic solutes, these will be trapped within the vesicles, which may then be transferred to fresh medium for measurement of the rate of efflux of solute through the bilayers. Alternatively, by reversing the procedure it is possible to measure the rate at which solutes diffuse from the medium into the interior of the vesicles. Observations on vesicles made from different phospholipids show that those phospholipids that form relatively condensed monolayers also form vesicles with low permeability to glycerol, glucose and other organic solutes (de Gier et al., 1968; Papahadjopoulos et al., 1973; Demel and de Kruyff, 1976). Thus, permeability increases with increasing unsaturation and decreasing length of the hydrocarbon chains. For example, permeability increases in the order di-18:0 < 18:0, 18:1 < di-18:1 < di-18:2 and in the order di-18:0 < di-16:0 < di-14:0 for liposomes of pure lecithins. When cholesterol, or other sterol with a free 3β-OH group and an intact side-chain, is incorporated into the bilayers of liposomes made from phospholipids that do not give fully condensed monolayers, the permeability of the liposomes is decreased, the effect of the sterol reaching a maximum at a sterol:phospholipid molar ratio of 1:1. Thus, the permeability of liposomes formed from 18:0; 18:1 lecithin is decreased ten-fold when the bilayers contain 50 moles of cholesterol %. On the other hand, cholesterol has no effect on the permeability of di-18:2 lecithin liposomes. The cholesterol-induced decrease in the permeability of liposomes with incompletely condensed bilayers is associated with changes in the X-ray diffraction pattern and NMR spectrum indicating decreased mobility of the hydrocarbon chains of the phospholipids, as discussed above.

4.2 Natural membranes

Although many aspects of the behaviour of natural membranes can now be understood in terms of interactions of cholesterol with membrane phospholipids and proteins, it must be remembered that the simplest living membrane is almost certainly more complex than any of the artificial systems that have been investigated, including the bilayers of phospholipid mixtures discussed above. Because living membranes are so complex, it is not always possible to interpret unequivocally the information obtained by physical methods such as NMR spectrometry, X-ray diffraction analysis and calorimetry. For example, though the NMR signals from artificial phospholipid bilayers can be assigned to the various chemical groupings in considerable detail, interpretation of the NMR spectrum of an intact red-cell membrane in relation to the fluidity of the hydrocarbon chains is still in dispute. These limitations should be borne in mind in the following discussion.

Several methods can be used to alter the amount and nature of the sterols in natural membranes. In animals fed the drug AY 9944, the Δ^7 double bond of the sterol ring system cannot be reduced and 7-dehydrocholesterol progressively replaces cholesterol in cell membranes throughout the body. A more versatile method, used extensively in the study of red-cell membranes, is to expose the cells *in vitro* to dispersions of lecithin in an isotonic medium (Bruckdorfer *et al.*, 1968). This results in a net flow of cholesterol from the outer layer of the membrane to the lecithin particles. By exposing the cholesterol-depleted cells to lecithin dispersions containing sterols other than cholesterol it is possible to replace about a third of the red-cell cholesterol with other sterols. Methods similar in principle to this may be used to bring about a marked reduction in the cholesterol content of the membranes of intact mitochondria. The application of these methods to the study of membrane function has shown that up to 30% of the cholesterol of human red cells can be removed without significant alteration in their osmotic fragility or permeability to non-ionic solutes, but that both are significantly increased if 35% of the membrane cholesterol is removed. These changes can be reversed in cholesterol-depleted red cells by animal sterols containing a 3β-OH group and planar ring system and, to a lesser extent, by some plant sterols, but not by sterols in which the 3-hydroxyl group is replaced by a keto group (Bruckdorfer *et al.*, 1969).

In cholesterol-fed guineapigs and in human subjects suffering from certain types of liver disease the concentration of cholesterol in the red-cell membranes increases markedly, the cholesterol:phospholipid molar ratio sometimes reaching values above 1.5 (see Chapter 18). In both instances the osmotic fragility of the red cells is decreased and ESR measurements suggest decreased mobility of the hydrocarbon chains (Kroes *et al.*, 1972). (At these very high cholesterol:phospholipid ratios it is likely that some cholesterol molecules in the membrane interact with each other.) Conversely, the low cholesterol:phospholipid molar ratio in the plasma membranes of leukaemic cells is associated with an increase in membrane fluidity (Inbar *et al.*, 1974).

All these observations are consistent with an effect of sterols on the permeability of intact cell membranes mediated by an effect on the fluidity of the hydrocarbon chains of the phospholipids, similar to that observed in phospholipid vesicles. In keeping with this interpretaion, examination of the bilayers formed from the lipids extracted from normal and cholesterol-depleted red cells shows an absence of any temperature-dependent phase transition in bilayers of the lipids from normal cells, but the presence of a transition between 2 °C and 20 °C in bilayers of the lipids of cholesterol-depleted cells (Gottlieb and Eanes, 1974). X-ray diffraction analysis of intact red-cell membranes also suggests that all the hydrocarbon chains are at least partially fluid at temperatures as low as 0 °C (Gottlieb and Eanes, 1974). Thus, it seems likely that the presence of cholesterol in the red-cell membrane prevents the hydrocarbon chains from crystallizing at body temperature, possibly maintaining them in the intermediate gel state.

Of special interest in relation to the effect of cholesterol on membrane fluidity are those membranes in which the cholesterol concentration is low. If sterols are of major importance in maintaining fluidity of the hydrocarbon chains of membrane phospholipids, it should be possible to demonstrate the presence of regional phase differences in membranes that do not contain enough sterol to interact with all the phospholipid molecules present, as discussed in Section 3.2. Temperature-dependent phase changes have indeed been observed in the membranes of animal mitochondria and cell nuclei and of the plasma membrane of the microorganism *Acholeplasma laidlawii*, all of which contain cholesterol at concentrations below 30 moles % (Chapman, 1973; de Kruyff *et al.*, 1974). The presence of phase changes has been taken to indicate that these membranes contain regions of phospholipid with no cholesterol. This does not necessarily mean that these regions are crystalline at the body temperature of warm-blooded animals since the phospholipids may contain polyunsaturated fatty-acid chains with low phase-transition temperatures.

More direct evidence that sterols help to control the fluidity of natural membranes has been obtained from the study of *Mycoplasma mycoides var. capri*. When the native strain is grown in the presence of cholesterol it incorporates cholesterol into its membranes. Under these conditions the membrane shows no thermotropic phase transition, as determined by calorimetry or fluorescence spectroscopy. However, in strains adapted to growth in the absence of cholesterol, the membrane is cholesterol-free and shows a well-defined phase transition. At temperatures above the transition temperature the membranes of the adapted organisms are more fluid than those of the native cells and the adapted organisms have increased permeability and are abnormally fragile (Rottem *et al.*, 1973*a*). The profound effect of changes in membrane fluidity on cell metabolism is illustrated by the fact that the adapted, cholesterol-free, cells are incapable of growth at temperatures below the phase transition (when the hydrocarbon chains are rigid), whereas the native cells grown in the presence of cholesterol can grow at these temperatures,

As well as influencing the physical state of the phospholipids of membranes, cholesterol also influences the biochemical properties of some membrane proteins, possibly by determining the physical state of the lipids in the immediate vicinity of the protein. The adapted strain of *M. mycoides*, mentioned above, provides an interesting example of this. Rottem *et al.* (1973*b*) have shown that the activity of the membrane-bound ATPase of the cholesterol-free strain changes sharply as the temperature is raised above the transition temperature. No such temperature-dependent change in enzyme activity is observed in the native strain. Other examples of an effect of cholesterol on membrane-bound enzymes are the decrease in activity of succinate-cytochrome reductase in cholesterol-depleted liver mitochondria (Graham and Green, 1970), the reversible inactivation of the ATPase of sarcoplasmic reticulum by cholesterol (Warren *et al.*, 1975) and the inhibition, by cholesterol, of the microsomal Na^+/K^+ ATPase of rabbit kidney (Kimelberg and Papahadjopoulos, 1974). An interaction of cholesterol with proteins in the outer layer of biological membranes may also account for the observation that there is more cholesterol in the outer side of the membrane of myelin than in the inner side. The possibility that the activity of HMG-CoA reductase is regulated by the amount of cholesterol in microsomal membranes is discussed in Chapter 8.

Observations on the plasma membranes of intact cells (Sachs, 1974) and on other biological membranes suggest that many proteins are free to move within the phospholipid bilayer, provided that the membrane lipids are in a suitably fluid state; a protein molecule in a living membrane has been likened to an iceberg floating in the sea. It also seems likely that rotational and lateral mobility of membrane proteins is essential for some of a cell's most important activities. It is possible, for example, that transport through membranes depends on the ability of specific carrier proteins 'floating' in a cell membrane to rotate about an axis parallel to the plane of the membrane (Cone, 1972), and that inhibition of the growth of cells by mutual contact depends upon the ability of specific proteins, capable of intercellular recognition, to diffuse laterally in the plasma membrane.

Membrane fluidity, sufficient to permit the lateral diffusion of proteins, must also be needed for the gathering together ('capping') of protein receptors in the plasma membrane of lymphocytes challenged by antibodies to their receptors, and may also be required for the adhesion of cells to one another in multicellular organisms (see Edelman, 1976). Since the amount of sterol in a membrane has a profound influence upon its fluidity, it is reasonable to suppose that changes in the cholesterol:phospholipid ratio of cell membranes could influence those activities of the cell that depend upon the maintenance of optimal mobility of membrane proteins. That this is indeed the case is suggested by the observation that leucocytes that have undergone malignant transformation by viral infection have abnormal plasma membranes, with a low cholesterol concentration, a pathological increase in fluidity and loss of contact inhibition (see Sachs, 1974). However, it should be noted that malignant transformation of cells in culture may occur without change in the lipid composition of their plasma membranes (Perdue *et al.*, 1971). For a review of membrane fluidity in relation to disease processes, see Wallach (1973).

5 DISTRIBUTION AND MOBILITY OF MEMBRANE CHOLESTEROL

Non-random distribution of cholesterol in artificial phospholipid bilayers containing phospholipids with very different transition temperatures has already been mentioned. Evidence from calorimetry, X-ray diffraction crystallography and other methods also indicates that 'clustering' of cholesterol occurs in natural membranes. Perhaps the most striking evidence for regional distribution of cholesterol in an intact cell membrane is that obtained by Murphy (1965), who showed by autoradiography with [^{3}H]cholesterol that the exchangeable cholesterol of the red-cell membrane is present predominantly at the periphery of the disc. If the concave region of the red-cell disc is virtually free of cholesterol and if, as X-ray diffraction and NMR spectrometry suggest, the red-cell membrane as a whole is in a partially fluid state, this would suggest that the bulk of the phosphlipids are above their transition temperatures at 37 °C. As mentioned in Section 2, evidence from X-ray diffraction suggests that in some natural membranes the concentration of cholesterol is higher in the outer than in the inner layer. However, this is a controversial question (Rothman and Lenard, 1977). In vesicles made by sonicating aqueous dispersions of some phospholipid-cholesterol mixtures, the concentration of cholesterol may be higher on the inside than on the outside of the bilayers, but this is due to the very small radius of curvature of the vesicles, favouring the presence of molecules occupying a smaller cross-sectional area on the inside.

Mobility of the molecules in a bilayer is of two kinds: lateral movement in the plane of the membrane and movement between the inner and outer layers. Lateral movement of phospholipid molecules in an artificial bilayer above T_c has been referred to above. In an

ESR study of single-bilayer vesicles with a spin-labelled marker, Kornberg and McConnell (1971a) have shown that lateral diffusion of lecithin takes place at a rate such that a lecithin molecule could diffuse from one end of a bacterium to the other in less than 5 minutes. Less attention has been paid to lateral diffusion of sterols in membranes though lateral diffusion of cholesterol has been demonstrated in artificial phospholipid monolayers (Stroeve and Miller, 1975) and there seems little doubt that it also occurs in the bilayers of natural membranes.

Movement of phospholipids between the two layers of a bilayer is much slower than lateral movement, because transmembrane movement involves a 180° change in the orientation of the long axis of the molecule, a process known as *flip-flop*. Kornberg and McConnell (1971b) estimate that flip-flop of lecithin molecules in a single-bilayer vesicle occurs with a half-life of longer than 6 hours at 30 °C.

The rate of flip-flop of cholesterol in bilayers is controversial. Poznansky and Lange (1976) have shown that the rate of exchange of cholesterol across a single bilayer of an artificial vesicle of a di-16:0 lecithin-cholesterol mixture is exceedingly slow, the half-life being at least 6 days. Exchange of cholesterol molecules across the two layers of the membrane of influenza virus appears to be equally slow (Lenard and Rothman, 1976). However, when human or dog red cells are labelled with [^{14}C]cholesterol *in vivo*, so that the cholesterol on both sides of the membrane is labelled, complete equilibration between red-cell cholesterol and plasm cholesterol occurs within a few hours during incubation of the labelled cells in plasma *in vitro* (Hagerman and Gould, 1951; Bruckdorfer and Graham, 1976). This could not occur if cholesterol molecules on the inner side of the red-cell membrane are virtually non-exchangeable owing to extreme slowness of flip-flop. The experiments of Lange *et al.* (1977), in which the sequential exchange of [^{3}H]cholesterol and [^{14}C]cholesterol between plasma and human red cells was investigated, also point to a rapid rate of transmembrane exchange of cholesterol in these cells, with a half-life possibly shorter than 50 minutes. Relatively rapid rates of transposition of phospholipid through the membranes of the red cells of rats have also been observed by Bloj and Zilversmit (1976) and by Renooij *et al.* (1976). These observations suggest that in at least some natural membranes there is a component, perhaps a protein spanning the width of the membrane, that facilitates the movement of cholesterol and phospholipid between the inner and outer leaflets. This may not be present in the red-cell membrane in all species since Bell and Schwartz (1971) have shown that when [^{3}H]cholesterol-labelled plasma lipoproteins are incubated with pig red cells, the specific radioactivity of the red-cell cholesterol is less than half that of the lipoprotein cholesterol at isotopic equilibrium.

6 EVOLUTIONARY SIGNIFICANCE OF MEMBRANE STEROLS

The ability of sterols to keep the hydrocarbon chains of phospholipid bilayers in a state of intermediate fluidity over a wide range of temperature is clearly advantageous to plants, and to animals that do not maintain a constant body temperature, since it must permit their cell membranes to function optimally in the face of changes in environmental temperature. During the evolution of plants and fungi, their sterols have been modified by the introduction of an alkyl group into the side-chain. It is not easy to see the selective advantage of this biochemical modification, since animal sterols, in which the 'primordial' side-chain (i.e., the one arising from the cyclization of squalene) is unmodified, are more readily incorporated into phospholipid bilayers than are plant sterols. Moreover, the animal sterols are at least as effective in maintaining normal permeability of natural membranes.

A mechanism for stabilizing cell membrane structure over a wide temperature range would not be of any obvious use to homeothermic animals, except possibly in skin cells. A clue to one of the functions of sterols in the cell membranes of warm-blooded animals may lie in the remarkable variability of the phospholipids present in the membranes of a given type of animal cell. The marked species variation in the phospholipid composition of red-cell membranes has been mentioned above. Wide variations in the degree of unsaturation of the fatty-acid chains of red-cell phospholipids in a given individual may also occur under physiological conditions. For example, Farquhar and Ahrens (1963) have shown that the proportion of 18:2 chains in the red-cell phospholipids of human subjects can be made to vary from 5% to 27% by changing the fatty acid composition of the diet. This reflects the exchangeability of red-cell phospholipids with plasma phospholipids, the fatty-acids of the latter being readily modified by dietary fat absorbed from the intestine. The presence of sterols in the plasma membrane would enable red cells, or any other cells bathed by interstitial fluid containing phospholipids, to maintain optimal fluidity of their plasma membranes despite variation in the length and unsaturation of their hydrocarbon chains due to exchange with extracellular phospholipids. This may enable the cells to tolerate considerable fluctuations in the lipid composition of their environment.

Observations on artificial membranes suggest that sterols may also diminish the effect of changes in the pH and cation concentrations of the aqueous medium on the physical state of phospholipid bilayers. This effect may help to maintain intracellular membranes in an optimal state of fluidity. Thus, given the appearance, during evolution, of a phospholipid bilayer as the fundamental component of cell membranes, the incorporation of a suitable amphiphile into the membrane would be expected to be favoured by natural selection. Owing to its size and shape, and to the position and configuration of its polar group, a Δ^5 sterol with a 3β-hydroxyl group would have been well-suited to act as a membrane stabilizer. The ability of certain membrane-bound enzymes to respond to changes in the amount of sterol present in their immediate vicinity may have arisen at a later stage in the evolution of the cell. For a discussion of the types of molecule that may have acted as membrane stabilizers before the evolutionary appearance of sterols in nature, see Bloch (1976), Ourisson *et al.* (1979) and Gibbons *et al.* (1982).

REFERENCES

Amar-Costesec, A., Wibo, M., Thinès-Sempoux, D., Beaufay, H. and Berthet, J. (1974). Analytical study of microsomes and isolated subcellular membranes from rat liver. IV. Biochemical, biophysical, and morphological modifications of microsomal components induced by digitonin, EDTA, and pyrophosphate. *Journal of Cell Biology*, **62**, 717–745.

Ashworth, L. A. E. and Green, C. (1966). Plasma membranes: phospolipid and sterol content. *Science*, **151**, 210–211.

Bell, F. P. and Schwartz, C. J. (1971). Exchangeability of cholesterol between swine serum lipoproteins and erythrocytes, *in vitro*. *Biochimica et Biophysica Acta*, **231**, 553–557.

Bleau, G., Bodley, F. H., Longpré, J., Chapdelaine, A. and Roberts, K. D. (1974). Cholesterol sulfate. I. Occurrence and possible biological function as an amphipathic lipid in the membrane of the human erythrocyte. *Biochimica et Biophysica Acta*, **352**, 1–9.

Bloch, K. On the evolution of a biosynthetic pathway. In: *Reflections on Biochemistry*. Ed. A. Kornberg, B. L. Horecker, L. Cornudella and J. Oró. Pergamon Press, Oxford, pp. 143–150, 1976.

Bloj, B. and Zilversmit, D. B. (1976). Asymmetry and transposition rates of phosphatidylcholine in rat erythrocyte ghosts. *Biochemistry*, **15**, 1277–1283.

Bretscher, M. S. (1973). Membrane structure: some general principles. *Science*, **181**, 622–629.

Bruckdorfer, K. R., Demel, R. A., De Gier, J. and van Deenen, L. L. M, (1969). The effect of partial replacements of membrane cholesterol by other steroids on the osmotic fragility and glycerol permeability of erythrocytes. *Biochimica et Biophysica Acta*, **183**, 334–345.

Bruckdorfer, K. R. and Graham, J. M. The exchange of cholesterol and phospholipids between cell membranes and lipoproteins. In: *Biological Membranes*, Vol. 3. Ed. D. Chapman and D. F. H. Wallach. Academic Press, London, pp. 103–152, 1976.

Bruckdorfer, K. R., Graham, J. M. and Green, C. (1968). The incorporation of steroid molecules into lecithin sols, β-lipoproteins and cellular membranes. *European Journal of Biochemistry*, **4**, 512–518.

Calvin, M. *Chemical evolution. Molecular evolution towards the origin of living systems on the earth and elsewhere.* Oxford University Press, Oxford, 1969.

Chapman, D. Some recent studies of lipids, lipid-cholesterol and membrane systems. In: *Biological Membranes*, Vol. 2. Ed. D. Chapman and D. F. H. Wallach. Academic Press, London, pp. 91–144, 1973.
Chapman, D., Gómez-Fernández, J. C. and Goñi, F. M. (1979). Intrinsic protein-lipid interactions. Physical and biochemical evidence. *FEBS Letters*, **98**, 211–223.
Chapman, D. and Wallach, D. F. H. Recent physical studies of phospholipids and natural membranes. In: *Biological Membranes. Physical Fact and Function*. Ed. D. Chapman. Academic Press, London, pp. 125–202, 1968.
Cone, R. A. (1972). Rotational diffusion of rhodopsin in the visual receptor membrane. *Nature (New Biology)*, **236**, 39–43.
Demel, R. A. and De Kruyff, B. (1976). The function of sterols in membranes. *Biochimica et Biophysica Acta*, **457**, 109–132.
Edelman, G. M. (1976). Surface modulation in cell recognition and cell growth. *Science*, **192**, 218–226.
Farquhar, J. W. and Ahrens, E. H. Jr. (1963). Effects of dietary fats on human erythrocyte fatty acid patterns. *Journal of Clinical Investigation*, **42**, 675–685.
Fisher, K. A. (1976). Analysis of membrane halves: cholesterol. *Proceedings of the National Academy of Sciences of the USA*, **73**, 173–177.
Gibbons, G. F., Mitropoulos, K. A. and Myant, N. B. *The Biochemistry of Cholesterol*. Elsevier, Amsterdam, 1982.
De Gier, J., Mandersloot, J. G. and van Deenen, L. L. M. (1968). Lipid composition and permeability of liposomes. *Biochimica et Biophysica Acta*, **159**, 666–675.
Gottfried, E. L. (1967). Lipids of human leukocytes: relation to cell type. *Journal of Lipid Research*, **8**, 321–327.
Gottlieb, M. H. and Eanes, E. D. (1974). On phase transitions in erythrocyte membranes and extracted membrane lipids. *Biochimica et Biophysica Acta*, **373**, 519–522.
Graham, J. M. and Green, C. (1970). The properties of mitochondria enriched *in vitro* with cholesterol. *European Journal of Biochemistry*, **12**, 58–66.
Hagerman, J. S. and Gould, R. G. (1951). The *in vitro* interchange of cholesterol between plasma and red cells. *Proceedings of the Society for Experimental Biology and Medicine*, **78**, 329–332.
Hesketh, T. R., Smith, G. A., Houslay, M. D., McGill, K. A., Birdsall, N. J. M., Metcalfe, J. C. and Warren, G. B. (1976). Annular lipids determine the ATPase activity of a calcium transport protein complexed with dipalmitoyllecithin. *Biochemistry*, **15**, 4145–4151.
Inbar, M., Shinitzky, M. and Sachs, L. (1974). Microviscosity in the surface membrane lipid liver layer of intact normal lymphocytes and leukaemic cells. *FEBS Letters*, **38**, 268–270.
Jain, M. K. and White, H. B. (1977). Long-range order in biomembranes. *Advances in Lipid Research*, **15**, 1–60.
Jost, P. C., Griffith, O. H., Capaldi, R. A. and Vanderkooi, G. (1973). Evidence for boundary lipid in membranes. *Proceedings of the National Academy of Sciences of the USA*, **70**, 480–484.
Kimelberg, H. K. and Papahadjopoulos, D. (1974). Effects of phospholipid acyl chain fluidity, phase transitions, and cholesterol on $(Na^+ + K^+)$-stimulated adenosine triphosphatase. *Journal of Biological Chemistry*, **249**, 1071–1080.
Kornberg, R. D. and McConnell, H. M. (1971a). Lateral diffusion of phospholipids in a vesicle membrane (spin-labeled phosphatidylcholine/nuclear resonance). *Proceedings of the National Academy of Sciences of the USA*, **68**, 2564–2568.
Kornberg, R. D. and McConnell, H. M. (1971b). Inside-outside transitions of phospholipids in vesicle membranes. *Biochemistry*, **10**, 1111–1120.
Kroes, J. Ostwald, R. and Keith, A. (1972). Erythrocyte membranes—compression

of lipid phases by increased cholesterol content. *Biochimica et Biophysica Acta*, **274**, 71–74.
De Kruyff, B., Van Dijck, P. W. M., Demel, R. A., Schuijff, A., Brants, F. and van Deenen, L. L. M. (1974). Non-random distribution of cholesterol in phosphatidylcholine bilayers. *Biochimica et Biophysica Acta*, **356**, 1–7.
Ladbrooke, B. D., Williams, R. M. and Chapman, D. (1968). Studies on lecithin-cholesterol-water interactions by differential scanning calorimetry and X-ray diffraction. *Biochimica et Biophysica Acta*, **150**, 333–340.
Lange, Y., Cohen, C. M. and Poznansky, M. J. (1977). Transmembrane movement of cholesterol in human erythrocytes. *Proceedings of the National Academy of Sciences of the USA*, **74**, 1538–1542.
Lenard, J. and Rothman, J. E. (1976). Transbilayer distribution and movement of cholesterol and phospholipid in the membrane of influenza virus. *Proceedings of the National Academy of Sciences of the USA*, **73**, 391–395.
Lucy, J. A. Theoretical and experimental models for biological membranes. In: *Biological Membranes. Physical Fact and Function*. Ed. D. Chapman. Academic Press, London, pp. 233–288, 1968.
Luzatti, V. X-ray diffraction studies of lipid-water systems. In: *Biological Membranes. Physical Fact and Function*. Ed. D. Chapman. Academic Press, London, pp. 71–123, 1968.
Madden, T. D., Chapman, D. and Quinn, P. J. (1979). Cholesterol modulates activity of calcium-dependent ATPase of the sarcoplasmic reticulum. *Nature*, **279**, 538–541.
Mitropoulos, K. A., Venkatesan, S., Balasubramaniam, S. and Peters, T. J. (1978). The submicrosomal localization of 3-hydroxy-3-methylglutaryl-coenzyme-A reductase, cholesterol 7α-hydroxylase and cholesterol in rat liver. *European Journal of Biochemistry*, **82**, 419–429.
Moore, B. M., Lentz, B. R. and Meissner, G. (1978). Effects of sarcoplasmic reticulum Ca^{2+}-ATPase on phospholipid bilayer fluidity: boundary lipid. *Biochemistry*, **17**, 5248–5255.
Murphy, J. R. (1965). Erythrocyte metabolism. VI. Cell shape and the location of cholesterol in the erythrocyte membrane. *Journal of Laboratory and Clinical Medicine*, **65**, 756–774.
Ourisson, G., Albrecht, P. and Rohmer, M. (1979). The hopanoids. Palaeochemistry and biochemistry of a group of natural products. *Pure & Applied Chemistry*, **51**, 709–729.
Papahadjopoulos, D., Jacobson, K., Nir, S. and Isac, I. (1973). Phase transitions in phospholipid vesicles. Fluorescence polarization and permeability measurements concerning the effect of temperature and cholesterol. *Biochimica et Biophysica Acta*, **311**, 330–348.
Perdue, J. F., Kletzien, R., Miller, K., Pridmore, G. and Wray, V. L. (1971). The isolation and characterization of plasma membranes from cultivated cells. II. The chemical composition of membrane isolated from uninfected and oncogenic RNA virus-converted parenchyma-like cells. *Biochimica et Biophysica Acta*, **249**, 435–461.
Phillips, M. C. and Finer, E. G. (1974). The stoichiometry and dynamics of lecithin-cholesterol clusters in bilayer membranes. *Biochimica et Biophysica Acta*, **356**, 199–206.
Poznansky, M. J. and Czekanski, S. (1979). Cholesterol exchange as a function of cholesterol/phospholipid mole ratios. *Biochemical Journal*, **177**, 989–991.
Poznansky, M. and Lange, Y. (1976). Transbilayer movement of cholesterol in dipalmitoyllecithin-cholesterol vesicles. *Nature (London)*, **259**, 420–421.
Renooij, W., van Golde, L. M. G., Zwaal, R. F. A. and van Deenen, L. L. M. (1976). Topological asymmetry of phospholipid metabolism in rat erythrocyte

membranes. Evidence for flip-flop of lecithin. *European Journal of Biochemistry*, **61**, 53–58.
Rothman, J. E. and Engelman, D. M. (1972). Molecular mechanism for the interaction of phospholipid with cholesterol. *Nature (New Biology)*, **237**, 42–44.
Rothman, J. E. and Lenard, J. (1977). Membrane asymmetry. *Science*, **195**, 743–753.
Rottem, S., Yashouv, J., Ne'eman, Z. and Razin, S. (1973a). Cholesterol in mycoplasma membranes. Composition, ultrastructure and biological properties of membranes from *mycoplasma mycoides var. capri* cells adapted to grow with low cholesterol concentrations. *Biochimica et Biophysica Acta*, **323**, 495–508.
Rottem, S., Cirillo, V. P., De Kruyff, B., Shinitzky, M. and Razin, S. (1973b). Cholesterol in mycoplasma membrane. Correlation of enzymic and transport activities with physical state of lipids in membranes of *mycoplasma mycoides var. capri* adapted to grow with low cholesterol concentrations. *Biochimica et Biophysica Acta*, **232**, 509–519.
Rouser, G., Nelson, G. J., Fleischer, S. and Simon, G. Lipid composition of animal cell membranes, organelles and organs. In: *Biological Membranes. Physical Fact and Function*. Ed. D. Chapman. Academic Press, London, pp. 5–69, 1968.
Sachs, L. (1974). Regulation of membrane changes, differentiation, and malignancy in carcinogenesis. *Harvey Lectures*, **68**, 1–35.
Stroeve, P. and Miller, I. (1975). Lateral diffusion of cholesterol in monolayers. *Biochimica et Biophysica Acta*, **401**, 157–167.
Vandenheuvel, F. A. (1971). Structure of membranes and role of lipids therein. *Advances in Lipid Research*, **9**, 161–248.
Wallach, D. F. H. The rôle of the plasma membrane in disease processes. In: *Biological Membranes*, Vol. 2. Ed. D. Chapman and D. F. H. Wallach. Academic Press, London, pp. 253–294, 1973.
Warren, G. B., Housley, M. D., Metcalfe, J. C. and Birdsall, N. J. M. (1975). Cholesterol is excluded from the phospholipid annulus surrounding an active calcium transport protein. *Nature (New Biology)*, **255**, 684–687.

Chapter 8

Cholesterol Synthesis in Animal Tissues

1	INTRODUCTION		341
2	MEASUREMENT OF CHOLESTEROL SYNTHESIS IN TISSUES		341
2.1	General		341
2.2	[^{14}C]Acetate		343
2.3	[^{14}C]Octanoic acid		345
2.4	[^{3}H]H$_2$O		346
2.5	The absolute rate of synthesis		349
3	THE CONTRIBUTIONS OF DIFFERENT TISSUES		350
3.1	Experimental approaches		350
3.2	Cholesterol synthesis in various tissues *in vitro*		352
3.2.1	General		352
3.2.2	Liver		353
3.2.3	Intestine		355
3.2.4	Skin		355
3.2.5	Arterial wall		356
3.2.6	White blood cells		356
3.2.7	Mevalonic acid metabolism in kidneys		357
4	REGULATION OF STEROL SYNTHESIS		358
4.1	General considerations		358
4.2	HMG-CoA reductase and the rate-limiting step		360
4.2.1	Review of the evidence		360
4.2.2	Some properties of HMG-CoA reductase		364
4.2.2.1	Effects of solubilization and of exposure to cold		364
4.2.2.2	Cyclic AMP and reversible phosphorylation		364
4.2.2.3	Other factors		367
4.3	Regulation in liver		368
4.3.1	Diurnal rhythm		368
4.3.2	Dietary cholesterol		371
4.3.3	Fasting		378
4.3.4	Fat feeding		379
4.3.5	Bile salts and the enterohepatic circulation		379

4.3.6	Hormones	381
4.3.7	Miscellaneous effects	383
4.4	Regulation in the intestinal wall	385
4.5	Regulation in other tissues.	386

Cholesterol Synthesis in Animal Tissues

1 INTRODUCTION

All metabolizing tissues in the animal body synthesize cholesterol *via* the pathway outlined in Chapter 4, although the rate of synthesis varies widely in different tissues and in a given tissue under different conditions. In this Chapter I shall consider the contributions of particular organs and tissues to cholesterol synthesis in the whole organism, the manner in which cholesterol synthesis is regulated in different tissues and, finally, the influence of various dietary, hormonal and pharmacological agents on cholesterol synthesis at the tissue or cell level. So much information about cholesterol metabolism in cells in culture and in other isolated cell systems has been collected in the recent past that it will be most convenient to deal with this topic in a separate chapter (Chapter 9), in which I shall also try to relate this information to the regulation of cholesterol metabolism *in vivo*. The turnover of cholesterol in the whole body, as determined by measurement of sterol balance or by analysis of the time-course of appearance and disappearance of isotopically labelled cholesterol in the plasma of intact animals, is dealt with in Chapter 10.

2 MEASUREMENT OF CHOLESTEROL SYNTHESIS IN TISSUES

2.1 General

Cholesterol synthesis may be measured in perfused organs or in incubations of tissue slices, biopsy specimens, freshly isolated cells, cells in culture or subcellular fractions of tissue homogenates. With few exceptions, the amount of cholesterol newly synthesized during the period of measurement is very small in comparison with the amount already present in the system. Hence, it is almost always necessary to estimate the rate of synthesis by measuring either the rate of incorporation of isotopically labelled precursors into cholesterol or, as in the most recent approach to the problem, the rate of accumulation of a sterol intermediate under conditions in which its further metabolism is blocked (see Section 2.5). Details of the methods used for the preparation and incubation of tissues, cells and subcellular fractions with labelled precursors of sterols, and for work with perfused livers, will be found in the references at the end of this Chapter. Measurement of the incorporation of a labelled precursor *in vitro* should always be made in the presence of the precursor at a concentration high enough to saturate the biosynthetic pathway and over a period during which incorporation is linear with respect to the time of incubation or perfusion. The lipids in the tissue or incubation system should be saponified to hydrolyse esterified cholesterol before extraction of the total non-saponifiable lipids into a suitable solvent.

With tissues or tissue fractions that synthesize cholesterol at a relatively rapid rate (e.g. liver slices), the carbon atoms of a labelled precursor that enters the biosynthetic pathway to cholesterol will be present predominantly in cholesterol itself at the end of an incubation continued for one or more hours. In this case, incorporation of the label into cholesterol may be estimated with sufficient accuracy for most purposes by measuring the amount of label incorporated into the digitonin-precipitable sterol fraction, even though analysis of this fraction may show the presence of small amounts of labelled C_{27} sterols other than cholesterol and of labelled C_{30} sterol. Only if one wishes to study the conversion of these intermediates into cholesterol is it necessary to separate the components of the digitonin-precipitable mixture and to measure incorporation into each component.

In some tissues, including sebaceous glands, artery and human circulating lymphocytes, the label accumulates predominantly in precursors of cholesterol, only a relatively small proportion of the label that enters the biosynthetic pathway reaching cholesterol even after incubation for several hours. According to the length of time for which the tissue has been incubated with the labelled precursor, the label may be present mainly in C_{27} sterols other than cholesterol, in C_{30} sterols, or, as in human white blood cells incubated in the presence of [^{14}C]mevalonate (Fogelman *et al.*, 1975), in squalene and farnesyl pyrophosphate. The accumulation of label in these intermediates suggests that in these tissues the capacity of the enzymes catalyzing certain of the later steps in sterol biosynthesis is low in comparison with the capacity of those catalyzing earlier steps. Whatever the reason may be, the presence of significant amounts of label in non-cholesterol C_{27} sterols and C_{30} sterols means that the incorporation of label into cholesterol cannot be estimated from the incorporation into digitonin-precipitable sterols without isolation of the cholesterol in this fraction. On the other hand, the object of an experiment on the incorporation of a labelled precursor into cholesterol is often to study changes in the rate of flow of carbon through the rate-limiting step leading to the formation of mevalonic acid. If this is the case, measurement of the total amount of label incorporated into intermediates beyond HMG-CoA may be more informative than measurement of incorporation only into cholesterol.

The problem of estimating the rate of synthesis of cholesterol from the rate of incorporation of a labelled precursor into cholesterol is dealt with in Sections 2.2 to 2.5.

2.2 [^{14}C]Acetate

Acetate labelled with ^{14}C at C-1 (carboxyl) or C-2 (methyl) has been used extensively for measuring the rate of synthesis of cholesterol in animal tissues and is still the precursor used most commonly for this purpose. The total amount of exogenous acetate converted into cholesterol during the incubation of the specimen may be calculated from the ^{14}C recovered in cholesterol and the specific radioactivity of the [^{14}C]acetate added to the medium. If it is assumed that the added [^{14}C]acetate is the sole source of the carbon used for cholesterol synthesis during the incubation, the mass of cholesterol synthesized may be calculated from the incorporation of ^{14}C; 12 µatoms of carboxyl carbon from acetate and 15 µatoms of methyl carbon are required for the synthesis of one µmole of cholesterol.

For measurement of the rate of cholesterol synthesis *in vitro*, labelled acetate has the important advantage that it enters the biosynthetic pathway before the rate-limiting step. Hence, changes in the capacity of this step will be reflected in changes in the rate of incorporation of ^{14}C from [^{14}C]acetate into cholesterol; as we shall see (Section 4.2), a great deal of information about the rate-limiting step in cholesterol biosynthesis has been obtained by parallel measurement of the incorporation of ^{14}C from [^{14}C]acetate and [^{14}C]mevalonate into cholesterol under conditions in which the rate of synthesis is varied. However, despite this advantage, labelled acetate has serious drawbacks as a precursor for the measurement *in vitro* of the absolute rate of synthesis of cholesterol or of the relative rates of synthesis under different experimental conditions. In non-ruminant mammals acetate is not the natural precursor of sterols. (In adult ruminants the major source of acetyl units for lipid synthesis, at least in the liver, is acetate formed by the breakdown of cellulose in the rumen.) The natural primary precursor is acetyl-CoA which is formed in the cytosol by the enzymic cleavage of citrate derived from the mitochondria (see

p. 185). When acetate is used as the precursor it must first be converted into acetyl-CoA by cytosolic acetate thiokinase ('acetate-activating enzyme'):

Acetate + CoA + ATP → Acetyl-CoA + AMP + PP

The acetyl-CoA so formed must then enter the pool of endogenous acetyl-CoA which provides acetyl carbon for sterol biosynthesis. The consequences of this are twofold.

In the first place, in conditions in which the conversion of acetate into cytosolic acetyl-CoA is rate-limiting for sterol biosynthesis from acetate, the rate of incorporation of ^{14}C from acetate into cholesterol would be determined by the capacity of the acetate-activation step. In which case, measurement of the rate of incorporation of acetate carbon into cholesterol would not provide valid information about the rate of synthesis of cholesterol from its normal precursor. While it is true that the capacity of acetate thiokinase is usually greater than that of the enzymes catalyzing the subsequent steps in the pathway to cholesterol, this may not always be so.

Secondly, since the pool of acetyl-CoA that supplies acetyl units for sterol biosynthesis is derived not only from exogenous acetate but also from endogenous sources, the absolute rate of synthesis of cholesterol in an intact cell or tissue preparation cannot be estimated from the ^{14}C incorporated from [^{14}C]acetate and the specific radioactivity of the added acetate. In so far as glucose, fatty acids and other sources of acetyl carbon contribute to the acetyl-CoA pool, the true rate of cholesterol synthesis will be underestimated when [^{14}C]acetate is used as labelled precursor. Furthermore, the magnitude of this error will vary according to the extent to which the specific radioactivity of the cytosolic acetyl-CoA pool is diluted by non-radioactive acetyl-CoA of endogenous origin. For example, an experimental procedure that increased the flux of free fatty acids into the liver could lead to an apparent decrease in hepatic synthesis of cholesterol merely by swamping the acetyl-CoA pool with non-radioactive acetyl-CoA derived from the β-oxidation of fatty acids.

Although the [^{14}C]acetate method has provided useful information about relative rates of synthesis of cholesterol in liver and other tissues in different experimental situations, a method for measuring the absolute rate, valid under all conditions, is clearly desirable. One approach has been to try to measure the specific radioactivity of the acetyl-CoA pool from which cholesterol is synthesized in liver preparations by measuring the specific radioactivity of the ketone bodies produced during the incubation. But this is invalid because ketone bodies are formed from an intramitochondrial pool of acetyl-CoA that is not in equilibrium with the cytosolic acetyl-CoA that supplies carbon for cholesterol synthesis. The use of [^{14}C]octanoic acid as precursor for cholesterol goes some way towards meeting this objection. It should be noted that although the main application of [^{14}C]acetate in this field has been in the measurement of cholesterol synthesis *in vitro*, [^{14}C]acetate has also been used to obtain an index of the rate of cholesterol synthesis in specific organs *in vivo* (see, for example, Edwards *et al.*, 1972).

2.3 [^{14}C]Octanoic acid

When liver slices are incubated in the presence of [1-^{14}C]octanoate, the labelled octanoate generates [1-^{14}C]acetyl-CoA within the mitochondria by β-oxidation. The intramitochondrial [1-^{14}C]acetyl-CoA supplies acetyl units for the synthesis of acetoacetate and also for the formation of acetyl-CoA in the cytosol *via* citrate and the citrate-cleavage enzyme. The cytosolic acetyl-CoA originating from octanoate must enter the pool from which cholesterol is synthesized, since ^{14}C from [1-^{14}C]octanoate is incorporated into cholesterol by liver slices. Dietschy and McGarry (1974) have suggested that if the incubation is carried out in the presence of high concentrations of [1-^{14}C]octanoate, the labelled octanoate may be the sole source of cytosolic acetyl-CoA. Under these conditions, the specific radioactivity of the acetyl-CoA from which cholesterol is synthesized should be the same as that of the acetyl-CoA from which acetoacetate is formed, provided that ketone bodies and cytosolic acetyl-CoA are in fact derived from a common intramitochondrial pool of acetyl-CoA. Hence, it should be possible to calculate the specific radioactivity of the acetyl units used for cholesterol synthesis by measuring that of the acetoacetate formed during the incubation.

On the basis of these assumptions Dietschy and McGarry have estimated the rate of synthesis of cholesterol in liver slices from normal rats using [1-^{14}C]octanoate or [1-^{14}C]acetate as precursors and have shown that the rate estimated by the octanoate method may be at least twice that estimated from the incorporation of [1-^{14}C]acetate without correction for dilution of the pool of cytosolic acetyl-CoA from endogenous sources of C_2. In principle, the octanoate method should provide a valid estimate of the absolute rate of incorporation of acetyl carbon into cholesterol in intact liver cells, and the only error in estimating the absolute rate of synthesis of cholesterol would be that due to contributions to cholesterol carbon from endogenous intermediates that enter the pathway other than *via* acetyl-CoA. However, not all the assumptions on which the octanoate method is based have been proved, nor has it been shown that octanoate at high concentration (1 mM) is without effect on cholesterol biosynthesis in liver cells. A serious limitation to the use of octanoate is, of course, the fact that it is applicable only to tissues that form ketone bodies.

2.4 [³H]H₂O

The use of isotopically labelled water in the study of cholesterol biosynthesis has a long history. Indeed, the observation that the cholesterol of animals given D₂O becomes heavily labelled with D (Rittenberg and Schoenheimer, 1937) was the first clue that cholesterol is synthesized from precursors of low molecular weight. This observation led initially to the use of D₂O as precursor for the measurement of the rate of synthesis of cholesterol *in vivo*, particularly in human subjects (see Chapter 10). For practical reasons, however, D₂O has now been largely replaced by [³H]H₂O in quantitative work on cholesterol synthesis, both *in vivo* and *in vitro*. The major advantage of [³H]H₂O as precursor is that the specific radioactivity of intracellular water is the same as that of the water in the medium and is not affected by the many metabolic factors that lead to variable dilution of the pool of cytosolic acetyl-CoA. However, apart from the objection that very large amounts of tritium are needed to give measurable incorporation into cholesterol, the use of [³H]H₂O as precursor has the serious drawback that the absolute rate of synthesis of cholesterol in a tissue preparation, perfused organ or intact animal cannot be deduced directly from the rate of incorporation of tritium into cholesterol, even though the specific radioactivity of the precursor pool can be ascertained without error. The reason for this is that although we know the *immediate* source of the hydrogen atoms of cholesterol (Chapter 4, Fig. 4.17) the number of hydrogen atoms incorporated into a cholesterol molecule from the water of an incubation medium in which cholesterol is being synthesized *de novo* will be influenced by several variables, including the extent to which the H of NADH and NADPH in the system is ultimately derived from water.

Owing to the complexity of the metabolic pathways through which the hydrogen of water enters cholesterol, the proportion of the total carbon-bound H atoms of cholesterol derived from water cannot be inferred from existing knowledge, but must be determined empirically. Rittenberg and Schoenheimer (1937) found that in mice fed D₂O for 60 days the D/H ratio in the total body cholesterol was 47% of the ratio in the body water. They concluded that about half the hydrogen atoms of cholesterol are derived from water. However, in retrospect it seems unlikely that this experiment was continued for long enough to permit complete turnover of all the cholesterol in the body.

The incorporation of ³H into cholesterol could be used to calculate the absolute rate of synthesis of cholesterol if one knew how many μg-atoms of hydrogen were incorporated from [³H]H₂O for each μg-atom of carbon incorporated from a ¹⁴C-labelled precursor which was the sole source of carbon for the cholesterol synthesized (the ³H/¹⁴C ratio) in the particular system under investigation. Jungas (1968) obtained a ^{3}H/^{14}C ratio of 0.87 in the fatty acids synthesized in pieces of adipose tissue in the presence of [^{3}H]H$_2$O, [U-^{14}C]glucose and sufficient insulin to inhibit completely the breakdown of intracellular glycogen. On the assumption that exogenous glucose was the only source of carbon for the fatty acids synthesized during the incubation, Jungas concluded that the rate of synthesis of fatty acids in adipose tissue could be estimated by measuring the incorporation of ^{3}H from [^{3}H]H$_2$O in the medium (µg-atoms of hydrogen/hour) and multiplying the value so obtained by 1/0.87 to give the absolute rate of synthesis of fatty acids (µg-atom of carbon/hour), whether or not insulin was present in the medium. Note that a correction for enzymic discrimination between ^{3}H and H is not required because the error due to the isotope effect would be the same in the experimental determination of the ^{3}H/^{14}C ratio and in the measurement of ^{3}H incorporated into the product in the test specimen.

The ^{3}H/^{14}C ratio for cholesterol cannot be estimated accurately by direct measurement because it is impossible to achieve conditions in which the ^{14}C-labelled precursor is the sole source of carbon for sterol synthesis. Brunengraber et al. (1972) have tried to overcome this difficulty by measuring simultaneously the incorporation of ^{3}H and ^{14}C into the fatty acids and cholesterol of rat livers perfused with a medium containing [^{14}C]glucose and [^{3}H]H$_2$O. Dilution of the pool of ^{14}C-labelled precursor for fatty acids by endogenous carbon was estimated from the observed ratio of ^{3}H to ^{14}C incorporated and the value of 0.87 obtained by Jungas (1968) for the true ^{3}H/^{14}C ratio (see above). On the assumption that fatty acids and cholesterol are synthesized in the liver from a common pool of precursor derived from glucose, the observed ratio of ^{3}H to ^{14}C incorporated into cholesterol was corrected for dilution of the precursor pool to give a value of 0.76 for the true ^{3}H/^{14}C ratio for cholesterol, i.e. the ratio that would have been observed if [^{14}C]glucose had been the sole source of carbon for cholesterol synthesis in the perfused liver.

Brunengraber et al. concluded that the rate of synthesis of cholesterol in the liver could be estimated by multiplying the rate of incorporation of [^{3}H]H$_2$O into cholesterol by 1/0.76. However, the assumptions that the ^{3}H/^{14}C ratio observed for fatty acids in adipose tissue is applicable to other tissues and that fatty acids and cholesterol are synthesized from a common pool of precursor are not necessarily valid. Moreover, it is questionable whether the rate of incorporation of ^{3}H from [^{3}H]H$_2$O into cholesterol in an intact cell is ever determined solely by the rate of synthesis of cholesterol. The carbon-bound hydrogen of cholesterol that is derived from water is incorporated into the cholesterol molecule by several routes. It may enter the biosynthetic pathway to cholesterol already bound to the methyl carbon of acetyl-CoA or to C-2 and C-4 of acetoacetyl-CoA. Opportunities for H from water to enter the pathway also occur during the isomerization of isopentenyl PP to dimethylallyl PP and of the Δ^8 double bond of lanosterol and at each of the reductive steps between lanosterol and cholesterol.

In an intact cell, the methyl group of acetyl-CoA could acquire H from water via fatty acid synthesis followed by β-oxidation, since the even-numbered carbons of fatty acids become labelled during synthesis in the presence of [^{3}H]H$_2$O (Jungas, 1968) and a methyl hydrogen would be introduced into acetyl-CoA from water during the thiolase reaction. The hydrogen of water could also enter the methyl group of acetyl-CoA via the glycolytic cycle, possibly by two routes. C-1 of the hexose carbon skeleton could pick up H from water during the isomerization of glucose 6-phosphate to fructose 6-phosphate and some of this H could appear on C-3 of glyceraldehyde phosphate, which becomes C-3 of pyruvate and the methyl carbon of acetyl-CoA. C-3 of pyruvate could also pick up H from water during the enzymic conversion of phosphoenolpyruvate into pyruvate (Robinson and Rose, 1972). During the non-enzymic interconversion of the keto and enol forms of acetoacetyl-CoA, C-2 might acquire H from the medium to an extent depending upon the mean life of acetoacetyl CoA molecules in the system.

At each of the reductions leading to saturation of a double bond, one of the carbon-bound hydrogen atoms would be derived from the medium and the other would be transferred stereospecifically from a reduced pyridine nucleotide; NADPH also supplies two hydrogen atoms for the reduction of HMG-CoA and one for the conversion of farnesyl PP into squalene. It is difficult to say how far H from water would become bound to NADP in an intact cell under given conditions, but NAD would certainly acquire H from the medium via C-1 of glyceraldehyde phosphate (which would pick up H at this position during the aldolase reaction) and some of this H could be transferred enzymically to NADP and thence to cholesterol.

From what has been said above it should be clear that the rate of incorporation of [^{3}H]H$_2$O into cholesterol in a cell, tissue or whole organism is unlikely to be determined solely by the absolute rate of synthesis of cholesterol. It must also depend upon the relative and absolute rates at which different metabolic pathways function and on the relative contributions of different sources of carbon to the cholesterol molecule under the particular conditions of observation. Nilsson (1975) observed a ^{3}H/^{14}C ratio of only 0.12 for cholesterol synthesized in rat hepatocytes with [^{14}C]mevalonate as the source of carbon for cholesterol. Taken in conjunction with the ^{3}H/^{14}C ratio of 0.76 deduced by Brunengraber *et al.* (1972) for cholesterol synthesized in perfused liver with glucose as substrate, Nilsson's observation suggests that about 6/7 of the hydrogen incorporated into cholesterol from water in liver cells is incorporated before mevalonate. If so, the major source of variation in the number of μg-atoms of H incorporated from water per μg-atom of carbon incorporated into cholesterol is likely to lie in the contribution from water to the stably-bound hydrogen of acetyl-CoA and acetoacetyl-CoA and perhaps also to the CH_2OH group of mevalonate.

Despite these theoretical drawbacks to the use of $[^3H]H_2O$ in the measurement of the rate of synthesis of cholesterol, the method usually gives results that are at least qualitatively consistent with those obtained with $[^{14}C]$acetate or $[^{14}C]$octanoate. Since the $[^3H]H_2O$ and $[^{14}C]$acetate methods are subject to independent errors, it is useful to use both methods simultaneously. If the apparent rate of synthesis of cholesterol changes in the same direction in response to an experimental modification when estimated by both methods, it may be assumed that the apparent change is a real one. However, the occasional report of contradictory results from the two methods indicates the need for a method free from error, against which isotopic methods can be tested.

2.5 The absolute rate of synthesis

The rate of synthesis of cholesterol could be measured without error due to dilution of radioactive intermediates from endogenous sources if one could measure the specific radioactivity of the precursor immediately preceding cholesterol during an incubation with $[^{14}C]$acetate. However, under normal conditions the steady-state concentration of cholesta-5,7-dien-3β-ol is too low for accurate measurement of its mass. An alternative approach is to block sterol synthesis at a point in the biosynthetic chain just before cholesterol and then to measure the rate of accumulation of the intermediate whose conversion into cholesterol is inhibited. Gibbons and Pullinger (1977) have shown that the absolute rate of synthesis of cholesterol in suspensions of hepatocytes can be estimated by measuring the rate at which desmosterol accumulates in the presence of triparanol, a drug that specifically inhibits the Δ^{24}-reductase. Although this method requires the use of very sensitive techniques for assaying desmosterol, it has great potential value as a reference method for validating isotopic methods. When used in combination with measurements of the incorporation of radioactive precursors into cholesterol, a method based on the above principle may also give information about the relative contributions of exogenous and endogenous sources of carbon to sterol biosynthesis (Gibbons, 1977; Gibbons and Pullinger, 1979).

3 THE CONTRIBUTIONS OF DIFFERENT TISSUES

3.1 Experimental approaches

The relative contributions made by different organs to cholesterol synthesis in the whole body may be investigated in several ways. The simplest and most direct is to measure the rate of incorporation of a labelled precursor into pieces of tissue *in vitro*. The problem of deducing the absolute rate of synthesis from the rate of incorporation has already been discussed. Added to this, it is by no means certain that the rate of synthesis of a tissue *in vitro* will be the same as that in the intact organ *in vivo*. Cholesterol synthesis may be altered by the handling of the tissue and by the unphysiological conditions under which oxygen and substrates from the incubation medium are supplied to the cells. When very small pieces of a tissue are used, a large and variable proportion of its cells may be damaged during the preparation of the specimen. This is especially apt to occur with biopsies weighing only a few milligrams and may account for the widely discrepant results obtained with needle biopsies of human liver and suction biopsies of human intestine; an example of the effect of mechanical damage upon cholesterol synthesis in intestinal villi *in vitro* is discussed below (p. 355).

Information about local synthesis under physiological conditions may be obtained by injecting the labelled precursor into the intact animal and then measuring incorporation into the tissue *in vivo* before the newly-synthesized cholesterol has had time to equilibrate with cholesterol elsewhere in the body. Using this approach, with D_2O as precursor, Waelsch et al. (1940) were able to show that lipid is synthesized *in vivo* by the brain of the immature rat. A similar approach, with $[^3H]H_2O$ and $[^{14}C]$acetate as precursors, has been used by Edwards et al. (1972) to demonstrate a diurnal rhythm in the rate of sterol synthesis in rat liver *in vivo*. However, this method cannot give reliable information about the relative rates of synthesis of sterol in different tissues unless one knows the extent to which the labelled precursor is diluted by endogenous metabolites in each tissue.

The activity of HMG-CoA reductase in different tissues might be expected to reflect relative rates of cholesterol synthesis, since this enzyme is generally considered to be the one responsible for catalyzing the rate-limiting step in the conversion of acetyl-CoA into cholesterol. In general, the activity of the enzyme is higher in tissues with high rates of sterol synthesis than in those with low rates, but there are serious drawbacks to the use of HMG-CoA reductase activity as an index of the rate of synthesis of sterol in a given tissue. The major objection is that enzyme activity assayed *in vitro* under optimal conditions is not necessarily the same as the activity of the enzyme under the conditions existing in the intact cell *in vivo* (for further discussion of this point, see p. 367).

Some information about the contribution of a particular organ to cholesterol synthesis in the whole body may be obtained by observing the effect of excluding the organ by surgical removal or by other means. Hotta and Chaikoff (1955) showed that turnover of cholesterol in the plasma of rats fed a cholesterol-low diet almost ceases when the liver and gastrointestinal tract are removed, but not when the gastrointestinal tract alone is removed. They concluded that in rats the liver is the main source of plasma cholesterol of endogenous origin. An analogous approach has been used by Wilson (Lindsey and Wilson, 1965; Wilson, 1968) to demonstrate the contributions of the liver and intestine to cholesterol synthesis in rats and monkeys, but in this case cholesterol from the liver was excluded by suppressing hepatic synthesis by feeding cholesterol and that derived from the intestine was excluded by diverting intestinal lymph from the blood circulation.

Analysis of plasma and tissue specific radioactivity curves after administration of radioactive cholesterol may give information of a limited kind about tissue synthesis of cholesterol *in vivo*. After a single intravenous injection of radioactive cholesterol, the specific radioactivity of the plasma cholesterol falls progressively, while that in the tissues rises to a maximum and then falls. If cholesterol synthesis in a tissue is negligible, the plasma and tissue specific radioactivity curves will be related to one another in a manner characteristic of a precursor and its product, the tissue curve reaching its maximum at the time when the two curves intersect (Zilversmit, 1960). If the tissue synthesizes a significant amount of cholesterol, the maximum will not occur at the point of intersection of the curves for plasma and tissue. Moutafis and Myant (1976) have used this method to show that cholesterol synthesis *in vivo* is negligible in skeletal muscle of monkeys. Observations on the specific radioactivity of cholesterol in tissues after continuous administration for long periods have also been used to evaluate local synthesis. For example, Newman and Zilversmit (1961) found that the specific radioactivity of the cholesterol in atheromatous plaques of rabbits fed [^{14}C]cholesterol for up to 87 days became nearly equal to the specific radioactivity of the plasma cholesterol. They concluded that the plaque cholesterol must have been derived almost entirely from the plasma, since any local synthesis from unlabelled precursors would have diluted the radioactive cholesterol derived from the plasma. This conclusion is valid in conditions in which the rate of equilibration between tissue and plasma cholesterol is slow, but may not be so if the rate of equilibration is rapid in comparison with the rate of synthesis. Thus, owing to very rapid equilibration, the specific radioactivity of liver cholesterol becomes equal to that of plasma cholesterol after prolonged feeding of radioactive cholesterol in the baboon (Wilson, 1970), even though liver synthesizes cholesterol very actively in primates.

3.2 Cholesterol synthesis in various tissues *in vitro*

In this section we shall consider quantitative aspects of cholesterol synthesis in various animal tissues, as revealed by measurements *in vitro*. We shall begin with a comparative survey before considering certain tissues of special interest in more detail. Cholesterol synthesis in brain and nervous tissue have been dealt with in Chapter 6.

3.2.1 General

Bloch *et al.* (1946) showed that deuterium-labelled acetate is incorporated into cholesterol by rat-liver slices but were unable to demonstrate cholesterol-synthesizing activity in several other tissues. However, Srere *et al.* (1950), using a more sensitive test for sterol synthesis, found that [^{14}C]acetate was incorporated into cholesterol *in vitro* in several extrahepatic tissues of the rat. Among the most active tissues was brain from immature animals. Table 8.1 summarizes some more recent observations on the incorporation of [^{14}C]acetate into digitonin-precipitable sterols in various tissues from rats, monkeys and guinea-pigs. In all cases the animals were fed a diet low in cholesterol

Table 8.1

Incorporation of ^{14}C from [^{14}C]acetate into digitonin-precipitable sterols in slices of tissue from rats, squirrel monkeys (Saimiri) and guinea-pigs. All animals were given a diet low in cholesterol. Values are expressed in nmoles of acetate incorporated per g fresh tissue per 2-hour incubation. A dash (—) means that no information is available

Tissue	Rat	Monkey	Guinea-pig
Liver	179	613	8
Small intestine	114	55	130
Colon	56	72	—
Skin	5	10	—
Kidney	4	6.5	—
Testis	9	—	—
Lung	7	3.5	22
Adrenal	5	1	13
Skeletal muscle	0.5	0.3	—
Brain (mature)	0.5	0.5	5
Spleen	3.5	3	11
Adipose tissue	—	5	—

Modified from Dietschy and Siperstein (1967), Dietschy and Wilson (1968), Swann *et al.* (1975).
Note that less than half the radioactive digitonin-precipitable sterol in skin is cholesterol and that a considerable proportion of that in guinea-pig intestine is lathosterol.

before the tissues were removed. Except for skin, almost all the radioactivity recovered in the digitonin-precipitable sterols of these tissues may be assumed to have been present as cholesterol. As we have seen, the true rate of synthesis of cholesterol is usually underestimated if calculated from the rate of incorporation of radioactive acetate. Hence, the values shown in Table 8.1 are likely to be lower than the true values. Nevertheless, the results obtained *in vitro* are consistent with observations made by other methods in showing that in rats and monkeys the most active cholesterol-synthesizing tissues are the liver and the gastrointestinal tract, other tissues contributing little in the mature animal. When the total mass of the organ is taken into account, the predominance of the liver and gastrointestinal tract is seen to be even more striking. In the squirrel monkey, synthesis in these two organs (as determined *in vitro*) accounts for about 97% of the cholesterol synthesized by all organs and tissues, the liver contributing about 80% of the total. A limited number of observations on dogs and man suggests that in these species also the liver contributes the bulk of the cholesterol synthesized in the whole body when the diet is low in cholesterol, though the intestine may be more important as a source of endogenous cholesterol in man than in some other species (Wilson and Lindsey, 1965). In the guinea-pig, on the other hand, cholesterol-synthesizing activity per g of fresh tissue in the liver is lower than that in several other tissues, including small intestine, lung and spleen.

The above conclusions are based largely on measurements of sterol synthesis or HMG-CoA reductase activity in tissues or homogenates *in vitro*. However, estimates based on the rate of incorporation of [^{3}H]H$_2$O into sterols *in vivo* suggest that the relative contribution of the liver to total sterol synthesis in the intact rat is less than that deduced from measurements *in vitro* (Jeske and Dietschy, 1980). To this extent, the values shown in Table 8.1 may give too much weight to the liver.

3.2.2 Liver

Liver from almost all vertebrate species that have been examined synthesizes cholesterol from acetate and other precursors very actively (see Table 8.1 for representative values from three species).

Synthesis may be observed in isolated perfused livers, in liver slices and in suspensions of hepatocytes prepared from pieces of liver perfused with collagenase. Hepatocytes may survive in suspension for several hours and are therefore useful for studying control mechanisms that operate by induction or repression of enzymes in the biosynthetic pathway to sterol. However, during the preparation of hepatocytes some surface protein may be removed from the plasma membrane. This could conceivably interfere with regulatory processes that depend upon the ability of liver cells to recognize specific substances in the external medium. Non-dividing monolayers of liver cells in culture, which may retain their specific biochemical functions for many days (Bissell *et al.*, 1973), offer a promising solution to this problem and are likely to be used increasingly in the study of cholesterol metabolism at the cell level.

Cell-free fractions of liver may also be used in the study of the incorporation of precursors into sterols. Bucher (1953) was the first to describe a method for preparing a liver homogenate that would incorporate the carbon of [^{14}C]acetate into cholesterol efficiently. An important factor in her success was probably the use of a method for breaking the liver cells without releasing mitochondrial HMG-CoA lyase, which would have hydrolyzed HMG-CoA as soon as it was formed in the incubation mixture. The introduction of an effective cell-free preparation was a landmark in the study of sterol biosynthesis since it opened the way to the study of problems such as the co-factor requirements and the mechanisms of enzyme regulation in the early stages of the pathway to cholesterol. In the original Bucher procedure, the liver is homogenized under precisely defined conditions in ice-cold phosphate buffer containing $MgCl_2$ and nicotinamide. The nuclei, cell debris and mitochondria are then removed by sequential ultracentrifugation. The supernatant remaining after centrifugation at 9000 × g, when incubated at 37 °C in the presence of O_2 and the necessary co-factors, converts acetate into cholesterol at a constant rate for at least two hours. Bucher and McGarrahan (1956) later showed that all the enzymes required for the complete sequence of steps from acetate to cholesterol are present either in the soluble supernatant fraction or in the RNA-poor fraction of the microsomes, rather than in the heavier, RNA-rich microsomal fraction. Liver homogenates prepared by the Bucher procedure are still used as the starting point for studies of the hepatic enzymes concerned in specific steps in the synthesis of cholesterol.

Sterol synthesis *in vitro* has been investigated in human liver in specimens obtained either during an abdominal operation or by needle biopsy. Values reported for incorporation of [^{14}C]acetate into digitonin-precipitable sterols in normal liver vary widely from one laboratory to another and even within the same laboratory (Miettinen, 1970). Results obtained from specimens removed at operation are likely to be influenced by the pre-operative fasting and the general anaesthetic. Variability in the results obtained with needle biopsies is very wide, reported values for normal subjects ranging from about 50 (Myant, 1970) to over 300 mmoles/g/2-hour incubation (Bhattathiry and Siperstein, 1963). Factors that must contribute to this variability include errors in weighing the fresh specimen without loss of water (total weight may be less than 5 mg), damage to liver cells and the presence of variable amounts of fat and connective tissue in the specimen.

3.2.3 Intestine

In the intestine of rats and squirrel monkeys cholesterol synthesis estimated *in vitro* varies at different levels of the intestinal tract. Incorporation of [^{14}C]acetate into sterols is relatively low in the jejunum, increases progressively down the ileum to reach a maximum in the lower ileum and then falls to a low level in the colon. Despite earlier claims to the contrary, the villi of the rat's intestine synthesize sterol as actively as the layer containing the crypts. The mucosal cells of the intestinal villi appear to be damaged very easily if they are separated from the underlying layers by scraping. This leads to diminished sterol-synthesizing activity when the cells are subsequently incubated with labelled precursor. If [^{14}C]acetate is injected into an intact rat and the animal is killed a short time later, the amount of ^{14}C incorporated into sterols is found to be as great in the villi as in the crypts (Muroya et al., 1977).

The rate of incorporation of [^{14}C]acetate into sterols by suction biopsies of human intestine is comparable with the rate observed in slices of rat intestine. In biopsies of intestine from human subjects fed diets with a normal or low cholesterol content, rates of incorporation reported by Myant (1970) and by Dietschy and Gamel (1971) varied from 32 to 135 nmoles/g/2 hours for jejunum, to 280 for lower ileum. The rate of incorporation of [^{14}C]acetate into sterols per g of fresh tissue in intestinal biopsies from patients with coeliac disease is higher than that in normal biopsies. This has been taken as evidence that intestinal villi do not synthesize sterol, since the villi are atrophied in coeliac disease. However, in view of the fragility of intestinal villi, as demonstrated by Muroya *et al.* (1977), it is possible that sterol synthesis in the villi of normal intestinal mucosa is depressed by damage sustained during the suction biopsy.

3.2.4 Skin

Estimated in terms of the incorporation of [^{14}C]acetate into digitonin-precipitable sterol *in vitro*, sterol synthesis by the whole skin of the squirrel monkey accounts for about 6% of the sterol synthesized by all organs and tissues. However, less than 20% of the radioactivity incorporated into sterol is in cholesterol itself, suggesting that the skin contributes only about 1% of the cholesterol synthesized in the whole body in this species.

Slices of fresh human skin incorporate ^{14}C into non-saponifiable lipids at a rapid rate when incubated with [^{14}C]acetate. Most of the radioactivity incorporated is present in squalene, probably synthesized in the sebaceous glands, but some is also present in digitonin-precipitable sterols synthesized in epidermal cells (Nicolaides et al., 1955). It should be noted that reproducible results are difficult to achieve with whole-thickness biopsies of skin and that results vary widely from one laboratory to another (compare, for example, the values reported by Mendelsohn and Mendelsohn (1972) with those of Brown et al. (1975)), probably because of the difficulty of preparing thin slices of uniform thickness and cell composition. For this reason small variations in sterol synthesis *in vitro* cannot be detected. The use of isolated epidermis obtained from suction blisters of human skin may partially overcome this problem (Hsiah et al., 1970).

3.2.5 Arterial wall

Although the rate of synthesis of sterols in arterial wall is very slow compared with that in tissues such as liver and intestine, incorporation of [^{14}C]acetate into digitonin-precipitable sterols has been demonstrated *in vitro* in arteries from pigeons, rats, rabbits, monkeys and man. Furthermore, the presence of all the enzymes catalyzing the conversion of acetyl-CoA into squalene has been demonstrated in arterial tissue (Slakey et al., 1973). A considerable proportion of the radioactivity incorporated into the total sterol fraction by arteries is present in sterols other than cholesterol (including 5α-cholestanol (Chobanian, 1968)), though incorporation into cholesterol itself has been demonstrated unequivocally by purification through the dibromide. In human and monkey aorta incubated with [^{14}C]acetate, more than half the ^{14}C incorporated into non-saponifiable lipid may be present in squalene, suggesting that the activity of the enzymes catalyzing the conversion of squalene into cholesterol is low in comparison with that of the enzymes catalyzing the formation of squalene.

Cholesterol synthesis in cultured arterial smooth-muscle cells is considered on p. 427. See also St. Clair (1976) for a general review.

3.2.6 White blood cells

Owing to their ready availability, circulating white blood cells are now used increasingly in investigations of sterol synthesis at the cellular level in man. Blood cells are particularly convenient for studies of sterol synthesis under different experimental conditions, since they can be obtained on repeated occasions from the same individual. As mentioned later, preparations of mononucleated white cells may also be useful in the diagnosis and investigation of inborn errors of cholesterol metabolism. Non-nucleated red blood cells do not synthesize cholesterol, but suspensions of total white cells, of partially purified lymphocytes and of partially purified monocytes from human blood all incorporate acetate into sterols at a measurable rate *in vitro*, though in the unstimulated state the rate of synthesis per mg of cell protein is far lower than that observed in liver cells or slices *in vitro*. The low rate of sterol synthesis in white blood cells is due to low enzyme activity rather than to damage to the cells during their isolation from blood, since the rate at which these cells incorporate [^{14}C]acetate added to whole blood before their separation from the red cells is no greater than the rate of incorporation by suspensions of isolated white cells.

Opinions differ as to the relative sterol-synthesizing capacity of different types of circulating human white cells, but it has been suggested that the capacity is greater in monocytes than in lymphocytes and that polymorphs make little contribution to sterol synthesis by mixed populations of white cells. Sterol synthesis has also been demonstrated in long-term suspension cultures of human lymphocytes (Kayden *et al.*, 1976) but does not appear to have been studied systematically in the precursors of white blood cells in marrow or lymphoid tissue.

The slow rate of synthesis of sterol in circulating white cells in the unstimulated state seems to be associated with a relative inefficiency of the later steps in the biosynthetic pathway. Hence, when freshly isolated lymphocytes are incubated with [^{14}C]acetate, much of the radioactivity in the unsaponifiable fraction of the cells is present in squalene, in C_{30} sterols and in C_{27} sterols other than cholesterol, unless the incubation is continued for several hours. This must be borne in mind in the choice of methods for assaying radioactivity incorporated into cholesterol and its precursors during the incubation.

3.2.7 Mevalonic acid metabolism in kidneys

Although the kidneys have only a limited capacity for synthesizing sterol from acetate (Table 8.1), they are the major site for the metabolism of the plasma mevalonic acid. Hellström *et al.* (1973) have shown that when [2-^{14}C]mevalonate is injected intravenously into rats, the uptake of ^{14}C in the kidneys, expressed in terms of the fraction of the dose taken up per gram of tissue, is at least twenty times that in any other organ. From the rate of turnover of the plasma mevalonate and the rate of synthesis of sterol in the liver, Hellström *et al.* estimate that about 5% of the mevalonate formed by the liver escapes into the circulation, to be metabolized largely by the kidneys.

Some of the plasma mevalonate taken up by the kidneys is converted into squalene, lanosterol and cholesterol, but a significant proportion is metabolized to acetoacetate and acetyl-CoA *via* the *trans*-methylglutaconate shunt (see Chapter 4). In rats, about 25% of the mevalonate that escapes from the liver and other tissues into the plasma is metabolized by the shunt pathway, the kidneys accounting for more than half the shunt (Popják, 1977). Wiley and coworkers (1977) have shown that the extent of the *trans*-methylglutaconate shunt in female rats is about twice that in male rats and that this sex difference is due to a difference in the ability of the kidneys to metabolize mevalonic acid through the shunt pathway. By measuring the recovery of $^{14}CO_2$ in the breath after an intravenous injection of $(3R)$-[5-^{14}C]mevalonate, Fogelman et al. (1975) have shown that the shunt accounts for up to 12% of the metabolism of mevalonate in normal human subjects. A pathway of this magnitude could conceivably participate in a mechanism for regulating sterol synthesis in the liver by diverting a variable proportion of the carbon of mevalonic acid from its flow along the pathway to sterol.

4 REGULATION OF STEROL SYNTHESIS

4.1 General considerations

In living systems the rates of metabolic processes are regulated* in accordance with the biological needs of the organism. In the mature animal, the general effect of metabolic regulation is to maintain homeostasis within each tissue and within the body as a whole. But homeostasis is by no means the only function of biochemical regulatory mechanisms. In some tissues, considerable deviations from the steady state may be essential to the success of the organism. An example of a long-term deviation is the marked increase in the rate of synthesis of cholesterol that occurs in the immature central nervous system during the deposition of myelin; once myelination is complete, the rate of synthesis falls irreversibly to a negligible level. Examples of short-term deviations from the steady state are the diurnal rhythm in cholesterol synthesis in the livers of some animals that feed intermittently (presumably, this is related to the need for bile acids in the intestine during the absorption of fat), and the very rapid increase in cholesterol synthesis in the adrenal glands in response to the need for a sudden increase in the secretion of steroid hormones.

The regulation of metabolic processes in a multicellular organism may be thought of in terms of two levels of complexity: that of the individual cell and that of the organism as a whole.

---

* The term 'regulation' (L. *regulare*, to direct or control), as used in relation to biological systems, is hard to define in a way that would satisfy all biologists. By derivation, the word implies a purposive process, since one would not control something without reference to some desirable or optimal state, though trying to define what is optimal for a particular system is, as Riggs (1967) has remarked in relation to feedback control, 'all too often an exercise in futility'. But if one discards altogether the idea of purpose from the meaning of regulation, one might as well not use the word at all in discussions about living systems. The word 'purpose', as used here, does not, of course, imply consciousness of the state that will result from regulation. Those who dislike any reference to purpose in a scientific context should note that few modern biologists have difficulty in accepting the possibility that purposive mechanisms could arise by natural selection in a purposeless universe.

The regulatory mechanisms inherent in the cell itself are primitive, in the sense that they are generally to be found in unicellular organisms. The regulation of sterol synthesis by control of the activity of HMG-CoA reductase, for example, seems to be very ancient since it is probably the means by which ergosterol synthesis is controlled in yeast cells (Kawaguchi, 1970) as well as being the control point in cholesterol synthesis in many mammalian tissues. The flow of metabolites along a metabolic pathway is usually regulated by control of the step catalyzed by the enzyme with the lowest capacity (the rate-limiting step); this step is often the one immediately after a branch point in the pathway. In unicellular organisms, control of the rate-limiting enzyme may be exerted by induction of the enzyme by its substrate (substrate induction), or by activation/inhibition or induction/repression mediated either by the end-product of the metabolic sequence (feedback control) or by a substance derived from an unrelated metabolic pathway. Examples suggestive of each of these types of primitive control are found in sterol biochemistry. The advantage to the cell of regulation of a complete metabolic sequence by means of a single control point is obvious. On the other hand, metabolic pathways in micro-organisms are sometimes regulated by the simultaneous induction or repression of two or more enzymes catalyzing sequential steps in the pathway (co-ordinate induction/repression). Co-ordinate induction occurs in the cells of mammals, though the mechanism by which it is brought about is probably different from that in micro-organisms. The biological value of co-ordinate induction is presumably that it enables the cell to respond maximally to a need for a very marked increase in end-product formation, as in the ACTH-stimulated adrenal gland (see p. 271). Co-ordinate repression, on the other hand, would enable the cell to avoid making unnecessary enzyme proteins when the need for end-product is minimal.

In higher organisms, the primitive control mechanisms are modulated by substances, such as hormones, which reach the cell from the external medium and whose actions serve to integrate the metabolism of different cells in the interests of the whole organism. The cells of many tissues possess surface receptors capable of recognizing specific constituents of the extra-cellular fluid. At least one such surface receptor plays an important role in the regulation of cholesterol metabolism in certain human cells (see Chapter 9). Although primitive control mechanisms probably contribute in some measure to the regulation of sterol metabolism in all mammalian cells, the manner in which these mechanisms are modulated differs widely in different tissues. For example, the regulation of cholesterol metabolism by gonadotrophic hormones does not occur in any tissue other than the gonads. Thus, it will be most convenient to deal first with regulation at the tissue or cell level in general terms and then to deal separately with tissues in which sterol metabolism is specialized. From a broader point of view we also have to consider regulation in terms of the whole body, but this is best dealt with under the general heading of whole-body turnover of sterols (see Chapter 10). In most animal tissues the intracellular content of total cholesterol (free plus esterified) is determined by the rate of intracellular synthesis and the balance between the rates of transport of cholesterol into and out of the cell. Only in the liver and the steroid-hormone-forming organs does catabolism play a significant role in the overall metabolism of cholesterol.

In many animal tissues the rate of sterol synthesis changes in response to a wide variety of experimental modifications, several of which are considered below. Some of these changes, such as the diurnal rhythm in hepatic synthesis of cholesterol in response to the feeding cycle, clearly reflect physiological regulation in the sense discussed in the preceding section. Others, such as the effects of X-irradiation or of pharmacological agents, clearly do not, although these effects often provide clues to physiological mechanisms and for this reason are included here. Between these two extremes are instances where it is hard to say whether or not one is dealing with a true control mechanism. The effects of thyroid hormone on sterol metabolism are a case in point. Cholesterol synthesis in the liver is depressed after thyroidectomy and is stimulated by injecting large doses of thyroxine into normal animals. But even if changes in plasma thyroxine concentration within the physiological range were shown to be capable of bringing about these effects, this would not prove that the thyroid gland *regulates* cholesterol metabolism in the liver in any meaningful sense of the word. To prove this, one would need evidence of a relevant response on the part of the thyroid gland itself, for example, a change in the rate of secretion of hormone in response to a physiological stimulus such as an alteration in the intake of dietary cholesterol. Until such evidence is forthcoming it would be unwise to regard the thyroid as a regulator of cholesterol metabolism in the liver, though the presence of thyroxine may be necessary for the operation of other mechanisms that do regulate cholesterol metabolism.

4.2 HMG-CoA reductase and the rate-limiting step

4.2.1 Review of the evidence

It is generally held that the rate-limiting reaction in the biosynthesis of cholesterol in animal tissues is the reduction of HMG-CoA to mevalonic acid, and that the rate of this reaction is determined by the capacity of HMG-CoA reductase. Most of the evidence for this is derived from the study of rat liver, but observations on other tissues and other species suggest that the site of the control point for sterol synthesis is common to many types of cell.

The probability that the rate-limiting step lies before mevalonic acid was first suggested by the observation that when the incorporation of [^{14}C]acetate into liver cholesterol is inhibited by a short period of cholesterol feeding, there is no change in the rate of incorporation of [^{14}C]mevalonate (Gould and Popják, 1957). Many other instances of a change in acetate incorporation into liver cholesterol without a concomitant change in mevalonate incorporation have since been observed, all indicating that under most conditions there are no rate-limiting steps beyond mevalonate. That the crucial step is in fact the reduction of HMG-CoA was first suggested by Siperstein and Fagan (1966), who showed that cholesterol feeding diminishes the rate of conversion of acetate into mevalonate in the liver, but not that of acetate into HMG.

Under conditions in which the inhibition of sterol synthesis is intense or prolonged, there may be a decrease in the capacity of some of the later steps in the biosynthetic sequence. For example, prolonged feeding with cholesterol may ultimately lead to decreased incorporation of mevalonate into farnesyl pyrophosphate and of farnesyl pyrophosphate into squalene in the liver (Gould and Swyryd, 1966). Slakey et al. (1972) have also demonstrated a marked fall in the activities of four enzymes catalyzing reactions beyond mevalonic acid in the livers of animals fasted for 48 hours, though in no case did the activity become lower than that of HMG-CoA reductase. It has been suggested that the steps catalyzed by these enzymes are secondary control points in segments of the biosynthetic pathway beyond mevalonate, though it should be noted that unless the capacity of one of these enzymes fell below that of HMG-CoA reductase it would not become rate-limiting for the overall flow of carbon from acetate to cholesterol. Gaylor (1974) has also suggested that there are additional control points in the pathway between lanosterol and cholesterol.

In keeping with the conclusion that the rate of sterol synthesis is determined by the capacity of HMG-CoA reductase, it has been shown that the activity of this enzyme, assayed in the microsomal fraction, rises or falls in parallel with changes in the rate of incorporation of [^{14}C]acetate into the cholesterol of liver slices brought about by many experimental procedures. Some of these experimentally-induced changes are discussed in the sections on the regulation of cholesterol synthesis in particular tissues. The close correlation between hepatic HMG-CoA reductase activity and cholesterol synthesis estimated by the octanoate method is illustrated in Fig. 8.1. It should also be noted that the activity of HMG-CoA reductase in the livers of normal and of cholesterol-fed and fasted rats is sufficient to account for the observed rate of conversion of acetate into cholesterol measured in subcellular fractions, but is much too low to account for the rate of conversion of mevalonate into cholesterol (Bucher et al., 1960; Slakey et al., 1972).

Strictly speaking, if the rate of synthesis of cholesterol in a given set of conditions is determined by the activity of HMG-CoA reductase, then in the intact cell the flow of carbon from HMG-CoA to mevalonate should be exactly equal to the flow of carbon from acetate

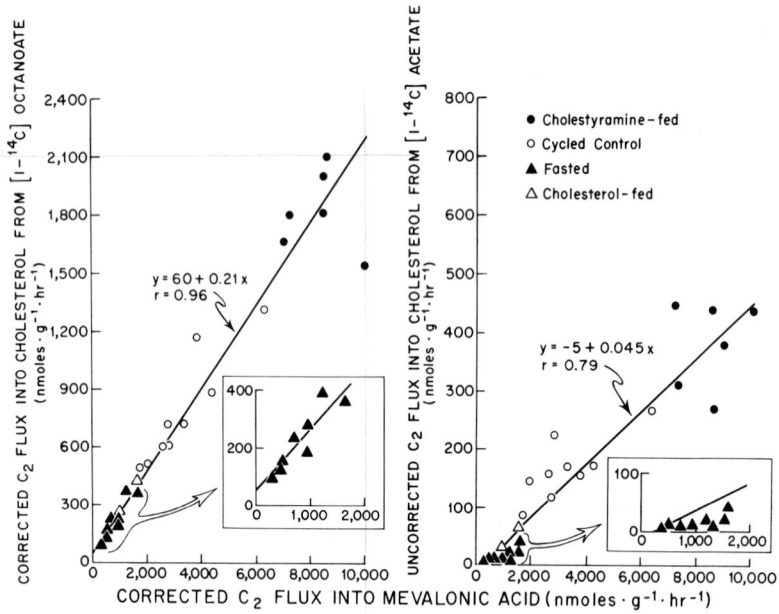

Figure 8.1
The rate of incorporation of acetyl carbon into the cholesterol of rat-liver slices as a function of microsomal HMG-CoA reductase activity, determined under conditions in which hepatic cholesterol synthesis was varied over a wide range by the agents shown in the right panel.

The flux of acetyl carbon into cholesterol was determined by the [^{14}C]octanoate method (left panel) and also by the [^{14}C]acetate method without correction for dilution of the acetyl-CoA pool from endogenous substrates (right panel). Note that the values determined by the [^{14}C]acetate method are less than half those determined by the [^{14}C]octanoate method. Note also that the activity of HMG-CoA reductase (a measure of the flux of C_2 into mevalonic acid under the conditions used for assaying the enzyme *in vitro*) was 3–4 times higher than the corrected estimate of C_2 flux into cholesterol (left panel). This discrepancy could be due to activation of the reductase during preparation of the microsomes (see Section 4.2.2) or to differences between the cofactor concentrations in the intact cell and in the incubation system used in the assay. 'Cycled control' rats were maintained under conditions of 12-hour light and dark cycles for one week before they were killed; the cholesterol-fed rats were given 1% of cholesterol in their diets for 48 hours before the experiment. (From Dietschy and Brown (1974), with the permission of the authors.)

to cholesterol. It is difficult to see how this can ever be tested rigorously because in order to assay HMG-CoA reductase it is necessary to prepare a microsomal fraction and to test the enzyme in the presence of concentrations of substrate and cofactors that may differ from those existing in the intact cell. Furthermore, the intrinsic activity of the enzyme may be altered during its preparation for assay (see below). Bucher *et al.* (1960) and Slakey *et al.* (1972) found reasonable agreement between the activity of HMG-CoA reductase and the rate of incorporation of acetate into cholesterol in subcellular fractions of liver. Dietschy and Brown (1974), on the other hand, found that over a wide range of rates of sterol synthesis in liver slices the capacity of HMG-CoA reductase, assayed in the microsomal fraction, was more than three times the rate of formation of cholesterol from acetate in the slices (determined by the octanoate method). This apparent anomaly could be due to overestimation of intracellular enzyme activity, for the reasons discussed on p. 367, but it does raise the possibility that the rate of reduction of HMG-CoA in the intact cell is not always determined by the capacity of the reductase. It is also possible that there is a potentially rate-limiting step before HMG-CoA. White and Rudney (1970) have, indeed, suggested that the rate of synthesis of mevalonate may under some conditions be determined by the supply of cytosolic HMG-CoA for the reductase. (For other examples of a dissociation between cholesterol synthesis and HMG-CoA reductase activity, see Johnston *et al.* (1979)).

The possibility that co-ordinate induction/repression of enzymes, analogous to that seen in micro-organisms, may occur in animal tissues has often been discussed. In true co-ordinate induction the co-ordination is controlled by a single gene, so that the rates of synthesis of the linked enzymes always change in parallel and to the same proportional extent. There seems to be nothing quite like this in the regulation of sterol biosynthesis, though parallel changes in the activities of several enzymes in the pathway to sterols (not necessarily due to induction or repression) have often been observed. Two examples, the effects of fasting and of prolonged cholesterol feeding, have already been mentioned. Another interesting example is the link between HMG-CoA reductase and cytosolic HMG-CoA synthase in the liver and adrenal cortex (see 4.3 and 4.5). The marked tendency of hepatic HMG-CoA reductase and cholesterol 7α-hydroxylase to respond in parallel to many physiological and non-physiological factors, and the functional significance of this co-ordination, have been discussed by Myant and Mitropoulos (1977).

An argument that has been used to support the view that the reduction of HMG-CoA is rate-limiting for sterol biosynthesis is the apparent position of this step at a point immediately after a branch in the pathway leading either to acetoacetate by cleavage or to mevalonate by reduction. But this argument is mistaken. We now know that selective regulation of the fate of HMG-CoA is achieved not by a favourable siting of the control point, but by the physical separation of the two pathways, the HMG-CoA synthase that provides substrate for ketone-body formation being confined to the mitochondria.

4.2.2 Some properties of HMG-CoA reductase

In this section we shall consider certain properties of HMG-CoA reductase, some of which are probably relevant to the validity of methods for assaying the enzyme or to its regulation under physiological conditions.

4.2.2.1 Effects of solubilization and of exposure to cold.

When microsomal HMG-CoA reductase is solubilized by procedures which separate the enzyme from the subcellular membrane with which it is associated, there may be a considerable increase in total activity. Treatment of the microsomes with deoxycholate, for example, may double enzyme activity. This effect could be due to a change in the configuration of the enzyme brought about by separating it from the lipids of the endoplasmic reticulum or to unmasking of catalytic sites normally buried in the membrane, or to removal of inhibitors.

Some procedures used for solubilizing the microsomal enzyme may also lead to changes in its sensitivity to temperature. Before separation from the microsomal fraction, the enzyme is relatively insensitive to cold, but after solubilization by freeze-thawing it loses activity very rapidly when incubated at 4 °C. Depending upon the procedure used for dissolving the enzyme, the loss of activity may be reversible (Heller and Gould, 1974) or irreversible (Brown et al., 1973). The mechanism responsible for cold inactivation is not understood, but it could well be related to the physiological mechanism responsible for the rapid changes in enzyme activity discussed in 4.3.2. Cold inactivation of solubilized HMG-CoA reductase also suggests a possible reason for the remarkably short half-life of the hepatic enzyme *in vivo*; Tormanen et al. (1977) have shown that the irreversible cold inactivation of the enzyme seen in some crude soluble extracts of liver microsomes is due to the presence, in these extracts, of a heat-labile inactivator (possibly an enzyme).

4.2.2.2 Cyclic AMP and reversible phosphorylation.

Several other factors which modify HMG-CoA reductase activity in intact cells or in cell-free systems have also been investigated with a view to their possible role in the normal regulation of cholesterol synthesis. Cyclic AMP (CAMP) added to slices or homogenates of liver decreases both the rate of synthesis of cholesterol and the activity of the reductase. These short-term effects of CAMP may be relevant to the role of reversible phosphorylation in the regulation of HMG-CoA reductase activity, as discussed below, though the extracellular concentrations of CAMP required to produce these effects are far above the physiological range.

Incubation of liver microsomes in the presence of ATP and Mg^{2+} also diminishes the activity of HMG-CoA reductase, and the inactivated enzyme can be re-activated by incubation at 37 °C in the presence of the cytosol (Beg et al., 1973). Re-activation of microsomal preparations of HMG-CoA reductase observed under certain conditions *in vitro* may be prevented by fluoride, an inhibitor of phosphatases (Berndt et al., 1976). The reactivating system has been shown by Nordstrom et al. (1977) to be a cytosolic enzyme (M.W. 30 000–35 000) effective with both microsomal and solubilized preparations of the inactivated reductase. These earlier observations may now be explained by the presence in liver cells of a complex system of enzymes capable of bringing about the inactivation and re-activation of HMG-CoA reductase by a phosphorylation-dephosphorylation mechanism similar in principle to that concerned in the regulation of some other enzymes. For a review of the information available in 1978, see Gibson and Ingebritsen (1978). Only a brief summary will be given here.

The microsomes of liver cells contain an ATP-dependent protein kinase ('reductase kinase') that inactivates HMG-CoA reductase by phosphorylating it, and the cytosol contains a phosphoprotein phosphatase that activates the reductase by dephosphorylating it (Ingebritsen et al., 1978). The phosphorylation of the reductase is accompanied by the incorporation of ^{32}P from $[\gamma$-$^{32}P]$ATP into the enzyme and the re-activation by phosphatase is accompanied by loss of ^{32}P from the ^{32}P-labelled inactive reductase (Beg et al., 1978). The reductase kinase is itself subject to modulation by reversible phosphorylation catalyzed by a microsomal ATP-dependent kinase ('reductase kinase kinase') and a cytosolic phosphoprotein phosphatase, the reductase kinase being *active* in the phosphorylated form (Beg et al., 1979).

Gibson and Ingebritsen (1978) have suggested that the activity of the phosphoprotein phosphatase is modulated by a phosphatase inhibitor which, in turn, is reversibly activated by a CAMP-dependent protein kinase, analogous to the reversible activation of the inhibitor of phosphorylase phosphatase ('inhibitor-1') in rabbit muscle (Nimmo and Cohen, 1978).

A sequence of interlocking phosphorylation cycles would provide the cell with a very sensitive mechanism for regulating the activity of HMG-CoA reductase by amplification of a signal such as a small change in the intracellular concentration of CAMP. Similar, and perhaps even more complex, control mechanisms are known to be responsible for modulating the activity of many enzymes that are activated or inactivated by phosphorylation. A scheme embodying what is already known about the regulation of hepatic HMG-CoA reductase by reversible phosphorylation, together with some speculations based on analogy with other regulatory systems, is shown in Fig. 8.2. In this scheme, a rise in CAMP concentration, for example, would tend to decrease the activity of HMG-CoA reductase by causing a net decrease in the rate of dephosphorylation of the phosphorylated reductase (inactive form) or by reducing the rate of dephosphorylation of the active form of reductase kinase. CAMP could also act directly by activating reductase kinase kinase and thus indirectly favouring the formation of the inactive form of HMG-CoA reductase. This scheme would provide a plausible explanation for the effects of some hormones on HMG-CoA reductase activity in intact cells. Ingebritsen *et al.* (1979) have, in fact, provided evidence that the stimulatory effect of insulin and the inhibitory effect of glucagon on HMG-CoA reductase activity in intact hepatocytes (see Chapter 9) are mediated partly by changes in the activity of the reductase kinase.

Thus, it is possible that those hormones that cause a change in

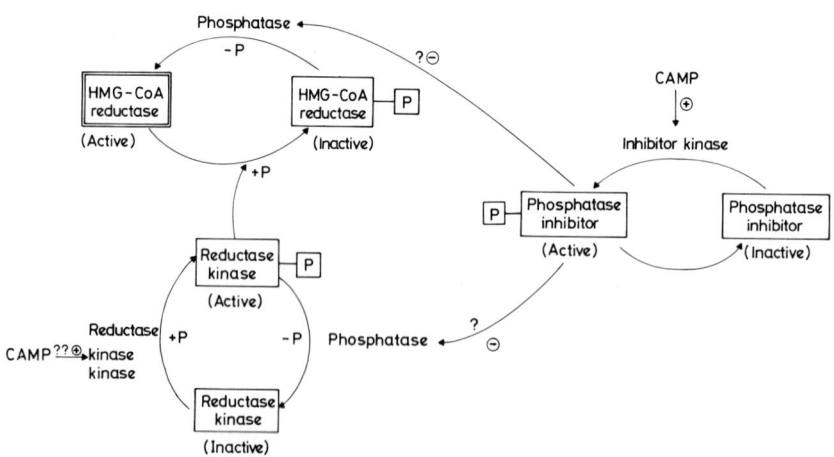

Figure 8.2
Scheme showing the reversible phosphorylation and dephosphorylation of hepatic HMG-CoA reductase. Phosphorylation, giving the inactive form of the enzyme, is catalyzed by *reductase kinase*. The reductase kinase is reversibly phosphorylated to the active form by another kinase (*reductase kinase kinase*). Dephosphorylation of phosphorylated reductase and of phosphorylated reductase kinase is catalyzed by cytosolic phosphoprotein phosphatase. The presence of a phosphatase inhibitor, subject to reversible phosphorylation by a CAMP-dependent inhibitor kinase, has been postulated but not proved. CAMP, cyclic AMP.

intracellular CAMP concentration may influence HMG-CoA reductase activity by altering the proportions of the active and inactive forms of the enzyme. However, there is no reason to suppose that this is the only mechanism through which the activity of the reductase is controlled. Reversible phosphorylation is clearly not responsible for the diurnal rhythm in hepatic reductase activity (see Section 4.3.1), since the ratio of active to inactive enzyme in the liver remains the same throughout the 24-hour cycle (Berndt et al., 1976). Nor is there any evidence to suggest that phosphorylation-dephosphorylation of the enzyme mediates changes in hepatic reductase activity brought about by fasting, cholesterol feeding or cholestyramine treatment (Brown et al., 1979). This is not surprising, since it is difficult to see the biological advantage to a liver cell of a mechanism capable of switching cholesterol synthesis on and off within minutes—a mechanism of the kind that would seem to be more appropriate for regulating the supply of substrates for rapidly changing energy requirements. Indeed, one has the suspicion that the reversible phosphorylation of HMG-CoA reductase in the liver may turn out to be a consequence of the incomplete specificity of enzyme systems that have evolved to fulfil a function other than that of regulating cholesterol synthesis.

Any further speculation as to the regulatory role of the reversible phosphorylation of HMG-CoA reductase under physiological conditions is likely to be overtaken by events. However, the existence of an activating system in the tissues has a practical bearing on the validity of methods for assessing the activity of the enzyme as it exists in the intact cell. Nordstrom et al. (1977) have shown that more than 80% of the HMG-CoA reductase normally present in rat liver is in the inactivated (phosphorylated) state, and that under the conditions commonly used for isolation of microsomes for assay of the enzyme, activation by enzymic dephosphorylation would be likely to occur. For this reason they suggest that the enzyme or microsomes should always be prepared for assay in the presence of NaF at a concentration high enough to inhibit phosphoprotein phosphatase present in the tissue. Philipp and Shapiro (1979) have also described a method for assaying the amounts of active and inactive enzyme in a tissue by measuring enzyme activity in microsomes prepared in the presence of NaF and after treatment with a purified potato phosphatase.

4.2.2.3 Other factors. Other natural substances that have been shown to modify HMG-CoA reductase activity *in vitro* include inhibitory factors, possibly proteins, in rat and ox bile and in the milk of several species (Rodwell et al., 1976). The influence of various hormones on HMG-CoA reductase is considered in the sections dealing with regulation in particular tissues (see especially Section 4.3.6 of this chapter and also Chapter 9). For *compactin* see page 735.

4.3 Regulation in liver

Regulation of sterol synthesis in the liver requires special consideration because of the unique role of the liver in the synthesis of bile acids and because in most mammalian species it contributes far more to the total exchangeable mass of cholesterol in the whole body than does any other organ or tissue.

4.3.1 Diurnal rhythm

When rats fed *ad libitum* are adapted to conditions in which a 12-hour period of light alternates with a 12-hour period of darkness, the activity of HMG-CoA reductase in their livers varies rhythmically, rising to a peak at about the mid-point of the dark phase (when the rats feed) and falling to a minimum during the light phase (when they sleep). When the animals are fully adapted to the light cycle, the activity of the enzyme at the peak is about five times that at the minimum. If the light cycle is reversed, the rhythmic rise and fall in HMG-CoA reductase activity is also reversed, the peak now occurring at the mid-point of the new dark phase. Reversal of the light cycle is often used in studies of the diurnal rhythm in the activity of HMG-CoA reductase and of other enzymes whose activity varies diurnally, since it is possible, by means of artificial lighting, to maintain one group of rats in the dark and another group in the light during a normal working day. A diurnal rhythm in HMG-CoA reductase activity also occurs in the crypt cells of the ileum (Shefer *et al.*, 1972) (Fig. 8.3), in some hepatomas (Goldfarb and Pitot, 1971) and in the adrenal cortex (Balasubramaniam *et al.*, 1977) of rats adapted to a 12-hour light/dark cycle, though the amplitude of the rhythm in these tissues is much smaller than that in the liver.

The rhythm in HMG-CoA reductase activity in both liver and intestine is accompanied by a parallel rhythmic variation in the incorporation of acetate, but not of mevalonate, into sterol, the increase in incorporation of acetate lagging about 2 hours behind the increase in enzyme activity (Edwards, Muroya and Gould, 1972). As discussed in Section 4.2, the association between acetate incorporation and HMG-CoA reductase activity during the diurnal cycle is an important part of the evidence that the reduction of HMG-CoA is rate-limiting for sterol synthesis under most physiological conditions. However, when rats are starved, the rhythm in enzyme activity continues, though with diminished amplitude, but the rhythm in the incorporation of exogenous acetate is abolished; this suggests that under these abnormal conditions some other step in the biosynthetic sequence becomes rate-limiting. HMG-CoA reductase appears to be the only enzyme in the pathway to sterols that undergoes a diurnal rhythm in activity in rat liver (Slakey *et al.*, 1972; Clinkenbeard *et al.*, 1975).

The immediate cause of the rise in enzyme activity in the liver is a marked increase in the rate of synthesis of enzyme protein, indicated by an increase in the incorporation of [^{3}H]leucine into the purified enzyme, beginning at about the time of the start of the dark period. If enzyme synthesis is blocked at any time before the peak by treating the animal with cycloheximide, enzyme activity begins to fall almost immediately with a half-life of about 2 hours. Once the peak has been reached, activity declines with the same 2-hour half-life and the rate of decline is unaffected by cycloheximide, indicating that synthesis of enzyme ceases completely at the mid-point of the dark cycle, the rate of degradation remaining unchanged. It is owing to the very short half-life of the enzyme that a diurnal rhythm in activity can be maintained solely by modulation of the rate of enzyme synthesis, without change in its rate of degradation or state of activation.

Despite intensive study of the problem, the basis of the rhythmic rise and fall in HMG-CoA reductase activity is still not completely understood. There are really two questions to be answered: 'What is the nature and mechanism of the stimulus to increased synthesis of enzyme protein?' and 'What causes the intensity of the stimulus to vary diurnally?'

The fact that the rhythm can be reversed by reversing the light

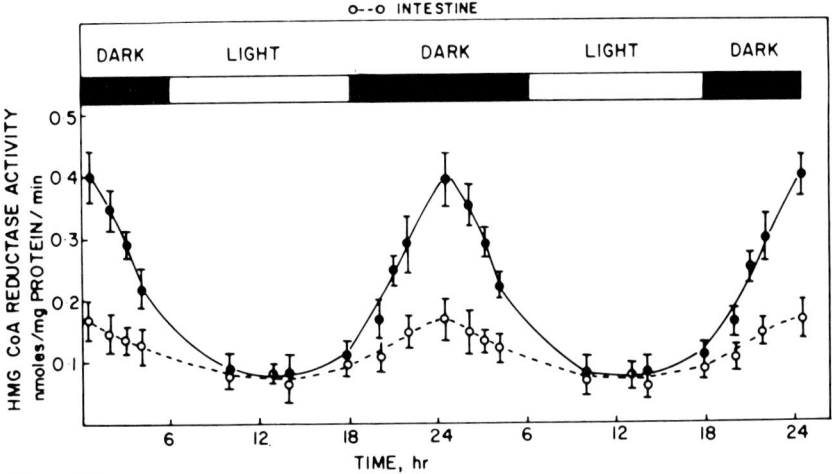

Figure 8.3
Diurnal rhythm of hepatic and intestinal HMG-CoA reductase activity in rats maintained under conditions of controlled lighting and feeding. Enzyme activity was measured in the liver (●) and crypts of the ileal mucosa (○) of rats killed at the intervals shown. Note the maximum value at about the mid-point of the dark phase of each diurnal cycle. (From Shefer *et al.*, 1972, with the permission of the authors.)

cycle in rats fed *ad libitum* shows that the time within the 24-hour cycle at which the peak in activity occurs is in some way determined by the time at which the animals feed. But it is equally clear that the rhythmic increase in enzyme activity is not simply a direct response to feeding, because, as mentioned above, the rhythm persists in fasted rats. Moreover, in rats adapted to meal-feeding during the dark phase, the rise in enzyme activity begins before the animals start feeding. Nor can the rhythm be due to cyclic repression by bile acids returning to the liver from the intestine (4.3.3) since it is retained, though with altered amplitude, in cholestyramine-fed or bile-fistula rats. It seems as though there is some process in the rat's body which 'ordains' that there shall be a rhythm in HMG-CoA reductase activity with a period of 24 hours, but that the phasing and amplitude of the oscillations can be modified by environmental and internal factors.

In the search for a rhythmic stimulus to the synthesis of HMG-CoA reductase in the liver, much attention has been given to the glucocorticoids. The plasma concentration of corticosterone varies diurnally in rats, reaching a maximum about six hours before the peak in HMG-CoA reductase activity. Since corticosteroids are known to induce many hepatic enzymes, the diurnal rhythm in plasma corticosterone concentration offers an attractive explanation for the diurnal rhythm in HMG-CoA reductase activity. However, experiments to test this have led to confusing and contradictory results. Removal of both adrenals has been reported to abolish the rhythm (Hickman *et al.*, 1972; Edwards, 1973), to diminish the amplitude of oscillation without abolishing the rhythm (Mitropoulos and Balasubramaniam, 1976) or to have no effect on it (Huber *et al.*, 1972). Observations on the influence of glucocorticoids on hepatic HMG-CoA reductase activity in rats have been equally contradictory and there is no agreement as to whether their major effect is to increase or to decrease reductase activity in intact animals.

According to several authors, the diurnal rhythm in HMG-CoA reductase activity is abolished in diabetes, but since the rhythm can be restored by giving injections of slow-release insulin it seems likely that insulin acts by permitting the liver to respond to some stimulus, other than insulin, which itself varies diurnally. Other hormones, including thyroid hormone, glucagon and the catecholamines, have been shown to influence hepatic HMG-CoA reductase activity or sterol synthesis in rats (see 4.3.6) but there is no evidence to suggest that their role in maintaining a normal diurnal rhythm is other than a permissive or potentiating one. The rhythm is abolished by hypophysectomy. This would be expected if the underlying rhythmic stimulus to the synthesis of HMG-CoA reductase cannot act in the absence of one or more of the hormones secreted by the pituitary.

Myant and Mitropoulos (1977) have discussed the possibility that the rise in HMG-CoA reductase activity during the dark phase of the 24-hour cycle is a direct consequence of the increased rate of catabolism of cholesterol to bile acids brought about by the concurrent increase in the activity of cholesterol 7α-hydroxylase. But this still leaves us with the unanswered question of the cause of the diurnal rhythm in cholesterol 7α-hydroxylase activity.

4.3.2 Dietary cholesterol

Suppression of cholesterol synthesis in the liver by dietary cholesterol was first demonstrated by Gould (1951), who showed that the incorporation of [^{14}C]acetate into cholesterol in the livers of dogs and rabbits is reduced to a few percent of the control value when cholesterol is added to the diet. This observation has since been extended in many laboratories and is still the model for much current investigation into the regulation of sterol synthesis in animal tissues in general.

Suppression of cholesterol synthesis by cholesterol feeding, loosely referred to as feedback inhibition, has now been shown to occur in many vertebrate species besides dogs and rabbits. These include human beings, subhuman primates, rats, guinea-pigs, mice, birds, reptiles, amphibia and fish (Siperstein, 1970). In most mammals, the inhibitory effect is confined almost entirely to the liver, though prolonged feeding with cholesterol may cause some inhibition of sterol synthesis in the intestinal wall and the adrenals. In guinea-pigs, on the other hand, marked feedback inhibition occurs in the intestine, lung and adrenals, as well as in the liver (Swann *et al.*, 1975). Inhibition by dietary cholesterol has also been reported in haematopoietic cells of rabbits and in lymph nodes of guinea-pigs (Siperstein, 1970).

Siperstein (1970) has shown that feedback inhibition is absent from all hepatomas of mice and rats, from the aflatoxin-induced hepatoma of the rainbow trout and from at least two human hepatomas. In each case, whereas the normal liver tissue shows almost complete suppression of cholesterol synthesis in response to cholesterol feeding, the hepatoma, even if well-differentiated, usually shows no response at all. The failure of hepatomas to respond to dietary cholesterol by suppression of cholesterol synthesis seems to be due to a diminished ability to take up and store cholesterol from the extracellular medium, rather than to an intrinsic inability of the hepatoma cells to regulate their sterol synthesis. When hepatoma cells are cultured *in vitro* they acquire the ability to suppress cholesterol synthesis when incubated in the presence of serum lipoproteins, and when transplanted back into the host they again fail to respond to cholesterol feeding (Beirne and Watson, 1976). Why hepatoma cells fail to take up cholesterol when the animal is fed cholesterol is not clear, but their behaviour in culture shows that their abnormal behaviour *in vivo* is not due to deletion of the normal intracellular mechanisms by which sterol synthesis is regulated in liver cells. It should also be noted that the physical and kinetic properties of HMG-CoA reductase from normal liver and hepatomas are identical (Rodwell *et al.*, 1976).

Feedback inhibition by dietary cholesterol is specific for sterol synthesis in so far as the oxidation of acetate to CO_2, the conversion of acetate into fatty acid and the general synthesis of protein in the liver are all unaffected by feeding cholesterol. As we have seen in connection with the rate-limiting step in sterol biosynthesis (4.2), suppression of acetate incorporation into liver cholesterol by dietary cholesterol is due primarily to a fall in the activity* of HMG-CoA reductase. In short-term feeding experiments there is a more or less simultaneous fall in acetate incorporation and HMG-CoA reductase activity in the liver, beginning within a few hours of feeding, with no significant change in the incorporation of mevalonate into cholesterol (Fig. 8.4) and without detectable change in the activities of other enzymes in the biosynthetic pathway from acetate to cholesterol. The fall in HMG-CoA reductase activity seems to be sufficient to account for the fall in cholesterol synthesis, as reflected in the incorporation of [^{14}C]acetate into sterol (Fig. 8.4). With more prolonged cholesterol feeding the activities of HMG-CoA synthase and of enzymes catalyzing steps beyond MVA may also decline. However, as discussed above, there is no evidence that any of the steps beyond the reduction of HMG-CoA becomes rate-limiting for sterol synthesis. It may be that the decreased activity of these post-mevalonate enzymes is due to repression of enzyme synthesis as a secondary adaptation to decreased concentrations of their substrates following the primary decrease in the rate of formation of mevalonate. As discussed in 4.1, this would enable the hepatocyte to economize in the synthesis of sterol-synthesizing enzymes.

Ever since the discovery of feedback inhibition of hepatic synthesis of cholesterol more than 25 years ago, a great deal of attention has been paid to the mechanism responsible for this inhibition. The finding that short-term feeding with cholesterol had no effect on the incorporation of mevalonate into hepatic sterol focused attention on the reduction of HMG-CoA as the probable sensitive step. In view of the rapidity with which hepatic synthesis of cholesterol in mice can be suppressed by intravenous injection of a very-low-density lipoprotein fraction obtained from the serum of cholesterol-fed chickens, Siperstein and Fagan (1964) concluded that HMG-CoA reductase is probably an allosteric enzyme and that the effect of dietary choles-

---

* In this context the term 'activity' refers to the rate of enzymic conversion (measured under specified conditions) of HMG-CoA into mevalonic acid/mg of microsomal protein.

Cholesterol Synthesis in Animal Tissues 373

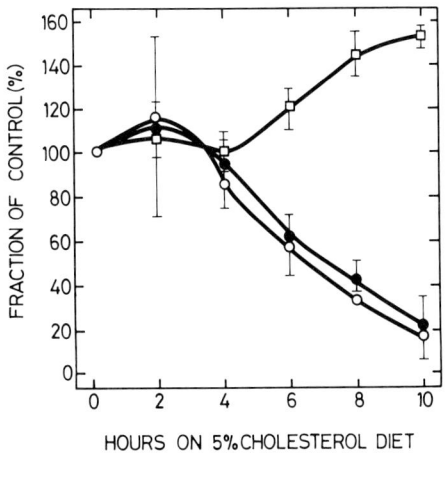

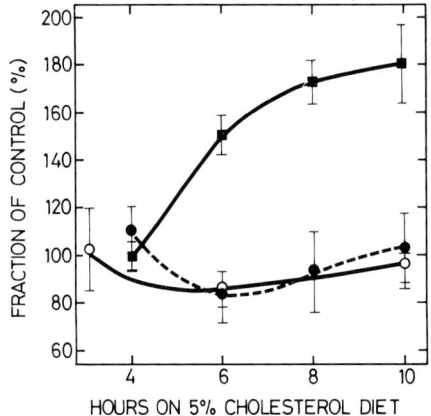

Figure 8.4
Time-course of the effect of cholesterol feeding on the activity of HMG-CoA reductase and the rate of incorporation of [^{14}C]acetate and [^{14}C]mevalonate into cholesterol in the liver. The rats were fed diets with 5% cholesterol, starting at 8 a.m. and their livers were analysed during the following 10 hours. All values are expressed as percentages of the values from rats fed normal diets.

Above; Incorporation of [^{14}C]acetate into cholesterol (●), HMG-CoA reductase activity (○), liver cholesterol content (□).

Below; Incorporation of [2-^{14}C]mevalonate into cholesterol (●), incorporation of [1-^{14}C]acetyl-CoA into HMG-CoA, liver cholesterol content (■). Cholesterol feeding causes a parallel fall in HMG-CoA reductase activity and acetate incorporation, beginning about 4 hours after the start of feeding, but has no effect on the incorporation of mevalonate into cholesterol. (From Shapiro and Rodwell, 1971, with the permission of the authors.)

terol is to cause allosteric inhibition of the hepatic enzyme. Against this view, however, it proved impossible to inhibit hepatic HMG-CoA reductase in broken-cell preparations by the addition of cholesterol in various physical forms, including cholesterol-carrying serum lipoproteins, to the incubation medium. It was also found that the K_m of the enzyme for HMG-CoA was similar in the livers of normal and cholesterol-fed rats. The latter observation led Rodwell *et al.* (1973) to conclude that HMG-CoA reductase is not an allosteric enzyme and that dietary feedback inhibition is mediated by repression of enzyme synthesis rather than by inhibition of pre-existing enzyme. In agreement with this, it had already been shown by Linn (1967) that the decreased activity of the hepatic enzyme prepared from cholesterol-fed rats cannot be restored by removal of bound lipid from the microsomes by extraction with organic solvents.

Although there can be no doubt that repression of enzyme synthesis contributes to the suppression of hepatic synthesis of cholesterol, more recent evidence, based on experiments timed in relation to the diurnal cycle in enzyme synthesis, suggests that the earliest effect of cholesterol feeding is to inhibit pre-existing enzyme. Thus, Higgins and Rudney (1973) have shown that when rats adapted to a light/dark cycle are fed cholesterol at the beginning of the dark phase, enzyme activity starts to decline several hours before there is any detectable change in the amount of enzyme protein, assayed by means of an immunoprecipitin to HMG-CoA reductase, or in the rate of enzyme synthesis, assayed by measuring incorporation of [^{3}H]leucine into the enzyme. After more prolonged feeding, both the quantity and rate of synthesis of the enzyme fall to very low levels. In agreement with this, Edwards and Gould (1974) have shown that if cholesterol is given to rats by intubation of the stomach at midnight, i.e. at the peak of enzyme activity, HMG-CoA reductase activity in the liver falls with a half-life (1.2 hours) shorter than that in rats fed a normal diet (2.2 hours). Since enzyme synthesis ceases completely at midnight (Section 4.3.1), this must mean either that the administered cholesterol inactivates pre-existing enzyme or that it increases the rate of degradation of the enzyme. That hepatic HMG-CoA reductase is subject to regulation by enzyme inhibition is clear from the observations of Edwards *et al.* (1977) and of Gould (1977) that the activity of HMG-CoA reductase in rat liver falls within minutes of an intragastric dose of mevalonate sufficient to raise the free-cholesterol content of hepatic microsomes.

Taken together, the observations discussed above suggest that the initial effect of cholesterol feeding is to inhibit hepatic HMG-CoA reductase, and that as the feeding is continued, synthesis of new enzyme protein is repressed.

There has been much discussion about the physicochemical form of the intracellular cholesterol responsible for suppressing hepatic synthesis of sterol in cholesterol-fed animals. Cholesterol feeding always increases the concentration of esterified cholesterol in the liver, and for this reason Siperstein (1970) suggested that suppression is brought about by an accumulation of esterified cholesterol in the membranes of the endoplasmic reticulum, already known to contain the bulk of the HMG-CoA reductase in rat liver. The inverse relationship between sterol synthesis and the concentration of cholesteryl ester in hepatic microsomes has also been emphasized by Harry et al. (1973). However, Gould (1958, 1959) has pointed out that cholesterol feeding also leads to an increase in the concentration of free cholesterol in the liver. Moreover, he has shown that there is an inverse linear relationship between the concentration of free cholesterol and the log of the rate of incorporation of acetate into cholesterol in liver slices over a wide range of free cholesterol concentration in the livers of rats fed different amounts of cholesterol or subjected to various experimental procedures. Gould suggested that cholesterol synthesis in the liver is regulated by the free cholesterol content of the microsomes, and in support of this he drew attention to the fact that the bulk of the cholesterol in microsomes is free and that the immediate product of the biosynthetic pathway to sterol is free cholesterol.

Sabine and James (1976) have shown that cholesterol feeding causes changes in the temperature-induced kinetics of hepatic HMG-CoA reductase that are consistent with an effect of the feeding on the fluidity of the membrane to which the enzyme is attached.

The Arrhenius plot (log of enzyme activity *versus* reciprocal of temperature) for HMG-CoA reductase in liver microsomes from normal rats shows a sharp decrease in slope when the temperature is raised above about 27 °C, indicating a decrease in activation energy of the enzyme above this temperature. Arrhenius plots also show that cholesterol feeding increases the activation energy of hepatic microsomal HMG-CoA reductase. Sabine and James suggest that the break in the Arrhenius plot for HMG-CoA reductase from normal liver reflects a change in the conformation of the enzyme, or in the interaction between its subunits, due to a temperature-induced change in the fluidity of the microsomal membrane. They also suggest that cholesterol feeding reduces enzyme activity by diminishing the fluidity of the membrane at a given temperature. These proposals have been developed by Mitropoulos and Venkatesan (1977), who suggest that cholesterol feeding decreases HMG-CoA reductase activity in the liver by raising the concentration of free cholesterol in a region of the membrane of the endoplasmic reticulum adjacent to the enzyme (see Chapter 7 for references to other membrane-bound enzymes whose activities are affected by changes in membrane fluidity). An effect of this kind would account for the very rapid suppression of cholesterol synthesis in the liver observed after cholesterol feeding or after oral administration of mevalonate, but it leaves unexplained the failure of cholesterol to diminish HMG-CoA reductase activity when added to microsomal preparations *in vitro*.

The idea that cholesterol feeding inhibits HMG-CoA reductase by changing the fluidity of membrane phospholipids is certainly an attractive one. However, it remains to be shown that dietary cholesterol does, in fact, cause the postulated change in fluidity in the region of the microsomal membrane in which the enzyme is embedded. Moreover, since breaks in the Arrhenius plot have been demonstrated with soluble enzymes (Dixon and Webb, 1964), it is clear that the break in the Arrhenius plot for HMG-CoA reductase could be due to something other than a change in membrane fluidity. A crucial test of the hypothesis of Sabine and James would be to observe the effect of temperature on the activation energy of HMG-CoA reductase separated from the microsomal membrane.

Observations on the effect of analogues of cholesterol on sterol synthesis in the livers of intact animals and in cultured cells *in vitro* have led to the suggestion that dietary cholesterol is converted into an active metabolite in the body and that this, rather than cholesterol itself, is responsible for suppressing cholesterol synthesis in the liver. While it seems possible that a metabolite of cholesterol is responsible for the short-term effects of cholesterol feeding, there is no reason to doubt that cholesterol itself is capable of repressing the synthesis of HMG-CoA reductase. Further discussion of the effects of oxygenated sterols on the biosynthesis of cholesterol will be found in Chapter 9 (Section 2.3).

It is not known whether dietary cholesterol represses the synthesis of HMG-CoA reductase before or after messenger RNA reaches the ribosomes on which the enzyme is synthesized. The time lag between cholesterol feeding and enzyme repression is consistent with an effect either on the formation or release of messenger RNA, or on a later stage in the control of protein synthesis. The observation of Gould (1977) that the chromatin of liver cells contains cholesterol, and that radioactive cholesterol fed to rats can be detected in their liver chromatin within two hours, raises the interesting possibility that cholesterol shares with other steroids the ability to influence the transcription of DNA into RNA.

The demonstration that a serum lipoprotein obtained from cholesterol-fed chickens suppresses hepatic synthesis of cholesterol *in vivo* has already been referred to. In the course of this work, Siperstein and coworkers (Sakakida *et al.*, 1963) noted that the equally hypercholesterolaemic serum of stilboestrol-treated chickens had no effect on cholesterol synthesis in the livers of mice. This suggested that the dietary cholesterol responsible for feedback inhibition is transported to the liver in lipoproteins of a particular class. Later work on rats has, indeed, shown that chylomicron remnants, the immediate products of the action of lipoprotein lipase upon the chylomicrons entering the circulation *via* the intestinal lymphatics, are selectively taken up by the liver and that the cholesterol present in the remnant particles exerts feedback inhibition of cholesterol synthesis in the liver. Andersen and Dietschy (1977) have shown that other serum lipoproteins are taken up by the liver slowly, if at all, when injected intravenously, and do not suppress cholesterol synthesis in the liver *in vivo*. (When chylomicrons are injected intravenously their cholesterol eventually enters the liver and suppresses cholesterol synthesis *in situ*, but only after they have been converted into remnants.) Andersen and Dietschy (1977) have also shown that chylomicron remnants are not taken up by tissues other than liver and do not suppress cholesterol synthesis in extrahepatic tissues when infused intravenously. The origin and fate of the cholesterol in chylomicrons and their remnants, and the possible reasons for the specific recognition of remnant particles by the liver, are discussed in Chapter 11. Here we need only note that the restriction of dietary feedback inhibition of cholesterol synthesis to the liver in rats, and probably in many other mammalian species, seems to be due to selective uptake of a specific cholesterol-carrying lipoprotein by the liver.

In animals whose natural diet contains cholesterol, feedback inhibition of sterol synthesis by dietary cholesterol has all the hallmarks of a true physiological regulatory mechanism. The mechanism is sensitive enough to function in response to very small variations in dietary intake of cholesterol, as little as 0.1% of cholesterol in a rat's diet producing a 50% inhibition of sterol synthesis in the liver. Feedback inhibition is also of obvious benefit to the animal, since it provides the body with a means of compensating for variations in the amount of cholesterol in the food. Although inhibition of hepatic sterol synthesis is not the only mechanism available to the rat for maintaining a constant amount of cholesterol in its whole body, feedback inhibition by dietary cholesterol must make a very substantial contribution to cholesterol homeostasis. If, for example, the liver of a rat synthesized 20 mg of cholesterol per day, the animal could compensate for an increase of 20 mg in the daily absorption of dietary cholesterol by completely suppressing cholesterol synthesis in its liver. In herbivorous animals, in which feedback inhibition occurs despite the absence of cholesterol from the diet, the biological function of the mechanism may be to compensate for variations in the amount of circulating cholesterol arising from reabsorption of biliary cholesterol and from synthesis in the intestinal wall during the absorption of fat. That reabsorbed endogenous cholesterol may, indeed, exert feedback inhibition is suggested by the fact that in rats fed a cholesterol-free diet, the rate of hepatic synthesis of cholesterol is only 30–40% of the maximum attainable by cannulation of the intestinal lymphatics (Weis and Dietschy, 1969).

4.3.3 Fasting

When rats are deprived of food for more than a few hours there is a marked decrease in the rate of synthesis of cholesterol in their livers, an effect first observed by Tomkins and Chaikoff (1952) and since confirmed by many other workers. Tomkins and Chaikoff estimated cholesterol synthesis from the incorporation of [^{14}C]acetate into the sterols of liver slices incubated *in vitro*, but Gould *et al.* (1959) subsequently reported a similar, though much less marked, effect of fasting when hepatic synthesis was estimated from the incorporation of [^{14}C]acetate or ^{3}H$_2$O into liver sterols *in vivo*. Others have noted a depression of incorporation of acetate into cholesterol by cell-free preparations of liver from fasted rats under conditions in which the supply of reductive hydrogen for sterol synthesis could not have been rate-limiting (Bucher *et al.*, 1959). In rats, the inhibitory effect of fasting on cholesterol synthesis seems to be confined largely to the liver; in particular, fasting has little effect on sterol synthesis in the intestinal wall (Dietschy and Siperstein, 1967).

Unless the fasting is prolonged, there is relatively little effect on the incorporation of mevalonate into sterols by liver homogenates. This, as noted in Section 4.2.1, was one of several observations responsible for the current view that the reduction of HMG-CoA to mevalonate is the rate-limiting step in sterol biosynthesis in animal tissues. In agreement with this, fasting has been shown to cause a marked fall in the activity of HMG-CoA reductase in liver microsomes (Bucher *et al.*, 1960), detectable as early as five hours after withholding food (Regen *et al.*, 1966). As we have already seen, fasting also causes a fall in the activities of several hepatic enzymes catalyzing steps in sterol biosynthesis beyond mevalonic acid, but not to the extent that these enzymes become rate-limiting. Since the incorporation of acetate into ketone bodies is not decreased by fasting, it is unlikely that cholesterol synthesis in the livers of fasted animals is limited by the supply of carbon from acetyl-CoA or acetoacetyl-CoA. There is, however, a fall in the activity of cytosolic HMG-CoA synthase in the livers of rats fasted for 48 hours (Clinkenbeard *et al.*, 1975), but there is no evidence that the fall is sufficiently rapid or profound for the supply of cytosolic HMG-CoA to become rate-limiting for cholesterol synthesis at any time.

The mechanism by which fasting decreases the activity of hepatic HMG-CoA reductase is not understood. The fact that several hours are required for the effect to become detectable, or to be reversed on re-feeding the animal after a fast, suggests repression of enzyme synthesis. In which case, the decrease in the activity of HMG-CoA reductase, and of other enzymes catalyzing steps in the pathway to cholesterol, may be a reflection of the tendency of fasting to cause repression of the synthesis of many inducible enzymes in the liver. On the other hand, fasting may also cause inhibition of pre-existing enzyme; in this connection it may be noted that liver homogenates from fasted rats have been reported to contain a substance capable of inhibiting the incorporation of acetate into cholesterol by normal liver (Migicovsky, 1955). An inhibitory effect would be consistent with the time-course of the suppression of HMG-CoA reductase activity during fasting if it takes time for the inhibitor to reach a critical concentration in the region of the smooth endoplasmic reticulum.

4.3.4 Fat feeding

The feeding of saturated or polyunsaturated fat to rats leads to a two- to threefold increase in the incorporation of acetate into liver sterols *in vivo* and *in vitro* (Linazasoro et al., 1958). Since fat feeding also suppresses fatty-acid synthesis in the liver by inhibiting acetyl-CoA carboxylase, the stimulation of cholesterol synthesis was at first attributed to diversion of acetyl-CoA away from fatty-acid synthesis and into the sterol pathway. However, this is unlikely to be a significant factor, since cholesterol synthesis in the livers of rats given corn oil by stomach tube does not begin to increase for at least 12 hours, whereas fatty-acid synthesis begins to decrease within one hour (Hill et al., 1960). Goldfarb and Pitot (1972) have shown that in rats adapted to regulated lighting and feeding, the isocaloric addition of corn oil to the diet results in an increase in hepatic HMG-CoA reductase activity beginning during the latter half of the fasting period and lasting throughout feeding. This, presumably, is the cause of the increase in cholesterol synthesis, though it is not known whether the effect of fat is to activate the enzyme or to increase its rate of synthesis. Bortz (1973) has suggested that plasma fatty acids taken up by the liver are inducers of HMG-CoA reductase. The possible co-ordination between cholesterol synthesis, triglyceride synthesis and protein synthesis in the formation and secretion of plasma lipoproteins by the liver is considered in Chapter 11.

4.3.5 Bile salts and the enterohepatic circulation

Interruption of the enterohepatic circulation of bile salts by means of a bile fistula, an ileal bypass or the feeding of cholestyramine enhances the rate of synthesis of cholesterol in the liver. The increase in cholesterol synthesis, first demonstrated by the observation that acetate incorporation into cholesterol is increased in the livers of bile-fistula dogs (Economu et al., 1958) and rats (Myant and Eder, 1961), is accompanied by a rise in the activity of hepatic HMG-CoA reductase (Back et al., 1969). In contrast to these effects, synthesis of cholesterol in the livers of rats decreases when cholic acid is added to the diet (Beher and Baker, 1959).

There are differences of opinion as to the mechanism responsible for the effects of these experimental procedures on sterol metabolism. Weis and Dietschy (1969) were able to reverse the effects of a bile fistula on hepatic synthesis of cholesterol in rats by intravenous infusions of chylomicrons, the form in which absorbed cholesterol enters the circulation via the intestinal lymphatics, but not by intravenous or intraduodenal infusions of bile salts. They concluded that bile salts influence cholesterol synthesis in the liver not by acting *in situ*, but by enhancing the transport of biliary and intestinal cholesterol into the circulation and thus promoting feedback inhibition of cholesterol synthesis. On this interpretation, the stimulatory effect of a bile fistula on hepatic HMG-CoA reductase activity is mediated by release from the inhibition normally exerted by cholesterol transported to the liver *via* the intestinal lymphatics, and the inhibitory effect of bile-salt feeding in intact animals is due to enhanced absorption of cholesterol. In support of the view that bile salts themselves do not suppress HMG-CoA reductase in the liver by an action *in situ*, Weis and Dietschy drew attention to the fact that hepatic synthesis of cholesterol is markedly increased by ligation of the bile duct (Fredrickson *et al.*, 1954), a procedure which increases the concentration of bile salts in whole liver.

Decreased absorption of cholesterol may well contribute to the effect of a bile fistula on sterol synthesis, since complete diversion of bile from the intestinal lumen is known to abolish the absorption of cholesterol from the intestine (Siperstein *et al.*, 1952). However, it is difficult to explain the effects of cholestyramine on hepatic synthesis of cholesterol simply in terms of an effect on absorption of cholesterol from the intestine, since cholestyramine acts by interfering specifically with the reabsorption of bile salts from the ileum and has generally been found to have little effect on the absorption of cholesterol. That bile salts have a direct effect on cholesterol synthesis in the liver is shown by the experiment of Hamprecht *et al.* (1971), who found that if rats with thoracic-duct fistulae are adapted to a regulated cycle of light and darkness, the subsequent administration of cholic acid by stomach tube decreases the activity of hepatic HMG-CoA reductase during the dark phase (when enzyme activity is maximal). Since all the cholesterol absorbed from the intestine is diverted by a thoracic-duct fistula, the inhibitory effect of cholic acid observed in these experiments cannot have been mediated by increased absorption of cholesterol. In an experiment in some ways analogous to that of Hamprecht *et al.*, Mosbach (1972) showed that in rats in which hepatic HMG-CoA reductase activity has been stimulated by feeding β-sitosterol (a plant sterol which interferes with the absorption of cholesterol), the further addition of taurocholate to the diet decreases the activity of the enzyme to the control level observed in animals not fed β-sitosterol. This result is difficult to explain other than by supposing that taurocholate decreases the activity of HMG-CoA reductase in the liver by an action *in situ*.

The effect of bile acids *in situ* upon hepatic HMG-CoA reductase is apparently not due to inactivation of preformed enzyme, since the addition of physiological amounts of taurocholate to the perfusing fluid of an isolated perfused rat liver has no immediate effect on the incorporation of [^{3}H]H$_2$O into liver sterols (Liersch *et al.*, 1973). In agreement with this, the activity of HMG-CoA reductase in liver homogenates is not inhibited by adding pure bile acids to the homogenate at physiological concentrations. This suggests that the modulation of HMG-CoA reductase activity in the liver by bile salts acting *in situ* is due to repression of enzyme synthesis. This could be wholly or in part the consequence of the effect of bile acids on the activity of cholesterol 7α-hydroxylase. By repressing this enzyme, bile acids might lead to an increase in the concentration of free cholesterol in the smooth endoplasmic reticulum (the substrate for cholesterol 7α-hydroxylase) which might, in turn, affect the activity of HMG-CoA reductase by one or other of the mechanisms discussed in Section 4.3.2. Additional evidence that bile salts act within liver cells to suppress the synthesis of HMG-CoA reductase has been obtained by Barth and Hillmar (1980), who showed that taurocholate at physiological concentrations inhibits the glucocorticoid-induced rise in HMG-CoA reductase activity in monolayer cultures of rat hepatocytes.

4.3.6 Hormones

Although there is an extensive literature on the effects of hormones upon sterol synthesis in the liver (see Rodwell *et al.* (1976) for references), much of it is contradictory and hard to interpret. Part of the difficulty arises from the complexity of the interactions between different hormones, which may be antagonistic, complementary or permissive, and also from the ability of some hormones to produce effects in one tissue as a result of an action in another tissue. These factors almost certainly account for many of the discrepancies between hormonal effects observed in intact animals, those observed in animals from which various endocrine glands have been removed and those observed in perfused livers or in other types of liver preparation.

All this is, of course, familiar to every experimental endocrinologist, but much of the early work on the effects of hormones on hepatic synthesis of cholesterol is questionable for two other reasons. First, in most of the work in this field carried out before about 1970, the experiments were designed without taking account of the diurnal rhythm in hepatic HMG-CoA reductase activity, itself capable of causing a five-fold variation in the rate of sterol synthesis. Secondly, in studies based on measurement of the rate of incorporation of [^{14}C]acetate into liver sterols, the results are subject to considerable error due to variable dilution of the acetyl-CoA pool from endogenous sources (see 2.2). Since several hormones (e.g.

glucagon, thyroid hormones and the catecholamines) mobilize free fatty acids from adipose tissue, the fatty acids giving rise to acetyl-CoA in the liver, the effects *in vivo* of some hormones on the incorporation of [^{14}C]acetate into hepatic sterols may well be influenced by the nutritional state of the animal. Furthermore, since insulin suppresses fatty-acid mobilization, the acetyl-CoA pool in the liver must be affected by the presence or absence of insulin in the intact animal. In view of this, the apparent rate of synthesis of cholesterol in the livers of diabetic animals, estimated from the incorporation of [^{14}C]acetate into cholesterol *in vitro*, could be influenced by the experimental conditions under which the diabetes is produced. This may help to account for the wide disagreement as to whether hepatic synthesis of cholesterol is increased (Hotta and Chaikoff, 1952) or decreased (Haft and Miller, 1958) in the livers of diabetic rats. These and other discrepancies in the literature point to the need for a re-examination of the effects of hormones on hepatic synthesis of sterols, using methods for measuring absolute rates of

Table 8.2
Effects of some hormonal alterations on the rate of synthesis of cholesterol or the activity of HMG-CoA reductase in the liver. In almost all cases the observations were made on rats

Hormonal alteration	Effect
Insulin (in intact or diabetic animal)	Stimulates HMG-CoA reductase; necessary for diurnal rhythm in cholesterol synthesis
Diabetes	Marked diminution in HMG-CoA reductase activity, with loss of diurnal rhythm. See text for effect on cholesterol synthesis
Glucagon	Antagonizes the stimulatory action of insulin in whole animals. No effect in isolated perfused liver
Thyroid hormone	Stimulates HMG-CoA reductase and is probably necessary for the action of insulin. May act partly by potentiating the action of catecholamines
Thyroidectomy	Depresses HMG-CoA reductase activity
Glucocorticoids	Effect in intact animal is controversial (see 4.3.1). Inhibits insulin-induced increase in HMG-CoA reductase activity in diabetic rats
Adrenalectomy	Effects controversial (see 4.3.1) and probably due to combined deficiency of glucocorticoids and catecholamines
Adrenaline and noradrenaline	Stimulate HMG-CoA reductase activity in intact animals
Hypophysectomy	Abolishes diurnal rhythm and lowers HMG-CoA reductase activity
Sex hormones	Cholesterol synthesis higher in female than male rats

synthesis, in conjunction with measurement of the activity of hepatic HMG-CoA reductase.

Table 8.2 (constructed mainly from the reviews of Bortz (1973) and Rodwell *et al.* (1976)) summarizes some of the effects of hormones on cholesterol synthesis in the liver for which the evidence is reasonably secure. In most cases the evidence is based on measurement of HMG-CoA reductase activity, but in some cases an effect at the reductase step has been deduced from the fact that the incorporation of acetate into sterol is less affected by excess or deficiency of the hormone than is that of mevalonate. Several of the hormonal effects listed in Table 8.2 have already been referred to in Section 4.3.1. From what has been said above it will be obvious that any tabulation of the available information in terms of single hormones is bound to be an oversimplification of the truth.

Little can be said with certainty about the mechanisms underlying any of the effects shown in the Table. Evidence discussed in Section 4.2.2 is consistent with the possibility that insulin stimulates hepatic synthesis of cholesterol by promoting the conversion of phosphorylated HMG-CoA reductase into the active, dephosphorylated, form and that glucagon has the opposite effect. It has also been suggested that the effects of these hormones on HMG-CoA reductase are mediated by the adenyl-cyclase system, but there is no experimental evidence to support this. Stimulation of HMG-CoA reductase activity by thyroid hormone and catecholamine in the intact animal could be mediated by the increased flux of plasma free fatty acids brought about by these hormones, since fatty acids enhance the activity of HMG-CoA reductase in perfused livers (Goh and Heimberg, 1977). It should also be borne in mind that cholesterol synthesis in the liver is to some extent linked with the synthesis and secretion of plasma lipoproteins. Hence, any hormonal influence on lipoprotein secretion is likely to have an indirect effect on cholesterol synthesis. Some hormonal effects on cholesterol synthesis in isolated hepatocytes are mentioned in Chapter 9.

4.3.7 Miscellaneous effects

Whole-body X-irradiation of rats or mice leads to a twenty- to thirtyfold increase in the rate of synthesis of cholesterol in the liver, shown by increased incorporation of [^{14}C]acetate into liver sterols *in vivo* and *in vitro*, and by increased activity of hepatic HMG-CoA reductase. Gould *et al.* (1959) noted that the rise in cholesterol synthesis is accompanied by a reciprocal fall in the concentration of cholesterol in the liver, suggesting to them that the immediate cause of the increased synthesis of cholesterol is a fall in liver free cholesterol concentration. Since the response of the liver is not detectable for several hours after X-irradiation and is blocked by puromycin, it is probably mediated by induction, rather than by activation, of HMG-CoA reductase. X-irradiation also causes an increase in cholesterol synthesis in the adrenals, accompanied by a sharp fall in adrenal cholesterol concentration, suggesting that X-irradiation acts like other forms of acute stress by stimulating the conversion of cholesterol into glucocorticoids in the adrenal cortex. It is difficult to explain the increased synthesis of cholesterol in the liver entirely in terms of increased output of hormones from the adrenal glands, since the stimulatory effect of catecholamines on hepatic cholesterol synthesis is not nearly as great as that of X-irradiation, and since corticosteroids are thought by most workers to have an inhibitory, rather than a stimulatory, effect on cholesterol synthesis in the liver.

At least one other form of acute stress—hind-limb ischaemia in the fasted rat—has been shown to stimulate cholesterol synthesis in the liver (De Matteis, 1969). This, too, cannot be mediated by a primary effect on the adrenal glands, since the rise in synthesis in the liver is not prevented by removal of the adrenals.

The intravenous injection of nonionic detergents such as Triton WR-1339 (a polyoxyethylene polymer) causes marked hypercholesterolaemia and an increased rate of sterol synthesis in the liver (Frantz and Hinkelman, 1955) and in many other tissues, particularly the adrenals (Andersen and Dietschy, 1977). The increase in sterol synthesis in the liver is accompanied by increased activity of HMG-CoA reductase (Bucher et al., 1960). Although the hypercholesterolaemia is due partly to accumulation of triglyceride-rich lipoproteins in the plasma owing to the inhibition of lipoprotein lipase by the detergent, it seems likely that there is also a redistribution of cholesterol from the liver into the plasma, since the liver cholesterol concentration falls while the rate of synthesis of cholesterol is rising (Hirsch and Kellner, 1956). If the redistribution involves a net loss of free cholesterol from the subcellular membranes to which HMG-CoA reductase is attached, this might be expected to lead to an increase in enzyme activity, as discussed in Section 4.3.2. A mechanism similar in principle to this could also be responsible for the observation of Jakoi and Quarfordt (1974) that intravenous infusions of lecithin into rats lead to a fall in the concentration of microsomal cholesterol in the liver, with a concomitant rise in hepatic HMG-CoA reductase activity.

The effects of some drugs on sterol synthesis in the liver may be mentioned briefly in this Section. Clofibrate (the ethyl ester of p-chlorophenoxyisobutyrate) and nicotinic acid are used clinically for lowering the plasma cholesterol concentration in hypercholesterolaemic patients. Both drugs inhibit cholesterol synthesis in the liver, but in neither case is this the complete explanation of the effect of the drug on the plasma cholesterol (for reviews see Steinberg (1970) and Gey and Carlson (1971)). Phenobarbital, a drug known to induce several enzymes associated with the endoplasmic reticulum of the liver, enhances hepatic synthesis of cholesterol from acetate (Jones and Armstrong, 1965), probably by induction of HMG-CoA reductase. The stimulatory effect of cholestyramine upon sterol synthesis in the liver has already been referred to (Section 4.3.5). β-Sitosterol, also used in the treatment of human hypercholesterolaemia, has a similar effect upon sterol synthesis in the liver by interfering with the absorption of dietary and endogenous cholesterol from the small intestine.

In the course of a general search for drugs likely to be of use in the treatment of hypercholesterolaemia, many compounds which inhibit various steps in the biosynthesis of cholesterol have been discovered. Although the great majority have been found to be unsuitable as therapeutic agents, usually because of their side-effects or because they are inactive in the whole organism, some have been useful in the study of sterol biosynthesis (see, for example, 2.5). Some of these inhibitors are discussed in a review by Dempsey (1969). Some other physiological factors that influence cholesterol synthesis in the liver are considered in the section dealing with developmental aspects of sterol metabolism (Chapter 6).

4.4 Regulation in the intestinal wall

A diurnal rhythm in HMG-CoA reductase activity is detectable in the rat's intestine (see Section 4.3.1).

In mammals, cholesterol synthesis in the small intestine differs from that in the liver in that intestinal synthesis is inhibited only to a small extent by fasting and is uninfluenced by cholesterol feeding, even if the feeding is prolonged for several weeks. In non-mammalian vertebrates, however, cholesterol feeding readily inhibits cholesterol synthesis in the intestine (Siperstein, 1970). Bile acids in the lumen of the gut inhibit the intestinal synthesis of cholesterol (see Wilson (1972) for review). In bile-fistula rats the rate of incorporation of [^{14}C]acetate into cholesterol in all segments of the small intestine is several times greater than that in intact animals and the increased rate of cholesterol synthesis in the bile-fistula animals is suppressed by intraduodenal infusion of whole bile or of taurocholate or other bile salts. A similar inhibitory effect of biliary bile acids on cholesterol synthesis in the wall of the small intestine occurs in man and in monkeys. Cholesterol synthesis in the wall of the rat's intestine increases after an intravenous injection of Triton 1339 or when the plasma lipoprotein concentration is lowered by administration of 4-aminopyrazolopyrimidine (4-APP). The possible relevance of these effects to the regulation of cholesterol synthesis under physiological conditions is discussed in Section 4.5.

Phenobarbital has a specific stimulatory effect on the incorporation of [^{14}C]acetate into cholesterol in the rat's small intestine *in vitro*, though the effect is less than that seen in the liver (Middleton and Isselbacher, 1969).

4.5 Regulation in other tissues

Investigations of the regulation of cholesterol synthesis in animal tissues carried out in the 1950's and 1960's were confined largely to the liver and intestine. Some attention was also paid to the adrenals and gonads at the intracellular level (see Chapter 5), but these tissues were rightly regarded as special cases in view of their need to regulate the production of steroid hormones in response to the variable stimuli of stress and reproduction. In most species, cholesterol synthesis in many tissues was found to be considerably lower than that in the liver and intestinal wall (see Table 8.1) and to show little if any response to various procedures which had a marked effect upon sterol synthesis in the liver or intestine. For example, in rats the feeding of cholesterol has little effect on sterol synthesis in any extrahepatic tissue, interference with the enterohepatic circulation of bile salts has little or no effect on tissues other than liver or intestine and the effects of fasting and of a diurnal rhythm are much more marked in the liver than in any other tissue. These and other differences in the responses of various tissues to physiological and unphysiological stimuli are listed in Table 8.3. The effects of several hormones (e.g. thyroxine, insulin and the catecholamines) on sterol synthesis have also been found to be generally more marked in the liver than in other tissues.

The view that emerged from these findings, and from the unique ability of the liver to metabolize cholesterol to bile acids at a variable rate, was that the regulation of the amount of cholesterol in the body as a whole is centred in the liver. The corollary to this was the idea that the extrahepatic tissues (with the possible exception of the intestine) receive from the liver the bulk of the cholesterol they need for maintenance of their membranes and that they lack the ability to synthesize their own sterol.

This view of the central role of the liver in cholesterol homeostasis is still broadly acceptable. As discussed above, the mechanisms which enable the liver to respond rapidly to changes in the amount of cholesterol absorbed from the diet by altering its rate of synthesis (Section 4.3.2, this chapter) or degradation (Section 1.4.2, Chapter 5) of cholesterol must help to maintain whole-body homeostasis of cholesterol under physiological conditions. However, the view that the cells of extrahepatic tissues other than the intestine are incapable of synthesizing cholesterol has had to be modified. This change of outlook came about primarily as a result of attempts to understand how cholesterol molecules move into and out of mammalian cells. It soon became clear, from studies *in vitro*, that nonhepatic cells of various types develop the capacity to synthesize cholesterol from acetate when they are suspended or cultured in a medium deficient in cholesterol-containing lipoproteins. This has led to the discovery of complex regulatory mechanisms by means of which the cells of some tissues, when maintained *in vitro*, adjust their

Table 8.3
The effects of some experimental procedures upon cholesterol synthesis in the liver, intestine and other tissues of rats

Procedure	Liver	Gut	Kidney	Lung	Adrenal	Ovary	Muscle	Adipose	Spleen	Skin
Cholesterol feeding	⇊	↑	↑	↑	↑		↑	↑	↑	↑
Bile fistula or cholestyramine	⇈	⇈	↑	↑	←	←	↑	↑	↑	↑
Fasting	⇊	→	→	↑	→	↑	↑	↑	↑	↑
Diurnal cycle (dark)	⇈	←	↑	↑	←	↑	↑	↑	↑	↑
Stress (including X-irradiation)	⇈	↑	↑	↑	⇈	↑	↑	↑	↑	↑
Chylomicron remnants	⇊	←	←	←	⇈	←	↑	↑	←	↑
Triton 1339	⇈	←	←	←	⇈		↑	←	←	←
4-APP	↑									

Double vertical arrow = marked effect; single vertical arrow = slight or moderate effect; horizontal arrow = no effect.

The Table is constructed from various sources referred to in the text. The evidence for most of the effects listed is based on changes in the rate of incorporation of [^{14}C]acetate or [^{3}H]H$_2$O into digitonin-precipitable sterols *in vitro* in tissues taken from animals given the various treatments *in vivo*. In many cases a change in HMG-CoA reductase activity was also observed.

Notes on the procedures listed:
(1) Effects of stress were usually observed in fasted animals and in some cases were not apparent in fed animals.
(2) Chylomicron remnants (see Chapter 11) were given by intravenous infusion.
(3) 4-APP = 4-aminopyrazolopyrimidine. The drug was given in doses sufficient to lower the plasma cholesterol concentration to less than 10% of the control value. Since the increase in cholesterol synthesis observed in gut, kidney, lung, adrenal, ovary and skin can be reversed by infusion of homologous or human plasma lipoproteins, the effect of the drug on tissue cholesterol synthesis is assumed to be mediated by a fall in plasma lipoprotein concentration.
(4) Effects of hormones are not included in the Table. For hormonal effects on cholesterol synthesis in the liver, see Section 4.3.6.

synthesis of cholesterol in accordance with the supply of cholesterol in the extracellular medium. In several types of human cell (Goldstein and Brown, 1977), the mouse adrenal cell (Faust *et al.*, 1977) and probably in several other types of animal cell, an essential part of this regulatory system is the ability to develop cell-surface receptors with high affinity for a specific lipoprotein.

When the plasma cholesterol concentration in rats is lowered by administration of the drug 4-APP, cholesterol synthesis and HMG-CoA reductase activity increase several-fold in a number of tissues other than the liver (Balasubramaniam *et al.*, 1976; Andersen and Dietschy, 1976), the increase being most marked in the adrenals. Of particular interest is the concomitant induction of HMG-CoA reductase and cytosolic HMG-CoA synthase in adrenal cortex of 4-APP-treated rats (Balasubramaniam *et al.*, 1977). In at least six of the tissues listed in the last line of Table 8.3, the increase in cholesterol synthesis brought about by treatment with 4-APP is reversed by intravenous infusion of a fraction of rat serum containing all the lipoproteins (density < 1.23 g/ml). This suggests that the effect of the 4-APP is to stimulate cholesterol synthesis in several extrahepatic tissues of the rat by lowering the concentration of plasma lipoproteins present in the interstitial fluid surrounding the surfaces of the tissue cells and, hence, that under physiological conditions cholesterol synthesis in these cells is normally suppressed. This possibility is considered in more detail in Chapter 9.

REFERENCES

Andersen, J. M. and Dietschy, J. M. (1976). Cholesterogenesis: depression in extrahepatic tissues with 4-aminopyrazolo[3,4-d]pyrimidine. *Science*, **193**, 903–905.

Andersen, J. M. and Dietschy, J. M. (1977). Regulation of sterol synthesis in 16 tissues of rat. 1. Effect of diurnal light cyclic, fasting, stress, manipulation of enterohepatic circulation, and administration of chylomicrons and triton. *Journal of Biological Chemistry*, **252**, 3646–3651.

Back, P., Hamprecht, B. and Lynen, F. (1969). Regulation of cholesterol biosynthesis in rat liver: diurnal changes of activity and influence of bile acids. *Archives of Biochemistry and Biophysics*, **133**, 11–21.

Balasubramaniam, S., Goldstein, J. L. and Brown, M. S. (1977). Regulation of cholesterol synthesis in rat adrenal gland through coordinate control of 3-hydroxy-3-methylglutaryl coenzyme A synthase and reductase activities. *Proceedings of the National Academy of Sciences of the USA*, **74**, 1421–1425.

Balasubramaniam, S., Goldstein, J. L., Faust, J. R. and Brown, M. S. (1976). Evidence for regulation of 3-hydroxy-3-methylglutaryl coenzyme A reductase activity and cholesterol synthesis in nonhepatic tissues of rat. *Proceedings of the National Academy of Sciences of the USA*, **73**, 2564–2568.

Barth, C. A. and Hillmar, I. (1980). Taurocholate inhibits the glucocorticoid-induced rise of 3-hydroxy-3-methylglutaryl-CoA reductase in primary culture of hepatocytes. *European Journal of Biochemistry*, **110**, 237–240.

Beg, Z. H., Allman, D. W. and Gibson, D. M. (1973). Modulation of 3-hydroxy-3-methylglutaryl coenzyme A reductase activity with cAMP and with protein fractions of rat liver cytosol. *Biochemical and Biophysical Research Communications*, **54**, 1362–1369.
Beg, Z. H., Stonik, J. A. and Brewer, H. B. (1978). 3-Hydroxy-3-methylglutaryl coenzyme A reductase: regulation of enzymatic activity by phosphorylation and dephosphorylation. *Proceedings of the National Academy of Sciences of the USA*, **75**, 3678–3682.
Beg, Z. H., Stonik, J. A. and Brewer, H. B. Jr. (1979). Characterization and regulation of reductase kinase, a protein kinase that modulates the enzymic activity of 3-hydroxy-3-methylglutaryl-coenzyme A reductase. *Proceedings of the National Academy of Sciences of the USA*, **76**, 4375–4379.
Beher, W. T. and Baker, G. D. (1959). Inhibition of cholesterol biosynthesis by cholic acid. *American Journal of Physiology*, **197**, 1339–1340.
Beirne, O. R. and Watson, J. A. (1976). Comparison of regulation of 3-hydroxy-3-methylglutaryl coenzyme A reductase in hepatoma cells grown *in vivo* and *in vitro*. *Proceedings of the National Academy of Sciences of the USA*, **73**, 2735–2739.
Berndt, J., Hegardt, F. G., Bove, J., Gaumert, R., Still, J. and Cardó, M.-T. (1976). Activation of 3-hydroxy-3-methylglutaryl-coenzyme A reductase *in vitro*. Hoppe-Seyler's Zeitschrift für physiologische Chemie, **357**, 1277–1282.
Bhattathiry, E. P. M. and Siperstein, M. D. (1963). Feedback control of cholesterol synthesis in man. *Journal of Clinical Investigation*, **42**, 1613–1618.
Bissell, D. M., Hammaker, L. E. and Meyer, U. A. (1973). Parenchymal cells from adult rat liver in nonproliferating monolayer culture. 1. Functional studies. *Journal of Cell Biology*, **59**, 722–723.
Bloch, K., Borek, E. and Rittenberg, D. (1946). Synthesis of cholesterol in surviving liver. *Journal of Biological Chemistry*, **162**, 441–449.
Bortz, W. M. (1973). On the control of cholesterol synthesis. *Metabolism*, **22**, 1507–1524.
Brown, M. S., Brannan, P. G., Bohmfalk, H. A., Brunschede, G. Y., Dana, S. E., Helgeson, J. and Goldstein, J. L. (1975). Use of mutant fibroblasts in the analysis of the regulation of cholesterol metabolism in human cells. *Journal of Cellular Physiology*, **85**, 425–436.
Brown, M. S., Dana, S. E., Dietschy, J. M. and Siperstein, M. D. (1973). 3-Hydroxy-3-methylglutaryl coenzyme A reductase. Solubilization and purification of a cold-sensitive microsomal enzyme. *Journal of Biological Chemistry*, **248**, 4731–4738.
Brown, M. S., Goldstein, J. L. and Dietschy, J. M. (1979). Active and inactive forms of 3-hydroxy-3-methylglutaryl coenzyme A reductase in the liver of the rat. *Journal of Biological Chemistry*, **254**, 5144–5149.
Brunengraber, H., Sabine, J. R., Boutry, M. and Lowenstein, J. M. (1972). 3-β-Hydroxysterol synthesis by the liver. *Archives of Biochemistry and Biophysics*, **150**, 392–396.
Bucher, N. L. R. (1953). The formation of radioactive cholesterol and fatty acids from C^{14}-labelled acetate by rat liver homogenates. *Journal of the American Chemical Society*, **75**, 498.
Bucher, N. L. R. and McGarrahan, K. (1956). The biosynthesis of cholesterol from acetate-1-C^{14} by cellular fractions of rat liver. *Journal of Biological Chemistry*, **222**, 1–15.
Bucher, N. L. R., McGarrahan, K., Gould, E. and Loud, A. V. (1959). Cholesterol biosynthesis in preparations of liver from normal, fasting, X-irradiated, cholesterol-fed, Triton, Δ^4-cholesten-3-one-treated rats. *Journal of Biological Chemistry*, **234**, 262–267.
Bucher, N. L. R., Overath, P. and Lynen, F. (1960). β-Hydroxy-β-methylglutaryl coenzyme A reductase, cleavage and condensing enzymes in relation to cholesterol formation in rat liver. *Biochimica et Biophysica Acta*, **40**, 491–501.

Chobanian, A. V. (1968). Sterol synthesis in the human arterial intima. *Journal of Clinical Investigation*, **47**, 595–603.
Clinkenbeard, K. D., Sugiyama, T., Reed, W. D. and Lane, M. D. (1975). Cytoplasmic 3-hydroxy-3-methylglutaryl Coenzyme A synthase from liver. Purification, properties, and role in cholesterol synthesis. *Journal of Biological Chemistry*, **250**, 3124–3135.
Dempsey, M. The effect of hypoglycemic agents on cholesterol biosynthesis. In: *Drugs Affecting Lipid Metabolism*. Ed. W. L. Holmes, L. A. Carlson and R. Paoletti. Plenum Press, New York, pp. 511–520, 1969.
Dietschy, J. M. and Brown, M. S. (1974). Effect of alterations of the specific activity of the intracellular acetyl CoA pool on apparent rates of hepatic cholesterogenesis. *Journal of Lipid Research*, **15**, 508–516.
Dietschy, J. M. and Gamel, W. G. (1971). Cholesterol synthesis in the intestine of man: regional differences and control mechanisms. *Journal of Clinical Investigation*, **50**, 872–880.
Dietschy, J. M. and McGarry, J. D. (1974). Limitations of acetate as a substrate for measuring cholesterol synthesis in liver. *Journal of Biological Chemistry*, **249**, 52–58.
Dietschy, J. M. and Siperstein, M. D. (1967). Effect of cholesterol feeding and fasting on sterol synthesis in seventeen tissues of the rat. *Journal of Lipid Research*, **8**, 97–104.
Dietschy, J. M. and Wilson, J. D. (1968). Cholesterol synthesis in the squirrel monkey: relative rates of synthesis in various tissues and mechanisms of control. *Journal of Clinical Investigation*, **47**, 166–174.
Dixon, M. and Webb, E. C. *Enzymes*. 2nd Edition, Longman, London, pp. 158–161, 1964.
Economu, S. G., Tews, B. J. and Taylor, C. B. and Cox, C. E. (1958). Studies on lipid metabolism in dogs with altered biliary physiology. *Surgical Forum*, **8**, 218–221.
Edwards, P. A. (1973). Effect of adrenalectomy and hypophysectomy on the circadian rhythm of β-hydroxy-β-methylglutaryl coenzyme A reductase activity in rat liver. *Journal of Biological Chemistry*, **248**, 2912–2917.
Edwards, P. A. and Gould, R. G. (1974). Dependence of the circadian rhythm of hepatic β-hydroxy-β-methylglutaryl coenzyme A on ribonucleic acid synthesis. A possible second site of inhibition by dietary cholesterol. *Journal of Biological Chemistry*, **249**, 2891–2896.
Edwards, P. A., Muroya, H. and Gould, R. G. (1972). In vivo demonstration of the circadian rhythm of cholesterol biosynthesis in the liver and intestine of the rat. *Journal of Lipid Research*, **13**, 396–401.
Edwards, P. A., Popják, G., Fogelman, A. M. and Edmond, J. (1977). Control of 3-hydroxy-3-methylglutaryl coenzyme A reductase by endogenously synthesized sterols *in vitro* and *in vivo*. *J. Biol. Chem.*, **252**, 1057–1063.
Faust, J. R., Goldstein, J. L. and Brown, M. S. (1977). Receptor-mediated uptake of low density lipoprotein and utilization of its cholesterol for steroid synthesis in cultured mouse adrenal cells. *Journal of Biological Chemistry*, **252**, 4861–4871.
Fogelman, A. M., Edmond, J. and Popják, G. (1975). Metabolism of mevalonate in rats and man not leading to sterols. *Journal of Biological Chemistry*, **250**, 1771–1775.
Fogelman, A. M., Edmond, J., Seager, J. and Popják, G. (1975). Abnormal induction of 3-hydroxy-3-methylglutaryl coenzyme A reductase in leukocytes from subjects with heterozygous familial hypercholesterolemia. *Journal of Biological Chemistry*, **250**, 2045–2055.
Frantz, I. D. and Hinkelman, B. T. (1955). Acceleration of hepatic cholesterol synthesis by Triton WR-1339. *Journal of Experimental Medicine*, **101**, 225–232.
Fredrickson, D. S., Loud, A. V., Hinkelman, B. T., Schneider, H. S. and Frantz, I. D. (1954). The effect of ligation of the common bile-duct on cholesterol synthesis in the rat. *Journal of Experimental Medicine*, **99**, 43–53.
Gaylor, J. L. Enzymes in sterol biosynthesis. In: *MTP International Review of Science*,

Biochemistry, Series One, Vol. 4, *Biochemistry of Lipids*. Ed. T. W. Goodwin. Butterworth, London, pp. 1–37, 1974.
Gey, K. F. and Carlson, L. A. Metabolic Effects of Nicotinic Acid and its Derivatives. Hans Huber, Bern, Switzerland, 1971.
Gibbons, G. F. and Pullinger, C. R. (1977) Measurement of the absolute rates of cholesterol biosynthesis in isolated rat liver cells. *Biochemical Journal*, **163**, 321–330.
Gibbons, G. F. and Pullinger, C. R. (1979). Utilization of endogenous and exogenous sources of substrates for cholesterol biosynthesis by isolated hepatocytes. *Biochemical Journal*, **177**, 255–263.
Gibson, D. M. and Ingebritsen, T. S. (1978). Minireview. Reversible modulation of liver hydroxymethylglutaryl CoA reductase. *Life Sciences*, **23**, 2649–2664.
Goh, E. H. and Heimberg, M. (1977). Effects of free fatty acids on activity of hepatic microsomal 3-hydroxy-3-methylglutaryl coenzyme A reductase. *Journal of Biological Chemistry*, **252**, 2822–2826.
Goldfarb, S. and Pitot, H. C. (1971). The regulation of β-hydroxy-β-methylglutaryl coenzyme A reductase in Morris hepatomas 5123C, 7800, and 9618A. *Cancer Research*, **31**, 1879–1882.
Goldfarb, S. and Pitot, H. C. (1972). Stimulatory effect of dietary lipid and cholestyramine on hepatic HMG CoA reductase. *Journal of Lipid Research*, **13**, 797–801.
Goldstein, J. L. and Brown, M. S. (1977). The low-density lipoprotein pathway and its relation to atherosclerosis. *Annual Review of Biochemistry*, **46**, 879–930.
Gould, R. G. (1951). Lipid metabolism and atherosclerosis. *American Journal of Medicine*, **11**, 209–227.
Gould, R. G. Biosynthesis of cholesterol. In: *Cholesterol. Chemistry, Biochemistry and Pathology.* Ed. R. P. Cook. Academic Press, New York, pp. 209–235, 1958.
Gould, R. G. The relationship between thyroid hormones and cholesterol biosynthesis and turnover. In: *Hormones and Atherosclerosis*. Ed. G. Pincus. Academic Press, New York, pp. 75–88, 1959.
Gould, R. G. Some aspects of the control of hepatic cholesterol biosynthesis. In: *Cholesterol Metabolism and Lipolytic Enzymes*. Ed. J. Polonovsky. Masson Publishing U.S.A., New York, pp. 13–38, 1977.
Gould, R. G., Bell, V. L. and Lilly, E. H. (1959). Stimulation of cholesterol biosynthesis from acetate in rat liver and adrenals by whole body X-irradiation. *American Journal of Physiology*, **196**, 1231–1237.
Gould, R. G. and Popják, G. (1957). Biosynthesis of cholesterol *in vivo* and *in vitro* from DL-β-hydroxy-β-methyl-δ-[2-^{14}C]-valerolactone. *Biochemical Journal*, **66**, 51P.
Gould, R. G. and Swyryd, E. A. (1966). Sites of control of hepatic cholesterol biosynthesis. *Journal of Lipid Research*, **7**, 698–707.
Haft, D. E. and Miller, L. L. (1958). Alloxan diabetes and demonstrated direct action of insulin on metabolism of isolated perfused rat liver. *American Journal of Physiology*, **192**, 33–42.
Hamprecht, B., Roscher, R., Waltinger, G. and Nüssler, C. (1971). Influence of bile acids on the activity of rat liver 3-hydroxy-3-methylglutaryl coenzyme A reductase. 2. Effect of cholic acid in lymph fistula rats. *European Journal of Biochemistry*, **18**, 15–19.
Harry, D. S., Dini, M. and McIntyre, N. (1973). Effect of cholesterol feeding and biliary obstruction on hepatic cholesterol biosynthesis in the rat. *Biochimica et Biophysica Acta*, **296**, 209–220.
Heller, R. A. and Gould, R. G. (1974). Reversible cold inactivation of microsomal 3-hydroxy-3-methylglutaryl coenzyme A reductase from rat liver. *Journal of Biological Chemistry*, **249**, 5254–5260.
Hellström, K. H., Siperstein, M. D., Bricker, L. A. and Luby, L. J. (1973). Studies of the

in vivo metabolism of mevalonic acid in the normal rat. *Journal of Clinical Investigation*, **52**, 1303–1313.

Hickman, P. E., Horton, B. J. and Sabine, J. R. (1972). Effect of adrenalectomy on the diurnal variation of hepatic cholesterogenesis in the rat. *Journal of Lipid Research*, **13**, 17–22.

Higgins, M. and Rudney, H. (1973). Regulation of rat liver β-hydroxy-β-methylglutaryl-CoA reductase activity by cholesterol. *Nature (New Biology)*, **246**, 60–61.

Hill, R., Webster, W. W., Linazosoro, J. M. and Chaikoff, I. L. (1960). Time of occurrence of changes in the liver's capacity to utilize acetate for fatty acid and cholesterol synthesis after fat feeding. *Journal of Lipid Research*, **1**, 150–153.

Hirsch, R. L. and Kellner, A. (1956). The pathogenesis of hyperlipemia induced by means of surface-active agents. II. Failure of exchange of cholesterol between the plasma and the liver in rabbits given Triton WR 1339. *Journal of Experimental Medicine*, **104**, 15–24.

Hotta, S. and Chaikoff, I. L. (1952). Cholesterol synthesis from acetate in the diabetic liver. *Journal of Biological Chemistry*, **198**, 895–899.

Hotta, S. and Chaikoff, I. L. (1955). The role of the liver in the turnover of plasma cholesterol. *Archives of Biochemistry*, **56**, 28–37.

Hsia, S. L., Fulton, J. E. Jr., Fulghum, D. and Buch, M. M. (1970). Lipid synthesis from acetate-1-^{14}C by suction blister epidermis and other skin components. *Proceedings of the Society for Experimental Biology and Medicine*, **135**, 285–291.

Huber, J., Hamprecht, B., Müller, O.-A. and Guder, W. (1972). Tageszeitlicher Rhythmus der Hydroxymethylglutaryl-CoA-Reduktase in der Rattenleber, II. *Hoppe Seyler's Zeitschrift für physiologische Chemie*, **353**, 313–317.

Ingebritsen, T. S., Geelen, M. J. H., Parker, R. A., Evensen, K. J. and Gibson, D. M. (1979). Modulation of hydroxymethylglutaryl-CoA reductase activity, reductase kinase activity, and cholesterol synthesis in rat hepatocytes in response to insulin and glucagon. *Journal of Biological Chemistry*, **254**, 9986–9989.

Ingebritsen, T. S., Lee, H.-S., Parker, R. A. and Gibson, D. M. (1978). Reversible modulation of the activities of both liver microsomal hydroxymethylglutaryl coenzyme A reductase and its inactivating enzyme. Evidence for regulation by phosphorylation-dephosphorylation. *Biochemical and Biophysical Research Communications*, **81**, 1268–1277.

Jakoi, L. and Quarfordt, S. H. (1974). The induction of hepatic cholesterol synthesis in the rat by lecithin mesophase infusions. *Journal of Biological Chemistry*, **249**, 5840–5844.

Jeske, D. J. and Dietschy, J. M. (1980). Regulation of rates of cholesterol synthesis *in vivo* in the liver and carcass of the rat measured using [^{3}H]water. *Journal of Lipid Research*, **21**, 364–376.

Johnston, D. and Cavenee, W. K., Ramachandran, C. K. and Melnykovych, G. (1979). Cholesterol biosynthesis in a variety of cultured cells. Lack of correlation between synthesis and activity of 3-hydroxy-3-methylglutaryl coenzyme A reductase caused by dexamethasone. *Biochimica et Biophysica Acta*, **572**, 188–192.

Jones, A. L. and Armstrong, D. T. (1965). Increased cholesterol biosynthesis following phenobarbital induced hypertrophy of agranular endoplasmic reticulum in liver. *Proceedings of the Society for Experimental Biology and Medicine*, **119**, 1136–1139.

Jungas, R. L, (1968). Fatty acid synthesis in adipose tissue incubated in tritiated water. *Biochemistry*, **6**, 3708–3717.

Kawaguchi, A. (1970). Control of ergosterol biosynthesis in yeast. *Journal of Biochemistry* (Tokyo), **67**, 219–227.

Kayden, H. J., Hatam, L. and Beratis, N. G. (1976). Regulation of 3-hydroxy-3-methylglutaryl coenzyme A reductase activity and the esterification of cholesterol in human long term lymphoid cell lines. *Biochemistry*, **15**, 521–528.

Liersch, M. E. A., Barth, C. A., Hackenschmidt, H. J., Ullmann, H. L. and Decker, K. F. A. (1973). Influence of bile salts on cholesterol synthesis in the isolated perfused rat liver. *European Journal of Biochemistry*, **32**, 365–371.
Linazasoro, J. M., Hill, R., Chevallier, F. and Chaikoff, I. L. (1958). Regulation of cholesterol synthesis in the liver: the influence of dietary fat. *Journal of Experimental Medicine*, **107**, 813–820.
Lindsey, C. A. and Wilson, J. D. (1965). Evidence for a contribution by the intestinal wall to the serum cholesterol of the rat. *Journal of Lipid Research*, **6**, 173–181.
Linn, T. C. (1967). The effect of cholesterol feeding and fasting upon β-hydroxy-β-methylglutaryl coenzyme A reductase. *Journal of Biological Chemistry*, **242**, 990–993.
de Matteis, F. (1969). Liver cholesterol metabolism following trauma. Evidence for increased rate of cholesterol synthesis and breakdown. *Biochimica et Biophysica Acta*, **187**, 422–434.
Mendelsohn, D. and Mendelsohn, L. (1972). The biosynthesis of cholesterol in human skin: a comparison between normal and hyperlipoproteinaemic subjects. *South African Medical Journal*, **46**, 229.
Middleton, W. R. J. and Isselbacher, K. J. (1969). The stimulation of intestinal cholesterogenesis in the rat by phenobarbital. *Proceedings of the Society for Experimental Biology and Medicine*, **131**, 1435–1437.
Miettinen, T. A. (1970). Detection of changes in human cholesterol metabolism. *Annals of Clinical Biochemistry*, **2**, 300–320.
Migicovsky, B. B. (1955). Inhibition of cholesterol formation by rat liver homogenates. *Canadian Journal of Biochemistry and Physiology*, **33**, 135–138.
Mitropoulos, K. A. and Balasubramaniam, S. (1976). The rôle of glucocorticoids in the regulation of the diurnal rhythm of hepatic β-hydroxy-β-methylglutaryl coenzyme-A reductase and cholesterol 7α-hydroxylase. *Biochemical Journal*, **160**, 49–55.
Mitropoulos, K. A. and Venkatesan, S. (1977). The influence of cholesterol on the activity, on the isothermic kinetics and on the temperature-induced kinetics of 3-hydroxy-3-methylglutaryl coenzyme A reductase. *Biochimica et Biophysica Acta*, **489**, 126–142.
Moutafis, C. D. and Myant, N. B. (1976). The distribution of [^{14}C]cholesterol in muscle and skin of Rhesus monkeys after intravenous injection. *Clinical Science and Molecular Medicine*, **50**, 307–310.
Mosbach, E. H. Regulation of bile acid synthesis. In: *Bile Acids in Human Diseases*, II. Ed. P. Back and W. Gerok. F. K. Schattauer Verlag, Stuttgart, pp. 89–96, 1972.
Muroya, H., Sodhi, H. S. and Gould, R. G. (1977). Sterol synthesis in intestinal villi and crypt cells of rats and guinea pigs. *Journal of Lipid Research*, **18**, 301–308.
Myant, N. B. The regulation of cholesterol metabolism as related to familial hypercholesterolaemia. In: *The Scientific Basis of Medicine Annual Reviews*, pp. 230–259, 1970.
Myant, N. B. and Eder, H. A. (1961). The effect of biliary drainage upon the synthesis of cholesterol in the liver. *Journal of Lipid Research*, **2**, 363–368.
Myant, N. B. and Mitropoulos, K. A. (1977). Cholesterol 7α-hydroxylase. *Journal of Lipid Research*, **18**, 135–153.
Newman, H. A. I. and Zilversmit, D. B. (1961). The origin of cholesterol and cholesterol ester of rabbit atheroma. *Federation Proceedings*, **20**, 92.
Nicolaides, N., Reiss, O. K. and Langdon, R. G. (1955). Studies of the *in vitro* lipid metabolism of the human skin. I. Biosynthesis in scalp skin. *Journal of the American Chemical Society*, **77**, 1535–1538.
Nilsson, Å. (1975). Increased cholesterol-ester formation during forced cholesterol synthesis in rat hepatocytes. *European Journal of Biochemistry*, **51**, 337–342.
Nimmo, G. A. and Cohen, P. (1978). The regulation of glycogen metabolism. Phosphorylation of inhibitor-1 from rabbit skeletal muscle, and its interaction with protein phosphatases -III and -II. *European Journal of Biochemistry*, **87**, 353–365.

Nordstrom, J. L., Rodwell, V. W. and Mitschelen, J. J. (1977). Interconversion of active and inactive forms of rat liver hydroxymethylglutaryl-CoA reductase. *Journal of Biological Chemistry*, **252**, 8924–8934.

Philipp, B. W. and Shapiro, D. J. (1979). Improved methods for the assay and activation of 3-hydroxy-3-methylglutaryl coenzyme A reductase. *Journal of Lipid Research*, **20**, 588–593.

Popják, G. (1977). 'As I remember it'. Research on biosynthesis of fatty acids, triglycerides, squalene, and cholesterol. *Journal of the American Oil Chemists' Society*, **54**, 647A–655A.

Regen, D., Riepertinger, C., Hamprecht, B. and Lynen, F. (1966). The measurement of β-hydroxy-β-methyl-glutaryl-CoA reductase in rat liver; effects of fasting and refeeding. *Biochemische Zeitschrift*, **346**, 78–84.

Riggs, D. S. Feedback: fundamental relationship or frame of mind? In: *Advances in Enzyme Regulation*, Vol. 5. Ed. G. Weber. Pergamon Press, Oxford, pp. 357–382, 1967.

Rittenberg, D. and Schoenheimer, R. (1937). Deuterium as an indicator in the study of intermediary metabolism. XI. Further studies of the biological uptake of deuterium into organic substances, with special reference to fat and cholesterol formation. *Journal of Biological Chemistry*, **121**, 235–253.

Robinson, J. L. and Rose, I. A. (1972). The proton transfer reactions of muscle pyruvate kinase. *Journal of Biological Chemistry*, **247**, 1096–1105.

Rodwell, V. W., McNamara, D. J. and Shapiro, D. J. (1973). Regulation of hepatic 3-hydroxy-3-methylglutaryl-coenzyme A reductase. *Advances in Enzymology*, **38**, 373–412.

Rodwell, V. W., Nordstrom, J. L. and Mitschelen, J. J. (1976). Regulation of HMG-CoA reductase. *Advances in Lipid Research*, **14**, 1–74.

Sabine, J. R. and James, M. J. (1976). The intracellular mechanism responsible for dietary feedback control of cholesterol synthesis. *Life Sciences*, **18**, 1185–1192.

St. Clair, R. W. (1976). Metabolism of the arterial wall and atherosclerosis. *Atherosclerosis Reviews*, **1**, 61–117.

Sakakida, H., Shediac, C. C. and Siperstein, M. D. (1963). Effect of endogenous and exogenous cholesterol on the feedback control of cholesterol synthesis. *Journal of Clinical Investigation*, **42**, 1521–1528.

Shapiro, D. J. and Rodwell, V. W. (1971). Regulation of hepatic 3-hydroxy-3-methylglutaryl coenzyme A reductase and cholesterol synthesis. *Journal of Biological Chemistry*, **246**, 3210–3216.

Shefer, S., Hauser, S., Lapar, V. and Mosbach, E. H. (1972). Diurnal variation of HMG-CoA reductase activity in rat intestine. *Journal of Lipid Research*, **13**, 571–573.

Siperstein, M. D. Regulation of cholesterol biosynthesis in normal and malignant tissues. In: *Current Topics in Cellular Regulation*, Vol. 2. Ed. B. L. Horecker and E. R. Stadtman. Academic Press, New York, pp. 65–100, 1970.

Siperstein, M. D., Chaikoff, I. L. and Reinhardt, W. O. (1952). C^{14}-Cholesterol. V. Obligatory function of bile in intestinal absorption of cholesterol. *Journal of Biological Chemistry*, **198**, 111–114.

Siperstein, M. D. and Fagan, V. M. (1964). Studies on the feed-back regulation of cholesterol synthesis. *Advances in Enzyme Regulation*, **2**, 249–264.

Siperstein, M. D. and Fagan, V. M. (1966). Feedback control of mevalonate synthesis by dietary cholesterol. *Journal of Biological Chemistry*, **241**, 602–609.

Slakey, L. L., Craig, M. C., Beytia, E., Briedis, A., Feldbruegge, D. H., Dugan, R. E., Qureshi, A. A., Subbarayan, C. and Porter, J. W. (1972). The effects of fasting, refeeding and time of day on the levels of enzymes effecting the conversion of β-hydroxy-β-methylglutaryl-coenzyme A to squalene. *Journal of Biological Chemistry*, **247**, 3014–3022.

Slakey, L. L., Ness, G. C., Qureshi, N. and Porter, J. W. (1973). Occurrence of the enzymes effecting the conversion of acetyl CoA to squalene in homogenates of hog aorta. *Journal of Lipid Research*, **14**, 485–494.

Srere, P. A., Chaikoff, I. L., Treitman, S. S. and Burstein, L. S. (1950). The extrahepatic synthesis of cholesterol. *Journal of Biological Chemistry*, **182**, 629–634.

Steinberg, D. Drugs inhibiting cholesterol biosynthesis, with special reference to clofibrate. In: *Atherosclerosis. Proceedings of the Second International Symposium*. Ed. R. J. Jones. Springer-Verlag, New York, pp. 500–508, 1970.

Swann, A., Wiley, M. H. and Siperstein, M. D. (1975). Tissue distribution of cholesterol feedback control in the guinea pig. *Journal of Lipid Research*, **16**, 360–366.

Tomkins, G. M. and Chaikoff, I. L. (1952). Cholesterol synthesis by liver I. Influence of fasting and of diet. *Journal of Biological Chemistry*, **196**, 569–573.

Tormanen, C. D., Srikantaiah, M. V., Hardgrave, J. E. and Scallen, T. J. (1977). Evidence for the presence of a natural inactivating factor of 3-hydroxy-3-methylglutaryl coenzyme A reductase in soluble extracts from rat liver microsomes. *Journal of Biological Chemistry*, **252**, 1561–1565.

Waelsch, H., Sperry, W. M. and Stoyanoff, V. A. (1940). A study of the synthesis and deposition of lipids in brain and other tissues with deuterium as an indicator. *Journal of Biological Chemistry*, **135**, 291–296.

Weis, H. J. and Dietschy, J. M. (1969). Failure of bile acids to control hepatic cholesterogenesis: evidence for endogenous cholesterol feedback. *Journal of Clinical Investigation*, **48**, 2398–2408.

White, L. W. and Rudney, H. (1970). Regulation of 3-hydroxy-3-methylglutarate and mevalonate biosynthesis by rat liver homogenates. Effects of fasting, cholesterol feeding, and triton administration. *Biochemistry*, **9**, 2725–2731.

Wiley, M. H., Howton, M. M. and Siperstein, M. D. (1977). Renal metabolism of mevalonate: a sex difference. *Federation Proceedings*, **36**, 817.

Wilson, J. D. (1968). Biosynthetic origin of serum cholesterol in the squirrel monkey: evidence for a contribution by the intestinal wall. *Journal of Clinical Investigation*, **47**, 175–187.

Wilson, J. D. (1970). The measurement of exchangeable pools of cholesterol in the baboon. *Journal of Clinical Investigation*, **49**, 655–665.

Wilson, J. D. (1972). The role of bile acids in the overall regulation of steroid metabolism. *Archives of Internal Medicine*, **130**, 493–505.

Wilson, J. D. and Lindsey, C. A. Jr. (1965). Studies on the influence of dietary cholesterol on cholesterol metabolism in the isotopic steady state in man. *Journal of Clinical Investigation*, **44**, 1805–1814.

Zilversmit, D. B. (1960). The design and analysis of isotope experiments. *American Journal of Medicine*, **29**, 832–848.

Chapter 9

Sterol Metabolism in Isolated Cells

1	INTRODUCTION	399
2	GENERAL ASPECTS OF STEROL METABOLISM	401
2.1	Sterol composition	401
2.2	Uptake and excretion of sterols	403
2.2.1	Methods	403
2.2.2	Effect of composition of the medium	404
2.2.3	Behaviour of macrophages	406
2.3	Synthesis of sterols	408
2.3.1	Effect of the composition of the medium	408
2.3.2	The sterol regulator of sterol synthesis	411
2.3.3	Effects of hormones	413
3	THE LDL RECEPTOR	414
3.1	Surface-binding and internalization of LDL	414
3.2	Properties of the LDL receptor	418
3.3	The LDL-receptor pathway in fibroblasts	423
3.4	The LDL pathway in cells other than human fibroblasts	427
3.5	LDL receptors in the liver	429
3.6	The role of the LDL pathway *in vivo*	430
3.6.1	Catabolism of LDL	430
3.6.2	Cholesterol synthesis	432
3.7	HDL and the LDL receptor	433
3.8	General significance of receptor-mediated endocytosis	434
4	REMOVAL OF CELL CHOLESTEROL *in vivo*	435
4.1	Reverse cholesterol transport	435
4.2	The acceptor for tissue cholesterol *in vivo*	436

Sterol Metabolism in Isolated Cells

1 INTRODUCTION

Sterol metabolism in homogeneous populations of mammalian cells *in vitro* may be studied either in cells maintained for many generations by sub-cultivation ('passage') after each successive phase of multiplication, or in suspensions of non-dividing cells isolated freshly from body fluids or tissues of the animal and kept alive *in vitro* for a limited period. The distinction between the two types of system is not clear cut, since cells such as macrophages or hepatocytes in monolayers (Bissell *et al.*, 1973) may remain alive for many days outside the body without multiplication if kept in a suitable medium. The term 'culture' is arbitrarily restricted to populations of cells, whether or not they are dividing, in which the majority remain alive *in vitro* for at least 24 hours (Paul, 1975).

Cells from most embryonic tissues can be cultured successfully, but many cells of postnatal animals tend to die out when maintained *in vitro* for more than a few days. The primary culture may be started from cells obtained by enzymic or sonic disaggregation of an organ such as the liver, or from the cells that grow out on to the surface of the container when a piece of tissue is placed in a culture medium. The cells maintained by subcultivation of the primary culture are known as a *primary cell line*. They are characterized by a stable diploid karyotype, the retention of many of the morphological and metabolic attributes of their cells of origin, the ability to survive only a limited number of passages (though they are immortal in the frozen state) and a tendency to 'contact inhibition', resulting in cessation of growth and division when the cells multiplying on the surface of their container have formed a single confluent layer. The cells of a primary culture may undergo 'transformation' into what is known as an *established cell line*, either spontaneously or as a result of treatment with a carcinogen or an oncogenic virus. The cells of an established line are characterized by an abnormal number of chromosomes, dedifferentiation as regards their morphology and metabolism, the ability to remain alive after an indefinite number of passages, and decreased or absent contact inhibition. Since the cells of an established line have several features in common with malignant cells, and since established cell lines can arise directly from explants of tumours, transformation *in vitro* is regarded by many as the equivalent of the transition to malignancy *in vivo*.

Cells in culture or short-term suspensions of cells are particularly suitable for the study of certain aspects of sterol metabolism that cannot be approached satisfactorily in the whole animal or in broken-cell preparations. They have been used extensively in the study of mechanisms concerned in the movement of sterols into and out of the cell and in the investigation of control systems for which an intact plasma membrane is required. Isolated cells are also of great potential value in the study of the complex processes involved in the elaboration, intracellular transport and secretion of sterol-containing lipoproteins by hepatocytes and intestinal cells. The study of isolated macrophages (see Section 2.2.3) has provided insight into the transmembrane transport of cholesterol that may well be relevant to this process in other types of cell. Since the composition of the culture or suspension medium can be altered, it is possible to examine the way in which intracellular sterol metabolism is affected by controlled changes in the concentrations of substances, such as hormones and lipoproteins, in the immediate vicinity of cell surfaces. The study of cells in culture may also help to uncover the basis of genetic errors of sterol metabolism.

Observations on isolated cells may supplement information obtained from the whole organism, from perfused organs and from subcellular systems. However, it should be noted that the behaviour of the isolated cell is not always directly relevant to the cell *in vivo*. For the preparation of suspensions of cells from an organ such as the liver it is usual to treat the tissue with an enzyme in order to separate the cells from one another; this may remove or damage cell-surface components that mediate effects of the extracellular environment upon the intracellular metabolism of sterols. A further limitation arises in the study of cultured cells. Many of the cell lines in which sterol metabolism has been investigated most extensively, such as the L-strain mouse fibroblast, are established lines. As we have seen, the metabolic behaviour of such cells may differ from that of normal cells *in vivo*. It should also be borne in mind that sterol metabolism may not reach a steady state within the relatively short period of an experiment on cells in culture. Hence, observations on cultured cells may fail to reflect long-term adaptive changes that occur in cells *in vivo*. An example of this is discussed elsewhere in this book in relation to the behaviour of cultured fibroblasts from patients with familial hypercholesterolaemia (Chapter 15).

In this chapter we shall consider various aspects of the biochemistry and physiology of sterols as seen in isolated cell systems. The relevance of this information to sterol metabolism in the whole body will become apparent in later chapters.

2 GENERAL ASPECTS OF STEROL METABOLISM

It is difficult to generalize about the quantitative aspects of sterol metabolism in cultured cells because there are substantial differences between different cell lines, and in a given cell line the sterol composition and the rate of metabolism of sterols may vary with the nature of the culture medium and the growth rate of the culture. Almost all animal cells in culture are capable of synthesizing cholesterol from precursors of low molecular weight. An interesting exception is the much-studied L-strain mouse fibroblast, which apparently lacks a Δ^{24}-reductase and therefore accumulates desmosterol rather than cholesterol when grown in a medium lacking cholesterol (Bates and Rothblat, 1974). Another exception to the general rule is a mutant cell line derived from hamster ovary which lacks lanosterol 14α-demethylase and is therefore incapable of synthesizing sterol intermediates beyond lanosterol (Chang *et al.*, 1977). Cholesterol, or a closely related sterol, is required for growth by all mammalian cells in culture. Hence, cultured cells cease to grow if cholesterol is absent from the medium and if, at the same time, cholesterol synthesis is suppressed by the presence of an inhibitor such as 7-ketocholesterol (see Section 2.4).

2.1 Sterol composition

With the exception of some specialized cells such as the cultured Y-1 mouse adrenal tumour, which converts cholesterol into C_{21} steroids in the presence of ACTH (Kowal, 1970), and hepatocytes cultured in conditions in which bile acids are formed, cells in culture do not metabolize cholesterol in significant amounts other than by esterification with long-chain fatty acids. Hence, the total cholesterol content of the great majority of cells in culture is a function of the rate of synthesis within the cell and the balance between uptake* and

---

* The term 'uptake' refers here to the movement of cholesterol from the medium to the inside of the cell. Elsewhere in this chapter the term is sometimes used to include surface-binding, as well as entry into the interior of the cell (internalization), of cholesterol-containing lipoproteins by cells in culture. In these cases the meaning should be clear from the context.

excretion into the medium. In most strains the bulk of the cholesterol is free and is present mainly in the various membranes of the cell, including the plasma membrane. However, esterified cholesterol is also present in cultured cells of many types, owing partly to uptake of serum lipoproteins, if these are present in the growth medium, and partly to intracellular esterification of free cholesterol by ACAT. Under certain abnormal conditions large amounts of esterified cholesterol may accumulate in cultured cells, as in the MAF strain of human fibroblasts grown in the presence of hypercholesterolaemic rabbit serum (Bailey and Keller, 1971) and in arterial smooth muscle cells grown in the presence of cationic human LDL (Goldstein et al. (1977a)).

Values for the sterol content of cultured cells of various lines will be found in the reviews by Rothblat (1969), Howard and Howard (1974) and Bailey (1977). When cells of a given strain are grown in a medium containing whole serum at different concentrations, the total cholesterol content of the cells usually remains more or less constant. This, presumably, is a consequence of the ability of cultured cells to maintain a balance between intracellular synthesis and their uptake and excretion of cholesterol, as discussed in Section 2.3. When the nature of the serum in the medium is changed, marked changes in cholesterol content of the cells may follow, irrespective of the concentration of cholesterol in the medium. Thus, Bailey (1977) has shown that the cholesterol content of cultured mouse lymphoblasts of the MB III strain may be made to vary sixfold by changing the source of the serum added to the medium. The cholesterol content of these cells grown in the presence of five types of serum is shown in Table 9.1. It may be seen that the cholesterol content of cells grown with normal rabbit serum is more than twice that of cells grown with normal

Table 9.1
Influence of the source of serum added to the medium upon the sterol content of cells in culture

Source of serum	Serum cholesterol concentration (mg/100 ml)	Cell cholesterol (% dry weight)
Normal human	199	3.60 ± 0.57
Atherosclerotic human	229	4.09 ± 0.86
Human placental cord	97	2.35 ± 0.23
Normal rabbit	86	7.8 ± 2.2
Hypercholesterolaemic rabbit	2148	22.2 ± 2.9

Cells of the MBIII strain of mouse lymphoblasts were grown for four days in the medium containing the serum diluted with one part of balanced saline solution. The hypercholesterolaemic rabbit serum was obtained from animals fed 2% of cholesterol in their diet. Values for cell cholesterol are means ±SD. (Modified from Bailey, 1977.)

human serum, although the cholesterol concentration of rabbit serum is less than half that of human serum. Cells of different strains grown under similar conditions also show marked differences in sterol content; in ten strains examined by Bailey (1977), including four from human tissues, the cholesterol content varied from 0.6% to 2.8% of the lipid-free dry weight. The transformation of a primary cell line into an established line does not appear to be associated with significant changes in total cholesterol content, expressed as a percentage of dry weight (Howard and Howard, 1974).

Since most cultured cells grown in the presence of serum obtain virtually all their cholesterol from the medium and do not synthesize their own, the differences in cholesterol content of cells grown in various types of serum, and of different strains of cells grown in the same serum, are probably due to differences in the net flux of cholesterol into the cells. As we shall see, the nature of the lipoproteins in the medium has a profound effect upon the uptake and excretion of cholesterol by cells in culture and could therefore influence cellular sterol content by determining the relative rates of influx and efflux. Differences in sterol content of different cell strains exposed to the same medium could conceivably be due to intrinsic differences in plasma-membrane components concerned in the uptake of lipoproteins and in the excretion of intracellular cholesterol into the medium.

2.2 Uptake and excretion of sterols

In this and the following section we shall consider the uptake, excretion and biosynthesis of sterols as general properties of mammalian cells in culture. The manner in which uptake and synthesis are co-ordinately regulated in some cultured cells by a complex sequence of events involving cell-surface receptors for plasma lipoproteins is dealt with in a separate section (Section 3). The factors that govern the uptake and excretion of cholesterol by cells in culture are relevant to the general question of the partition of cholesterol between the tissues and the extracellular fluids *in vivo*. But they are also of interest in relation to two other more specific problems: the mechanism by which cholesterol in extrahepatic tissues is transported to the liver for metabolism or excretion, and the process leading to the formation or regression of atherosclerotic lesions. Both of these questions are considered below (Section 4).

2.2.1 Methods

Uptake and excretion of sterol may be studied either by measuring changes in the mass of sterol in the cells and the medium during a period of incubation, or by observing the movement of labelled sterol from the medium into the cells or from pre-labelled cells into the medium. Both approaches have their limitations. If there is no sterol in the growth medium, the appearance of sterol in the medium during an incubation clearly indicates net transport from the inside to the outside of the cell, but if sterol is present initially in the medium there could be a flux into and out of the cell without net change in the sterol content of the medium. A two-way flux without net change in intracellular or extracellular mass would be detected with labelled sterol, but the movement of labelled sterol molecules across the plasma membrane may merely reflect a molecule-for-molecule exchange between cells and medium and does not necessarily indicate a net flow in either direction. A combination of the two approaches was used by Bailey (1961) to demonstrate excretion of sterol, in the presence of uptake from the medium, by MB-III-strain mouse lymphoblasts. Another interesting approach is that of Bates and Rothblat (1974), who have exploited the inability of L-strain mouse fibroblasts to reduce the Δ^{24} double bond in the biosynthesis of cholesterol. When these cells are cultured in a medium containing cholesterol, the rate at which cholesterol accumulates within the cells provides an index of the net rate of sterol influx and the rate at which desmosterol accumulates in the medium provides an index of the rate of sterol efflux.

2.2.2 Effect of composition of the medium

The investigations of Rothblat (1972) and of Bailey (1977) on the uptake of cholesterol by various types of cell in culture have shown that uptake is favoured by the presence of high cholesterol:protein and cholesterol:phospholipid ratios in the growth medium. The nature of the protein with which cholesterol is complexed also influences the rate of uptake. In Rothblat's experiments with cultured mouse fibroblasts (Bates and Rothblat, 1975), uptake at a given concentration of free cholesterol in the medium was greater when the cholesterol was carried in human LDL than when it was carried in human HDL. Esterified cholesterol added to the medium in the form of lipoprotein complexes is also taken up by mouse fibroblasts. Once inside the fibroblast the cholesteryl esters are hydrolysed to free cholesterol, presumably by the mechanism discussed in Section 3.

The excretion of cholesterol from cultured cells into the medium has been demonstrated by labelling the cells, either with labelled cholesterol added to the medium or by allowing them to synthesize cholesterol from a radioactive precursor, and then transferring them to fresh medium. The cholesterol lost from the cells is excreted as free cholesterol, cultured cells being apparently unable to excrete cholesterol in esterified form, and the rate at which sterol leaves the cell is influenced by the composition of the medium. Working with mouse lymphoblasts, Bailey (summarized in Bailey, 1977) found that pre-labelled cells lose labelled free cholesterol at a rapid rate when the medium contains whole human serum, but that excretion ceases when the serum is removed from the medium. Excretion is resumed when various serum lipoproteins are added back, the most effective being α-lipoprotein (the HDL discussed in Chapter 11). Since the mass of sterol in cells and medium was not measured in these experiments, the efflux of free cholesterol observed in the presence of cholesterol-containing lipoproteins in the medium may have been balanced by an equal flow into the cells. These observations certainly cannot be taken as proof that HDL preferentially causes a net removal of cholesterol, since it is possible that plasma membranes exchange their free cholesterol with some lipoproteins more readily than with others; the rate of exchange could, for example, be influenced by the surface area per unit mass of lipoprotein.

There is, however, abundant evidence that a net loss of cholesterol from cells in culture can indeed occur, provided that the medium contains a suitable acceptor for free cholesterol.

Evidence for net efflux from cells has been obtained by demonstrating the movement of labelled free cholesterol from prelabelled cells into a medium containing no cholesterol, or by showing a net decrease in the mass of cell cholesterol when the cells are incubated in a medium which may or may not be free of sterol. Experiments of this kind with a variety of cell types, including mouse lymphoblasts, ascites tumour cells, arterial smooth-muscle cells, human fibroblasts and isolated rat hepatocytes (see Stein *et al.*, 1975, 1976) have shown that net efflux of cholesterol occurs if the medium contains serum from which the lipoproteins have been removed by ultracentrifugation (lipoprotein-deficient serum) or serum from which the triglycerides and cholesterol have been removed by solvent extraction (lipid-depleted serum). Net excretion of cholesterol from cells also occurs if the medium contains complexes formed by sonicating phospholipids with the whole protein of HDL, with the individual components of HDL protein or with plasma albumin. Under certain conditions, native HDL added to a culture medium containing no protein may also promote a net efflux of cholesterol from cells (Stein *et al.*, 1976).

In all these experimental conditions the acceptor for cholesterol is probably a phospholipid layer capable of incorporating free cholesterol, either because it contains no cholesterol (as in the vesicles and bilaminar discs formed by sonicating phospholipid-protein mixtures) or because the cholesterol:phospholipid molar ratio in the acceptor is lower than that in the outer layer of the plasma membranes of the cells. All that is required for the transfer of cholesterol from the cell to the phospholipid acceptor is a brief collision between the phospholipid-containing particle in the medium and the surface of the cell. As free cholesterol molecules move off the outer layer of the cell membrane, free cholesterol would tend to move by flip-flop (see Chapter 7) from the inner to the outer layer, thus promoting a flow of cholesterol from the inside to the outside of the cell. This process may be thought of as a movement of cholesterol molecules down a concentration gradient and is similar to the mechanism by which the cholesterol content of red-cell membranes can be diminished by incubating the cells with phospholipid vesicles. It has been suggested that free cholesterol may also move from inside the cell to the outer layer of the plasma membrane by a reversal of endocytosis, which would bring the inner layer of the lysosomal bilaminar membrane to the outer surface of the cell, thus allowing lysosomal cholesterol to be picked up by cholesterol acceptors in the medium (Small, 1977). Although there is no direct evidence for this process, there is reason to believe that at least some of the plasma membrane taken into the cell during the formation of endocytotic vesicles eventually returns to the cell surface. Further discussion of the mechanisms by which cholesterol leaves cells will be found in the section dealing with the acceptors for tissue cholesterol *in vivo* (4.1).

2.2.3 Behaviour of macrophages

The uptake and excretion of cholesterol by non-dividing mouse peritoneal macrophages in cultue has been studied in considerable detail by Werb and Cohn (1971a,b; 1972). The behaviour of macrophages towards cholesterol, especially when present in particulate form, is in some respects peculiar to cells capable of phagocytosis, but some of the findings of Werb and Cohn are undoubtedly of wider relevance.

When macrophages are incubated in calf serum in which the lipoproteins contain [^{3}H]-labelled free cholesterol in non-particulate form, the free cholesterol of the plasma membrane and of intracellular membranes (mainly lysosomal) becomes labelled, eventually reaching a specific activity nearly equal to that of the free cholesterol in the culture medium. Since there is no change in the free cholesterol contact of the cells or culture medium and no significant esterification of the labelled cholesterol, labelling of the macrophage cholesterol must be due to exchange. When the labelled cells are transferred to fresh medium, labelled cholesterol leaves the cells, again without change in cholesterol content, at a rate expressed by two exponentials, one with a half-life of about 2 hours and the other with a half-life of about 15 hours. By a combination of morphological analysis of the cells and kinetic analysis of the radioactivity curves, Werb and Cohn showed that the rapid component of the radioactivity curve represents exchange of free cholesterol between the plasma membrane and the medium, while the slow component represents exchange between lysosomal cholesterol, most of which is present in the lysosomal membrane, and cholesterol in the medium. Since the exchange of free cholesterol between cells and medium is unaffected by inhibition of endocytosis or immobilization of the lysosomes, the exchange between lysosomal membranes and acceptors in the medium cannot be mediated by bulk transfer of plasma-membrane cholesterol to and from the lysosomal membranes, as would occur during endocytosis and exocytosis. It is much more likely that the whole process consists of a sequence of steps in which cholesterol molecules exchange between the lysosomal membrane and the cytosol, then between the cytosol and the plasma membrane and, finally, between the plasma membrane and the medium (presumably by the mechanism discussed in Section 2.2.2 above). Werb and Cohn suggest that the rate-limiting step responsible for the slow component of the whole exchange process is the transfer of cholesterol, possibly by means of a saturable protein carrier, between the lysosomal membrane and the plasma membrane.

When mouse macrophages are incubated with free cholesterol in particulate form, either in red-cell ghosts or in emulsions of an albumin-cholesterol complex, the particles are ingested by phagocytosis and the cholesterol accumulates in lysosomes, leading to a net increase in the sterol content of the cells. If the cholesterol-loaded cells are transferred to fresh particle-free medium containing serum, the cholesterol is excreted from the cells with a half-life of about 20 hours. This suggests that net outflow of cholesterol into the medium is mediated by the process (discussed above) that is responsible for exchange of non-particulate cholesterol between the lysosomes and the medium, one or other of the phospholipid-containing components of the serum acting as acceptor for cellular free cholesterol. Whether or not the outward component of the exchange process exceeds the inward component presumably depends upon the relation between the capacity of the serum in the medium for accepting free cholesterol and the free cholesterol content of the cells.

If the cells are incubated with emulsions of an albumin-cholesteryl ester complex, the particles are phagocytosed and the cholesteryl esters that accumulate in the lysosomes are hydrolyzed to free cholesterol, which is then excreted when the cells are transferred to fresh medium containing serum.

Mouse macrophages and other cells of the macrophage class, including human monocytes and guinea-pig Kupffer cells, have been shown to take up and degrade chemically acetylated LDL (acetyl-LDL) by a process that involves high-affinity binding to the cell surface, followed by internalization and lysosomal digestion (Goldstein et al., 1979a). In contrast to the receptor-mediated endocytosis of native LDL discussed in Section 3, uptake of acetyl-LDL by macrophages is not regulated by the cholesterol content of the cell. Hence, uptake, if allowed to continue for many hours, leads to the massive accumulation of cholesteryl ester within the cells, converting them into foam cells. Goldstein et al. (1979a) suggest that the macrophage uptake system may be responsible for the formation of foam cells in the tissues of patients with familial hypercholes- terolaemia, perhaps by facilitating the uptake of LDL that has been altered *in vivo* in a manner such that it is recognized by the acetyl- LDL receptors on macrophages. Other aspects of cholesterol metab- olism in macrophages are discussed in Chapter 5, Section 4.6.

2.3 Synthesis of sterols

The ability of mammalian cells in culture to synthesize all the sterol they need for the formation and maintenance of membranes is shown by the fact that they can grow and multiply in artificial media containing no lipid. Under these conditions of culture the principal sources of carbon from which sterols are synthesized are acetate and glucose. Bailey (1964) showed that when serum is added to a lipid- free medium in which mouse fibroblasts are growing, sterol synthesis is suppressed, the cells now satisfying essentially all their sterol requirement by net uptake from the medium. Thus, cells in culture exhibit feedback control of sterol synthesis mediated by sterol reach- ing the interior of the cell from the external medium.

2.3.1 Effect of the composition of the medium

When cultured cells are transferred from a medium containing normal serum to one containing delipidated serum, the rate of incorporation of [^{14}C]acetate or of [^{14}C]glucose, but not of [^{14}C]mevalonic acid, into sterol increases several-fold within a few hours. When normal serum is added back to the lipid-deficient medium there is a rapid suppression of the incorporation of carbon from acetate and glucose into sterol, usually detectable within one or two hours. Marked suppression is also observed when free cholesterol emulsified in Tween is added to the medium. Howard et al. (1974) deduced that the short-term effect of the removal or addition of normal serum upon acetate incorporation into sterol by mouse fibroblasts of the L strain is due to reversible activation-inhibition of acetyl-CoA synthetase. Others, however, have concluded that the rate- limiting step in sterol biosynthesis in most mammalian cells in culture, including primary and established lines of non-malignant cells and cells from malignant tissues, is the reduction of HMG-CoA by HMG- CoA reductase. (See Howard and Howard (1974) for a review of earlier work on this question, and Section 3 below for regulation in human skin fibroblasts in culture.)

Fig. 9.1 shows the effect of incubating human skin fibroblast cultures in a medium containing delipidated serum upon the ability of the fibroblasts to incorporate radioactive acetate into lipids. When fibroblasts previously grown in the presence of normal serum are incubated for 18 hours in a medium in which normal serum is replaced by delipidated serum, incorporation of acetate into sterol is markedly stimulated, whereas incorporation into fatty acids is only moderately increased. The extent of the stimulation depends upon the concentration of delipidated serum protein in the medium. No stimulation occurs in the absence of protein, but as the concentration of protein is increased there is a progressive increase in the rate of incorporation of acetate into sterol. As shown in Section 3, the increased rate of incorporation of acetate into sterols by the fibroblasts is due to derepression of HMG-CoA reductase. The effect of increasing concentrations of delipidated serum is presumably due to an effect on the excretion of cholesterol from the cells into the medium, leading to derepression of HMG-CoA reductase.

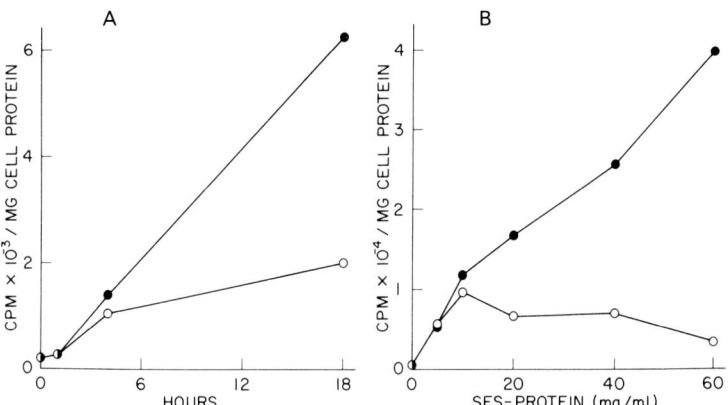

Figure 9.1
The effect of a medium containing lipid-deficient serum on the incorporation of [³H]acetate into sterols (●) and fatty acids (○) by cultured human skin fibroblasts previously grown in a medium containing 10% fetal calf serum.

Panel A. After growth in the medium containing calf serum the cells were incubated for various periods (0–18 hours) in a medium containing human serum (10 mg/ml) delipidated by extraction with lipid solvent. [³H]Acetate was then added to the medium for measurement of the incorporation of ³H into lipids during a further 2-hour incubation.

Panel B. After growth in the medium containing calf serum the cells were incubated for a standard 18-hour period in a medium containing delipidated human serum at various concentrations (shown on the horizontal axis). Incorporation of [³H]acetate into lipids was then measured during a further 2-hour incubation.

SES—protein, solvent—extracted serum protein.
(From Williams and Avigan (1972), with the permission of the authors.)

Experiments designed to elucidate the effect of serum upon cholesterol synthesis in cultured cells in terms of the effects of specific lipoprotein fractions have led to contradictory results. For example, Williams and Avigan (1972) observed inhibition of cholesterol synthesis when HDL was added to cultures of human skin fibroblasts preincubated in a medium containing lipid-depleted serum. Bates and Rothblat (1974), on the other hand, observed stimulation of sterol synthesis in mouse L-cell cultures when human HDL was added to the medium. Breslow *et al.* (1977) also noted a stimulatory effect of human HDL upon HMG-CoA reductase activity in primary cell cultures of rat liver. Cells of different types may also respond quite differently to a given lipoprotein. Thus, human LDL, which suppresses HMG-CoA reductase activity in cultured human fibroblasts (see Section 3), has no effect on HMG-CoA reductase activity in rat-hepatocyte cultures (Breslow *et al.*, 1977).

The most likely explanation for these apparent inconsistencies is that the influence of different lipoproteins, or of mixtures of lipoproteins, on cholesterol synthesis in cells in culture is determined by the net effect of the lipoproteins on the amount of free cholesterol in the whole cell or in a restricted pool that is responsible for regulating the activity or rate of synthesis of HMG-CoA reductase. The effect upon the free cholesterol content of the cells will, in turn, depend upon the balance between uptake of cholesterol from the cells by the lipoproteins in the medium and their ability to deliver cholesterol to the interior of the cells. As we have already seen, the ability to enhance cholesterol excretion by cultured cells varies from one lipoprotein to another. Furthermore, the delivery of cholesterol to the cell interior may be mediated by at least three processes: non-specific fluid endocytosis (pinocytosis), uptake facilitated by specific lipoprotein receptors, and the exchange of free cholesterol between lipoproteins and cell membranes discussed above. The relative importance of each of these processes is likely to differ according to the nature of the cell and of the lipoprotein under investigation. It is also possible that the effect of a given lipoprotein on the cholesterol content of a cell in culture is influenced by the extent to which the cell has already been loaded with cholesterol by its previous treatment. In view of these complexities, it is hardly surprising that there have been inconsistencies in the findings obtained under different experimental conditions.

The behaviour of hepatocytes provides a striking example of the way in which components in the incubation medium may influence cholesterol synthesis in isolated cells by modifying their cholesterol content. When rat hepatocytes in suspension are incubated in a sterol-free medium containing albumin and lecithin, cell cholesterol is taken up by the medium and the activity of HMG-CoA reductase increases, the rise in enzyme activity being directly proportional to the amount of cholesterol lost from the cells during the early part of the incubation (Edwards et al., 1976).

Further evidence for the importance of intracellular cholesterol content as a determinant of sterol synthesis in isolated cells is considered in Section 3. It should be noted, however, that the influence of particular lipoproteins or lipoprotein mixtures on sterol synthesis in cultured cells cannot always be explained in terms simply of their effect on sterol content of the cells, whatever the mechanism by which this effect is mediated. Bates and Rothblat (1974, 1975), for example, found that human LDL suppresses sterol synthesis in mouse L cells pre-incubated with delipidated calf serum, whereas human HDL, adjusted to give an equal free-cholesterol concentration in the medium, stimulates sterol synthesis even though the two lipoproteins have the same effect on cell uptake of cholesterol from the medium and on the sterol content of the cells. Since HDL promotes a greater efflux of sterol from L cells than does LDL it is possible that HDL selectively depletes a small pool of intracellular sterol responsible for suppressing sterol synthesis. Alternatively, this hypothetical regulatory pool of sterol may be more accessible to cholesterol delivered to the interior of the cell *via* LDL than to that delivered *via* HDL.

2.3.2 The sterol regulator of sterol synthesis

When cholesterol feeding was first shown to lead to inhibition of hepatic synthesis of cholesterol in parallel with an accumulation of cholesterol in the liver, it was tacitly assumed that cholesterol itself, whether free or esterified, is the intracellular steroid regulator of sterol synthesis. However, it was later shown that several analogues of cholesterol, such as cholest-4-en-3-one and cholesta-4,6-dien-3-one, inhibit sterol synthesis *in vivo* or in cells in culture. This raised the possibility that the biologically active steroid is a metabolite of cholesterol rather than cholesterol itself. In support of this, Kandutsch and Chen (1973, 1974) have shown that whereas unpurified cholesterol complexed with albumin selectively inhibits sterol synthesis in mouse L cells and mouse liver cells in culture, chromatographically pure cholesterol added in the same form has no inhibitory effect in cultured mouse liver cells (purified cholesterol has some inhibitory effect in mouse L cells, but only after incubation for 20 hours). A search for the active contaminant of preparations of unpurified cholesterol showed that several analogues of cholesterol containing an additional oxygen function in positions 6, 7, 20, 22, 24 or 25 are potent inhibitors of acetate incorporation into sterol, and of HMG-CoA reductase activity, in mouse fibroblasts and liver cells in culture. These analogues include 7-ketocholesterol, 7α-hydroxycholesterol, 7β-hydroxycholesterol and 25-hydroxycholesterol. Since some of these compounds are present in unpurified specimens of cholesterol obtained from animal tissues, possibly arising by autoxidation *in vivo* or during the extraction and isolation of cholesterol, Kandutsch and Chen suggested that they are responsible for the inhibitory effect of unpurified cholesterol on sterol synthesis in cultured cells and that one or other compound is responsible for the inhibitory effect of purified cholesterol in L cells after prolonged incubation. Kandutsch *et al.* (1978) suggest that the inhibitory effect of these sterols is due to repression of enzyme synthesis because they have no effect when added to microsomal suspensions containing the enzyme and because enzyme activity declines with a half-life of about 1 hour when the inhibitor is added to a cell culture.

The relevance of these observations to the physiological steroid regulator of sterol synthesis is not at all obvious, since it is unlikely that a biological control mechanism would be dependent upon the formation of an effector by non-enzymic autoxidation. It should be noted, however, the 7α-hydroxycholesterol is formed enzymically from cholesterol in the liver and that 20α-hydroxycholesterol is an intermediate in the conversion of cholesterol into steroid hormones. These products of cholesterol might therefore play a physiological role in the regulation of HMG-CoA reductase activity in the liver and in steroid-hormone-forming tissues. In other tissues it is possible that hydroxylated intermediates in the conversion of lanosterol into cholesterol, such as lanosterol derivatives with an oxygen function at C-32, act as regulators of cholesterol synthesis by inhibiting HMG-CoA reductase (Schroepfer *et al.*, 1978; Gibbons *et al.*, 1980). Bell *et al.* (1976) have shown that HMG-CoA reductase activity is suppressed when freshly prepared human serum or human LDL, free from autoxidation products of cholesterol, is added to a culture of rat hepatoma cells pre-incubated in a lipoprotein-deficient medium. Since the suppression of enzyme activity takes place in association with uptake of cholesterol, Bell *et al.* conclude that the inhibitory effect of whole serum or LDL is mediated by cholesterol itself rather than by a product of its metabolism. They suggest that the effectiveness of cholesterol as an inhibitor of sterol synthesis in cells in culture depends upon the form in which the cholesterol is added to the culture medium. From a consideration of the effect of human serum and of some inhibitory analogues of cholesterol upon the half-life of HMG-CoA reductase in hepatoma cells in culture, Bell *et al.* conclude that cholesterol inhibits mainly by decreasing the rate of synthesis of the enzyme and that inhibitory analogues (particularly 25-hydroxycholesterol) act by increasing its rate of inactivation. The latter effect seems to be due to a change in the structure of the enzyme rather than to an increase in its rate of degradation (Beirne *et al.*, 1977). This, of course, would be consistent with inhibition mediated by allosteric modification, but would not exclude reversible inactivation by phosphorylation.

Although these highly inhibitory analogues of cholesterol have not been proved to be physiological regulators of sterol synthesis, their potential value for experimental purposes should not be overlooked. The fact that some oxygenated sterols inhibit cholesterol synthesis in intact experimental animals raises the question of their possible value in the treatment of hypercholesterolaemia.

2.3.3 Effects of hormones

Insulin has been shown to stimulate cholesterol synthesis and to increase HMG-CoA reductase activity when added at physiological concentrations to cultures of several primary cell lines including human fibroblasts and rabbit aortic cells. In two transformed cell lines (mouse L cells and cells of a rat hepatoma) tested by Avigan (1977) insulin had no effect on seterol synthesis. The effect of insulin on sterol synthesis in diploid cells in culture is selective in so far as the proportional increase in incorporation of [^{14}C]acetate into sterol is several times that into fatty acids and protein. The increase in HMG-CoA reductase activity in response to insulin has a lag period of several hours and is prevented by cycloheximide, suggesting that insulin stimulates sterol synthesis in diploid cells in culture by induction of enzyme synthesis. Although insulin is known to stimulate growth and proliferation of mammalian cells in culture, its effect on sterol synthesis may occur in the absence of any increase in DNA synthesis in confluent cultures of fibroblasts.

Glucagon prevents the induction of HMG-CoA reductase by insulin in primary cultures of rat hepatocytes, but a similar anti-insulin effect cannot be demonstrated in cultures of human fibroblasts (Avigan, 1977). Dexamethasone, a compound with the hormonal properties of a glucocorticoid, increases HMG-CoA reductase activity in primary cell lines derived from human and animal tissues. Like that of insulin, the effect of dexamethasone has a prolonged lag period and is prevented by inhibitors of protein synthesis, again suggesting an action mediated by enzyme induction rather than by activation of pre-existing molecules of HMG-CoA reductase.

Cells in culture have provided a good deal of relevant information as to the possible role of cyclic AMP in the regulation of sterol synthesis. As we have already seen (Chapter 8, Section 4.2), observations on the behaviour of partially purified preparations of HMG-CoA reductase have led to the suggestion that cyclic AMP influences the activity of the enzyme *in vivo* by promoting its reversible conversion into an inactive, phosphorylated form. However, several observations on diploid cells in culture (summarized by Avigan, 1977) are difficult to reconcile with this idea. In particular, dibutyryl cyclic

AMP does not decrease HMG-CoA reductase activity in cultured human fibroblasts; nor does prostaglandin E_1 have any effect on sterol synthesis in cultured fibroblasts when added to the culture medium at a concentration sufficient to raise the intracellular cyclic AMP concentration by nearly one hundredfold.

3 THE LDL RECEPTOR

In this section we shall consider how some mammalian cells in culture take up cholesterol from serum in the medium by means of specific receptors for LDL, the lipoprotein of density 1.019–1.063 g/ml present in normal plasma. The composition, structure and general metabolism of LDL are dealt with fully in Chapter 11. Here it is sufficient to note that LDL is the major carrier of cholesterol in normal human plasma and that the human LDL particle consists of a sphere 200–250 Å in diameter, containing a single protein component (apoB) and esterified cholesterol as the predominant lipid. Although there is evidence for the presence of LDL receptors in a variety of human and non-human cells, our understanding of their nature and function is based largely upon studies of cultured skin fibroblasts from normal human subjects and from patients with familial hypercholesterolaemia (FH). LDL receptors were, in fact, discovered in human skin fibroblasts by Brown and Goldstein (1974) in the course of a search for the underlying genetic defect in FH.

3.1 Surface-binding and internalization of LDL

The first hint that fibroblasts might possess LDL receptors came from the observation that LDL (but not HDL) suppressed HMG-CoA reductase activity in cultured normal fibroblasts pre-incubated in a medium containing lipoprotein-deficient serum, but had essentially no effect on enzyme activity in similarly treated fibroblasts from a patient with homozygous FH (Goldstein and Brown, 1973). Since the kinetic properties of the enzyme from normal and FH fibroblasts are identical, and since cholesterol delivered to the inside of the cell from an ethanolic solution of cholesterol is capable of suppressing HMG-CoA reductase in FH cells, these findings suggested that the FH gene does not affect the structure of the enzyme or the intracellular mechanisms responsible for its regulation. This line of reasoning raised the possibility that the product of the normal gene at the FH locus in some way enables LDL in the external medium to influence the activity of intracellular HMG-CoA reductase. Subsequent work on the binding of ^{125}I-labelled LDL by cultured normal fibroblasts revealed the presence of cell-surface receptors which specifically bind

LDL with high affinity and transfer it to the inside of the cell, thus mediating the regulation of HMG-CoA reductase in fibroblasts *in vitro* by LDL cholesterol delivered to the cell interior. Although the LDL receptor is almost certainly the immediate product of the normal allele corresponding to the FH gene, this remains to be proved.

High-affinity binding of LDL by fibroblasts can be demonstrated by measuring uptake (surface-binding plus internalization) of ^{125}I-LDL as a function of LDL concentration by cultured fibroblasts in which LDL receptors have been developed by pre-incubating the cells in a medium containing lipoprotein-deficient serum for 24 hours. Fig. 9.2 shows the results of an experiment in which monolayer cultures of pre-incubated cells from a normal subject and from a homozygous FH patient were incubated for 6 hours at 37 °C in the presence of ^{125}I-LDL at increasing concentrations. After incubation, the monolayers were washed with an albumin-containing buffer and assayed for radioactivity. With normal cells there was a steep linear increase in the total amount of cell-associated ^{125}I-LDL as the LDL concentration was increased to about 50 μg of LDL protein/ml, followed by a much less steep increase when the LDL concentration was raised progressively to 200 μg of protein/ml or higher. With the FH cells, the steep increase in uptake at low LDL concentrations was not apparent. Goldstein and Brown interpreted these curves in terms of two processes: uptake mediated by a high-affinity process that requires binding to specific LDL receptors on the cell surfaces and is saturated at a concentration of about 50 μg of LDL protein/ml; a low-affinity process not approaching saturation at the highest concentration tested. Since uptake by the FH cells was linear from zero concentration and parallel to the less steep component of the uptake curve for the normal cells, FH cells were assumed to lack the high-affinity process. On these assumptions, a curve for the high-affinity process can be constructed by subtracting the low-affinity component from the experimental curves obtained with normal cells, to give curves such as that shown in Fig. 9.2c. The curve shows saturation at 50 μg of protein/ml and half-saturation at about 10 μg/ml. The high-affinity component of the uptake of LDL may also be determined as the difference between the uptake of ^{125}I-LDL in the absence of unlabelled LDL and in the presence of unlabelled LDL at a concentration many times that sufficient to saturate the high-affinity process.

In experiments in which total uptake of ^{125}I-LDL is measured at 37 °C, binding at the cell surface may be obscured by the presence of ^{125}I-LDL that has been transferred to the inside of the cell. For example, in a 6-hour incubation at this temperature the bulk of the cell-associated ^{125}I-LDL would be inside the cells (see Fig. 9.3). Goldstein *et al.* (1976) have shown that ^{125}I-LDL specifically bound to

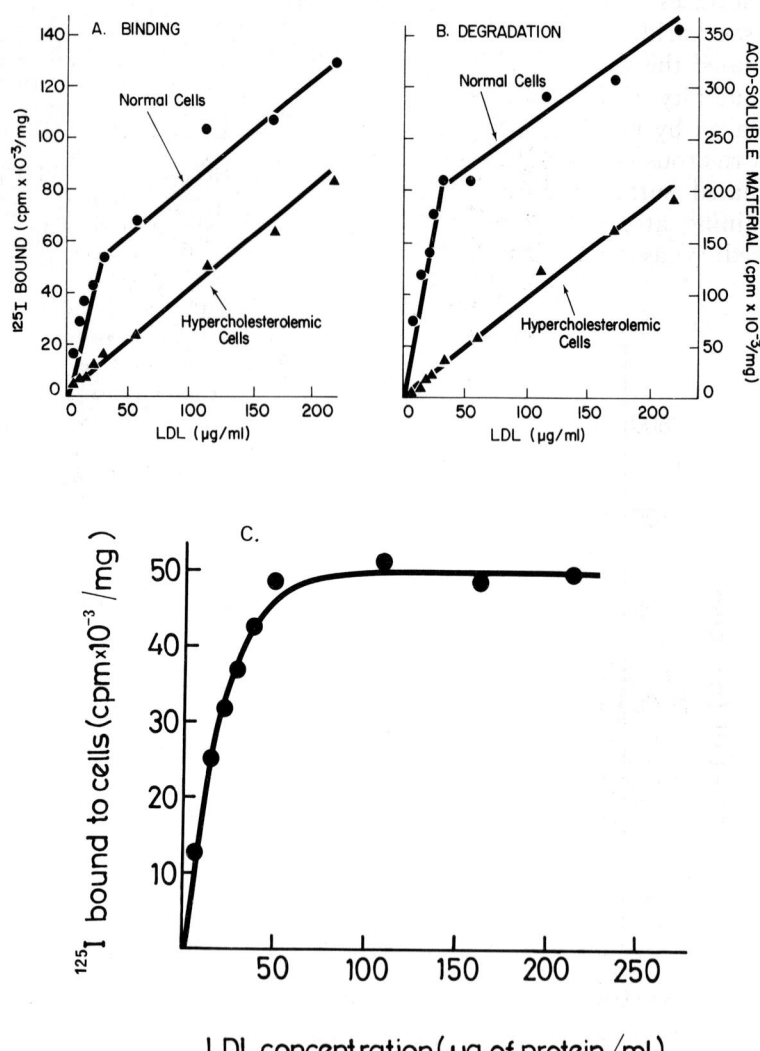

Figure 9.2
Binding A. and degradation B. of ^{125}I-labelled normal human LDL, as a function of LDL concentration in the medium, by cultured skin fibroblasts from a normal subject (●) and from a subject with familial hypercholesterolaemia in the homozygous form (▲).
 C, high-affinity component of binding of ^{125}I-labelled LDL, as a function of LDL concentration, by cultured fibroblasts from a normal subject. The curve was obtained by subtracting the low-affinity component (lower curve in A) from the curve for total binding (upper curve in A).
 (From Goldstein and Brown (1974), with the permission of the authors.)

Sterol Metabolism in Isolated Cells 417

the surfaces of cultured fibroblasts can be displaced by sulphated polysaccharides such as heparin or dextran sulphate, and they have estimated the amount of ^{125}I-LDL bound to the cell surfaces by the high-affinity process, i.e. by the LDL receptors, as the amount displaced by heparin after removal of loosely adherent radioactivity by a rigorous washing procedure. Others (Bierman *et al.*, 1974) have estimated surface-bound ^{125}I-LDL (defined as the labelled LDL remaining attached to the cell surfaces after a specified washing procedure) as the amount that can be displaced from the washed cells

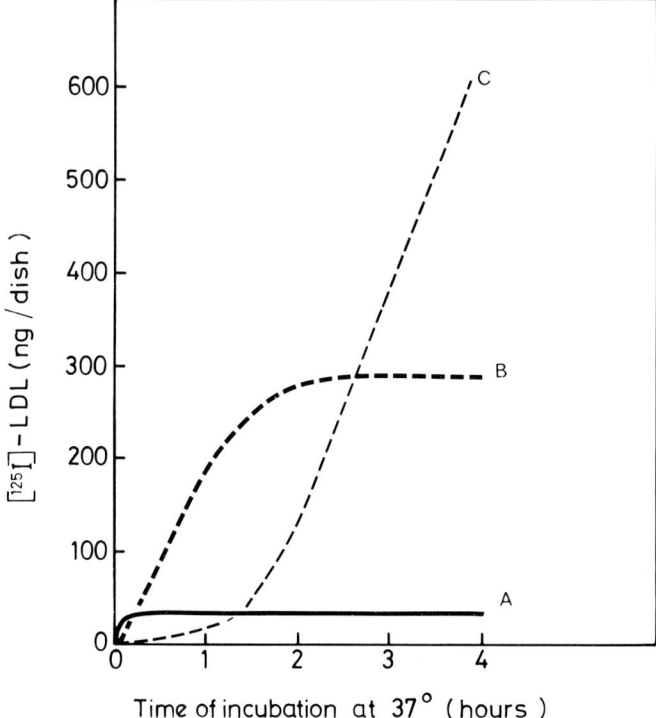

Time of incubation at 37° (hours)

Figure 9.3
Idealized representation of the time-course of surface-binding, internalization and proteolytic degradation of ^{125}I-labelled LDL by cultured human fibroblasts in which LDL receptors have been maximally induced by pre-incubating the fibroblasts in a medium containing lipoprotein-deficient serum for 18–24 hours at 37 °C. After pre-incubation, ^{125}I-labelled LDL (925 μg of protein/ml) was added to the medium and the incubation was continued at 37 °C. Surface-bound ^{125}I-LDL was determined from the amount releasable by heparin; internalized ^{125}I-LDL was estimated from the total uptake of ^{125}I minus that releasable by heparin. Degradation of labelled LDL protein was determined as the amount of trichloroacetic-acid soluble radioactivity in the medium.

A, surface-bound; B, inside cell; C, trichloroacetic-acid soluble. (From Goldstein and Brown (1976), with the permission of the authors.)

by a brief incubation with trypsin. There is some doubt as to how far results obtained by the two methods are comparable. Discrepancies between results from different laboratories could be due to differences in the washing procedure used to remove unbound ^{125}I-LDL, since LDL tends to stick to surfaces of all kinds by non-specific association, raising the practical problem of removing this non-specifically attached ^{125}I-LDL from the cells without displacing the specifically bound material. On the other hand, it is possible that, in addition to high-affinity receptors, fibroblasts possess low-affinity receptors from which LDL is not equally displaceable by heparin and trypsin. The possibility that fibroblasts possess low-affinity binding sites for LDL, in addition to LDL receptors, is of interest in relation to the mechanism by which LDL is taken up by the low-affinity process (see Fig. 9.2A). It is not yet clear whether this process is mediated by surface receptors with low affinity and high capacity for LDL, or whether it merely reflects the uptake of droplets of the medium by bulk-phase pinocytosis. In either case, the term '*LDL receptor*' should be restricted to the physical unit presumed to be responsible for high-affinity surface-binding and internalization of LDL by fibroblasts and other cells.

3.2 Properties of the LDL receptor

Using the heparin-release method for assaying LDL receptors, in combination with methods for measuring total cell-uptake of ^{125}I-LDL, Goldstein and Brown have examined the behaviour of the receptors in human cultured fibroblasts in considerable detail. Some of the properties they have deduced are listed in Table 9.2. References to the experimental evidence for these properties will be found in the review from which this Table has been constructed (Goldstein and Brown, 1977). Only the briefest notes are included in this section.

The receptor is probably a protein or glycoprotein, since its activity can be reversibly abolished by trypsin or pronase, and since recovery of receptor activity after exposing the cells to proteolytic enzymes can be prevented by cycloheximide. In view of the nature of the interaction between LDL and heparin (Iverius, 1972) and of the ability of heparin to displace LDL from LDL receptors on fibroblasts, it seems likely that the receptor possesses negatively charged groups which interact ionically with positively charged amino groups on the apoB of LDL. This non-covalent interaction is such that once a molecule of ^{125}I-LDL has been bound to its receptor, it cannot be displaced by unlabelled LDL, even at high concentrations, though labelled and unlabelled molecules compete for receptors if added to the medium together. In this respect the interaction of LDL with its receptor differs from that of insulin with the insulin receptor (Zeleznik and

Roth, 1978), possibly because each particle of LDL is bound simultaneously by more than one receptor or because of its very rapid internalization.

Although the biological function of the LDL receptor is probably to bind LDL in the extracellular fluid and thus to initiate the sequence of events discussed below (Section 3.3), the binding specificity of the receptor is not absolute. VLDL also binds to the receptors on fibroblasts, presumably because about half the protein of VLDL is apoB. However, Mahley and co-workers (Mahley et al., 1978; Pitas et al., 1979) have shown that two lipoproteins that contain apoE but no apoB also bind to LDL receptors on cultured human fibroblasts. These apoE-rich lipoproteins are the HDL_c of cholesterol-fed animals and human HDL-I, a small subfraction of the d 1.063–1.125 fraction of normal HDL. Moreover, HDL_c is 100 times more effective than LDL at displacing ^{125}I-labelled LDL from LDL receptors, a property that is due partly to the fact that each HDL_c particle binds to 4 times as many receptors as each LDL particle. The binding of LDL and of apoE-containing lipoproteins to the LDL receptor can be prevented by selective blocking of a proportion either of the arginyl residues by cyclohexanedione or of the lysyl residues by reductive methylation.

Table 9.2
A summary of some of the properties of the LDL receptor of human fibroblasts

Chemical composition	Probably a glycoprotein.
Binding affinity	Half-saturation at about 10 µg of LDL protein/ml of medium at 37 °C; at about 2 µg of protein/ml at 4 °C.
Binding capacity	Saturated at about 50 µg of LDL protein/ml.
Number of receptors per cell	When fully derepressed: equivalent to 15 000–70 000 LDL molecules at 37 °C or 7500–15 000 at 4 °C.
Rate of internalization of receptor-bound LDL	Half-life, about 3 minutes at 37 °C.
Binding specificity	Binds LDL, VLDL and apoE-containing lipoproteins with high affinity; affinity for LDL more than 200 times that for HDL. Fails to bind apoB- or apoE-containing lipoproteins in which a limited number of the arginyl or lysyl residues have been blocked.
Requirements in medium	Ca^{2+} (EDTA inhibits binding); optimum pH, 7.5.
Interaction with LDL	Probably ionic, between anionic groups in receptor and cationic groups in apoB of LDL.
Rate of turnover of receptors	Half-life about 20 hours.
Agents that displace LDL from receptors	Heparin, dextran sulphate, polyphosphates of chain-length greater than 4.

Modified from Goldstein and Brown (1977).

This suggests that apoB and apoE share arginine- and lysine-rich segments that are essential for the recognition of LDL receptors by lipoproteins containing these two apoproteins.

The properties of the LDL receptor we have discussed so far were deduced by Brown and Goldstein from observations on cultured fibroblasts that had been incubated for 24 hours in a medium containing lipoprotein-deficient serum. Under these conditions, normal fibroblasts develop a maximal number of receptors. If, however, LDL is added to the lipoprotein-deficient medium the number of receptors per cell declines, owing to repression of receptor synthesis. For example, in the presence of LDL at a concentration of 10 µg of protein/ml, the number of receptors per cell falls to about $\frac{1}{3}$ of the initial value in 20 hours. When the LDL is removed from the medium, receptor number returns to the maximum. The half-life of LDL receptors in cultured fibroblasts, calculated from the rate at which the number decreases when cycloheximide is added to the medium containing lipoprotein-deficient serum, is about 20 hours. Feedback repression of receptor synthesis by LDL in the medium depends upon the ability of LDL to increase the amount of free cholesterol in the cell (probably at a critical site) by the mechanism described in Section 3.3. Receptor synthesis is also repressed by the addition of free cholesterol or 25-hydroxycholesterol to the medium. As we shall see (Section 3.6), feedback repression of receptor synthesis in the presence of LDL at concentrations well below the level required to saturate receptors raises the question of the extent to which receptors are present in various tissues *in vivo*.

The distribution of LDL receptors on the fibroblast surface has been studied by electron-microscopic observation of the uptake of ferritin-labelled LDL. The plasma membranes of fibroblasts and of other cells capable of absorbing proteins have indented regions, 3000–5000 Å in diameter. These specialized regions are known as *coated pits* because their cytoplasmic surfaces are coated with material giving the region a fuzzy appearance on electron microscopy. The cytoplasmic coat consists largely of a specific protein, of molecular weight 180 000, named *clathrin*. Clathrin can be isolated from bovine brain and used as an antigen for the preparation of a specific antibody. Using an immunofluorescence technique with antibody to clathrin, Anderson *et al.* (1978) have shown that the coated pits of cultured skin fibroblasts are arranged linearly in parallel with the alignment of intracellular actin-containing fibres. When fibroblasts in culture are incubated with ferritin-labelled LDL at 4 °C, the labelled LDL can be seen to be bound mainly to the sides of the coated pits, 60–70% of the bound material being localized in an area occupying less than 2% of the cell surface. If the fibroblasts are then warmed to 37 °C, the coated pits rapidly invaginate and become pinched off from the plasma membrane, forming endocytotic vesicles which enclose the ferritin-labelled LDL particles originally attached to the surface. Since these vesicles are formed by invagination of the plasma-membrane bilayer, the outer layer of the vesicle is derived from the inner, clathrin-coated layer of the coated pits. Three stages in this process are shown in Fig. 9.4.

The behaviour of fibroblasts obtained by Goldstein et al. (1977b) from the members of a family carrying an unusual mutation affecting the LDL receptor suggests that the receptor is a single protein molecule with two functional components, one that binds LDL and the other that mediates the internalization of the receptor and its bound LDL. The index patient from this family is a genetic compound whose fibroblasts carry two different sets of mutant receptors, the two mutations occurring at different mutable sites on the gene specifying the whole receptor molecule. One set, specified by the allele inherited from the patient's father, binds LDL with normal kinetics but cannot internalize it and the other set (inherited from the patient's mother) cannot bind LDL (see Chapter 15 for further details). Electron microscopy of the fibroblasts from this patient shows that the receptors capable of binding ferritin-labelled LDL are not clustered at the coated regions, but are scattered at random over the cell surface. This suggests that the function of the receptor component other than the one responsible for binding LDL is to facilitate the movement of the receptor into the coated regions. In the light of this suggestion, Goldstein and Brown (1979) have speculated that receptors, either newly synthesized or re-utilized, are continually being transferred from the cytoplasm to the plasma membrane, where they take up a position as trans-membrane proteins with the binding component projecting into the external medium. Having reached the plasma membrane they drift laterally through the liquid-crystalline bilayer, to be concentrated in the coated regions, the internalization component perhaps enabling the clathrin in the coated regions to recognize a receptor. Once a receptor has become incorporated into a coated region it would automatically be carried inside the cell by adsorptive endocytosis due to the continuous formation and invagination of the coated pit, which must occur once every few minutes.

At present, LDL receptors can only be detected by their ability to bind LDL under specified conditions. However, the isolation of receptors from their associated plasma membranes would clearly be of great help in the study of receptor function and should eventually make it possible to establish their chemical composition. As a step towards this goal, Brown and Goldstein and their coworkers (Basu et al., 1978; Kovanen et al., 1979a) have developed a method for assaying the high-affinity binding of LDL by mixtures of membrane fragments prepared from homogenates of human fibroblast cultures,

422 The Biology of Cholesterol and Related Steroids

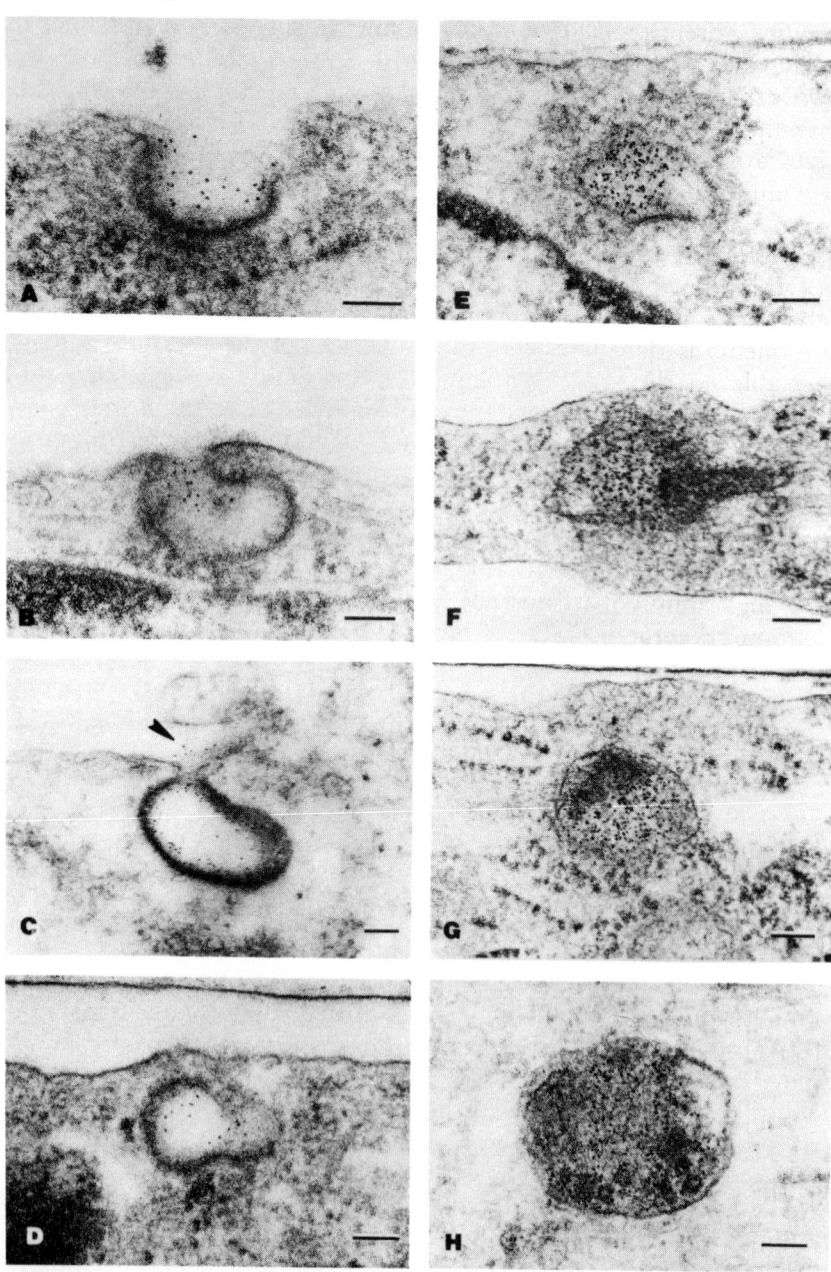

Figure 9.4
Electron micrograph showing representative stages in the endocytosis of ferritin-labelled LDL by cultured normal human fibroblasts, with subsequent appearance in a lysosome. The fibroblasts were incubated with the labelled LDL at 4 °C to permit surface binding, washed to remove unbound labelled LDL and then warmed at 37 °C for various times.

bovine adrenal-cortex cells and bovine ovarian corpus luteum. The behaviour of these membranes exhibits several features in common with that of LDL receptors on intact cells *in vitro*. In particular, the binding of human ^{125}I-labelled LDL by isolated cell membranes is saturated at low LDL concentrations and is competitively inhibited by unlabelled human LDL but not by cyclohexanedione-treated LDL or by human HDL. Furthermore, membranes prepared from skin fibroblasts of a patient with homozygous FH show greatly diminished LDL-binding capacity. These findings strongly suggest that the selective binding of LDL by mixed populations of cell-membrane fragments is due to the presence of the high-affinity receptors detectable on the surfaces of several types of intact cell *in vitro* (see Table 9.3). It is reasonable to suppose that the membranes responsible for this binding are derived from the plasma membranes of the homogenized cells.

Using membranes derived from cultured human fibroblasts and from bovine adrenal cortex (a tissue with an unusually high LDL-receptor activity), Schneider *et al.* (1979) have succeeded in solubilizing high-affinity LDL-receptor activity with octyl-β-D-glucoside, a nonionic detergent. Receptor activity is associated with a protein that can be precipitated by 50% ammonium sulphate or by dilution of the detergent. It is to be hoped that this technique will open the way to the purification of the LDL receptor in quantities sufficient for direct analysis of its physical properties and chemical composition.

3.3 The LDL-receptor pathway in fibroblasts

The binding and internalization of LDL by LDL receptors is the first of a series of steps that Goldstein and Brown (1977) have termed the

---

A. A typical coated pit (seen after 1 min at 37 °C) (× 77 500).
B. A coated pit being transformed into a vesicle enclosing labelled LDL particles (seen after 1 min at 37 °C) (× 65 000).
C. Formation of a coated vesicle by complete invagination of the coated pit (seen after 1 min at 37 °C) (× 43 500).
D. A fully-formed coated vesicle that appears to be losing its cytoplasmic coat on one side (arrow) (seen after 2 min at 37 °C) (× 60 000).
E. An endocytotic vesicle that has completely lost its cytoplasmic coat (seen after 2 min at 37 °C) (× 60 000).
F. An irregularly shaped endocytotic vesicle that contains more labelled LDL than a typical coated vesicle and also has a region of increased electron density within the lumen (arrow) (seen after 6 min at 37 °C) (× 60 000).
G. An endocytotic vesicle similar to F (seen after 6 min at 37 °C) (× 55 000).
H. A secondary lysosome that contains labelled ferritin (seen after 8 min at 37 °C) (× 60 000).

(From Anderson *et al.* (1977), with the permission of the authors.)

LDL pathway for the uptake and intracellular metabolism of cholesterol from the external medium by human fibroblasts and other cells. From the functional point of view, Goldstein and Brown see the LDL pathway as a mechanism that has evolved to enable cells to acquire the cholesterol they need for growth and maintenance without calling upon their capacity to synthesize their own sterol. The pathway appears to be regulated by the amount of free cholesterol (or related sterol) in certain critical regions of the cell, rather than by the concentration of LDL in the external medium. Current ideas on the LDL pathway have been developed from several experimental approaches, including the study of LDL uptake by fibroblasts from

Table 9.3
References to published work providing evidence for the presence of high-affinity LDL receptors in various human and animal cells other than cultured fibroblasts

	Cell system	Reference
Human	Long-term cultures of lymphocytes	Kayden *et al.* (1976); Ho *et al.* (1976*b*)
	Fresh lymphocytes pre-incubated in LPDS*	Ho *et al.* (1976*a*)
	Aortic s.m.c.† in culture	Bierman and Albers (1975); Goldstein and Brown (1975)
	Cultured umbilical-vein endothelial cells	Stein and Stein (1976)
	Freshly isolated adipocytes	Angel *et al.* (1979)
	Fibroblasts transformed by SV40 virus	Quoted in Goldstein and Brown (1976)
	Cell membranes from fibroblasts and lymphocytes	Basu *et al.* (1978)
Non-human	Cultured rat s.m.c.	Bierman *et al.* (1974)
	Cultured pig s.m.c.	Weinstein *et al.* (1976)
	Cultured bovine s.m.c.	Vlodavsky *et al.* (1978)
	Non-confluent bovine arterial endothelium in culture	Vlodavsky *et al.* (1978)
	Mouse fibroblasts of the L strain	Beirne and Watson (1976)
	Rat hepatoma (HTC) in culture	Kirsten and Watson (1974)
	Mouse Y-1 adrenal tumour in culture	Faust *et al.* (1977)
	Cultured bovine adrenal-cortex cells	Kovanen *et al.* (1979*c*)
	Cell membranes from various animal tissues (possibly including rat liver)	Kovanen *et al.* (1979*a,b*)

* Lipoprotein-deficient serum.
† Smooth-muscle cells.

patients with single-gene mutations affecting specific steps in the pathway and by fibroblasts treated with selective inhibitors of lysosomal function. A particularly useful inhibitor is chloroquine, a drug that is ingested by lysosomes, in which it induces a pH too high for the catalytic activity of lysosomal hydrolases. Compactin, a very powerful selector inhibitor of HMG-CoA reductase (see Chapter 15, Section 3.6), has also been of use in the study of the regulation of cholesterol synthesis by the LDL pathway in cultural fibroblasts (Brown et al., 1978).

After receptor-bound LDL has been internalized by the process described above, the subsequent steps in the LDL pathway in fibroblasts are thought to be as follows: The endocytotic vesicles formed by the invagination of the coated pits form secondary lysosomes by fusing with primary lysosomes containing hydrolases capable of hydrolyzing the apoB and cholesteryl esters of the ingested LDL (see Chapter 17, Section 1). The amino acids resulting from the digestion of apoB diffuse into the medium. The free cholesterol, including that brought into the cell as a component of LDL and that formed by the hydrolysis of LDL cholesteryl esters, leaves the lysosomes to enter extralysosomal pools of free cholesterol, presumably present in membranes. The free cholesterol released from the lysosomes exerts three regulatory influences within the cell. It represses the synthesis of HMG-CoA reductase and thus suppresses sterol synthesis; it activates ACAT, thus promoting its own esterification with long-chain fatty acids; it represses the synthesis of LDL receptors and thus suppresses the further receptor-mediated uptake of LDL by the fibroblast. The net effect of the intracellular hydrolysis and re-esterification of the esterified cholesterol of LDL is to change the fatty-acid pattern of the incoming cholesteryl esters from one in which linoleate predominates to one in which the major fatty acid is oleate, the preferred substrate for ACAT.

The relative rates of the initial steps in the LDL pathway are shown in Fig. 9.3. The curves illustrate, in idealized form, the time-course of surface-binding, internalization and proteolytic degradation of ^{125}I-LDL by human cultured fibroblasts pre-incubated in lipoprotein-deficient serum. As soon as the labelled LDL is added to the medium it is taken up by the receptors and is then transferred to the interior of the cell. The amount of ^{125}I-LDL bound to the cell surface at any instant reaches a plateau after about 15 minutes, when the rate at which labelled molecules are internalized has become equal to the rate at which they are taken up from the medium. After a brief lag period the protein of the internalized labelled LDL begins to be degraded by lysosomal hydrolysis, as shown by the appearance of labelled amino acids in the medium. When the rate of hydrolysis becomes equal to the rate at which labelled LDL reaches the inside of the cell, the amount of internalized labelled LDL (total uptake minus surface-bound) remains constant. At this point, most of the total cell-associated ^{125}I-LDL is inside the cells.

Each of the three effects produced by receptor-mediated uptake of LDL can also be brought about by adding an ethanolic solution of free cholesterol or of an oxygenated sterol analogue to the medium. Furthermore, cholesterol synthesis in normal and FH fibroblasts is suppressed by cationized LDL, a modified LDL that can be internalized by adsorptive endocytosis not involving the receptor. On the other hand, LDL taken up by the low-affinity process (Section 3.1) has no effect on cholesterol synthesis or esterification in cultured fibroblasts, as shown by the failure of LDL at high concentrations to affect either of these activities in fibroblasts from patients homozygous for FH (whose cells lack receptors).

These apparently contradictory properties of cultured fibroblasts raise questions that cannot yet be answered. Possibly, LDL cholesterol taken up by the low-affinity process fails to suppress cholesterol synthesis or to stimulate cholesterol esterification because it does not reach a specific compartment of the intracellular pool of cholesterol that initiates the signal for repression of the synthesis of HMG-CoA reductase and activation of ACAT. But if this is the case it is difficult to see why the uptake of cationized LDL, which also bypasses the LDL-receptor route into the cell, should suppress cholesterol synthesis in both normal and FH fibroblasts.

The characteristics of the LDL pathway in cultured fibroblasts grown to confluency are such that cholesterol metabolism can be made to oscillate between two quite different steady states. In State 1, which occurs when the cells are incubated in a medium containing lipoprotein-deficient serum but no LDL, LDL-receptors are maximally developed, cholesterol is synthesized at a high rate, ACAT activity is negligible and the cells are depleted of cholesteryl ester. When LDL is added to the medium, cell metabolism changes over a period of about 24 hours to a new steady state (State 2) in which the number of receptors is low or negligible, cholesterol synthesis is suppressed and the cholesteryl-ester content of the cells is high. In both steady states there must, of course, be a balance between the total input of cholesterol into the cell by uptake from the medium and intracellular synthesis, and the total efflux of cholesterol by excretion into the medium. In State 1 the rate of efflux must be very nearly equal to the rate of synthesis. While the cells are changing from State 1 to State 2, their total cholesterol content (free plus esterified) may increase by nearly twofold. This increase is due, presumably, to an influx of LDL cholesterol greater than the decrease in intracellular synthesis. However, until something is known about the absolute rate of efflux during the transition between the two states and during State

2 we cannot exclude the possibility that the cholesterol content of the fibroblasts changes partly as a result of a change in the rate of efflux. Quantitative information about cholesterol efflux under defined conditions is essential if we are to draw up a complete balance sheet for cholesterol in normal fibroblasts in culture and would also be of interest in view of the suggestion that FH cells 'leak' cholesterol.

3.4 The LDL pathway in cells other than human fibroblasts

Although the protein specified by a gene is not necessarily synthesized in all cells of the body, it would be surprising if fibroblasts were the only mammalian cells capable of forming the LDL receptors. In fact, there is now satisfactory evidence for the presence of the LDL receptor in a wide variety of cells other than human fibroblasts. Since LDL receptors cannot yet be identified by chemical or immunological methods, proof of their presence in a human or animal tissue must be based on indirect evidence. In essence, this means demonstrating that the tissue in question exhibits LDL-receptor functions with properties similar to those listed in Table 9.2. Of these properties, the ones that carry the most weight are a high and specific affinity for apoB- and apoE-containing plasma lipoproteins, loss of binding when a limited number of the arginyl or lysyl residues of the apoprotein has been blocked (cyclohexanedione treatment, acetylation or reductive methylation), together with the expected changes in intracellular cholesterol metabolism when the binding is observed under conditions in which surface receptors can be internalized. Additional criteria are the inducibility of the putative receptors by incubation in a lipoprotein-deficient medium, their suppression by 25-hydroxycholesterol and (only in the case of human receptors) their absence from cells obtained from patients with receptor-negative homozygous FH.

On the basis of some or all of these criteria, human lymph cells and arterial smooth-muscle cells have been shown to be capable of developing receptors under the appropriate conditions. Subconfluent cultures of endothelial cells from the human umbilical vein also bind and degrade LDL at a significant rate, probably *via* the LDL pathway (Stein and Stein, 1976). Freshly isolated human lymphocytes show little or no receptor activity (Reichl *et al.*, 1976), but if they are incubated at 37 °C in a medium containing lipoprotein-deficient serum they develop LDL receptors within 72 hours (Ho *et al.*, 1976a). Freshly isolated human adipocytes appear to possess functioning LDL receptors which bind and internalize LDL without pre-incubation of the cells in the presence of lipoprotein-deficient serum (Angel *et al.*, 1979). It may also be noted that human fibroblasts transformed by the SV40 virus retain their ability to develop LDL receptors (see Table 9.2), but that cholesterol synthesis in human leukaemic cells is not suppressed by LDL in the external medium (Betteridge et al., 1979).

As regards animal cells, there is good evidence for the presence of receptors for LDL in cultural vascular smooth-muscle and endothelial cells, in cultured mouse adrenal tumour cells of the Y-1 strain, and in cultured bovine adrenal-cortex cells. There are also reasonable grounds for assuming the presence of LDL receptors in cultured mouse fibroblasts of the L strain and in cultures of the rat hepatoma 7288C (HTC cells). In addition to evidence from the study of intact cells, the study of membranes isolated from disrupted cells has provided suggestive evidence for the presence of LDL receptors in several bovine tissues, particularly the adrenal-cortex and the corpus luteum (see Section 3.2).

References to work suggesting the presence of LDL receptors in the human and animal cells discussed above are listed in Table 9.3. In most cases, the evidence for receptor activity is based at least on the ability of LDL at low concentrations specifically to suppress cholesterol synthesis or HMG-CoA reductase activity in cells pre-incubated in a lipoprotein-deficient medium containing acceptors for cell cholesterol. In human lymphocytes and arterial smooth-muscle cells the evidence is strengthened by the ability of the normal cells to regulate receptor activity in a manner similar to that seen in fibroblasts, and by the absence of activity attributable to receptors in the cells obtained from FH homozygotes. Not surprisingly, the functional activity and mode of regulation of receptors are not the same in all cells. Of particular interest is the observation of Vlodavsky et al. (1978) that in contact-inhibited monolayer cultures of arterial endothelial cells, LDL receptors are present but cannot internalize their bound LDL and are not repressed when LDL at saturating concentrations is added to the culture medium. Non-confluent endothelial cells, on the other hand, behave like fibroblasts with respect to their LDL receptors. Thus, it seems likely that the LDL pathway in arterial endothelial cells *in vivo* is regulated, not by the concentration of LDL in the external medium, but by cell-cell contact, which may perhaps determine the ability of the receptors to move into the coated regions by influencing the fluidity of the plasma membrane.

Additional evidence for the presence of LDL-receptor activity in particular tissues or in the whole body *in vivo* has been obtained by studying the effects *in vivo* of modifications known to influence receptor-mediated uptake of LDL by cells *in vitro*. Such evidence is bound to be somewhat indirect, but it may strengthen or supplement the more detailed observations that can be made on *in vitro* systems. Examples are the effect of lowering the plasma cholesterol concentration on HMG-CoA reductase activity in various tissues of rats (see Section 3.6), the effect of blocking arginyl residues on the catabolism of LDL by perfused livers from oestrogen-treated rats (see Section 3.5) and the effect of blocking lysyl or arginyl residues on LDL catabolism in whole animals or human subjects (see Chapter 15, Section 3.4.3). The special case of the liver is considered in the next section (3.5).

In addition to LDL receptors, there is growing evidence to suggest the presence of receptors with specific affinity for HDL in the tissues of some animal species, particularly those, such as the rat, in which the concentration of HDL in the plasma is much higher than that of LDL (see Brown *et al.*, 1979; Kovanen *et al.*, 1979c).

3.5 LDL receptors in the liver

The importance of establishing whether or not the liver makes a significant contribution to LDL catabolism *in vivo* by the LDL-receptor pathway is considered in Chapter 15 (Section 3.6). Apart from the general interest of this question in relation to the sites of catabolism of LDL in the whole body, there is the important practical point that transplantation of a normal liver into a patient with homozygous FH would be worth attempting if, but only if, we can be sure that the liver normally catabolizes substantial amounts of circulating LDL *via* receptor-mediated uptake.

Observations on the behaviour of liver cells in culture or in suspension have been contradictory. Kirsten and Watson (1974) deduced that HMG-CoA reductase activity in cultured rat hepatomas is regulated by lipoproteins in the medium in a manner similar to that seen in human fibroblasts in culture. However, the lipoprotein fraction responsible for this regulation was not identified. Breslow *et al.* (1977) failed to observe suppression of HMG-CoA reductase activity in non-dividing cultures of normal rat hepatocytes when lipoproteins from normal rat or human serum were added to the culture medium. However, they did observe suppression by an apoE-rich lipoprotein fraction, with β mobility on electrophoresis, obtained from the serum of cholesterol-fed rats. Thus, studies of intact hepatocytes have not provided evidence for the presence of LDL receptors on liver cells. On the other hand, there is growing evidence to suggest that rat hepatocytes *in vitro* take up and degrade both chylomicron remnant particles (Florén and Nilsson, 1977) and rat HDL (Ose *et al.*, 1979) by saturable mechanisms probably involving surface binding followed by internalization and lysosomal digestion. Sherrill *et al.* (1980) have also shown that perfused rat livers take up dog lipoproteins containing only apoE (HDL$_c$) by a high-affinity saturable mechanism.

The remarkable effect of oestrogenic hormones on lipoprotein metabolism in rats has suggested a different approach to the question of LDL receptors in liver tissue. It has been known for some years that when rats are given large doses of oestrogenic hormone there is a profound fall in plasma cholesterol concentration accompanied by a marked increase in the rate of catabolism of LDL by perfused livers removed from the treated animals. Kovanen *et al.* (1979*b*) have shown that membranes prepared from the livers of oestrogen-treated rats show saturable binding of human ^{125}I-labelled LDL and that this binding is inhibited competitively by native human LDL but not by acetylated or methylated LDL or by human HDL. In contrast, saturable and specific binding of human LDL by liver membranes from normal rats could not be demonstrated convincingly. These results are consistent with the possibility that LDL receptors, similar to those present on human fibroblasts, are present in the livers of rats, that the number of receptors is greatly increased by oestrogen treatment and that this leads to increased catabolism of LDL by the liver, with a consequent fall in plasma LDL-cholesterol concentration. In agreement with this interpretation, Chao *et al.* (1979) have shown that perfused livers of oestrogen-treated rats have a greatly enhanced capacity for catabolizing both human LDL and apoE-containing fractions of rat HDL (known to have a high affinity for classical LDL receptors), but do not catabolize cyclohexanedione-treated human LDL or human HDL at an increased rate. If LDL receptors are present on rat-liver cells, it is reasonable to suppose that they play a significant role in the catabolism of LDL, and perhaps of HDL (the major cholesterol-carrying lipoprotein of rat plasma), in the bodies of rats under physiological conditions. However, the affinity for human LDL shown by the LDL-binding sites on rat-liver membranes (half saturation at a concentration of 280 µg of LDL protein/ml at 37 °C) is many times lower than that of the LDL receptors on human fibroblasts or bovine adrenal-cortex cells in culture (about 10 µg of LDL protein/ml at 37 °C). Thus, the presence of functional high-affinity receptors for LDL in rat liver cannot yet be regarded as proven.

3.6 The role of the LDL pathway *in vivo*

3.6.1 Catabolism of LDL

A normal human subject catabolizes at least 500 mg of plasma LDL protein per day. The tissues in which this occurs have not been identified with certainty, but there is reason to think that even if the liver is an important site for the final disposal of LDL, extra-hepatic tissues have a considerable capacity for degrading the apoB of LDL in the living animal (see Chapter 11). This raises the question of the physiological function of the LDL receptors demonstrated in fibroblasts and other mammalian cells in culture. In view of the marked and specific increase in plasma LDL concentration that occurs in FH, a disease characterized by the presence of a single mutation causing the virtual absence of LDL receptors in the homozygous state, the conclusion that receptor-mediated degradation of LDL normally occurs to a significant extent *in vivo* is inescapable. Nevertheless, it is not a simple matter to deduce, from a consideration of the behaviour of cells in culture, how LDL receptors *in vivo* would behave in the steady state in cells bathed by extravascular interstitial fluid or (in the case of blood cells and arterial endothelium) by blood plasma.

The LDL circulating in the plasma reaches the extravascular fluid space (Reichl *et al.*, 1977*b*) and thus becomes accessible to a variety of tissue cells. Furthermore, the apoB-containing lipoprotein of density 1.019–1.063 g/ml in peripheral lymph (lymph LDL) induces a characteristic receptor-mediated response in cultured fibroblasts from normal human subjects, but not in fibroblasts from FH homozygotes (Reichl *et al.*, 1978), thus demonstrating that an LDL molecule retains its ability to interact with receptors after it has crossed the walls of the blood capillaries.

The capacity of a particular type of cell for degrading LDL by the LDL pathway *in vivo* will depend upon the concentration of LDL in the immediate vicinity of the cell surface and the extent to which the cell develops receptors under physiological conditions. The concentration of lymph LDL in human peripheral lymph is between 70 and 100 µg of protein per ml (Reichl *et al.*, 1977*a*). At this concentration, at least half the uptake of degradation of LDL by fibroblasts would be receptor-mediated if their receptors were maximally developed. Steinberg *et al.* (1976) have also pointed out that if fibroblasts *in vivo* behave like cultured fibroblasts in which receptors have been induced to the maximum by pre-incubation in the presence of lipid-deficient serum, then the rate of degradation per unit mass of fibroblasts would be greater than that per unit mass of the whole body, even if the LDL concentration in the interstitial fluid were only 5 µg of protein/ml. Similar calculations, based on the behaviour of cells in culture, suggest that the endothelial and smooth-muscle cells of the cardiovascular system could make a very substantial contribution to the total degradation of LDL *in vivo*.

These calculations would be physiologically relevant only if we knew the extent to which LDL receptors are, in fact, developed by the cells in the living body. High-affinity surface binding of LDL is almost completely suppressed in freshly isolated human lymphocytes (Reichl *et al.*, 1976; Ho *et al.*, 1976*a*). This is to be expected in view of the very high LDL concentration in human plasma (500–1000 µg of protein/ml), though there may be factors other than the plasma LDL that repress receptor formation in circulating lymphocytes, since high-affinity binding of LDL by these cells may also be suppressed in abetalipoproteinaemia (an inherited disorder in which LDL is absent from the plasma) (Reichl *et al.*, 1978). Quantitative information about receptor activity in skin fibroblasts *in vivo* is not available. However, the concentration of LDL in peripheral lymph is considerably higher than the concentration at which LDL receptors on cultured fibroblasts are saturated. If, therefore, lymph is representative of interstitial fluid, one would expect that in the steady state *in vivo* fibroblast receptors would be largely suppressed and, hence, that receptor-mediated catabolism of LDL by fibroblasts would take place only at a very low rate. A similar argument holds for any cells in which receptor formation is regulated in the same way as in cultured fibroblasts.

How, then, can we explain the undoubted operation of the LDL pathway under normal conditions *in vivo*? One possibility is that in some tissues receptors are expressed and are able to internalize LDL even in the continued presence of quite high concentrations of LDL in the interstitial fluid. That receptor function is not regulated in the same way in all tissues is suggested by the behaviour of arterial endothelial cells grown to confluency in culture (see Section 3.4) and, possibly, by the behaviour of freshly isolated adipocytes. The latter, it appears, have functional receptors *in vivo* even though the concentration of LDL to which they are exposed is likely to be high enough to repress receptor formation in fibroblasts.

The ability to develop LDL receptors in many types of cell also raises the question as to how far the LDL pathway could contribute to the homeostatic regulation of the plasma LDL concentration. This is part of the more general question of the regulation of plasma lipoprotein metabolism discussed in Chapter 11. At this point we need only note that the 'down-regulation' of LDL receptors by LDL in the medium would prevent the cells from increasing receptor-mediated catabolism of LDL in response to a rise in plasma LDL concentration. Pinocytosis, on the other hand, would favour homeostasis since the absolute amount of LDL engulfed with each droplet of extracellular fluid would increase in proportion to the plasma LDL concentration.

3.6.2 Cholesterol synthesis

As we have seen in Chapter 8, in adult mammals of most species cholesterol is synthesized at a relatively low rate in tissues other than liver and intestine. This would be expected if, under normal conditions, HMG-CoA reductase activity in the cells of many extrahepatic tissues is suppressed by receptor-mediated uptake of LDL cholesterol. Balasubramaniam *et al.* (1976, 1977*a*,*b*) have shown that cholesterol synthesis in the lungs, kidneys and adrenal glands of rats is specifically increased when the plasma cholesterol concentration is lowered by 4-APP, a drug that inhibits the secretion of lipoproteins by the liver. These observations, which have been confirmed and extended by Andersen and Dietschy (1976), are consistent with the hypothesis that cholesterol synthesis is regulated in some tissues by cholesterol taken up by the cells from the extracellular medium. If this uptake were mediated by the LDL pathway, one would expect that cholesterol synthesis would be markedly increased in the cells of extra-hepatic tissues of homozygous FH subjects, who have no LDL receptors, and of abetalipoproteinaemic patients, who have no LDL. The evidence now available suggests that cholesterol synthesis is not increased in the tissues of FH patients and that in abetalipoproteinaemia it is increased only moderately, if at all. How this might be reconciled with receptor-mediated regulation of cholesterol synthesis in the extra-hepatic tissues of normal human subjects *in vivo* is considered in the relevant sections in Chapters 15 and 16.

3.7 HDL and the LDL receptor

Human HDL, the lipoprotein of density 1.063–1.21 g/ml present in normal human plasma, has generally been found to have little effect on the surface-binding, uptake and degradation of LDL by cultured fibroblasts in which receptors have been developed by pre-incubation in a lipoprotein-deficient medium. Indeed, Goldstein and Brown (1977) concluded, from studies of the competition between LDL and HDL, that the affinity of LDL for the LDL receptor is at least 200 times that of HDL. Nevertheless, as Steinberg *et al* (1976) have pointed out, binding of HDL to the receptor, even to a very small extent, could have a finite effect on LDL uptake by cells *in vivo*. Cultured endothelial cells (Stein and Stein, 1976) and smooth-muscle cells from the arterial wall (Carew *et al.*, 1976) bind almost as much HDL as LDL to their surfaces, but the surface-bound HDL is internalized and degraded much more slowly than is surface-bound LDL. The nature of the surface-binding of HDL by these cells is not fully understood, but there does appear to be some competition between HDL and LDL for LDL receptors, since the uptake and degradation of LDL at low concentrations is partially inhibited when HDL is added to the culture medium. HDL is also surface-bound by cultured human fibroblasts, largely by a low-affinity process that is not destroyed by pronase and is unaffected by the presence of the FH gene. However, a small fraction, perhaps less than 5%, of the HDL that is surface-bound by fibroblasts competes with LDL for LDL receptors. The magnitude of this competition is such that the high-affinity binding and internalization of LDL is reduced by about 25% when the HDL:LDL molar ratio is 25:1 (protein ratio ≃5:1) (Miller *et al.*, 1977).

The net effect of the competition between HDL and LDL for

surface binding, with relatively little internalization of the bound HDL, is to diminish the increase in cell-cholesterol content that normally occurs when LDL is added to a medium containing cultured fibroblasts that have been depleted of cholesterol by pre-incubation in the absence of lipoprotein. The consequences of this HDL-LDL interaction *in vivo* are difficult to predict, since the inhibition of LDL uptake by a lipoprotein that does not itself deliver cholesterol to fibroblasts in significant amounts would tend to diminish the delivery of extracellular cholesterol to cells that use the LDL pathway, but at the expense of interfering with their capacity to catabolize LDL protein. There is also the possibility that, in the long term, a rise in HMG-CoA reductase activity would offset the decrease in receptor-mediated uptake of LDL cholesterol. A further difficulty in transposing observations on cells in culture to the whole body arises from uncertainty as to the relative concentrations of HDL and LDL in the interstitial fluid. The concentrations of apoB and apoA-I (the major apoproteins of plasma LDL and plasma HDL respectively) measured in human peripheral lymph suggest that the HDL:LDL molar ratio in the interstitial fluid could be as high as 10:1, which should result in a significant effect on LDL uptake by fibroblasts and other cells with functional LDL receptors. However, Mahley *et al.* (1978) have shown that human and animal lipoproteins obtained from plasma by ultracentrifugation at the HDL density range (1.063–1.21 g/ml) do not compete with LDL for LDL receptors unless these lipoproteins contain apoE. HDL from which the apoE-containing subpopulation has been selectively removed by heparin-manganese precipitation does not interact with the LDL receptor and therefore does not inhibit receptor-mediated uptake of LDL. In view of these findings, we shall not be in a position to assess the physiological significance of the HDL-LDL interaction at receptor sites *in vitro* until we know more about the apoE content of different subfractions of the plasma HDL and until we have some information about the apoE content of interstitial fluid.

3.8 General significance of receptor-mediated endocytosis

In the previous sections of this chapter the discussion has been concerned mainly with receptor-mediated uptake of LDL. However, this is only one instance of a general mechanism by which animal cells satisfy their requirements for substances carried in specific transport proteins present in the extracellular medium, or for the proteins themselves (see Goldstein *et al.*, 1979*b*, for review and references). Other proteins known to be taken into cells by receptor-mediated endocytosis include egg-yolk proteins, epidermal growth factor, transferrin and insulin. In several cases it is known that the receptors cluster on the coated pits and that the internalized protein is degraded within lysosomes. Thus, the continual invagination of coated pits, with the formation of coated vesicles which may fuse with lysosomes, provides the cell with a means of transporting extracellular proteins into its interior. In at least two instances (LDL and epidermal growth factor) independent regulation of the uptake of a particular protein species is achieved by control of the number of specific receptors on the cell surface. In view of the considerable number of proteins that are already known to be internalized by receptor-mediated endocytosis (thirteen are listed by Goldstein *et al*., 1979*b*), it is reasonable to expect that other lipoproteins besides LDL will be found to be taken up by this process. It is possible, for example, that the high rate of uptake of HDL by the adrenal gland of the rat (Gwynne *et al*., 1976) and the uptake of chylomicron remnant particles by hepatocytes (Florén and Nilsson, 1977) are mediated by a sequence of specific binding on coated pits followed by internalization.

4 REMOVAL OF CELL CHOLESTEROL *IN VIVO*

4.1 Reverse cholesterol transport

With few exceptions, the extra-hepatic tissues of the animal body synthesize cholesterol *in vivo*. Furthermore, as discussed in Chapter 11, the peripheral tissues make a substantial contribution to the total degradation of LDL *in vivo*, presumably by the mechanism involving surface-binding and internalization described in Section 3 above. There must therefore be a continuous input of cholesterol into the cells by endogenous synthesis and uptake of LDL, and since the peripheral tissues are in general unable to catabolize cholesterol, this input must be balanced by efflux from the cells at an equal rate if a steady state is to be maintained. Since the liver is the major site for removal of cholesterol from the body by catabolism or excretion, the cholesterol transferred continuously from the cells to the extracellular fluid must ultimately be transported to the liver. This *reverse cholesterol transport* raises the question of the nature of the extracellular lipoprotein acceptor or acceptors for intracellular cholesterol under physiological conditions, a question that prompted much of the work discussed in Section 2.2 above. Extracellular acceptor molecules for cholesterol must also be involved under non-steady-state conditions in which there is a net flow of cholesterol from the tissues to the liver, for example, during the resolution of skin xanthomas or of atheromatous lesions in the arteries. Work with isolated cells has contributed so much to this field that it will be convenient to consider reverse cholesterol transport, including some of its broader aspects, in this chapter.

4.2 The acceptor for tissue cholesterol *in vivo*

As we have seen, observations on isolated cell systems have shown that phospholipids complexed with one or more of a variety of different proteins derived from plasma are capable of picking up free cholesterol from cells, either by exchange or by a process involving a net transfer of cholesterol from the inside to the outside of the cell. Indeed, it is likely that any protein, whether or not it is a constituent of plasma, could take up free cholesterol from animal cells, provided that it is capable of forming a suitable complex with phospholipid. However, a *physiological* acceptor for tissue cholesterol, in addition to being a natural constituent of the body, would have to meet certain requirements in order to function efficiently. It must reach the interstitial fluids (except in the case of cells in direct contact with the plasma); it must be capable of increasing its load of total cholesterol (free plus esterified) per particle; it must deliver its cholesterol, directly or indirectly, to the liver. The problem is to identify a lipoprotein that can act as preferential acceptor for free cholesterol in the presence of other lipoproteins present in plasma and interstitial fluid. From this point of view, information obtained from experiments on the uptake of cholesterol from cells *in vitro* by isolated lipid/protein complexes may be of limited value.

Circumstantial evidence, derived mainly from some of the observations discussed above (Section 2.2), suggests that HDL is the lipoprotein primarily concerned in reverse cholesterol transport. In keeping with this, apoA-I, the major apoprotein of HDL, is present in peripheral lymph at a concentration more than twice that of apoB (Reichl and Myant, 1978). There is also experimental evidence to suggest that a significant proportion of the circulating HDL is taken up and degraded by the liver (Rachmilewitz *et al.*, 1972). That HDL is concerned in the net removal of cholesterol from the tissues is also consistent with the current view that a high plasma HDL concentration protects against coronary atherosclerosis (see Chapter 13). In Tangier disease, a condition in which HDL is almost completely absent from the plasma, cholesterol accumulates in certain tissues. This has been taken as evidence that HDL is necessary for reverse cholesterol transport, but it should be noted that the deposition of cholesterol in Tangier disease is not generalized, and that in some tissues there is no excess of cholesterol (Assmann *et al.*, 1977).

As we shall see (Chapter 11), the HDL particle consists essentially of a sphere with an apolar core of esterified cholesterol surrounded by a polar shell consisting of a phospholipid/free-cholesterol monolayer with which the apoproteins are associated. The initial step in the net transfer of cholesterol from a tissue cell to an HDL particle must be the incorporation of free cholesterol from the cell into the surface layer of the particle. But this process would be limited by the capacity of a liquid-crystalline phospholipid monolayer to incorporate cholesterol; the cholesterol:phospholipid molar ratio can hardly exceed 1:1. Glomset (1968) has proposed a mechanism that would overcome this theoretical limitation to the ability of HDL to take up cholesterol. He suggests that the unesterified cholesterol taken up by HDL is continually esterified by the LCAT reaction and transferred to the core of the particle, thus freeing the surface for uptake of more cholesterol. LCAT is present in the interstitial fluid, so that the esterification of newly-incorporated free cholesterol in the HDL particle could take place at or near the cell surface, though the mechanism could still function if HDL particles moved to and fro between the plasma and the interstitial fluid, and were acted upon by LCAT only while they were in the plasma. Glomset's mechanism for the transfer of cholesterol from cells to native HDL has not been demonstrated with isolated cells *in vitro*, though Murphy (1962) has shown that the capacity of HDL to take up cholesterol from red cells is increased if the HDL is preincubated in the presence of LCAT. Nor is there any direct evidence that the LCAT mechanism promotes the removal of tissue cholesterol *in vivo*, though there is no doubt that it plays an essential role in the disposal of free cholesterol within the plasma. The accumulation of free cholesterol in certain tissues of patients with familial LCAT deficiency (see Chapter 16) is not conclusive proof that LCAT is concerned in the normal removal of cholesterol from tissues, since the excess of free cholesterol in the tissues of these patients could be derived from the redundant surface material of triglyceride-rich lipoproteins that is normally disposed of by the LCAT reaction within the plasma, as discussed in Chapter 11. In any case, the abnormal deposits of free cholesterol in LCAT-deficient patients are found mainly in the reticulo-endothelial system.

In the above discussion of the possible natural acceptor for tissue cholesterol, we have treated HDL as if it were homogeneous, consisting of a single population of particles, all with the same size and chemical composition. But HDL is far from being a homogeneous lipoprotein. The HDL fraction isolated from normal human plasma contains particles varying continuously in size and lipid:protein ratio over the density range from 1.063–1.21 g/ml. At least two subpopulations within the HDL class have been identified. These are designated HDL_2 and HDL_3. The particles in the HDL_2 subclass are larger, and have a higher lipid:protein ratio, than the HDL_3 particles (Tables 11.3 and 11.4). Furthermore, HDL present in the circulation arises by the action of LCAT upon 'nascent' HDL particles secreted by the liver and intestine into the plasma. As we shall see in more detail in Chapter 11, the nascent particle is a disc consisting mainly of a phospholipid/free-cholesterol bilayer. During the conversion of these discs into mature spherical HDL particles by LCAT, the cholesterol content of each particle increases markedly by esterification of free cholesterol continuously taken up by the particle from other plasma constituents.

Thus, nascent HDL, together with LCAT, is an extremely efficient system for taking up free cholesterol and converting it into cholesteryl ester by a mechanism similar in principle to that proposed by Glomset for the removal of cholesterol from tissue cells. Nascent HDL would therefore be ideal as the acceptor for free cholesterol in reverse cholesterol transport. However, nascent HDL particles are not normally detectable in human plasma, other than in the splanchnic circulation (Turner et al., 1979), presumably because they react with LCAT as soon as they leave the liver. Hence, they are unlikely to survive long enough to reach the interstitial fluid at the surfaces of cells of the peripheral tissues.

It is possible that the immediate product of the action of LCAT on nascent HDL is the small spherical particle present in HDL_3 of normal plasma and that HDL_3 is converted into a more lipid-rich particle present in the HDL_2 density fraction, perhaps by the further action of LCAT in conjunction with the uptake of free cholesterol derived from triglyceride-rich lipoproteins (see Chapter 11 for details) or from the plasma membranes of tissue cells. If HDL_3 is indeed a precursor of a lipid-enriched component of HDL_2, it is of interest to calculate how much additional cholesterol could be accommodated by an HDL_3 particle. HDL_3 (mean m.w. 1.9×10^5) contains, on average, about 35 molecules of esterified cholesterol and about 15 of free cholesterol per particle, whereas HDL_2 (mean m.w. 3.9×10^5) contains an average of about 100 molecules of esterified cholesterol and about 50 of free cholesterol per particle. This corresponds to a net difference of some 100 molecules of total cholesterol per HDL particle. This calculation only provides a minimum estimate of the amount of cholesterol that could be accepted by HDL, since there is a continual mass transfer of newly-formed cholesteryl ester from HDL to VLDL and thence to LDL (see Chapter 11, Section 5.4). Thus, it is likely that much of the cholesteryl ester formed on HDL recycles to other lipoproteins, only a relatively small proportion being deposited in the liver as a consequence of the catabolism of HDL by liver cells.

Recycling of HDL cholesteryl ester, some of which may be derived from tissue free cholesterol, raises the question as to how far HDL can act *directly* as a 'reverse-transport' lipoprotein responsible for the transfer of cholesterol from the tissues to the liver. It is not easy to design a decisive experiment *in vivo* to test the assumption that HDL can act as an acceptor for tissue cholesterol. The obvious approach is to label tissue pools of cholesterol and then to look for evidence of selective uptake of labelled tissue free cholesterol by one or other of the lipoprotein fractions in plasma. Nestel and Miller (1978) labelled the adipose-tissue cholesterol in obese human subjects and then measured the specific activity of the cholesterol in HDL and LDL in plasma during a period of rapid weight loss accompanied by the mobilization of cholesterol from adipocytes. During calorie restriction there was a marked increase in cholesterol specific activity in HDL, but not in LDL. In an attempt to identify the lipoprotein acceptor for tissue cholesterol in direct contact with cell surfaces, Reichl *et al.* (1980) measured the specific activity of the free cholesterol in apoB-containing and apoA-I-containing lipoproteins in peripheral lymph from human subjects whose tissue cholesterol had been pre-labelled. In most cases the results suggested that an apoA-I-containing lipoprotein (presumably HDL) was the primary acceptor, though in at least one subject the predominant acceptor appeared to be LDL. It is possible, therefore, that different lipoproteins can act as cholesterol acceptor, depending upon such factors as the relative concentrations of HDL, LDL and other lipoproteins in the interstitial fluid. It should also be noted that evidence based on the use of labelled cholesterol may be hard to interpret owing to exchange of free cholesterol between lipoproteins and plasma membranes, which could be more rapid with some lipoproteins than with others.

REFERENCES

Andersen, J. M. and Dietschy, J. M. (1976). Cholesterogenesis: derepression in extrahepatic tissues with 4-aminopyrazolo[3,4-d]pyrimidine. *Science*, **193**, 903–905.

Anderson, R. G. W., Brown, M. S. and Goldstein, J. L. (1977). Role of the coated endocytic vesicle in the uptake of receptor-bound low density lipoprotein in human fibroblasts. *Cell*, **10**, 351–364.

Anderson, R. G. W., Vasile, E., Mello, R. J., Brown, M. S. and Goldstein, J. L. (1978). Immunocytochemical visualization of coated pits and vesicles in human fibroblasts: relation to low density lipoprotein receptor distribution. *Cell*, **15**, 919–933.

Angel, A., D'Costa, M. A. and Yuen, R. (1979). Low density lipoprotein binding, internalization, and degradation in human adipose cells. *Canadian Journal of Biochemistry*, **57**, 578–587.

Assmann, G., Simantke, O., Schaefer, H-E. and Smootz, E. (1977). Characterization of high density lipoproteins in patients heterozygous for Tangier disease. *Journal of Clinical Investigation*, **60**, 1025–1035.

Avigan, J. Studies on the effects of hormones on cholesterol synthesis in mammalian cells in culture. In: *Cholesterol Metabolism and Lipolytic Enzymes*. Ed. J. Polonowski. Marron Publishing U.S.A. Inc., New York, pp. 1–11, 1977.

Bailey, J. M. (1961). Lipid metabolism in cultured cells. I. Factors affecting cholesterol uptake. *Proceedings of the Society for Experimental Biology and Medicine*, **107**, 30–34.
Bailey, J. M. (1964). Lipid metabolism in cultured cells. V. Comparative lipid nutrition in serum and in lipid-free chemically defined medium. *Proceedings of the Society for Experimental Biology and Medicine*, **115**, 747–750.
Bailey, J. M. Cultured cells. In: *Lipid Metabolism in Mammals*, Vol. 2. Ed. F. Snyder. Plenum Press, New York, pp. 323–352, 1977.
Bailey, P. J. and Keller, D. (1971). The deposition of lipids from serum into cells cultured *in vitro*. *Atherosclerosis*, **13**, 33–343.
Balasubramaniam, S., Goldstein, J. L. and Brown, M. S. (1977a). Regulation of cholesterol synthesis in rat adrenal gland through coordinate control of 3-hydroxy-3-methylglutaryl coenzyme A synthase and reductase activities. *Proceedings of the National Academy of Sciences of the USA*, **74**, 1421–1425.
Balasubramaniam, S., Goldstein, J. L., Faust, J. R. and Brown, M. S. (1976). Evidence for regulation of 3-hydroxy-3-methylglutaryl coenzyme A reductase activity and cholesterol synthesis in nonhepatic tissues of rat. *Proceedings of the National Academy of Sciences of the USA*, **73**, 2564–2568.
Balasubramanian, S., Goldstein, J. L., Faust, J. R., Brunschede, G. Y. and Brown, M. S. (1977b). Lipoprotein-mediated regulation of 3-hydroxy-3-methylglutaryl coenzyme A reductase activity and cholesteryl ester metabolism in the adrenal gland of the rat. *Journal of Biological chemistry*, **252**, 1771–1779.
Basu, S. K., Goldstein, J. L. and Brown, M. S. (1978). Characterization of the low density lipoprotein receptor in membranes prepared from human fibroblasts. *Journal of Biological Chemistry*, **253**, 3852–3856.
Bates, S. R. and Rothblat, G. H. (1974). Regulation of cellular sterol flux and synthesis by human serum lipoproteins. *Biochimica et Biophysica Acta*, **360**, 38–55.
Bates, S. R. and Rothblat, G. (1975). Effect of mixtures of human serum lipoproteins on cellular sterol metabolism. *Artery*, **1**, 480–494.
Beirne, O. R., Heller, R. and Watson, J. A. (1977). Regulation of 3-hydroxy-3-methylglutaryl coenzyme A reductase in minimal deviation hepatoma 7288C. Immunological measurements in hepatoma tissue culture cells. *Journal of Biological Chemistry*, **252**, 950–954.
Beirne, O. R. and Watson, J. A. (1976). Comparison of regulation of 3-hydroxy-3-methylglutaryl coenzyme A reductase in hepatoma cells from *in vivo* and *in vitro*. *Proceedings of the National Academy of Sciences of the USA*, **73**, 2735–2739.
Bell, J. J., Sargeant, T. E. and Watson, J. A. (1976). Inhibition of 3-hydroxy-3-methylglutaryl coenzyme A reductase activity in hepatoma tissue culture cells by pure cholesterol and several cholesterol derivatives. *Journal of Biological Chemistry*, **251**, 1745–1758.
Betteridge, D. J., Krone, W., Ford, J. M. and Galton, D. J. (1979). Regulation of sterol synthesis in leukaemia blast cells: a defect resembling familial hypercholesterolaemia. *European Journal of Clinical Investigation*, **9**, 439–441.
Bierman, E. L. and Albers, J. J. (1975). Lipoprotein uptake by cultured human arterial smooth muscle cells. *Biochimica et Biophysica Acta*, **388**, 198–202.
Bierman, E. L., Stein, O. and Stein, Y. (1974). Lipoprotein uptake and metabolism by rat aortic smooth muscle cells in tissue culture. *Circulation Research*, **35**, 136–150.
Bissell, D. M., Hammaker, L. E. and Meyer, U. A. (1973). Parenchymal cells from adult rat liver in nonproliferating monolayer culture. 1. Functional studies. *Journal of Cell Biology*, **59**, 722–734.
Breslow, J. L., Lothrop, D. A., Clowes, A. W. and Lux, S. E. (1977). Lipoprotein regulation of 3-hydroxy-3-methylglutaryl coenzyme A reductase activity in rat liver cell cultures. *Journal of Biological Chemistry*, **252**, 2726–2733.

Brown, M. S., Faust, J. R., Goldstein, J. L., Kaneko, I. and Endo, A. (1978). Induction of 3-hydroxy-3-methylglutaryl coenzyme A reductase activity in human fibroblasts incubated with compactin (ML-236B), a competitive inhibitor of the reductase. *Journal of Biological Chemistry*, **253**, 1121–1128.

Brown, M. S. and Goldstein, J. L. (1974). Familial hypercholesterolemia: defective binding of lipoproteins to cultured fibroblasts associated with impaired regulation of 3-hydroxy-3-methylglutaryl Coenzyme A reductase activity. *Proceedings of the National Academy of Sciences of the USA*, **71**, 788–792.

Brown, M. S., Kovanen, P. T. and Goldstein, J. L. Receptor-mediated uptake of lipoprotein-cholesterol and its utilization for steroid synthesis in the adrenal cortex. In: *Recent Progress in Hormone Research, Vol. 35.* Ed. R. O. Greep. Academic Press, New York, pp. 215–257, 1979.

Carew, T. E., Koschinsky, T., Hayes, S. B. and Steinberg, D. (1976). A mechanism by which high-density lipoproteins may slow the atherogenic process. *Lancet*, **1**, 1315–1317.

Chang, T. Y., Telakowski, C., Heuvel, W. V., Alberts, A. W. and Vagelos, P. R. (1977). Isolation and partial characterization of a cholesterol-requiring mutant of Chinese hamster ovary cells. *Proceedings of the National Academy of Sciences of the USA*, **74**, 832–836.

Chao, Y-S., Windler, E. E., Chen, G. C. and Havel, R. J. (1979). Hepatic catabolism of rat and human lipoproteins in rats treated with 17α-ethinyl estradiol. *Journal of Biological Chemistry*, **254**, 11360–11366.

Edwards, P. A., Fogelman, A. M. and Popják, G. (1976). A direct relationship between the amount of sterol lost from rat hepatocytes and the increase in activity of HMG-CoA reductase. *Biochemical and Biophysical Research Communications*, **68**, 64–69.

Faust, J. R., Goldstein, J. L. and Brown, M. S. (1977). Receptor-mediated uptake of low density lipoprotein and utilization of its cholesterol for steroid synthesis in cultured mouse adrenal cells. *Journal of Biological Chemistry*, **252**, 4861–4871.

Florén, C-H. and Nilsson, Å. (1977). Binding, interiorization and degradation of cholesteryl ester-labelled chylomicron-remnant particles by rat hepatocyte monolayers. *Biochemical Journal*, **168**, 483–494.

Gibbons, G. F., Pullinger, C. R., Chen, H. W., Cavenee, W. K. and Kandutsch, A. A. (1980). Regulation of cholesterol biosynthesis in cultured cells by probable natural precursor sterols. *Journal of Biological Chemistry*, **255**, 395–400.

Glomset, J. A. (1968). The plasma lecithin:cholesterol acyltransferase reaction. *Journal of Lipid Research*, **9**, 151–167.

Goldstein, J. L., Anderson, R. G. W. and Brown, M. S. (1979b). Coated pits, coated vesicles, and receptor-mediated endocytosis. *Nature*, **279**, 679–685.

Goldstein, J. L., Anderson, R. G. W., Buja, L. M., Basu, S. K. and Brown, M. S. (1977a). Overloading human aortic smooth muscle cells with low density lipoprotein-cholesteryl esters reproduces features of atherosclerosis *in vitro*. *Journal of Clinical Investigation*, **59**, 1196–1202.

Goldstein, J. L., Basu, S. K., Brunschede, G. Y. and Brown, M. S. (1976). Release of low density lipoprotein from its cells surface receptor by sulfated glycosaminoglycans. *Cell*, **7**, 85–95.

Goldstein, J. L. and Brown, M. S. (1973). Familial hypercholesterolemia: Identification of a defect in the regulation of 3-hydroxy-3-methylglutaryl coenzyme A reductase activity associated with overproduction of cholesterol. *Proceedings of the National Academy of Sciences of the USA*, **70**, 2804–2808.

Goldstein, J. L. and Brown, M. S. (1974). Binding and degradation of low density lipoproteins by cultured human fibroblasts. Comparison of cells from a normal subject and from a patient with homozygous familial hypercholesterolemia. *Journal of Biological Chemistry*, **249**, 5153–5162.

Goldstein, J. L. and Brown, M. S. (1975). Lipoprotein receptors, cholesterol metabolism, and atherosclerosis. *Archives and Pathology*, **99**, 181–184.

Goldstein, J. L. and Brown, M. S. The LDL pathway in human fibroblasts: a receptor-mediated mechanism for the regulation of cholesterol metabolism. *Current Topics in Cellular Regulation*, Vol. *11*. Ed. B. Horecker and E. R. Stadtman. Academic Press, New York, pp. 147–181, 1976.

Goldstein, J. L. and Brown, M. S. (1977). The low-density lipoprotein pathway and its relation to atherosclerosis. *Annual Review of Biochemistry*, **46**, 897–930.

Goldstein, J. L. and Brown, M. S. (1979). The LDL receptor locus and the genetics of familial hypercholesterolemia. *Annual Review of Genetics*, **13**, 259–289.

Goldstein, J. L., Brown, M. S. and Stone, N. J. (1977*b*). Genetics of the LDL receptor: evidence that the mutations affecting binding and internalization are allelic. *Cell*, **12**, 629–641.

Goldstein, J. L., Ho, Y. K., Basu, S. K. and Brown, M. S. (1979*a*). Binding site on macrophages that mediates uptake and degradation of acetylated low density lipoprotein, producing massive choleterol deposition. *Proceedings of the National Academy of Sciences of the USA*, **76**, 333–337.

Gwynne, J. T., Mahaffee, D., Brewer, H. B. and Ney, R. L. (1976). Adrenal cholesterol uptake from plasma lipoproteins: regulation by corticotropin. *Proceedings of the National Academy of Sciences of the USA*, **73**, 4329–4333.

Ho, Y. K., Brown, M. S., Bilheimer, D. W. and Goldstein, J. L. (1976*a*). Regulation of low density lipoprotein receptor activity in freshly isolated human lymphocytes. *Journal of Clinical Invetigation*, **58**, 1465–1474.

Ho, Y. K., Brown, M. S., Kayden, H. J. and Goldstein, J. L. (1976*b*). Binding, internalization, and hydrolysis of low density lipoprotein in long-term lymphoid cell lines from a normal subject and a patient with homozygous familial hypercholesterolemia. *Journal of Experimental Medicine*, **144**, 444–455.

Howard, B. V. and Howard, W. J. (1974). Lipid metabolism in cultured cells. *Advances in Lipid Research*, **12**, 51–96.

Howard, B. V., Howard, W. J. and Bailey, J. M. (1974). Acetyl coenzyme A synthetase and the regulation of lipid synthesis from acetate in cultured cells. *Journal of Biological Chemistry*, **249**, 7912–7921.

Iverius, P-H. (1972). The interaction between human plasma lipoproteins and connective tissue glycosaminoglycans. *Journal of Biological Chemistry*, **247**, 2607–2613.

Kandutsch, A. A. and Chen, H. W. (1973). Inhibition of sterol synthesis in cultured mouse cells by 7α-hydroxycholesterol, 7β-hydroxycholesterol, and 7-ketocholesterol. *Journal of Biological Chemistry*, **248**, 8408–8417.

Kandutsch, A. A. and Chen, H. W. (1974). Inhibition of sterol synthesis in cultured mouse cells by cholesterol derivatives oxygenated in the side chain. *Journal of Biological Chemistry*, **249**, 6057–6061.

Kandutsch, A. A., Chen, H. W. and Heiniger, H-J. (1978). Biological activity of some oxygenated sterols. *Science*, **201**, 498–501.

Kayden, H. J., Hatam, L. and Beratis, N. G. (1976). Regulation of 3-hydroxy-3-methylglutaryl coenzyme A reductase activity and the esterification of cholesterol in human long term lymphoid cell lines. *Biochemistry*, **15**, 521–528.

Kirsten, E. S. and Watson, J. A. (1974). Regulation of 3-hydroxy-3-methylglutaryl coenzyme A reductase in hepatoma tissue culture cells by serum lipoproteins. *Journal of Biological Chemistry*, **249**, 6104–6109.

Kovanen, P. T., Basu, S. K., Goldstein, J. L. and Brown, M. S. (1979*a*). Low density lipoprotein receptors in bovine adrenal cortex. II. Low density lipoprotein binding to membranes prepared from fresh tissue. *Endocrinology*, **104**, 610–616.

Kovanen, P. T., Brown, M. S. and Goldstein, J. L. (1979*b*). Increased binding of low density lipoprotein to liver membranes from rats treated with 17α-ethinylestradiol. *Journal of Biological Chemistry*, **254**, 11367–11373.

Kovanen, P. T., Faust, J. R., Brown, M. S. and Goldstein, J. L. (1979c). Low density lipoprotein receptors in bovine adrenal cortex. I. Receptor-mediated uptake of low density lipoprotein and utilization of its cholesterol for steroid synthesis in cultured adrenocortical cells. *Endocrinology*, **104**, 599–609.

Kovanen, P. T., Schneider, W. J., Hillman, G. M., Goldstein, J. L. and Brown, M. S. (1979). Separate mechanisms for the uptake of high and low density lipoproteins by mouse adrenal gland *in vivo*. *Journal of Biological Chemistry*, **254**, 2498–2505.

Kowal, J. (1970). ACTH and the metabolism of adrenal cell cultures. *Recent Progress in Hormone Research*, **26**, 623–676.

Mahley, R. W., Weisgraber, K. H., Bersot, T. P. and Innerarity, T. L. Effects of cholesterol feeding on human and animal high density lipoproteins. In: *High Density Lipoproteins and Atherosclerosis*. Ed. A. M. Gotto Jr., N. E. Miller and M. F. Oliver. Elsevier, Amsterdam, pp. 149–176, 1978.

Miller, N. E., Weinstein, D. B., Carew, T. E., Koschinsky, T. and Steinberg, D. (1977). Interaction between high density and low density lipoproteins during uptake and degradation by cultured human fibroblasts. *Journal of Clinical Investigation*, **60**, 78–88.

Murphy, J. R. (1962). Erythrocyte metabolism. III. Relationship of energy metabolism and serum factors to the osmotic fragility following incubation. *Journal of Laboratory and Clinical Medicine*, **60**, 86–109.

Nestel, P. J. and Miller, N. E. Mobilization of adipose tissue cholesterol in high density lipoprotein during weight reduction in man. In: *High Density Lipoproteins and Atherosclerosis*. Ed. A. M. Gotto Jr., N. E. Miller and M. F. Oliver. Elsevier, Amsterdam, pp. 51–54, 1978.

Ose, L., Ose, T., Norum, K. R. and Berg, T. (1979). Uptake and degradation of ^{125}I-labelled high density lipoproteins in rat liver cells *in vivo* and *in vitro*. *Biochemica et Biophysica Acta*, **574**, 521–535.

Paul, J. *Cell And Tissue Culture*, 5th edition. Churchill Livingstone, Edinburgh, 1975.

Pitas, R. E., Innerarity, T. L., Arnold, K. S. and Mahley, R. W. (1979). Rate and equilibrium constants for binding of ape-E HLD$_c$ (a cholesterol-induced lipoprotein) and low density lipoproteins to human fibroblasts: Evidence for multiple receptor binding of apo-E HDL$_c$. *Proceedings of the National Academy of Sciences of the USA*, **76**, 2311–2315.

Rachmilewitz, D., Stein, O., Roheim, P. S. and Stein, Y. (1972). Metabolism of iodinated high density lipoproteins in the rat. II. Autoradiographic localization in the liver. *Biochimica et Biophysica Acta*, **270**, 414–525.

Reichl, D. and Myant, N. B. Lipoproteins of human peripheral lymph. In: *Protides of the Biological Fluids, Proceedings of the Twenty-Fifth Colloquium*. Ed. H. Peeters. Pergamon Press, Oxford, pp. 189–192, 1978.

Reichl, D., Myant, N. B., Brown, M. S. and Goldstein, J. L. (1978). Biologically active low density lipoprotein in human peripheral lymph. *Journal of Clinical Investigation*, **61**, 64–71.

Reichl, D., Myant, N. B. and Lloyd, J. K. (1978). Surface binding and catabolism of low-density lipoprotein by circulating lymphocytes from patients with abetalipoproteinaemia, with observations on sterol synthesis in lymphocytes from one patient. *Biochimica et Biophysica Acta*, **530**, 124–131.

Reichl, D., Myant, N. B. and Pflug, J. J. (1977a). Concentration of lipoproteins containing apolipoprotein B in human peripheral lymph. *Biochimica et Biophysica Acta*, **429**, 98–105.

Reichl, D., Myant, N. B., Rudra, D. N. and Pflug, J. J. (1980). Evidence for the presence of tissue-free cholesterol in low-density- and high-density-lipoproteins of human peripheral lymph. *Atherosclerosis*, **37**, 489–495.

Reichl, D., Myant, N. B., Pflug, J. J. and Rudra, D. N. (1977b). The passage of apoproteins from plasma lipoproteins into the lipoproteins of peripheral lymph in man. *Clinical Science and Molecular Medicine*, **53**, 221–226.

Reichl, D., Postiglione, A. and Myant, N. B. (1976). Uptake and catabolism of low density lipoprotein by human lymphocytes. *Nature*, **260**, 634–635.

Rothblat, G. H. (1969). Lipid metabolism in tissue culture cells. *Advances in Lipid Research*, **7**, 135–163.

Rothblat, G. H. Cellular sterol metabolism. In: *Growth, Nutrition and Metabolism of Cells in Culture*, Vol. 1. Ed. G. H. Rothblat and V. J. Cristofalo. Academic Press, New York, pp. 297–325, 1972.

Schneider, W. J., Basu, S. K., McPhaul, M. J., Goldstein, J. L. and Brown, M. S. (1979). Solubilization of the low density lipoprotein receptor. *Proceedings of the National Academy of Sciences of the USA*, **76**, 5577–5581.

Schroepfer, G. J., Pascal, R. A. Jr., Shaw, R. and Kandutsch, A. A. (1978). Inhibition of sterol biosynthesis by 14α-hydroxymethyl sterols. *Biochemical and Biophysical Research Communications*, **83**, 1024–1031.

Sherrill, B. C., Innerarity, T. L. and Mahley, R. W. (1980). Rapid hepatic clearance of the canine lipoproteins containing only the E apoprotein by a high affinity receptor. *Journal of Biological Chemistry*, **255**, 1804–1807.

Small, D. M. (1977). Cellular mechanisms for lipid deposition in atherosclerosis. *New England Journal of Medicine*, **297**, 873–877, 924–929.

Stein, O. and Stein, Y. (1976). High density lipoproteins reduce the uptake of low density lipoproteins by human endothelial cells in culture. *Biochimica et Biophysica Acta*, **431**, 363–368.

Stein, O., Vanderhoek, J. and Stein, Y. (1976). Cholesterol content and sterol synthesis in human skin fibroblasts and rat aortic smooth muscle cells exposed to lipoprotein-depleted serum and high density apolipoprotein/phospholipid mixtures. *Biochimica et Biophysica Acta*, **431**, 347–358.

Stein, Y., Glangeaud, M. C., Fainaru, M. and Stein, O. (1975). The removal of cholesterol from aortic smooth muscle cells in culture and Landschutz ascites cells by fractions of human high density apolipoprotein. *Biochimica et Biophysica Acta*, **380**, 106–118.

Steinberg, D., Carew, T. E., Weinstein, D. B. and Koschinsky, T. Binding, uptake, and catabolism of low density (LDL) and high density lipoproteins (HDL) by cultured smooth muscle cells. In: *Lipoprotein Metabolism*. Ed. H. Greten. Springer-Verlag, Berlin, pp. 90–98, 1976.

Turner, P., Miller, N., Chrystie, I., Coltart, J., Mistry, P., Nicoll, A. and Lewis, B. (1979). Splanchnic production of discoidal plasma high-density lipoprotein in man. *Lancet*, **1**, 645–647.

Vlodavsky, I., Fielding, P. E., Fielding, C. J. and Gospodarowicz, D. (1978). Role of contact inhibition in the regulation of receptor-mediated uptake of low density lipoprotein in cultured vascular endothelial cells. *Proceedings of the National Academy of Sciences of the USA*, **75**, 356–360.

Weinstein, D. B., Carew, T. E. and Steinberg, D. (1976). Uptake and degradation of low density lipoprotein by swine arterial smooth muscle cells with inhibition of cholesterol biosynthesis. *Biochimica et Biophysica Acta*, **424**, 404–421.

Werb, Z. and Cohn, Z. A. (1971a). Cholesterol metabolism in the macrophage. I. The regulation of cholesterol exchange. *Journal of Experimental Medicine*, **134**, 1545–1569.

Werb, Z. and Cohn, Z. A. (1971b). Cholesterol metabolism in the macrophage. II. Alteration of subcellular exchangeable cholesterol compartments and exchange in other cell types. *Journal of Experimental Medicine*, **134**, 1570–1590.

Werb, Z. and Cohn, Z. A. (1972). Cholesterol metabolism in the macrophage. III. Ingestion and intracellular fate of cholesterol and cholesterol esters. *Journal of Experimental Medicine*, **135**, 21–44.

Williams, C. D. and Avigan, J. (1972). *In vitro* effects of serum proteins and lipids on lipid synthesis in human skin fibroblasts and leukocytes grown in culture. *Biochimica et Biophysica Acta*, **260**, 413–423.

Zeleznik, A. J. and Roth, J. (1978). Demonstration of the insulin receptor *in vivo* in rabbits and its possible rôle as a reservoir for the plasma hormone. *Journal of Clinical Investigation*, **61**, 1363–1374.

Chapter 10

Cholesterol Metabolism in the Whole Body

1	INTRODUCTION	449
2	EXCHANGEABLE CHOLESTEROL IN THE WHOLE BODY.	449
2.1	Investigation by pulse-labelling or labelling to isotopic equilibrium	449
2.2	Measurement of the turnover and mass of exchangeable cholesterol.	453
2.2.1	Definitions	453
2.2.2	Measurement of turnover by sterol balance	454
2.2.3	Measurement of turnover and mass by analysis of plasma specific activity-time curves	455
3	CHOLESTEROL SYNTHESIS IN THE WHOLE BODY	459
3.1	Methods of measurement	459
3.1.1	Specific activity-time curves	459
3.1.2	Sterol balance	460
3.1.3	Incorporation of labelled precursors	460
3.2	Rates of cholesterol synthesis in the whole body.	463
4	CHOLESTEROL ABSORPTION	466
4.1	Definition.	466
4.2	The sources of absorbed cholesterol	466
4.3	The routes of absorption	467
4.4	The mechanism of absorption	467
4.4.1	The luminal phase.	467
4.4.2	The mucosal phase	470
4.5	Sterols other than cholesterol	471
4.6	Methods of measurement	473
4.6.1	Non-isotopic sterol balance	473
4.6.2	Combined chemical and isotopic balance	473
4.6.3	Faecal excretion of a single labelled oral dose.	474
4.6.4	Plasma radioactivity after oral labelling.	474
4.6.5	The isotope-ratio method	474
4.6.6	Recovery of cholesterol from a lymph-duct fistula	475
4.6.7	Absorption of endogenous cholesterol and the method of intestinal perfusion	475

448 The Biology of Cholesterol and Related Steroids

4.7	The rate of absorption	476
4.7.1	Normal rates in man and experimental animals	476
4.7.2	Factors influencing cholesterol absorption	479
5	CHANGES IN WHOLE-BODY METABOLISM	480
5.1	Dietary cholesterol	480
5.1.1	Absorption as a regulatory mechanism	481
5.1.2	Responses to changes in cholesterol absorption	481
5.2	Polyunsaturated fat	484
5.3	Other dietary factors	487
5.4	Hyperlipidaemia and obesity	491
5.5	Drugs and operative procedures	492
5.5.1	Bile-acid binding resins	492
5.5.2	Thyroid hormones	494
5.5.3	Clofibrate, nicotinic acid and neomycin	494
5.5.4	Operative procedures	496

Cholesterol Metabolism in the Whole Body

1 INTRODUCTION

The synthesis, uptake and excretion of cholesterol by the cells of animal tissues were discussed in Chapters 8 and 9. In this chapter the metabolism and distribution of cholesterol are considered from the point of view of the body as a whole. Various aspects of the turnover of the plasma cholesterol, including its esterification and its transport between different lipoprotein fractions, are considered in the next chapter.

2 EXCHANGEABLE CHOLESTEROL IN THE WHOLE BODY

2.1 Investigation by pulse-labelling or labelling to isotopic equilibrium

The plasma cholesterol is part of an exchangeable mass which includes the bulk of the cholesterol in the extravascular tissues. This is apparent from the familiar observation that when radioactive cholesterol is injected intravenously into an adult animal, the cholesterol in virtually all the tissues other than the central nervous system becomes labelled.

After a single intravenous injection of plasma lipoprotein labelled with radioactive free cholesterol,* the specific activity-time curve of the plasma cholesterol exhibits an initial rapid fall which merges with

---

* After an intravenous injection of an *emulsion* of radioactive free cholesterol the injected dose is removed from the circulation very rapidly, mainly by the Kupffer cells in the liver (Nilsson and Zilversmit, 1972), subsequently reappearing in the plasma lipoproteins as free cholesterol.

a log-linear phase. In human subjects the log-linear phase begins about 6 weeks after the injection, but in most experimental animals the transition to log-linearity is earlier than this. Detailed analysis of the early part of the curve obtained by frequent plasma sampling during the first 2–3 days shows that the initial phase can be resolved into at least three components, possibly reflecting equilibration of the dose with liver cholesterol, red-cell cholesterol and plasma esterified cholesterol (Porte and Havel, 1961). Thus, the form of the specific activity-time curve indicates the presence of multiple pools of cholesterol which equilibrate with the plasma cholesterol at different rates.

The existence of multiple pools may also be demonstrated by observing the rise in specific activity of the cholesterol in different tissues after an intravenous injection of radioactive cholesterol. Such observations show that the times taken to reach maximum specific activity vary from a few hours to periods measured in days or weeks. In man, for example, the plasma free cholesterol equilibrates with cholesterol in the liver in less than 3 hours (Gould et al., 1955), whereas equilibration with adipose-tissue cholesterol takes several weeks (Schreibman and Dell, 1975). Observations on the specific activity of the cholesterol in tissues taken at various times after a single dose of [^{14}C]cholesterol in rats (Avigan et al., 1962) and human subjects (Gould et al., 1955; Field et al., 1960; Chobanian and Hollander, 1962) indicate that the plasma cholesterol exchanges relatively rapidly with the cholesterol in liver, red cells, spleen, lung and intestine, more slowly with that in skeletal muscle, adipose tissue, skin and kidney, and even more slowly with the cholesterol of the arterial wall. In tissues in which the fractional rate of turnover of the exchangeable cholesterol is slower than that of the plasma cholesterol, the specific activity at long intervals after an intravenous injection of radioactive cholesterol may be several times higher than that of the plasma cholesterol. This has been shown both in man (Moutafis and Myant, 1969; Schreibman and Dell, 1975) and animals (Avigan et al., 1962; Moutafis and Myant, 1976), as shown in Fig. 10.1.

Another method of studying exchange between the cholesterol of plasma and tissues (the isotopic equilibrium method) has been discussed in considerable detail by Chevallier (1967). If an animal or human subject is fed radioactive cholesterol of constant specific activity for long periods of time, the specific activity of the plasma cholesterol eventually reaches a plateau and then remains constant as long as the feeding is continued. When the plateau has been reached, isotopic equilibrium should have been achieved throughout the exchangeable mass of cholesterol in the whole body. Under these conditions, the fraction of the total exchangeable cholesterol that is derived from the diet will be equal to the ratio of the specific activity of the plasma cholesterol to that of the dietary cholesterol; in the

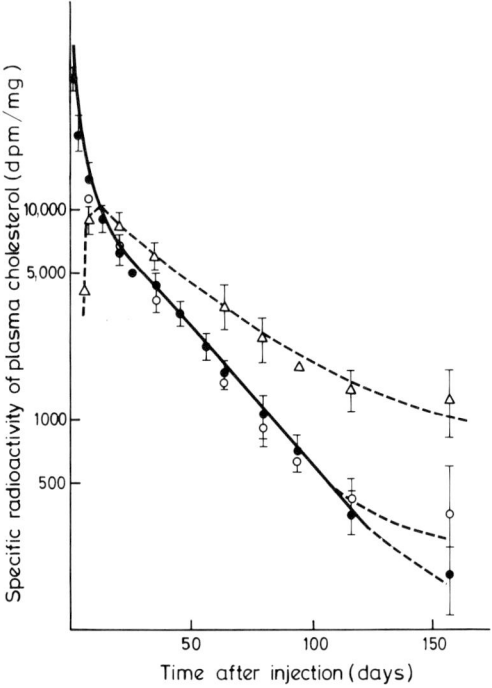

Figure 10.1
Time-course of the changes in specific radioactivity of the cholesterol in plasma (●), muscle (△) and skin (○) of monkeys after a single intravenous injection of [4-^{14}C]cholesterol. Note that the peak specific radioactivity in muscle cholesterol occurs at the point where the plasma and muscle specific-activity curves intersect, indicating a precursor-product relationship between plasma cholesterol and muscle cholesterol. (From Moutafis and Myant, 1976.)

extreme case, if all the exchangeable cholesterol in the body were of dietary origin the specific activity of the plasma cholesterol at isotopic equilibrium would be equal to that of the cholesterol in the diet. Furthermore, at isotopic equilibrium the proportion of the total cholesterol in the body that is exchangeable with the plasma cholesterol may be estimated as the ratio: mean specific activity of whole-body cholesterol ÷ specific activity of plasma cholesterol. According to Chevallier (1967), this ratio, estimated in rats fed radioactive cholesterol for 25 weeks, is about 0.70, i.e. about 70% of all the cholesterol in a rat's body is exchangeable with the plasma cholesterol.

During the approach to isotopic equilibrium the specific activity of the cholesterol in different tissues rises at widely different rates. In liver, red cells, lungs and spleen, for example, the rise in specific activity closely parallels that in the plasma, indicating rapid exchange between the cholesterol of these tissues and the plasma cholesterol. In other tissues, including muscle, kidney and aorta, the rise is considerably slower, in keeping with the slow exchange of the cholesterol in these tissues observed after pulse-labelling of the plasma. In most organs the specific activity of the total cholesterol eventually reaches a value equal to, or very close to, that of the plasma cholesterol, indicating that all their cholesterol is exchangeable. In some tissues, however, the specific activity never reaches that in the plasma, even after long periods of feeding the radioactive cholesterol. Morris and Chaikoff (1959), for example, found that when rats were fed [^{14}C]cholesterol for six weeks the specific activity of the cholesterol in the testis was only 38% of that in plasma, whereas the specific activities in the adrenal and plasma were virtually identical. Failure to achieve equal specific activities in plasma and tissue under these conditions could be due either to continual synthesis of cholesterol within the tissue at a rapid rate in relation to the rate at which cholesterol exchanges between the tissue and the plasma, or to the presence of non-exchangeable cholesterol in the tissue. A distinction between these two possibilities is difficult to make in practice, but experiments combining the use of pulse-labelling with labelling to isotopic equilibrium suggest that certain tissues, in addition to the central nervous system, contain cholesterol that does not undergo significant exchange with the plasma cholesterol during the lifetime of an adult animal. These include skin, colon, testis and bone (Wilson, 1970).

Thus, the total exchangeable mass of cholesterol comprises many pools equilibrating with the plasma cholesterol at different rates. Furthermore, there may be more than one pool within a given tissue, within a given cell and (since compartmentation of cholesterol has been demonstrated in liver microsomes) within a given subcellular fraction. Mixing throughout the exchangeable mass is a complex process to which several factors contribute. These include the exchange of free cholesterol between plasma lipoproteins and cell surfaces, the net cellular uptake of lipoprotein cholesterol with net excretion of the internalized cholesterol, and the mixing of cholesterol within the cell, a process which may be mediated by the formation of soluble cholesterol-carrier complexes. The enterohepatic circulation of cholesterol must also contribute to the mixing of cholesterol molecules between plasma, liver, bile and intestinal wall.

The exchangeable cholesterol in the whole body is in a state of flux owing to continual removal from the body by *excretion* and *catabolism*, with replacement by *endogenous synthesis* and, in animals whose diet contains cholesterol, by *absorption* from the food. In the steady state, output from the exchangeable mass is, by definition, exactly balanced by input. To understand the physiology of exchangeable cholesterol in the organism as a whole we need, at the very least, to be able to measure the flux or turnover (g/day) of the whole exchangeable mass, the relative contributions of newly-synthesized and dietary cholesterol to the total turnover and finally, the total mass of all cholesterol that is exchangeable with the plasma cholesterol. More detailed information about the amounts of cholesterol in the various pools of exchangeable cholesterol and about the rates of flow into and out of these pools is also desirable; as discussed above, a limited amount of such information is already available.

In Section 2.2 I shall consider the measurement of the turnover and mass of the exchangeable cholesterol, with particular reference to living human subjects in the steady state and under non-steady-state conditions such as those induced by drugs or dietary factors. In Section 3 I shall consider the measurement of the rate of synthesis of cholesterol in the whole organism. The contribution of dietary cholesterol to total turnover is considered in Section 4 as part of a general discussion of the absorption of cholesterol from the intestine.

2.2 Measurement of the turnover and mass of exchangeable cholesterol

2.2.1 Definitions

In this section and throughout the subsequent discussion of whole-body turnover and absorption of cholesterol, the following definitions are used:

The *total exchangeable mass* of cholesterol is the mass that equilibrates with the plasma cholesterol within a period of time that is long in relation to the life of the animal. The actual equilibration time taken as a basis for the definition is to a certain extent arbitrary. The observations of Samuel and Lieberman (1973) suggest a limit of 50–66 weeks in man, though it is possible that there are very slowly exchanging pools of cholesterol in the human body that do not equilibrate completely even within this period. As discussed below, it may be acceptable for practical purposes to define the total exchangeable mass of cholesterol in man in terms of much shorter equilibration times (see Goodman, Noble and Dell, 1973).

The term *faecal neutral steroids* refers to the cholesterol, together with the steroids resulting from its bacterial modification, excreted in the faeces. The term includes all the neutral steroids derived from endogenous cholesterol (as defined below) and from unabsorbed dietary cholesterol, but arbitrarily excludes plant sterols and the products of their modification by intestinal bacteria.

The term *endogenous cholesterol* refers to all the cholesterol in the exchangeable mass, including that derived from synthesis within the body and that derived from absorption of dietary cholesterol. Hence, *faecal neutral steroids of endogenous origin* are the faecal neutral steroids derived from endogenous cholesterol secreted into the lumen of the intestine *via* the bile duct or the intestinal wall. Note that the term *endogenous cholesterol* is restricted by some authors to the cholesterol synthesized within the body.

The *production rate* in a pool of exchangeable cholesterol is the rate of entry of cholesterol into that pool, excluding cholesterol that has re-entered the pool after reversible transfer into other pools (Gurpide *et al.*, 1964). An alternative definition is the rate at which cholesterol molecules enter the pool for the first time.

The term *steady state*, when used in relation to cholesterol metabolism in the whole organism, refers to a state in which (1) the rates of absorption and whole-body synthesis of cholesterol are constant and (2) there is no net transfer of exchangeable cholesterol to or from the tissues. If both these conditions are satisfied, the total exchangeable mass of cholesterol remains constant. In the steady state, the plasma cholesterol concentration is constant, the rate of excretion of total endogenous steroids (neutral plus acidic) is constant and there is no growth or change in body weight.

Turnover of cholesterol refers to the absolute rate at which exchangeable cholesterol is lost from the body and replaced by synthesis and absorption of dietary cholesterol. In the absence of dietary cholesterol, synthesis is equal to turnover.

2.2.2 Measurement of turnover by sterol balance

If it is assumed that excretion *via* the intestine is the only route for exit of cholesterol and its metabolites from the exchangeable mass, the total turnover of cholesterol (g/day) in the steady state should be equal to the sum of endogenous neutral steroids and bile acids excreted in the faeces (g/day). In a human subject whose plasma cholesterol has been labelled by an intravenous injection of radioactive cholesterol, daily excretion of endogenous neutral steroids may be estimated as: [total radioactivity in the faecal neutral steroid fraction] ÷ [specific activity of the plasma cholesterol 1–2 days previously]. Daily excretion of bile acids may be estimated by GLC (Chapter 2, Section 6.3). Total radioactivity in the acidic steroid fraction should be corrected for variations in faecal flow by means of an unabsorbed marker (Davignon *et al.*, 1968) and, in subjects taking liquid-formula diets, degradation of the sterol ring system by intestinal bacteria should be corrected for by measuring the recovery of an oral dose of β-sitosterol, a plant sterol that is essentially unabsorbed from the human intestine but is degraded by intestinal bacteria to the same extent as is cholesterol (Grundy *et al.*, 1968).

A satisfactory estimate of cholesterol turnover by the balance method may be made in 3–4 weeks by analysing six 4-day faecal collections. In so far as small amounts of exchangeable cholesterol may be excreted through the skin (Bhattacharyya et al., 1970) or may be converted into steroid hormones that are ultimately excreted in the urine, total turnover is underestimated by the sterol balance method. However, this error is unlikely to amount to much more than 100 mg/day (see Nikkari et al., 1974).

2.2.3 Measurement of turnover and mass by analysis of plasma specific activity-time curves

Early attempts to estimate total turnover of exchangeable cholesterol from the plasma specific activity-time curve obtained after an intravenous injection of radioactive cholesterol were based on the assumption that the initial fall was due to mixing of the dose within a single pool and that the log-linear phase reflected turnover of the cholesterol in this pool. On these assumptions total exchangeable mass was estimated from the specific activity obtained by extrapolating the log-linear portion of the curve to zero time, and the rate of turnover was estimated from the total exchangeable mass and the half-life of the log-linear phase of the curve (Chobanian et al., 1962; Lewis and Myant, 1967). Rates of turnover estimated by this method in normal and hyperlipidaemic human subjects were nearly twice as high as the rates estimated from the faecal excretion of bile acids and endogenous neutral steroids in the same subject (Lewis and Myant, 1967). Estimates of the total exchangeable mass of cholesterol were also much higher than is now considered reasonable. There are several reasons for these discrepancies, but the most important is undoubtedly the erroneous assumption that the specific activity-time curve reflects mixing and turnover in a single pool of cholesterol.

Goodman and Noble (1968) showed that the curves obtained by sampling the plasma at intervals of a few days during the first 10 weeks after an injection of radioactive cholesterol could be interpreted more satisfactorily by compartmental analysis, using the method of Gurpide et al. (1964) applicable to a two-pool system. In the model proposed by Goodman and Noble, cholesterol exchanges between two pools (Fig. 10.2). Pool A, which includes the plasma and is therefore the pool into which the labelled cholesterol is introduced, turns over rapidly, while pool B turns over more slowly. It should be understood that neither pool of cholesterol corresponds to a physical entity, since a given organ or tissue may contain cholesterol in both pools. Moreover, interpretation of the plasma specific activity curve in terms of two pools is clearly an over-simplification since, as we have already seen, the plasma cholesterol is known to exchange with many pools of cholesterol whose rates of turnover differ widely. Nevertheless, despite the presence of multiple pools of exchangeable cholesterol in the body, the plasma specific activity curves obtained from human subjects over a 10-week period can always be resolved into two

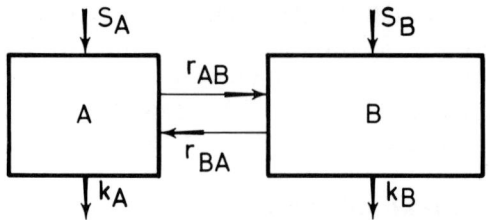

Figure 10.2
The two-pool model proposed by Goodman and Noble (1968) for the distribution and turnover of cholesterol in man. A is a rapidly-turning-over pool that includes the cholesterol in plasma, and B is a pool with slow turnover that includes cholesterol in skeletal muscle and adipose tissue. S_A and S_B are the rates of entry (g/day) of cholesterol into A and B from outside the system; K_A and K_B are the rate constants for the removal of cholesterol from pool A and pool B, and r_{AB} and r_{BA} are rate constants for the transfer of cholesterol from A to B and from B to A, respectively. See the text for discussion of the parameters that can be estimated from the plasma cholesterol specific activity curve obtained after a single intravenous injection of [^{14}C]cholesterol on the basis of various assumptions. (From Goodman and Noble, 1968; after Gurpide *et al.*, 1964.)

exponential components (Goodman and Noble, 1968), possibly because the various pools that equilibrate within this period fall broadly into two groups, one group containing pools which turn over relatively rapidly and the other containing pools with slower rates of turnover. Goodman and Noble suggest that pool A comprises the cholesterol in liver, bile, plasma, red cells and small intestine, together with some of the cholesterol in several other viscera, while pool B contains most of the cholesterol in skeletal muscle, adipose tissue, skin and arterial wall.

By analysing the plasma specific activity curve in terms of this model it is possible to estimate several quantities that are relevant to cholesterol turnover in the whole body. If no assumptions are made about k_B or S_B (a quantity equivalent to the rate of synthesis of cholesterol in pool B), it is possible to estimate the mass of pool A and the production rate of pool A. If it is assumed that the only route for the exit of cholesterol from the whole system is *via* pool A, then k_B becomes zero and the production rate of pool A becomes equal to S_A + S_B. This corresponds to the total rate of entry of cholesterol into the system from synthesis and absorption of dietary cholesterol, and is thus equivalent to the rate of turnover of the whole exchangeable mass in the steady state. Even if k_B is assumed to be zero, the mass of pool B cannot be estimated from parameters deducible from the specific activity-time curve. However, it is possible to calculate a lower limit on the additional assumption that no cholesterol is synthesized in pool B (i.e. that both k_B and S_B are zero) and an upper limit on the assumption that no synthesis occurs in pool A and, hence, that all the cholesterol entering pool A is derived from the diet or from synthesis in pool B.

On the basis of these assumptions Nestel *et al.* (1969) have estimated the production rate, the mass of pool A and the mean of the maximum and minimum values for the mass of pool B (M_{BM}) in a group of adult human subjects from whom plasma specific activity-time curves were obtained over a 10-week period after injection of [^{14}C]cholesterol. The production rate ranged from 0.73 to 1.68 g/day, the mean value for the mass of pool A was 22.7 g and the mean value for M_{BM} was 42.4 g, suggesting that the total mass of cholesterol that equilibrates with the plasma cholesterol within 10 weeks is about 65 g or, in round figures, about 1 g/kg body weight. In the group of subjects studied by Nestel *et al.*, neither the production rate nor the mass of pool B was correlated with the plasma cholesterol concentration, but both were positively correlated with excess body weight. From the regression of production rate on excess body weight, Nestel *et al.* estimated that the production rate of an adult of ideal body weight for height, weighing 60 kg, would be 1.1 g/day.

In man, the mass of exchangeable cholesterol cannot be measured directly *in vivo*. In animals, on the other hand, it is possible to estimate the exchangeable mass by analysing the plasma specific activity-time curve obtained after labelling with radioactive cholesterol and then to compare the value so obtained with the value determined directly, after killing the animal (total radioactivity in the whole body ÷ specific activity of the plasma cholesterol at death). In baboons (Wilson, 1970) and squirrel monkeys (Lofland *et al.*, 1970) estimates based on analysis in terms of a two-pool model agree closely with the values determined *post mortem* by direct measurement. This might suggest that the two-pool model is valid for man. However, when the daily turnover of cholesterol is estimated in the same human subject by the sterol-balance method (Section 2.2.2) and by analysis of the 10-week specific activity-time curve in terms of the two-pool model, the values obtained by compartmental analysis are 15% higher than those derived from sterol balance (Grundy and Ahrens, 1969). This discrepancy could, in theory, be due to loss of cholesterol from the exchangeable mass other than *via* the faeces, leading to underestimation of turnover by the sterol-balance method. However, Samuel and his colleagues have shown that if the plasma specific activity curves are followed for much longer than the standard period of 10–12 weeks, the curves obtained from some subjects exhibit a third component with a slower rate of fall beginning 20–30 weeks after the injection of radioactive cholesterol. This suggests the presence of a third pool, or group of pools, that does not equilibrate with the plasma cholesterol within 10 weeks. Samuel and Lieberman (1973) have shown that when the specific activity curves are continued for 50–66 weeks, estimates of cholesterol turnover are about 14% less, and of total exchangeable mass are about 26% greater, than estimates based on 10- or 12-week curves. Moreover, they have shown that when the total exchangeable mass and the mass of pool B are estimated from curves obtained over these longer periods, the values for both are increased in hypercholesterolaemia. In view of the good agreement between the estimates of cholesterol turnover based on plasma specific activity-time curves continued for 50–66 weeks and the values obtained by the sterol balance method, it seems likely that the relatively large estimates of total exchangeable mass based on long-term curves are nearer to the true value than those based on a two-pool model.

A method for measuring the total exchangeable mass of cholesterol that takes about one year, the subject remaining in a steady state with respect to cholesterol metabolism throughout the whole period, is clearly impracticable except in very special circumstances. Common sense might suggest that it would be inherently impossible to measure the total exchangeable mass within a period appreciably less than the time taken for the whole mass to equilibrate completely with the plasma cholesterol. However, Samuel et al. (1978) have proposed an ingenious method for estimating the total mass of exchangeable cholesterol (M) within 12 weeks. The value of M is calculated from the equation:

$$M = I_T \times \bar{t}_p$$

where I_T (g/day) is the rate of input of cholesterol into the exchangeable mass (corresponding to the daily turnover) and $\bar{t}_p$ (days) is the mean transit time through the body of all the molecules of cholesterol in the injected radioactive dose. I_T is measured directly within 3–4 weeks by the sterol balance method and $\bar{t}_p$ is calculated from a 12-week specific activity-time curve by a method (input-output analysis) that does not require the fitting of exponentials to the experimental curves. In a group of 17 human subjects, Samuel et al. (1978) found that the mean value for M obtained by the combined method (1.32 g/kg body weight) agreed closely with that obtained by input-output analysis of curves continued for 50–66 weeks (1.43 g/kg).

In conclusion, it should be noted that with the methods now available for estimating exchangeable cholesterol *in vivo*, a relatively large change in the mass of cholesterol in a small subpool could easily escape detection. For example, a selective increase in the cholesterol content of the arterial wall, though clinically significant, might not increase the value of M estimated in a living subject.

3 CHOLESTEROL SYNTHESIS IN THE WHOLE BODY

In the investigation of many aspects of cholesterol metabolism, both in experimental animals and in man, one needs to be able to measure the rate of synthesis of cholesterol in the whole body. This need arises, for example, in the study of the homeostatic mechanisms responsible for regulating the total amount of cholesterol in the body and in clinical studies of the mechanism of hypercholesterolaemia. Information about whole-body synthesis of cholesterol is also desirable in the study of the mode of action of clinical procedures for lowering the plasma cholesterol concentration. Although none of the methods available for measurement of whole-body synthesis of cholesterol is entirely free from theoretical limitations, a good approximation to the true value can usually be obtained under steady-state conditions, and even under non-steady-state conditions qualitative information about changes in the rate of synthesis can sometimes be obtained by combinations of more than one approach.

3.1 Methods of measurement

3.1.1 Specific activity-time curves

If there is no cholesterol in the diet, turnover of the exchangeable mass must be due solely to synthesis of cholesterol. Hence, in the absence of dietary cholesterol the rate of synthesis in the whole body is equal to the rate of turnover. The latter, as we have seen (Section 2.2.3), may be estimated by compartmental or input-output analysis of the plasma specific activity-time curve after labelling the plasma cholesterol, though the estimate will tend to be erroneously high unless the curve is continued for considerably longer than 12 weeks. With any method based on analysis of plasma specific activity curves, newly-synthesized cholesterol that equilibrates with the plasma cholesterol, but is excreted by routes other than the intestine, will be included in the estimate. However, cholesterol synthesized in the intestinal mucosa and excreted in the faeces without equilibration with the plasma cholesterol will not be included. This error may be substantial in rats (Chevallier, 1967), but is probably negligible in man, since Wilson and Lindsey (1965) have shown that little or no cholesterol is secreted by the human intestinal mucosa without equilibration with the plasma cholesterol.

If cholesterol is present in the diet, whole-body synthesis of cholesterol cannot be estimated from plasma specific activity curves unless the contribution of absorbed dietary cholesterol to total turnover can be estimated at the same time. This may be achieved by estimating the fraction of the total exchangeable cholesterol that is derived from the diet, using the isotopic equilibrium method (Section 2.1), or by direct estimation of the rate of absorption of dietary cholesterol by one or other of the methods described below. In either case, radioisotopic cholesterol other than that used for the specific activity-time curves will be required.

3.1.2 Sterol balance

In the absence of dietary cholesterol, whole-body synthesis may be estimated as [*daily output of faecal neutral steroids and bile acids*]. If cholesterol is present in the diet, synthesis may be estimated as [*daily output of faecal neutral steroids plus bile acids*] minus [*daily intake of cholesterol*] or, alternatively, as [*daily output of faecal endogenous neutral steroids plus bile acids*] minus [*daily absorption of dietary cholesterol*]. Daily absorption may be measured by one of the methods discussed below. In all sterol balance methods for estimating cholesterol synthesis, greater accuracy will be achieved if bile acid output is corrected for variations in faecal flow by means of an unabsorbable marker and if neutral steroid output is corrected for possible degradation of the steroid ring system in the intestinal lumen.

Sterol balance methods are valid only if the subject is in a steady state with respect to cholesterol metabolism throughout the whole period of measurement. Clearly, if there is net deposition of cholesterol in the tissues in the period during which synthesis is measured, the rate of synthesis will be underestimated; conversely, if there is net mobilization of cholesterol from the tissues, estimates of synthesis will be erroneously high.

3.1.3 Incorporation of labelled precursors

Methods for measuring whole-body synthesis of cholesterol that are based on analysis of plasma specific-activity curves or on estimation of sterol balance are only applicable under steady-state conditions and are therefore unsuited to the measurement of synthesis during a rapid change from one steady state to another.

As we have seen, when a tracer dose of radioactive acetate is given by mouth or by intravenous injection to a human subject, radioactivity appears rapidly in the plasma free cholesterol, the specific activity reaching a maximum within a few hours. In so far as the rate of synthesis of cholesterol is determined by the flow of carbon at the rate-limiting step, one would expect to find a positive correlation between whole-body synthesis of cholesterol and some parameter (such as the rate of rise of the ascending limb or the value at the maximum) of the plasma cholesterol specific activity curve obtained after an injection of radioactive acetate, since acetate lies before the rate-limiting step. In keeping with this, Gould *et al.* (1955) observed a greatly diminished appearance of ^{14}C in the plasma cholesterol after oral [^{14}C]acetate in patients with myxoedema, a condition in which hepatic synthesis of cholesterol is depressed.

Subsequent experience has tended to show that the incorporation of radioactive acetate into the plasma cholesterol provides a very inadequate reflection of the rate of synthesis of cholesterol in the whole body under different conditions. This is not surprising, since the proportion of a trace of radioactive acetate incorporated into cholesterol by the tissues must be influenced by many factors besides the rate at which cholesterol is synthesized during the few hours after the administration of the dose. Probably the most important of these factors are the extent to which other metabolic pathways compete for the radioactive acetate and the extent to which the specific activity of the exogenous acetyl-CoA formed from the radioactive acetate is diluted by unlabelled acetyl-CoA derived from endogenous sources of acetyl carbon. There may also be variable dilution of the specific activity of intermediates further along the biosynthetic chain, including those beyond mevalonate. Variable dilution of precursor pools beyond mevalonate may be corrected for by simultaneous measurement of the incorporation, into the plasma cholesterol, of radioactive acetate and radioactive mevalonate labelled with different isotopes. Miettinen (1970) has proposed using, as an index of cholesterol synthesis in human subjects *in vivo*, the ratio of ^{14}C to ^{3}H in the plasma cholesterol after administration of a mixture of [^{14}C]acetate and [^{3}H]mevalonate. He has shown that the ratios observed are increased in several conditions in which cholesterol synthesis is known to be increased, and are diminished by fasting the subject. However, the ^{14}C/^{3}H ratio method cannot correct for the considerable variation in acetate incorporation that must occur between different normal individuals and within the same individual at different times. Furthermore, since the mass of the acetyl-CoA pool from which sterol is synthesized is likely to vary rapidly at different stages of the 24-hour cycle, the incorporation of a single dose of labelled acetate into the plasma cholesterol is unlikely to reflect the mean rate of synthesis of cholesterol over a 24-hour period. Nor can it, of course, provide an estimate of the absolute rate of synthesis of exchangeable cholesterol.

Miettinen (1970) has pointed out that if the capacities of the enzymes catalysing the steps in sterol biosynthesis beyond mevalonate remain more or less constant, then the tissue concentrations of sterol precursors beyond mevalonate should increase when the rate-limiting step is stimulated and should decrease when it is depressed. Furthermore, it might be expected that such changes in tissue concentration would be reflected in parallel changes in plasma concentration. Miettinen (1969) has shown that the plasma concentration of methyl sterols (including lanosterol) is decreased by fasting and is increased in at least two conditions—obesity and cholestyramine treatment—in which cholesterol synthesis in the whole body is known to be increased. However, the plasma methyl sterol concentration was also increased in patients with primary hypercholesterolaemia investigated by Miettinen, although cholesterol synthesis estimated by the sterol balance method in these patients was subnormal. This suggests that in some circumstances the amount of methyl sterol in the plasma merely reflects the concentration of the plasma lipoproteins in which it is carried.

Squalene is also present in human plasma, though at a concentration less than 1 µmol/l in normal subjects. Miettinen (1970) could find no consistent increase in the plasma squalene concentration in patients in whom cholesterol synthesis was stimulated by treatment with cholestyramine. Nestel and Kudchodkar (1975), on the other hand, observed an increase in plasma squalene concentration when cholesterol synthesis was stimulated by colestipol and a decrease when cholesterol synthesis was depressed by cholesterol feeding.

Although measurement of the plasma squalene concentration may have little value as an index of cholesterol synthesis, the fact that squalene is an obligatory precursor of cholesterol has been exploited by Liu *et al.* (1975) in their development of a new method for measuring the absolute rate of synthesis of cholesterol *in vivo*. The principle of the method is to measure the rate of synthesis of squalene in the whole body and to equate this to the rate of synthesis of cholesterol, on the assumption that all the squalene labelled by a single dose of radioactive mevalonate is converted into cholesterol. The steps in the method are as follows:

(a) The subject, who should be on a squalene-free diet, is given an intravenous injection of a mixture of [^{3}H]cholesterol and $(3R,3S)$-[^{14}C]mevalonate. This results in the rapid appearance of ^{14}C in the plasma squalene, the specific activity (dpm/mg) reaching a maximum in about 2 h and then declining exponentially with a half-life of about 7 h. Concurrently, ^{14}C appears in the plasma cholesterol, the specific activity rising to a peak and then falling slowly in parallel with the specific activity of the plasma [^{3}H]cholesterol.

(b) The absolute rate of turnover, or synthesis, of squalene (mg/day) is estimated as [total ^{14}C (dpm) in the squalene pool from which cholesterol is synthesized] ÷ [area under the plasma squalene specific activity-time curve (dpm/mg × days) from zero time to infinity].

(c) The total ^{14}C introduced into the squalene pool from the dose of [^{14}C]mevalonate is calculated from the radioactivity in the injected dose of $(3R)$-mevalonate and the proportion of this dose that is converted into squalene. The latter is estimated as:

[plasma [¹⁴C]cholesterol:plasma [³H]cholesterol specific-activity ratio (adjusted for differences in doses of $(3R)$-[¹⁴C]mevalonate and [³H]cholesterol) three weeks after the injection].

In addition to the assumption that the rate of squalene synthesis is identical with the rate of cholesterol synthesis, calculation of the rate of synthesis of squalene from the plasma squalene specific activity-time curve is based on the assumption that the plasma squalene is in isotopic equilibrium with the squalene synthesized in the tissues from exogenous mevalonate. These assumptions remain to be tested. However, the method seems to be promising, since the rates of cholesterol synthesis estimated in the same human subjects by the squalene method and by the sterol balance method differ by an average of less than 10% (Liu et al., 1975). If the squalene method can be validated it would be superior to all other methods for measuring whole-body synthesis of cholesterol, since it provides an estimate of the rate of synthesis during a period of about 10 hours after the injection. Hence, apart from the advantage that the whole procedure takes less than four weeks to complete, the method is applicable to the non-steady state.

Nestel and Kudchodkar (1975) have proposed a simplified procedure for obtaining an index of the rate at which squalene is converted into cholesterol *in vivo*. The subject is given a continuous intravenous infusion of [¹⁴C]mevalonate until a plateau in the plasma squalene specific activity curve is achieved. Under these conditions, the rate of appearance of ¹⁴C in the plasma free cholesterol is linear. The rate of transfer of ¹⁴C from squalene to free cholesterol is increased when cholesterol synthesis is stimulated by colestipol or by a reduction in the cholesterol content of the diet.

3.2 Rates of cholesterol synthesis in the whole body

The rates of whole-body synthesis of cholesterol estimated by the sterol balance method in more than 100 human adults have now been published. In every series of subjects in whom cholesterol synthesis may be considered to be within the normal range, the mean rate has been found to lie between 10 and 15 mg/kg/day, with rates per whole body ranging from about 450 to about 1000 mg/day in different individuals of both sexes. Table 10.1 shows the values obtained from a total of 65 subjects investigated in four different laboratories. Subjects who were obese, those who had moderate or marked hypertriglyceridaemia and those whose diet contained large amounts of cholesterol have been omitted from the Table. On the other hand, patients with primary hypercholesterolaemia have been included, since there appears to be no significant correlation between whole-body synthesis

Table 10.1

Whole-body synthesis of cholesterol in men and women estimated in four laboratories by the sterol balance method

Laboratory	Conditions	Cholesterol synthesis (mg/kg/day) Mean	Range
Grundy and Ahrens (1969)	Liquid-formula diet with cholesterol content ranging from ≃ zero to 577 mg/day. Series included primary hyperlipidaemic patients and two normocholesterolaemics.	11.9	7.0–21.6
Grundy and Ahrens (1970)		10.4	6.6–13.6
Quintão et al. (1971a)		10.7	8.9–14.6
Connor et al. (1969)	Cholesterol-free corn-oil liquid-formula diet. Six normal men.	11.1	8.8–16.9
Miettinen (1971)	Low-cholesterol solid diet. Five normal men and five normal women.	11.3 (♀) 13.6 (♂) 12.4 (♀+♂)	7.7–16.5
Nestel and Poyser (1976)	Solid diet with cholesterol from 103 to 338 mg/day. Two normals and 7 with moderate hyperlipidaemia.	8.6	6.4–11.3
Whyte et al. (1977)	Twelve Papuans eating habitual diet (cholesterol intake ≃ zero).	12.4	7.0–17.5
	Six normal Australian men on solid diet (cholesterol <80 mg/day).	11.3	

Table 10.2
Whole-body synthesis of cholesterol in rats, dogs and non-human primates

Species	Reference	Method	mg/day	mg/kg/day
Rat	Wilson (1964)	Faecal steroid excretion by isotopic balance with zero cholesterol intake	6	40
Squirrel monkey	Lofland et al. (1972)	Faecal bile acids (GLC) plus endogenous neutral steroids (isotopic balance) minus cholesterol absorbed	35	35
Squirrel monkey	Eggen (1974)	Faecal total steroids (isotopic balance) with low cholesterol intake	33	52
Cebus monkey	Lofland et al. (1968)	Faecal steroid excretion by isotopic balance (uncorrected for absorption)	142	61
Dog	Pertsemlidis et al. (1973)	Sterol balance	325	12
Rhesus monkey	Eggen (1974)	Faecal total steroids (isotopic balance) with low cholesterol intake	42	10
Baboon	Eggen (1974)	As above	196	9

and plasma cholesterol concentration in adults. The few observations that have been published on cholesterol synthesis in children (Carter et al., 1975; Martin and Nestel, 1979) suggest rates of whole-body synthesis close to those observed in normal adults (10–15 mg/kg/day).

Whole-body synthesis of cholesterol in man under abnormal conditions is discussed in Section 5 below.

The methods for measuring turnover and synthesis discussed in Sections 2.2 and 3.1, though developed primarily for the investigation of human subjects, are applicable in principle to experimental animals. Cholesterol synthesis has been measured in rats, in dogs and in several species of non-human primates by chemical and isotopic balance methods, or by various combinations of the two methods. Some representative values obtained for cholesterol synthesis in animals are listed in Table 10.2. It should be noted that the isotopic balance method for estimating the faecal excretion of endogenous neutral steroids is not valid in rats, since in this species a considerable proportion of the faecal neutral steroid fraction is formed in the intestinal wall and is excreted without equilibration with the plasma cholesterol (Chevallier, 1967). In some of these studies the turnover of whole-body cholesterol and the mass of the exchangeable pools have been estimated by isotopic methods discussed in Section 2.2.3.

4 CHOLESTEROL ABSORPTION

4.1 Definition

Although simple exchange of cholesterol between the intestinal lumen and the mucosal cells must obviously be distinguished from true *absorption*, the term absorption could arguably be used to include total transport of cholesterol into the mucosal cells by the physiological processes discussed below, even if some of the cholesterol so 'absorbed' returns to the intestinal lumen without reaching the lymphatic system. However, I shall follow the current practice by which cholesterol absorption is defined, explicitly or implicitly, as the overall process by which cholesterol is transported from the lumen of the intestine into the intestinal lymphatics. Thus, on this definition absorption includes all the processes by which cholesterol is taken into the mucosal cells, incorporated into triglyceride-rich lipoprotein particles within the cells and secreted thence into the lymphatics.

4.2 The sources of absorbed cholesterol

Cholesterol available for absorption from the intestine is derived from three sources: the food, the bile and, to a small extent, the wall of the intestine itself. Cholesterol discharged directly from the intestinal wall into the lumen arises by synthesis *de novo* in the mucosal cells (Wilson and Reinke, 1968) and by continual desquamation of these cells. Since cholesterol absorption does not occur to any significant extent beyond the distal end of the jejunum, cholesterol entering the lumen directly from the ileum and colon is not available for reabsorption. It is generally assumed that dietary and biliary cholesterol mix completely in the duodenum and jejunum and, hence, that equal proportions of the cholesterol from these two major sources are absorbed. This assumption is reasonable since cholesterol exchanges freely between the mixed micelles formed in the intestinal lumen. However, it is conceivable that biliary cholesterol, which is wholly unesterified, tends to be absorbed at a higher level in the small intestine than esterified dietary cholesterol, which must be hydrolysed before incorporation into micelles.

4.3 The route of absorption

Borgström (1960), using a method which enabled him to analyse the contents of successive segments of the human small intestine, showed that absorption of an oral dose of cholesterol is completed above the distal end of the jejunum. Observations on the uptake of labelled cholesterol by the small intestine of the rat *in vivo* (Swell *et al.*, 1958*a*) suggest that in this species, also, the proximal region of the small intestine is the major site of cholesterol absorption. Cholesterol absorbed from the intestine enters the mesenteric lymph ducts, reaching the blood circulation *via* the thoracic duct. Estimates of the recovery of absorbed labelled cholesterol in thoracic-duct lymph of rats (Biggs *et al.*, 1951) and human subjects (Hellman *et al.*, 1960) indicate that in both species the intestinal lymphatic system is essentially the only route by which absorbed cholesterol reaches the circulation.

4.4 The mechanism of absorption

4.4.1 The luminal phase

The small amount of esterified cholesterol present in the diet (usually less than 5% of the total dietary cholesterol) is hydrolysed by pancreatic cholesteryl-ester esterase in the lumen of the small intestine, the bile salts possibly acting as cofactors for the enzyme or as detergents by means of which the water-insoluble substrate is brought into solution (Treadwell and Vahouny, 1968). The cholesterol of cholesteryl esters cannot be absorbed without hydrolysis in the intestinal lumen, as is shown by the fact that esters resistant to the hydrolytic action of cholesteryl-ester hydrolase are not absorbed. The free cholesterol resulting from the hydrolysis of dietary cholesteryl esters, together with that already present in the diet and the bile, is incorporated into mixed ('expanded') micelles containing conjugated bile acids, phospholipids, 2-monoglycerides, fatty acids and small amounts of 1,2-diglycerides. The micelles present in the intestinal lumen during the digestion of fat are spherical particles, less than 10 mµ in diameter, in which the amphipathic molecules are oriented with their polar regions at the surfaces of the particles and the apolar regions forming a fluid core. At the pH and temperature of the intestinal lumen the micelles are quite stable.

Conjugated bile salts, when present at concentrations above their critical micellar concentration, form micelles that are capable of dissolving free cholesterol but the amount of cholesterol so dissolved is very small—less than 1 molecule of cholesterol per 40 molecules of bile salt (see Hofmann and Small, 1967). The capacity of the micelles for dissolving free cholesterol is greatly increased by the addition of phospholipid, monoglyceride and fatty acid. In an expanded micelle the free cholesterol molecules probably interdigitate between the detergent molecules, with their hydroxyl groups at the micelle/water interface, or are dissolved in the interior of the micelle.

If the intestinal fluid obtained during the digestion of a fat-containing meal is submitted to high-speed centrifugation, three layers are formed: an upper oily layer containing the triglycerides and diglycerides undergoing hydrolysis by pancreatic lipase, a clear infranatant layer containing the micellar components, and an insoluble sediment. Cholesterol, fat soluble vitamins and other lipids are partitioned between the oil phase and the micellar phase. According to the present view as to how lipids are absorbed, the monoglycerides and fatty acids released during the enzymic hydrolysis of triglyceride present in the emulsified oil phase are transferred to the aqueous phase, where they are incorporated into the expanded micelles in which cholesterol and other water-insoluble amphipaths are dissolved. The components of the micellar phase are then taken into the interior of the mucosal cells of the microvilli, the process continuing until all the products of the digestion of triglyceride have been absorbed *via* the micellar phase.

Although the formation of micelles in the intestinal lumen is known to be essential for cholesterol absorption, there is some doubt as to how cholesterol molecules are taken up by the mucosal cells. It is unlikely that intact micelles are carried across the plasma membrane into the interior of the cells and that the bile salts then return directly to the lumen of the intestine. Rather, it seems that the function of the micelles is to facilitate the movement of cholesterol and other lipids across the layer of 'unstirred' water that overlies the luminal surface of the mucosa and through which the movement of solute molecules cannot occur by convection. Although the unstirred layer of water covering the microvilli *in vivo* is probably less than 0.5 mm thick, it constitutes a major diffusion barrier to the absorption of relatively insoluble substances such as cholesterol. Indeed, Dietschy (1978) has estimated that micelle formation increases the intestinal uptake of cholesterol about 145-fold by facilitating the passage of cholesterol molecules across the unstirred water layer up to the cell-membrane surface. The final step in the uptake of cholesterol could consist in the collision of a micelle with the plasma membrane of a mucosal cell, followed by the movement of free cholesterol into the cell membrane and thence into the interior of the cell; this would be analogous to the mechanism thought to be responsible for exchange of cholesterol between cell membranes and plasma lipoproteins (see Fig. 11.10). Alternatively, absorption might occur by passive diffusion, across the cell membrane, of cholesterol molecules dissolved in monomolecular form at very low concentration in the water immediately adjacent to the cell surface. Since these molecules are in rapid equilibrium with the cholesterol in the micelles, they would be continually replaced by movement of other molecules out of the micelles, as long as these were present (see Fig. 10.3). For reasons discussed by Dietschy (1978), the latter mechanism seems the more likely.

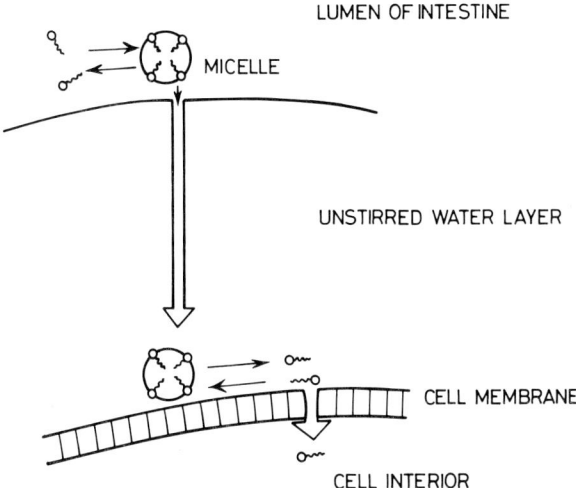

Figure 10.3
The probable mechanism by which cholesterol is taken up by intestinal mucosal cells. Cholesterol enters mixed micelles in the intestinal lumen and is carried across the unstirred water layer to the cell surface. Cholesterol molecules dissolved as monomers at very low concentration in the water at the surface of the mucosal cells enter the cell interior by passive diffusion through the plasma membrane. Cholesterol molecules taken up by the cells are continually replaced by molecules leaving the micelles. Note that the unstirred layer and the plasma membrane are not drawn to scale. (Modified from Dietschy, 1978.)

Although triglycerides are absorbed completely under normal conditions, cholesterol is incompletely absorbed even at the lowest concentrations present in the intestinal lumen. Borgström (1960) has suggested that this selectivity of absorption is partly a function of the partition of cholesterol between the oil phase and the micellar phase. He has shown that during the absorption of cholesterol from the human intestine the partition coefficient favours solution in the oil phase. Hence, the cholesterol in the total system is incompletely absorbed by the time that all the triglyceride has been absorbed. Another possibility is that monoglycerides and fatty acids leave the micelles in the unstirred layer and enter the mucosal cells more rapidly than cholesterol. This could cause disruption of the micelles, leading to precipitation of some of the micellar cholesterol, which would then be unavailable for absorption. In favour of this possibility, Simmonds et al. (1967) have shown that when a solution of micelles containing bile salts, monoglycerides and [^{14}C]cholesterol is perfused through the jejunum of a human subject, absorption of monoglyceride is virtually complete, whereas only 70–75% of the labelled cholesterol is absorbed.

4.4.2 The mucosal phase

The free cholesterol that enters the mucosal cells is esterified with long-chain fatty acids before incorporation into triglyceride-rich lipoproteins, 80–90% of the cholesterol in the chylomicrons of intestinal lymph being in esterified form. In the lymph of fasting rats the predominant fatty acids with which cholesterol is esterified are oleate, palmitate and linoleate. During fasting, most of the palmitate and oleate is probably synthesized in the intestine itself. However, fatty acids derived from the fed fat can also be incorporated into the cholesteryl esters of chylomicrons. When fat is fed, the fatty-acid composition of the intestinal-lymph cholesteryl esters is a function of the composition of the dietary fat and the preference of the mucosal cholesterol-esterifying enzyme for oleate as substrate.

At one time it was believed that the esterification of free cholesterol within the mucosal cells is catalyzed by pancreatic cholesteryl-ester esterase acting in reverse (see Treadwell and Vahouny (1968) for discussion of this point). However, it now seems more likely that the intramucosal esterification of cholesterol is catalyzed by ACAT, since Norum et al. (1977) have shown that the mucosal cells of the guinea-pig's intestine contain ACAT and that the activity of the enzyme is sufficient to account for the observed rate of esterification of cholesterol during its transport across the intestinal wall.

When a dose of cholesterol labelled with [^{14}C]cholesterol is given orally to rats (Swell et al., 1958a) or human subjects (Hellman et al., 1960), the total cholesterol content of thoracic-duct lymph rises to a peak within a few hours and then falls rapidly. [^{14}C]Cholesterol, however, continues to appear in the lymph for many hours. Swell et al. (1958b) have shown that this rather puzzling phenomenon is due to the presence of a pool of free cholesterol in the mucosal cells which turns over relatively slowly (about once every 24 hours in rats). Free cholesterol transferred from the intestinal lumen into the mucosa mixes with the pool of endogenous free cholesterol from which cholesterol is transported to the intracellular site where esterification occurs. The presence of this intracellular pool explains why, after an oral dose of radioactive cholesterol, the specific activity of intestinal-lymph cholesterol is lower than that of the cholesterol in the lumen.

The cholesteryl esters formed in the endoplasmic reticulum by the action of ACAT are incorporated into nascent VLDL and chylomicrons at some stage in their synthesis, assembly and export into the intestinal lymphatics. These processes have been discussed in several reviews (see Soutar and Myant, 1979). The formation and secretion of triglyceride-rich lipoproteins by the intestinal mucosa must be essential for cholesterol absorption, as defined in Section 4.1 above, since cholesterol is not absorbed in conditions in which apoB-containing lipoproteins cannot be formed, as in familial abetalipoproteinaemia (Chapter 16, Section 4).

4.5 Sterols other than cholesterol

The extent to which the intestine can absorb analogues of cholesterol is of interest from the point of view of the structural features required for efficient absorption of a sterol. Of all sterols that have been tested, cholesterol is absorbed with the greatest efficiency by the mammalian intestine. However, other sterols must be absorbed to some extent, since β-sitosterol, stigmasterol and campesterol are detectable in human plasma. Early work on the absorption of sterols other than cholesterol, estimated by sterol balance methods, led to the conclusion that plant sterols are absorbed with considerable efficiency, but the low faecal recoveries of fed sterol observed in these experiments were probably due to extensive bacterial modification in the intestine rather than to absorption. More recent work, in which absorption of an oral dose of radioactive plant sterol has been estimated from the amount recovered in plasma or intestinal lymph in human subjects (Gould et al., 1956; Salen et al., 1970) and rats (Swell et al., 1959), indicate that less than 5% of a standard dose is absorbed. Plant sterols are not absorbed in the absence of bile salts in the intestine and their absorption is confined to the lymphatic route, suggesting that they are taken up by the mucosal cells of the intestine by a mechanism similar to that responsible for the uptake of cholesterol. Plant sterols are esterified in the intestinal wall to a much smaller extent than is cholesterol (Swell et al., 1959; Kuksis and Huang, 1962).

The fate of absorbed β-sitosterol has been investigated in man by Salen *et al.* (1970). In subjects given intravenous injections of radioactive β-sitosterol and cholesterol, the β-sitosterol disappears from the plasma more rapidly than the cholesterol. The more rapid rate of disappearance of β-sitosterol is due in part to selective uptake by the liver, with secretion in the bile as neutral sterol. β-Sitosterol absorbed from the diet may also be converted into cholic and chenodeoxycholic acids in the liver (Salen *et al.*, 1970) and into corticosteroids in the adrenal cortex (Werbin and Chaikoff, 1961).

5α-Cholestanol is absorbed from the intestine, though only about half as efficiently as cholesterol. After oral administration of radioactive 5α-cholestanol to rats about 80% of the radioactive sterol in the intestinal lymph is esterified (Chapman and Chaikoff, 1959). Coprostanol, the 5β isomer of 5α-cholestanol, is not absorbed, but lathosterol (5α-cholest-7-en-3β-ol) and 7-dehydrocholesterol (provitamin D_3) are absorbed, to a limited extent, from the rabbit's intestine. Vitamin D_3 is absorbed from the rat's intestine, probably after incorporation into mixed micelles (Thompson *et al.*, 1969), and appears in the intestinal lymph in unesterified form (Schachter *et al.*, 1964). Epicholesterol (the 3α-hydroxy epimer of cholesterol) is absorbed, but with only half the efficiency of cholesterol and without esterification during transit through the mucosa (Hernandez *et al.*, 1954).

Taken together, these rather limited observations suggest that the efficient absorption of a sterol requires the presence of a 3β-hydroxyl group, a double bond in the Δ^5 position, the absence of additional double bonds in ring B and the absence of a substituent at C-24. It is not known whether this specificity is related to the transport of the sterol into the mucosal cells, its intracellular esterification, the incorporation of the esterified sterol into triglyceride-rich lipoproteins or some other event in the overall process of absorption. Specificity is unlikely to be related to the formation of micelles in the intestinal lumen, since β-sitosterol and cholesterol have the same partition coefficients between the oil and micellar phases of intestinal contents (Borgström, 1967).

The ability of the intestinal mucosa to select cholesterol in preference to other sterols, including those which differ from cholesterol only in having a substituent at C-24, suggests that the absorption of cholesterol subserves an important biological function. This could be to make use of the biliary cholesterol for the formation of lipoproteins in the intestinal wall during the absorption of fat, and thus to conserve endogenous cholesterol. The presence of a specific mechanism for absorbing cholesterol would lead inevitably to the absorption of dietary cholesterol. The secretion of cholesterol in bile could have evolved to provide the intestinal mucosa with some of the cholesterol it needs for fat absorption. On the other hand, the presence of free cholesterol in bile may simply be a consequence of the solvent effect of the bile salts on the plasma membranes of the cells lining the bile canaliculi.

4.6 Methods of measurement

The difficulty in measuring the intestinal absorption of a substance that undergoes extensive enterohepatic circulation is reflected in the number of methods that have been proposed for estimating cholesterol absorption. The principal methods that have been used for the quantitative study of cholesterol absorption are considered in this section.

4.6.1 Non-isotopic sterol balance

In much of the early work on the absorption of cholesterol in man and experimental animals (summarized in Cook 1958), absorption was estimated from the recovery of digitonin-precipitable sterols in the faeces after a single large oral dose of cholesterol. The estimates obtained with this method are now known to have been erroneously high and did not include reabsorption of the endogenous cholesterol secreted in the bile.

4.6.2 Combined chemical and isotopic balance

Methods for estimating the daily absorption of dietary cholesterol over periods of several weeks in human subjects in the metabolic steady state have been developed by Grundy and Ahrens (1969). The subject is given a liquid-formula diet providing a constant daily intake of cholesterol. Absorbed cholesterol is estimated as the difference between intake and daily faecal excretion of unabsorbed dietary cholesterol. Unabsorbed dietary cholesterol may be estimated as the difference between total faecal neutral steroids (estimated by GLC) and faecal neutral steroids of endogenous origin, estimated by the isotopic balance method after labelling the plasma with a single intravenous dose of radioactive cholesterol (Method I of Grundy and Ahrens). Alternatively, unabsorbed dietary cholesterol may be estimated from specific-activity measurements made after continuous labelling of the dietary cholesterol (Method II of Grundy and Ahrens). With both methods the estimates of faecal neutral steroid excretion are corrected for losses due to degradation of sterol in the intestine.

In principle, it is also possible to calculate absorption from the total turnover of exchangeable cholesterol, estimated from the daily faecal excretion of bile acids and neutral steroids of endogenous origin, and the fraction of the exchangeable cholesterol derived from the diet, estimated by the isotopic equilibrium method discussed in Section 2.1

above. However, this method appears to be unreliable, largely because of the difficulty of achieving isotopic equilibrium in human subjects, even after feeding radioactive cholesterol continuously for many weeks.

Combined chemical and isotopic methods have been used for measuring cholesterol absorption in non-human primates (Lofland et al., 1972; Wilson, 1972).

4.6.3 Faecal excretion of a single labelled oral dose

Borgström (1969) has described a simple and rapid method for measuring the absorption of cholesterol in human subjects eating a normal diet. A single dose of radioactive cholesterol is given by mouth and the cumulative excretion of radioactivity in the faeces is measured over the next six days. Radioactivity recovered over this period represents the unabsorbed fraction of the administered dose. A correction for loss of unabsorbed cholesterol due to bacterial degradation of sterol in the intestine may be made by measuring the recovery, in the faeces, of a single dose of [^{3}H]β-sitosterol. Borgström concludes that in most subjects virtually all the unabsorbed fraction of the dose appears in the faeces within six days and that there can be little or no re-excretion of the absorbed fraction during this period. The method is suitable for estimating cholesterol absorption in animals.

4.6.4 Plasma radioactivity after oral labelling

Semi-quantitative information about sterol absorption may be obtained by measuring the radioactivity appearing in the plasma after a single oral dose of the radioactive sterol. This method was used by Gould et al. (1956) in their study of β-sitosterol absorption. Since one measures what is absorbed rather than what is not absorbed, errors due to intestinal degradation are eliminated. The method is useful for comparing the relative absorbabilities of two different sterols by observing the appearance of ^{14}C and ^{3}H in the plasma after feeding a mixture of a ^{14}C-labelled and a ^{3}H-labelled sterol. However, the absolute amount of radioactive sterol absorbed cannot be estimated accurately because absorbed radio-sterol begins to leave the plasma before absorption of the dose is complete.

4.6.5 The isotope-ratio method

Zilversmit (1972) has proposed a dual-isotope method for estimating the absorption of cholesterol in rats. If an oral dose of [^{14}C]cholesterol and an intravenous injection of an emulsion of [^{3}H]cholesterol are given intravenously to a rat, the proportion of the oral dose absorbed will be equal to the dose-standardized ^{14}C/^{3}H specific-activity ratio of the plasma cholesterol measured at a suitable time after the test doses, provided that absorbed and injected cholesterol are metabolized and distributed identically. Zilversmit and Hughes (1974) have shown that this assumption is valid if the intravenous dose of cholesterol is given as an emulsion in physiological saline. They have also shown that absorption estimated from the isotope ratio 48 hours after the two doses agrees closely with estimates based on the percentage of the oral radioactive cholesterol recovered in the faeces over 4 days.

The advantages of the method are that it requires only a single blood sample, without collection of faeces, and that it is not sensitive to errors due to intestinal degradation of the oral dose. Samuel *et al.* (1978) have shown that the method is applicable to human subjects and that satisfactory measurements can be made in the same individual at intervals of 3–4 weeks.

4.6.6 Recovery of cholesterol from a lymph-duct fistula

Experimental animals with intestinal-lymph-duct or thoracic-duct fistulas have been used estensively for quantitative studies of cholesterol absorption (see Treadwell and Vehouny, 1968, for references). Recovery of cholesterol (estimated chemically) in the lymph over a 24-hour period provides an estimate of total cholesterol absorption (dietary plus endogenous), and if the animal is given oral radioactive cholesterol the contribution of dietary cholesterol to the total absorbed may be estimated from the total lymph radioactivity and the lymph cholesterol/dietary cholesterol specific-activity ratio (Sylvén and Borgström, 1968). Borgström *et al.* (1970) have used the lymph method to measure cholesterol absorption in human subjects with thoracic-duct fistulas, but it is clearly not applicable to man as a routine procedure.

4.6.7 Absorption of endogenous cholesterol and the method of intestinal perfusion

With the exception of the lymph-duct-fistula method (Section 4.6.6), all the methods described above provide direct information only about the absorption of exogenous cholesterol, given either as a single test dose or fed continuously in the diet. But we also need to know the rate of secretion of endogenous cholesterol into the lumen of the intestine and the amount of this endogenous cholesterol that is reabsorbed. This is particularly important in relation to the study of cholesterol absorption in man in view of the controversy as to the maximal capacity of the human intestine for absorbing cholesterol (see below).

One approach to the problem is to deduce the rate of secretion indirectly from the percentage absorption of an oral dose of radioactive cholesterol and the daily faecal excretion of total neutral steroids (Stanley and Cheng, 1956) or of neutral steroids of endogenous origin

(Grundy et al., 1969), on the assumption that equal proportions of endogenous and exogenous cholesterol are absorbed. For example, if P is the proportion of exogenous cholesterol absorbed and N (mg/day) is the daily faecal excretion of endogenous neutral steroids, secretion of endogenous cholesterol (mg/day) = N ÷ (1 − P).

Alternatively, secretion may be determined more directly by intestinal intubation or perfusion. Borgström (1960) estimated the rate of secretion from the dilution of the specific activity of radioactive cholesterol in a test meal during its digestion in the jejunum. In normal human subjects the mean rate of secretion of endogenous cholesterol was 610 mg during a 3- to 4-hour digestion period. Grundy and Metzger (1972) have described an improved method based on a combination of perfusion and aspiration. A liquid diet containing a marker is infused at a constant rate above the opening of the common bile duct. Intestinal contents are then aspirated from a point distal to the entry of bile into the duodenum and the rate of secretion of cholesterol is calculated from the rate of infusion of the marker and the ratio of cholesterol to marker in the aspirate. Endogenous secretion can be measured continuously for many hours. The method is therefore well suited to the study of short-term changes in secretion in response to diet, drugs and other agents. Values obtained with this method average about 40 mg/h (1 g/day). Grundy and Mok (1977) have adapted and extended this method to the direct estimation of the rate of absorption of total cholesterol (exogenous + endogenous) from the jejunum of human subjects. A liquid-formula diet containing varying amounts of cholesterol and an unabsorbable marker is infused into the duodenum. Absorption of total cholesterol is estimated from the disappearance of cholesterol relative to the marker from a 100-cm segment of the jejunum.

A potentially important outcome of the use of this method is the suggestion that significant exchange occurs between radioactive cholesterol in the lumen of the jejunum and the jejunal mucosa. In so far as exchange takes place, absorption of dietary cholesterol must be over-estimated by any method which depends upon the use of labelled cholesterol (see Mok et al., 1979).

4.7 The rate of absorption

4.7.1 Normal rates in man and experimental animals

There has been much disagreement as to the rate at which dietary cholesterol can be absorbed by the human intestine. Kaplan et al. (1963), using a method based on the continuous feeding of [^{14}C]cholesterol until isotopic equilibrium is achieved, concluded that in normal human subjects the maximal capacity for absorbing dietary cholesterol is about 300 mg/day. Wilson and Lindsey (1965), who also used an isotopic-equilibrium method, reached a similar conclusion. Kaplan *et al.*, suggested that the much higher values reported previously for the absorption of a single large oral dose of cholesterol were not representative of the rates of absorption that could be sustained under conditions of continued daily feeding, and that the intake of cholesterol from the average American diet (about 500 mg/day) was sufficient to saturate the mechanism for absorbing exogenous cholesterol. However, Quintão *et al.* (1971*a,b*), using the combined chemical and isotopic balance methods (Section 4.6.2 above) with which a constant intake is maintained for weeks, found that 30–40% of the dietary cholesterol is absorbed in most subjects over a range of intake from 40 mg/day to more than 2 g/day, some individuals absorbing over 1 g/day at the highest intakes tested. Comparable results have been reported by others (Connor and Lin, 1974; Whyte *et al.*, 1977). Borgström (1969), using a single-dose method (Section 4.6.3), also observed a more or less linear relation between intake and absorption in normal subjects given doses of 150 mg to 1.9 g of cholesterol; one subject studied by Borgström absorbed a total of 1.52 g of dietary cholesterol in a single day.

In view of these more recent findings it seems unlikely that the maximal capacity for absorbing dietary cholesterol is reached when the daily intake is equal to that provided by a typical Western diet. The much lower values for absorption obtained with isotopic-equilibrium methods may have been due to failure to achieve complete isotopic equilibrium, leading to underestimation of the contribution of exogenous cholesterol to the plasma cholesterol. It is difficult to say how far an increase in the absorption of dietary cholesterol leads to an increase in the *total* amount of cholesterol absorbed from the human intestine. Borgström *et al.* (1970) found little or no increase in the amount of cholesterol excreted through a thoracic-duct fistula in human subjects when 1.63 g of cholesterol was given by mouth. They concluded that the absorptive capacity of the human intestine for cholesterol is already saturated by the endogenous load, and that absorption of exogenous cholesterol can only occur at the expense of endogenous cholesterol. However, it is difficult to believe that there is no increase in total absorption when dietary cholesterol is absorbed, in view of the well-established evidence that the addition of moderate amounts of cholesterol to the diet may lead to a rise in plasma cholesterol concentration and to deposition of cholesterol in the tissues in man. Moreover, Grundy and Mok (1977) have shown by direct measurement (Section 4.6.7) that an increase in the input of exogenous cholesterol into the jejunum leads to a net increase in cholesterol absorption in human subjects.

The capacity of the rat's intestine for absorbing cholesterol has been examined in many laboratories with a variety of methods, including thoracic-duct cannulation (Swell et al., 1958b; Sylvén and Borgström, 1968), faecal recovery of a single oral dose (Borgström, 1968), isotopic-balance methods (Chevallier, 1967; Wilson, 1964) and the isotope-ratio method (Zilversmit, 1972). Reported values for the efficiency of absorption have varied widely, ranging from less than 10% to over 80%. Despite these discrepancies, due partly to differences in method of measurement and partly to differences in the form in which the cholesterol is given, it seems clear that the rat can absorb dietary cholesterol in substantial amounts, and that the apparent resistance of this species to atherosclerosis by cholesterol feeding is not due to failure to absorb dietary cholesterol. With continuous feeding of cholesterol to rats, Wilson (1964) found that 70% of the dietary cholesterol was absorbed when the daily intake was low, the efficiency of absorption falling to less than 50% at high intakes. Borgström (1968), however, found that when rats were given single oral doses of cholesterol in triolein, a constant fraction of the dose was absorbed (about 50%) when the oral load was varied over a wide range. Using the isotope-ratio method, Zilversmit (1972) obtained essentially similar results. Measurements of the net rate of absorption of cholesterol (dietary plus endogenous) in rats with thoracic-duct fistulas indicate that absorption of dietary cholesterol is accompanied by increased total absorption (Swell et al., 1958b), though only up to a certain level of intake. With increasing oral doses greater than about 20 mg, the net rate of absorption reaches a plateau, although the rate of absorption of the dietary cholesterol continues to increase (Sylvén and Borgström, 1968). The efficiency of absorption of dietary cholesterol by the rabbit's intestine, which averaged 30% in the experiments of Rudel et al. (1972), is no greater than that of the rat's intestine, indicating that the ease with which atheroma can be produced in rabbits by cholesterol feeding is not due to an exceptional capacity for absorbing cholesterol in these animals.

In non-human primates, dietary cholesterol is absorbed with about the same efficiency as that generally reported for man, 40–50% of the daily intake being absorbed by baboons, rhesus monkeys and squirrel monkeys (Eggen, 1974). Under conditions of continued feeding with cholesterol, adult baboons can absorb at least 600 mg of dietary cholesterol/day (Wilson, 1972), a rate equivalent to more than 2 g/day in a human subject if expressed in terms of body weight. Dogs seem to be able to absorb dietary cholesterol with greater efficiency than human subjects or non-human primates, at both high and low levels of intake. Efficiencies of 80% or more have been observed in dogs, even when the daily intake of cholesterol is increased to more than 1 g/day (Abell et al., 1956; Pertsemlidis et al., 1973).

4.7.2 Factors influencing cholesterol absorption

The amounts of endogenous and dietary cholesterol absorbed from the intestine are increased by the feeding of fat. This effect has been demonstrated in human subjects and in rats (see Treadwell and Vahouny, 1968), and is probably due mainly to facilitation of micelle formation by the products of triglyceride hydrolysis in the jejunal lumen (see Section 4.4.1), though increased provision of exogenous fatty acid for the esterification of cholesterol in the intestinal mucosa may be an additional factor. The ability of dietary polyunsaturated fat to lower the plasma cholesterol concentration in man has led to considerable interest in the relation between the fatty-acid composition of the dietary fat and the efficiency of absorption of cholesterol. Much of the experimental work on this question is difficult to interpret because of inadequacy of the methods used for estimating cholesterol absorption. There is certainly no evidence to support the view that polyunsaturated fats decrease the absorption of endogenous or dietary cholesterol in man (see Grundy and Ahrens (1970) and McGill (1979) for discussion).

The possibility that dietary fibre lowers the plasma cholesterol concentration (see Section 5.3) led Raymond *et al.* (1977) to test the effect of mixed plant fibres on the absorption of cholesterol in human subjects. When the fibre content of the diet was increased to five times that of the typical American diet, daily absorption of cholesterol was not significantly affected.

Plant sterols have long been known to diminish the absorption of cholesterol in animals and birds, an effect that is presumably due to competition with cholesterol for incorporation into micelles or for transport across the intestinal wall. In view of this effect, β-sitosterol has been used as a therapeutic agent for lowering the plasma cholesterol level in hypercholesterolaemic patients. It has usually been given in doses of 10–20 g/day. However, Grundy and Mok (1977) have shown that maximal inhibition of cholesterol absorption in man is achieved with much smaller doses. When the diet contains 3 g of β-sitosterol per day, absorption of dietary cholesterol is reduced by 50%, and no further reduction occurs when the dose of β-sitosterol is increased. β-Sitosterol infused into the duodenum in micellar solution is capable of inhibiting cholesterol absorption even when the concentration of β-sitosterol is less than that of cholesterol. This raises the possibility that differences in the normal consumption of plant sterols could contribute to differences in the plasma cholesterol concentration in different human populations.

An obvious approach to the treatment of hypercholesterolaemia is to try to diminish the absorption of dietary and endogenous cholesterol. When it was discovered that bile salts are necessary for the absorption of cholesterol, attempts were made to inhibit absorption by feeding unabsorbable substances that interfere with the lipid-solubilizing action of bile salts in the lumen of the jejunum. Judged by their ability to lower the plasma cholesterol concentration, the most effective of these agents are cholestyramine and other bile-salt-binding resins, already discussed in Chapter 5. However, although cholestyramine given in large doses markedly diminishes the total amount of cholesterol absorbed *via* the intestinal lymphatics in rats (Hyun *et al.*, 1963), doses that are clinically effective in man have little effect on the absorption of dietary cholesterol (Miettinen, 1970). (For further discussion of the effects of cholestyramine on cholesterol absorption, see Section 5.5.)

The absorption of dietary cholesterol is diminished in rabbits and in human subjects by an operation for bypass of the ileum (Buchwald, 1964). The effects of this operation on whole-body cholesterol metabolism in man are discussed in Section 5.5.4.

5 CHANGES IN WHOLE-BODY METABOLISM

Changes in the metabolism and distribution of cholesterol in the body as a whole occur in response to variations in the intake of cholesterol and other dietary constituents. They may also occur in various diseases affecting lipid or lipoprotein metabolism and in response to the administration of drugs or other procedures used for therapeutic purposes. Some of these changes are considered in the following sections, with special emphasis on man. Changes in whole-body metabolism and distribution of cholesterol may also occur during post-natal development and, in some human populations, during ageing.

5.1 Dietary cholesterol

Several mechanisms are available to the body for adjusting to changes in the dietary intake of cholesterol. The relative contributions of different mechanisms appear to vary from one species to another. There are also considerable species differences in the success of these mechanisms as a whole in maintaining homeostasis. For example, in rats and dogs the feeding of moderate amounts of cholesterol has little or no influence on the plasma cholesterol concentration or the amount of cholesterol in the whole body, whereas cholesterol feeding in rabbits leads rapidly to the accumulation of cholesterol in the plasma and tissues. There is also some evidence to suggest that differences in plasma cholesterol concentration *between* apparently normal human populations are due partly to differences in the efficiency of cholesterol-homeostasis mechanisms. As discussed below, the evidence for this interesting possibility is still insecure, but it raises the question as to how far person-to-person variability in the efficiency of cholesterol homeostasis may also contribute to the wide range in plasma cholesterol concentration observed *within* a given human population.

5.1.1 Absorption as a regulatory mechanism

Incomplete absorption of dietary or endogenous cholesterol is not in itself regulatory, but it does contribute to homeostasis by decreasing the additional load of exchangeable cholesterol that has to be disposed of when cholesterol intake is increased. The decreased efficiency of absorption that occurs at high intakes of dietary cholesterol is in effect a regulatory mechanism though not, of course, one that could play any part in homeostasis in herbivorous animals under natural conditions. There is little evidence to suggest that variations in the efficiency of cholesterol absorption contribute to the variability in plasma cholesterol concentration within normal human populations, or that an increased capacity for absorbing cholesterol is ever a cause of hypercholesterolaemia. However, hypocholesterolaemia may occur in human malabsorption.

5.1.2 Responses to changes in cholesterol absorption

When cholesterol is added to the diet, the increase in net absorption of cholesterol leads to a decrease in the rate of synthesis in the whole body. In rats and dogs, suppression of synthesis may be complete, as shown by the finding that the specific activity of the plasma cholesterol becomes virtually equal to that of the dietary cholesterol after prolonged feeding with radioactive cholesterol. In these species, synthesis in extra-hepatic tissues must make little or no contribution to the total turnover of exchangeable cholesterol when hepatic synthesis is suppressed by cholesterol feeding. However, in non-human primates cholesterol feeding does not lead to complete suppression of whole-body synthesis, possibly because in primates cholesterol synthesized in the intestinal wall and other extrahepatic tissues contributes significantly to total turnover in the presence of dietary cholesterol (see Dietschy and Wilson, 1970, for references). The response to dietary cholesterol in man is considered below.

The addition of cholesterol to the diet of an animal adapted to a cholesterol-free diet may be fully compensated for by decreased synthesis, provided that the rate of absorption of dietary cholesterol does not exceed the rate at which the liver synthesizes cholesterol in the absence of dietary cholesterol. Above this limit, cholesterol must accumulate in the body unless other compensatory mechanisms are brought into play.

In rats (Wilson, 1964) and dogs (Abell *et al.*, 1956), cholesterol feeding leads to increased synthesis of bile acids, the output of bile acids rising at high intakes of dietary cholesterol to three times the basal level in rats and to an even greater extent in dogs. Cholesterol balance measurements have shown that rats (Wilson, 1964) and dogs (Pertsemlidis *et al.*, 1973) are able to maintain zero balance of cholesterol in the presence of very high dietary intakes by a combination of suppression of whole-body synthesis of cholesterol and increased bile-acid formation. The efficiency of these mechanisms is such that cholesterol-rich diets cause little or no increase in plasma cholesterol concentration in these species unless the compensatory increase in bile-acid synthesis is blocked by making the animals hypothyroid. The ability to increase bile-acid synthesis in response to cholesterol feeding has been demonstrated in squirrel monkeys (Lofland *et al.*, 1972) and rhesus monkeys (Eggen, 1974) though this mechanism appears to be much less effective in non-human primates than in rats and dogs. In rabbits, cholesterol feeding has no effect on the rate of synthesis of bile acids (Hellström, 1965).

At this point it will be useful to consider separately the effect of dietary cholesterol on whole-body metabolism of cholesterol in man, since this has been the subject of controversy, especially as regards the extent to which cholesterol synthesis in the human body is suppressible. Studies in which cholesterol metabolism was investigated by the isotopic equilibrium method suggested initially that cholesterol feeding has little effect on whole-body synthesis in man (Kaplan *et al.*, 1963; Wilson and Lindsey, 1965), though it soon became clear that the synthesis of cholesterol in the human liver, estimated from the incorporation of radioactive acetate into cholesterol in needle biopsies, is almost completely inhibited when the daily intake of cholesterol is increased to 3 g/day (see Dietschy and Wilson, 1970). This apparent anomaly was explained on the grounds that in man the liver makes a relatively small contribution to the pool of exchangeable cholesterol in the absence of cholesterol in the diet, and that the human intestine has such a limited capacity for absorbing dietary cholesterol that homeostasis can be maintained without the need for an efficient regulatory mechanism. However, later work has shown that considerable amounts of dietary cholesterol can, in fact, be absorbed in man (see Section 4.7.1) and that feedback inhibition of cholesterol synthesis in the whole body is capable of compensating for quite substantial increases in the rate of absorption of dietary cholesterol, in both normal and hypercholesterolaemic human subjects (Quintão *et al.*, 1971*b*; Nestel and Poyser, 1976). That cholesterol synthesis in man is under feedback control by absorbed cholesterol is also shown by the observation that whole-body synthesis is increased when cholesterol absorption is selectively blocked by feeding β-sitosterol (Grundy et al., 1969).

It has been shown repeatedly that the feeding of cholesterol, even in doses as high as 3 g/day, has no effect on bile-acid synthesis in man. However, the human liver has a considerable capacity for increasing the rate at which absorbed cholesterol is re-excreted in the bile as neutral sterol (Quintão et al., 1971b). Since biliary cholesterol is incompletely re-absorbed, this mechanism results in an increased rate of faecal excretion of neutral steroids of endogenous origin in response to increased absorption of cholesterol in the diet.

In most normal human subjects and in most patients with moderate hypercholesterolaemia, variations in dietary intake within a range of about 250 mg/day to 750 mg/day can be largely compensated for by changes in whole-body synthesis or in re-excretion of absorbed cholesterol, or by a combination of both mechanisms (Nestel and Poyser, 1976). In some subjects, however, a prolonged increase in the intake of dietary cholesterol leads to the accumulation of cholesterol in the body, as estimated from sterol balance measurements (Quintão et al., 1971b). This appears to be due to the presence, in some individuals, of a partial inadequacy of one or other of the compensatory mechanisms available to the body for adjusting to changes in cholesterol intake. How far this person-to-person variability is responsible for the variability in plasma cholesterol concentration in free-living populations can only be established by observing the metabolic response to a challenge of increased dietary cholesterol in groups of individuals whose natural plasma cholesterol levels are known. An interesting pointer to the situation that may exist in human populations is the finding of Lofland et al. (1972) that within populations of squirrel monkeys some individuals show no change in plasma cholesterol concentration when their cholesterol intake is increased, whereas others become hypercholesterolaemic. In the former group there is an immediate increase in bile-acid synthesis in response to the dietary cholesterol; in the latter the increase is delayed and is less marked.

Ho et al. (1971) have suggested that the reason why the Masai (a pastoral community living in East Africa) have low plasma cholsterol concentrations, despite a high intake of dietary cholesterol, is that they differ from the people of 'Western' countries in being able to suppress cholesterol synthesis in response to absorbed dietary cholesterol. This suggestion was based on the finding that cholesterol synthesis in the Masai, estimated by a method requiring the feeding of radioactive cholesterol to isotopic equilibrium, appeared to be controlled by feedback inhibition, whereas feedback inhibition seemed to play little or no role in cholesterol homeostasis in North American adults. It would be unwise to disregard the possibility that there are racial differences in the efficiency of compensatory mechanisms for maintaining cholesterol homeostasis. However, the suggestion of Ho et al., has lost some of its force since more recent observations made with the chemical sterol balance method have shown that as a general rule, people from Western countries do, in fact, suppress cholesterol synthesis when cholesterol is present in the diet and that this mechanism operates efficiently over the range of cholesterol intakes typical of Western diets (see, in particular, Nestel and Poyser, 1976). It is possible that non-genetic factors, such as dietary constituents other than cholesterol and fat, the amount of physical exercise taken or other special features of the way of life of the Masai, are more important then genetic constitution in maintaining their plasma cholesterol concentration at an unusually low level.

Finally, it should be noted that an increase in the dietary intake of cholesterol usually causes some rise in plasma cholesterol concentration in normal and hyperlipidaemic human subjects (Connor et al., 1961; Keys et al., 1965a; Quintão et al., 1971b). Mattson et al. (1972) concluded that in normal men an increase of 100 mg of cholesterol per 1000 dietary calories causes, on average, a rise in plasma cholesterol concentration of 12 mg/100 ml. However, there is considerable person-to-person variation in the response to a given increase in cholesterol intake, some individuals showing little or no rise in plasma cholesterol concentration when the intake is increased to more than 2 g/day.

5.2 Polyunsaturated fat

Unsaturated vegetable oils, when added to the diet, have long been known to lower the plasma cholesterol concentration (Kinsell et al., 1952). However, it is now generally recognized that the effect of a given neutral fat on the plasma cholesterol concentration does not depend upon whether the fat is of animal or vegetable origin, but upon the chain length and degree of unsaturation of its component fatty acids. Keys et al. (1965b), who made a detailed study of the effects of different fats on the plasma cholesterol of normal human subjects, came to the following conclusions: (1) saturated fatty acids with more than 12 but less than 18 carbon atoms raise the plasma cholesterol concentration; (2) fatty acids with two or more double bonds (polyunsaturated) have an opposite, but weaker, effect, about 2 g of polyunsaturated fat being required to counteract the effect of 1 g of saturated fat; (3) mono-unsaturated fatty acids have no effect on the plasma cholesterol concentration. Keys et al. (1965b) have proposed a formula relating the change in plasma cholesterol concentration to the change in cholesterol content of the diet and in the percentages of total dietary calories contributed by polyunsaturated fatty acids and saturated fatty acids of chain length C_{12} to C_{16}. However, the Keys formula has been criticized by Vergroesen and Gottenbos (1975), who have drawn attention to the possible effects of elaidic acid (the *trans*-isomer of oleic acid), and to our lack of information on the effects of fatty acids with 20 or more carbon atoms, on the plasma cholesterol.

Investigation of the mechanisms by which these effects of dietary fat are brought about has led to contradictory results. In much of the earlier clinical work, the methods used for estimating turnover, excretion and synthesis of cholesterol were almost certainly inadequate, but discrepant results have since been reported from different laboratories in all of which the methods introduced by Ahrens and his collaborators were used.

Three groups of workers, using the isotope balance method, have reported increases in the faecal excretion of bile acids and endogenous neutral steroids during the feeding of polyunsaturated-fat diets in adult human subjects with normal plasma cholesterol concentrations (Wood *et al.*, 1966; Moore *et al.*, 1968; Connor *et al.*, 1969). Increased faecal excretion of bile acids has also been reported in infants when soy-bean milk, which contains a high ratio of polyunsaturated to saturated fat, is substituted for cow's milk (Potter and Nestel, 1976). In two of these studies, the cumulative increase in the faecal excretion of total steroids was greater than the amount of cholesterol lost from the plasma. This suggests that, in addition to increased removal of cholesterol from the plasma, there was mobilization and excretion of tissue cholesterol, though it does not exclude the possibility that the fall in plasma cholesterol concentration led to increased cholesterol synthesis, and that this was in part responsible for the increased faecal excretion of steroids.

In contrast to these observations, Avigan and Steinberg (1965) and Grundy and Ahrens (1970) found no consistent change in faecal excretion of bile acids or neutral steroids in patients of whom the majority were hyperlipidaemic. Although there were increases in the excretion either of bile acids or of neutral steroids in at least four of these patients, a marked fall in plasma cholesterol concentration during corn-oil feeding occurred in the majority without significant increase in steroid excretion. Grundy and Ahrens (1970) concluded that the fall in plasma cholesterol concentration induced by polyunsaturated fat in their patients was probably due to a shift of cholesterol from the plasma into the tissues, a suggestion previously made by Spritz and Mishkel (1969). It is consistent with this idea that Lindstedt *et al.* (1965) found that a decrease in plasma cholesterol concentration could occur in the absence of any increase in the absolute rate of turnover of cholic acid in patients or normal subjects fed polyunsaturated-fat diets.

Grundy and Ahrens (1970) pointed out that if some of the cholesteriol lost from the plasma during polyunsaturated-fat feeding were transferred to the liver, it might subsequently be excreted in the bile as bile acid or neutral sterol, some of which would then be lost in the faeces; if this process were spread out over a long time it might not cause a detectable increase in the daily excretion of faecal steroids. It should be noted that a decrease in plasma cholesterol concentration without any increment in faecal steroid excretion could be caused by a decrease in the rate of synthesis of cholesterol by the liver. However, suppression of cholesterol synthesis should cause a decrease in the slope of the specific activity-time curve for plasma cholesterol obtained after pulse-labelling with radioactive cholesterol. This was not observed in any of the patients studied by Grundy and Ahrens when polyunsaturated fat was fed. This, incidentally, provides a good illustration of the way in which additional information about whole-body metabolism of cholesterol can be obtained by combining the results of balance measurements with observations on plasma specific-activity curves.

A possible clue to the discrepancies between the findings from different laboratories is the fact that almost all the *normal* subjects tested have shown a marked increase in faecal steroid excretion in response to polyunsaturated-fat feeding, whereas most of the subjects in whom the fall in plasma cholesterol concentration was not accompanied by increased steroid excretion were hyperlipidaemic. This suggests that at least two mechanisms are involved in the response to polyunsaturated fat—a stimulation of the mechanisms by which plasma cholesterol is excreted from the body, and a redistribution of cholesterol from plasma to tissues, which may or may not be followed by a detectable increase in elimination of cholesterol and its metabolites in the faeces—and that both mechanisms need not operate if a fall in plasma cholesterol concentration is to occur. Judging from the clinical status of the hyperlipidaemic patients who have been investigated, it seems that a fall in plasma cholesterol concentration without stimulation of cholesterol excretion tends to occur in familial hypercholesterolaemia, but that patients with hypertriglyceridaemia often show very substantial increases in the faecal excretion of neutral steroids or of bile acids, or of both, when fed polyunsaturated fat (see Grundy (1975) for discussion and extensive list of references).

In normal subjects and in patients with essential hypercholesterolaemia, the fall in plasma total cholesterol concentration that occurs when polyunsaturated fat is fed is due to a fall in plasma LDL concentration. This suggests that one effect of the polyunsaturated fat might be to change the properties of LDL in a manner such as to facilitate its uptake and degradation by extravascular tissues. In this connection it may be relevant that the fatty-acid composition of the cholesteryl esters of LDL is altered by changing the fatty acids of the dietary fat. Increased elimination of cholesterol from the body could be brought about by decreased reabsorption of cholesterol and its metabolites from the intestine, or by increased secretion in the bile. That increased biliary secretion may be an important factor is suggested by the observation of Grundy (1975) that the output of cholesterol in the bile was increased by polyunsaturated fat in some of his hypertriglyceridaemic patients.

In view of the widespread use of polyunsaturated fat in the treatment of hypercholesterolaemia it is clearly important to collect more information about the mechanisms by which the effect on plasma cholesterol concentration is mediated. In particular, there is a need for investigation of the effect of dietary fat on the amount of exchangeable cholesterol in the whole body and in individual tissues, including, of course, the arterial wall. There is also the question of the possible effects of increased biliary excretion of cholesterol on the formation of gallstones. Finally, we need to know much more about the effect of polyunsaturated fat on the metabolism of specific lipoproteins.

5.3 Other dietary factors

Animal experiments carried out primarily to test the atherogenic potency of different diets have shown that several dietary constituents other than cholesterol and neutral fat influence the plasma cholesterol concentration. These include protein, carbohydrate, vegetable fibre, plant sterols and other minor components of the diet. A limited amount of information is also available about the effect of some of these constituents on the plasma cholesterol concentration in man, and this information is supplemented by epidemiological observations on the relation between plasma cholesterol concentration and the composition of the diet in different human populations. There has been little attempt to explain the effects of these dietary factors on plasma cholesterol in terms of effects on the whole-body metabolism of cholesterol. Much of the rather confusing literature on the subject dealt with in this section has been reviewed by Kritchevsky (1976).

The nature and amount of protein in the diet has been shown to influence the plasma cholesterol concentration in several species, apparently by interaction between protein and other dietary constituents. In rabbits, for example, the hypercholesterolaemia induced by cholesterol feeding is enhanced by adding protein to the diet, animal protein (especially casein) having a greater effect than vegetable protein (Carroll and Hamilton, 1975). Broadly similar effects of protein have been observed in pigeons (Lofland et al., 1961) and monkeys (Middleton et al., 1967). The effect of defined protein constituents in the diet on human cholesterol metabolism has not been investigated systematically, but the epidemiological evidence suggests that there is a positive correlation between plasma cholesterol concentration and the percentage of dietary calories due to animal protein in different populations; this could, however, merely reflect the association between animal protein and saturated fat in the diet.

Since there is, in general, a positive correlation between plasma cholesterol concentration and sugar consumption in different human populations, it has been suggested that the high sucrose intake of people living in Westernized communities is a major cause of their relatively high plasma cholesterol concentrations. In support of this, it has been reported that isocaloric substitution of sucrose for starch in the diet of hyperlipidaemic patients increases their plasma cholesterol and triglyceride concentrations (see Grande *et al.*, 1974). However, the epidemiological evidence does not prove that the relation between *per capita* consumption of refined sugar and plasma cholesterol concentration is a causal one. Indeed, it is likely that the high plasma cholesterol levels usually found in communities whose consumption of refined sugar is high are due to other associated factors, such as a high intake of saturated fat or of total calories, or a low intake of certain types of dietary fibre; it is noteworthy that in Caribbean populations, whose consumption of sucrose is the highest in the world, the mean plasma cholesterol concentration is strikingly low. Furthermore, sucrose is without significant effect on the plasma cholesterol concentration of normal men tested under experimental conditions (Grande *et al.*, 1974).

The effects of changing the nature of the dietary carbohydrate on plasma cholesterol levels in animals are confusing and hard to interpret. The effects of a given type of carbohydrate are influenced by the presence or absence of other dietary constituents, particularly cholesterol and unabsorbable food residue. For example, in rabbits and chickens the substitution of sucrose for glucose increases the plasma cholesterol concentration if the diet contains cholesterol, but not if it is cholesterol-free (Grant and Fahrenbach, 1959). There are also species differences in the response to a given type of dietary carbohydrate. Lang and Barthel (1972), for example, found that in the presence of dietary cholesterol the substitution of dextrin (a complex polysaccharide) for sucrose increased the plasma cholesterol concentration in Rhesus monkeys but not in Cebus monkeys.

The possible influence of dietary fibre on cholesterol absorption in man has already been mentioned briefly (Section 4.7.2). This is a convenient point at which to say something more about the relation between dietary fibre and cholesterol metabolism in general. Current interest in this question stems partly from animal experiments on the effects of synthetic, residue-free, diets on the metabolism of cholesterol and bile acids, and partly from a consideration of the possible effects of the low fibre content of modern Western diets on human health. In the present state of knowledge dietary fibre is best defined, not in chemical terms, but as the total indigestible residue remaining after digestion of vegetable matter in the human intestinal tract. It consists essentially of the semi-rigid material of plant cell walls and comprises several complex substances, including cellulose, hemi-celluloses, pectin and lignin (see Cummings, 1973; Eastwood, 1973). The composition of fibre varies widely from one type of plant to another. It should also be noted that the chemical and physical properties of the components of dietary fibre may be changed during their isolation and purification and, therefore, that the results of experiments on the effects of chemically defined fibre components on cholesterol metabolism under experimental conditions may not be relevant to the possible effects of the fibre in natural diets.

Dietary experiments on birds and animals carried out in the 1950's and 1960's showed that semi-purified, high-fat, diets with a low fibre content tended to cause hypercholesterolaemia and to be more atherogenic than stock diets with the same fat content but with normal amounts of fibre. It was also shown that these effects could be counteracted by supplementing the semi-purified diets with fibre from various sources. Vegetable fibres from different sources differed widely in their ability to lower the plasma cholesterol concentration, wheat straw, pectin and alfalfa being much more effective than cellulose; mucilaginous gums from several sources have also been shown to lower the plasma cholesterol concentration in cholesterol-fed rats (see Kritchevsky, 1976, for references).

Part of the effect of dietary fibre on cholesterol metabolism in animals seems to be due to interference with the absorption of cholesterol from the intestine, but a more important factor is probably the stimulation of bile-acid excretion in the faeces (Portman, 1960; Gustafsson and Norman, 1969). Increased bile-acid excretion may be mediated partly by an effect of the dietary fibre on the intestinal microflora (see Myant, 1975), but fibre may also act directly by binding bile acids in the intestinal lumen and thus preventing their reabsorption from the ileum. Conjugated bile acids are bound by dietary fibre *in vitro*, and there is a rough correlation between the capacity of fibres from different plant sources to bind taurocholate *in vitro* and their ability to lower the plasma cholesterol concentration in rats (Kritchevsky *et al.*, 1975). The mechanism of the binding probably differs with different types of fibre. Some fibres may possibly act as anion-exchangers, but most dietary fibres, including cellulose and lignin have no ionizable groups and therefore cannot bind in this way. These fibres probably act either as non-ionic adsorbers or by imbibing water in which bile-acids are trapped. Whatever the mechanism, interference with the reabsorption of bile acids would tend to release bile-acid synthesis from feedback inhibition and thus to stimulate the catabolism of cholesterol.

Experimental work on the effects of dietary fibre on human cholesterol metabolism has led to a good deal of controversy (see Eastwood, 1975). Everyone who has worked on the problem agrees that cellulose, even given in very large amounts, has no effect on the plasma cholesterol concentration or the faecal excretion of steroids. On the other hand, some, though not all, workers who have investigated the effect of pectin on cholesterol metabolism in man have observed a significant fall in plasma cholesterol concentration (see Kay *et al.*, 1978, for references) with, in some instances, an increase in the faecal excretion of bile acids. Claims with regard to the effects of wheat bran on cholesterol metabolism in man have been equally contradictory. Bengal gram, a fibre-rich legume, has been shown to lower the plasma cholesterol concentration when added to the diet of normal men (Mathur *et al.*, 1968).

In the human experiments of Raymond *et al.* (1977) mentioned in Section 4.7.2, wheat bran, pectin and other vegetable fibres were added to the diet of normal men over 4-week periods in amounts equivalent to the quantities eaten in many primitive populations. In no case was there a detectable effect on the plasma cholesterol concentration or on the absorption of cholesterol or its elimination from the body. Hence, it is unlikely that a high intake of dietary fibre is a contributory cause of the low plasma cholesterol concentrations observed in primitive peoples, though it remains possible that in free-living populations a high intake of fibre maintained over many years does affect cholesterol metabolism in a way that is not apparent during short experimental periods. It is also possible that fibre affects cholesterol metabolism indirectly by interacting in some way with other dietary constituents not present in the diets of Western countries.

As we have seen (Section 4.7.2), plant sterols interfere with the absorption of cholesterol in animals and human subjects. β-Sitosterol, the major sterol of most plants, diminishes cholesterol absorption from the human intestine when infused into the duodenum in amounts comparable with the quantities present in some human diets. Observations on the effects of much larger intakes of β-sitosterol in man have shown that although the decreased cholesterol absorption is partially balanced by increased whole-body synthesis, the net effect is usually to lower the plasma cholesterol concentration. In the light of these facts it is worth considering the possibility that variations in the dietary intake of plant sterols make some contribution to the variability in plasma cholesterol concentration between different populations.

References to some of the rather controversial literature on the possible influence of trace elements and vitamins on plasma cholesterol concentration will be found in the reviews by Kritchevsky (1976) and Keys (1975), and in Davidson et al. (1979).

5.4 Hyperlipidaemia and obesity

In hypertriglyceridaemic patients the output of bile acids (Kottke, 1969; Einarsson and Hellström, 1972) and the synthesis of cholesterol in the whole body (Sodhi and Kudchodkar, 1973) are often increased, the increase being especially marked in patients with the type V plasma lipoprotein pattern. Sodhi and Kudchodkar (1973) suggest that the increased rate of synthesis of cholesterol in these patients is a consequence of increased hepatic synthesis of VLDL. However, hypertriglyceridaemia can occur in the presence of normal rates of cholesterol and bile-acid synthesis (Grundy, 1975), and in the hypertriglyceridaemic patients investigated by Miettinen (1970) with the sterol balance method, neither bile-acid output nor cholesterol turnover was significantly increased when the values were expressed in terms of body weight.

Some of the published reports on cholesterol metabolism in hypercholesterolaemic patients are difficult to interpret because of insufficient clinical information. Bile-acid synthesis tends to be below normal in essential hypercholesterolaemia in general (Einarsson et al., 1974) and was markedly diminished in the affected members of a single family with familial hypercholesterolaemia studied by Miettinen et al. (1967). However, cholesterol turnover is usually within normal limits in familial hypercholesterolaemia (for further discussion of this question, see Chapter 15). In a group of 22 human subjects studied by Nestel et al. (1969), there was no correlation between plasma cholesterol concentration and the production rate of cholesterol or the exchangeable mass (minus that in the plasma), estimated by analysis of plasma specific activity-time curves in terms of a two-pool system. Failure to detect any increase in the extravascular exchangeable mass of cholesterol in hypercholesterolaemic subjects is perhaps surprising in view of their tendency to deposit cholesterol in skin, tendons and other tissues. As noted in Section 2.2.3, Samuel and Lieberman (1973) found a significant correlation between plasma cholesterol concentration and the mass of pool B estimated from specific-activity curves continued for long enough to take account of very slowly-exchanging pools of cholesterol. A positive correlation between the amounts of cholesterol in the plasma and the extravascular pools has also been observed in cholesterol-fed Cebus monkeys (Lofland et al., 1968).

In obesity there is an increase in the rate of whole-body synthesis of cholesterol, determined by the sterol balance method (Miettinen, 1971; Nestel et al., 1973), and in the mass of pool B determined by the method of Goodman and Noble (1968). Cholesterol synthesis is most closely related to the excess of body weight over the ideal weight for height, the rate of synthesis/day increasing by about 20 mg for each kg of surplus body weight. When an obese subject loses weight, cholesterol synthesis falls towards the normal rate. The site of the increased synthesis of cholesterol in obese subjects is not known, but is unlikely to be the adipose tissue itself, since human adipocytes have a very low capacity for synthesizing cholesterol (see Schreibman and Dell, 1975).

5.5 Drugs and operative procedures

In this section I shall consider how whole-body metabolism of cholesterol is affected by drugs and operative procedures used for treating hypercholesterolaemia. The clinical aspects of these forms of treatment are discussed in Chapter 15.

5.5.1 Bile-acid-binding resins

Cholestyramine and other anion exchangers that bind bile salts have already been referred to in this chapter and in Chapter 5. The main action of cholestyramine when given to human subjects in therapeutic doses is to stimulate the conversion of cholesterol into bile acids by preventing the reabsorption of bile salts from the ileum. This leads to a reduction in the plasma cholesterol concentration, due mainly to a fall in plasma LDL concentration. There may also be an increase in the fractional catabolic rate of LDL apoB (Langer et al., 1969). The decrease in effective concentration of bile salts in the intestinal lumen diminishes the absorption of cholesterol in some patients, but in many this effect is not observed (Miettinen, 1970). Increased catabolism of cholesterol induces a compensatory increase in whole-body synthesis of cholesterol. If the administration of cholestyramine to hypercholesterolaemic patients is continued for long periods, a new steady state is achieved in which whole-body synthesis and production rate of cholesterol are maintained at a rate several times that in the untreated state. This is reflected in an increase in the slope of the plasma cholesterol specific-activity curve after pulse-labelling. The increase in whole-body synthesis is due to stimulation of synthesis in the liver (Myant, 1972) and intestinal wall (Grundy et al., 1971). If the fall in plasma cholesterol concentration is maintained for many months, cholesterol may be transferred to the plasma from slowly-exchanging pools of cholesterol in the tissues, as shown by a gradual decrease in the size of skin xanthomas in some hypercholesterolaemic patients. In some cases, the stimulation of cholesterol synthesis leads to a temporary increase in plasma VLDL concentration (Jones and

Dobrilovic, 1970), accompanied by an increased flux of VLDL cholesterol into the plasma (Clifton-Bligh et al., 1974). This could reflect increased hepatic synthesis and secretion of VLDL particles in response to the increased synthesis of cholesterol. Some of these effects are shown in Fig. 10.4.

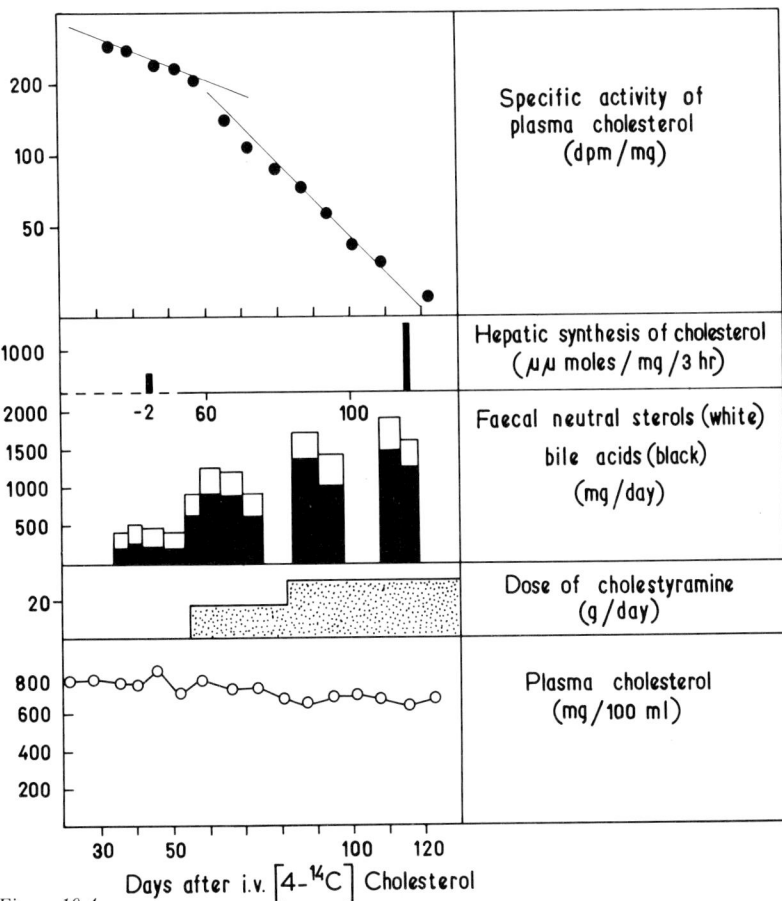

Figure 10.4
The effect of daily treatment with cholestyramine (16–30 g/day) on cholesterol metabolism in a 10-year-old boy with familial hypercholesterolaemia in the homozygous form.
The plasma cholesterol was labelled by an intravenous injection of [^{14}C]cholesterol at day 0 and cholestyramine treatment was started on day 55. Cholesterol treatment (1) increased the slope of the plasma cholesterol specific-activity curve, (2) stimulated hepatic synthesis of cholesterol (estimated from the rate of incorporation of [^{14}C]acetate into cholesterol in liver biopsies in vitro) and (3) increased faecal bile acid excretion. Though there was a fall in plasma cholesterol concentration during the treatment period, the concentration remained above 600 mg/100 ml even when the dose was increased to 30 g/day. (From the observations of C. D. Moutafis, P. W. Adams, N. B. Myant and V. Wynn (Myant, 1972), with the permission of Plenum Press, New York.)

5.5.2 Thyroid hormones

The natural thyroid hormones lower the plasma cholesterol concentration in human subjects with myxoedema or primary hypercholesterolaemia. Owing to the potentially harmful effects of the natural hormones on the heart, neither L-thyroxine nor L-tri-iodothyronine can be used to treat primary hypercholesterolaemia, but D-thyroxine given in conjunction with a β-blocking agent has been used in the treatment of this condition. Thyroid hormone given to myxoedematous subjects (Miettinen, 1968) and D-thyroxine given to those with familial hypercholesterolaemia (Simons and Myant, 1974) increase the faecal output of total steroids of endogenous origin, due apparently to increased removal of circulating cholesterol together with mobilization and excretion of tissue cholesterol. The increase in faecal steroid excretion is usually due predominantly to increased excretion of neutral steroids, but there may also be a rise in bile-acid output, suggesting that the effect of thyroid hormone is in some way to facilitate the entry of plasma lipoprotein cholesterol into the hepatocytes rather than to stimulate some specific intracellular mechanism concerned either in the secretion of cholesterol into the bile or in the conversion of cholesterol into bile acids.

5.5.3 Clofibrate, nicotinic acid and neomycin

Clofibrate, the ethyl ester of p-chlorophenoxyisobutyrate, is used extensively in the treatment of hyperlipidaemia. The effects of clofibrate on whole-body lipid metabolism in man, and the possible mechanisms underlying these effects, have been reviewed by Havel and Kane (1973). The most striking clinical response to the drug is a fall in plasma VLDL concentration in hypertriglyceridaemic patients, but the plasma LDL concentration may also be diminished in primary hypercholesterolaemia. The initial response to clofibrate in hyperlipidaemic patients is an increase in the rate of secretion of cholesterol in the bile and a net increase in the faecal excretion of endogenous steroids, without a compensatory increase in whole-body synthesis of cholesterol. If the drug treatment is continued for months or years, a new steady state is achieved in which cholesterol synthesis is maintained at a normal or reduced level and the mass of exchangeable cholesterol in slowly-exchanging pools is decreased.

The possibility that the prolonged administration of clofibrate may lead to undesirable side-effects is discussed in Chapter 13, Section 4.9.

Experimental work on rats has shown that clofibrate affects many biochemical processes concerned in lipid metabolism. In the present state of knowledge it is impossible to explain all these effects in terms of a single action of the drug at the cellular or sub-cellular level. Moreover, it is likely that some of the enzymic changes seen in the livers of rats treated with large doses of clofibrate are not relevant to the therapeutic properties of the drug. In rats, clofibrate has been shown to affect several metabolic events in a manner that would be expected to decrease the rate of synthesis of triglycerides in the liver and, hence, to diminish the synthesis and secretion of hepatic VLDL. These effects include a reduced rate of mobilization of fatty acids from adipose tissue, descreased fatty-acid synthesis in the liver and increased activity of hepatic α-glycerophosphate dehydrogenase (which would tend to diminish the supply of α-glycerophosphate for esterification with fatty acid). Inhibition of cholesterol synthesis in the liver and increased activity of lipoprotein lipase in adipose tissue have also been observed in clofibrate-treated rats. It is not clear which, if any, of these effects underlies the actions of clofibrate on lipid metabolism in man. In so far as VLDL is the precursor of LDL, the major carrier of the plasma cholesterol in man, a diminished output of VLDL from the liver would tend to lower the plasma cholesterol concentration. However, the experimental evidence available is not consistent with the view that clofibrate diminishes hepatic VLDL secretion in man. In fact, the major effect of clofibrate on VLDL metabolism in human subjects seems to be to increase the efficiency of removal of VLDL from the plasma. None of the effects that have been described in rats explains the increased biliary secretion of cholesterol observed in man.

Nicotinic acid lowers the plasma cholesterol concentration in human subjects and in some experimental animals, including monkeys and rabbits. Extensive investigation of the effects of nicotonic acid on cholesterol metabolism in intact animals and animal tissues (see Kritchevsky (1971) and Myant (1981)) has not provided a fully adequate explanation of the hypocholesterolaemic action of this drug in man. Nicotinic acid inhibits hepatic synthesis of cholesterol in rats (Gamble and Wright, 1961) and monkeys (Magide and Myant, 1974) and in some hypercholesterolaemic patients undergoing treatment with cholestyramine (Moutafis *et al.*, 1971). Increased faecal excretion of endogenous neutral steroids has been observed in some hypercholesterolaemic patients given nicotinic acid, but not in all. The earliest observable change in lipid metabolism in response to nicotinic acid in man (Carlson *et al.*, 1968) and monkeys (Magide and Myant, 1974) is a fall in plasma free-fatty-acid concentration. This is followed by a fall in plasma triglyceride concentration with, finally, a fall in plasma cholesterol concentration. This sequence of events is consistent with a primary effect on the mobilization of fatty acids from adipose tissue, leading to decreased hepatic synthesis and secretion of VLDL with a consequent fall in the rate of production of LDL. In keeping with this, nicotinic acid has been shown to decrease the incorporation of labelled threonine into VLDL protein in monkeys

(Magide et al., 1975), and to decrease the rate of production of LDL-apoB in patients with familial hypercholesterolaemia (Langer and Levy, 1971). Observations on the effect of long-term treatment with nicotinic acid on exchangeable pools of cholesterol in man have not been reported, but Magide and Myant (1975) have shown that repeated injections of nicotinic acid cause a net loss of cholesterol from skeletal muscle and skin in monkeys.

Neomycin, an unabsorbable polybasic antibiotic, lowers the plasma cholesterol concentration in man, probably by intefering with the absorption of bile salts and cholesterol. Analysis of plasma radioactivity curves after labelling with radioactive cholesterol shows that long-term treatment with neomycin reduces the mass of cholesterol in the rapidly exchanging extravascular pool (Samuel et al., 1968).

5.5.4 Operative procedures

An operation for by-pass of a third or more of the ileum usually causes a sustained fall in plasma cholesterol concentration in patients with moderate hypercholesterolaemia (Buchwald et al., 1974). The effects of this procedure on whole-body metabolism of cholesterol are analogous to those of cholestyramine, though the mechanism is not quite the same. Since the ileum is the major site of the reabsorption of bile salts, by-pass of the ileum leads to a substantial decrease in the efficiency of absorption of bile salts, with increased faecal output of acidic steroids and a compensatory increase in hepatic synthesis of cholesterol and bile acids. Since there is a net fall in the quantity of bile salts available for the formation of micelles in the jejunum, cholesterol absorption is usually diminished. Kinetic analysis of plasma cholesterol specific-activity curves reveals a situation similar to that seen during treatment with cholestyramine. The rate of fall in specific activity of the plasma cholesterol is greatly increased and there is an increase in the production rate of cholesterol due to increased cholesterol synthesis. In the long term, the mass of cholesterol in slowly-exchanging pools may decrease, as shown by analysis of plasma cholesterol specific-activity curves (Moore et al., 1969) and by the slow disappearance of xanthomatous deposits in some hypercholesterolaemic patients (Miettinen, 1970). Similar changes in whole-body metabolism of cholesterol occur after resection of the ileum (Moutafis et al., 1968).

Anastomosis of the portal vein to the inferior vena cava causes a marked fall in plasma cholesterol concentration in some patients with familial hypercholesterolaemia. It has been suggested that this effect is due to decreased synthesis and secretion of hepatic VLDL, leading to decreased production of LDL. However, there is no experimental evidence to support this supposition. Observations on the effects of a portacaval anastomosis in rats and sub-human primates have not been very informative, the effects of the operation on plasma lipoprotein concentration being small and variable. It seems likely that total diversion of portal blood from the liver decreases both LDL production, by diminishing VLDL output, and LDL degradation, the net effect on plasma LDL concentration in different species depending upon the balance between these two effects. It is also possible that the abnormal hepatic secretion of LDL that occurs in the severer form of familial hypercholesterolaemia (see Chapter 15) makes patients with this disease unusually susceptible to the hypocholesterolaemic action of portacaval anastomosis.

REFERENCES

Abell, L. L., Mosbach, E. H. and Kendall, F. E. (1956). Cholesterol metabolism in the dog. *Journal of Biological Chemistry*, **220**, 527–536.
Avigan, J. and Steinberg, D. (1965). Sterol and bile acid excretion in man and the effects of dietary fat. *Journal of Clinical Investigation*, **44**, 1845–1856.
Avigan, J., Steinberg, D. and Berman, M. (1962). Distribution of labeled cholesterol in animal tissues. *Journal of Lipid Research*, **3**, 216–221.
Bhattacharyya, A. K., Connor, W. E. and Spector, A. A. (1970). Excretion of sterols from the skin of man: implications for sterol balance studies. *Clinical Research*, **18**, 621.
Biggs, M. W., Friedman, M. and Byers, S. O. (1951). Intestinal lymphatic transport of absorbed cholesterol. *Proceedings of the Society for Experimental Biology and Medicine*, **78**, 641–643.
Borgström, B. (1960). Studies on intestinal cholesterol absorption in the human. *Journal of Clinical Investigation*, **39**, 809–815.
Borgström, B. (1967). Absorption of fats. *Proceedings of the Nutrition Society*, **26**, 34–46.
Borgström, B. (1968). Quantitative aspects of the intestinal absorption and metabolism of cholesterol and β-sitosterol in the rat. *Journal of Lipid Research*, **9**, 473–481.
Borgström, B. (1969). Quantification of cholesterol absorption in man by fecal analysis after feeding of a single isotope-labeled meal. *Journal of Lipid Research*, **10**, 331–337.
Borgström, B., Radner, S. and Werner, B. (1970). Lymphatic transport of cholesterol in the human being. Effect of dietary cholesterol. *Scandinavian Journal of Clinical and Laboratory Investigation*, **26**, 227–235.
Buchwald, H. (1964). Lowering of cholesterol absorption and blood levels by ileal exclusion. Experimental basis and preliminary clinical report. *Circulation*, **29**, 713–720.
Buchwald, H., Moore, R. B. and Varco, R. L. (1974). Surgical treatment of hyperlipidemia. *Circulation*, **49**, Supplement I, I-1–I-37.
Carlson, L. A., Orö, L. and Ostman, J. (1968). Effect of nicotinic acid on plasma lipids in patients with hyperlipoproteinemia during the first week of treatment. *Journal of Atherosclerosis*, **8**, 667–677.
Carroll, K. K. and Hamilton, R. M. G. (1975). Effects of dietary protein and carbohydrate on plasma cholesterol levels in relation to atherosclerosis. *Journal of Food Science*, **40**, 18–23.
Carter, G. A., Connor, W. E. and Bhattacharyya, A. K. (1975). Cholesterol turnover and balance studies in normal, heterozygous and homozygous type II children. *Circulation*, **51** and **52**, *Supplement II*, II-270.

Chapman, D. D. and Chaikoff, I. L. (1959). The manner of absorption of 3-β-cholestanol and Δ⁴-cholestenone by the rat. *Journal of Biological Chemistry*, **234**, 273–275.
Chevallier, F. (1967). Dynamics of cholesterol in rats, studied by the isotopic equilibrium method. *Advances in Lipid Research*, **5**, 209–239.
Chobanian, A. V., Burrows, B. A. and Hollander, W. (1962). Body cholesterol metabolism in man. II. Measurement of the body cholesterol miscible pool and turnover rate. *Journal of Clinical Investigation*, **41**, 1738–1744.
Chobanian, A. V. and Hollander, W. (1962). Body cholesterol metabolism in man. I. The equilibration of serum and tissue cholesterol. *Journal of Clinical Investigation*, **41**, 1732–1737.
Clifton-Bligh, P., Miller, N. E. and Nestel, P. J. (1974). Increased plasma cholesterol esterifying activity during colestipol resin therapy in man. *Metabolism*, **23**, 437.
Connor, W. E., Hodges, R. E. and Bleiler, R. E. (1961). The serum lipids in men receiving high cholesterol and cholesterol-free diets. *Journal of Clinical Investigation*, **40**, 894–901.
Connor, W. E. and Lin, D. S. (1974). The intestinal absorption of dietary cholesterol by hypercholesterolemic (type II) and normocholesterolemic humans. *Journal of Clinical Investigation*, **53**, 1062–1070.
Connor, W. E., Witiak, D. T., Stone, D. B. and Armstrong, M. L. (1969). Cholesterol balance and fecal neutral steroid and bile acid excretion in normal men fed dietary fats of different fatty acid composition. *Journal of Clinical Investigation*, **48**, 1363–1375.
Cook, R. P. *Cholesterol. Chemistry, Biochemistry and Pathology*. Ed. R. P. Cook. Academic Press, New York, 1958.
Cummings, J. H. (1973). Dietary fibre. *Gut*, **14**, 69–81.
Davidson, S., Passmore, R., Truswell, A. S. and Brock, J. F. *Human Nutrition and Dietics*, 7th edn. Churchill-Livingstone, Edinburgh, 1979.
Davignon, J., Simmonds, W. J. and Ahrens, E. H. Jr. (1968). Usefulness of chromic oxide as an internal standard for balance studies in formula-fed patients and for assessment of colonic function. *Journal of Clinical Investigation*, **47**, 127–138.
Dietschy, J. M. General principles governing movement of lipids across biological membranes. In: *Disturbances in Lipid and Lipoprotein Metabolism*. Ed. J. M. Dietschy, A. M. Gotto Jr. and Ontko, J. A. American Physiological Society, Bethesda, Maryland, pp. 1–28, 1978.
Dietschy, J. M. and Wilson, J. D. (1970). Regulation of cholesterol metabolism. *New England Journal of Medicine*, **282**, 1128–1138, 1179–1183, 1241–1249.
Eastwood, M. A. (1973). Vegetable fibre: its physical properties. *Proceedings of the Nutrition Society*, **32**, 137–143.
Eastwood, M. A. (1975). The role of vegetable dietary fibre in human nutrition. *Medical Hypotheses*, **1**, 46–53.
Eggen, D. A. (1974). Cholesterol metabolism in rhesus monkey, squirrel monkey, and baboon. *Journal of Lipid Research*, **15**, 139–145.
Einarsson, K. and Hellström, K. (1972). The formation of bile acids in patients with three types of hyperlipoproteinaemia. *Journal of Clinical Investigation*, **2**, 225–230.
Einarsson, K., Hellström, K. and Kallner, M. (1974). Bile acid kinetics in relation to sex, serum lipids, body weights, and gallbladder disease in patients with various types of hyperlipoproteinemia. *Journal of Clinical Investigation*, **54**, 1301–1311.
Field, H., Swell, L., Schools, P. E. and Treadwell, C. R. (1960). Dynamic aspects of cholesterol metabolism in different areas of the aorta and other tissues in man and their relationship to atherosclerosis. *Circulation*, **22**, 547–558.
Gamble, W. and Wright, L. D. (1961). Effect of nicotinic acid and related compounds on incorporation of mevalonic acid into cholesterol. *Proceedings of the Society for Experimental Biology and Medicine*, **107**, 160–162.

Glomset, J. A. and Norum, K. R. (1973). The metabolic role of lecithin:cholesterol acyltransferase: perspectives from pathology. *Advances in Lipid Research*, **11**, 1–65.

Goodman, D. S. and Noble, R. P. (1968). Turnover of plasma cholesterol in man. *Journal of Clinical Investigation*, **47**, 231–241.

Goodman, D. S., Noble, R. P. and Dell, R. B. (1973). Three-pool model of the long-term turnover of plasma cholesterol in man. *Journal of Lipid Research*, **14**, 178–188.

Gould, R. G., LeRoy, G. V., Okita, G. T., Kabara, J. J., Keegan, P. and Bergenstal, D. M. (1955). The use of C^{14}-labeled acetate to study cholesterol metabolism in man. *Journal of Laboratory and Clinical Medicine*, **46**, 372–384.

Gould, R. G., Lotz, L. V. and Lilly, E. M. Absorption and metabolism of dihydrocholesterol and beta-sitosterol. In: *Biochemical Problems of Lipids*. Ed. G. Popják and E. Le Breton. Butterworths, London, pp. 353–358, 1956.

Grande, F., Anderson, J. T. and Keys, A. (1974). Sucrose and various carbohydrate-containing foods and serum lipids in man. *American Journal of Clinical Nutrition*, **27**, 1043–1051.

Grant, W. C. and Fahrenbach, M. J. (1959). Effect of dietary sucrose and glucose on plasma cholesterol in chicks and rabbits. *Proceedings of the Society for Experimental Biology and Medicine*, **100**, 250–252.

Grundy, S. M. (1975). Effects of polyunsaturated fats on lipid metabolism in patients with hypertriglyceridemia. *Journal of Clinical Investigation*, **55**, 269–282.

Grundy, S. M. and Ahrens, E. H. Jr. (1969). Measurements of cholesterol turnover, synthesis, and absorption in man, carried out by isotope kinetic and sterol balance methods. *Journal of Lipid Research*, **10**, 91–107.

Grundy, S. M. and Ahrens, E. H. Jr. (1970). The effects of unsaturated dietary fats on absorption, excretion, synthesis, and distribution of cholesterol in man. *Journal of Clinical Investigation*, **49**, 1135–1152.

Grundy, S. M., Ahrens, E. H. Jr. and Davignon, J. (1969). The interaction of cholesterol absorption and cholesterol synthesis in man. *Journal of Lipid Research*, **10**, 304–315.

Grundy, S. M., Ahrens, E. H. Jr. & Salen, G. (1968). Dietary β-sitosterol as an internal standard to correct for cholesterol losses in sterol balance studies. *Journal of Lipid Research*, **9**, 374–387.

Grundy, S. M., Ahrens, E. H. Jr. and Salen, G. (1971). Interruption of the enterohepatic circulation of bile acids in man: comparative effects of cholestyramine and ileal exclusion on cholesterol metabolism. *Journal of Laboratory and Clinical Medicine*, **78**, 94–121.

Grundy, S. M. and Metzger, A. L. (1972). A physiological method for estimation of hepatic secretion of biliary lipids in man. *Gastroenterology*, **62**, 1200–1217.

Grundy, S. M. and Mok, H. Y. I. (1977). Determination of cholesterol absorption in man by intestinal perfusion. *Journal of Lipid Research*, **18**, 263–271.

Gurpide, E., Mann, J. and Sandberg, E. (1964). Determination of kinetic parameters in a two-pool system by administration of one or more tracers. *Biochemistry*, **3**, 1250–1255.

Gustafsson, B. E. and Norman, A. (1969). Influence of the diet on the turnover of bile acids in germ-free and conventional rats. *British Journal of Nutrition*, **23**, 429–442.

Havel, R. J. and Kane, J. P. (1973). Drugs and lipid metabolism. *Annual Review of Pharmacology*, **13**, 287–308.

Hellman, L., Frazell, E. L. and Rosenfeld, R. S. (1960). Direct measurement of cholesterol absorption via the thoracic duct in man. *Journal of Clinical Investigation*, **39**, 1288–1294.

Hellström, K. (1965). On the bile acid and neutral fecal steroid excretion in man and rabbits following cholesterol feeding. Bile acids and steroids. 150. *Acta Physiologica Scandinavica*, **63**, 21–35.

Hernandez, H. H., Chaikoff, I. L., Dauben, W. G. and Abraham, S. (1954). The absorption of C^{14}-labeled epicholesterol in the rat. *Journal of Biological Chemistry*, **206**, 757–765.
Ho, K. J., Biss, K., Mikkelson, B., Lewis, L. A. and Taylor, C. B. (1971). The Masai of East Africa: some unique biological characteristics. *Archives of Pathology*, **91**, 387–410.
Hofmann, A. F. and Small, D. M. (1967). Detergent properties of bile salts: correlation with physiological function. *Annual Review of Medicine*, **18**, 333–376.
Hyun, S. A., Vahouny, G. V. and Treadwell, C. R. (1963). Effect of hypocholesterolemic agents on intestinal cholesterol absorption. *Proceedings of the Society for Experimental Biology and Medicine*, **112**, 496–501.
Jones, R. J. and Dobrilovic, L. (1970). Lipoprotein lipid alterations with cholestyramine administration. *Journal of Laboratory and Clinical Medicine*, **75**, 953–966.
Kaplan, J. A., Cox, G. E. and Taylor, C. B. (1963). Cholesterol metabolism in man. Studies on absorption. *Archives of Pathology*, **76**, 359–368.
Kay, R. M., Judd, P. A. and Truswell, A. S. (1978). The effect of pectin on serum cholesterol. *American Journal of Clinical Nutrition*, **31**, 562–563.
Keys, A. (1975). Coronary heart disease—the global picture. *Atherosclerosis*, **22**, 149–192.
Keys, A., Anderson, J. T. and Grande, F. (1965a). Serum cholesterol response to changes in the diet. II. The effect of cholesterol in the diet, *Metabolism*, **14**, 759.
Keys, A., Anderson, J. T. and Grande, F. (1965b). Serum cholesterol response to changes in the diet. I. Iodine value of dietary fat versus 2S-P. *Metabolism*, **14**, 747–758.
Kinsell, L. W., Partridge, J., Boling, L., Margen, S. and Michaels, G. (1952). Dietary modification of serum cholesterol and phospholipid levels. *Journal of Clinical Endocrinology*, **12**, 909–913.
Kottke, B. A. (1969). Differences in bile acid excretion. Primary hypercholesterolemia compared to combined hypercholesterolemia and hypertriglyceridemia. *Circulation*, **40**, 13–20.
Kritchevsky, D. Effect of nicotinic acid and its derivatives on cholesterol metabolism: A review. In: *Metabolic Effects of Nicotinic Acid and Its Derivatives*. Ed. K. F. Gey and L. A. Carlson. Hans Huber Publishers, Bern, pp. 541–566, 1971.
Kritchevsky, D. (1976). Diet and atherosclerosis. *American Journal of Pathology*, **84**, 615–632.
Kritchevsky, D., Tepper, S. A. and Story, J. A. (1975). Nonnutritive fiber and lipid metabolism. *Journal of Food Science*, **40**, 8–11.
Kuksis, A. and Huang, T. C. (1962). Differential absorption of plant sterols in the dog. *Canadian Journal of Biochemistry*, **40**, 1493–1504.
Lang, C. M. and Barthel, C. H. (1972). Effects of simple and complex carbohydrates on serum lipids and atherosclerosis in nonhuman primates. *American Journal of Clinical Nutrition*, **25**, 470–475.
Langer, T. and Levy, R. I. The effect of nicotinic acid on the turnover of low density lipoproteins in Type II hyperlipoproteinemia. In: *Metabolic Effects of Nicotinic Acid and Its Derivatives*. Ed. K. F. Gey and L. A. Carlson. Hans Huber Publishers, Bern, pp. 641–647, 1971.
Langer, T., Levy, R. I. and Fredrickson, D. S. (1969). Dietary and pharmacologic perturbation of beta lipoprotein (BLP) turnover. *Circulation*, **40**, *Suppl. III*, III-14.
Lewis, B. and Myant, N. B. (1967). Studies in the metabolism of cholesterol in subjects with normal plasma cholesterol levels and in patients with essential hypercholesterolaemia. *Clinical Science*, **32**, 201–213.
Lindstedt, S., Avigan, J., Goodman, De W. S., Sjovall, J. and Steinberg, D. (1965). The effect of dietary fat on the turnover of cholic acid and on the composition of the biliary bile acids in man. *Journal of Clinical Investigation*, **44**, 1754–1765.

Liu, G. C. K., Ahrens, E. H. Jr., Schreibman, P. H., Samuel, P., McNamara, D. J. and Crouse, J. P. (1975). Measurement of cholesterol synthesis in man by isotope kinetics of squalene. *Proceedings of the National Academy of Sciences of the USA*, **72**, 4612–4616.

Lofland, H. B. Jr., Clarkson, T. B. and Bullock, B. C. (1970). Whole body sterol metabolism in squirrel monkeys (*Saimiri sciureus*). *Experimental and Molecular Pathology*, **13**, 1–11.

Lofland, H. B., Clarkson, T. B. and Goodman, H. O. (1961). Interactions among dietary fat, protein, and cholesterol in atherosclerosis-susceptible pigeons. Effects on serum cholesterol and aortic atherosclerosis. *Circulation Research*, **9**, 919–924.

Lofland, H. B. Jr., Clarkson, T. B., St. Clair, R. W. and Lehner, N. D. M. (1972). Studies on the regulation of plasma cholesterol levels in squirrel monkeys of two genotypes. *Journal of Lipid Research*, **13**, 39–47.

Lofland, H. B. Jr., Clarkson, T. B., St. Clair, R. W., Lehner, N. D. M. and Bullock, B. C. (1968). Atherosclerosis in *Cebus albifrons* monkeys. 1. Sterol metabolism. *Experimental and Molecular Pathology*, **8**, 302–313.

Magide, A. A. and Myant, N. B. (1974). Effect of nicotinic acid on cholesterol metabolism in monkeys. *Clinical Science and Molecular Medicine*, **46**, 527–538.

Magide, A. A. and Myant, N. B. (1975). Loss of cholesterol from muscle and skin of monkeys treated with nicotinic acid. *Atherosclerosis*, **21**, 273–281.

Magide, A. A., Myant, N. B. and Reichl, D. (1975). The effect of nicotinic acid on the metabolism of the plasma lipoproteins of Rhesus monkeys. *Atherosclerosis*, **21**, 205–215.

Martin, G. M. and Nestel, P. (1979). Changes in cholesterol metabolism with dietary cholesterol in children with familial hypercholesterolaemia. *Clinical Science*, **56**, 377–380.

Mathur, K. S., Khan, M. A. and Sharma, R. D. (1968). Hypocholesterolaemic effect of Bengal gram: a long-term study in man. *British Medical Journal*, **1**, 30–31.

Mattson, F. H., Erickson, B. A. and Kligman, A. M. (1972). Effect of dietary cholesterol on serum cholesterol in man. *American Journal of Clinical Nutrition*, **25**, 589–594.

McGill, H. C. (1979). The relationship of dietary cholesterol to serum cholesterol concentration and to atherosclerosis in man. *American Journal of Clinical Nutrition*, **32**, 2664–2702.

Middleton, C. C., Clarkson, T. B., Lofland, H. B. and Prichard, R. W. (1967). Diet and atherosclerosis of squirrel monkeys. *Archives of Pathology*, **83**, 145–153.

Miettinen, T. A. (1968). Mechanism of serum cholesterol reduction by thyroid hormones in hypothyroidism. *Journal of Laboratory and Clinical Medicine*, **71**, 537–547.

Miettinen, T. A. (1969). Serum squalene and methyl sterols as indicators of cholesterol synthesis *in vivo*. *Life Sciences*, **8**, 713–721.

Miettinen, T. A. (1970). Detection of changes in human cholesterol metabolism. *Annals of Clinical Research*, **2**, 300–320.

Miettinen, T. A. (1971). Cholesterol production in obesity. *Circulation*, **44**, 842–850.

Miettinen, T. A., Pelkonen, R., Nikkilä, E. A. and Heinonen, O. (1967). Low excretion of fecal bile acids in a family with hypercholesterolemia. *Acta Medica Scandinavica*, **182**, 645–650.

Mok, H. Y. I., von Bergmann, K. and Grundy, S. M. (1979). Effects of continuous and intermittent feeding on biliary lipid outputs in man: application for measurements of intestinal absorption of cholesterol and bile acids. *Journal of Lipid Research*, **20**, 389–398.

Moore, R. B., Anderson, J. T., Taylor, H. L., Keys, A. and Frantz, I. D. Jr. (1968). Effect of dietary fat on the fecal excretion of cholesterol and its degradation products in man. *Journal of Clinical Investigation*, **47**, 1517–1534.

Moore, R. B., Frantz, I. D. Jr. and Buchwald, H. (1969). Changes in cholesterol pool size, turnover rate, and fecal bile acid and sterol excretion after partial ileal bypass in hypercholesteremic patients. *Surgery*, **65**, 98–108.
Morris, M. D. and Chaikoff, I. L. (1959). The origin of cholesterol in liver, small intestine, adrenal gland and testis of the rat: dietary *versus* endogenous contributions. *Journal of Biological Chemistry*, **234**, 1095–1097.
Moutafis, C. D. and Myant, N. B. (1969). The metabolism of cholesterol in two hypercholesterolaemic patients treated with cholestyramine. *Clinical Science*, **37**, 443–454.
Moutafis, C. D. and Myant, N. B. (1976). The distribution of [^{14}C]cholesterol in muscle and skin of Rhesus monkeys after intravenous injection. *Clinical Science and Molecular Medicine*, **50**, 307–310.
Moutafis, C. D., Myant, N. B., Mancini, M. and Oriente, P. (1971). Cholestyramine and nicotinic acid in the treatment of familial hyperbetalipoproteinaemia in the homozygous form. *Atherosclerosis*, **14**, 247–258.
Moutafis, C. D., Myant, N. B. and Tabaqchali, S. (1968). The metabolism of cholesterol after resection or by-pass of the lower small intestine. *Clinical Science*, **35**, 537–545.
Myant, N. B. Effects of drugs on the metabolism of bile acids. In: *Pharmacological Control of Lipid Metabolism*. Ed. W. L. Holmes, R. Paoletti and D. Kritchevsky. Plenum Press, New York, pp. 137–154, 1972.
Myant, N. B. (1975). The influence of some dietary factors on cholesterol metabolism. *Proceedings of the Nutrition Society*, **34**, 271–278.
Myant, N. B. (1981). In: Acido Nicotinico e Derivati nella Prevenzione dell'Arteriosclerosi. *Farmaci*, Supplement.
Myant, N. B. and Mitropoulos, K. A. (1977). Cholesterol 7α-hydroxylase. *Journal of Lipid Research*, **18**, 135–153.
Nestel, P. J. and Kudchodkar, B. (1975). Plasma squalene as an index of cholesterol synthesis. *Clinical Science and Molecular Medicine*, **49**, 621–624.
Nestel, P. J. and Poyser, A. (1976). Changes in cholesterol synthesis and excretion when cholesterol intake is increased. *Metabolism*, **25**, 1591–1599.
Nestel, P. J., Schreibman, P. H. and Ahrens, E. H. Jr. (1973). Cholesterol metabolism in human obesity. *Journal of Clinical Investigation*, **52**, 2389–2397.
Nestel, P. J., Whyte, H. M. and Goodman, D. S. (1969). Distribution and turnover of cholesterol in humans. *Journal of Clinical Investigation*, **48**, 982–991.
Nikkari, T., Schreibman, P. H. and Ahrens, E. H. Jr. (1974). *In vivo* studies of sterol and squalene secretion by human skin. *Journal of Lipid Research*, **15**, 563–573.
Nilsson, Å. and Zilversmit, D. B. (1972). Fate of intravenously administered particulate and lipoprotein cholesterol in the rat. *Journal of Lipid Research*, **13**, 32–38.
Norum, K. R., Lilljeqvist, A. C. and Drevon, C. A. (1977). Coenzyme-A-dependent esterification of cholesterol in intestinal mucosa from guinea-pig. Influence of diet on the enzyme activity. *Scandinavian Journal of Gastroenterology*, **12**, 281–288.
Pertsemlidis, D., Kirchman, E. H. and Ahrens, E. H. Jr. (1973). Regulation of cholesterol metabolism in the dog. I. Effects of complete bile diversion and of cholesterol feeding on absorption, synthesis, accumulation, and excretion rates measured during life. *Journal of Clinical Investigation*, **52**, 2353–2367.
Porte, D. and Havel, R. J. (1961). The use of cholesterol-4-C^{14} labeled lipoproteins as a tracer for plasma cholesterol in the dog. *Journal of Lipid Research*, **2**, 357–362.
Portman, O. W. (1960). Nutritional influences on the metabolism of bile acids. *American Journal of Clinical Nutrition*, **8**, 462–470.
Potter, J. M. and Nestel, P. J. (1976). Greater bile acid excretion with soy bean than with cow milk in infants. *American Journal of Clinical Nutrition*, **29**, 546–551.
Quintão, E., Grundy, S. M. and Ahrens, E. H. Jr. (1971a). An evaluation of four methods for measuring cholesterol absorption by the intestine of man. *Journal of Lipid Research*, **12**, 221–232.

Quintão, E., Grundy, S. M. and Ahrens, E. H. Jr. (1971b). Effects of dietary cholesterol on the regulation of total body cholesterol in man. *Journal of Lipid Research*, 12, 233–247.
Raymond, T. L., Connor, W. E., Lin, D. S., Warner, S., Fry, M. M. and Connor, S. L. (1977). The interaction of dietary fibers and cholesterol upon the plasma lipids and lipoproteins, sterol balance, and bowel functions in human subjects. *Journal of Clinical Investigation*, 60, 1429–1437.
Rudel, L. L., Morris, M. D. and Felts, J. M. (1972). The transport of exogenous cholesterol in the rabbit. I. Role of cholesterol ester of lymph chylomicra and lymph very low density lipoproteins in absorption. *Journal of Clinical Investigation*, 51, 2686–2692.
Salen, G., Ahrens, E. H. Jr. and Grundy, S. M. (1970). Metabolism of β-sitosterol in man. *Journal of Clinical Investigation*, 49, 952–967.
Samuel, P., Crouse, J. R. and Ahrens, E. H. Jr. (1978). Evaluation of an isotope ratio method for measurement of cholesterol absorption in man. *Journal of Lipid Research*, 19, 82–93.
Samuel, P., Holtzman, C. M., Meilman, E. and Perl, W. (1968). Effect of neomycin on exchangeable pools of cholesterol in the steady state. *Journal of Clinical Investigation*, 47, 1807–1818.
Samuel, P. and Lieberman, S. (1973). Improved estimation of body masses and turnover of cholesterol by computerized input-output analysis. *Journal of Lipid Research*, 14, 189–196.
Samuel, P., Lieberman, S. and Ahrens, E. H. Jr. (1978). Comparison of cholesterol turnover by sterol balance and input-output analysis, and a shortened way to estimate total exchangeable mass of cholesterol by the combination of the two methods. *Journal of Lipid Research*, 19, 94–102.
Schachter, D., Finkelstein, J. D. and Kowarski, S. (1964). Metabolism of vitamin D. I. Preparation of radioactive vitamin D and its intestinal absorption in the rat. *Journal of Clinical Investigation*, 43, 787–796.
Schreibman, P. H. and Dell, R. B. (1975). Human adipocyte cholesterol. Concentration, localization, synthesis, and turnover. *Journal of Clinical Investigation*, 55, 986–993.
Simmonds, W. J., Hofmann, A. F. and Theodor, E. (1967). Absorption of cholesterol from a micellar solution: intestinal perfusion studies in man. *Journal of Clinical Investigation*, 46, 874–890.
Simons, L. A. and Myant, N. B. (1974). The effect of D-thyroxine on the metabolism of cholesterol in familial hyperbetalipoproteinaemia. *Atherosclerosis*, 19, 103–117.
Sodhi, H. S. and Kudchodkar, B. J. (1973). Correlating metabolism of plasma and tissue cholesterol with that of plasma-lipoproteins. *Lancet*, 1, 513–519.
Soutar, A. K. and Myant, N. B. Plasma lipoproteins. In: *Chemistry of Macromolecules IIB. Macromolecular Complexes*. International Review of Biochemistry, Vol. 25. Ed. R. E. Offord. University Park Press, Baltimore, pp. 55–119, 1979.
Spritz, N. and Mishkel, M. A. (1969). Effects of dietary fats on plasma lipids and lipoproteins: an hypothesis for the lipid-lowering effect of unsaturated fatty acids. *Journal of Clinical Investigation*, 48, 78–86.
Stanley, M. M. and Cheng, S. H. (1956). Cholesterol exchange in the gastrointestinal tract in normal and abnormal subjects. *Gastroenterology*, 30, 62–74.
Swell, L., Trout, E. C. Jr., Hopper, J. R., Field, H. Jr. and Treadwell, C. R. (1958a). Mechanism of cholesterol absorption. 1. Endogenous dilution and esterification of fed cholesterol-4-C^{14}. *Journal of Biological Chemistry*, 232, 1–8.
Swell, L., Trout, E. C., Hopper, J. R., Field, H. and Treadwell, C. R. (1958b). Mechanism of cholesterol absorption. II. Changes in free and esterified cholesterol pools of mucosa after feeding cholesterol-4-C^{14}. *Journal of Biological Chemistry*, 233, 49–53.
Swell, L., Trout, E. C., Field, H. and Treadwell, C. R. (1959). Absorption of H^3-β-

sitosterol in the lymph fistula rat. *Proceedings of the Society for Experimental Biology and Medicine*, **100**, 140–142.

Sylvén, C. and Borgström, B. (1968). Absorption and lymphatic transport of cholesterol in the rat. *Journal of Lipid Research*, **9**, 596–601.

Thompson, G. R., Ockner, R. K. and Isselbacher, K. J. (1969). Effect of mixed micellar lipid on the absorption of cholesterol and vitamin D_3 into lymph. *Journal of Clinical Investigation*, **48**, 87–95.

Treadwell, C. R. and Vahouny, G. V. Cholesterol absorption. In: *Handbook of Physiology*, Sec. 6, Vol. 3. Ed. C. F. Code. American Physiology Society, Washington, pp. 1407–1438, 1968.

Vergroesen, A. J. and Gottenbos, J. J. The role of fats in human nutrition: an introduction. In: *The Role of Fats in Human Nutrition*. Ed. A. J. Vergroesen. Academic Press, London, pp. 1–41, 1975.

Werbin, H. and Chaikoff, I. L. (1961). Utilization of adrenal gland cholesterol for synthesis of cortisol by the intact normal and the ACTH-treated guinea pig. *Archives of Biochemistry and Biophysics*, **93**, 476–482.

Whyte, M., Nestel, P. and MacGregor, A. (1977). Cholesterol metabolism in Papua New Guineans. *European Journal of Clinical Investigation*, **7**, 53–60.

Wilson, J. D. (1964). The quantification of cholesterol excretion and degradation in the isotopic steady state in the rat: the influence of dietary cholesterol. *Journal of Lipid Research*, **5**, 409–417.

Wilson, J. D. (1970). The measurement of exchangeable pools of cholesterol in the baboon. *Journal of Clinical Investigation*, **49**, 655–665.

Wilson, J. D. (1972). The relation between cholesterol absorption and cholesterol synthesis in the baboon. *Journal of Clinical Investigation*, **51**, 1450–1458.

Wilson, J. D. and Lindsey, C. A. Jr. (1965). Studies on the influence of dietary cholesterol on cholesterol metabolism in the isotopic steady state in man. *Journal of Clinical Investigation*, **44**, 1805–1814.

Wilson, J. D. and Reinke, R. T. (1968). Transfer of locally synthesized cholesterol from intestinal wall to intestinal lymph. *Journal of Lipid Research*, **9**, 85–92.

Wood, P. O. S., Shioda, R. and Kinsell, L. W. (1966). Dietary regulation of cholesterol metabolism. *Lancet*, **2**, 604–607.

Zilversmit, D. B. (1972). A single blood sample dual isotope method for the measurement of cholesterol absorption in rats. *Proceedings of the Society for Experimental Biology and Medicine*, **140**, 862–865.

Zilversmit, D. B. and Hughes, L. B. (1974). Validation of a dual-isotope plasma ratio method for measurement of cholesterol absorption in rats. *Journal of Lipid Research*, **15**, 465–473.

Chapter 11

The Plasma Cholesterol: Composition and Metabolism

1	INTRODUCTION	507
2	CONCENTRATION AND COMPOSITION	507
3	THE PLASMA LIPOPROTEINS	510
3.1	Classification and composition of normal lipoproteins.	510
3.2	Abnormal lipoproteins of human plasma	513
3.2.1	LP-X	514
3.2.2	β-VLDL	514
3.3	The lipoproteins of animal plasma	514
3.4	The structure of normal plasma lipoproteins	515
3.4.1	General features	515
3.4.2	HDL	517
3.4.3	LDL	517
3.4.4	Triglyceride-rich lipoproteins	520
3.5	Biogenesis and metabolic transformations	521
3.5.1	The origin of HDL	521
3.5.2	The origin of VLDL and chylomicrons	523
3.5.3	Metabolic transformations of lipoproteins within the plasma	524
3.6	The metabolism of LDL	528
3.6.1	Methods for measuring LDL turnover *in vivo*	528
3.6.2	LDL turnover in man	530
3.6.3	The site of catabolism of LDL	534
3.7	The metabolism of HDL	535
4	THE ORIGIN AND TURNOVER OF THE PLASMA ESTERIFIED CHOLESTEROL	538
4.1	Origin	538
4.1.1	Man	538
4.1.2	Rats	540
4.2	Turnover	540
4.2.1	Methods of measurement	541
4.2.2	The rate of turnover *in vivo* and *in vitro*	543

506 The Biology of Cholesterol and Related Steroids

5	EXCHANGE OF LIPOPROTEIN CHOLESTEROL	547
5.1	Exchange of unesterified cholesterol	547
5.2	Exchange with mass transfer	550
5.3	The mechanism of exchange of free cholesterol	552
5.4	Exchange of esterified cholesterol	554
6	LIPOPROTEIN CHOLESTEROL METABOLISM: QUANTITATIVE ASPECTS	555
6.1	Turnover in plasma in relation to whole-body turnover	555
6.2	The pathways from plasma to liver	558

The Plasma Cholesterol: Composition and Metabolism

1 INTRODUCTION

Although all the free and esterified cholesterol in plasma forms part of the exchangeable mass discussed in the previous chapter, certain aspects of the physiology and biochemistry of cholesterol must be considered specifically in relation to the plasma. This is so because the pathways through which endogenous cholesterol is transported between the extravascular tissues, and through which dietary cholesterol is carried to the liver from the intestine, intersect within the plasma. While cholesterol is in transit through the vascular system it is carried in lipoproteins, the lipoproteins acting as vehicles for the passage of cholesterol through the aqueous medium of the plasma and the unesterified cholesterol acting as an essential stabilizing component of the lipoprotein particles. Furthermore, cholesterol undergoes a complex series of interchanges from one lipoprotein fraction to another, including the esterification of free cholesterol by the LCAT reaction and the redistribution of the cholesteryl esters so formed. In order to understand these aspects of cholesterol metabolism it will be necessary to consider the nature and origin of the plasma lipoproteins, their interconversions within the plasma and their extravascular metabolism.

These topics are considered in the present chapter, together with an introductory summary of the concentration and composition of the plasma cholesterol in man and other mammalian species. Chapters 12 to 16 deal with other aspects of the plasma cholesterol.

2 CONCENTRATION AND COMPOSITION

In most communities in Westernized countries the mean plasma cholesterol concentration lies between 200 and 250 mg/100 ml in healthy adults, but in many under-developed or agricultural populations the mean concentration in adults is well below 200 mg/100 ml (see Chapter 12 for details). In most animal species, the plasma cholesterol concentration is much lower than in man. For example, in animals eating a standard diet, the concentration of total cholesterol is about 50 mg/100 ml in rats and rabbits and between 100 and 150 mg/100 ml in non-human primates. There are also marked species differences in the proportions of the total plasma cholesterol carried in the different lipoprotein fractions. In the plasma of adult human subjects in the fasting state, at least 60% of the total cholesterol is carried in LDL, whereas in many animal species the amount carried in HDL may equal or exceed that carried in LDL (see Table 11.1 for representative values for man, rhesus monkeys and rats, and see the reviews by Mills (1976) and Calvert (1976) for comparative aspects of the plasma lipoprotein cholesterol). During the absorption of a fatty meal the lipoprotein distribution of cholesterol may change, owing to the entry, into the plasma, of triglyceride-rich lipoproteins of density <1.006 g/ml, carrying cholesterol absorbed from the food or synthesized in the intestinal wall. Other effects of diet on the plasma cholesterol are considered below.

In all mammalian species in which the plasma cholesterol has been investigated, about two thirds of the total cholesterol in plasma is esterified with long-chain fatty acids, the remaining third being free, or unesterified. In man the ratio of esterified to total cholesterol in the lipoproteins of 'fasting' plasma is highest in HDL, lowest in VLDL and intermediate in LDL (Table 11.1).

Table 11.1
The cholesterol concentration (mg/100 ml) in whole plasma and plasma lipoprotein fractions of fasting adult human subjects, rhesus monkeys and rats

Plasma or lipoprotein	Man Total cholesterol[a]	Esterified cholesterol[b] (% total)	Monkey Total cholesterol[c]	Rat Total cholesterol[d]
Whole plasma	194	64–72	151	47
VLDL	17	60	10	5
LDL	126	71	81	12
HDL	51	79	60	30

[a] From Fredrickson and Levy (1972), values for human subjects aged 30–39.
[b] Modified from Goodman and Shiratori (1964).
[c] From Magide et al. (1975).
[d] Modified from Gidez et al. (1965).

VLDL, very-low-density lipoprotein (density <1.006 g/ml); LDL, low-density lipoprotein (density 1.006–1.063 or 1.019–1.063 g/ml); HDL, high-density lipoprotein (density 1.063–1.210 g/ml).

The fatty-acid composition of the cholesteryl esters in whole plasma and in individual lipoprotein fractions has aroused much interest in view of the light that it may throw on the origin of the plasma esterified cholesterol. In man and other mammalian species (see Goodman, 1965, for a general review) the cholesteryl esters of plasma obtained in the fasting state contain a high proportion of fatty acids with two or more double bonds. There are, however, species differences in the fatty-acid pattern. For example, under normal dietary conditions the predominant fatty acid of the plasma cholesteryl esters in man is linoleate (18:2) and in rats is arachidonate (20:4) (Table 11.2). In both species, this pattern differs markedly from the fatty-acid pattern of the esterified cholesterol in the liver, in which oleate (18:1) predominates. In fasting man, the fatty-acid pattern is very similar in the cholesteryl esters of all three major lipoprotein fractions, but in rats the cholesteryl esters of VLDL resemble those of the liver in having oleate as their predominant fatty acid (Table 11.2). The effects of dietary fat on the composition of human plasma cholesteryl esters depend upon the duration of the fat-feeding. After a single fatty meal, the composition of the VLDL cholesteryl esters changes towards that of the fed fat, but there is little change in the fatty acids of the cholesteryl esters of LDL or HDL (Kayden et al., 1963). This is what one would expect, since the absorption of fat is accompanied by the intestinal secretion of triglyceride-rich particles containing cholesteryl esters in which the fatty-acid pattern tends towards that of the fed fat, whereas the cholesteryl esters of HDL and LDL are formed by the

Table 11.2

Fatty acid composition of the major cholesteryl esters of human and rat plasma. Values for human and rat liver are shown for comparison

	Lipoprotein or tissue	16:0	18:1	18:2	20:4
Man	VLDL	12	26	52	6
	LDL	11	22	55	7
	HDL	11	22	55	6
	Liver	24	37	16	3
Rat	VLDL	16	38	25	10
	LDL	12	15	34	34
	HDL	10	5	35	46
	Liver	17	39	25	7

Values for fasting human plasma are from Goodman and Shiratori (1964) and for rat plasma are from Gidez et al. (1965). Abbreviations are the same as in Table 11.1 except that the density of the human VLDL was <1.1019 g/ml. Fatty acid numbers refer to chain length and number of double bonds.

LCAT reaction (Section 4, below). After a prolonged change in the fatty-acid composition of the diet, there are marked changes in the fatty-acid pattern of the LDL cholesteryl esters, accompanied by changes in the fatty acids at the β-position of the phospholipids of LDL (Spritz and Mishkel, 1969).

3 THE PLASMA LIPOPROTEINS

A comprehensive account of the lipoproteins of human and animal plasma, some of which have already been mentioned here, is beyond the scope of this book. Nevertheless, the normal physiology of the plasma cholesterol cannot be understood without reference to the lipoproteins in which all of it is carried. Moreover, we now recognize that an abnormal plasma cholesterol concentration usually reflects an underlying change in the concentration of a specific lipoprotein. This has led to a far more fruitful approach to the classification and investigation of disorders of cholesterol metabolism than was possible a few years ago. It is also becoming clear that the cholesterol carried in different lipoproteins does not have equal significance in relation to atherosclerosis and, hence, that epidemiological and experimental work in this field must now be focused upon the concentration of cholesterol in specific lipoprotein fractions of the plasma. Thus, from the point of view of both the normal and abnormal physiology of the plasma cholesterol, a brief discussion of the composition, structure and metabolism of the plasma lipoproteins is essential. More detailed accounts will be found in the reviews by Jackson *et al.* (1976) and by Soutar and Myant (1979).

3.1 Classification and composition of normal lipoproteins

The plasma lipoproteins are usually defined as lipid-protein complexes of density < 1.21 g/ml present in normal or abnormal plasma. The lipoproteins of normal human plasma are most conveniently classified in terms of their hydrated density, as determined in the preparative ultracentrifuge. Four classes of lipoprotein particle, characterized by their density range, are present in the plasma of normal fasting human subjects. Particles of a fifth class, the *chylomicrons*, appear in the plasma a few hours after a fatty meal and are gradually cleared from the circulation by the mechanism described below. Table 11.3 shows the five classes of normal human plasma lipoprotein, including the two subclasses of HDL (HDL$_2$ and HDL$_3$), together with their electrophoretic mobilities on zonal electrophoresis and their major physical and chemical characteristics. Particle diameters range from less than 100 Å in the HDL class to about 10^4 Å

Table 11.3
The lipoproteins of normal human plasma

Designation	Density (g/ml)	Electrophoretic mobility	Diameter (Å)	Molecular weight	Protein (% dry weight)	Lipid (% dry weight)
Chylomicrons	<0.95	Origin	10^3–10^4	10^9–10^{10}	1.5–2.5	97–99
VLDL	0.95–1.006	pre-β	250–750	5×10^6–10^7	5–10	90–95
IDL	1.006–1.019	β or pre-β	250	4.5×10^6	15–20	80–85
LDL	1.019–1.063	β	200–250	2.0–2.5×10^6	20–25	75–80
HDL₂	1.063–1.120	α_1	70–120	3.9×10^5	40–45	55
HDL						
HDL₃	1.120–1.210	α_1	50–100	1.9×10^5	50–55	45

VLDL, very-low-density lipoprotein; IDL, intermediate-density lipoprotein; LDL, low-density lipoprotein; HDL, high-density lipoprotein. Note that in the older literature IDL was usually referred to as LDL₁ or was included within the VLDL class. Alternative names in common use are: VLDL, pre-β-lipoprotein; LDL, β-lipoprotein; HDL, α-lipoprotein.

Table 11.4
Protein and lipid composition of normal human plasma lipoproteins

Lipoprotein	Protein constituents			Lipid constituents (% dry weight of lipoprotein)			
	Major	Minor	Trace	Triglyceride	Phospholipid	Esterified cholesterol	Free cholesterol
Chylomicrons	ApoB and apoC	apoE	apoA-I and apoA-II	85–90	10	3–5	1–3
VLDL	ApoB and apoC	apoE	apoA-I and apoA-II	50–65	20	15	5–10
IDL	ApoB and apoE	apoC	—	30	22	22	8
LDL	ApoB	—	apoC	7–10	20–22	35–40	7–10
*HDL$_2$	ApoA-I and apoA-II (A-I:A-II = 3.5:1)	apoC	apoE and apoD	5	30	16	5
*HDL$_3$	ApoA-I and apoA-II (A-I:A-II = 2:1)	apoC	apoE and apoD	4	23	12	3–4

Values for lipid composition are rounded averages for all particles throughout the density range of each class. For references, see Soutar and Myant (1979).
* Values for the molar ratios of apo-I to apoA-II in HDL subclasses are from Cheung and Albers (1977).

($1\,\mu$) in the chylomicrons. Molecular weights determined in the analytical ultracentrifuge range from about 200 000 to 10^{10} daltons. As particle density increases, protein content increases from less than 2% of total dry weight in chylomicrons to 50–55% in HDL_3, the lipid content decreasing as protein content increases.

Table 11.4 shows the protein and lipid composition of the lipoproteins in greater detail.

At least eight distinct proteins (apoproteins) have been identified in the lipoproteins of human plasma and are usually denoted by a system of capital letters. Two of the apoproteins, apoC-III and apoE, each exist in three or more polymorphic forms. ApoA-I and apoA-II are the two major proteins of HDL; aopB is the major protein of LDL and also comprises about half the protein of VLDL; apoC-I, apoC-II and apoC-III are low-molecular-weight proteins present in VLDL and, to a minor extent, in HDL; apoD is a minor constituent of HDL; apoE (formerly known as 'arginine-rich protein') is a constituent of VLDL and is also detectable in HDL. ApoA-IV, an apoprotein first identified in the HDL of rat plasma (Swaney et al., 1974), is also detectable in normal human plasma, though the bulk of the circulating apoA-IV in normal human subjects is not associated with lipoproteins of any class (Green et al., 1980).

With regard to lipid composition, points of interest to note are the marked difference between the triglyceride contents of VLDL and LDL, the high cholesterol content of LDL and the higher proportion of total cholesterol in HDL_2 than in HDL_3. These differences in percentage composition are more striking when particle mass is taken into account. Thus, if one particle of LDL corresponds to one of VLDL, each VLDL particle must contain 10–15 times as much triglyceride as each LDL particle, and if one HDL_2 particle corresponds to one of HDL_3, each particle of HDL_2 must contain 2–3 times as much total cholesterol as one of HDL_3.

3.2 Abnormal lipoproteins of human plasma

In addition to the normal lipoproteins discussed in the previous section, abnormal lipoproteins may appear in the plasma of patients suffering from various disorders of metabolism. These include lipoprotein-X (LP-X), a lipoprotein referred to as 'floating β-lipoprotein' or 'β-VLDL', and a variety of abnormal lipoproteins present in the plasma of patients with familial LCAT deficiency. Other abnormal plasma lipoproteins include an abnormal component in the HDL fraction of the plasma of patients with Tangier disease and an HDL with abnormal apoprotein composition in patients with abetalipoproteinaemia, but these are not of sufficient relevance to the plasma cholesterol to be worth considering here. In this section we shall consider LP-X and β-VLDL. The abnormal lipoproteins of LCAT deficiency are dealt with in Chapter 16.

3.2.1 LP-X

The d 1.006–1.063 fraction of the plasma of patients with biliary obstruction often contains peculiar particles, which appear on electron microscopy as stacked bilaminar discs of diameter 400–600 Å, and much larger bilaminar structures arranged in coils ('myelin figures'). These particles are known as LP-X. The protein consists of plasma albumin and one or more of the apoC proteins. The lipid component consists almost entirely of phospholipid and free cholesterol. (See Chapter 18, Section 2.1.1. for further details).

3.2.2 β-VLDL

The term *β-VLDL* refers to an abnormal lipoprotein first observed in the plasma fraction of density < 1.006 g/ml in patients suffering from a form of essential hyperlipidaemia often designated 'broad β disease' because of the characteristic lipoprotein distribution observed on paper electrophoresis of the plasma (Fredrickson *et al.*, 1967). In terms of the system of classification of the hyperlipidaemias recommended by the WHO (Beaumont *et al.*, 1970), the plasma lipoprotein pattern characteristic of broad β disease is denoted type III. Although the β-VLDL in patients with the type III lipoprotein pattern is present in all plasma fractions of density < 1.019 g/ml, it is present in greatest quantity in the IDL fraction (density 1.006–1.019 g/ml). Moreover, the protein and lipid composition of the abnormal lipoprotein is broadly similar to that of the small quantity of IDL present in normal human plasma. In particular, both β-VLDL and normal IDL have a higher cholesterol:triglyceride ratio than has VLDL and both are rich in apoE. These similarities have led to the suggestion that the presence of β-VLDL in broad β disease reflects an abnormal accumulation of a normal lipoprotein (IDL). However, this seems unlikely since the apoE protein of β-VLDL is abnormal in that it lacks at least one of the subfractions of normal apoE (Utermann *et al.*, 1975).

3.3 The lipoproteins of animal plasma

Lipoproteins similar in protein and lipid composition to human plasma lipoproteins have been demonstrated in the plasma of many mammals, birds and lower vertebrates. The plasma of most mammals contains lipoproteins analogous to normal human lipoproteins, though the relative concentrations of the lipoproteins of animal plasma differ from those of human plasma. In most mammalian species the relative and absolute concentrations of lipoprotein corresponding to human LDL are lower, and the proportion of HDL is much greater, than in man. An interesting exception is the guinea-pig, in which HDL is barely detectable in the plasma. The concentration of VLDL in the plasma of most non-human mammals is far lower than in man, but may be considerable in some birds and fish (Mills, 1976). It should also be noted that a given lipoprotein of an animal plasma does not necessarily extend over the same density range as its counterpart in human plasma. A well-studied example is the plasma lipoprotein pattern in dogs. Normal dog plasma contains four lipoproteins separable by a combination of ultracentrifugation and electrophoresis:—VLDL (density <1.006 g/ml), an apoB-containing lipoprotein of density 1.006–1.087 g/ml, corresponding to human LDL, and two apoA-I-containing lipoproteins in the HDL fraction designated HDL_1 and HDL_2 by Mahley and Weisgraber (1974), but not corresponding precisely with the HDL sub-fractions of human plasma (see Table 11.3). Canine HDL_1 extends over the density range 1.025 to 1.10 g/ml and has α_2 mobility; canine HDL_2 extends over the density range 1.070 to 1.21 g/ml, has α_1 mobility and carries 85% of the total cholesterol in whole plasma. See Mahley (1978) for review.

Various abnormal lipoproteins appear in the plasma of animals made hypercholesterolaemic by feeding cholesterol-rich diets. In guinea-pigs, these include discoidal particles about 250 Å in diameter and much larger discs 800–1100 Å in diameter, both particles containing a high proportion of unesterified cholesterol (Sardet et al., 1972). Two abnormal lipoproteins, containing esterified cholesterol as their major lipid, have been described by Mahley and his co-workers in the plasma of cholesterol-fed rats, dogs, monkeys and pigs (Mahley, 1978). One of these is similar in protein and lipid composition to human β-VLDL. The other, known as HDL_c, is an α_2-migrating lipoprotein, usually isolated in the density range 1.006–1.060 g/ml. The protein of HDL_c consists of apoE, with variable amounts of apoA-I and the apoC proteins, but no apoB. The lipoproteins at the lower end of the HDL_c density range (1.006–1.020 g/ml) contain 50–60% of cholesterol by weight.

3.4 The structure of normal plasma lipoproteins

3.4.1 General features

From the point of view of their structural organization, it is useful to divide the lipids of lipoproteins into the apolar, or hydrophobic, and the amphipathic (*Gr., feeling both*). The apolar lipids, comprising the triglycerides and cholesteryl esters, are immiscible with water because they lack a polar (hydrophilic) group. The amphipathic lipids, of which the most important are unesterified cholesterol and the phospholipids, have a polar and an apolar region and are therefore capable of interacting with both the aqueous medium and the apolar lipids of the lipoprotein particle. In unesterified cholesterol the polar group is the 3β-hydroxyl group and in the phospholipids it is the phosphoryl residue.

Evidence derived from several independent approaches points to a basic structure common to all the lipoproteins of normal human plasma (see Soutar and Myant (1979) for a survey of the methods used for investigating lipoprotein structure). According to the current view, each particle is roughly spherical and consists of an inner core containing the apolar lipids and an outer shell, about 22 Å thick, consisting of a monolayer of amphipathic lipids. The lipids of the outer shell are arranged with their long axes parallel, with the polar groups in contact with the aqueous medium and the apolar groups in contact with the core lipids, as shown in Fig. 11.1. In VLDL and

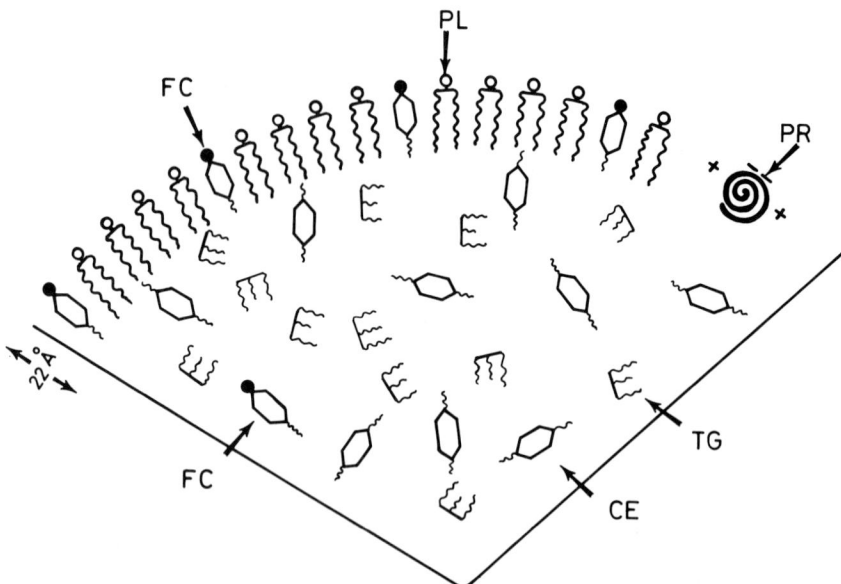

Figure 11.1
Diagrammatic representation of a typical plasma lipoprotein particle. A segment of the spherical particle is seen in cross-section. The polar groups of the phospholipid (○) and free cholesterol (●) molecules face towards the aqueous medium; the fatty-acyl chains of the phospholipids and the side-chains of free cholesterol are in contact with the apolar core. The fatty-acyl chains of the phospholipids are shown in a liquid (mobile) state; the apolar molecules in the core are completely disordered. A portion of a helical segment of a protein molecule is shown end-on. The phospholipid:free cholesterol molar ratio is shown arbitrarily as 3:1. Note the presence of a small number of free cholesterol molecules in the core. FC, free cholesterol; PL, phospholipid; PR, protein; CE, cholesteryl ester; TG, triglyceride.

LDL, a small percentage of the total free cholesterol is thought to be held in solution in the apolar lipids of the core. In the idealized lipoprotein depicted in Fig. 11.1, the core lipids are in a completely fluid state, but investigations of human and animal plasma lipoproteins by scanning calorimetry and analysis of the X-ray scattering patterns have shown that under some conditions the cholesteryl esters are in a partially ordered state (see Section 3.4.3 below).

The proteins of the lipoprotein particle are known to be surface components, but the manner in which the protein chains interact with lipids in the outer shell is not fully understood. Three-dimensional models of the human apoproteins whose amino-acid sequences have been determined (apoA-I, apoA-II and the three apoC proteins) have revealed the presence of α-helical segments in which one side of the helix contains only positively or negatively charged amino-acid residues and the other side contains only hydrophobic amino-acid residues. These unusual structures have been termed *amphipathic helices* by Gotto and his co-workers. It is thought that amphipathic helical regions are the sites at which the protein chains interact with the surface lipids. In the light of current evidence, the most plausible arrangement is one in which the long axes of the helical segments are parallel to the surface of the particle, the polar faces interacting with the aqueous medium and the hydrophobic faces interacting non-ionically with the fatty-acyl chains of the phospholipids, as in Fig. 11.1.

In general, the apoproteins of the plasma lipoproteins are of two kinds:—those that are essential for the formation of a stable particle and those that can move from one lipoprotein to another by exchange or net flux without disorganization of the particle. The distinction between 'structural' and 'non-structural' apoprotein components is not absolute, but it seems likely that apoB, apoA-II and possibly apoA-I, are structural apoproteins and that the apoC and apoE proteins are relatively loosely associated with the lipoprotein particles of which they are a part.

3.4.2 HDL

The physical, chemical and immunochemical properties of the native HDL in the circulation are fully consistent with the general structure shown in Fig. 11.1. Scanning calorimetry of human HDL over the temperature range 10–40 °C shows no evidence of a change of phase from the liquid-crystalline to the liquid state, indicating that the lipids of the core are fluid at body temperature.

3.4.3 LDL

Although it is now agreed that the constituents of the LDL particle are arranged more or less in the manner shown in Fig. 11.1, there is some uncertainty about the molecular organization of the surface layer, particularly with regard to the orientation of the protein chains. The study of apoB has been hampered by its insolubility in water. Its amino-acid sequence has not been determined and estimates of the subunit molecular weight have ranged from 8000 to 275 000, the higher values probably reflecting the marked tendency of apoB to aggregate even in the presence of detergents. Nor do we know whether apoB corresponds to one or to more than one species of protein molecule. Until these uncertainties have been resolved, the three-dimensional structure of apoB and its orientation in the surface layer of the native LDL particle must remain in doubt. ApoB is a glycoprotein containing 5–9% of carbohydrate by weight, with the oligosaccharide chains linked to the protein at an asparagine residue. Since native LDL reacts with concanavalin A (Shore and Shore, 1973), the sugar residues of apoB are probably exposed to the surface of the particle. The likelihood that an arginine-containing region of apoB is necessary for the recognition of LDL by the LDL receptor has already been mentioned (Section 3, Chapter 9).

Variations in the lipid composition of LDL are of considerable interest in relation to the fluidity of the lipids in the surface layer and the core.

The free cholesterol:phospholipid molar ratio in the LDL of normal plasma is between 0.7 and 0.8, but in familial hypercholesterolaemia the ratio may increase to values approaching unity (Shattil *et al.*, 1977). Increased ratios may also be observed in the LDL of primates fed atherogenic diets (Howard *et al.*, 1972). As we have already seen (Section 2 above) changes in the fatty-acid composition of the diet may also lead to changes in the degree of unsaturation of the fatty acids of the LDL phospholipids. From what we know of the influence of unesterified cholesterol and of the number of double bonds in the fatty-acyl chains of the phospholipids upon the fluidity of a phospholipid monolayer, these changes in the composition of the surface components of LDL might be expected to alter the physical state of LDL particles at body temperature.

Of potentially greater significance is the effect of triglyceride on the molecular arrangement of the cholesteryl esters in the apolar core of LDL. Small and his coworkers (Deckelbaum *et al.*, 1977) have shown that when native LDL is cooled or warmed, it undergoes a reversible thermal transition due to a change in the arrangement of the cholesteryl esters from a smectic liquid-crystalline state, in which the molecules are stacked in layers 36 Å thick, to a more disordered state in which the molecules are almost completely unrestricted (Fig. 11.2). This change is not a sharp one, but takes place over a range of temperature from about 20 °C to about 40 °C, with a peak at about 30 °C. In samples of LDL from different human subjects, the temperature at which the liquid crystals in the core melt to a near-fluid state is inversely proportional to the percentage of triglyceride in the core of the LDL particles. In other words, the lower the triglyceride:cholesteryl ester ratio the less fluid is the LDL at a given temperature within the range 20 °C to 40 °C. The reason why the phase transition takes place over a relatively wide range of temperature is not clear. It may be either because any sample of LDL contains particles of different lipid composition, each particle melting within its own narrow range, or because there are domains within the core of each particle which melt at different temperatures. In either case, the range of temperature over which the transition occurs and the effect of triglyceride content upon the peak temperature of the transition suggest that small changes in the triglyceride:cholesteryl ester ratio of the LDL lipids could have a significant effect on the mean fluidity of the circulating LDL particles at body temperature. Tall *et al.* (1977) have also shown that under some experimental conditions the peak temperature of the transition from liquid crystal to liquid may be increased by increasing the degree of saturation of the fatty acids of the LDL cholesteryl esters.

In at least two conditions associated with premature atherosclerosis

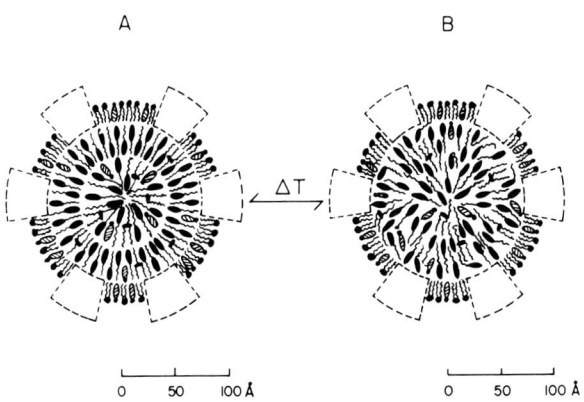

Figure 11.2
Schematic representation of the distribution of lipids in human LDL.

Phospholipids, ●⁓⁓ ; free cholesterol, ●⫞⫞⫞ ; cholesteryl esters, ⁓⫞⫞⫞ ; triglycerides, ⁓⌒⁓ .

A shows the probable structure of the particle at 10 °C (i.e. below the transition temperature). The cholesteryl esters in the core of the particle are arranged in two concentric layers.

B shows the probable structure at 45 °C (above the transition temperature). The layered arrangement of the cholesteryl esters is lost. All the LDL triglyceride and about 15% of the free cholesterol are dissolved in the inner apolar core. The outer shell is formed by phospholipid, free cholesterol and apoprotein. (From Deckelbaum *et al.* (1977), with the permission of the authors.)

(human familial hypercholesterolaemia and the hypercholesterolaemia of cholesterol-fed pigs) the cholesteryl-ester:triglyceride ratio of LDL increases, a change that leads to decreased fluidity of the core components of LDL at body temperature. It has been suggested that this alteration in the physical state of the LDL lipids in some way enhances the atherogenic potency of the plasma LDL. One possibility is that the cholesteryl esters of LDL particles that enter the arteries from the circulation cannot be hydrolyzed because their rigid conformation decreases their accessibility to cholesteryl-ester hydrolase in the arterial wall. This could interfere with the removal of the intracellular esterified cholesterol. Deckelbaum *et al.* (1978) have also discussed the possibility that changes in the physical state of the core lipids could affect the surface of the particle in such a way as to modify its ability to interact with tissue cells.

Some of the early confusion about the nature of human apoB has now been resolved by Kane *et al.* (1980), who have identified four species of apoB in the lipoproteins of human plasma and thoracic-duct lymph. One apoB species (designated B-100) has a molecular weight of about 549 000 and is the major appB of LDL and VLDL, but is also a minor component of the apoB of chylomicrons in plasma and lymph. Two other lower-molecular-weight species (designated B-74 and B-26) are also present in the LDL of many normal subjects and are probably complementary fragments of B-100. The fourth species (MW about 264 000 and designated B-48) is the major component of the apoB of chylomicrons and is essentially absent from LDL. Comparison of the amino-acid composition of the four types of apoB indicates that B-48 is not a component of B-100. Kane *et al.* (1980) suggest that B-48 is synthesized in the intestine.

3.4.4 Triglyceride-rich lipoproteins

The physical and chemical properties and the electron-microscopic appearance of VLDL and chylomicrons are consistent with a structural organization consisting of a lipid droplet surrounded by a monolayer of polar lipids and apoproteins. In agreement with such an arrangement for the components of VLDL, Sata *et al.* (1972) have shown that, over a wide range of particle size, the relation between the ratio of polar and apolar constituents and the volume of the particle is consistent with a model in which the apolar lipids are surrounded by a polar shell 21.5 Å thick containing essentially all the polar constituents. A similar relationship holds for chylomicrons, though the larger chylomicrons have more free cholesterol than is likely to be accommodated in the shell, suggesting that some of their free cholesterol is dissolved in the apolar core. Phase transitions in triglyceride-rich lipoprotein particles are not observed over the temperature range 10–45 °C (Deckelbaum *et al.*, 1977), indicating that the cholesteryl esters in the apolar core are fluid at body temperature, probably because the large amount of triglyceride in the core is sufficient to dissolve all the cholesteryl ester in the particle.

3.5 Biogenesis and metabolic transformations

The mature lipoprotein particles present in the plasma arise partly from synthesis and secretion by the liver and intestine, and partly by modification or catabolism of lipoproteins that have entered the blood circulation. The metabolic changes undergone by lipoproteins in the plasma are very complex, and there is still a good deal of uncertainty about the origin of the components of some lipoprotein fractions, particularly of those isolated within the density range 1.063–1.21 g/ml, and about the mechanisms by which they acquire their final form by transfer of lipids and proteins between fractions of different density. In this section I shall deal briefly with the manner in which normal circulating lipoproteins are now thought to arise. The intracellular synthesis of the separate components of plasma lipoproteins, the assembly of these components into nascent particles and the secretion of nascent particles into the interstitial fluid are discussed in the review by Soutar and Myant (1979).

Much of our understanding of the biogenesis of plasma lipoproteins is based on information derived from the study of animals. However, it is becoming increasingly clear that the intravascular phase of lipoprotein metabolism differs from one species to another, at least as regards the relative importance of different pathways. Moreover, there are discrepancies between the currently accepted view of plasma lipoprotein metabolism and the effects of certain human genetic disorders in which one or other specific lipoprotein is missing from the plasma (see Chapters 15 and 16). Hence, it is probable that the present view of human plasma lipoprotein metabolism will have to be modified, in detail though not in essentials, in the light of future clinical studies.

3.5.1 The origin of HDL

The spherical cholesteryl-ester-rich particles present in the d 1.063–1.21 fraction of normal human plasma are not secreted as such into the circulation. A clue to the mechanism by which the spherical particles of HDL are generated came from the early attempts of Nichols and his co-workers to reconstruct HDL from its purified components. Forte *et al.* (1971) showed that sonication of mixtures of phospholipid, free cholesterol and HDL protein leads to the formation of bilayer discs which can be converted subsequently into spheres by incubation with a plasma fraction containing LCAT. Observations on perfused rat livers in which LCAT is inhibited have since shown that the liver of the rat secretes discoidal particles, similar in electron-microscopic appearance to the 'recombinant' discs described by Forte *et al.* and consisting of phospholipid, free cholesterol, apoE and apoA-I, with essentially no esterified cholesterol. Each particle consists of a phospholipid-cholesterol bilayer 45 Å thick and 150–250 Å in diameter with the protein molecules forming an annulus around the periphery of the disc (Fig. 11.3). Similar discoidal particles are present in the plasma of human subjects with familial LCAT deficiency (Forte *et al.*, 1974), in rat intestinal lymph collected in the presence of an LCAT inhibitor (Green *et al.*, 1978) and in the HDL$_2$ of normal human splanchnic blood plasma (Turner *et al.*, 1979). When these bilayer discs are incubated with LCAT, the free choles-

A

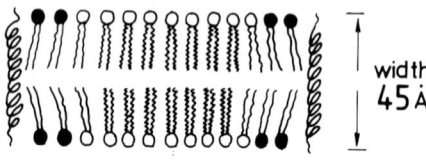

transverse section

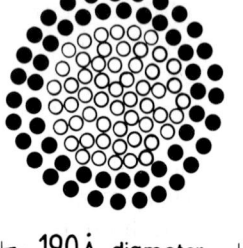

|←— 190 Å diameter —→|
View from above

B

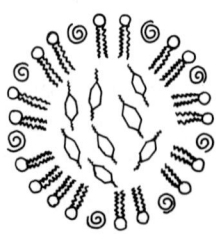

transverse section

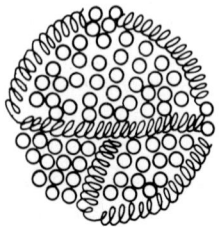

View from above

Figure 11.3
Structure of HDL, showing the possible orientation of the apoproteins.

A, possible structure of the complex reassembled *in vitro* from phospholipids and HDL apoproteins. The phospholipids form a bilayer disc with the protein round the periphery, oriented so that the long axes of the amphipathic helices are parallel to the fatty acyl chains.

B, possible structure of native HDL. The spherical particle is composed of an apolar core containing cholesteryl esters surrounded by a monolayer of polar lipids and proteins. The proteins are arranged on the surface of the sphere with the long axes of the amphipathic helices perpendicular to the fatty acyl chains. (Free cholesterol not shown.)

terol is esterified by the LCAT reaction and the discs are converted into spheres containing an apolar core of cholesteryl esters. The spherical particles produced by the action of LCAT on naturally-formed bilayer discs are similar in size and shape to the particles present in the HDL fraction of human or rat plasma.

On the basis of these observations it is now believed that the liver and intestine secrete bilaminar discoidal particles consisting almost entirely of phospholipid, free cholesterol and the apoE or apoA proteins, and that these discs of nascent HDL are converted into mature HDL particles immediately they reach the circulation. From what is known of the conversion of artificial recombinant discs into spherical particles *in vitro*, it is likely that an important step in the formation of HDL particles *in vivo* is the esterification of free cholesterol in the bilayer by the LCAT reaction, with the continuous transfer of the esterified cholesterol into the potential space between the two sides of the disc, thus forcing the disc to assume a spherical micellar structure of the kind shown in Fig. 11.1 and Fig. 11.3. LCAT is necessary for this process, but there is a good deal more to the conversion of nascent into mature HDL than the esterification of the free cholesterol present in newly-secreted particles. This can be seen by comparing the composition of the nascent HDL present in the plasma of LCAT-deficient human subjects with that of the mature HDL present in normal human plasma. In nascent HDL virtually the only lipids present are phospholipid and free cholesterol, the major apoprotein is apoE, and apoA-II is present in greater concentration than apoA-I. In the HDL of normal plasma, on the other hand, 15% of the total lipoprotein mass is esterified cholesterol, triglyceride is present in significant amounts, apoA-I is the predominant apoprotein and apoC proteins are present as minor constituents of the protein component. ApoE is present in circulating human HDL only as a constituent of a minor subfraction of HDL_2 (Weisgraber and Mahley, 1980), but is present in significant quantities in rat HDL. Thus, when nascent HDL is converted into normal HDL, in addition to the esterification of free cholesterol, the nascent particles acquire triglyceride, apoC proteins and additional apoA-I, and they lose apoE. These changes, and other changes resulting in the redistribution of lipids between different lipoprotein fractions, will be easier to understand when we have considered the origin and metabolism of the triglyceride-rich lipoproteins. As we shall see, it now seems possible that the nascent HDL secreted by the liver and intestine is not the only source of the circulating HDL of normal plasma.

3.5.2 The origin of VLDL and chylomicrons
Both VLDL and chylomicrons are synthesized in the intestinal wall and are secreted into the bloodstream via the intestinal lymphatics

and the thoracic duct during the absorption of fat. VLDL is also secreted continuously by the liver into the space of Disse and thence into the blood circulation. The intestinal wall is capable of synthesizing all the lipid components of the triglyceride-rich lipoproteins, including the cholesteryl esters, which are formed by the esterification of dietary or endogenous cholesterol by ACAT. The human intestine can also synthesize apoB, apoA-I, ap-A-II and apoA-IV, but is apparently unable to synthesize apoC or apoE proteins (see Green et al., 1979, for references). The liver, on the other hand, synthesizes apoA-I, apoA-II, apoB, the three apoC proteins and apoE.

The nascent triglyceride-rich lipoproteins secreted by the intestinal mucosa have their full complement of apoB and are enriched with apoA-I, apoA-IV and (in man) apoA-II. Comparisons between the lipoproteins in plasma and those in mesenteric lymph, thoracic-duct lymph or the urine of human subjects with chyluria, suggest that as soon as nascent intestinal VLDL and chylomicrons enter the plasma they acquire apoC and apoE, probably from HDL, and lose the bulk of their apoA proteins (see Tall et al., 1979; Green et al., 1979). In rats the apoA-I and apoA-IV are transferred to HDL; in man apoA-I moves to HDL but apoA-IV is transferred predominantly to the non-lipoprotein fraction of plasma (d >1.21 g/ml). Nascent VLDL secreted by the liver contains some apoC proteins, but it takes up additional apoC from HDL in the space of Disse or in the circulation. In rats, VLDL and chylomicrons secreted by the intestine contain esterified cholesterol formed by intestinal ACAT, and the VLDL secreted by the liver contains esterified cholesterol formed by ACAT in the hepatocytes. Indirect evidence suggests that cholesteryl esters are also present in the nascent VLDL and chylomicrons secreted by the human intestine, but nascent VLDL secreted by the human liver probably does not contain esterified cholesterol (see Section 4 below).

3.5.3 Metabolic transformations of lipoproteins within the plasma

As soon as the newly-secreted VLDL and chylomicrons have entered the circulation and have acquired apoC proteins from HDL, their triglyceride core is rapidly hydrolyzed by lipoprotein lipase on the luminal surface of the endothelium of the blood capillaries, apoC-II acting as activator for the enzyme. The hydrolytic activity of lipoprotein lipase results in the removal of 80–90% of the triglyceride in the particle, with a consequent reduction in the volume of the core, so that much of the polar surface material becomes redundant. This leads to the release of apoC proteins, phospholipid and free cholesterol, leaving a residue or *remnant* which contains all the apoB of the original triglyceride-rich particle, most of the cholesteryl ester and a reduced amount of apoC and of the polar lipids. The remnant particle, which has a density corresponding to that of IDL, is also relatively enriched with apoE, but it is not known whether this is derived from nascent HDL (which must lose apoE during its maturation) or whether it represents apoE originally present in the mature triglyceride-rich lipoproteins and retained by these particles during their hydrolysis.

Glomset and Norum (1973) have suggested that apoC and the polar lipids are released as a single unit from the surface of the triglyceride-rich particle, and that the constituents of this unit are then incorporated into HDL in the presence of LCAT. In keeping with this, Norum et al. (1975) have shown that the d 1.063–1.21 fraction of the plasma of LCAT-deficient patients contains small spherical particles rich in phospholipid and free cholesterol, as well as the large discs already referred to in Section 3.5.1, and that when LCAT is added to the plasma in vitro, the small particles and the large discs disappear and are converted into particles having the composition and appearance of normal HDL. Eisenberg and Olivecrona (1979) have also shown that incubation of VLDL with purified lipoprotein lipase in the absence of HDL results in the release of discoidal particles consisting of phospholipid, free cholesterol and apoC proteins. These observations might suggest that the maturation of HDL normally requires a supply of phospholipid and free cholesterol generated by the catabolism of VLDL and chylomicrons, in addition to LCAT. However, it seems unlikely that this is the only mechanism whereby mature HDL is formed in the circulation, since the composition of the circulating HDL is not grossly abnormal in abetalipoproteinaemia (when VLDL and chylomicrons are never formed) or in the fasting state (when the production of triglyceride-rich lipoproteins is greatly diminished). Possibly, mature HDL may also be formed in vivo by an alternative or additional mechanism in which nascent HDL takes up free cholesterol, perhaps in association with phospholipid, from the surfaces of tissue cells and that this is then esterified by LCAT, as discussed in Chapter 9, Section 4.2.

The fate of the remnants resulting from the partial breakdown of triglyceride-rich particles varies from species to species, as exemplified by differences in the metabolism of VLDL remnants in man and the rat (see Eisenberg and Levy (1975) for review). In both species, the hydrolysis of VLDL triglyceride in the capillary bed proceeds as far as the formation of particles with the chemical composition of IDL and it then ceases, or slows down considerably, possibly owing to loss of apoC-II (the activator for non-hepatic lipoprotein lipase) from VLDL. Thereafter, the pathway for VLDL catabolism differs markedly in the two species.

In rats, the bulk of the esterified cholesterol and more than 90% of the apoB of VLDL remnants is rapidly and efficiently removed by the liver, less than 10% of the apoB appearing in the circulating LDL. It is possible that hepatic uptake of remnants is mediated by interaction of apoE in the remnant particles with specific receptors on the surfaces of liver cells, the presence of apoC-III in triglyceride-rich lipoproteins (which also contain apoE) preventing this interaction (see Grundy and Kern, 1980). In normal man, most of the apoB of circulating VLDL is transferred to LDL *via* IDL, the IDL presumably corresponding to remnant particles. The fact that in rats only a very small fraction of the circulating VLDL is converted into LDL may explain why the plasma LDL concentration is so much lower in rats then in man. In normal human subjects the rate of secretion of VLDL-apoB is sufficient to account for the observed absolute rate of turnover of LDL-apoB. This might suggest that VLDL is the sole source of LDL-apoB in man. However, it should be noted that during the absorption of 100 g of fat per day, some 200–500 mg of apoB would be secreted each day in chylomicrons. If all the remnant particles formed from chylomicrons are converted into LDL without loss of apoB, this could account for up to one third of the total daily turnover of LDL. However, although the potential contribution of chylomicrons to the total pool of LDL is considerable, their actual contribution is probably small (Schaefer *et al.*, 1978). The possibility that LDL may be secreted *directly* into the circulation under abnormal conditions is considered in Chapter 15.

As we have seen, the maturation of HDL under normal conditions *in vivo* is closely related to events occurring during the catabolism of triglyceride-rich lipoproteins, the surface elements released during the action of lipoprotein lipase contributing to the formation of the mature HDL present in the circulation. The LCAT-mediated formation of mature HDL is not essential for the action of lipoprotein lipase upon VLDL, since the triglycerides of VLDL are hydrolyzed by lipoprotein lipase *in vitro* when no HDL is present to act as acceptor for the surface material released by shrinkage of the VLDL particles (see, for example, Glangeaud *et al.*, 1977). Nevertheless, observations on LCAT-deficient human plasma (Norum *et al.*, 1975) suggest that the LCAT reaction, with nascent HDL as substrate, does influence the course of VLDL and chylomicron catabolism in whole plasma. In particular, when LCAT is added to LCAT-deficient human plasma, the conversion of nascent HDL into mature HDL is accompanied by a transfer of apoE and cholesteryl esters from the HDL density fraction to VLDL or LDL and a change towards normal composition and electron-microscopic appearance of the lipoproteins in the LDL density fraction. This has led to the suggestion that the LCAT reaction promotes the net transport of cholesteryl esters (formed during the maturation of HLD) into VLDL and that apoE acts as a carrier in this process. Norum *et al.* (1975) have suggested that the

The Plasma Cholesterol: Composition and Metabolism   527

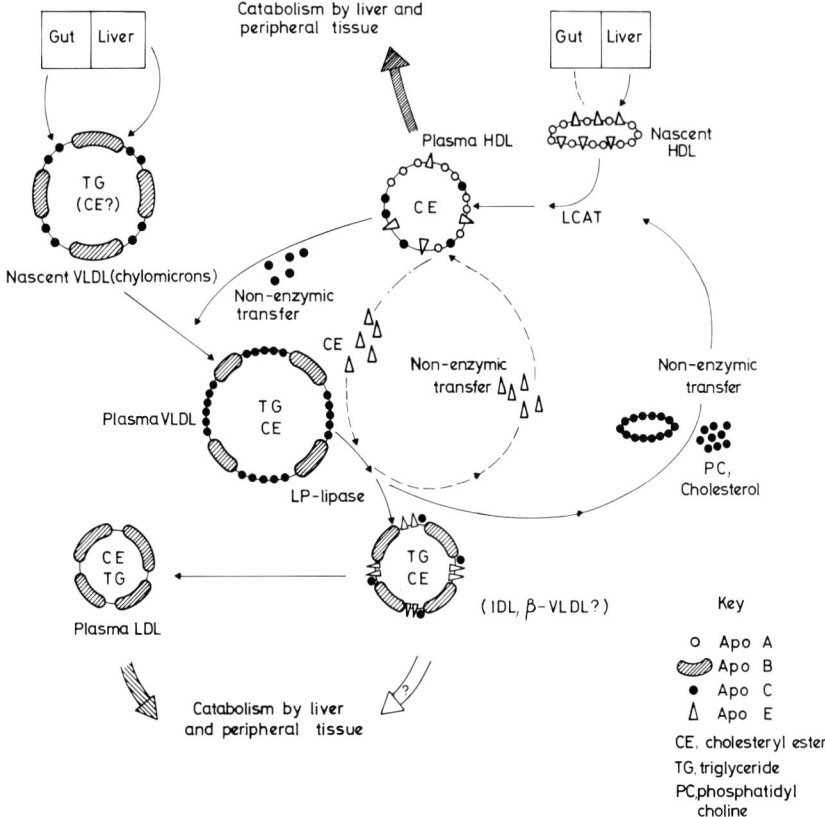

Figure 11.4
Diagrammatic representation of some transformations undergone by lipoproteins and their apoproteins in the plasma. Pathways for which there is good evidence are shown as thick lines; other pathways are shown by broken lines. Nascent triglyceride-rich lipoproteins (top left) aquire additional apoC proteins and, possibly, cholesteryl esters, from HDL. Mature chylomicrons and VLDL are acted upon by lipoprotein lipase (LP-lipase) with the formation of lipoproteins of intermediate density (IDL). During the formation of IDL, the triglyceride-rich particles lose about 95% of their triglyceride and much of their phospholipid, cholesterol and apoC protein; they retain all their apoB and acquire apoE, probably from HDL. Phospholipid, free cholesterol and apoC released by the action of LP-lipase (centre right) may be associated as lipoprotein complexes that can be converted into HDL by the action of LCAT. IDL is catabolized in the liver (bottom centre) or is converted into LDL (possibly in the liver). LDL is catabolized partly in extrahepatic tissues by the receptor pathway. HDL particles, secreted into the plasma in nascent form containing apoE and apoA protein (top right), are converted into mature spherical particles by the action of LCAT. During their metabolism in the circulation, HDL particles act as reservoirs for apoC and apoE recycled during the intravascular metabolism of triglyceride-rich lipoproteins. (From Soutar and Myant (1979), with the permission of University Park Press.)

transfer of apoE from nascent HDL and VLDL in some way facilitates the normal fragmentation of VLDL to IDL and, subsequently, to LDL. However, the stage in the biogenesis and metabolism of triglyceride-rich particles at which they acquire apoE from nascent HDL is far from clear. Moreover, cholesteryl-ester transfer proteins other than apoE have been demonstrated in the d >1.21 fraction of human plasma (see Section 5.4).

In conclusion, it may be helpful to bring together some of the points discussed in this section by summarizing the multiple functions of HDL in the metabolism of the plasma lipoproteins. As well as acting as a source of apoE for triglyceride-rich particles, HDL acts as a reservoir of the apoC required for the conversion of nascent VLDL and chylomicrons into mature particles. In this capacity, HDL may be regarded as a means of conserving apoC within the circulation, accepting apoC from VLDL and chylomicrons during their catabolism, and then returning it to the nascent triglyceride-rich particles secreted by the liver and intestine. In view of the addition of apoA-I to HDL during its maturation and possible return of some HDL-apoA-I to newly-secreted triglyceride-rich lipoproteins (Havel, 1978), HDL may also act as a reservoir of apoA-I. In addition to its role in relation to apoprotein metabolism, HDL also acts as a generator of cholesteryl esters from free cholesterol *via* the LCAT reaction, the free cholesterol arising from triglyceride-rich particles and, possibly, from the cells of extra-hepatic tissues. In so far as HDL acts as an acceptor for tissue free cholesterol it performs an important role in the 'reverse transport' discussed in Chapter 9 (Section 4) and in Section 6 of this chapter. The biological function of the LCAT reaction is considered more fully in the section on familial LCAT deficiency (Chapter 16).

Some of the metabolic transformations discussed above are summarized in Fig. 11.4.

3.6 The metabolism of LDL

3.6.1 Methods for measuring LDL turnover *in vivo*

The degradation of the protein of LDL (LDL-apoB) in intact animals can be studied by measuring the rate at which protein-bound radioactivity in the circulation declines after an intravenous injection of autologous radioiodine-labelled LDL. The fraction of the circulating LDL-apoB catabolized in unit time (the fractional catabolic rate or FCR) and the fraction of the total exchangeable LDL that is in the circulation may be estimated by analysing the plasma radioactivity curve in terms of the two-pool system shown in Fig. 11.5 (Matthews, 1957). In this model system it is assumed that the total exchangeable mass of LDL is distributed between the plasma and an extravascular pool, and that when LDL is labelled with radioiodine, the radioiodine can leave the whole system only through the plasma compartment. It is important to note that the method of analysis proposed by Matthews gives an estimate of the fractional rate of catabolism of the circulating LDL-apoB, and not of that of the LDL-apoB in the whole system. If the thyroidal uptake of the radioiodide released by the catabolism of LDL-apoB is blocked by administration of KI, all the radioiodide will be excreted in the urine. A semi-independent estimate of the FCR may then be obtained by measuring the proportion of the total radioactivity in the circulation that is excreted in the urine each day. This is known as the urine/plasma (U/P) ratio method for estimating FCR. The U/P ratio method has the advantages that it does not require measurements of plasma radioactivity during the first few hours after the injection of labelled LDL and that it can be used to measure FCR when LDL metabolism is not in the steady state. Results obtained by the two methods from the same animal or human subject are usually in reasonable agreement, though the U/P ratio method tends to give lower values than

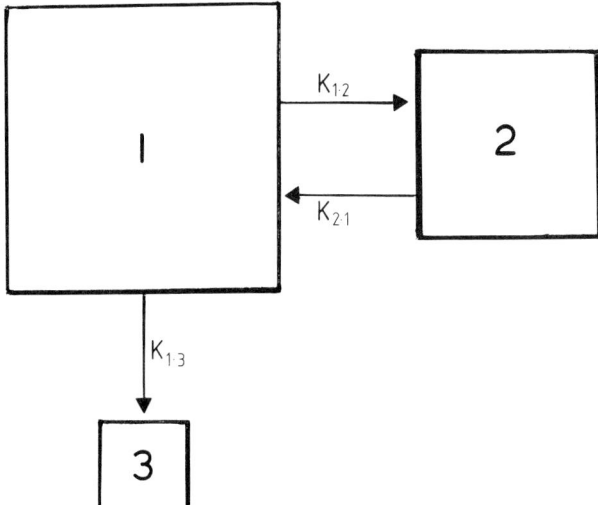

Figure 11.5
Two-pool system for analysis of plasma LDL kinetics after an intravenous injection of radioiodine-labelled LDL. Compartment 1 is the intravascular mass of LDL in equilibrium with a smaller exchangeable mass in the extravascular extracellular fluid space (compartment 2). The radioiodide released by the catabolism of the labelled LDL is excreted irreversibly from compartment 1 into the urine (compartment 3). $K_{1.2}$ and $K_{2.1}$ are the rate constants for the flow of labelled LDL from 1 to 2 and from 2 to 1 respectively. $K_{1.3}$ is the rate constant for the excretion of radioiodide from compartment 1. It is a condition of this model that LDL-apoB can enter the system only through 1 and that all radioiodide leaves the system through 1.

the method using analysis of the plasma radioactivity curve in terms of two linked pools.

The absolute rate of catabolism of LDL-apoB may be estimated from the FCR and the mass of LDL-apoB in the circulation. Under steady-state conditions, the rate of synthesis of LDL-apoB is, by definition, equal to the rate of catabolism. If LDL metabolism is not in the steady state, the amount of LDL-apoB synthesized on a given day may be estimated by summing the amount catabolized and the increment or decrement in the mass of circulating LDL-apoB on the same day (Thompson et al., 1977).

If the injected LDL is labelled with ^{131}I, a gamma-ray-emitting isotope of iodine, the daily decrement in radioactivity in the whole body may be measured with a whole-body gamma counter. The amount of LDL-apoB catabolized on a given day may then be estimated from the specific activity of the plasma LDL-apoB and the loss of radioactivity from the whole body. The use of a whole-body counter is particularly valuable if one wishes to obtain a record of the relative amounts of radioactive LDL-apoB inside and outside the blood circulation at successive intervals after an injection of radioactive LDL.

3.6.2 LDL turnover in man

Figure 11.6 shows a typical plasma radioactivity curve obtained after an intravenous injection of ^{125}I-labelled autologous LDL into a normal adult human subject. During the first three or four days there is a relatively rapid decline in plasma radioactivity. The curve then merges with a log-linear phase which lasts until the final plasma sample, obtained 16 days after the injection. Interpreted in terms of the two-pool system shown in Fig. 11.5, the initial phase of the disappearance curve reflects mixing of the labelled LDL molecules with LDL in the extravascular compartment and their concurrent removal from the system by catabolism; the log-linear phase reflects removal of the equilibrated ^{125}I-labelled LDL from the system. The half-life of the log-linear phase in this subject was 3.1 days and the half-life of the line obtained by subtracting the extrapolated portion of the log-linear curve from the observed values was 0.9 days (see Fig. 11.6). Analysis of the plasma radioactivity curve by the method of Matthews showed that the FCR was 0.34 of the intravascular pool of LDL-apoB/day and that the fraction of the total LDL-apoB in the circulation was 65.2%.

In most normal human subjects the FCR is between 0.3 and 0.5/day and the intravascular pool of LDL-apoB comprises 65–75% of the total LDL-apoB in the combined intravascular and extravascular pools. Since the plasma LDL-apoB concentration in normal men is usually between 50 and 100 mg/100 ml, an FCR of 0.3–

0.5/day is equivalent to an absolute rate of LDL-apoB catabolism of 10–15 mg/Kg/day (assuming that the plasma volume is 4.5% of body mass), or to some 0.75 to 1.0 g of LDL-apoB catabolized per day in a whole man. Since the ratio of total cholesterol to protein in LDL is about 1.6, this corresponds very roughly to the release of 1.0–1.5 g of cholesterol/day from the catabolism of LDL. These values are, of course, approximate, but they give some idea of the quantities of protein and cholesterol involved in the daily breakdown of LDL in a normal adult man.

Since LDL is the major carrier of cholesterol in human plasma, changes in the rate of production or catabolism of LDL would be

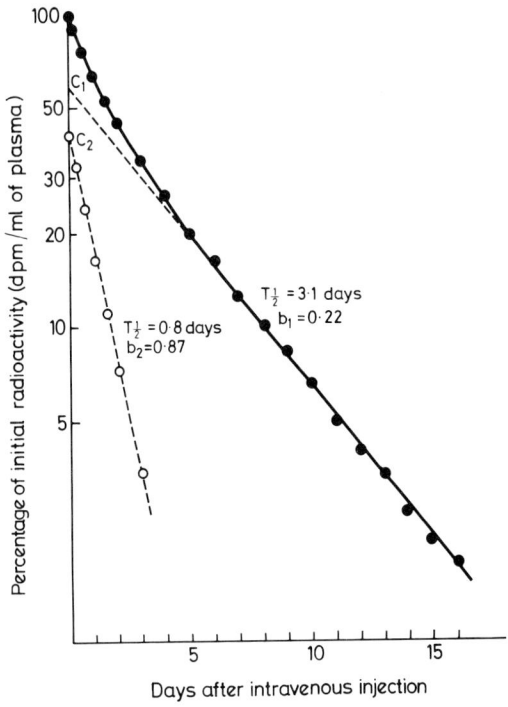

Figure 11.6
The turnover of LDL in a 54-year-old normal man, as shown by the fall in plasma radioactivity (●) after an intravenous injection of 25 μCi of ^{125}I-labelled autologous LDL (density 1.019–1.063 g/ml). The log-linear portion of the curve ($T_{\frac{1}{2}} = 3.1$ days) was extrapolated to zero time; the lower curve ($T_{\frac{1}{2}} = 0.8$ days) was derived by subtracting the extrapolated line from the observed values. The FCR was calculated from the equation:

$$FCR = [C_1/b_1 + C_2/b_2]^{-1},$$

where C_1 and C_2 are the intercepts shown on the vertical axis, and b_1 and b_2 are the rate constants of the two exponential curves (calculated as $\log_e 2 \div T_{\frac{1}{2}}$). (For further details of the method of calculation, see Matthews, 1957.)

expected to have a marked influence on the plasma cholesterol concentration. For this reason, a good deal of attention has been paid to the effects of diet, drugs and hormones upon the metabolism of the plasma LDL in man. The effects of some of these agents on the metabolism of LDL-apoB are listed in Table 11.5. (LDL metabolism is modified profoundly in familial hypercholesterolaemia, but this is dealt with at length in Chapter 15). Although some of the effects shown in Table 11.5 may be accompanied by changes in the cholesterol:protein ratio of LDL, such changes are usually small, so that the plasma LDL-apoB concentration closely reflects LDL cholesterol concentration under most conditions.

Diets low in cholesterol and rich in polyunsaturated fat lower the plasma LDL concentration by increasing the FCR of LDL-apoB. The mechanism by which this increase in LDL catabolism is brought about is not understood, but it could conceivably be due to an effect on the lipid composition of LDL such that the LDL particles interact more readily with those cells in which they are catabolized, as discussed in Section 3.4.3 above. Cholestyramine and nicotinic acid both lower the plasma LDL concentration, though by different mechanisms. Cholestyramine increases the FCR by stimulating LDL catabolism, but nicotinic acid depresses the synthesis of LDL-apoB without affecting its catabolism. Since LDL-apoB is derived from VLDL, and since nicotinic acid decreases VLDL secretion by the

Table 11.5
The effects of diet, drugs and hormones on the metabolism of the plasma LDL-apoB in human subjects

Condition	Plasma LDL-apoB		Synthesis*
	Concentration	FCR (fraction of IV pool/day)	
Diet low in cholesterol and high in P/S	↓	↑	→
Nicotinic acid (4–5 g/day)	↓	→	↓
Cholestyramine (20–30 g/day)	↓	↑	→
Myxoedema	↑	↓	↓
Thyrotoxicosis	↓	↑	↑

* The rate of synthesis (mg of LDL-apoB synthesized/kg/day) is assumed to be equal to the absolute rate of catabolism (estimated from the mass of LDL-apoB in the intravascular pool and the FCR determined in the steady state). ↓ = decrease; ↑ = increase; → = no significant change; P/S = ratio of polyunsaturated to saturated fat.

Results for diet and drugs obtained mainly from patients with primary hyperbetalipoproteinaemia (Type II) (see Eisenberg and Levy (1975) and Walton et al. (1965)).

liver, it is possible that the effect of nicotinic acid on LDL-apoB synthesis is mediated by an effect on the secretion of VLDL (see Carlson and Walldius (1972) and Chapter 10, Section 5.5 for discussion of this point).

In myxoedema, both the rate of synthesis of LDL-apoB and the FCR are decreased; in thyrotoxicosis the opposite occurs (Walton et al., 1965). Thompson et al. (1980) have compared the rates of catabolism of native LDL and cyclohexanedione-treated LDL (see Chapter 15, Section 3.4.3.3) in a myxoedematous patient before and after treatment with thyroxine. Their findings suggest that the low FCR of LDL in myxoedema is due predominantly to a reversible defect in the receptor-mediated pathway for LDL catabolism. However, it should be noted that there is also a decrease in the rate of catabolism of plasma albumin (Rothschild et al., 1957) and total body protein (Crispell et al., 1956) in myxoedema, suggesting that a nonspecific effect on protein metabolism makes some contribution to the low FCR of LDL in this disorder. The plasma LDL concentration falls in the presence of increased secretion of thyroid hormone and rises in the presence of diminished secretion, presumably because in both states the effect on FCR is greater than that on synthesis of LDL-apoB.

There is a disagreement about the effects of sex hormones on LDL metabolism. Walton et al. (1965) found that the rate of synthesis and the FCR of LDL-apoB were both higher in women than in men, but Langer et al. (1972) failed to observe these sex differences. In diabetes, hyperlipidaemia is often present, though the abnormal lipoprotein pattern underlying the raised plasma lipid concentration is variable. The limited amount of information available suggests that in diabetics with increased plasma LDL concentration but normal VLDL concentration (type II hyperlipoproteinaemia, as defined in Chapter 15) the hyperlipidaemia is associated with increased synthesis of LDL-apoB with no significant change in FCR (Scott et al., 1970). The hyperlipidaemia of the nephrotic syndrome also appears to be accompanied by increased synthesis of LDL protein (Scott et al., 1970). The effect of clofibrate on LDL metabolism is variable. In primary type II hyperlipoproteinaemia, clofibrate usually has little or no effect on the plasma lipid concentration, but in a few patients with this plasma abnormality, clofibrate in maximal doses depresses the rate of synthesis of LDL-apoB without altering the FCR (Scott and Hurley, 1969), the net effect being a fall in plasma LDL concentration. In some patients with increased plasma VLDL concentration, treatment with clofibrate leads not only to a fall in VLDL concentration but also to a temporary rise in LDL concentration (Strisower et al., 1968). This paradoxical response to clofibrate may be explained by a combination of inhibition of VLDL output from the liver and stimulation of VLDL catabolism in the circulation. Since VLDL is the precursor of LDL, the effect of this dual mechanism would be to cause an initial increase in the rate of production of LDL, followed by a new steady state in which LDL production was diminished. Reciprocal changes in the plasma concentrations of LDL and VLDL have also been noted during weight reduction, when plasma VLDL concentration usually falls, and during the taking of a carbohydrate-rich diet, when plasma VLDL concentration rises (Wilson and Lees, 1972). These reciprocal changes may be explained in terms of effects on the rate of catabolism of VLDL.

3.6.3 The site of catabolism of LDL

If we are to understand the part played by LDL in the movement of cholesterol between the liver and the extrahepatic tissues, we need to know which tissues are responsible for the uptake and catabolism of LDL. In so far as some of the lipids of LDL may be transferred to other lipoproteins by exchange or net transport (see Sections 4 and 5 below), it is, of course, possible that the different components of an LDL particle are not all taken up initially by the same tissues. Nevertheless, the work described in Chapter 9 shows that the cells of many tissues are capable of taking up whole LDL particles, including their lipid and protein components. To this extent, the initial steps in the disposal of the circulating LDL must be reflected in the uptake and catabolism of LDL-apoB. However, despite the importance of the question, there is disagreement as to which tissues are mainly responsible for catabolizing LDL-apoB in the intact animal or human subject.

The perfused rat liver catabolizes the apoB of LDL at a rate at least equal to the rate of catabolism observed *in vivo* (Hay *et al.*, 1971), suggesting that the liver is the main site of catabolism of LDL in the intact animal. In keeping with this, a larger proportion of an intravenous dose of ^{125}I-LDL is recoverable from the liver than from any other organ in rats (Eisenberg *et al.*, 1973) and pigs (Sniderman *et al.*, 1975) killed at various times after the injection. This suggests that most of the extravascular pool of LDL is in the liver and is therefore within, or adjacent to, the hepatocytes. However, the capacity of an isolated liver to degrade LDL does not necessarily reflect the rate of catabolism of LDL by the liver in the presence of other tissues in the intact animal, several of which are known to be capable of degrading LDL *in vitro*. Indeed, Sniderman *et al.* (1974) have shown that the rate of catabolism of the apoB of autologous LDL in pigs is not diminished by removal of the liver. This might suggest that catabolism takes place predominantly in the extrahepatic tissues. It is consistent with this that LDL-like lipoproteins derived from the plasma are present in the d <1.063 fraction of lymph draining the human foot (Reichl et al., 1973; 1978), demonstrating that at least a part of the extravascular pool of LDL is in the interstitial fluids of the peripheral tissues, where it would be accessible to fibroblasts and other non-hepatic cells capable of taking up and degrading LDL particles. However, as discussed in Chapter 9, in the absence of any information about the extent to which LDL receptors are expressed by cells *in vivo* it is impossible to deduce the contribution of extra-hepatic cells to LDL degradation in the living animal merely from a consideration of the behaviour of cells in culture under conditions in which receptor activity is maximal. It should also be noted that the physiological relevance of experiments on LDL catabolism in totally hepatectomized animals has been questioned by van Tol *et al.* (1978), who have shown that in rats the rate of catabolism of the apoB of LDL is considerably reduced by *partial* hepatectomy. This suggests that the liver does, in fact, make a significant contribution to LDL catabolism in the whole body. Further support for this has been obtained from experiments on the cumulative uptake of labelled LDL in the tissues of intact animals. Pittman *et al.* (1979) have shown that when LDL labelled with covalently-linked [^{14}C]sucrose is injected intravenously, the [^{14}C]sucrose accumulates in the lysosomes of tissues in which LDL is taken up and catabolized. Using this technique they have shown that up to 40% of a dose of labelled LDL injected into a pig is catabolized in the liver.

Uptake and catabolism of LDL by the liver raises the question as to which cell type (whether hepatocytes, Kupffer cells or endothelial cells of the sinusoids) is responsible for this process. For a discussion of the probable site of uptake of LDL and of other lipoproteins by the rat's liver, see Kuusi *et al.* (1979).

There is no clinical or experimental evidence as to the sites of catabolism of LDL in man, though we know that human fibroblasts, aortic smooth-muscle cells and vascular endothelial cells can degrade LDL (see Chapter 9). The ability of intact human liver cells to take up and degrade human LDL *in vitro* does not seem to have been studied, but is clearly a question of considerable interest in relation to LDL catabolism in man. The role of LDL receptors in the catabolism of LDL in the living human body is discussed in Chapter 15.

3.7 The metabolism of HDL

The turnover of the plasma HDL can be investigated by methods similar in principle to those described for LDL in Section 3.6.1 above. Measurement of the turnover of the protein of HDL is complicated by the presence of several apoproteins in HDL, all of which become labelled when the lipoprotein is labelled with radioiodine. This difficulty can be overcome in two ways. In the method of Blum *et al.*

(1977) all the proteins of the sample of HDL to be injected intravenously are labelled by labelling the unfractionated HDL. Radioactivity is then measured serially in the apoA-I and apoA-II isolated from the subject's HDL by column chromatography. Alternatively, apo-A-I or apoA-II in the injected HDL can be labelled selectively by labelling the purified apoprotein and then incorporating it into native unlabelled HDL by exchange (Shepherd et al., 1978). Observations on the turnover of labelled apoC proteins in HDL do not provide information about the true rate of catabolism of HDL since apoC proteins equilibrate rapidly between HDL and VLDL, as described in Section 3.5.3.

In normal human subjects given an intravenous injection of ^{125}I-labelled HDL the specific activities of apoA-I and apoA-II decline in parallel, with an initial rapid fall merging into an exponential phase with a half-life of 5 to 6 days. Analysis of the plasma and urinary radioactivity curves in terms of a two-compartment model of the distribution and catabolism of apoA-I and apoA-II (Blum et al., 1977) shows that about 40% of the total exchangeable HDL protein is extravascular and that the net rate of synthesis of apoA-I plus apoA-II is about 8 mg/kg/day in normal subjects. Furthermore, when the FCR of HDL protein is increased by carbohydrate feeding or is decreased by treatment with nicotinic acid, the proportional changes in the catabolism of apoA-I and apoA-II are virtually identical, indicating that the two major apoproteins of HDL are catabolized together as a unit. However, when the apoA-I and apoA-II of HDL are labelled by exchange, the FCR of apoA-I is higher than that of apoA-II (Shepherd et al., 1978).

Until recently, much less attention was paid to the metabolism of HDL than to that of LDL. However, increasing evidence to suggest that the plasma HDL protects against atherosclerosis is beginning to arouse interest in various intrinsic and environmental factors that influence the plasma HDL cholesterol concentration in man. Some of these are discussed in Chapter 12. As yet, we have only a limited amount of information about the mechanisms by which changes in plasma HDL concentration are brought about. The fall that tends to occur during carbohydrate feeding is accompanied by an increase in the FCR of the circulating pool of apoA-I and apoA-II, whereas the increase induced by nicotinic acid treatment is associated with a decrease in FCR (Blum et al., 1977). Shepherd et al. (1978) have also shown that the rate of synthesis of HDL apoA-I is decreased by diets rich in polyunsaturated fat; this may help to explain the fall in plasma HDL cholesterol concentration observed by some, though not all, workers in human subjects fed polyunsaturated-fat diets. During carbohydrate feeding there is an increase in plasma VLDL concentration, in addition to the fall in HDL concentration. This reciprocal relationship may possibly be explained in terms of the contribution of VLDL surface components to the genesis of mature HDL within the circulation, as discussed in Section 3.5.3 above. Other examples of reciprocal changes in VLDL and HDL cholesterol concentration have been discussed by Wilson and Lees (1972). But it should be noted that reciprocity is by no means the rule; alcohol, for example, tends to increase the plasma concentration of both VLDL and HDL.

The liver is generally considered to be the major site of the catabolism of HDL, though none of the evidence for this view is decisive. Rachmilewitz *et al.* (1972) have shown that the livers of rats injected with ^{125}I-labelled rat HDL accumulate a larger proportion of the injected dose in trichloroacetic acid-precipitable form than does any other tissue. This in itself does not prove that the liver catabolizes HDL. However, Rachmilewitz *et al.* were able to show that much of the radioactivity taken up by the liver is adjacent to secondary lysosomes within the parenchymal cells and, furthermore, that the intrahepatic ^{125}-I-labelled protein rapidly loses its immunoreactivity to antibody to rat HDL. These observations strongly suggest that the labelled HDL in the liver does, indeed, undergo proteolytic degradation by lysosomal proteases. That the liver plays a significant role in the degradation of HDL is also suggested by the observations of Nakai *et al.* (1976), who have shown that isolated rat-liver parenchymal cells take up and degrade rat HDL_3 (the lipoprotein of d 1.10–1.21 g/ml), apparently by a mechanism requiring specific cell-surface receptors for HDL. Experiments showing that a broken cell preparation of liver can hydrolyze the protein component of HDL are not strictly relevant to the site of degradation of HDL *in vivo*, since they beg the question as to how far liver cells are capable of taking up and internalizing HDL molecules in the plasma. The possibility that HDL is catabolized in extrahepatic tissues cannot be excluded, since several types of human cell in culture, including aortic smooth-muscle cells (Bierman and Albers, 1975), vascular endothelial cells (Stein and Stein, 1976) and fibroblasts (Miller *et al.*, 1977) take up and catabolize HDL at a measurable rate. The observations of Carew *et al.* (1976) that the FCR of HDL protein in pigs does not decrease after an operation for portacaval anastomosis also suggests that the liver is not the only site of HDL catabolism.

In conclusion, in view of the heterogeneity of HDL (which may well turn out to be even greater than is now recognized), one should not assume that all lipoprotein particles within what is operationally defined as the HDL fraction are metabolized identically. Indeed, there is growing evidence to suggest that the apoE-rich subfraction of HDL is taken up avidly by the liver via high-affinity apoE receptors, presumed to be present on the surfaces of the hepatocytes (see, for example, Quarfordt *et al.*, 1980 and Sherrill *et al.*, 1980).

4 THE ORIGIN AND TURNOVER OF THE PLASMA ESTERIFIED CHOLESTEROL

The plasma cholesteryl esters have been mentioned at several points in this chapter in relation to the chemical composition, biogenesis and intravascular metabolism of the plasma lipoproteins. We must now turn more specifically to the origin of the cholesteryl esters within each lipoprotein fraction and to their turnover within the plasma.

4.1 Origin

4.1.1 Man

In human subjects in the fasting state (when the intestinal secretion of triglyceride-rich lipoproteins is minimal) the bulk of the esterified cholesterol in the plasma is probably formed, directly or indirectly, by the LCAT reaction within the circulation. The evidence for this, discussed in detail by Glomset (1968) and Myant (1971), may be summarized as follows:

(1) The fatty-acid pattern of the cholesteryl esters of the HDL, LDL and VLDL of human plasma obtained in the fasting state is similar to the fatty-acid pattern at C-2 of the plasma lecithin (predominantly 18:2 under normal dietary conditions) and is different from the pattern that would result from esterification by ACAT (mainly 18:1).

(2) The rate of esterification of free cholesterol by the LCAT reaction in human plasma *in vitro* is sufficient to account for the rate of turnover of the plasma cholesteryl esters measured in normal human subjects *in vivo* (see Section 4.2 for method of measurement).

(3) The relative initial rates of esterification of the free cholesterol in the different lipoprotein fractions of human plasma are the same *in vitro* as *in vivo*; in both cases the initial rates decrease in the order HDL > VLDL > LDL. This would be expected if the cholesteryl esters are formed primarily by the action of LCAT on the free cholesterol of HDL and are then transferred to other lipoproteins, as discussed below.

(4) Esterified cholesterol is almost completely absent from the 'fasting' plasma of patients with inherited deficiency of LCAT. The small quantity of esterified cholesterol in plasma taken from these patients in the fasting state probably enters the circulation in the VLDL secreted by the intestine, since this esterified cholesterol becomes labelled when radioactive free cholesterol is given by mouth, but is not labelled after an intravenous injection of radioactive mevalonate (Norum and Gjone, 1967).

Since VLDL and LDL are relatively poor substrates for LCAT *in vitro*, it has been suggested that the cholesteryl esters of human plasma in the fasting state originate primarily in HDL by the action of LCAT on nascent HDL, and that they are then transferred to VLDL. In agreement with this, Nichols and Smith (1965) have shown that when whole human serum is incubated at 37 °C, cholesteryl esters are transferred in bulk from HDL to VLDL in exchange for triglyceride, and that this bulk transfer of cholesteryl ester continues when the LCAT in the serum is inhibited. Since each VLDL particle contains more than enough cholesteryl ester to account for the amount of cholesteryl ester in an LDL particle, all the esterified cholesterol in human LDL could be derived from VLDL, though the possibility that some esterification of cholesterol occurs in LDL cannot be excluded, since LCAT can use LDL as substrate (Glomset, 1968). A mechanism by which the cholesteryl esters of LDL are derived mainly from HDL *via* VLDL and IDL would explain the observation that when radioactive free cholesterol is injected intravenously into a fasting man, the specific radioactivity of esterified cholesterol in each of the three lipoprotein fractions rises in the manner shown in Fig. 11.8. However, it is possible that VLDL itself may act to a limited extent as substrate for LCAT *in vivo*, since the rate of formation of esterified cholesterol by LCAT in whole plasma is increased when the VLDL concentration is raised. The formation of esterified cholesterol with VLDL as substrate could also explain the curious anomaly that the fractional rate of esterification of cholesterol in the plasma of patients with Tangier disease (a condition in which HDL is absent from the plasma) may be nearly normal (Assmann *et al.*, 1978).

In the fed state the situation differs considerably from that discussed above, in that cholesteryl esters formed by ACAT in the intestinal wall enter the circulation in VLDL and chylomicrons. These esters have oleate as their predominant fatty acid. Hence, the fatty-acid pattern of the VLDL cholesteryl esters changes markedly during the absorption of fat. It is perhaps worth noting that, contrary to what was thought a few years ago, cholesteryl esters exchange between the lipoproteins of plasma, though at a slower rate than the rate at which free cholesterol exchanges (see Section 5 below). This exchange probably accounts for the fact that although the fatty-acid pattern of the HDL cholesteryl esters is similar to that of the C-2 fatty acids of lecithin, the two patterns are not identical. In particular, the HDL cholesteryl esters have more 16:1 and less 20:4 fatty acid than the C-2 of lecithin (Goodman, 1965). This would be expected if there is some molecule-for-molecule exchange of esterified cholesterol between HDL and the VLDL secreted in the fed state. Thus, the fatty-acid pattern of the cholesteryl esters present in HDL during the fasting state must be influenced by that of the cholesteryl esters of VLDL previously secreted during the absorption of dietary fat.

4.1.2 Rats

LCAT activity has been demonstrated in the plasma of many vertebrates, including reptiles and amphibians (Gillett, 1978). However, what we know about the origin of the plasma cholesteryl esters of rats suggests that the LCAT reaction is not as important a source of plasma esterified cholesterol in non-human species as it appears to be in man.

The plasma LCAT is probably responsible for the formation of the cholesteryl esters of rat HDL, since their fatty-acid pattern is similar to that of the fatty acids on C-2 of the plasma lecithin (predominantly 20:4) and is different from that of the fatty-acid pattern of the cholesteryl esters of rat liver (mainly 18:1); in keeping with this, the pattern of the fatty acids transferred *in vitro* to radioactive free cholesterol by the LCAT in rat plasma (20:4 > 18:2 > 18:1) (Portman and Sugano, 1964) is similar to the fatty-acid pattern of the cholesteryl esters of rat HDL (Table 11.2). On the other hand, the composition of the VLDL cholesteryl esters in the plasma of fasting rats (18:1 the predominant fatty acid) is not consistent with formation by the LCAT reaction and suggests, rather, that these cholesteryl esters are formed in the liver, presumably by ACAT. That the VLDL particles secreted by the rat's liver do indeed contain esterified cholesterol is indicated by the observation of Mahley *et al.* (1969) that nascent VLDL particles isolated from the Golgi apparatus of rat liver contain cholesteryl ester in roughly the same proportion as that found in the circulating VLDL (about 10% of the total lipid). Since ACAT is a microsomal enzyme and is therefore very close to the enzymes concerned in the synthesis and assembly of other components of VLDL, it is understandable that, at any rate in rats, esterified cholesterol should be incorporated into the VLDL particle at some stage in its formation. The cholesteryl esters of the triglyceride-rich particles secreted by the rat's intestine during the absorption of fat are formed by ACAT and therefore contain oleate (18:1) as their predominant fatty acid.

4.2 Turnover

Under steady-state conditions the whole mass of plasma cholesteryl esters turns over at a constant rate owing to their continual formation by the esterification of free cholesterol and their removal at an equal rate, largely as a consequence of the catabolism of plasma lipoproteins. In rats, the main site of catabolism is probably the liver, where the bulk of the cholesteryl esters of IDL and, possibly, HDL are catabolized. In man, however, the liver may play a smaller role in the hydrolysis of plasma esterified cholesterol than those extra-hepatic tissues in which LDL is taken up and catabolized.

Turnover of the plasma esterified cholesterol may be expressed either as the fraction of the total pool replaced in unit time (*fractional rate of turnover*) or as the total mass replaced in unit time (*absolute rate of turnover*). It is also meaningful to consider the fractional and absolute rates of turnover of the cholesteryl esters within a particular lipoprotein fraction and within a particular fatty-acid class (e.g. the esters with 20:4 fatty acids *versus* those with 18:2 fatty acids). Quantitative information about the turnover of the plasma cholesteryl esters is essential for a full understanding of the transport and metabolism of cholesterol in the body as a whole under physiological conditions and in many disorders of lipid metabolism. In this section we shall consider dynamic aspects of the plasma esterified cholesterol.

4.2.1 Methods of measurement

As described below, the rate of esterification of the plasma free cholesterol may be estimated *in vivo* from the time-course of the incorporation of labelled cholesterol, or of a labelled precursor of cholesterol, into the plasma esterified cholesterol. If these estimates are combined with measurements *in vitro* of LCAT activity and of the net rate of esterification of free cholesterol in the whole plasma, it is often possible to deduce whether differences in the rate of esterification measured *in vivo* under different conditions are due to differences in the concentration of active enzyme or in the concentration or accessibility of the substrate. In this connection it may be noted that when abnormal lipoproteins, such as LP-X, are present in the plasma it may be difficult to estimate the rate of esterification of cholesterol *in vitro* with a method depending on the use of labelled exogenous free cholesterol, owing to uncertainty as to how far the labelled substrate equilibrates with the free cholesterol in the abnormal lipoprotein. In such cases, it may be better to measure the rate of esterification *in vitro* with a non-isotopic method (see Chapter 5, Section 3.4).

If a single dose of radioactive acetate or mevalonate is injected intravenously into a normal human subject, the specific radioactivities of the total free and total esterified cholesterol in the plasma rise and fall in the manner shown in Fig. 11.7. The labelled free cholesterol, synthesized in the liver during a brief period after the pulse of labelled precursor, enters the plasma mainly by exchange with the free cholesterol in plasma lipoproteins, the specific radioactivity of the plasma free cholesterol rising to a maximum in 4–6 hours and then falling as the radioactive molecules are replaced by unlabelled ones. As the radioactive free cholesterol is esterified, radioactivity begins to appear in the plasma cholesteryl esters, rising to a maximum at the point where the radioactivity curves for free and esterified cholesterol intersect (usually 2–3 days after the injection). The two curves then decline in parallel, the curve for esterified cholesterol remaining slightly higher than that for free cholesterol. If the reasonable assumption is made that the plasma cholesteryl esters are synthesized from the plasma free cholesterol, or from a pool of free cholesterol in rapid equilibrium with that in the plasma, the fractional rate of turnover of the plasma esterified cholesterol may be calculated from the two specific radioactivity curves by the method described by Zilversmit (1960) for calculating the fractional rate of turnover of a labelled product derived from a labelled precursor *in vivo* (Nestel and Monger, 1967) (see Fig. 11.7 legend). The absolute rate of turnover may then be calculated from the fractional rate and the total amount of esterified cholesterol in the whole plasma volume. In so far as there may be a small amount of esterified cholesterol in

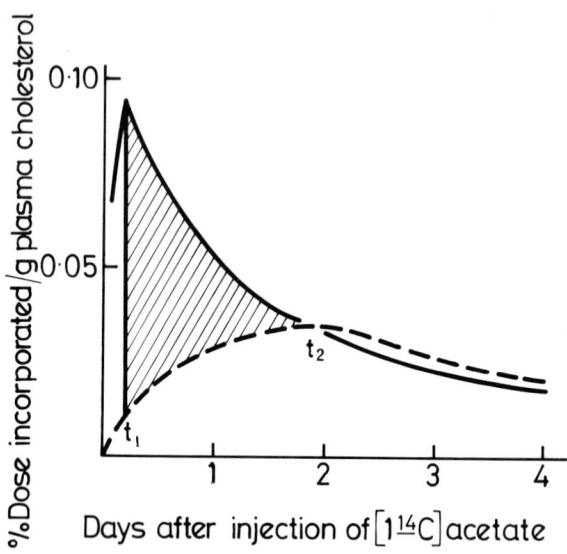

Figure 11.7
Time-course of the incorporation of ^{14}C into free (———) and esterified (-----) plasma total cholesterol after an intravenous injection of [1-^{14}C]acetate into a normal human subject. The two specific activity curves intersect at the maximum of the curve for esterified cholesterol.

The fractional rate of turnover (FRT) of the total mass of esterified cholesterol in the plasma may be calculated from the equation:

$$\mathrm{FRT} = \frac{(\mathrm{SA})_2 - (\mathrm{SA})_1}{A},$$

where $(\mathrm{SA})_1$ and $(\mathrm{SA})_2$ are the specific activities of the plasma esterified cholesterol at times t_1 and t_2, and A is the area enclosed by the two curves between t_1 and t_2 (shaded area). The quotient gives a fraction per unit of time and is usually expressed as the fraction of the total circulating esterified cholesterol that is replaced per hour or per day. (After Nestel and Monger, 1967.)

the liver in equilibrium with that in the plasma, estimates of the absolute rate of turnover of the plasma esterified cholesterol in man are not without error.

A method similar in principle to this may be used to measure the fractional and absolute rates of turnover of the esterified cholesterol in HDL, LDL and VLDL of human plasma *in vivo*, though such measurements are subject to error due to exchange of the labelled cholesteryl esters between the lipoprotein fractions. The relative rates of turnover of cholesteryl esters of different fatty-acid classes may also be measured by observing the time-course of incorporation of radioactive free cholesterol into cholesteryl esters separated by TLC on the basis of the number of double bonds in their fatty acyl residues.

The methods outlined above for measurement of the turnover of plasma cholesteryl esters in man cannot be applied to rats and other experimental animals in which a substantial fraction of the esterified cholesterol in the plasma is not derived from plasma free cholesterol. Sugano and Portman (1964) have obtained an approximate estimate of the rate of esterification of the plasma free cholesterol in rats *in vivo* by relating the amount of an intravenous dose of [^{14}C]cholesterol incorporated into the plasma cholesteryl esters to the mean specific activity of the plasma free cholesterol during the period of incorporation.

4.2.2 The rate of turnover *in vivo* and *in vitro*

In normal human subjects 2–3% of the whole plasma pool of esterified cholesterol is removed and resynthesized each hour (Nestel and Monger, 1967). In a 70-kg man with a normal plasma cholesteryl-ester concentration this would correspond to the esterification of about 100 mg of plasma free cholesterol/hour. Values for the rate of esterification of free cholesterol in human plasma *in vitro* have varied widely from one laboratory to another, partly because some workers have measured rates of esterification under conditions in which the substrate for LCAT was not rate-limiting, whereas others have measured net rates of esterification in the whole plasma without adjusting the substrate concentration. Most reported values for the rates of esterification in normal human plasma *in vitro* lie between 60 µmoles (23 mg) and 100 µmoles (39 mg) of cholesterol esterified/litre of plasma/hour, corresponding to the esterification of 80–130 mg of cholesterol/hour in the whole plasma of a 70-kg man. This is in surprisingly good agreement with the values estimated *in vivo* and is, of course, consistent with the hypothesis that the bulk of the plasma cholesteryl esters are formed by the esterification of free cholesterol within the plasma. In plasma from a given normal individual the rate measured *in vitro* under conditions of enzyme-saturation with substrate is usually higher than the rate measured in the subject's whole plasma with no adjustment of substrate concentration (Blomhoff, 1974). This suggests that the LCAT in the plasma *in vivo* is not saturated with substrate. However, this it not necessarily the case under abnormal conditions in which the capacity of the plasma LCAT is diminished.

Goodman has shown that all the cholesteryl esters in human plasma as a whole turn over at the same fractional rate *in vivo* irrespective of their fatty-acid composition, but that the fractional rate is different in the three major lipoprotein fractions, being highest in HDL, lowest in LDL and intermediate in VLDL. These differences in turnover may be seen by observing the initial appearance of radioactivity in the esterified cholesterol in the three lipoprotein fractions after an intravenous injection of [^{14}C]mevalonate (Fig. 11.8). The initial rate of rise of the specific radioactivity of esterified cholesterol increases in the order LDL < VLDL < HDL. Once the specific radioactivity of the cholesteryl esters has become equal in all three lipoproteins, owing to hydrolysis and re-esterification and to exchange between lipoproteins within the plasma, these differences can no longer be observed (usually at two to three days after the injection of labelled precursors). It should be noted that the rate at which esterified choles-

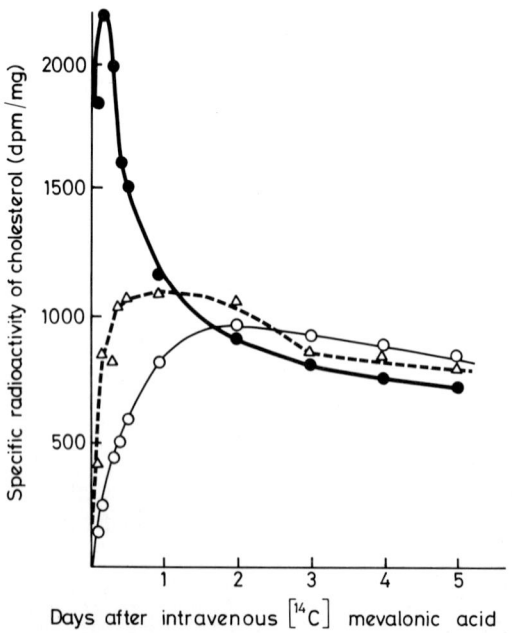

Fig. 11.8
Time-course of the incorporation of ^{14}C into plasma LDL free cholesterol (●) and into plasma esterified cholesterol in LDL (○) and HDL (△) after an intravenous injection of [2-^{14}C]mevalonate into a normal human subject. (From Myant *et al.*, 1973.)

terol molecules become randomized throughout the plasma by exchange must be slow in comparison with their rate of turnover. Unless this were so, it would be impossible to detect differences in the specific radioactivity of the cholesteryl esters in different lipoproteins during the first few hours after a single pulse of a radioactive precursor of cholesterol, as shown in Fig. 11.8.

In rats, the turnover of plasma esterified cholesterol differs in certain respects from that in man. The fractional rate of turnover of cholesteryl esters is higher in VLDL than in HDL or LDL. There also appear to be differences in the fractional rates of turnover of different cholesteryl esters in the whole plasma of rats. Goodman and Shiratori (1964) found a higher fractional rate in the 18:1 esters than in the esters with saturated or 20:4 fatty acids. They suggested that this reflected the relatively rapid turnover of VLDL cholesteryl esters synthesized in the liver by ACAT. However, Sugano and Portman (1964) have described observations suggesting that in rats the 20:4 cholesteryl esters in whole plasma turn over at a higher fractional rate than the esters with saturated or monounsaturated fatty acids.

Variations in the turnover of the plasma cholesteryl esters in health and disease have attracted a good deal of attention, but many of the conclusions drawn from observations *in vivo* and *in vitro* are contradictory or have not been generally confirmed. Two groups of workers have observed a positive correlation between the plasma free cholesterol concentration and the rate of esterification of cholesterol per ml of plasma *in vitro* in normal and hyperlipidaemic subjects (Monger and Nestel, 1967; Marcel *et al.*, 1971). As discussed elsewhere in this book, this correlation does not hold in the presence of severe liver disease or familial LCAT deficiency and is unlikely to hold in familial hypercholesterolaemia. Miller and Thompson (1973) have suggested that in so far as there is a correlation between free cholesterol concentration and rate of esterification *in vitro*, this is due to a correlation between free cholesterol concentration and the capacity of the plasma LCAT, and that this reflects a physiological mechanism by which the concentration of LCAT in the plasma rises or falls in parallel with the concentration of free cholesterol. Such a mechanism would go some way towards explaining the fact that under most conditions the ratio of esterified to total cholesterol in human plasma shows little or no variation over a very wide range of cholesterol concentrations.

In keeping with the idea that the plasma LCAT is in some way regulated in accordance with the load of substrate presented to it, the cholesterol-esterifying activity of the plasma *in vitro* (Nestel *et al.*, 1974) and the rate of turnover of the plasma esterified cholesterol *in vivo* (Sodhi, 1974) have been shown to be correlated with the flux of total cholesterol through the plasma (the 'production rate' discussed in Chapter 10). However, it must be pointed out that Blomhoff (1974) was unable to demonstrate a positive correlation between plasma free cholesterol concentration and rate of esterification of cholesterol *in vitro* under conditions in which the LCAT was saturated with substrate, though he was able to show a positive correlation when the rate of esterification was measured by the method of Stokke and Norum (1971), a method with which LCAT is not necessarily saturated. Hence, the tendency reported by some workers for net esterification to increase with increasing concentrations of plasma free cholesterol may merely reflect increasing saturation of LCAT at the higher concentrations of free cholesterol.

There is general agreement that the rate of esterification of the plasma cholesterol *in vivo* and *in vitro* is positively correlated with the plasma concentrations of triglyceride and VLDL in man. Nestel *et al.* (1974) have suggested that this reflects a correlation between the rate at which free cholesterol enters the blood circulation in triglyceride-rich lipoproteins and the activity of LCAT. In support of this, they have shown that the turnover of the plasma cholesteryl esters increases when the influx of newly-synthesized cholesterol into the plasma, secreted as VLDL, is stimulated by the administration of colestipol (a bile-acid sequestrant that stimulates hepatic synthesis of cholesterol by an action similar to that of cholestyramine). The mechanism responsible for the association between cholesteryl-ester turnover and the plasma VLDL concentration is not clear. Marcel and Vezina (1972) have shown that the rate of esterification of free cholesterol by human plasma *in vitro* is increased when the plasma concentration of triglyceride-rich lipoproteins is raised by adding VLDL or chylomicrons to the plasma *in vitro* or by giving the subject a fatty meal before taking blood for preparation of the plasma. However, it is impossible to tell whether this stimulatory effect is due to an increase in the supply of substrate for LCAT by the transfer of lecithin and free cholesterol from the surfaces of the triglyceride-rich particles to HDL, or to increased supply of the protein activators of LCAT (apoA-I and apoC-I). Nevertheless, these observations bring home the point that the conditions under which LCAT is assayed in plasma differ from those under which cholesterol is esterified in the circulation *in vivo*. In the former case, the system contains a limited supply of substrate, whereas in the latter case the substrate components in HDL are continually replenished from what amounts to an inexhaustible supply of surface components of triglyceride-rich particles.

In Section 3.5.3 above we considered the role of the LCAT reaction in catalyzing the esterification of the free cholesterol released from the surfaces of chylomicrons and VLDL particles during their catabolism within the circulation. Glomset and Norum (1973) have discussed the quantitative aspects of this process. In particular, they have considered the question as to how far the rate of esterification of plasma free cholesterol by LCAT *in vivo* matches the rate at which free cholesterol is released into the plasma during the catabolism of triglyceride-rich lipoproteins. A major difficulty in trying to answer this question is our lack of information about the rate of secretion of VLDL cholesterol into the circulation. However, by making several plausible assumptions, Glomset and Norum conclude that the rate at which free cholesterol is released into the circulation from chylomicrons and VLDL in a 70-kg man, eating 100 g of triglyceride/day, would be between 2.3 and 4.2 g/day, and that his rate of esterification of free cholesterol in the plasma and intestinal fluids would be between 2.8 and 5.6 g/day. These approximations suggest that the capacity of the LCAT reaction in human plasma *in vivo* is at least equal to the daily amount of free cholesterol released into the plasma from the triglyceride-rich lipoproteins. However, the above calculations do not take account of the free cholesterol secreted as HDL, or of the esterified cholesterol taken into the extra-hepatic tissues during the uptake and catabolism of LDL and HDL, and then released from the cells after intracellular hydrolysis. The problem of estimating how much cholesterol is recycled by this route is discussed in Section 6 below.

5 EXCHANGE OF LIPOPROTEIN CHOLESTEROL

5.1 Exchange of unesterified cholesterol

The unesterified cholesterol in plasma exchanges freely between the different lipoproteins and between lipoproteins and red cells. Exchange must also occur between the free cholesterol of plasma lipoproteins and that of the plasma membranes of all cells that are in contact with the intravascular or extravascular pools of plasma lipoprotein. These cells include the white blood cells, platelets, the cells of the vascular endothelium and, presumably, those of the liver and other tissues in which cholesterol exchanges rapidly with the plasma cholesterol. The exchange of free cholesterol between lipoproteins and red blood cells has been investigated in considerable detail (see Bruckdorfer and Graham, 1976), but we have little information about exchange of lipoprotein cholesterol with the plasma membranes of other cells under normal and pathological conditions.

The exchange of plasma free cholesterol with red-cell cholesterol, all of which is unesterified, was first demonstrated *in vitro* by Hagerman and Gould (1951), who showed that when dog red cells labelled with [^{14}C]cholesterol are incubated with unlabelled dog plasma, the specific activity of the free cholesterol in the red cells falls, while that in the plasma rises, the specific activities in the two components eventually becoming equal. Hagerman and Gould concluded that all the free cholesterol in plasma and red cells is exchangeable and, since the approach to complete equilibration was mono-exponential, that the cholesterol of red cells comprises a single pool. When the incubations were carried out at 37 °C, the rate of isotopic equilibration, expressed as a half-life (the time taken to reach half-equilibration), was 1.1 hours, corresponding to a turnover time of 1.6 hours. In so far as plasma and red-cell free cholesterol exchanges at the same rate *in vivo* as *in vitro*, this would mean that a mass of red-cell cholesterol equal to the amount present in the whole circulation is replaced by exchange with the plasma cholesterol about 15 times every 24 hours. It should be noted that although the free-cholesterol:phospholipid ratio is higher in red cells than in plasma lipoproteins, there is no net transfer of cholesterol between red cells and plasma during a 4-hour incubation. Thus, the term 'equilibration' in the present context refers to the achievement of equal specific activities in the two components of the plasma red-cell system, without change in the ratio of the concentrations of free cholesterol in plasma and red cells. Conditions under which net transfer does take place are considered below.

Exchange of free cholesterol between plasma, liver and red cells *in vivo* may be observed by following the changes in specific activity of the free cholesterol in these three components during the first few hours after an intravenous injection of a radioactive precursor of cholesterol. Fig. 11.9 shows, in an idealized form, the specific activity-time curves for free cholesterol obtained by Eckles *et al.* (1955) in dogs given injections of [^{14}C]acetate. The specific activity of free cholesterol rises most rapidly in the liver, reaching a maximum in less than 1 hour. Then, as free cholesterol newly synthesized in the liver exchanges with plasma free cholesterol, the specific activity of the free cholesterol in the liver falls and that in the plasma rises, reaching a maximum at about $1\frac{1}{2}$ hours. Lastly, radioactive cholesterol appears in the red cells owing to exchange with plasma free cholesterol, the specific activity reaching a maximum 3–8 hours after the injection. By making certain simplifying assumptions, the rate at which free cholesterol exchanges between plasma and liver, and between plasma and red cells, may be estimated from the rates at which the specific activities in the three compartments approach equality. Eckles *et al.* (1955) estimated that in their dogs the plasma free cholesterol equilibrated with liver free cholesterol with a half-life of about 20 minutes, and with red-cell cholesterol with a half-life of about 1.4 hours. Comparable observations on human subjects suggest that the rate of exchange of free

The Plasma Cholesterol: Composition and Metabolism 549

cholesterol between plasma and red cells *in vivo* is somewhat slower in man than in dogs (Gould *et al.*, 1955).

Gould's observations have been largely confirmed by other workers (see, for example, Porte and Havel, 1961) and have been extended to human blood. As in dog red cells, all the cholesterol of human red cells appears to behave as a single pool exchangeable with the free cholesterol in plasma. This is consistent with the conclusion of Lange *et al.* (1977) that flip-flop of cholesterol molecules between the two leaflets of the plasma membrane of the human red cell is relatively rapid. If this were not so, the cholesterol in the human red-cell membrane would behave as if it were separated into two compartments and the equilibration of labelled cholesterol between red cells and plasma would not be mono-exponential. There is some doubt as to how far the behaviour of the red-cell cholesterol in other species is similar to that in dogs and man. d'Hollander and Chevallier (1972) have concluded that rat red cells contain at least two pools of exchangeable cholesterol and, as discussed in Chapter 7, a substantial fraction of the cholesterol of pig red cells behaves as if it were non-exchangeable, or only very slowly exchangeable

Since free cholesterol exchanges between lipoproteins of different classes (Goodman, 1962; Roheim *et al.*, 1963), the exchange between red cells and whole plasma is clearly the net result of lipoprotein–

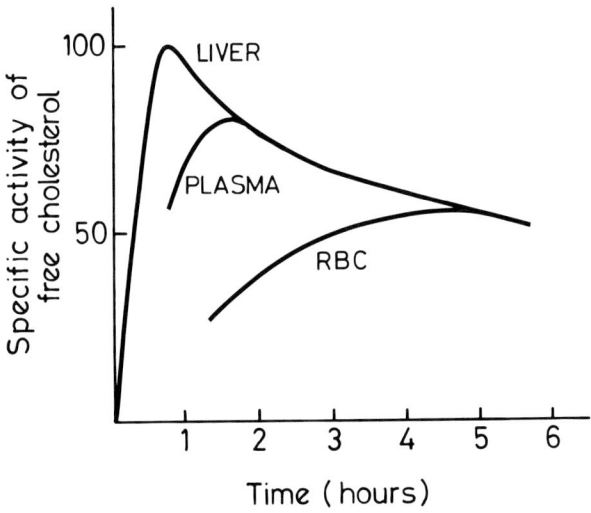

Figure 11.9
Time-course of the rise and fall in specific activity of free cholesterol in the liver, plasma and red blood cells of a dog given a single intravenous injection of [^{14}C]acetate. The relations between the three curves suggest that the free cholesterol of liver is the precursor of that in plasma, and that the free cholesterol of plasma is the precursor of that in red blood cells. (Based on the observations of Eckles *et al.*, 1955.)

lipoprotein and red cell-lipoprotein exchanges. The study of these multiple exchanges in mixtures of the isolated components in buffered solutions (Ashworth and Green, 1964; Quarfordt and Hilderman, 1970) has shown that exchange of free cholesterol occurs between LDL and HDL and between both these lipoproteins and red cells, and that equilibration between the two lipoproteins is more rapid than that between red cells and either lipoprotein.

5.2 Exchange with mass transfer

In the above experiments, and in the earlier work of Hagerman and Gould (1951), exchange occurred without change in the mass of free cholesterol in the red cells or lipoproteins, despite the fact that in some cases the concentration of lipoprotein free cholesterol relative to that of red-cell cholesterol was varied over a considerable range. However, under certain conditions, reversible bulk transfer of free cholesterol may occur at the same time as exchange. For example, if red cells are incubated with whole plasma at 37 °C for 24 hours, the red cells lose up to 40% of their cholesterol and the plasma cholesteryl ester concentration increases (Murphy, 1962). If the cholesterol-depleted cells are then incubated with cholesterol-enriched serum, the cholesterol content of the cells increases. The explanation of the initial loss of cholesterol from the cells is that during prolonged incubation in normal plasma, LCAT esterifies a substantial fraction of the plasma free cholesterol, causing a net movement of free cholesterol from the red-cell membranes to the free-cholesterol-depleted lipoproteins. Reversible mass transfer of free cholesterol, together with exchange, also occurs when rat-liver mitochondria are incubated with serum lipoproteins. In this case, however, the net movement is from lipoproteins to mitochondria, resulting in a considerably increased cholesterol:phospholipid ratio in the inner and outer mitochondrial membranes (Graham and Green, 1970).

Changes in the cholesterol content of the circulating red cells, apparently due to net uptake of plasma free cholesterol by the cells, also occur in several pathological conditions. In cholesterol-fed guinea-pigs (Sardet *et al.*, 1972) and in human subjects with familial LCAT deficiency (Gjone *et al.*, 1968) or obstructive jaundice (Cooper, 1977), the plasma contains abnormal lipoproteins enriched with unesterified cholesterol and this abnormality is accompanied by a marked increase in the cholesterol:phospholipid ratio of the red-cell membranes and in their cholesterol content. The consequent changes in the physical properties of these red cells are discussed in Chapters 16 and 18. When the abnormal red cells are incubated in normal plasma, they lose their excess of cholesterol to the lipoproteins in the medium and their cholesterol:phospholipid ratio returns to the normal level. In human familial abetalipoproteinaemia, and in the abetalipoproteinaemia of rats treated with orotic acid, the cholesterol:phospholipid ratio of the red-cell membranes is significantly increased (McBride and Jacob, 1970). This change in the lipid composition of the red cells must be due to the absence of LDL in the plasma, since it can be reversed by incubating the abnormal cells in normal plasma or in abetalipoproteinaemic plasma to which LDL has been added. The lipid composition of the red cells of patients with FH has been reported to be normal, despite the considerable increase in the concentration of LDL free cholesterol and in the LDL free cholesterol:phospholipid ratio that occurs in these patients; there is, however, a significant increase in the cholesterol:phospholipid ratio of the plasma membranes of the platelets in FH (Shattil *et al.*, 1977).

The conditions required for bulk transfer of free cholesterol, as distinct from molecule-for-molecule exchange, between plasma lipoproteins and cell membranes are not entirely clear. A change in the concentration of free cholesterol in the plasma may not, by itself, be sufficient to bring about a net transfer of cholesterol, since the cholesterol content of normal red cells is not changed by incubating the cells in plasma from patients with FH (Shattil *et al.*, 1977), in whom the plasma concentration of free cholesterol may be 2-3 times the normal level. However, net transfer, involving a redistribution of cholesterol, seems to occur invariably to or from the cells when red cells are exposed to plasma containing lipoproteins with a free cholesterol:phospholipid ratio widely different from that in the red-cell membrane, as in LCAT-deficient plasma *in vivo* or in plasma in which LCAT has been allowed to act for several hours *in vitro*.

Thus, with respect to the free cholesterol in a system containing lipoproteins and cell membranes, it is necessary to distinguish *exchange equilibration* from what may be called *partition equilibration*. Partition equilibration does not lead to a steady state in which the free cholesterol:phospholipid ratio is uniform throughout the system, because different biological membranes have different optimal free cholesterol:phospholipid ratios, the optimal ratio for a given species of membrane presumably depending upon the nature of its phospholipids and proteins. For example, red cells are capable, within limits, of maintaining a cholesterol:phospholipid ratio different from that in their environment, as may be seen from the fact that circulating red cells, while exchanging their cholesterol with the free cholesterol of the plasma lipoproteins, maintain a free cholesterol:phospholipid ratio higher than that in any of the lipoproteins of normal plasma, and that the ratio in the red cells of FH patients remains normal despite the increase in the free cholesterol:phospholipid ratio in LDL. How far these considerations apply to the interaction between plasma lipoproteins and cells other than the red cell is a matter for conjecture. The high cholesterol content of the red cells in abetalipoproteinaemia suggests that the LDL in normal plasma may act as an acceptor for red-cell cholesterol.

5.3 The mechanism of exchange of free cholesterol

Exchange of free cholesterol between plasma lipoproteins and red cells does not require metabolic energy, since complete and rapid exchange takes place between lipoproteins and red-cell ghosts. Nor is there any convincing evidence to suggest that the transfer of free cholesterol between lipoproteins and red cells, or between different lipoproteins, is mediated by a water-soluble cholesterol carrier. Perhaps the most plausible mechanism for exchange, first proposed in detail by Gurd (1960), is the formation of a transient complex at the point of contact between the outer leaflet of a cell plasma membrane and the surface lipids of a lipoprotein particle during a brief collision between cell and lipoprotein. As pointed out by Bruckdorfer and Graham (1976), fusion of the lipoprotein surface monolayer with the outer leaflet of a red-cell membrane would orientate the polar lipids in the manner shown in Fig. 11.10, leaving a hydrophobic channel lined by non-polar acyl chains through which cholesterol molecules would diffuse in both directions. Phospholipid molecules, being more polar, would not diffuse in this way, but could exchange more slowly by lateral diffusion through the fused monolayers. The core lipids of the lipoprotein would diffuse into the hydrophobic channel, but would cross the inner leaflet of the red-cell membrane only very slowly.

Presumably, the normal difference in the cholesterol:phospholipid ratios of red cells and lipoproteins is maintained at the site of the collision complex by the presence of the proteins and slowly-exchanging phospholipids in the red-cell membrane and the lipoprotein surface layer. A net transfer of free cholesterol, as in the conditions discussed in Section 5.2 above, could be mediated by the formation of a collision complex, the flux of molecules in the hydrophobic channel in one direction exceeding that in the opposite direction. It should be noted that the rate of exchange of free cholesterol between red cells and lipoproteins is probably not limited by the rate of collision between particles and cells, since the flux of cholesterol between red cells and plasma lipoproteins *in vitro* remains constant over a wide range of lipoprotein concentration (Quarfordt and Hilderman, 1970). A net movement of free cholesterol from plasma into the interior of fibroblasts and other cells must also occur during the internalization of lipoprotein particles by the mechanisms considered in Chapter 9.

The Plasma Cholesterol: Composition and Metabolism 553

For a discussion of the alternative possibility that free cholesterol exchanges between lipoproteins and between lipoproteins and cell surfaces by diffusion through the aqueous medium, see Phillips *et al.* (1980).

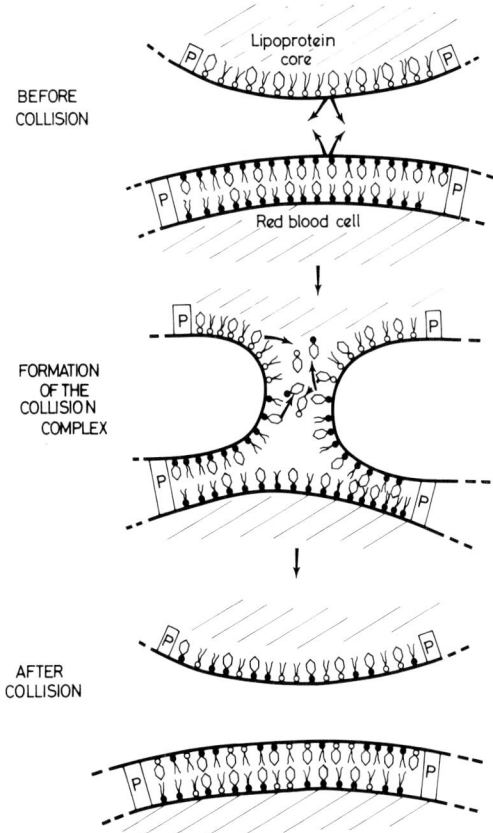

Figure 11.10
Possible mechanism by which free cholesterol exchanges between a lipoprotein particle and the plasma membrane of a red blood cell by the momentary formation of a collision complex. The fusion of the polar shell of the lipoprotein particle with the outer leaflet of the red-cell plasma membrane leads to the formation of a channel of non-polar lipid in which cholesterol molecules diffuse in both directions and are re-inserted at random into the two monolayers before separation of the particle from the red cell.

Phospholipid, ⊝⁓ , ●⁓
Cholesterol, ⊝⊐ , ●⊐
○ – originally in lipoprotein; ● = originally in red cell.

(From Bruckdorfer and Graham, 1976.)

5.4 Exchange of esterified cholesterol

The movement of esterified cholesterol between lipoprotein classes, analogous to that of free cholesterol, is negligible in rat plasma (Roheim *et al.*, 1963). As we saw in Section 4.2.2, exchange of cholesteryl esters between the lipoproteins of human plasma must also be comparatively slow, both *in vivo* and *in vitro*, since it would not otherwise be possible to detect differences between the rates of turnover of cholesteryl esters in HDL, LDL and VLDL by isotopic methods. However, contrary to the earlier view that cholesteryl esters do not undergo appreciable exchange between human plasma lipoproteins, more recent work has shown that there is both molecule-for-molecule exchange and bulk transfer of cholesteryl esters between the lipoproteins of whole plasma from man and other species in the presence of one or more cholesteryl-ester transfer proteins.

Zilversmit *et al.* (1975) showed that normal rabbit plasma contains a globulin capable of transferring esterified cholesterol between LDL and lipoproteins in the plasma fraction of density <1.019 g/ml from cholesterol-fed rabbits. Pattnaik *et al.* (1978) have also shown that a non-enzymic exchange of esterified cholesterol occurs between HDL and LDL in the presence of a protein isolated from the d >1.25 fraction of human plasma. This exchange is not associated with any net transfer of esterified cholesterol from one lipoprotein class to the other. Chajek and Fielding (1978) have described a transfer protein, present in the d >1.063 fraction of human plasma but distinct from apoE, that facilitates the bulk transfer of cholesteryl esters from HDL to VLDL and LDL. During the transfer of cholesteryl ester, triglyceride is transported from VLDL to HDL. A similar transfer protein in the d >1.25 fraction of human plasma had been described by Marcel *et al.* (1980). A mass transfer of cholesteryl esters from HDL_3 to VLDL during alimentary lipaemia has also been demonstrated in human subjects *in vivo* by Rose and Juliano (1979).

The transfer protein in human plasma is presumably responsible for the bulk movement of esterified cholesterol from HDL to VLDL in whole human plasma *in vitro*, described some years ago by Nichols and Smith (1965), and for the continuous redistribution of cholesteryl esters from HDL to VLDL and, indirectly, to LDL during the LCAT reaction *in vivo*. It is not known whether the exchange protein in human plasma described by Pattnaik *et al.* is or is not the same as the protein that brings about the bulk transfer of cholesteryl esters from HDL to VLDL. As mentioned in Section 6, Sniderman *et al.* (1978) have shown that cholesteryl esters are transferred in bulk from LDL to VLDL in the human splanchnic circulation *in vivo*, but the mechanism of this transfer has not been elucidated. A comparative study of plasma factors capable of effecting the transfer of cholesteryl esters between plasma lipoprotein fractions (Barter and Lally, 1979) has shown that an exchange or transfer protein is present in the d > 1.21 fraction of serum from rabbits, human subjects and guinea pigs but is not present in rat serum. Absence of an exchange protein from rat serum explains why cholesteryl esters do not exchange between the lipoproteins of rat plasma and suggests that in this respect the rat is the exception rather than the rule.

The transfer of cholesteryl esters between lipoprotein particles must involve the movement of cholesteryl-ester molelcules from the non-polar core of one particle to that of another. Pattnaik *et al.* (1978) suggest that one of the functions of the exchange protein they have described is to facilitate the passage of cholesteryl ester across the polar shell of a lipoprotein particle.

6 LIPOPROTEIN CHOLESTEROL METABOLISM: QUANTITATIVE ASPECTS

In this and the previous two chapters we have dealt with the metabolism of cholesterol and of lipoproteins to some extent as separate processes. In the final section of this chapter we shall consider how far the flow of cholesterol between different organs and tissues can be explained in terms of what is known of the rates and directions of flow of each class of plasma lipoprotein.

6.1 Turnover in plasma in relation to whole-body turnover

Figure 11.11 shows in diagrammatic form the major routes generally assumed to be followed by cholesterol molecules entering the plasma by synthesis or absorption of dietary cholesterol in man. The true state of affairs is, of course, much more complex than that shown in Fig. 11.11. In particular, net transfer of cholesterol between lipoprotein classes is ignored, other than the transfer of free cholesterol from triglyceride-rich lipoproteins to HDL that occurs as a result of the combined actions of lipoprotein lipase and LCAT; the redistribution of esterified cholesterol between lipoproteins and the hepatic uptake of IDL cholesteryl esters are shown in Fig. 11.12, which complements Fig. 11.11.

If it is assumed that the system as a whole is in the steady state and that the sole exit pathway from the system is by excretion of neutral steroids and bile acids via the bile into the intestine, then the rate of excretion of endogenous steroid (END) equals the production rate, or the total input of cholesterol into the system $(S_L + S_T + S_I + A)$. Cholesterol enters the plasma, in a net sense, in VLDL and HDL secreted by the liver and intestine, and in chylomicrons secreted by the intestine. In a normal human adult, the production rate of cholesterol is about 1 g/day, i.e. about 1 g of cholesterol must enter and leave the system each day. However, in the presence of a normal intake of fat, say 100 g/day, the intestine must secrete into the plasma about 3 g of cholesterol per day in chylomicrons (calculated from the cholesterol:triglyceride ratio in human chylomicrons and 100 g of triglyceride), plus additional amounts of cholesterol secreted in

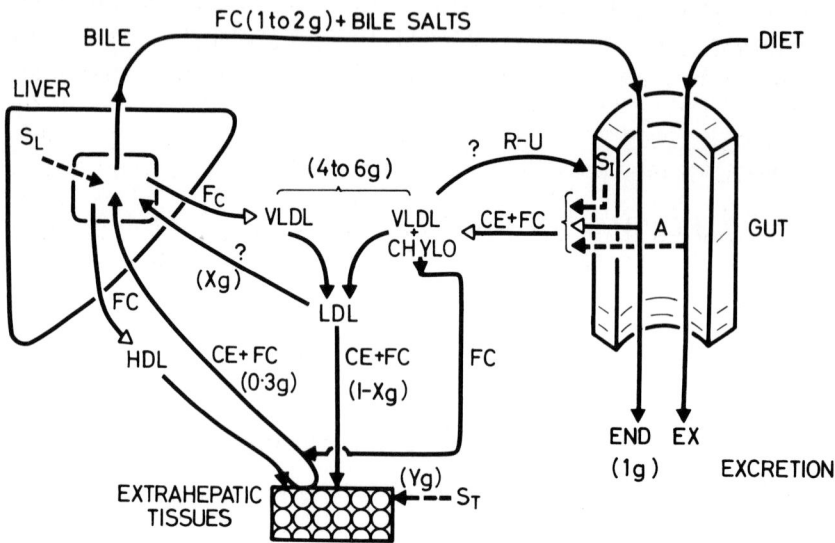

Figure 11.11
A diagrammatic representation of the main routes by which cholesterol enters and leaves the plasma of a normal human subject.

S_L, S_T, S_I; synthesis in liver, peripheral tissues and intestine.
A; absorbed dietary cholesterol.
CE; cholesteryl esters.
FC; free cholesterol.
R-U; re-utilized cholesterol.
END; faecal excretion of bile acids and endogenous neutral steroids.
EX; faecal excretion of unabsorbed dietary cholesterol.
---▶ ; net addition of cholesterol to the total system by synthesis or absorption of exogenous cholesterol.

The square box in the liver shows the entry of cholesterol into hepatic cholesterol pools derived from plasma lipoproteins and from synthesis *in situ*.
Values in parentheses show approximate rates of flow in g/day.
Assumptions: (1) A healthy 70-kg man in the steady state with respect to cholesterol, eating 100 g of fat/day.
(2) All loss of cholesterol from the system is by faecal excretion of bile acids or neutral steroid.
Ignored: (1) Net transfer between lipoproteins other than that of FC from chylomicrons to HDL.
(2) Conversion of cholesterol into steroid hormones.

VLDL and HDL. The total amount of cholesterol secreted in hepatic intestinal HDL is not known, but that secreted in VLDL is unlikely to be much less than 0.8 g/day and could be as high as 3 g/day (see Glomset and Norum, 1973). For convenience we may make the reasonable assumption that cholesterol synthesis in tissues other than liver and intestine is very small. Thus, the total amount of cholesterol entering the plasma in the presence of a normal fat intake probably lies between 4 and 6 g/day. Since this is considerably higher than the rate at which cholesterol leaves the whole system, there must be reutilization of cholesterol, a given cholesterol molecule entering the plasma (other than by simple exchange) on average more than once during its life in the body. Re-utilization could occur in the liver by incorporation of plasma lipoprotein cholesterol into nascent VLDL and HDL. It must also occur in the intestinal wall in so far as biliary cholesterol derived ultimately from plasma lipoproteins is partially reabsorbed and incorporated into the triglyceride-rich particles secreted by the intestine. Direct uptake of plasma cholesterol by

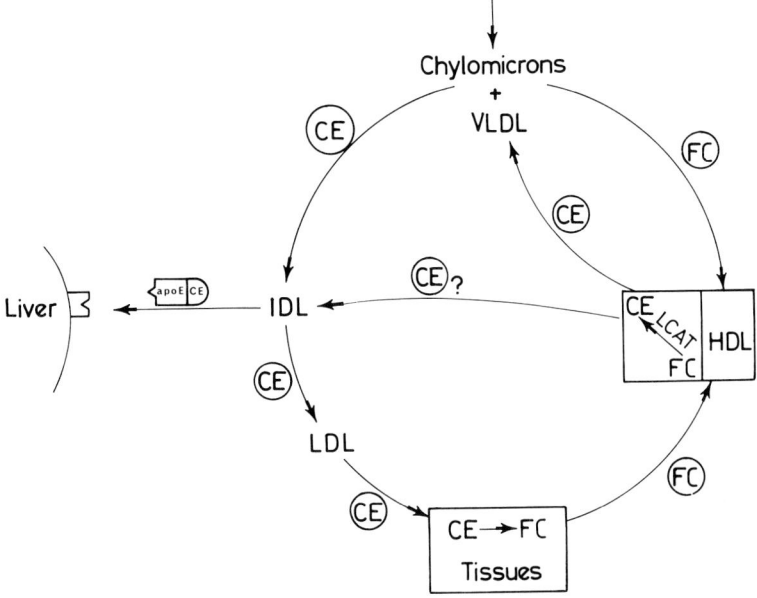

Figure 11.12
Diagram to show recycling of cholesterol between triglyceride-rich particles, HDL and extrahepatic tissues, with a possible leak of esterified cholesterol from IDL to the liver. Uptake of LDL and HDL by the liver and of HDL by extrahepatic tissues are ignored. A receptor for apoE is shown on the liver.

HDL, high-density lipoprotein; VLDL, very-low-density lipoprotein; IDL, intermediate-density lipoprotein; LDL, low-density lipoprotein; CE, cholesteryl ester; FC, free cholesterol; LCAT, lecithin:cholesterol acyltransferase. (Based on Glomset, 1979).

the intestine and its ultilization for lipoprotein synthesis cannot be excluded, but there is no evidence that this occurs in man.

Re-utilization of plasma cholesterol for hepatic synthesis of plasma lipoprotein raises the question of compartmentation of cholesterol in human liver. In rats, bile acids are derived preferentially from newly-synthesized hepatic free cholesterol (see Myant and Mitropoulos, 1977). However, Schwartz et al. (1978a, 1978b) have described experiments on the transfer of labelled cholesterol into biliary lipids in bile-fistula patients which suggest that in man the biliary cholesterol and bile acids are derived preferentially from a pool of hepatic free cholesterol to which HDL is the major contributor. This does not exclude the possibility that HDL cholesterol is also used for lipoprotein synthesis, but it is of considerable interest in relation to the site of uptake of HDL cholesterol in man (see below).

6.2 The pathways from plasma to liver

As well as the apparent discrepancy between the rate at which cholesterol enters the plasma and the rate at which it leaves the whole system, there is the question of the routes by which cholesterol secreted into the plasma finds it way to the liver.

In a normal man the catabolism of LDL (equivalent to 10–15 mg of apoB degraded/kg/day) must release at least 1 g of cholesterol per day. As discussed in Chapter 9, our knowledge of the site of catabolism of LDL is incomplete, but we do know that human extrahepatic tissues possess a specialized mechanism for the uptake and internalization of LDL, including its free and esterified cholesterol, and that extra-hepatic tissues of pigs have a capacity for uptake and degradation of LDL in vivo about equal to that of the liver (Pittman et al., 1979). Moreover, human fibroblasts and arterial smooth-muscle cells in culture have a limited capacity for uptake and degradation of HDL. Hence, even if we assume that a significant fraction of the circulating LDL is taken up and catabolized by the liver in man (equivalent to the hepatic uptake of X g of LDL cholesterol per day in Fig. 11.11), we still have to account for the transport, to the liver, of a substantial amount of LDL cholesterol deposited in extrahepatic tissues (1-X g/day in Fig. 11.11), in addition to (1) the small amount of cholesterol entering the extrahepatic tissues by synthesis in situ (Y g/day), (2) cholesterol deposited in tissues as a consequence of the extrahepatic catabolism of HDL, (3) the esterified cholesterol of VLDL and chylomicrons that does not end up in LDL and (4) the substantial amounts of free cholesterol released from the surfaces of triglyceride-rich particles. Although this last fraction of the plasma cholesterol, which may well amount to more than 3 g/day (see Glomset and Norum, 1973), is transferred to HDL and thence to other lipoproteins as cholesteryl ester, it must eventually be transported to the liver.

In Chapter 9 we considered the possibility that HDL, by taking up free cholesterol from extrahepatic tissues and transporting it to the liver, could contribute to 'reverse transport' of cholesterol. However, the rate of degradation of HDL (equivalent to about 10 mg of apoA-I plus apoA-II degraded/kg/day) is such that not more than 300 mg of cholesterol would be deposited in the liver as a result of HDL catabolism, even if the liver were the sole site of the catabolism of HDL in man. The observations of Schwartz et al. (1978a,b) indicate that at least some of the plasma HDL delivers its cholesterol directly into the hepatic pool from which bile acids are synthesized, but they do not provide quantitative information from which one could deduce the rate at which HDL is taken up irreversibly by the liver. However, even if it is assumed that all HDL is catabolized in the liver, there remains a considerable discrepancy between the amount of cholesterol entering the plasma and the amount that could be deposited in the liver by the catabolism of HDL and LDL. This raises the possibility that HDL or LDL, or both, act as shuttles for the plasma cholesterol, delivering cholesterol to the liver and returning to the plasma without degradation of their apoproteins. If this occurred, the rate of delivery of cholesterol to the liver would be greater than the rate of catabolism of the lipoprotein determined from the rate of turnover of its protein component. In an attempt to test this possibility, Sniderman et al. (1978) measured the plasma cholesterol concentration in the lipoproteins of aortic and hepatic-venous blood of human subjects. They found a positive A-V difference of about 8 mg of LDL cholesterol per 100 ml of plasma, but no A-V difference for LDL-apoB or for total cholesterol or for HDL cholesterol. They concluded that a net transfer of cholesterol from LDL to VLDL occurs somewhere in the splanchnic bed, and they suggested that this takes place by uptake of LDL cholesterol by the liver or intestine, with re-secretion of this cholesterol in VLDL. More recently, Sniderman and Teng (1980) have suggested that cholesteryl ester is transferred from LDL to nascent VLDL in the space of Disse, probably through the mediation of the cholesteryl-ester exchange protein.

Another shuttle mechanism, involving IDL, has been discussed in the light of growing evidence that the liver has specific receptors for apoE, a major component of IDL protein (see Glomset, 1979). As shown in the hypothetical scheme depicted in Fig. 11.12, the metabolism of free and esterified cholesterol within the plasma may be visualized in terms of two interlocked cycles linked together through HDL and the LCAT reaction. In one cycle (upper right of Fig. 11.12), cholesterol moves from triglyceride-rich lipoproteins to HDL in unesterified form and then returns to VLDL as esterified cholesterol with the co-operation of the cholesteryl-ester transfer protein. In the other cycle, esterified cholesterol from triglyceride-rich lipoproteins is deposited in extrahepatic tissues as a consequence of the cellular uptake of LDL; the intracellular cholesterol is then taken up as free cholesterol by HDL, re-esterified by LCAT and returned to VLDL by the cholesteryl-ester transfer protein. Neither of these cycles would contribute to the net removal of cholesterol from the plasma. However, if human liver resembles rat liver in possessing specific receptors for apoE, a proportion of the esterified cholesterol of IDL could be taken up by the liver as part of an apoE-cholesteryl ester complex, leaving the remainder of the IDL particle to form a particle of LDL (see Fig. 11.12). Operating in conjunction with the two cycles, this could provide a pathway for the net outflow of cholesterol from the plasma. In keeping with this scheme, the amount of esterified cholesterol in each triglyceride-rich particle is greater than that in each particle of LDL (Eisenberg and Levy, 1975). Furthermore, the observations of Janus *et al.* (1980) suggest that in normal human subjects not all the apoB in VLDL ends up in LDL. Finally, it should be noted that an important unknown in the equation relating input of plasma cholesterol to output is the fate of remnants derived from chylomicrons. It is conceivable that a substantially higher proportion of chylomicron remnants than of VLDL remnants is taken up irreversibly by the liver without conversion into LDL.

REFERENCES

Ashworth, L. A. E. and Green, C. (1964). The transfer of lipids between human α-lipoprotein and erythrocytes. *Biochimica et Biophysica Acta*, **84**, 182–187.

Assmann, G., Schmitz, G. and Heckers, H. (1978). The role of high density lipoproteins in lecithin:cholesterol acyltransferase activity: perspectives from Tangier disease. *Scandinavian Journal of Clinical and Laboratory Investigation*, **38**, Supplement 150, 98–102.

Barter, P. J. and Lally, J. I. (1979). *In vitro* exchanges of esterified cholesterol between serum lipoprotein fractions: studies of humans and rabbits. *Metabolism*, **28**, 230–236.

Beaumont, J. L., Carlson, L. A., Cooper, G. R., Fejfar, Z., Fredrickson, D. S. and Strasser, T. (1970). Classification of hyperlipidaemias and hyperlipoproteinaemias. *Bulletin of the World Health Organization*, **43**, 891–915.

Bierman, E. L. and Albers, J. J. (1975). Lipoprotein uptake by cultured human arterial smooth muscle cells. *Biochimica et Biophysica Acta*, **388**, 198–202.

Blomhoff, J. P. (1974). *In vitro* determination of lecithin:cholesterol acyltransferase in plasma. *Scandinavian Journal of Clinical and Laboratory Investigation*, **33**, Supplement 137, 35–43.

Blum, C. B., Levy, R. I., Eisenberg, S., Hall, M. III., Goebel, R. H. and Berman, M. (1977). High density lipoprotein metabolism in man. *Journal of Clinical Investigation*, **60**, 795–807.

Bruckdorfer, K. R. and Graham, J. M. The exchange of cholesterol and phospholipids between cell membranes and lipoproteins. In: *Biological Membranes*, Vol. 3. Ed. D. Chapman and D. F. H. Wallach. Academic Press, London, pp. 103–152, 1976.

Calvert, G. D. Mammalian low density lipoproteins. In: *Low Density Lipoproteins*. Ed. C. E. Day and R. S. Levy. Plenum Press, New York, pp. 281–319, 1976.

Carew, T. E., Saik, R. P., Johansen, K. H., Dennis, C. A. and Steinberg, D. (1976). Low density and high density lipoprotein turnover following portocaval shunt in swine. *Journal of Lipid Research*, **17**, 441–450.

Carlson, L. A. and Walldius, G. Serum and tissue lipid metabolism and effect of nicotinic acid in different types of hyperlipidemia. In: *Pharmacological Control of Lipid Metabolism. Proceedings of the Fourth International Symposium on Drugs Affecting Lipid Metabolism*. Ed. W. L. Holmes, R. Paoletti and D. Kritchevsky. Plenum Press, New York, pp. 165–178, 1972.

Chajek, T. and Fielding, C. J. (1978). Isolation and characterization of a human serum cholesteryl ester transfer protein. *Proceedings of the National Academy of Sciences of the USA*, **75**, 3445–3449.

Cheung, M. C. and Albers, J. J. (1977). The measurement of apolipoprotein A-I and A-II levels in men and women by immunoassay. *Journal of Clinical Investigation*, **60**, 43–50.

Cooper, R. A. (1977). Abnormalities of cell-membrane fluidity in the pathogenesis of disease. *New England Journal of Medicine*, **297**, 371–377.

Crispell, K. R., Parson, W., Hollifield, G. and Brent, S. (1956). A study of the rate of protein synthesis before and during the administration of L-triiodothyronine to patients with myxedema and healthy volunteers using N-15 glycine. *Journal of Clinical Investigation* **35**, 164–169.

Deckelbaum, R. J., Shipley, G. G., Tall, A. R. and Small, D. M. Lipid distribution and interaction in human plasma low density and very low density lipoproteins. Lipid core fluidity and surface properties. In: *Protides of the Biological Fluids*. Proceedings of the Twenty-Fifth Colloquium. Ed. H. Peeters. Pergamon Press, Oxford, pp. 91–98, 1978.

Deckelbaum, R. J., Tall, A. R. and Small, D. M. (1977). Interaction of cholesterol ester and triglyceride in human plasma very low density lipoprotein. *Journal of Lipid Research*, **18**, 164–168.

Eckles, N. E., Taylor, C. B., Campbell, D. J. and Gould, R. G. (1955). The origin of plasma cholesterol and the rates of equilibration of liver, plasma, and erythrocyte cholesterol. *Journal of Laboratory and Clinical Medicine*, **46**, 359–371.

Eisenberg, S. and Levy, R. I. (1975). Lipoprotein metabolism. *Advances in Lipid Research*, **13**, 1–89.

Eisenberg, S. and Olivecrona, T. (1979). Very low density lipoprotein. Fate of phospholipids, cholesterol, and apolipoprotein C during lipolysis *in vitro*. *Journal of Lipid Research*, **20**, 614–623.

Eisenberg, S., Windmueller, H. G. and Levy, R. I. (1973). Metabolic fate of rat and human lipoprotein apoproteins in the rat. *Journal of Lipid Research*, **14**, 446–458.

Forte, T. M., Nichols, A. V., Gong, E. L., Lux, S. and Levy, R. I. (1971). Electron microscopy study on reassembly of plasma high density apoprotein with various lipids. *Biochimica et Biophysica Acta*, **248**, 381–386.

Forte, T., Nichols, A., Glomset, J. and Norum, K. (1974). The ultrastructure of plasma lipoproteins in lecithin:cholesterol acyltransferase deficiency. *Scandinavian Journal of Clinical and Laboratory Investigation*, **33**, Supplement **137**, 121–132.

Fredrickson, D. S. and Levy, R. I. Familial hyperlipoproteinemia. In: *The Metabolic Basis of Inherited Disease*, Third edition. Ed. J. B. Stanbury, J. B. Wyngaarden and D. S. Fredrickson. McGraw-Hill, New York, pp. 545–614, 1972.

Fredrickson, D. S., Levy, R. I. and Lees, R. S. (1967). Fat transport in lipoproteins—an integrated approach to mechanisms and disorders. *New England Journal of Medicine*, **276**, 34–44, 148–156, 215–225, 273–281.
Gidez, L. I., Roheim, P. S. and Eder, H. A. (1965). Effect of diet on the cholesterol ester composition of liver and of plasma lipoproteins in the rat. *Journal of Lipid Research*, **6**, 377–382.
Gillett, M. P. T. (1978). Comparative studies of lecithin:cholesterol acyltransferase reaction in the plasma of reptiles and amphibians. *Scandinavian Journal of Clinical and Laboratory Investigation*, **38**, Supplement **150**, 32–39.
Gjone, E., Torsvik, H. and Norum, K. R. (1968). Familial plasma cholesterol ester deficiency. A study of the erythrocytes. *Scandinavian Journal of Clinical and Laboratory Investigation*, **21**, 327–332.
Glangeaud, M. C., Eisenberg, S. and Olivecrona, T. (1977). Very low density lipoprotein dissociation of apolipoprotein C during lipoprotein lipase induced lipolysis. *Biochimica et Biophysica Acta*, **486**, 23–35.
Glickman, R. M. and Green, P. H. R. (1977). The intestine as a source of apolipoprotein A. *Proceedings of the National Academy of Sciences of the USA*, **74**, 2569–2573.
Glickman, R. M., Green, P. H. R., Lees, R. S. and Tall, A. (1978). Apoprotein A-I synthesis in normal intestinal mucosa and in Tangier disease. *New England Journal of Medicine*, **299**, 1424–1427.
Glomset, J. A. (1968). The plasma lecithin:cholesterol acyltransferase reaction. *Journal of Lipid Research*, **9**, 155–167.
Glomset, J. A. (1979). Lecithin:cholesterol acyltransferase. An exercise in comparative biology. *Progress in Biochemical Pharmacology*, **15**, 41–66.
Glomset, J. A. and Norum, K. R. (1973). The metabolic role of lecithin:cholesterol acyltransferase: perspectives from pathology. *Advances in Lipid Research*, **11**, 1–65.
Goodman, DeW. S. (1962). The metabolism of chylomicron cholesterol ester in the rat. *Journal of Clinical Investigation*, **41**, 1886–1896.
Goodman, DeW. S. (1965). Cholesterol ester metabolism. *Physiological Reviews*, **45**, 747–839.
Goodman, D. S. and Shiratori, T. (1964). Fatty acid composition of human plasma lipoprotein fractions. *Journal of Lipid Research*, **5**, 307–313.
Gould, R. G., LeRoy, G. V., Okita, G. T., Kabara, J. J., Keegan, P. and Bergenstal, D. M. (1955). The use of C^{14}-labelled acetate to study cholesterol metabolism in man. *Journal of Labatory and Clinical Medicine*, **46**, 372–384.
Graham, J. M. and Green, C. (1970). The properties of mitochondria enriched *in vitro* with cholesterol. *European Journal of Biochemistry*, **12**, 58–66.
Green, P. H. R., Glickman, R. M., Riley, J. W. and Quinet, E. (1980). Human apolipoprotein A-IV. Intestinal origin and distribution in plasma. *Journal of Clinical Investigation*, **65**, 911–919.
Green, P. H. R., Glickman, R. M., Saudek, C. D., Blum, C. B. and Tall, A. R. (1979). Human intestinal lipoproteins. Studies in chyluric subjects. *Journal of Clinical Investigation*, **64**, 233–242.
Green, P. H. R., Tall, A. R. and Glickman, R. M. (1978). Rat intestine secretes discoid high density lipoprotein. *Journal of Clinical Investigation*, **61**, 528–534.
Grundy, S. M. and Kern, F. (1980). Workshop on regulation of hepatic cholesterol and bile acid metabolism. *Journal of Lipid Research*, **21**, 496–500.
Gurd, F. R. N. Some naturally occurring lipoprotein systems. In: *Lipide Chemistry*. D. J. Hanahan. John Wiley and Sons, New York, pp. 260–325, 1960.
Hagerman, J. S. and Gould, R. G. (1951). The *in vitro* interchange of cholesterol between plasma and red cells. *Proceedings of the Society for Experimental Biology and Medicine*, **78**, 329–332.
Havel, R. J. Origin of HDL. In: *High Density Lipoproteins and Atherosclerosis*. Ed.

A. M. Gotto, Jr., N. E. Miller and M. F. Oliver. Elsevier/North-Holland Biomedical Press, Amsterdam, pp. 21–35, 1978.
Hay, R. V., Pottenger, L. A., Reingold, A. L., Getz, G. S. and Wissler, R. W. (1971). Degradation of ^{125}I-labelled serum low density lipoprotein in normal and oestrogen-treated male rats. *Biochemical and Biophysical Research Communications*, **44**, 1471–1477.
d'Hollander, F. and Chevallier, F. (1972). Mouvements de cholestérol *in vitro* entre les α- et les β-lipoprotéines plasmatiques du rat et entre chacune d'elles et les globules rouges. *Biochimica et Biophysica Acta*, **260**, 110–132.
Howard, A. N., Blaton, V., Gresham, G. A., Vandamme, D. and Peeters, H. The lipoproteins in hyperlipidaemic primates as a model for human atherosclerosis. In: *Protides of the Biological Fluids*. Proceedings of the Nineteenth Colloquium. Ed. H. Peeters. Pergamon Press, Oxford and New York, pp. 341–344, 1972.
Jackson, R. L., Morrisett, J. D. and Gotto, A. M. Jr. (1976). Lipoprotein structure and metabolism. *Physiological Reviews*, **56**, 259–316.
Janus, E. D., Nicoll, A. M., Turner, P. R., Magill, P. and Lewis, B. (1980). Kinetic bases of the primary hyperlipidaemias: studies of apolipoprotein B turnover in genetically defined subjects. *European Journal of Clinical Investigation*, **10**, 161–172.
Kane, J. P., Hardman, D. A. and Paulus, H. E. (1980). Heterogeneity of apolipoprotein B: isolation of a new species from human chylomicrons. *Proceedings of the National Academy of Sciences of the USA*, **77**, 2465–2469.
Kayden, H. J., Karmen, A. and Dumont, A. (1963). Alterations in the fatty acid composition of human lymph and serum lipoproteins by single feedings. *Journal of Clinical Investigation*, **42**, 1373–1381.
Kuusi, T., Nikkilä, E. A., Virtanen, I. and Kinnunen, P. K. J. (1979). Localization of the heparin-releasable lipase *in situ* in the rat liver. *Biochemical Journal*, **181**, 245–246.
Lange, Y., Cohen, C. M. and Poznansky, M. J. (1977). Transmembrane movement of cholesterol in human erythrocytes. *Proceedings of the National Academy of Sciences of the USA*, **74**, 1538–1542.
Langer, T., Strober, W. and Levy, R. I. (1972). The metabolism of low density lipoprotein in familial type II hyperlipoproteinemia. *Journal of Clinical Investigation*, **51**, 1528–1536.
McBride, J. A. and Jacob, H. S. (1970). Abnormal kinetics of red cell membrane cholesterol in acanthocytes: studies in genetic and experimental abetalipoproteinaemia and in spur cell anaemia. *British Journal of Haematology*, **18**, 383–397.
Magide, A. A., Myant, N. B. and Reichl, D. (1975). The effect of nicotinic acid on the metabolism of the plasma lipoproteins of Rhesus monkeys. *Atherosclerosis*, **21**, 205–215.
Mahley, R. W. Alterations in plasma lipoproteins induced by cholesterol feeding in animals including man. In: *Disturbances in Lipid and Lipoprotein Metabolism*. Ed. J. M. Dietschy, A. M. Gotto, Jr. and J. A. Ontko. American Physiological Society, Bethesda, pp. 181–197, 1978.
Mahley, R. W., Hamilton, R. L. and Lequire, V. S. (1969). Characterization of lipoprotein particles isolated from the Golgi apparatus of rat liver. *Journal of Lipid Research*, **10**, 433–439.
Mahley, R. W. and Weisgraber, K. H. (1974). Canine lipoproteins and atherosclerosis. 1. Isolation and characterization of plasma lipoproteins from control dogs, *Circulation Research*, **35**, 713–721.
Marcel, Y. L., Fabien, H. D. and Davignon, J. (1971). Net esterification *in vitro* of plasma cholesterol in human primary hyperlipidemia. *Lipids*, **6**, 722–726.
Marcel, Y. L. and Vezina, C. (1972). Lecithin:cholesterol acyltransferase of human plasma. Role of chylomicrons, very low, and high density lipoproteins in the reaction. *Journal of Biological Chemistry*, **248**, 8254–8259.

Marcel, Y. L., Vezina, C., Teng, B. and Sniderman, A. (1980). Transfer of cholesterol esters between human high density lipoproteins and triglyceride-rich lipoproteins controlled by a plasma protein factor. *Atherosclerosis*, **35**, 127–133.

Matthews, C. M. E. (1957). The theory of tracer experiments with ^{131}I-labelled plasma proteins. *Physics in Medicine and Biology*, **2**, 36–53.

Miller, J. P. and Thompson, G. R. (1973). Plasma cholesterol esterification in patients with secondary hypocholesterolaemia. *European Journal of Clinical Investigation*, **3**, 401–406.

Miller, N. E., Weinstein, D. B. and Steinberg, D. (1977). Binding, internalization, and degradation of high density lipoprotein by cultured normal human fibroblasts. *Journal of Lipid Research*, **18**, 438–450.

Mills, G. L. Lipoproteins in animals. In: *Handbuch der Inneren Medizin*, Vol. 7. Ed. G. Schettler, H. Greten, G. Schlierf and D. Seidel. Springer-Verlag, Berlin, pp. 173–195, 1976.

Monger, E. A. and Nestel, P. J. (1967). Relationship between the concentration and the rate of esterification of free cholesterol by the plasma esterification system. *Clinica Chimica Acta*, **15**, 269–273.

Murphy, J. R. (1962). Erythrocyte metabolism. III. Relationship of energy metabolism and serum factors to the osmotic fragility following incubation. *Journal of Laboratory and Clinical Medicine*, **60**, 86–109.

Myant, N. B. The transport and turnover of the plasma cholesterol. In: *Plasma Lipoproteins*. Biochemical Society Symposium No. 33. Ed. R. M. S. Smellie. Academic Press, London, pp. 99–121,1971.

Myant, N. B. and Mitropoulos, K. A. (1977). Cholesterol 7α-hydroxylase. *Journal of Lipid Research*, **18**, 135–153.

Nakai, T., Otto, P. S., Kennedy, D. L. and Whayne, T. F. Jr. (1976). Rat high density lipoprotein subfraction (HDL$_3$) uptake and catabolism by isolated rat liver parenchymal cells. *Journal of Biological Chemistry*, **251**, 4914–4921.

Nestel, P. J., Miller, N. E. and Clifton-Bligh, P. (1974). Plasma cholesterol esterification *in vivo* in man. *Scandinavian Journal of Clinical and Laboratory Investigation*, **33**, Supplement **137**, 157–160.

Nestel, P. J. and Monger, E. A. (1967). Turnover of plasma esterified cholesterol in normocholesterolemic and hypercholesterolemic subjects and its relation to body build. *Journal of Clinical Investigation*, **46**, 967–974.

Nichols, A. V. and Smith, L. (1965). Effect of very low-density lipoproteins on lipid transfer in incubated serum. *Journal of Lipid Research*, **6**, 206–210.

Norum, K. R. and Gjone, E. (1967). Familial plasma lecithin:cholesterol acyltransferase deficiency. Biochemical study of a new inborn error of metabolism. *Scandinavian Journal of Clinical and Laboratory Investigation*, **20**, 231–243.

Norum, K. R., Glomset, J. A., Nichols, A. V., Forte, T., Albers, J. J., King, W. C., Mitchell, C. D., Applegate, K. R., Gong, E. L., Cabana, V. and Gjone, E. (1975). Plasma lipoproteins in familial lecithin:cholesterol acyltransferase deficiency: effects of incubation with lecithin:cholesterol acyltransferase *in vitro*. *Scandinavian Journal of Clinical and Laboratory Investigation*, Supplement **142**, 31–55.

Pattnaik, N. M., Montes, A., Hughes, L. B. and Zilversmit, D. B. (1978). Cholesteryl ester exchange protein in human plasma: isolation and characterization. *Biochimica et Biophysica Acta*, **530**, 428–438.

Phillips, M. C., McLean, L. R., Stoudt, G. W. and Rothblat, G. H. (1980). Mechanism of cholesterol efflux from cells. *Atherosclerosis*, **36**, 409–422.

Pittman, R. C., Attie, A. D., Carew, T. E. and Steinberg, D. (1979). Tissue sites of degradation of low density lipoprotein: application of a method for determining the fate of plasma proteins. *Proceedings of the National Academy of Sciences of the USA*, **76**, 5345–5349.

Porte, D. and Havel, R. J. (1961). The use of cholesterol-4-C^{14} labelled lipoproteins

as a tracer for plasma cholesterol in the dog. *Journal of Lipid Research*, 2, 357–362.
Portman, O. W. and Sugano, M. (1964). Factors influencing the level and fatty acid specificity of cholesterol esterification activity in human plasma. *Archives of Biochemistry and Biophysics*, 105, 532–540.
Quarfordt, S., Hanks, J., Jones, R. S. and Shelburne, F. (1980). The uptake of high density lipoprotein cholesteryl ester in the perfused rat liver. *Journal of Biological Chemistry*, 255, 2934–2937.
Quarfordt, S. H. and Hilderman, H. L. (1970). Quantitation of the *in vitro* free cholesterol exchange of human red cells and lipoproteins. *Journal of Lipid Research*, 11, 528–535.
Rachmilewitz, D., Stein, O., Roheim, P. S. and Stein, Y. (1972). Metabolism of iodinated high density lipoproteins in the rat. II. Autoradiographic localization in the liver. *Biochimica et Biophysica Acta*, 270, 414–425.
Reichl, D., Myant, N. B., Brown, M. S. and Goldstein, J. L. (1978). Biologically active low density lipoprotein in human peripheral lymph. *Journal of Clinical Investigation*, 61, 64–71.
Reichl, D., Simons, L. A., Myant, N. B. Pflug, J. J. and Mills, G. L. (1973). The lipids and lipoproteins of human peripheral lymph, with observations on the transport of cholesterol from plasma and tissues into lymph. *Clinical Science and Molecular Medicine*, 45, 313–329.
Roheim, P. S., Haft, D. E., Gidez, L. I., White, A. and Eder, H. A. (1963). Plasma lipoprotein metabolism in perfused rat livers. II. Transfer of free and esterified cholesterol into the plasma. *Journal of Clinical Investigation*, 42, 1277–1285.
Rose, H. G. and Juliano, J. (1979). Regulation of plasma lecithin:cholesterol acyltransferase in man. III. Role of high density lipoprotein cholesteryl esters in the activating effect of a high-fat test meal. *Journal of Lipid Research*, 20, 399–407.
Rothschild, M. A., Bauman, A., Yalow, R. S. and Berson, S. A. (1957). The effect of large doses of desiccated thyroid on the distribution and metabolism of albumin-I[131] in euthyroid subjects. *Journal of Clinical Investigation*, 36, 422–428.
Sardet, T. C., Hansma, H. and Ostwald, R. (1972). Characterization of guinea pig plasma lipoproteins: the appearance of new lipoproteins in response to dietary cholesterol. *Journal of Lipid Research*, 13, 624–639.
Sata, T., Havel, R. J. and Jones, A. L. (1972). Characterization of subfractions of triglyceride-rich lipoproteins separated by gel chromatography from blood plasma of normolipemic and hyperlipemic humans. *Journal of Lipid Research*, 13, 757–768.
Schaefer, E. J., Jenkins, L. L. and Brewer, H. B. Jr. (1978). Human chylomicron apolipoprotein metabolism. *Biochemical and Biophysical Research Communications*, 80, 405–412.
Schwartz, C. C., Berman, M., Vlahcevic, Z. R., Halloran, L. G., Gregory, D. H. and Swell, L. (1978*a*). Multi-compartmental analysis of cholesterol metabolism in man: Characterization of the hepatic bile acid and biliary cholesterol precursor sites. *Journal of Clinical Investigation*, 61, 408–423.
Schwartz, C. C., Halloran, L. G., Vlahcevic, Z. R., Gregory, D. H. and Swell, L. (1978*b*). Preferential utilization of free cholesterol from high-density lipoproteins for biliary cholesterol secretion in man. *Science*, 200, 62–64.
Scott, P. J. and Hurley, P. J. (1969). Effect of clofibrate on low-density lipoprotein turnover in essential hypercholesterolaemia. *Journal of Atherosclerosis Research*, 9, 25–34.
Scott, P. J., White, B. M., Winterbourn, C. C. and Hurley, P. J. (1970). Low density lipoprotein peptide metabolism in nephrotic syndrome: A comparison with patterns observed in other syndromes characterised by hyperlipoproteinaemia. *Australasian Annals of Medicine*, 19, 1–15.

Shattil, S. J., Bennett, J. S., Colman, R. W. and Cooper, R. A. (1977). Abnormalities of cholesterol-phospholipid composition in platelets and low-density lipoproteins of human hyperbetalipoproteinemia. *Journal of Laboratory and Clinical Medicine*, **89**, 341–353.

Shepherd, J., Packard, C. J., Gotto, A. M. Jr. and Taunton, O. D. (1978). A comparison of two methods to investigate the metabolism of human apolipoproteins A-I and A-II. *Journal of Lipid Research*, **19**, 656–661.

Sherrill, B. C., Innerarity, T. L. and Mahley, R. W. (1980). Rapid hepatic clearance of the canine lipoproteins containing only the E apoprotein by a high affinity receptor. *Journal of Biological Chemistry*, **255**, 1804–1807.

Shore, V. G. and Shore, B. (1973). Heterogeneity of human plasma very low density lipoproteins. Separation of species differing in protein components. *Biochemistry*, **12**, 502–507.

Sniderman, A. D., Carew, T. E., Chandler, J. G. and Steinberg, D. (1974). Paradoxical increase in rate of catabolism of low-density lipoproteins after hepatectomy. *Science*, **183**, 526–528.

Sniderman, A. D., Carew, T. E. and Steinberg, D. (1975). Turnover and tissue distribution of ^{125}I-labelled low density lipoprotein in swine and dogs. *Journal of Lipid Research*, **16**, 293–299.

Sniderman, A. and Teng, B. The liver and cholesterol ester transfer amongst lipoprotein—one suggested model. In: *Proceedings of the Fifth International Symposium on Atherosclerosis*. Ed. A. M. Gotto Jr., L. C. Smith and B. Allen. Springer-Verlag, New York, pp. 596-599, 1980.

Sniderman, A., Teng, B., Vezina, C. and Marcel, Y. L. (1978). Cholesterol ester exchange between human plasma high and low density lipoproteins mediated by a plasma protein factor. *Atherosclerosis*, **31**, 327–333.

Sniderman, A., Thomas, D., Marpole, D. and Teng, B. (1978). Low density lipoprotein. A metabolic pathway for return of cholesterol to the splanchnic bed. *Journal of Clinical Investigation*, **61**, 867–875.

Sodhi, H. S. (1974). Current concepts of cholesterol metabolism and their relationship to lecithin:cholesterol acyltransferase. *Scandinavian Journal of Clinical and Laboratory Investigation*, **33**, Supplement **137**, 161–163.

Soutar, A. K. and Myant, N. B. Plasma lipoproteins. In: *Chemistry of Macromolecules IIB. Macromolecular Complexes*. International Review of Biochemistry, Vol. 25. Ed. R. E. Offord. University Park Press, Baltimore, pp. 55–119, 1979.

Spritz, N. and Mishkel, M. A. (1969). Effects of dietary fats on plasma lipids and lipoproteins: an hypothesis for the lipid-lowering effect of unsaturated fatty acids. *Journal of Clinical Investigation*, **48**, 78–86.

Stein, O. and Stein, Y. (1976). High density lipoproteins reduce the uptake of low density lipoproteins by human endothelial cells in culture. *Biochimica et Biophysica Acta*, **431**, 363–368.

Stokke, K. T. and Norum, K. R. (1971). Determination of lecithin:cholesterol acyltransfer in human blood plasma. *Scandinavian Journal of Clinical and Laboratory Investigation*, **27**, 21–27.

Strisower, E. H., Adamson, G. and Strisower, B. (1968). Treatment of hyperlipidemias. *American Journal of Medicine*, **45**, 488–501.

Sugano, M. and Portman, O. W. (1964). Fatty acid specificities and rates of cholesterol esterification *in vivo* and *in vitro*. *Archives of Biochemistry and Biophysics*, **107**, 341–351.

Swaney, J. B., Reese, H. and Eder, H. A. (1974). Polypeptide composition of rat high density lipoprotein: characterization by SDS-gel electrophoresis. *Biochemical and Biophysical Research Communications*, **59**, 513–519.

Tall, A. R., Atkinson, D., Small, D. M. and Mahley, R. W. (1977). Characterization

of the lipoproteins of atherosclerotic swine. *Journal of Biological Chemistry*, **252**, 7288–7293.
Tall, A. R., Green, P. H. R., Glickman, R. M. and Riley, J. W. (1979). Metabolic fate of chylomicron phospholipids and apoproteins in the rat. *Journal of Clinical Investigation*, **64**, 977–989.
Tall, A., Rudel, L., Small, D. and Atkinson, D. (1978). Structure of atherogenic low density lipoprotein (LDL). *Circulation, Part II*, **58**, *Abstract* 656.
Thompson, G. R., Soutar, A. K. and Myant, N. B. (1980). Congenital and acquired defects of receptor-mediated low density lipoprotein (LDL) catabolism. *Circulation*, **62**, *Supplement 3*, III-44.
Thompson, G. R., Spinks, T., Ranicar, A. and Myant, N. B. (1977). Non-steady-state studies of low-density lipoprotein turnover in familial hypercholesterolaemia. *Clinical Science and Molecular Medicine*, **52**, 361–369.
van Tol, A., van Gent, T. and van't Hooft, F. M. Low density lipoprotein catabolism in the liver: decrease of fractional catabolic rate after partial hepatectomy. In: *Protides of the Biological Fluids*. Proceedings of the Twenty-Fifth Colloquium. Ed. H. Peeters. Pergamon Press, Oxford, pp. 197–200, 1978.
Turner, P., Miller, N., Chrystie, I., Coltart, J., Mistry, P., Nicoll, A. and Lewis, B. (1979). Splanchnic production of discoidal plasma high-density lipoprotein in man. *Lancet*, **1**, 645–647.
Utermann, G., Jaeschke, M. and Menzel, J. (1975). Familial hyperlipoproteinemia type III: deficiency of a specific apolipoprotein (apoE-III) in the very-low-density lipoproteins. *FEBS Letters*, **56**, 352–355.
Walton, K. W., Scott, P. J., Dykes, P. W. and Davies, J. W. L. (1965). The significance of alterations in serum lipids in thyroid dysfunction. II. Alterations of the metabolism and turnover of ^{131}I-low-density lipoproteins in hypothyroidism and thyrotoxicosis. *Clinical Science*, **29**, 217–238.
Weisgraber, K. H. and Mahley, R. W. (1980). Subfractionation of human high density lipoproteins by heparin-sepharose affinity chromatography. *Journal of Lipid Research*, **21**, 316–325.
Wilson, D. E. and Lees, R. S. (1972). Metabolic relationships among the plasma lipoproteins. Reciprocal changes in the concentrations of very low and low density lipoproteins in man. *Journal of Clinical Investigation*, **51**, 1051–1057.
Zilversmit, D. B. (1960). The design and analysis of isotope experiments. *American Journal of Medicine*, **29**, 832–848.
Zilversmit, D. B., Hughes, L. B. and Balmer, J. (1975). Stimulation of cholesterol ester exchange by lipoprotein-free rabbit plasma. *Biochimica et Biophysica Acta*, **409**, 393–398.

Chapter 12

The Epidemiology of the Plasma Cholesterol

1	INTRODUCTION	571
2	THE SELECTION OF STATISTICAL POPULATIONS	572
3	METHODOLOGY	573
4	VARIABILITY WITHIN POPULATIONS AND WITHIN INDIVIDUALS	574
4.1	Frequency distributions	574
4.2	Influence of environment, age and sex	576
4.2.1	Total cholesterol	576
4.2.2	Lipoprotein cholesterol	579
5	GENETIC INFLUENCES	585
5.1	Methods of estimation	585
5.2	Observations on families	585
5.3	Observations on twins	589
5.4	Critical summary and conclusions	590
5.5	Genetics of plasma cholesterol in animals	592
5.6	Mechanisms of gene-mediated effects	593
6	VARIABILITY BETWEEN POPULATIONS	594
6.1	Plasma cholesterol in different geographical, racial and social groups	594
6.2	The basis of inter-population variability	596

The Epidemiology of the Plasma Cholesterol

1 INTRODUCTION

In this chapter I shall discuss differences in plasma cholesterol concentration within and between human populations, particularly in relation to ischaemic heart disease (IHD). Hypercholesterolaemia will not be considered here except in so far as it bears on the nature of the link between plasma cholesterol concentration and premature cardiovascular disease in the general population.

Our approach to the study of the plasma cholesterol in human disease has changed radically since it became clear that all the cholesterol in plasma is carried in lipoproteins, which, as we saw in Chapter 11, comprise several classes of particle differing from one another in composition, structure and metabolic fate. Not surprisingly, we now find that as regards human health the significance of a change in plasma total cholesterol concentration depends largely upon the underlying change in plasma lipoprotein pattern. Hence, in recent years there has been a shift of emphasis in work on the atherosclerosis problem, away from measurement of total plasma cholesterol concentration and towards the study of plasma lipoproteins, including their lipid and protein composition as well as their concentration. This trend is certain to become more pronounced as simpler methods are developed for the mass-scale investigation of plasma lipoproteins and their separate components. To this extent, the enormous volume of work already carried out on the epidemiological aspects of the plasma cholesterol in the fifties and sixties may come increasingly to seem dated. Indeed, it could be argued that in relation to cardiovascular disease the plasma cholesterol is of interest only as a means to the measurement of the concentrations of the plasma lipoproteins, its advantage over other lipoprotein constituents being the ease and accuracy with which it can be assayed.

However, this would be a one-sided view. In the first place, cholesterol plays a special role in the development of atherosclerotic lesions in that it is the only bulk constituent of plasma lipoproteins that cannot be metabolized in tissues other than the liver and the steroid-hormone-forming organs. Secondly, despite current interest in HDL cholesterol as a negative *risk factor* (for a definition see Chapter 13) for IHD, the earlier conclusion that plasma total cholesterol concentration is a positive risk factor remains valid in all essentials. This is so because plasma LDL cholesterol is a positive risk factor and, under most conditions, the plasma total cholesterol concentration closely reflects the concentration of LDL, in which the bulk of the cholesterol in human plasma is carried. Thus, what we now know about the importance of HDL in relation to atherosclerosis does not nullify the earlier work on plasma cholesterol. Nor does it mean that measurement of plasma total cholesterol concentration has ceased to be of use in epidemiological studies or in clinical practice, though it does mean that much of the older work can now be interpreted in a wider framework. I mention these points at this stage in order to forestall the possible objection that it is inconsistent to discuss the epidemiological aspects of plasma total cholesterol concentration in the ensuing section, after emphasizing the importance of plasma lipoproteins as carriers of the plasma cholesterol.

2 THE SELECTION OF STATISTICAL POPULATIONS

Information about the plasma cholesterol concentration in human communities is derived from a variety of sources. In making use of this information one should bear in mind the fact that the basis on which a group of subjects is selected for study (a 'population' in the statistical sense) differs according to the purpose of the investigation. The criteria adopted for selection will not be the same in a study of the plasma cholesterol as a risk factor for first attacks of IHD, an investigation of the heritability of hypercholesterolaemia and a case-control study of the relation between plasma cholesterol and a previous heart attack.

For some purposes, as in the construction of standard frequency-distribution curves for use in the diagnosis of hypercholesterolaemia, the ideal population would be a completely representative sample of all the individuals in the community of the same age and sex as the patient. In most cases, however, the method of choosing a representative population has to be a compromise between the ideal and the practicable, as in the use of civil servants, army conscripts (of both sexes in Israel) or employees at a local factory. It is worth noting how very difficult it is to obtain an unbiassed sample from any population.

Even in the carefully designed Framingham study of male and female adults who had not had a heart attack, some unavoidable bias may have been introduced by selecting for people who responded to a written request and who were able to attend the clinic for blood sampling. Before one uses published values to deduce the range of plasma cholesterol concentrations in any community it is worth while reading the small print in the Methods section, to see how the study population was chosen. It will often be found that the sampling procedure has involved selection for or against some characteristic that may be related to plasma cholesterol concentration. Perhaps the nearest to an ideal sample is that of Glueck *et al.* (1971), who measured plasma cholesterol concentration in the cord blood of 1800 consecutive infants born in a hospital. Finally, it may be noted that an interesting sampling problem arises in a region containing an immigrant community originating in a country where plasma cholesterol concentrations differ significantly from those in the host country. This raises the question as to the appropriate standard with which one should compare the plasma cholesterol concentration in an immigrant patient.

3 METHODOLOGY

When blood samples are taken for diagnostic purposes or in epidemiological studies it is essential to make sure that the conditions of sampling are standardized. Details of the precautions that should be taken will be found in the paper by Beaumont *et al.* (1970) and in Chapter 9 of Lewis (1976). Ideally, the blood sample should be taken 12–14 hours after the last meal, although this is not usually regarded as essential unless the sample is to be used for determination of the plasma triglyceride concentration in addition to cholesterol concentration. (In many population surveys, plasma cholesterol concentration was determined in samples not taken in the fasting state.) The subject should have been eating his normal diet for the previous two weeks, he should not be losing or gaining weight, and he should not be taking any drugs known to influence cholesterol metabolism. He should not have had a recent acute illness or a major operation, since either may lower the plasma cholesterol concentration for several weeks. Of particular interest from the point of view of the design of case-control studies of the relation between plasma cholesterol and IHD is the effect of a myocardial infarct. The plasma cholesterol concentration usually falls significantly within 3 days of an infarct and may not return to the basal level for 8 weeks (Watson *et al.*, 1963).

Either plasma or serum may be used for determination of total cholesterol or of cholesterol in the separate lipoprotein fractions.

Throughout this chapter I refer to plasma as a source of cholesterol and plasma lipoproteins in a general sense, though in many studies the determinations were carried out on serum rather than plasma. Whether serum or plasma is used makes very little difference to the results obtained; the concentration of total cholesterol is only about 3% higher in plasma than in serum.

Only a few general points about analytical methods need to be made here. The methods available for determination of cholesterol were discussed in Chapter 2, where I drew attention to the need for standardization and quality control of analytical procedures in epidemiological studies, particularly in those involving several centres. In any investigation of the plasma cholesterol on a community scale, an automated method for the determination of cholesterol is essential. To appreciate this one has only to consider that a single sample of plasma will generate at least four determinations in duplicate if total cholesterol and cholesterol in VLDL, LDL and HDL are measured. Automation of the separation of lipoproteins in the preparative ultracentrifuge is not possible and zonal electrophoresis is not quantitative. However, the cholesterol concentration in VLDL, LDL and HDL may be measured by the much simplified 'beta quantification' procedure of Fredrickson et al. (1967) in which VLDL is removed by a single centrifugation, followed by precipitation of LDL in the subnatant with heparin and manganese chloride. With more recent precipitation methods it is possible to separate all three major lipoprotein classes without the use of an ultracentrifuge (see Lewis (1976) for details).

4 VARIABILITY WITHIN POPULATIONS AND WITHIN INDIVIDUALS

4.1 Frequency distributions

The plasma total cholesterol concentration varies widely between different individuals in any human population. Fig. 12.1 shows the distribution of plasma total cholesterol concentrations in all the men and women aged 35 to 64 in the Framingham study population. The shape of the curves is typical for human populations in general, provided that the sample is reasonably representative. In particular, all the curves in Fig. 12.1 show a single peak with skewing to the right of the modal value and a wide scatter on either side of the mode. Because of the skewness of the distribution in most populations, a mean with standard deviation is not always a suitable statistic for describing the plasma cholesterol concentration in a human population. Distributions are usually described in terms of a mean or

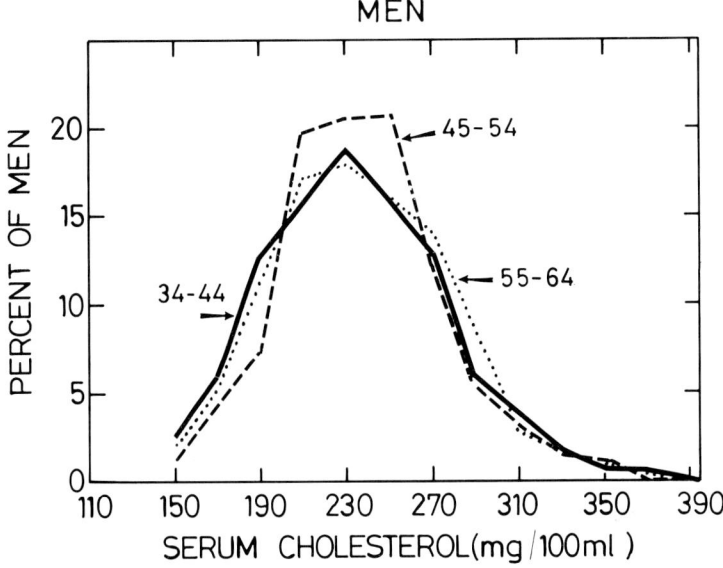

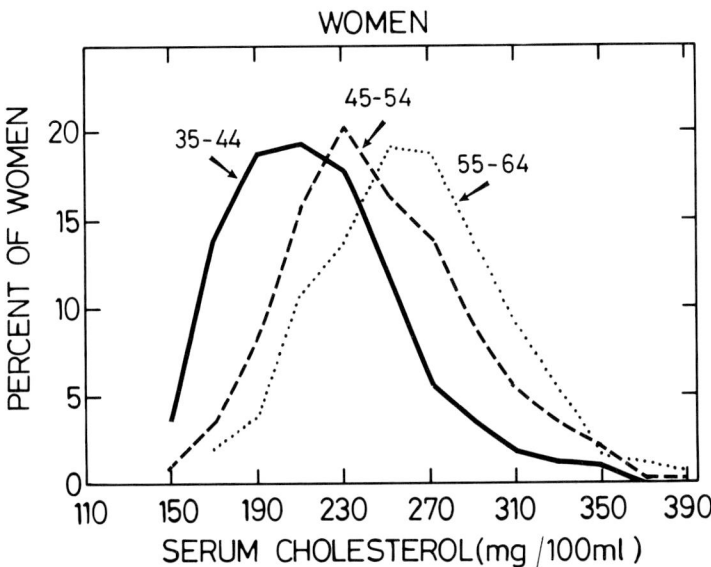

Figure 12.1
Distributions of serum cholesterol concentration in 1875 men and 2256 women by age. Values taken from the Framingham study (Examination IV). (From Kannel (1971), with the permission of the author.)

median, with an upper limit expressed as the upper 90th or 95th percentile, i.e. the value that cuts off the top 10% or 5% of the whole distribution.

4.2 Influence of environment, age and sex

Intra-population variability of plasma cholesterol level is due to a combination of environmental and genetic factors and of age. In this section we shall consider the influence of environment, age and sex.

4.2.1 Total cholesterol

The effect of changes in the diet on plasma total cholesterol under experimental conditions suggests that one of the environmental causes of variability in free-living populations is the habitual diet eaten by different individuals, particularly with regard to total calories, cholesterol, saturated *versus* polyunsaturated fat, alcohol and indigestible food residue. However, it has been surprisingly difficult to demonstrate a significant correlation between plasma cholesterol concentration and any dietary constituent in a free-living population (for references see McGill (1979)), though the plasma level may deviate widely from the general mean in special groups eating atypical diets. For example, the mean plasma cholesterol concentration is below that in the general population in Trappist monks (Groen *et al.*, 1962), lacto-ovo-vegetarians of the Seventh-day Adventist sect (Walden *et al.*, 1964) and the members of North American communes subsisting on a 'macrobiotic' diet (Sacks *et al.*, 1975). However, it should be noted that diet is not by any means the only atypical feature of the way of life of these groups. For a discussion of the anomalous lack of correlation between plasma cholesterol concentration and dietary composition within populations, see McGill (1979); for a more general discussion of the complex relationship between inter- and intra-population correlations, see Robinson (1950).

Differences in the habitual diet eaten by different individuals is unlikely to be the major cause of the wide range of plasma cholesterol concentrations within free-living populations, such as that shown in Fig. 12.1. This is illustrated by the fact that when groups of individuals are given a standard diet in a metabolic ward, inter-individual variability of plasma cholesterol concentration remains considerable; according to Stamler (1973), the standard deviation of the mean in such groups is about ± 30 mg/100 ml. It is also worth noting that in primary trials of the effect of 'cholesterol-lowering' diets on the incidence of first attacks of IHD, the plasma cholesterol concentrations in the subjects given the standard diet do not converge to a common value, but remain widely scattered (see Miettinen *et al.*, 1972).

Other non-genetic factors that may influence the plasma cholesterol concentration in different individuals within a population include smoking, habitual amount of exercise taken, mental stress and drugs or toxic agents such as phenobarbital, oestrogen-containing contraceptives, certain anticonvulsants and the chlorinated hydrocarbon insecticides. Pregnancy and the secondary hyperlipidaemias discussed in Chapter 15 will also contribute to the variability encountered in a representative sample of the population. In a given individual, the plasma cholesterol concentration determined on a single occasion may be influenced by the recent intake of dietary cholesterol, as illustrated by the rather extreme instance shown in Fig. 12.2, and there may also be seasonal variations, the concentration tending to be higher in winter than summer (Carlson and Lindstedt, 1969). Although sustained physical training has been found to lower the plasma total cholesterol concentration (see Wong and Johnson (1977) for references), an immediate change after intensive exercise has not been demonstrated.

In addition to the above factors, age- and sex-related differences in plasma cholesterol concentration will also contribute to the total variability in populations not selected for age or sex. Plasma total cholesterol concentration is influenced by age before and after adolescence, and in adults it is influenced by sex. In the plasma of cord

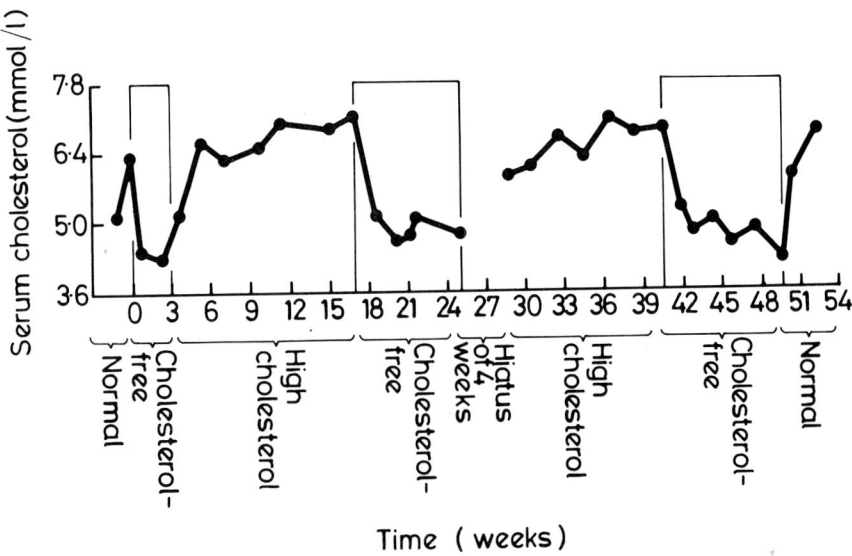

Figure 12.2
Effect of dietary cholesterol (2.4 g/day as egg yolk) on serum cholesterol concentration in a normal man. Periods of cholesterol feeding alternated with periods of cholesterol-free diet. The whole experiment lasted one year. (From Connor and Connor (1972), with the permission of the authors.)

578 The Biology of Cholesterol and Related Steroids

blood of infants from many parts of the world the concentration is very low, most reported mean values lying within the range 60–90 mg/100 ml. Non-genetic variations in the maternal plasma cholesterol level seem to be essentially without influence on the cord-blood level. In the first week of life there is a rapid increase to about twice the level at birth. During the subsequent few months there is a further increase, the increase being more marked in infants fed breast milk than in those fed cow's milk or artificial milks enriched with polyunsaturated fat (Tsang *et al.*, 1974). Studies of children of preschool and school age in America (Lee, 1967; Owen *et al.*, 1974; Lauer *et al.*,

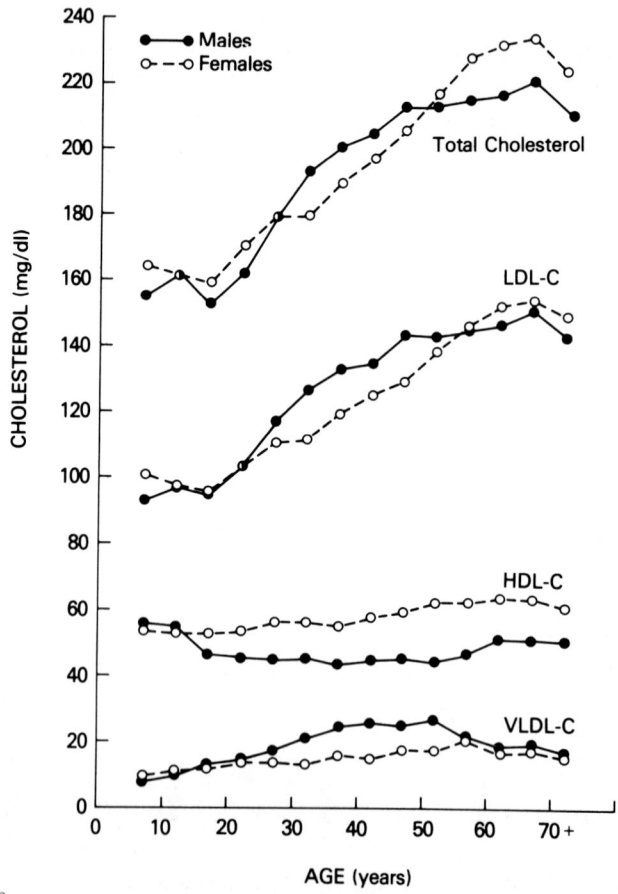

Figure 12.3
Mean plasma total, LDL-, HDL- and VLDL-cholesterol levels by five-year age groups. Lipid Research Clinics Programme, Visit 2, Random Sample (North American Prevalence Study). (With the permission of Dr. B. M. Rifkind, Lipid Metabolism Branch, Division of Heart and Vascular Diseases, National Heart and Lung Institute, Bethesda, Maryland.)

1975) suggest that there is little or no further increase from age 2 until adolescence in either sex, though in the schoolchildren from an Australian town there was a progressive increase in the median plasma cholesterol concentration from 160 mg/100 ml at age 6 to above 180 at age 17 (Godfrey et al., 1972).

The changes that occur between birth and adolescence are probably physiological, in the sense that they are a reflection of natural growth and development, since they appear to take place in all human populations, irrespective of race or environment. Subsequent changes depend upon environmental conditions and, to a smaller extent, upon sex.

In affluent industrial communities the mean plasma total cholesterol concentration rises more or less continuously from the immediate post-adolescent period until the fifth or sixth decade. In men the rise ceases at about age 50 and is followed by a fall after age 70, due possibly to selective death of men with high plasma cholesterol concentrations. In women the increase in mean concentration is less steep than in men until about age 50; thereafter the increase continues into the sixties. The net result of these complex changes is that in women the mean concentration is slightly but significantly lower than in men until about age 50, after which the level in women exceeds that in men. These trends are illustrated in the relevant parts of Fig. 12.3, which shows the mean plasma cholesterol concentration by 5-year age groups for males and females in a random sample of the participants in a North American epidemiological study. Table 12.1 shows the mean and upper limits of plasma cholesterol concentration, by various age groups, in male and female employees in a London factory and in a selected population of healthy Americans. Both sets of values in this Table have been used as standards of 'normality' in clinical practice. The mean values in the British factory employees are somewhat higher than those shown for adults of comparable age in Fig. 12.3, but are similar to those in the American adults shown in Table 12.2.

4.2.2 Lipoprotein cholesterol

The wide range of plasma total cholesterol concentration within populations is due to an underlying variability in cholesterol concentration in each of the lipoprotein fractions. As may be seen from the upper limits shown in Table 12.1, in absolute terms the major contribution to total variability is from LDL cholesterol. However, the smaller absolute variability in the concentration of the other two lipoproteins, particularly that in HDL, may be very important in relation to IHD (see below). In so far as there is a contribution from the diet to intra-population variability in plasma cholesterol level, this is probably mediated largely through LDL, since the major effect

Table 12.1

Means and arbitrary upper limits of cholesterol concentration in whole plasma and in lipoprotein fractions in selected populations in Britain and the United States

Sex		Age (years)	Mean cholesterol concentration (mg/100 ml)				
			Total	VLDL	LDL	HDL Male	HDL Female
Britain[a]	Male	20–39	214 (252)		138 (184)		
		40–69	234 (291)		160 (215)		
	Female	20–39	211 (260)		127 (168)		
		40–69	245 (305)		168 (230)		
United States[b]	Both sexes combined except HDL	0–19	175 (230)	12 (25)	103 (170)	51 (65)	54 (70)
		20–29	180 (240)	16 (25)	112 (170)	49 (70)	56 (75)
		30–39	205 (270)	17 (35)	126 (190)	46 (65)	57 (80)
		40–49	225 (310)	19 (35)	134 (190)	48 (65)	65 (85)
		50–59	245 (330)	25 (40)	161 (210)	42 (65)	49 (85)

[a] Values from Lewis et al. (1974).
[b] Values from Fredrickson et al. (1978).
Values in parentheses are upper limits set at the upper 95th percentile.
For details of methods of assay and selection of the populations, see the original papers.

of dietary cholesterol and of polyunsaturated fat on plasma lipoproteins is on LDL. For example, in the vegetarian communes investigated by Sacks et al. (1975) the mean plasma LDL cholesterol concentration in the vegetarians was 73 mg/100 ml compared with 118 mg/100 ml in the control population, whereas the plasma HDL cholesterol concentration was only 6 mg/100 ml lower in the vegetarians than in the controls.

In view of current interest in HDL as a negative risk factor for IHD, much attention is now being given to environmental and 'host' factors that influence the plasma HDL cholesterol concentration. Those for which the evidence is reasonably strong are listed in Table 12.2. Several of these factors must contribute to the variability in plasma HDL cholesterol level encountered in the population at large. Of special interest from the point of view of IHD are sex (discussed below) and physical exercise. Plasma HDL cholesterol concentration is higher in male skiers (Carlson and Mossfeldt, 1964), trained runners (Wood et al., 1976) and lumberjacks (Nikkilä, 1978) than in the general population. The increase due to exercise is apparent within a few weeks of a period of physical training (Lopez-S et al., 1974).

The age- and sex-related differences in plasma total cholesterol concentration discussed above are, of course, due to differences in lipoprotein cholesterol concentration. In cord blood about half the

Table 12.2
Factors influencing plasma HDL cholesterol concentration in man

Factor	Effect	Reference
Female (over age 14)	↑	Russ et al. (1955); Rifkind et al. (1978)
Oestrogenic contraceptives (over age 30–40)	↑	Rifkind et al. (1978)
Exercise	↑	Carlson and Mossfeldt (1964) and see text
Alcohol	↑	Johansson and Medhus (1974)
Weight loss	↑	Wilson and Lees (1972)
Clofibrate	↑	Nichols et al. (1968)
Nicotinic acid	↑	Blum et al. (1977)
Cholesterol feeding	↑	Mahley et al. (1978)
Male (over age 14)	↓	Russ et al. (1955); Rifkind et al. (1978)
Obesity	↓	Wilson and Lees (1972)
Hypertriglyceridaemia	↓	Wilson and Lees (1972)
Carbohydrate feeding	↓	Wilson and Lees (1972)
Polyunsaturated fat feeding	↓	Nichaman et al. (1967) (controversial)
Diabetes	↓	Barr et al. (1951)
Smoking	↓	Garrison et al. (1978)

↑ = increase; ↓ = decrease compared with the mean value in the general population.

total cholesterol in plasma is carried in HDL (Tsang *et al.*, 1974). During the first few days of life there is a rapid rise in the concentration of cholesterol in LDL, with little change in that in HDL. The subsequent changes in lipoprotein cholesterol level that occur from childhood into old age in industrialized communities are illustrated in Fig. 12.3 and 12.4. After about age 20, LDL cholesterol concentration rises in both sexes, but more steeply in males than in females. After age 50, LDL cholesterol in females exceeds that in males. Until age 14–15 HDL cholesterol concentration is the same in both sexes (about 53 mg/100 ml). In females the level begins to rise in the early twenties, reaching a peak (65 mg/100 ml) at about age 65, and then

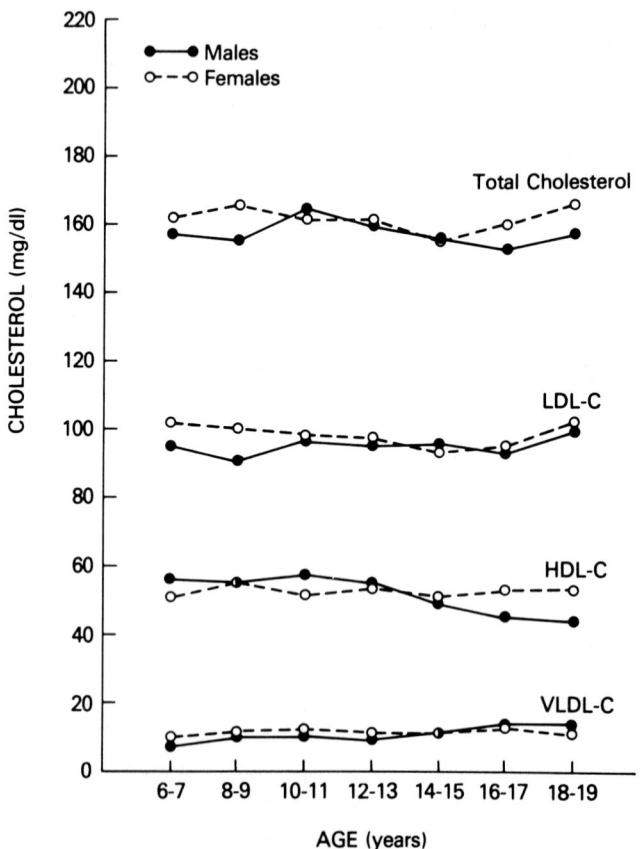

Figure 12.4
Mean plasma total, LDL-, HDL- and VLDL-cholesterol levels by two-year age groups for participants aged 6–19 years. Lipid Research Clinics Programme, Visit 2, Random Sample (North American Prevalence Study). (With the permission of Dr. B. M. Rifkind, Lipid Metabolism Branch, Division of Heart and Vascular Diseases, National Heart and Lung Institute, Bethesda, Maryland.)

falls slightly. In males, on the other hand, there is a sharp fall at age 15 to about 45 mg/100 ml with no further change until the fifties, when there is a moderate increase. The VLDL cholesterol concentration begins to increase at least as early as age 20, the rise being steeper in males than in females until age 40. In women using oestrogenic hormones (Fig. 12.5), total cholesterol is higher up to age 50, HDL cholesterol is higher after age 40 (but not before) and VLDL cholesterol is higher at all ages up to age 60, than in non-users of oestrogens. Since oestrogens are widely used as contraceptives in the reproductive period or as replacement therapy after the menopause,

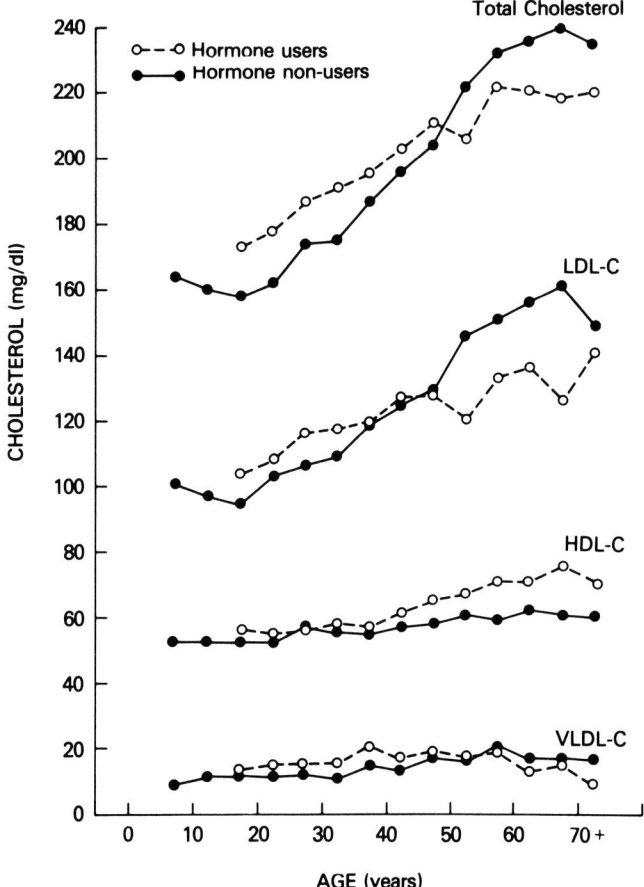

Figure 12.5
Mean plasma total, LDL-, HDL- and VLDL-cholesterol levels by five-year age groups—in female user and non-users of sex hormones. Lipid Research Clinics Programme, Visit 2, Random Sample (North American Prevalence Study). (With the permission of Dr. B. M. Rifkind, Lipid Metabolism Branch, Division of Heart and Vascular Diseases, National Heart and Lung Institute, Bethesda, Maryland.)

these effects must be taken into account in epidemiological surveys of the plasma cholesterol in which women are included.

Two points are worth noting about the age- and sex-related changes described above. First, the sex difference in plasma HDL cholesterol concentration, though small in absolute terms is proportionally quite substantial. Thus, by age 50 the mean level is at least 30% higher in women than in men. Secondly, the changes in total cholesterol are dominated by the changes in LDL cholesterol. As a consequence of this, the very significant proportional difference in HDL cholesterol between the sexes is hidden by the much larger absolute differences, in an opposite sense, in LDL cholesterol concentration up to age 50. An analogous situation arises in relation to the effect of chronic exercise on the plasma cholesterol level. The rise in HDL cholesterol level is masked by a fall in the level of VLDL cholesterol and, possibly, of LDL cholesterol, so that there may be a net fall in total cholesterol concentration. Failure to appreciate the point that changes in HDL cholesterol concentration are not usually reflected in changes in total cholesterol concentration is one reason for the prolonged neglect of HDL in work on the atherosclerosis problem.

A general discussion of the mechanisms by which the various factors listed in Table 12.2 affect the plasma HDL cholesterol concentration is beyond the scope of this chapter. As discussed in Chapter 11, some of them are probably mediated by an influence on the metabolism of the HDL apoproteins. Another possibility is suggested by the fact that the products of VLDL catabolism are an important source of HDL. Nikkilä (1978) has drawn attention to the frequent reciprocal relation between VLDL and HDL cholesterol concentrations, as in female sex, habitual physical exercise and hypertriglyceridaemia, and has suggested that one of the determinants of plasma HDL concentration is the efficiency of the catabolic mechanisms for VLDL. It should be noted that any explanation of the manner in which the plasma HDL concentration is regulated must take into account the fact that differences in HDL cholesterol concentration are in most cases due largely to differences in the concentration of cholesterol in the HDL_2 fraction, with little or no difference in HDL_3; for example, the difference between men and women with respect to HDL cholesterol concentration is due almost entirely to a difference in HDL_2 (Cheung and Albers, 1977). In cholesterol-fed human subjects, the increase observed in HDL cholesterol concentration occurs mainly in an electrophoretically distinct apoE-rich species designated HDL-I by Mahley et al. (1978).

We do not know how far the numerous factors known to influence the plasma HDL concentration interact with one another. But if their effects are additive, then perhaps from the point of view of the plasma HDL concentration the ideal person would be a lean non-smoking alcoholic 40-year-old female Marathon runner, taking oral contraceptives and with four nonagenarian grandparents (see next section).

5 GENETIC INFLUENCES

5.1 Methods of estimation

The variability in plasma cholesterol concentration within any population is due to a combination of *genetic* factors and of all those other factors, such as diet, physical exercise and smoking habits, which may be called *environmental*. We need to know the relative contributions from these two sources if only because the genetic component represents the residual variability that will remain whatever is done to modify natural environmental influences acting upon the population as a whole. In other words, genetically determined variability limits the extent to which we can change the frequency distribution of plasma cholesterol concentrations in any population by, for example, bringing about a change in dietary habits. A simple example will illustrate this point. For any two pairs of monozygotic twins there would be differences in plasma cholesterol concentration within and between each pair. If all four twins were placed in an environment identical with respect to all those environmental factors that influence the plasma cholesterol, the difference within pairs would disappear, but there would remain a difference between pairs, due to their different genetic make-up.

Evidence for a genetic influence on the concentration of cholesterol in whole plasma and in the separate lipoprotein fractions is derived from two complementary types of observation. First, one may measure the degree of concordance for plasma cholesterol concentration in randomly selected families or in the families of index subjects whose plasma cholesterol concentration deviates markedly from the population mean. Secondly, one may compare the degree of concordance within and between monozygotic and dizygotic co-twins. A recent development, combining features from both approaches, is to study the progeny of monozygotic twins, whose genetic relationship is that of half-sibs (Nance *et al.*, 1974).

5.2 Observations on families

'I have as much of my father in me as you.'
(Orlando to his brother Oliver, in As You Like It)

In first-degree relatives, on average, the genes at 50% of gene loci are derived from the same ancestral genes, i.e. they are identical by descent. Hence, the probability that the genes at a given locus in first-degree relatives have identical descent is 0.5. This may be expressed by saying that the *genetic relatedness* between first-degree relatives is 0.5. That between monozygotic twins (who have all their genes in common) is 1.0, that between first cousins is 0.125 ($\frac{1}{8}$) and that between unrelated spouses is zero. The corollary to this is that a given person has a 50% chance of carrying a rare mutant gene present by inheritance in a first-degree relative and a 12.5% chance of carrying one inherited by a third-degree relative (e.g. a cousin). It also follows that if the variability of plasma cholesterol concentration in the general population is entirely genetic in origin, the correlation between sibs who are not monozygotic twins and between parents and their children should be 0.5, while that between spouses should approach zero. It should be noted that genetic relatedness used in the above sense refers to the average proportion of genes that are identical *by virtue of their descent*. At some loci the genes will be *chemically* identical in most individuals in a given population, whether or not they are related. For example, in a British population the gene for the β chain of haemoglobin will be chemically identical in most people because heterozygosity at this locus is comparatively rare in Britain.

Table 12.3 shows the correlation coefficients for plasma total cholesterol concentration observed by Adlersberg et al. (1957) in 201 families chosen at random from a New York white population. The correlation between spouses was not significantly different from zero, but there were significant positive parent-child and sib-sib correlations. These results suggest a strong genetic influence on plasma cholesterol. The correlation between sibs is consistent with the conclusion that 74% (0.37/0.50) of the total variability for plasma cholesterol concentration in the population examined by Adlersberg et al. was genetic in origin. The higher correlation between mother and child than between father and child also suggests that the relative

Table 12.3
Correlation coefficients for plasma cholesterol concentration in families; all concentrations adjusted for age and sex to equivalent levels determined in males aged 20

Relation	Correlation	P
Mother–father	0.0056	>0.2
Father–child	0.2101	<0.001
Mother–child	0.3646	<0.001
Sib–sib	0.3701	<0.001

P is the probability that the correlation coefficient was zero. (From Adlersberg et al., 1957.)

importance of genes *versus* environment in determining plasma cholesterol level is greater for the female than for the male parent. However, members of a family living together share more of their environment with each other than with members of the general population, so that some familial aggregation would be expected even if there is no genetic contribution to the intra-population variability. Furthermore, if children share more of their environment with their mother than with their father, the mother-child correlation would be higher than the father-child correlation. Adlersberg *et al.* argued that the familial aggregation they had observed in their New York population could not have been due solely to environmental factors because of the absence of a correlation between spouses who, presumably, shared much of their environment with their children. But this argument is not decisive, since parents only share their family environment as adults. Results similar to those of Adlersberg *et al.* were obtained by Godfrey *et al.* (1972) in their study of school children and their parents in an Australian town. Significant correlations were found between parents and children throughout the whole range of plasma cholesterol levels, suggesting some degree of polygenic inheritance of variability in plasma cholesterol level. However, as with the New York population, it was not possible to exclude similarities in the family environment as a cause of the resemblances within families.

Deutscher *et al.* (1966) tried to get round this problem by measuring familial aggregation at different ages in nearly 90% of the total population of the town of Tecumseh. They found that the resemblance for plasma cholesterol concentration between sibs was highest in children, falling after age 16 and then rising again at age 40. They concluded that the familial aggregation observed in children was due to a combination of environmental and genetic factors, that the environmental contribution tends to be lost as the children leave the family, and that genes with delayed penetration are responsible for the reappearance of familial aggregation later in life. As in the Australian study, the family aggregation was as high at the lower end of the distribution of plasma cholesterol concentration as at the upper end, again suggesting that the major genetic contribution to familial resemblance in plasma cholesterol is due to polygenic factors, rather than to inheritance of the single gene for familial hypercholesterolaemia.

In contradistinction to these and other population-based studies in America, all of which have shown significant familial aggregation, Brunner *et al.* (1971) found no correlations within the families of communal settlements in Israel. Since the children in these communes did not eat with their parents, Brunner *et al.* concluded that the resemblances between plasma cholesterol concentration observed in other studies on families living together were due entirely to environmental factors. However, it is possible that in the Israeli study, genetic influences on the plasma cholesterol concentration were masked by the very marked differences in the environments of the children and their parents. Thus, although the design of this study was such as to minimize familial aggregation due to non-genetic factors, minor genetic influences could have remained undetected. Had there been any families with familial hypercholesterolaemia in the study population, they would presumably have been detected.

Using a different approach, Patterson and Slack (1972) measured the plasma cholesterol concentration in first-degree relatives of survivors of a myocardial infarction who had hyperlipidaemia, defined as an age- and sex-adjusted plasma cholesterol or triglyceride concentration more than 2 SD above the means determined in a group of control subjects. The mean plasma cholesterol concentration in the relatives was significantly higher than that in the controls. Since the whole distribution of cholesterol scores for the first-degree relatives was shifted to the right, without any evidence of bimodality, Patterson and Slack (1972) concluded that in so far as there was a genetic basis to the hypercholesterolaemia in the index patients and their relatives, this was predominantly polygenic rather than monogenic. Goldstein *et al.* (1973) have also examined the relatives of hyperlipidaemic survivors of myocardial infarction and have found evidence for heritability of the hyperlipidaemia in the index patients. The distribution of hypercholesterolaemia and hypertriglyceridaemia in the relatives led them to postulate the presence of three genetic forms of hypercholesterolaemia in the patients and their relatives: the monogenic form of familial hypercholesterolaemia discussed in Chapter 15, a previously unrecognised monogenic form designated 'combined hyperlipidaemia' and a polygenically determined hypercholesterolaemia. Goldstein *et al.* deduced that only a small fraction of the genetically determined hypercholesterolaemia associated with myocardial infarction in their index patients was polygenic. This is not inconsistent with the conclusion, derived from population-based family studies, that the main genetic contribution to variability in plasma cholesterol level in the general population is polygenic, since it is quite possible that single-gene effects, some of which may be expressed at birth, are more conducive to atherosclerosis than polygenic effects, which may act later in life and with less intensity. It should also be noted that the index patients in one sub-group in the study of Goldstein *et al.* were selected for having at least one hyperlipidaemic relative. This may possibly have introduced bias in favour of patients with monogenically inherited hyperlipidaemia.

Another finding of interest in relation to the question of genetic influences on the plasma cholesterol concentration is that of Glueck *et al.* (1977), who have demonstrated familial aggregation of high

The Epidemiology of the Plasma Cholesterol 589

plasma HDL-cholesterol concentrations in the first-degree relatives of octogenarians. For discussion of this, see Chapter 13, Section 3.6. Feinleib *et. al.* (1976) have also noted a significant clustering of *low* plasma HDL cholesterol concentrations in the children of parents who have had a heart attack.

5.3 Observations on twins

The proportion of the total intra-population variability of plasma cholesterol concentration that is due to heredity (the *heritability*) is difficult to estimate from family studies of the kind discussed above because of the problem of distinguishing between genetic and environmental influences. This arises particularly in relation to polygenic factors, which are probably the main genetic cause of minor variations close to the population mean. The best method of approaching this problem is by the study of twins. If there is a genetic contribution to population variability, then one may predict that intra-pair variance would be smaller for monozygotic twins (in whom relatedness is 1.0) than for like-sex dizygotic twins (in whom relatedness is only 0.5) and that intra-pair variance would be smaller than inter-pair variance in all twin groups. One may also predict that if there is an environmental component, the variance for twins living together would be smaller than for twins living apart.

Table 12.4 shows the variances for plasma total cholesterol concentration in 102 pairs of adult twins examined by Osborne *et al.* (1959). In each comparison for which twins were available, the variance was greater for dizygotic than for monozygotic twins and also for those living apart than for those living together. These findings indicate the presence of both genetic and environmental contributions to total variability in the population from which these

Table 12.4
Intra-pair variance of plasma total cholesterol concentration in monozygotic and like-sex dizygotic twins living apart and together

	Monozygotic	Dizygotic
Male, together	280	694
Male, apart	340	—
Female, together	206	366
Female, apart	602	869

The variance is $\Sigma x^2/2n$, where x is the difference between the members of a pair of co-twins in mg/100 ml and n is the number of pairs.
(Modified from Osborne *et al.*, 1959.)

twins were drawn. Since hypercholesterolaemic twins were excluded, it is unlikely that the single gene for familial hypercholesterolaemia made any contribution to the total genetic influence on plasma cholesterol level observed in this study. In one pair of male monozygotic twins living apart, the difference in plasma cholesterol concentration was 31 mg/100 ml, a striking illustration of the extent to which environmental factors may influence the plasma cholesterol.

Since the investigation of Osborne *et al.* there have been at least nine other twin studies of the variability of plasma cholesterol concentration and in some cases the lipoprotein fractions were examined, as well as the whole plasma (for references, see Heiberg, 1974). In all but two of these studies the authors concluded that there was a significant genetic contribution to intra-population variability for total cholesterol concentration, and in the Norwegian twins examined by Heiberg (1974) there was evidence for some heritability of LDL cholesterol and HDL cholesterol. Estimates of heritability of cholesterol concentration vary widely in different studies. For example, the heritability in males, calculated by applying the formula of Falconer (1965) to the published observations, was 0.38 in the Finnish twins examined by Pikkarainen *et al.* (1966) and 0.66 in Heiberg's twins. At the other extreme, there was no consistent evidence for heritability in the Scottish twins studied by Rifkind *et al.* (1968) or in the American twins examined in the National Heart and Lung Institute twin study (Feinleib, 1975), though in the latter study the variance within monozygotes was significantly smaller than that within dizygotes.

5.4 Critical summary and conclusions

Almost all workers agree that a significant proportion of the intra-population variability of plasma cholesterol concentration is genetic in origin and that most of the genetic variation seen in unselected human populations is polygenic rather than monogenic. However, there is much disagreement about the quantitative importance of genetically determined variability. One reason for this is that different methods have been used for calculating heritability (see Weinberg *et al.* (1976) for critical comments) and for selecting the subjects to be examined; in twin studies, for example, estimates of heritability are very sensitive to the presence of a small number of twin pairs carrying the gene for familial hypercholesterolaemia. It is also worth noting that in twin studies a surprisingly large number of pairs is required if statistical significance is to be achieved. In several of the published studies, too few twins were examined.

However, over and above these methodological sources of disagreement, the relative contribution of genetic factors to total variability is likely to differ from one population to another. For example, heritability would be bound to increase in any population or subpopulation in which the force of environmental factors was decreased. Since this fact is often ignored, a few words about heritability in general may be helpful at this point. Because the intensity with which the environment acts upon any trait may vary considerably under different conditions, the heritability of a variable trait is not something that is fixed in time and space. Two examples should make this clear.

Both genetic and environmental factors can contribute to the development of rickets in a given individual, though the frequency of genes causing rickets is rare in the population as a whole. In the smoky industrial towns of 19th century England, rickets due to a combination of nutritional deficiency and lack of sunlight was rife. Hence, the genetic contribution to the prevalence of rickets must have been very largely submerged by the environmental contribution, and the estimated heritability of the clinical condition in urban communities determined, for example, by family studies would have been close to zero. In present-day England environmental causes of rickets have been almost completely eliminated, except possibly among the women of some immigrant communities. Rickets has therefore become an uncommon disease due, in the majority of cases, to the inheritance of inborn errors affecting the metabolism of calcium or phosphorus; as a consequence of this change the heritability of rickets in most English communities is probably close to unity. Thus, a change in the environment may radically alter the relative contribution of genetic factors, expressed numerically in terms of heritability, within a few generations in a given geographical region.

The heritability of plasma cholesterol concentration illustrates the effect of differences in the environment in different populations at a given time. In populations, such as those of most Westernized countries, where the mean plasma cholesterol concentration is relatively high, environmental factors (especially diet) must make a substantial contribution to the high prevalence of hypercholesterolaemia compared with that in populations where, owing to the lower intensity of these environmental factors, the mean plasma cholesterol level is so much lower. Hence, heritability of plasma cholesterol level is likely to be much lower in Westernized countries than in underdeveloped countries. Indeed, one could imagine a population living under conditions in which the strength of the environmental contribution is so weak that hypercholesterolaemia is due almost entirely to monogenically or polygenically inherited factors. In such a population, the heritability of hypercholesterolaemia would be very high. The same considerations apply to subpopulations within the community and may help to explain why the heritability of plasma cholesterol concentration has been found to be higher in females than in males in several studies. The relative importance of polygenic and monogenic inheritance is also likely to vary between different subpopulations. For example, if monogenic hypercholesterolaemia specifically increases the risk of IHD, the relative contribution of monogenic inheritance to total variability of plasma cholesterol concentration will be higher in families of an IHD index patient than in the general population.

Slack (1974) has drawn attention to the predictions that can be made from an estimate of heritability. If, for example, the heritability of plasma cholesterol concentration in the males of a particular population is 0.38, then the children of a man whose plasma cholesterol concentration is one SD above the population mean will, on average, have an age-adjusted concentration that is 0.19 (0.38/2) of one SD above the population mean. In the example given by Slack, the SD of the population mean was 42 mg/100 ml; therefore the mean elevation in the children would be 8 mg/100 ml. It should be noted that these calculations are valid only if the inheritance is polygenic. If our hypothetical index subject is a carrier of the single gene for familial hypercholesterolaemia, in which case his plasma cholesterol concentration would be more than one SD above the population mean, his children would inherit the gene according to Mendel's laws, half having concentrations similar to the index subject's and the other half having concentrations distributed about the population mean.

5.5 Genetics of plasma cholesterol in animals

In keeping with what is generally observed in human populations, genetic factors have been shown to influence the plasma cholesterol concentration in several species of animal under experimental conditions, including rats (Kohn, 1950), mice (Bruell, 1963), rabbits (Roberts *et al.*, 1974), cattle (Stufflebean and Lasley, 1969), monkeys (Clarkson *et al.*, 1971), chickens (Estep *et al.*, 1963) and pigeons (Patton *et al.*, 1974). In most cases, inheritance of plasma cholesterol level seems to be polygenic, estimates of heritability ranging from less than 0.3 to over 0.6. However, Clarkson *et al.* (1971) have described a response to cholesterol feeding in squirrel monkeys which they believe to be monogenically inherited. In some monkeys of a captive population the plasma cholesterol concentration increases markedly when cholesterol is fed (hyper-responders) while in others (hypo-responders) there is little or no increase. Breeding experiments suggest that the type of response is determined by a single gene. The existence of this gene in monkeys gives rise to an interesting situation of possible relevance to variability in human populations (see below). In unselected populations of squirrel monkeys given a cholesterol-rich diet, the variability of plasma cholesterol concentration is very considerable (from less than 200 mg/100 ml to more than 1000 mg/100 ml), but in the same population given a normal vegetarian diet this potential variability is not expressed.

5.6 Mechanisms of gene-mediated effects

With regard to the mechanism of gene-mediated effects on the plasma cholesterol, we have a good deal of information about the underlying biochemical abnormalities in the familial hyperlipidaemias and hypolipidaemias, all of which are generally believed to be monogenic (see Chapters 15 and 16). However, these single-gene effects account for only a small fraction of the inherited variability of plasma cholesterol concentration in the general population and are responsible mainly for the more extreme variations at either end of the distribution. We know little about the way in which polygenic effects contribute to the relatively small differences that we see on each side of the population mean. Since the plasma concentrations of cholesterol and of its lipoprotein carriers are influenced directly or indirectly by many metabolic processes, all of which must be subject to some degree of genetic control, polygenic effects could be very complex. Some polygenic systems could act by modifying the efficiency of intrinsic regulatory mechanisms, such as the receptor-mediated catabolism of LDL (though there is no evidence for this particular example). Others could influence the efficiency of the body's response to environmental stimuli. According to Clarkson *et al.* (1971) the difference between hypo-responder and hyper-responder monkeys is due to an inherited difference in their ability to respond to increased dietary cholesterol by increasing bile-acid synthesis. There is no evidence that a similar cause of inherited variability of plasma cholesterol concentration exists in human populations, but it is a possibility worth considering in relation to human communities with a high intake of cholesterol. It is not difficult to think of ways in which the ability to respond to other dietary factors which affect the plasma cholesterol could be modified by polygenic systems.

One mechanism by which genes could modify the plasma cholesterol level is by influencing the rate of production or degradation of specific apolipoproteins. Indeed, this is thought to be the genetic basis of at least some of the familial abnormalities in human plasma lipoprotein concentration (familial hypercholesterolaemia, abetalipoproteinaemia, Tangier disease and, possibly, familial broad beta disease). However, the extent to which polygenically determined variations in plasma lipoprotein concentration are mediated in this way is not known. Of interest in this connection is the observation of Berg (1978) that 0.5 to 0.6 of the variability of plasma apoA-I concentration in adults living in the Oslo area is heritable.

Statistically significant correlations between plasma cholesterol concentration and certain polymorphic antigens, including those of the ABO, Rh and Lp(a) systems, have been observed in human populations (see Morton, 1976, for review). For example, Oliver et al. (1969) have shown that group A individuals have, on average, higher plasma cholesterol concentrations than group O, B or AB individuals and Dahlén and Berg (1977) have observed higher plasma total- and LDL-cholesterol concentrations in Lp(a+) than in Lp(a−) individuals. These correlations have not, as yet, thrown any light on the biochemical mechanisms underlying polygenic inheritance of plasma cholesterol concentration, but they can be exploited in epidemiological investigations and in studies of genetic linkage.

6 VARIABILITY BETWEEN POPULATIONS

6.1 Plasma cholesterol in different geographical, racial and social groups

In many populations living under economically backward conditions or in regions where subsistence is based mainly on agriculture or fishing, the mean plasma cholesterol concentration in adults is much below that in affluent industrialized communities. Since these economically 'primitive' groups often live in parts of the world where the climate is pleasing and the scenery picturesque, they have attracted the attention of many epidemiologists interested in the atherosclerosis question (see Jones, 1970, for references). Table 12.5 lists, by geographical region, the plasma cholesterol concentration in a few of the large number of these communities on which we have information. Some of the older values may no longer be accurate because the mean concentration in adults of underdeveloped populations may increase within a matter of years if there is a rise in living standards. It should also be noted that the differences between some population means shown in Table 12.5 may be due as much to inter-laboratory errors of measurement as to genuine biological variability (see Chapter 2, Section 6.1). However, it is clear that none of the values listed, all of which are derived from adult males, exceeds the mean concentration in the children of North American or British populations. Evidently, the post-adolescence increase that occurs in affluent populations does not take place in populations living under comparatively primitive social conditions.

It is generally agreed that these inter-population differences in plasma total cholesterol concentration are due mainly to differences in LDL concentration, but there is growing evidence to suggest that there are also differences in HDL cholesterol concentration between different populations. A striking example is the much higher plasma HDL concentration in Greenland Eskimos than in Danes living in Denmark (Bang et al., 1971).

Most inter-population surveys of plasma cholesterol concentration have been restricted to adults. The few comparative studies that have been made on cord plasma suggest that the plasma cholesterol level at birth is much the same in all parts of the world and is unaffected by race or economic status. Thus, cord plasma concentrations in low-income and high-income groups in Guatemala (Méndez et al., 1959) do not differ significantly and are similar to those reported for Britain and the United States; similar values have also been reported for South African whites and Bantus (Bersohn and Wayburne, 1956), two groups which differ markedly in standard of living as well as racially. However, observations on children from different countries (Golubjatnikov et al., 1972) and from different social classes within the same town (Baker et al., 1967) indicate that inter-population differences in plasma cholesterol concentration may develop before adolescence (see Uppal, 1974, for references).

In addition to the above differences between affluent and economically backward populations, there are also quite substantial variations in the mean plasma cholesterol concentrations from one affluent population to another. See, for example, the differences between men aged 40 to 59 in East Finland, West Finland and the town of Zutphen (Fig. 13.7).

Table 12.5
Plasma total cholesterol concentration in some free-living populations in which mean or median values are significantly lower than in Britain and North America

Population	Mean or median cholesterol (mg/100 ml)	Reference
Dalmation villages (men, 40–59)	186	Keys (1970)
Jews' (immigrants from Yemen) (men)	146	Toor et al. (1960)
Ushibuka, Japan (men, 40–59)	140	Keys (1970)
Pukapuka, South Pacific (men, 40–50)	178	Prior and Evans (1970)
New Guinea (men, 20–45)	176	Whyte et al. (1977)
Uganda Africans (men 40)	145	Shaper and Jones (1959)
Bantu Africans (men)	152	Antonis and Bersohn (1962)
Navajo Indians, North America (young men)	178	Page et al. (1956)
Tarahumara Indians, Mexico (men)	120	Connor et al. (1978)

6.2 The basis of inter-population variability

It would not be surprising to find some racial differences in plasma cholesterol concentration in man, analogous to the inherited differences observed by Bruell (1963) in different strains of mice. However, although some genetic contribution to inter-population variability cannot be ruled out, the bulk of the available evidence favours the view that the main causes are environmental. Perhaps the most telling argument for this is the effect of migration from one geographical region to another, particularly when there is a racial difference between host and immigrant population. When people emigrate from a country in which the plasma cholesterol concentration in adults is low to one in which it is high, they often acquire the concentration characteristic of the host population. Examples are Neapolitans who have emigrated to Boston (Miller et al., 1958), Yemenite Jews who have emigrated to Israel (Brunner, 1968) and Japanese born in Japan and living in Hawaii or the United States (Keys et al., 1958). Keys and his coworkers found that in Japanese men matched for age and relative fatness, the plasma cholesterol concentration increased in the order Shine (a Japanese town) < Honolulu < Los Angeles. The mean value for Japanese men living in Los Angeles was similar to that of the local white men.

When there are marked differences between different racial groups living in the same region, this can usually be explained by differences in economic status or cultural habits associated with race. A good example of this is the difference between plasma cholesterol concentrations in Bantu and white populations in South Africa. In the free-living state, the concentration in Bantu men (see Table 12.5) is about 60 mg/100 ml lower than that in white men of European origin. However, the concentrations become indistinguishable in Bantu and white prisoners eating the same diet and taking the same amount of physical exercise (Antonis and Bersohn, 1962). In keeping with this, the plasma cholesterol concentration is similar in American urban blacks and whites of comparable social class. Conversely, populations of similar racial origin but different social class, living within the same country may have different plasma cholesterol levels. Keys et al. (1954, 1955), for example, found higher levels in business men than in working-class men in Naples, and in men of similar social class in North Italy than in South Italy.

Much of the geographical variation in plasma cholesterol concentration may be explained by differences in habitual diet eaten by different populations. Of all the dietary components that have been investigated on a world-wide scale, the percentage of total calories provided by saturated fat seems to be the one most closely correlated with the mean plasma cholesterol level in adult populations. Fig. 13.7 shows the correlation obtained by Keys (1970) in his study of 14 communities in seven different countries. All cholesterol determinations were carried out at a single centre, but the questionnaire method used for assessing the composition of the diets must have been subject to considerable error. If inter-population differences in plasma cholesterol level are due solely to differences in dietary fat, the observed differences should be consistent with the known effects of a change in dietary fat under experimental conditions. Keys concluded that the inter-population differences in plasma cholesterol concentration that he was able to observe were about 20 mg/100 ml greater than would have been predicted from the differences in the intake of saturated fat and cholesterol. This indicates that other aspects of the environment contribute to inter-population differences in plasma total cholesterol concentration. Some of these additional factors could be dietary, such as the intake of total calories, cholesterol, fibre or plant sterols. But other non-dietary factors, such as physical exercise and smoking habits, may be equally important. It is also possible that the plasma cholesterol concentration is influenced by environmental factors that we do not recognize at present.

Epstein (1971) has drawn attention to the existence of primitive communities in which the plasma cholesterol level in adults is considerably lower than that in affluent communities, despite a high intake of saturated fat. Examples are the inhabitants of Pukapuka, whose diet is rich in coconut oil, and the Masai of Central Africa, who eat large quantities of beef fat. In so far as dietary fat is not the only determinant of the plasma cholesterol concentration in human populations, one would expect to find exceptions to the general correlation between saturated fat intake and cholesterol level. In primitive societies, a combination of low total caloric intake and a high level of physical activity may outweigh the effects of a high intake of saturated fat. Another possibility is that the fatty acids in some of these high-fat diets differ in chain length from the saturated fatty acids that cause a rise in plasma cholesterol level under experimental conditions.

The much-quoted example of the Eskimos, who obtain up to 50% of their total calories as animal fat but who have comparatively low plasma cholesterol concentrations (Bang and Dyerberg, 1972), may be explained by the presence of considerable quantities of polyunsaturated fat, particularly of the linolenate ($\omega 3$) class. The diet of the Eskimos of the West coast of Greenland consists largely of seals, small whales and fish (Sinclair, 1953), all of which are rich in polyunsaturated fats. An Eskimo commonly eats as much as 4 kg of raw meat at a single meal—hence the name given to these people by neighbouring Indians (Cree: *aski*, raw; *mow*, he eats).

REFERENCES

Adlersberg, D., Schaefer, L. E. and Steinberg, A. G. (1957). Studies on genetic and environmental control of serum cholesterol level. *Circulation*, **16**, 487–488.

Antonis, A. and Bersohn, I. (1962). The influence of diet on serum lipids in South African white and Bantu prisoners. *American Journal of Clinical Nutrition*, **10**, 484–499.

Baker, H., Frank, O., Feingold, S., Christakis, G. and Ziffer, H. (1967). Vitamins, total cholesterol, and triglycerides in 642 New York City school children. *American Journal of Clinical Nutrition*, **20**, 850–857.

Bang, H. O. and Dyerberg, J. (1972). Plasma lipids and lipoproteins in Greenlandic west coast eskimos. *Acta Medica Scandinavica*, **192**, 85–94.

Bang, H. O., Dyerberg, J. and Nielsen, A. B. (1971). Plasma lipid and lipoprotein pattern in Greenland West-coast Eskimos. *Lancet*, **1**, 1143–1145.

Barr, D. P., Russ, E. M. and Eder, H. A. (1951). Protein-lipid relationships in human plasma. II. In atherosclerosis and related conditions. *American Journal of Medicine*, **11**, 480–493.

Beaumont, J. L., Carlson, L. A., Cooper, G. R., Fejfar, Z., Fredrickson, D. S. and Strasser, T. (1970). Classification of hyperlipidaemias and hyperlipoproteinaemias. *Bulletin of the World Health Organization*, **43**, 891–915.

Berg, K. Genetic influence on variation in serum high density lipoprotein. In: *High Density Lipoproteins and Atherosclerosis*. Ed. A. M. Gotto Jr., N. E. Miller and M. F. Oliver. Elsevier, Amsterdam, pp. 207–211, 1978.

Bersohn, I. and Wayburne, S. (1956). Serum cholesterol concentration in new-born African and European infants and their mothers. *American Journal of Clinical Nutrition*, **4**, 117–123.

Blum, C. B., Levy, R. I., Eisenberg, S., Hall, M. III. Goebel, R. H. and Berman, M. (1977). High density lipoprotein metabolism in man. *Journal of Clinical Investigation*, **60**, 795–807.

Bruell, J. H. (1963). Additive inheritance of serum cholesterol level in mice. *Science*, **142**, 1664–1665.

Brunner, D. Effect of Western diet on serum cholesterol in Yemenite Jews in Israel. In: *Progress in Biochemical Pharmacology, Vol. 4*. Ed. C. J. Miras, A. N. Howard and R. Paoletti. S. Karger, Basel, p. 52, 1968.

Brunner, D., Altman, S., Posner, L., Bearman, J. E., Loebl. K. and Lewin, C. S. (1971). Heredity, environment, serum lipoproteins and serum uric acid. A study in a community without familial eating pattern. *Journal of Chronic Diseases*, **23**, 763–773.

Carlson, L. A. and Lindstedt, S. (1969). The Stockholm Prospective Survey. The initial values for plasma lipids. *Acta Medica Scandinavica, Supplement* 493.

Carlson, L. A. and Mossfeld, T. F. (1964). Acute effects of prolonged heavy exercise on the concentration of plasma lipids and lipoproteins in man. *Acta Physiologica Scandinavica*, **62**, 51–59.

Castelli, W. P., Coorer, G. R., Doyle, J. T., Garcia-Palmieri, M., Gordon, T., Hames, C., Hulley, S. B., Kagan, A., Kuchmak, M., McGee, D. and Vicic, W. J. (1977). Distribution of triglyceride and total, LDL and HDL cholesterol in several populations: a cooperative lipoprotein phenotyping study. *Journal of Chronic Diseases*, **30**, 147–169.

Cheung, M. C. and Albers, J. J. (1977). The measurement of apolipoprotein A-I and A-II levels in men and women by immunoassay. *Journal of Clinical Investigation*, **60**, 43–50.

Clarkson, T. B., Lofland, H. B., Bullock, B. C. and Goodman, H. O. (1971). Genetic

control of plasma cholesterol. Studies on squirrel monkeys. *Archives of Pathology*, **92**, 37–45.
Connor, W. E. and Connor, S. L. (1972). The key role of nutritional factors in the prevention of coronary heart disease. *Preventive Medicine*, **1**, 49–83.
Connor, W. E., McMurry, M., Cerqueira, M. and Solis, D. (1978). The effects of dietary cholesterol upon the plasma lipoproteins, cholesterol synthesis, and absorption in the Tarahumara Indians. *Circulation*, **58**, Supplement II, II–171.
Dahlén, G. and Berg, K. Studies indicating metabolic differences between Lp(a+) and Lp(a−) individuals. In: *Atherosclerosis IV. Proceedings of the Fourth International Symposium*. Ed. G. Schettler, Y. Goto, Y. Hata and G. Klose. Springer-Verlag, Berlin, 1977.
Duetscher, S., Epstein, F. H. and Kjelsberg, M. O. (1966). Familial aggregation of factors associated with coronary heart disease. *Circulation*, **33**, 911–924.
Epstein, F. H. (1971). Epidemiologic aspects of atherosclerosis. *Atherosclerosis*, **14**, 1–11.
Estep, G. D., Fanguy, R. C. and Ferguson, T. M. (1963). The effect of age and heredity upon serum cholesterol levels in chickens. *Poultry Science*, **48**, 1908–1911.
Falconer, D. S. (1965). The inheritance of liability to certain diseases estimated from the incidence among relatives. *Annals of Human Genetics*, **29**, 51–76.
Feinleib, M. Twin studies. In: *Task Force on Genetic Factors in Atherosclerotic Disease*. DHEW Publication No. (NIH) 76-922. National Institutes of Health, Bethesda, pp. 59–81, 1975.
Feinleib, M., Kannel, W. B., Garrison, R. J., McNamara, P. and Castelli, W. P. (1976). Relation of parental history of coronary heart disease to risk factors in young adults. The Framingham offspring study. *Circulation*, **54**, Supplement II, II–52.
Fredrickson, D. S., Goldstein, J. L. and Brown, M. S. The familial hyperlipoproteinemias. In: *The Metabolic Basis of Inherited Disease*, 4th edition. Ed. J. B. Stanbury, J. B. Wyngaarden and D. S. Fredrickson. McGraw Hill, New York, pp. 604–655, 1978.
Fredrickson, D. S., Levy, R. I. and Lees, R. S. (1967). Fat transport in lipoproteins—an integrated approach to mechanisms and disorders. *New England Journal of Medicine*, **276**, 34–44, 94–103, 148–156, 215–225, 273–281.
Garrison, R. J., Kannel, W. B., Feinleib, M., Castelli, W. P., McNamara, P. M. and Padgett, S. J. (1978). Cigarette smoking and HDL cholesterol. The Framingham offspring study. *Atherosclerosis*, **30**, 17–25.
Glueck, C. J., Gartside, P. S., Steiner, P. M., Miller, M., Todhunter, T., Haaf, J., Pucke, M., Terrana, M., Fallat, R. W. and Kashyap, M. L. (1977). Hyperalpha- and hypobeta-lipoproteinemia in octogenarian kindreds. *Atherosclerosis*, **27**, 387–406.
Glueck, C. J., Heckman, F., Schoenfeld, M., Steiner, P. and Pearce, W. (1971). Neonatal familial Type II hyperlipoproteinemia: cord blood cholesterol in 1800 births. *Metabolism*, **20**, 597–608.
Godfrey, R. C., Stenhouse, N. S., Cullen, K. J. and Blackman, V. (1972). Cholesterol and the child: studies of the cholesterol levels of Busselton school children and their parents. *Australian Paediatric Journal*, **8**, 72–78.
Goldstein, J. L., Hazzard, W. R., Schrott, H. G., Bierman, E. L. and Motulsky, A. G. (1973). Hyperlipidemia in coronary heart disease. I. Lipid levels in 500 survivors of myocardial infarction. *Journal of Clinical Investigation*, **52**, 1533–1543.
Golubjatnikov, R., Paskey, T. and Inhorn, S. L. (1972). Serum cholesterol levels of Mexican and Wisconsin school children. *American Journal of Epidemiology*, **96**, 36–39.
Groen, J. J., Tijong, K. B., Koster, M., Willebrands, A. F., Verdonck, G. and Pierloot, M. (1962). The influence of nutrition and ways of life on blood

cholesterol and the prevalence of hypertension and coronary heart disease among Trappist and Benedictine monks. *American Journal of Clinical Nutrition*, **10**, 456–470.

Heiberg, A. (1974). The heritability of serum lipoprotein and lipid concentrations. A twin study. *Clinical Genetics*, **6**, 307–316.

Johansson, B. G. and Medhus, A. (1974). Increase in plasma α-lipoproteins in chronic alcoholics after acute abuse. *Acta Medica Scandinavica*, **195**, 273–277.

Jones, R. J. Environmental and host factors in coronary heart disease, including risk factors: an epidemiological view. In: *Atherosclerosis. Proceedings of the Second International Symposium*, Section X. Springer-Verlag, New York, 1970.

Kannel, W. B. Normal limits for serum cholesterol. In: *Treatment of the Hyperlipidemic States*. Ed. H. R. Casdorph. Charles C. Thomas, Springfield, Illinois, pp. 36–45, 1971.

Keys, A. *Coronary Heart Disease in Seven Countries. Circulation*, Vol. XLI, No. 4, Suppl. 1, Monograph No. 29. Ed. A. Keys. American Heart Association, 1970.

Keys, A., Fidanza, F. and Keys, H. M. (1955). Further studies on serum cholesterol of clinically healthy men in Italy. *Voeding*, **16**, 492.

Keys, A., Fidanza, F., Scardi, V., Bergami, G., Keys, M. H. and Di Lorenzo, F. (1954). Studies on serum cholesterol and other characteristics of clinically healthy men in Naples. *Archives of Internal Medicine*, **93**, 328–336.

Keys, A., Kimur, A. N., Kusukawa, A., Bronte-Stewart, B., Larsen, N. and Keys, M. H. (1958). Lessons from serum cholesterol studies in Japan, Hawaii and Los Angeles. *Annals of Internal Medicine*, **48**, 83–94.

Kohn, H. I. (1950). Changes in plasma of the rat during fasting and influence of genetic factors upon sugar and cholesterol levels. *American Journal of Physiology*, **163**, 410–417.

Lauer, R. M., Connor, W. E., Leaverton, P. E., Reiter, M. A. and Clarke, W. R. (1975). Coronary heart disease risk factors in school children: the Muscatine study. *Journal of Pediatrics*, **86**, 697–706.

Lee, V. A. (1967). Individual trends in the total serum cholesterol of children and adolescents over a ten-year period. *American Journal of Clinical Nutrition*, **20**, 5–12.

Lewis, B. *The Hyperlipidaemias. Clinical and Laboratory Practice*. Blackwell Scientific Publications, Oxford, 1976.

Lewis, B., Chait, A., Wootton, I. D. P., Oakley, C. M., Krikler, D. M., Sigurdsson, G., February, A., Maurer, B. and Birkenhead, J. (1974). Frequency of risk factors for ischaemic heart-disease in a healthy British population with particular reference to serum-lipoprotein levels. *Lancet*, **1**, 141–146.

Lopez-S, A., Vial, R., Balart, L. and Arroyave, G. (1974). Effect of exercise and physical fitness on serum lipids and lipoproteins. *Atherosclerosis*, **20**, 1–9.

Mahley, R. W., Innerarity, T. L., Bersot, T. P., Lipson, A. and Margolis, S. (1978). Alterations in human high-density lipoproteins, with or without increased plasma-cholesterol, induced by diets high in cholesterol. *Lancet*, **2**, 807–809.

McGill, H. C. (1979). The relationship of dietary cholesterol to serum cholesterol concentration and to atherosclerosis in man. *American Journal of Clinical Nutrition*, **32**, 2664–2702.

Méndez, J., Savits, B. S., Flores, M. and Scrimshaw, N. S. (1959). Cholesterol levels of maternal and fetal blood at parturition in upper and lower income groups in Guatemala city. *American Journal of Clinical Nutrition*, **7**, 595–598.

Miettinen, M., Turpeinen, O., Karvonen, M. J., Elosuo, R. and Paavilainen, E. (1972). Effect of cholesterol-lowering diet on mortality from coronary heart-disease and other causes. A twelve-year clinical trial in men and women. *Lancet*, **2**, 835–838.

Miller, D. C., Trulson, M. F., McCann, M. B., White, P. D. and Stare, F. J. (1958).

Diet, blood lipids and health of Italian men in Boston. *Annals of Internal Medicine*, **49**, 1178–1200.
Morton, N. E. (1976). Genetic markers in atherosclerosis: a review. *Journal of Medical Genetics*, **13**, 81–90.
Nance, W. E., Nakata, M., Paul, T. D. and Yu, P. The use of twin studies in the analysis of phenotypic traits in man. In: *Congenital Defects. New Directions in Research.* Ed. D. T. Janerich, R. G. Skalko and I. H. Porter. Academic Press, New York, pp. 23–49, 1974.
Nichaman, M. Z., Sweeley, C. C. and Olson, R. E. (1967). Plasma fatty acids in normolipemic and hyperlipemic subjects during fasting and after linoleate feeding. *American Journal of Clinical Nutrition*, **20**, 1057–1069.
Nichols, A. V., Strisower, E. H., Lindgren, F. T., Adamson, G. L. and Poggiola, E. L. (1968). Analysis of change in ultracentrifugal lipoprotein profiles following heparin and ethyl-*p*-chlorophenoxyisobutyrate administration. *Clinica Chimica Acta*, **20**, 277–283.
Nikkilä, E. A. Metabolic and endocrine control of plasma high density lipoprotein concentration. In: *High Density Lipoproteins and Atherosclerosis.* Ed. A. M. Gotto Jr., N. E. Miller and M. F. Oliver. Elsevier, Amsterdam, pp. 177–192, 1978.
Oliver, M. F., Geizerova, H., Cumming, R. A. and Heady, J. A. (1969). Serum-cholesterol and ABO and rhesus blood groups. *Lancet*, **2**, 605–606.
Osborne, R. H., Adlersberg, D., DeGeorge, F. V. and Wang, C. (1959). Serum lipids, heredity and environment. A study of adult twins. *American Journal of Medicine*, **26**, 54–59.
Owen, G. M., Krim, K. M., Garry, P. J., Lowe, J. E. and Lubin, A. H. (1974). A study of nutritional status of preschool children in the United States. 1968–1970. *Pediatrics*, **53**, 597–646.
Page, I. H., Lewis, L. A. and Gilbert, J. (1956). Plasma lipids and proteins and their relationship to coronary disease among Navajo Indians. *Circulation*, **13**, 675–679.
Patterson, D. and Slack, J. (1972). Lipid abnormalities in male and female survivors of myocardial infarction and their first-degree relatives. *Lancet*, **1**, 393–399.
Patton, N. M., Brown, R. V. and Middleton, C. C. (1974). Familial cholesterolemia in pigeons. *Atherosclerosis*, **19**, 307–314.
Pikkarainen, J., Takkunen, J. and Kuonen, E. (1966). Serum cholesterol in Finnish twins. *American Journal of Human Genetics*, **18**, 115–126.
Prior, I. A. M. and Evans, J. G. Current developments in the Pacific. In: *Atherosclerosis. Proceedings of the Second International Symposium.* Ed. R. J. Jones. Springer-Verlag, Berlin, pp. 335–342, 1970.
Rifkind, B. M., Boyle, J. A., Gale, M., Greig, W. and Buchanan, W. W. (1968). Study of serum lipid levels in twins. *Cardiovascular Research*, **2**, 148–156.
Rifkind, B. M., Tamir, I. and Heiss, G. Preliminary high density lipoprotein findings. The lipid research clinic program. In: *High Density Lipoproteins and Atherosclerosis.* Ed. A. M. Gotto Jr., N. E. Miller and M. F. Oliver. Elsevier, Amsterdam, pp. 109–119, 1978.
Roberts, D. C. K., West, C. E., Redgrave, T. G. and Smith, J. B. (1974). Plasma cholesterol concentration in normal and cholesterol-fed rabbits. Its variation and heritability. *Atherosclerosis*, **19**, 369–380.
Robinson, W. S. (1950). Ecological correlations and the behaviour of individuals. *American Sociological Review*, **15**, 351–357.
Russ, E. M., Eder, H. A. and Barr, D. P. (1955). Influence of gonadal hormones on protein-lipid relationships in human plasma. *American Journal of Medicine*, **19**, 4–24.
Sacks, F. M., Castelli, W. P., Donner, A. and Kass, E. H. (1975). Plasma lipids and lipoproteins in vegetarians and controls. *New England Journal of Medicine*, **292**, 1148–1151.

Shaper, A. G. and Jones, K. W. (1959). Serum-cholesterol, diet, and coronary heart-disease in Africans and Asians in Uganda. *Lancet*, **2**, 534–537.

Sinclair, H. M. (1953). The diet of the Canadian Indians and Eskimos. *Proceedings of the Nutrition Society*, **12**, 69–82.

Slack, J. (1974). Genetic differences in liability to atherosclerotic heart disease. *Journal of the Royal College of Physicians of London*, **8**, 115–126.

Stamler, J. (1973). Epidemiology of coronary heart disease. *Medical Clinics of North America*, **57**, 5–46.

Stufflebean, C. E. and Lasley, J. F. (1969). Hereditary basis of serum cholesterol level in beef cattle. *Journal of Heredity*, **60**, 15–16.

Toor, M., Katchalsky, A., Agmov, J. and Allalouf, D. (1960). Atherosclerosis and related factors in immigrants to Israel. *Circulation*, **22**, 265–279.

Tsang, R. C., Fallat, R. W. and Glueck, C. J. (1974). Cholesterol at birth and age 1: comparison of normal and hypercholesterolemic neonates. *Pediatrics*, **53**, 458–470.

Uppal, S. C. *Coronary Heart Disease. Risk Pattern in Dutch Youth. A Pilot Study in Westland Schoolchildren.* New Rhine Publishers, Leiden, 1974.

Walden, R. T., Schaefer, L. E., Lemon, F. R., Sunshine, A. and Wynder, E. L. (1964). Effect of environment on the serum cholesterol-triglyceride distribution among Seventh-day Adventists. *American Journal of Medicine*, **36**, 269–276.

Watson, W. S., Buchanan, K. D. and Dickson, C. (1963). Serum cholesterol levels after myocardial infarction. *British Medical Journal*, **2**, 709–712.

Weinberg, R., Avet, L. M. and Gardner, M. J. (1976). Estimates of the heritability of serum lipoprotein and lipid concentrations. *Clinical Genetics*, **9**, 588–592.

Whyte, M., Nestel, P. and MacGregor, A. (1977). Cholesterol metabolism in Papua New Guineans. *European Journal of Clinical Investigation*, **7**, 53–60.

Wilson, D. E. and Lees, R. S. (1972). Metabolic relationships among the plasma lipoproteins. Reciprocal changes in the concentrations of very low and low density lipoproteins in man. *Journal of Clinical Investigation*, **51**, 1051–1057.

Wong, H. Y. C. and Johnson, F. B. The effect of strenuous exercise on plasma lipids and atherosclerosis in cholesterol-fed cockerels. In: Atherosclerosis IV. *Proceedings of the Fourth International Symposium.* Ed. G. Schettler, Y. Goto, Y. Hata and G. Klose. Springer-Verlag, Berlin, pp. 263–268, 1977.

Wood, P. D., Haskell, W., Klein, H., Lewis, S., Stern, M. P. and Farquhar, J. W. (1976). The distribution of plasma lipoproteins in middle-aged male runners. *Metabolism*, **25**, 1249–1257.

Chapter 13

Cholesterol and Atherosclerosis

1	INTRODUCTION	605
2	THE ATHEROSCLEROTIC LESION	605
2.1	The normal artery	605
2.2	The fatty streak.	607
2.3	The fibrous plaque	609
2.4	The complicated lesion	609
2.5	The relation between lesions	610
2.6	The origin of the cholesterol in the lesions.	611
3	EXPERIMENTAL ATHEROSCLEROSIS.	616
3.1	Introduction	616
3.2	Dietary atherosclerosis	617
3.2.1	Effects of fat content	617
3.2.2	Species differences.	617
3.2.3	Non-human primates	618
3.3	The mechanism of action of atherogenic diets	621
3.4	Regression of dietary atherosclerosis	625
4	THE PLASMA CHOLESTEROL AND ISCHAEMIC HEART DISEASE	627
4.1	The search for causes	627
4.2	The case-control approach	628
4.3	The risk-factor concept	628
4.4	The plasma cholesterol as a positive risk factor	630
4.5	Plasma cholesterol and the prediction of IHD	639
4.6	The plasma HDL as a negative risk factor.	641
4.7	The significance of plasma cholesterol and HDL as risk factors	646
4.7.1	General conclusions	646
4.7.2	The plasma cholesterol as a 'cause' of IHD in man	647
4.7.3	Does HDL protect against IHD?	650
4.8	The dietary fat hypothesis.	652
4.9	The plasma cholesterol in relation to total mortality and non-IHD mortality.	654
5	THE CLONAL HYPOTHESIS OF ATHEROGENESIS	657

Cholesterol and Atherosclerosis

1 INTRODUCTION

A full account of the pathology, causes and clinical consequences of atherosclerotic lesions in the arterial wall would take us far beyond the proper limits of a book on cholesterol. Nevertheless, there has been so much discussion of the plasma cholesterol in relation to ischaemic heart disease* (IHD) that we cannot ignore atherosclerosis altogether. Whether or not the current preoccupation with cholesterol as a possible cause of IHD will turn out to have been wholly justified, it is undeniable that cholesterol is a major component of the lipids of all atherosclerotic lesions and that the plasma cholesterol concentration is, in a statistical sense, predictive of heart attacks. In this chapter I shall consider the morphology and chemistry of the lesions of human arteries, the experimental production and regression of lesions in animals, the role of the plasma cholesterol in the development of atherosclerosis and the mechanisms by which the plasma cholesterol acts as a risk factor for IHD in man. Throughout, the emphasis will be on the coronary arteries, since IHD is by far the most serious outcome of atherosclerosis. So as to avoid confusion between *risk factors* and *causes* of IHD, these two aspects of the atherosclerosis question are considered separately.

2 THE ATHEROSCLEROTIC LESION

2.1 The normal artery

Fig. 13.1A shows, in diagrammatic form, the main features of a normal medium-sized artery, such as the coronary artery, of a young human

* In the context of this chapter the term *IHD* is preferable to the more usual *coronary heart disease* because the study of the plasma cholesterol as a risk factor for heart disease in man is concerned largely with clinically detectable ischaemia of the myocardium and not with the underlying coronary atherosclerosis (which is present in many apparently healthy adults).

being. The luminal surface of the intima is covered by a continuous sheet of interdigitating endothelial cells. In young arteries the subendothelial space contains few connective tissue elements, little or no extracellular lipid and very few cells, most of which are modified smooth-muscle cells (SMC) (see Geer and Haust, 1972).

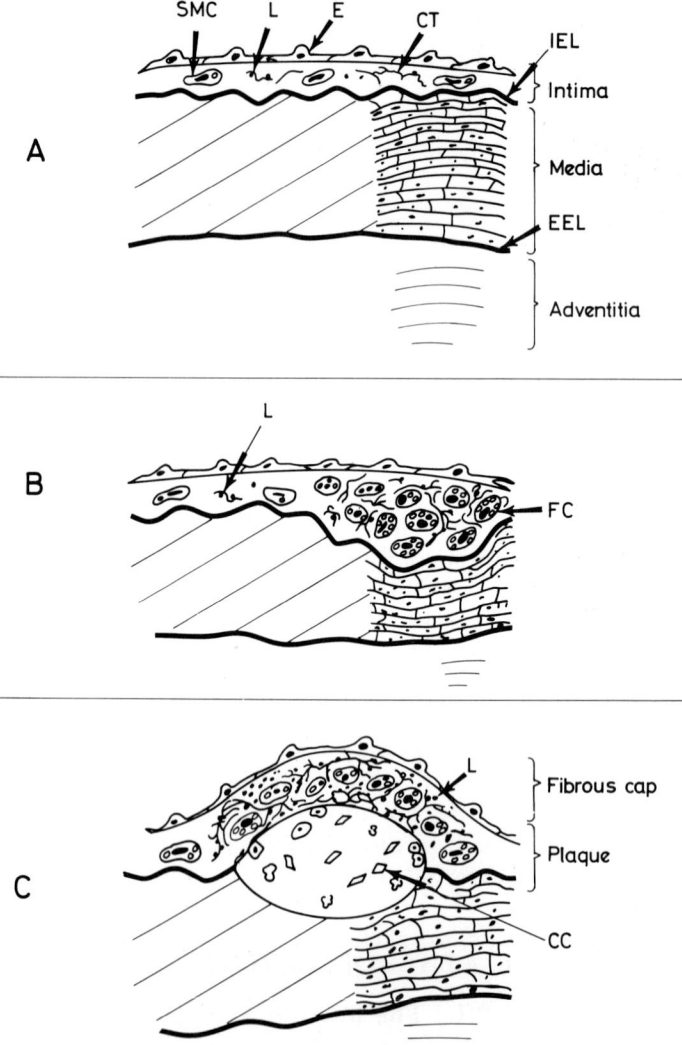

Figure 13.1
Diagram of the wall of a normal artery (A), a fatty streak (B) and a fibrous plaque (C). E, endothelial cell; SMC, smooth-muscle cell; CT, connective tissue; L, extracellular lipid droplet associated with connective tissue; IEL, internal elastic lamina; EEL, external elastic lamina; FC, foam cell; CC, crystal of unesterified cholesterol in an encapsulated lipid pool containing dead and dying cells.

A word or two about the connective tissue of the arterial intima will be helpful at this point because of its role in the development of atherosclerotic lesions. In addition to collagen and elastic fibres, the sub-endothelial connective tissue matrix contains two other types of macromolecule: mucopolysaccharides (MPS) and sialic acid-containing glycoproteins. MPS, also known as *glycosaminoglycans* (GAG), are a heterogeneous group of polymers all of which contain a hexosamine as the main repeating unit and most of which are sulphated. MPS in connective tissue are bound covalently to proteins to form *proteoglycans*. The proteoglycans in the arterial wall are present as a chain network which may exert a sieving effect on large molecules. Furthermore, owing to the presence of their sulphate and carboxyl groups, sulphated MPS may bind reversibly to positively charged macromolecules, including LDL and VLDL (Iverius, 1972).

With increasing age there is a progressive generalized thickening of the intima of all human arteries. In the coronary arteries, for example, the intima may equal the media in thickness by the third decade. This natural increase in intimal thickness is due to proliferation of SMC and increased formation, probably by these cells, of all the major connective tissue elements. There is also a progressive increase in the amount of extracellular lipid in the intima. The extracellular lipid consists largely of droplets of esterified and unesterified cholesterol adsorbed to MPS and other components of the intimal connective tissue, with linoleate as the major cholesteryl-ester fatty acid (Smith and Smith, 1976).

In addition to these generally-distributed intimal changes, which are usually regarded as part of the normal process of ageing, focal atherosclerotic lesions occur in the large and medium-sized arteries. For descriptive purposes these may be classified as *fatty streaks* or *dots, fibrous plaques* and *complicated lesions*.

2.2 The fatty streak

As seen with the naked eye, fatty lesions (Fig. 13.1B) are flat or slightly raised yellowish streaks or dots on the luminal surface of the artery. Microscopically, the lesion consists of an accumulation of fat-laden SMC between the endothelium and the internal elastic lamina, with increased amounts of connective tissue and, in the more advanced lesions, lipid droplets along the fibres of the intimal connective tissue. The intracellular lipid is present as spherical inclusions, about 2 µ in diameter, which may occupy most of the cytoplasm of the SMC, converting them into foam cells. These cells are generally thought to be derived from smooth-muscle cells and are therefore referred to as 'myogenic', as distinct from the 'histiocytic' foam cells derived from macrophages (but see Chapter 15, Section 3.4.3.2 for discussion of this point). The major lipid of the foam-cell droplets is esterified cholesterol,

Table 13.1
Lipid composition of human atherosclerotic lesions (taken from Katz et al., 1976)

Types of lesion	Cholesteryl ester	Free cholesterol	Phospholipid	Triglyceride	Sphingomyelin/lecithin
Fatty streaks (13)	77.0	9.6	10.1	2.8	1.2
Fibrous plaques (27)	55.5	22.5	16.8	5.2	3.5
Gruel plaques* (24)	47.2	31.5	15.3	6.0	3.4

Values show percentages of the total lipid in the lesion.
The number of lesions analyzed in each class is shown in brackets.
* Advanced plaques containing pools of atheromatous lipid.

of which the predominant fatty acid is oleate, together with smaller amounts of unesterified cholesterol, phospholipid and triglyceride (Table 13.1). Examination of the intracellular droplets by crystallographic methods shows that at room temperature most of them exhibit positive birefringence and other optical properties characteristic of esterified cholesterol in a smectic liquid-crystalline state (Hata et al., 1974). According to Katz et al. (1976) the lipid in many of the droplets of a fatty streak remains in a liquid-crystalline state when the temperature is raised to 37 °C; this is consistent with the relatively high transition temperature of cholesteryl oleate from liquid crystal to liquid (Small, 1970). The unesterified cholesterol of the droplets is probably dissolved in phospholipid lamellae (which are capable of incorporating up to 1 mole of cholesterol per mole of phospholipid) and does not appear as crystals (Katz et al., 1976).

2.3 The fibrous plaque

Fig. 13.1C shows the main features of a fibrous plaque. The intima is thickened by increased connective tissue and an accumulation of myogenic and histiocytic foam cells, forming a fibrous cap which to the naked eye appears as a raised white or greyish patch on the luminal surface of the artery. Within the fibrous cap there is a considerable amount of extracellular lipid, of which the major component is esterified cholesterol with linoleate as the predominant fatty acid. Beneath the cap is an encapsulated mass of extracellular lipid containing dead and dying cells. The lipid in the plaque consists mainly of free and esterified cholesterol, with linoleate as the major fatty acid, together with phospholipid and some triglyceride (Table 13.1). A consideration of the chemical composition and crystallographic properties of the lipids of fibrous plaques has led Katz et al. (1976) to conclude that in most cases the plaque lipids are present as a three-phase system at body temperature: (1) a true liquid phase consisting of esterified cholesterol saturated with unesterified cholesterol and containing small amounts of triglycerides in solution, (2) a liquid-crystalline lamellar phase of phospholipid and free cholesterol in which some esterified cholesterol is dissolved and (3) a crystalline phase of cholesterol monohydrate. The failure of the cholesteryl esters of most plaques to form liquid crystals at body temperature is probably due to the high proportion of polyunsaturated fatty acids in these esters; the phase-transition temperature of the cholesteryl ester mixture in the plaque lipids could well be below 37 °C (see Small, 1970).

2.4 The complicated lesion

Fibrous plaques may undergo a variety of degenerative and inflammatory changes. In such complicated lesions there is gross fibrous thickening of the intima, with ulceration of the intimal surface and subintimal haemorrhages. The large lipid-filled plaque is surrounded by media in various stages of degeneration and there may be areas of calcification in the plaque and adjacent medial tissue. In arteries of the size of the coronaries the lumen is often narrowed or almost completely occluded at the site of the lesion by successive mural thrombi in various stages of organization, sometimes giving the appearance of concentric laminae. In the coronary arteries of a person who has died shortly after a myocardial infarction, the lumen at the site of a complicated lesion may be blocked by fresh thrombus. As in the fibrous plaque, the predominant lipid is cholesterol, both free and esterified, and the major fatty acid of the esterified cholesterol in linoleate. Crystals of cholesterol monohydrate are almost always present in the plaque lipids of complicated lesions.

2.5 The relation between lesions

Although there is a progressive increase in complexity from fatty streaks, through fibrous plaques and complicated lesions to the final occlusive event that gives rise to an infarct, there is no direct evidence that in man the fatty streak is the precursor of the more advanced lesions (see McGill (1974) for discussion).

Fatty streaks appear in the aortic intima in young children of all populations and all races, increasing in extent until the fourth decade. In different populations the frequency and extent of fatty streaks in young individuals appear to be unrelated to the frequency and extent of fibrous plaques in older people, to the prevalence of clinical IHD, or to the presence of risk factors for IHD in the population. There is also a marked difference in the effect of sex on the frequency of fatty streaks compared with fibrous plaques. In all populations, young females have more aortic fatty streaks than young males, but fibrous plaques are more extensive in older males than in older females (Tejada et al., 1968). Fibrous plaques begin to appear in the aorta and coronary arteries about 10 years later than fatty streaks and their incidence in different populations is closely correlated with the prevalence of IHD and with the intensity of risk factors in the population, including plasma cholesterol concentration, smoking and blood pressure (Strong et al., 1972). There are also differences in the localization of fatty streaks and fibrous plaques within the arterial tree. Whereas fatty streaks in the aorta appear predominantly in the ascending and thoracic segments, fibrous plaques and complicated lesions are usually most extensive in the abdominal region.

These facts show clearly that the relation between fatty streaks and fibrous plaques is not simply one of invariable progression from the fatty streak to the advanced lesion. Indeed, there are those who argue that fatty streaks and advanced atherosclerotic lesions develop independently of one another. However, all the above observations are compatible with the hypothesis that fatty streaks arise at an early age in all individuals, that in the absence of risk factors the majority of lesions do not progress (or may even regress), but that in the presence of risk factors the fatty streaks in certain regions of the arterial system are converted into fibrous lesions which may progress to complicated lesions if the unfavourable influences are maintained throughout adult life. On this view, all fibrous plaques are derived from fatty streaks but not all fatty streaks become fibrous plaques. It should be noted that in this general formulation no assumptions need be made as to the mechanism by which the fatty streaks in certain areas are converted into fibrous plaques, or as to whether or not the lesions are monoclonal. Definitive evidence on the relation between fatty streaks and fully developed lesions in man would obviously be very difficult to obtain, but the question is important because it bears on the relevance of experimental atherosclerosis in animals, in which the fatty streak is often the only lesion observed, to the naturally occurring advanced lesions in man.

2.6 The origin of cholesterol in the lesions

It is generally agreed that almost all the cholesterol in atherosclerotic lesions is derived from the plasma rather than from synthesis *in situ* or release of lipid from blood cells such as the platelets of mural thrombi. This view is based partly on the negative observation that the cells of the arterial wall have only a limited capacity for synthesizing cholesterol (see Dayton and Hashimoto, 1970; St. Clair, 1976) and partly on the demonstration that cholesterol and lipoproteins are capable of crossing from the plasma into the subendothelial layers of the artery.

Several groups of workers have shown that the cholesterol of normal and atherosclerotic areas of the arterial wall becomes labelled when the plasma cholesterol is labelled, both in experimental animals and birds (Newman and Zilversmit, 1962; Dayton and Hashimoto, 1966; Lofland and Clarkson, 1970) and in human subjects given the labelled cholesterol at various intervals before death (Field *et al.*, 1960; Chobanian and Hollander, 1962; Gould *et al.*, 1963). The observations of Newman and Zilversmit (1962) on rabbits fed an atherogenic diet containing [^{14}C]cholesterol suggest that virtually all the cholesterol that accumulates in aortic lesions is derived from the plasma and that the rate of influx of cholesterol into the artery increases as the severity of the atherosclerosis increases. It has generally been found that, relative to the plasma concentration, the rate of influx of labelled free cholesterol is much greater than that of labelled esterified cholesterol. This has been taken as evidence that plasma free cholesterol can enter the artery other than as a constituent of an intact lipoprotein molecule, perhaps by molecule-for-molecule exchange. Some exchange of free cholesterol between plasma lipoproteins and the arterial wall would certainly be expected (see Chapter 11 for general discussion of this point). However, Stender *et al.* (1978), on the basis of experiments on pigs given injections of LDL containing labelled phospholipid and labelled cholesterol, have suggested that much of the difference between the apparent rates of influx of free and esterified cholesterol is due to rapid hydrolysis of the esterified cholesterol in the artery.

Several plasma proteins, including albumin, fibrinogen, LDL and HDL, have been identified in the intima of normal and atherosclerotic human arteries by immunofluorescence *in situ*, by identification of intravenous labelled protein in the arterial wall, by direct immunoelectrophoresis of pieces of artery or by examination of tissue fluid obtained from the artery (for review see Smith, 1974; Walton, 1978). The immunofluorescence studies have, in general, shown that LDL apoprotein is present in all types of atherosclerotic lesion and that most of it is extravascular (see Hoff *et al.*, 1974). Methods for detecting plasma lipoproteins on the basis of their immunochemical properties can provide direct information only about the amount and localization of the protein components. However, Walton and Williamson (1968), using a combination of immunofluorescence and lipid staining, have shown that the immunoreactive LDL protein in human atherosclerotic lesions is closely associated with lipid. This suggests that intact LDL molecules are present in the arterial wall, though it does not exclude the possibility that lipoproteins undergo some change in lipid composition during their passage across the endothelium. In keeping with the idea that more or less intact LDL molecules are present in the intima, lipoproteins with the density and the electrophoretic and immunological properties of LDL have been identified in extracts of arterial tissue. It would, perhaps, be surprising if plasma lipoproteins did not reach the subendothelial layer of the arterial wall, since biologically active LDL is present in the interstitial fluid of the human foot (Reichl *et al.*, 1977 and 1978), a clear demonstration of the ability of LDL molecules to cross a layer of capillary endothelial cells without detectable modification.

Smith and Slater (1972) measured the concentration of LDL in *post mortem* specimens of normal human aortic intima by direct immunoelectrophoresis. They found that the intimal concentration of LDL was roughly proportional to the plasma cholesterol concentration measured before death and that the LDL/albumin concentration ratio in the intima was several times that in plasma. A relative enrichment of the intimal fluid with LDL (a much larger molecule than albumin) cannot be explained in terms of any known mechanism for transendothelial transport of plasma proteins. Rather, it suggests that there is selective reversible binding of LDL to intimal connective-tissue elements, such as proteoglycans (see Section 2.1), or selective removal of albumin by filtration across the internal elastic lamina with eventual removal *via* the lymphatic channels draining towards the adventitia. It is consistent with these possibilities that LDL, as demonstrated in the arterial wall by immunofluorescent antibodies to LDL protein, is localized chiefly in extracellular perifibrous regions (Woolf and Pilkington, 1965; Walton and Williamson, 1968), and that LDL does not normally penetrate into the deeper layers of the media of the perfused rat aorta (Stein and Stein, 1973), whereas albumin penetrates from the bloodstream into all layers of the arterial wall, including the adventitia (Adams *et al.*, 1968).

The concentration of LDL in atherosclerotic lesions seems to be rather unpredictable. In the intima of fatty streaks the concentration is lower than in adjacent normal intima; in early fibrous lesions the concentration is increased, but in fully developed lesions with underlying pools of lipid it is decreased (Smith, 1974). One would not expect to find a simple relationship between intimal LDL concentration and the pathology of the lesion, since the steady-state concentration of LDL must be determined by several factors, such as the rate of entry from the plasma, the extent of binding to connective tissue, the rate of efflux and the rate at which LDL is degraded *in situ*. Thus, the low concentration in fatty streaks could be due to rapid uptake and degradation by SMC, as discussed below, and the high concentration in early fibrous lesions could be due to a combination of increased influx and increased binding by connective tissue. The amount of cholesterol in all lesions is far greater than that which can be accounted for by the amount of readily-extractable LDL present. This discrepancy may be due partly to the presence of LDL bound irreversibly to extracellular elements in a manner such that it can only be released by mild proteolysis, but a more important factor must be the release of LDL cholesterol within the arterial wall by the proteolysis of LDL protein, as discussed below.

The evidence outlined above has led to the current view that the bulk of the extracellular and intracellular cholesterol in atherosclerotic lesions, and the cholesterol that accumulates in the normal intima of ageing arteries, is derived from LDL that has entered the arterial wall from the plasma. Since most of the cholesterol in the lesion as a whole, and all of that in the pools of plaque lipid, is not associated with protein (see Sections 2.2 and 2.3), most of the protein of intra-arterial LDL must ultimately undergo proteolytic digestion. Some of this digestion probably takes place outside cells, though we know very little about the nature and source of extracellular proteolytic enzymes in the arterial wall. LDL must also undergo proteolysis within SMC, presumably by lysosomal digestion of LDL taken up by receptor-mediated endocytosis or by low-affinity uptake (see Chapter 9). In keeping with this, cultured SMC from human arteries have been shown to take up and degrade LDL *in vitro* (Bierman and Albers, 1975) and Goldstein *et al.* (1977) have been able to produce typical myogenic foam cells, containing droplets of esterified cholesterol in a liquid-crystalline state, by incubating cultured human SMC in the presence of cationized LDL.

With regard to the esterified cholesterol of the artery, the fatty-acid pattern of the extracellular cholesteryl esters of atherosclerotic lesions and of the ageing intima is similar to that of cholesteryl esters of the plasma LDL. This suggests that the extracellular esters are the unhydrolyzed esters of LDL transported into the artery from the plasma. The intracellular cholesteryl esters, on the other hand, have oleate as their predominant fatty acid. They probably arise by hydrolysis of LDL cholesteryl esters by lysosomal ester hydrolases, followed by re-esterification by microsomal ACAT with oleyl-CoA as the preferred substrate. As discussed in Chapter 5, both ACAT and acid ester hydrolases are present in the arterial wall. Furthermore, the activity of ACAT in atherosclerotic lesions of many species, including man, is considerably increased (St. Clair, 1976; Day and Wilkinson, 1967).

No account of the origin of the cholesterol in atherosclerotic plaques would be complete without some discussion of the mechanism by which plasma lipoproteins reach the subendothelial layers of the arterial wall. Electron-microscopic observations have shown that in normal blood capillaries with a continuous endothelium, molecules of diameter 100 Å or more are transported across endothelial cells in both directions by plasmalemmal vesicles, of diameter 400–1000 Å, formed by invagination of the plasma membrane. The formation of these vesicles requires energy but their passage through the cytoplasm of an endothelial cell can be explained by Brownian movement (see Simionescu *et al.*, 1976). The mean time for loading, movement across the cell and discharge of contents from the opposite face has been estimated to be about 5 seconds (Casley-Smith, 1976) or about 25 seconds (Simionescu *et al.*, 1976). Simionescu *et al.* (1975) have also described transendothelial channels, formed by the fusion of a chain of vesicles and allowing molecules up to 100 Å in diameter to cross from one surface of the cell to the other. In fenestrated capillaries, molecules larger than 100 Å in diameter may cross the capillary wall directly through pores and it is also possible that relatively large macromolecules cross *via* intercellular channels under conditions in which endothelial cells are stimulated to contract (see Schwartz *et al.*, 1977, for discussion).

The endothelium of a normal artery is continuous (Fig. 13.1A) and is rich in plasmalemmal vesicles similar in size to those in capillary endothelial cells. Schwartz et al. (1977) have shown that ferritin particles (diameter, 110 Å) injected intravenously into pigs are transported rapidly into the subendothelial space of the aorta by plasmalemmal vesicles and do not pass through intercellular junctions (Fig. 13.2). In view of this and other observations discussed by Stein and Stein (1973), it is reasonable to assume that HDL (diameter 100 Å) and LDL (diameter 200–250 Å) are transported across the endothelium of a normal artery by plasmalemmal vesicles, some HDL particles possibly crossing *via* transendothelial channels. If this is, in fact, the route by which plasma lipoproteins reach the subendothelial layers of an artery with a normal endothelium, factors which influence the activity of the vesicular transport system could help to determine the rate at which plasma lipoproteins accumulate in the

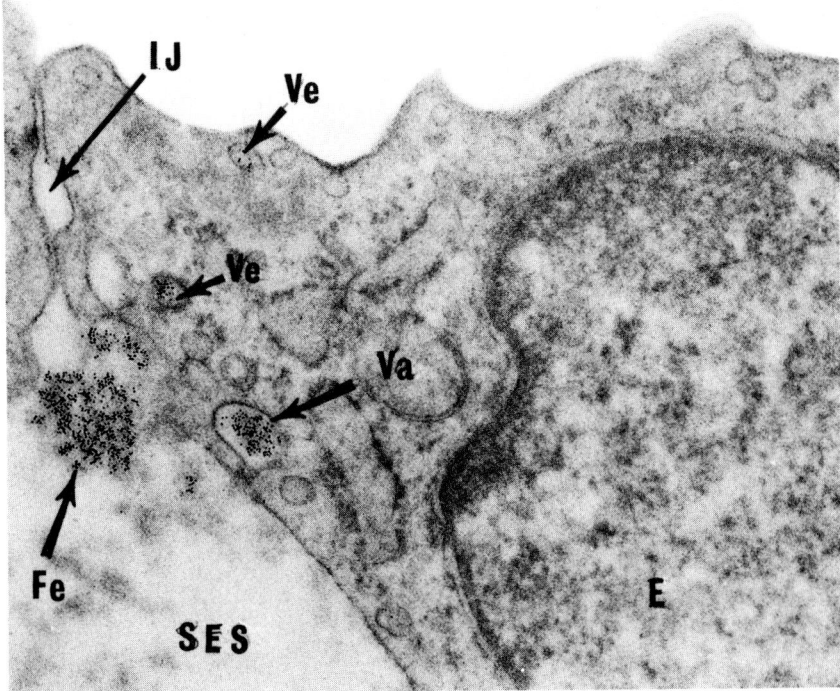

Figure 13.2
Transmission electronmicrograph of an unstained section through the subendothelial space (SES) of pig aortic arch taken 15 minutes after an intravenous injection of ferritin. Numerous ferritin granules (Fe) are visible in the extracellular space, in vesicles (Ve) and in large vacuoles (Va) in undifferentiated subendothelial cells (E). Note the absence of ferritin granules in intercellular junctions (IJ). × 62 500. (From Schwartz *et al.* (1977), with the permission of the authors.)

arterial wall. There is also evidence to suggest that vesicular activity, as revealed by the transendothelial flux of intravenous ferritin, is increased in the patches of increased endothelial permeability that are present in most normal arteries (see Schwartz et al. (1977) and Section 3.3 of this chapter).

Human vascular endothelial cells in culture resemble human fibroblasts in that they bind LDL by the specific receptor mechanism and incorporate it into endocytotic vesicles which fuse with lysosomes. In view of this it may seem surprising that the plasmalemmal vesicles do not also fuse with lysosomes and thus abandon their load of lipoprotein molecules to the attentions of lysosomal hydrolytic enzymes. Presumably, the plasmalemmal vesicles have some special surface properties which hinder fusion with lysosomes.

3 EXPERIMENTAL ATHEROSCLEROSIS

3.1 Introduction

The observation of Anitschkow (1913) that cholesterol-fed rabbits develop aortic lesions with some resemblance to those of human atherosclerosis has generated an enormous amount of work on the production of atherosclerosis in animals and birds by dietary means, or by combinations of diet with various types of injury to the vascular system. Although the study of atherosclerosis in animals cannot be a substitute for the study of the natural disease in man, the experimental approach does have several distinct advantages. In particular, it is possible to observe the progress of the lesion in experimental animals from the initial stages to the most advanced, in response to a single controlled atherogenic stimulus, and to observe the steps by which the lesions regress or heal when the stimulus is withdrawn. It is also much easier to study the time-course of events in the arterial wall at the cellular and subcellular levels in experimental animals than in human subjects. Nevertheless, there are two serious limitations to the value of work on experimentally produced atherosclerosis. In the first place, by far the most frequent lesion produced by cholesterol feeding in many species is the fatty streak; as discussed in Section 2, it is by no means certain that this is an obligatory stage in the development of fibrous plaques in man. Secondly, the feeding of cholesterol-rich diets to animals tends to lead to the appearance of abnormal lipoproteins in the plasma which may influence the nature and severity of the atherosclerotic lesions produced experimentally and which are not present in the plasma of the great majority of human beings who develop atherosclerosis. Some of these lipoproteins were mentioned briefly in Chapter 11; a fuller account of them will be found in the reviews by Mahley (1978) and Sirtori et al. (1978).

Spontaneous atherosclerosis of the aorta has been reported in a wide range of reptiles, birds and mammals (see Fox (1933) and Adams (1964) for reviews). Spontaneous atherosclerosis has also been reported in several species of non-human primate under captivity and in the wild state; the naturally-occurring lesions are predominantly fatty streaks, but fibrous plaques have also been observed in the aortas of wild baboons (see Gresham and Howard, 1965, for review). Some species or sub-species (e.g. the White Carneau pigeon) have a marked tendency to develop atherosclerosis of the aorta and coronary arteries when fed natural diets. A high incidence of spontaneous lesions does, of course, limit the value of a species in the study of experimental atherosclerosis. The presence of spontaneous atherosclerosis in passerine birds (Adams, 1964) raises the interesting question as to how far the feeding of garden birds with pieces of animal fat is likely to shorten their lives through induction of premature heart disease.

3.2 Dietary atherosclerosis

3.2.1 Effect of fat content

In every species of animal that has been tested, cholesterol feeding has been shown to lead to the development of atherosclerotic lesions. Cholesterol-rich diets containing a high proportion of saturated fats, such as butter and lard, are usually more atherogenic than those in which the fat is polyunsaturated. An exception is peanut oil, which, though containing a high proportion of polyunsaturated fatty acids, is very atherogenic when fed with cholesterol to rats (Gresham and Howard, 1960) or rabbits (Kritchevsky et al., 1971). A possible reason for the atherogenic potency of peanut oil is its high content of arachidic (20:0) and behenic (22:0) acids. Although most diets used in the study of experimental atherosclerosis contain added cholesterol, semi-purified cholesterol-free diets, low in fibre and containing various types of animal protein, cause hypercholesterolaemia and aortic atherosclerosis in rabbits (see Carroll and Hamilton, 1975).

3.3.2 Species differences

There are marked species differences in susceptibility to atherogenic diets. For example, rabbits develop extensive lesions when fed cholesterol, whereas it is difficult to induce atherosclerosis in rats unless the diet is supplemented with cholic acid and an antithyroid drug in addition to cholesterol. Pigs and non-human primates are much less susceptible to cholesterol-rich diets than rabbits, but are not as resistant as rats. These species differences are related to some extent to the degree of hypercholesterolaemia produced by cholesterol feeding. Thus, the addition of 2% of cholesterol to the diet raises the plasma cholesterol concentration to more than 1000 mg/100 ml in rabbits within a few weeks, but may have little effect on the plasma cholesterol in rats. Another factor contributing to species differences may be the nature of the lipoproteins that accumulate in the plasma during cholesterol feeding. It is conceivable that some lipoproteins are more damaging to the arterial wall, or have a greater effect on platelet behaviour, than others, irrespective of their contribution to plasma total cholesterol concentration.

As well as differences in susceptibility to atherogenic diets in different species, there are also differences in the nature and distribution of the lesions produced. The gross histological features and the anatomical distribution of the lesions that develop in response to cholesterol-rich diets in rats, rabbits, chickens, pigs and non-human primates, together with those that develop spontaneously in man, have been discussed by Wissler and Vesselinovitch (1974) and are summarized in Table 13.2. In man, atherosclerosis is largely confined to the large and medium-sized arteries and its severity usually decreases in the order: abdominal aorta > thoracic aorta > coronary arteries > renal and mesenteric arteries. In the cholesterol-fed rabbit the lesions are more extensive in the thoracic than in the abdominal aorta and are widely distributed throughout the arterial system, including the small arteries; histologically, the lesions consist predominantly of histiocytic foam cells and are accompanied by a generalized fatty infiltration of the reticuloendothelial system. Fibrous plaques do not develop in rabbits unless the cholesterol feeding is prolonged or is combined with some other atherogenic stimulus (Constantinides, 1965; and see Section 3.3). In pigs, the lesions are present predominantly in the larger arteries and may become fibrous after prolonged feeding (Scott *et al.*, 1972).

3.2.3 Non-human primates

Experimental lesions in non-human primates are of particular interest because of their resemblance to human atherosclerosis. Extensive atherosclerosis has been produced by feeding 'hypercholesterolaemic' diets to non-human primates of many species including baboons (*Papio sp.*), rhesus, cynomolgus and squirrel monkeys (*Macaca mulatta, Macaca irus* and *Saimiri sciureus*), stump-tailed macaques (*Macaca arctoides*) and cebus and African green monkeys (*Cebus albifrons* and *Cercopithecus aethiops*). A detailed account of the production of dietary atherosclerosis in rhesus monkeys, and of the distribution and histology of the lesions produced in these animals, will be found in Cox *et al.* (1958) and Taylor *et al.* (1962); for references to atherosclerosis in other non-human primates, see Lehner *et al.* (1977) and Wissler and Vesselinovitch (1974).

There are some striking differences in the regional distribution and intensity of the lesions produced in different primate species (Lehner

Table 13.2

Some characteristics of the atherosclerotic lesions produced by feeding atherogenic diets to rabbits, rats, chickens, pigs and monkeys, and of lesions occurring spontaneously in man. (Modified from Wissler and Vesselinovitch, 1974)

Species	Distribution in aorta	Coronaries affected	Usual type of lesion	Loading of RE system
Rabbit*	Thoracic > abdominal	Uncommon	Mainly foam cells	Marked
Rat	Mainly ascending	Uncommon	Mainly foam cells	Usually minor
Chicken	Mainly lower abdominal	Uncommon	Mainly foam cells	Marked
Pig	Abdominal > thoracic	Described, but uncommon	Foam cells and fibrous plaques	None
Squirrel monkey	Abdominal = thoracic	Common	All human types from fatty streaks to complicated	None
Rhesus monkey	Abdominal = thoracic	Common	All human types	None†
Man	Abdominal > thoracic	Common	All human types	None†

* Lesions closely resembling advanced lesions of man may be produced in the arteries of rabbits (including the coronaries) by a combination of hypercholesterolaemia with immunological injury (Minick, 1976).
† Some RE loading may occur if hypercholesterolaemia is marked and prolonged.

et al., 1977). In general, however, the feeding of cholesterol-rich diets containing a high proportion of saturated fat for periods of many months produces lesions mainly in the aorta and medium-sized arteries, including the coronary arteries, with little involvement of small arteries and no fat-loading of the reticulo-endothelial system (though Taylor *et al.* (1963) have reported the development of skin xanthomas in two rhesus monkeys given a cholesterol-rich diet for two years). The nature of the lesions produced depends to some extent upon the type of diet fed and the time-course of feeding (whether prolonged and whether continuous or intermittent). When rhesus monkeys are given a cholesterol diet for 12 weeks, they develop intimal lesions resembling the fatty streaks of human arteries and occurring predominantly in the thoracic aorta. If the feeding is continued for months or years, gross intimal thickening develops, with the formation of fibrous plaques, destruction of the internal elastic lamina and media, accumulation of extracellular lipid in the sub-intimal layers of the arteries and, eventually, narrowing of the lumen by focal thickening of the intima and the formation of luminal thrombi. The lesions appear first in the aorta and carotid arteries, but after prolonged feeding they also appear in the coronary arteries (Taylor *et al.*, 1962). The severity and extent of the lesions produced by cholesterol feeding varies markedly from one rhesus monkey to another and seems to be related to individual variation in the degree of hypercholesterolaemia that occurs in response to the diet. In the monkeys studied by Taylor and his co-workers, atherosclerosis did not develop unless the plasma cholesterol concentration remained continuously above about 250 mg/100 ml, and in most of the animals which developed complicated lesions with marked narrowing of the arterial lumen, the plasma cholesterol level was above 400 mg/100 ml for a year or longer. Only one of these monkeys developed a fatal myocardial infarction while on the cholesterol diet, but myocardial lesions during cholesterol feeding have been reported in cholesterol-fed cynomolgus monkeys with serum cholesterol concentrations in the range 350–400 mg/100 ml (Kramsch *et al.*, 1970).

As regards the relevance of these experiments to human atherosclerosis, it is worth noting that the type of hyperlipidaemia produced in rhesus monkeys by cholesterol feeding is broadly similar to the Type II pattern in human hyperlipidaemia (see Chapter 15), though the plasma of the cholesterol-fed rhesus monkey contains increased amounts of IDL and VLDL (Sirtori *et al.*, 1978). It should also be noted that although the proportion of cholesterol in most experimental atherogenic diets is greater than that in normal human diets, Wissler *et al.* (1971) have produced atherosclerotic lesions in monkeys by feeding them 'average' American human diets.

By examining the arteries at different times after putting animals on an atherogenic diet it is possible to gain some idea as to how the lesions progress. According to Shimamoto (1974), within a few hours of feeding cholesterol, the endothelial cells of the rabbit's aorta contract and allow lipoprotein molecules to reach the sub-endothelial layer of the intima through the widened intercellular junctions. Shimamoto suggests that the lipoproteins trapped in the intima stimulate proliferation of SMC and cause other changes characteristic of the atherosclerotic lesion. Increased mitosis (indicated by increased incorporation of [^{3}H]thymidine) has also been demonstrated in aortic endothelium and SMC of rabbits within weeks of giving them a cholesterol diet (Stary, 1967). In terms of a longer time scale, Taylor et al. (1962) concluded that in cholesterol-fed rhesus monkeys the sequence of events at the site of formation of a lesion is probably as follows. The first histologically detectable change is a diffuse deposition of lipid droplets in the extracellular matrix of the intima, apparent within four months of the beginning of the cholesterol feeding. The presence of intimal lipid then stimulates the proliferation of mesenchymal cells (presumably SMC), which ingest the lipid to become foam cells, this process taking 7–9 months of feeding. Subsequent changes include the degeneration of foam cells, leading to reactive fibrosis in the intima, disruption of the internal elastic lamina and, after many months of cholesterol feeding, replacement of the media at the site of the lesion by lipid droplets. Focal loss of patches of endothelium, amounting to more than 5% of the total surface of the aorta and iliac arteries, has also been observed in monkeys made hypercholesterolaemic for 9 months or longer (Ross and Harker, 1976).

3.3 The mechanism of action of atherogenic diets

The observations discussed in the previous section show beyond any doubt that a dietary regimen which raises the plasma cholesterol concentration can be a sufficient cause of focal atherosclerosis in animals, and that in some species lesions indistinguishable from those of human atherosclerosis may be found if the hyperlipidaemia is prolonged and intense enough. This raises two questions. 'What is the causal chain that leads from the feeding of the atherogenic diet to the formation of fully developed lesions, and why are the lesions focal?'.

Experimental and observational evidence built up over the past two decades has led to the widely held view that atherosclerosis begins in the intima and that at least two processes contribute to the development of the lesions: (1) a proliferative reaction in which SMC multiply in the intima and secrete connective-tissue elements and (2) an accumulation of intracellular and extracellular cholesterol-rich lipid, derived largely from the plasma and localized at first in the intima. We still do not know with certainty how the proliferative reaction is initiated under natural conditions or in the cholesterol-fed animal. However, evidence derived from the study of the consequences of deliberate injury to the arterial wall *in vivo*, and from observations on the behaviour of arterial-wall cells in culture, suggests very strongly that an essential step in the initiation of the lesion is the formation of a patch of injured or desquamated endothelium, and that the proliferative reaction in the intima requires the presence of normally functioning platelets in the circulation. This evidence (reviewed by Ross and Glomset, 1976, and by Moore *et al.*, 1977) has led to the working hypothesis that atherosclerosis is essentially a response to local injury, the extent and intensity of the response depending upon the strength of various modifying factors in the circulation (including the concentration of plasma lipoproteins) and in the arterial wall itself.

In brief, localized injury to the arterial endothelium, produced, for example, by means of an intraluminal catheter, is followed within minutes by the formation of platelet microthrombi at the site of the injury and, within weeks, by SMC proliferation in the intima, leading to intimal thickening and fibrosis; if the platelets are prevented from sticking to the damaged arterial wall by treating the animal with antibodies to platelets or with an inhibitor of platelet function, intimal lesions are not formed. The proliferative response to injury seems to be due to the action of a non-dialyzable mitogen released from platelets attached to the injured intima; the mitogenic factor stimulates multiplication of cultured SMC from the arteries of monkeys, but has no effect on cultured endothelial cells. Provided that the injury is not repeated and that the animal is otherwise normal, the intimal lesions regress and the area of damaged endothelium is replaced by new endothelial cells that grow in from the edge of the lesion; repair of the endothelial surface is very slow and may take up to one year. If, however, the injury is repeated or if the animal is made hyperlipidaemic by cholesterol feeding, regression of the intimal lesion and healing of the endothelial surface are delayed or incomplete and the lesion may progress to a fibrous plaque.

Atherosclerotic lesions similar to those occurring spontaneously in man have been produced experimentally in animals of several species by a combination of injury with dietary hyperlipidaemia under conditions in which neither the injury nor the hyperlipidaemia alone produces a fibrous plaque similar to the human lesion. Examples of the type of injury that produce atherosclerotic lesions in the presence, but not in the absence, of hyperlipidaemia are: immunological injury to the arterial wall in baboons (Howard *et al.*, 1971), a cutting injury to a large area of the rabbit's aorta (Björkerud, 1974), and a single balloon-catheter injury in monkeys (Harker *et al*, 1976).

It is not known how hypercholesterolaemia interacts with mechanical or immunological injury to the artery to produce progressive atherosclerotic lesions, but several possibilities are worth considering, all of them supported by some experimental evidence.

The combination of a raised plasma lipoprotein concentration with a defective barrier to the entry of lipoprotein molecules into the subendothelial layers of the artery could lead to a net accumulation of lipoprotein within the arterial wall. In conjunction with the platelet mitogen this could, in turn, stimulate the proliferation of SMC and the formation of foam cells. In support of the idea that plasma lipoproteins and their lipid components may enhance SMC proliferation, an apoB-containing fraction of the plasma LDL of cholesterol-fed monkeys has been shown to stimulate mitosis in cultured aortic SMC (Fischer-Dzoga and Wissler, 1977) and cholesterol and its fatty-acid esters have been shown to promote local fibrosis when implanted under the skin of rats (Abdulla et al., 1967). As already mentioned in the previous section, prolonged hypercholesterolaemia produced by cholesterol feeding may result in focal damage to the arterial endothelium. This could be due to a primary effect of the hypercholesterolaemia on normal endothelial cells. In support of this, Shimamoto (1974) has described electron-microscopic abnormalities in endothelial cells of the arteries of rabbits given a cholesterol-containing meal. Alternatively, hypercholesterolaemia could lead indirectly to focal loss of endothelium by inhibiting the repair of areas of damaged endothelium that result from the normal wear and tear of the arterial wall, as discussed below.

As well as influencing the arterial wall itself, dietary hyperlipidaemia could enhance the effects of injury by modifying one or other of the blood constituents concerned in the development of atherosclerotic lesions. For example, there is evidence to suggest that the feeding of atherogenic diets increases blood coagulability and the sensitivity of platelets to thrombin-induced aggregation (Mustard et al., 1974). It should be noted, however, that most diets used for producing hypercholesterolaemia in animals are rich in saturated fat and that some saturated fatty acids stimulate blood coagulation and platelet aggregation (see Mustard et al., 1974); there is also the possibility that unusual fatty acids present in some atherogenic diets are injurious to the arterial wall.

Thus, there is clearly more than one way in which hypercholesterolaemia could promote the formation of fibrous plaques once the luminal surface of the arterial wall is damaged or destroyed by artificial means. Nor is it difficult to imagine that the continued accumulation of lipoproteins in the exposed intima would eventually lead to necrosis of SMC overloaded with lipid, release of lysosomal enzymes from these cells, reactive fibrosis in the surrounding tissue and progression to the fully-developed complicated lesion. However, we still need an explanation for the production of complicated lesions in the arteries of monkeys and other animals fed cholesterol diets for very long periods *without* deliberate damage to the arterial wall at any stage of the experiment. One possibility is that the hyperlipidaemia provides both the initial injury (which exposes the subendothelial intima to circulating platelets) and the continuing stimulus to the formation of lesions. As already mentioned, there is some reason to think that hypercholesterolaemia is capable of damaging endothelial cells. An alternative explanation is that the arterial wall is always subject to recurrent focal damage by haemodynamic stresses, that in the presence of a normal plasma cholesterol concentration the damaged areas heal completely, but that in the presence of dietary hypercholesterolaemia they progress to atherosclerotic lesions by the sequence of events suggested above.

It is consistent with this explanation that the arterial wall of normal animals contains patches of functionally abnormal endothelium revealed by a focal distribution of supravital staining with dyes. Björkerud and Bondjers (1972) have shown that the endothelial cells in the dye-stained areas of the normal rabbit's aorta are characterized by histological changes suggesting a response to injury. Furthermore, patches of high permeability to labelled plasma proteins and labelled free and esterified cholesterol, and of high uptake of albumin-bound Evans blue, have been demonstrated in the arteries of dogs, rabbits, pigs and monkeys. It has also been shown that cholesterol feeding accentuates the differences between these regions and the remaining areas of the arterial endothelium (see Schwartz *et al.*, 1977, for review). However, it should be noted that although areas of high endothelial permeability tend to occur at probable sites of haemodynamic stress, the coincidence between areas of maximum permeability or dye uptake and maximum formation of fatty streaks in response to cholesterol feeding is far from perfect (see Armstrong *et al.*, 1978, for discussion of this complex but very important question).

Fig. 13.3 shows the way in which some of the effects of cholesterol feeding discussed above might interact to produce atherosclerotic lesions in animals.

The reason why atherosclerotic lesions in cholesterol-fed animals (and in human beings) are focal rather than general has often been discussed, but the problem seems to have been much exaggerated. If injury due to mechanical stress is an important, if not an essential, factor in the development of lesions, one would not expect atherosclerosis to be generally distributed throughout the arterial system or to have the same distribution in all species. Indeed, it is easier to provide a plausible explanation for the focal distribution of atherosclerosis than for the very characteristic distribution of skin lesions in some of the common fevers and the vitamin deficiencies.

LUMEN   WALL

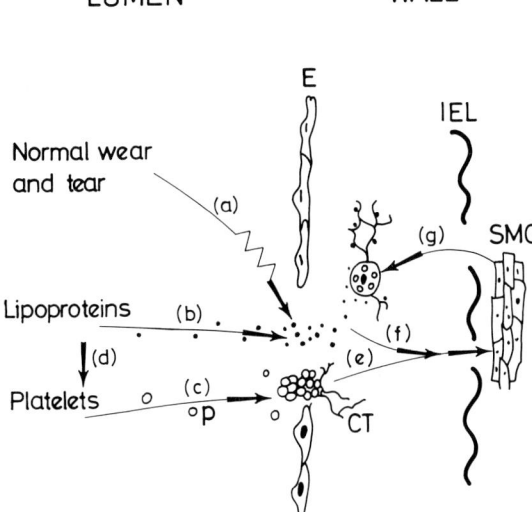

Figure 13.3
Possible mechanisms by which an increased concentration of plasma lipoproteins produced by cholesterol feeding leads to the formation of a fibrous lesion in an artery. E, endothelium, showing an area denuded of endothelial cells; IEL, internal elastic lamina; P, platelet; SMC, smooth-muscle cells; CT, connective tissue.

Suggested stages in the formation of the lesion are:—(a) damaging effect of mechanical stress; (b) lipoproteins in excess cause direct damage to the endothelium or interfere with normal endothelial repair; lipoproteins accumulate in the sub-endothelial layers of the artery, where they potentiate the mitogenic action of the platelet mitogen and provide lipid for the formation of foam cells from SMC; (c) platelets, possibly altered by the presence of hypercholesterolaemia (d), form microthrombi by sticking to exposed subendothelial components of the intima and release a mitogenic factor; (e) the mitogenic factor, in combination with intimal plasma lipoproteins, stimulates SMC in the media to multiply and migrate through the IEL into the intima (g), where they secrete connective tissue elements and become foam cells by ingesting lipoproteins.

Note that in the absence of hyperlipidaemia the accumulation of plasma lipoproteins in the intima in response to injury may be a biologically useful mechanism for providing the regenerating tissue with an immediate supply of cholesterol for cell-membrane formation.

3.4 Regression of dietary atherosclerosis

Under certain conditions, almost always associated with a reduction in plasma cholesterol concentration, atherosclerotic lesions may undergo favourable morphological changes which result in decreased thickening of the intima and widening of the lumen of the artery. This is usually referred to as *regression*, though the changes included within the term are not necessarily a mere retracing or reversal of the steps by which the lesion was formed. As Armstrong (1976) has said, 'After successful regression regimens, arteries that contain larger, more advanced lesions are improved conduits for the circulating blood, but they are histologically abnormal;'. In this section we shall be concerned with regression of lesions induced by atherogenic diets in animals.

Since the claim of Anitschkow (1928) that the atherosclerotic lesions of cholesterol-fed rabbits undergo a change ('Rückbildungsvorgänge') when the animals are given a normal cholesterol-free diet, regression of dietary atherosclerosis has been studied in many species. Some degree of regression has been achieved in all species investigated. However, the extent and nature of the response to a change from an atherogenic to a normal diet has been found to vary widely according to the stage to which the lesions have progressed when the atherogenic diet is withdrawn, the duration of cholesterol feeding and the species of experimental animal. In general, fatty streaks regress more rapidly and completely than fibrous lesions, and the longer the time for which the atherogenic diet has been fed the longer the time required to induce regression by feeding a cholesterol-free diet; Vesselinovitch and Wissler (1977) concluded, from a survey of published reports, that the time required for regression is at least as long as the time taken to induce atherosclerosis. Despite the early observations of Anitschkow (1928), the rabbit is now considered to be unusually resistant to measures designed to induce regression of dietary atherosclerosis. Indeed, some workers have observed continued cell proliferation and lipid accumulation in the lesions of cholesterol-fed rabbits after the plasma cholesterol concentration has been lowered by returning the animals to a cholesterol-free diet, though there is usually some shrinkage of the lesions (see Armstrong, 1976). However, Vesselinovitch and Wissler (1968) have been able to induce regression of advanced diet-induced lesions in rabbits by a combination of a low-fat, low-cholesterol diet with cholestyramine or increased atmospheric O_2 pressure.

It is generally agreed that in most species the plasma cholesterol concentration must be reduced to below about 150 mg/100 ml if regression is to be achieved, but Bond et al. (1977) have succeeded in bringing about a reduction in the amount of lipid in diet-induced lesions in monkeys by maintaining their plasma cholesterol concentration at about 200 mg/100 ml for two years, a plasma cholesterol level comparable with the lowest levels achieved in the treatment of human hyperlipidaemia.

Of greatest relevance to the possible regression of spontaneous atherosclerosis in man is the growing body of work on regression of dietary atherosclerosis in non-human primates, especially that concerned with experimentally-induced advanced lesions, similar to human complicated lesions, in the coronary arteries of rhesus monkeys. Armstrong *et al.* (1970) have shown that advanced lesions produced in rhesus monkeys by cholesterol feeding for 17 months regress when the animals are fed a cholesterol-free diet for 40 months. Regression of the lesions occurs in the aorta and coronaries and in the arteries supplying the limbs and viscera, but not in the cerebral arteries, and seems to require a sustained reduction of the plasma cholesterol concentration to 130–150 mg/100 ml. The regression observed by Armstrong *et al.* (1970) was characterized by widening of the arterial lumen, decreased intimal thickening, loss of stainable lipid and, possibly, repair of damaged media and internal elastic lamina. The histological changes underlying the gross morphological changes seen in lesions that have undergone regression have been discussed by Armstrong (1976) and by Stary *et al.* (1977). Among the more obvious changes are decreased cell proliferation, loss of extracellular lipid and of intracellular lipid droplets, with eventual necrosis and loss of foam cells.

Chemical analysis of the lesions shows that the loss of lipid is due predominantly to loss of esterified and free cholesterol. During regression there is a decrease in collagen content, but not all of the excess collagen formed during the cholesterol feeding disappears from the lesion. The mechanisms involved in the regression of advanced lesions must be of considerable complexity. Presumably, they include the enzyme-catalyzed hydrolysis of complex lipids and connective-tissue components and the removal of the products of enzymic digestion from the arterial wall. The role of plasma lipoproteins in the removal of free cholesterol from tissues has been discussed in Chapter 9. Observations on human arteries *in vitro* suggest that the cholesterol of atherosclerotic lesions may be removed preferentially by HDL (Bondjers and Björkerud, 1975).

4 THE PLASMA CHOLESTEROL AND ISCHAEMIC HEART DISEASE

4.1 The search for causes

The striking increase in death rate from heart disease in Western countries, which seems to have begun in the 1920's, has led to an intensive search for factors in the environment and in the 'host' that are associated with IHD in individuals or populations. In epidemiological investigations of this kind it is usually possible to demonstrate associations which are statistically significant, but which on grounds of ordinary common sense can be rejected as having no relevance to the cause or pathogenesis of the disease in question. Of particular interest in relation to the atherosclerosis problem are associations which, in the light of what we know about the nature of the human lesion and about the way in which lesions can be induced experimentally in animals, seem likely to play a causal role in the initiation or progression of IHD in man.

In parenthesis, it should be noted that few now believe that the development of coronary atherosclerosis, culminating in some people in a myocardial infarct, is due to a single sufficient and necessary cause (as is chicken-pox in a non-immune person). The epidemiological evidence collected from all over the world during the past three decades shows clearly that human coronary atherosclerosis is almost always multifactorial. That is to say, in most individuals it develops as the result of interactions between several factors; only in some instances, as in severe familial hypercholesterolaemia, is a single cause sufficient to bring about fatal IHD. The interaction between contributory causes seems to be complex, some factors acting only when others have reached a certain minimum level of intensity; for example, there is evidence to suggest that cigarette smoking does not increase the risk of IHD unless the plasma cholesterol concentration exceeds a certain level (Gordon et al., 1974; Robertson et al., 1977a,b). What is known of the pathogenesis of myocardial infarction in man suggests that it is usually due to the formation of an occlusive thrombus and that the thrombus forms at the site of a fibrous or complicated atherosclerotic lesion (Davies et al., 1979). Hence, as regards the aetiology of myocardial infarction we have to explain why the atherosclerotic lesion develops in the coronary artery and why the lumen becomes occluded by a thrombus. The two processes are not necessarily influenced to the same extent by all the factors which together contribute to the development of clinically apparent IHD. It is possible, for example, that the plasma cholesterol plays a part in the formation of the lesion, as discussed in Section 3, but that other factors, such as emotional stress, are more important in thrombus formation. There is no clear evidence to support this speculation, but something of the sort must occur if we are to explain why most middle-aged men living in affluent societies have coronary atherosclerosis but only a small proportion die from IHD before age 60 years. Indeed, if coronary atherosclerosis were invariably fatal, few such men would survive beyond the age of 40. Although this section is concerned with the plasma cholesterol in relation to IHD, it is obvious from what has been said above that this question needs to be considered in the wider context of a multifactorial aetiology.

4.2 The case-control approach

The first systematic approach to the search for causes of IHD in the general population was to compare the plasma lipid concentration in patients with clinical evidence of IHD with that in healthy subjects (the case control method). Special attention was paid to the plasma cholesterol because it was already known that patients with hypercholesterolaemia due to various causes tend to die from premature heart disease, that cholesterol is a major component of advanced atherosclerotic lesions, and that atherosclerosis can be induced in animals by cholesterol feeding. By the end of the 1940's it had become clear that the plasma cholesterol concentration tends to be higher in patients with overt IHD than in matched controls (see Gertler *et al.*, 1950, for references), though it was equally clear that in many IHD patients the concentration is within the normal range for the healthy subjects from the same population. Case-control observations on the cholesterol-carrying plasma lipoproteins of survivors of myocardial infarction also showed that the concentration of S_f 10–20 lipoprotein (Gofman *et al.*, 1950) and of β-lipoprotein (LDL) (Barr *et al.*, 1951) is, on average, higher in IHD patients than in normal control subjects. Barr *et al.* (1951) also noted that a common finding in their IHD patients was a relative and absolute reduction in the concentration of α-lipoprotein (HDL). In some cases this was so marked that the plasma total cholesterol concentration was within the normal range, despite an increase in β-lipoprotein concentration.

All the above observations were consistent with the hypothesis that a raised plasma cholesterol concentration in one or other of the lower-density lipoprotein fractions is a contributory cause of IHD, but they left open the possibility that the plasma lipid abnormality is merely a consequence of the clinical event. To exclude this, it is necessary to show that the increase in plasma lipid concentration precedes the heart attack. This requires the organization of *prospective* studies in which plasma lipid levels are measured in groups of healthy individuals (none of whom has had a heart attack) drawn from stable and relatively homogeneous populations. The subjects are then observed over periods of years so that the initial plasma lipid measurement can be related to the subsequent development of coronary atherosclerosis. Since it is not practicable to assess the extent of atherosclerosis in the coronaries of normal subjects during life, it is necessary to continue the follow-up until the number of clinical events (angina pectoris, myocardial infarction, death from a heart attack or other unequivocal signs of IHD) is sufficient for the calculation of statistical significance. The results of such studies are discussed in Section 4.4.

4.3 The risk-factor concept

Prospective studies based on the principles discussed in the previous section are never designed solely with the object of testing the hypothesis that there is a positive correlation between IHD and the antecedent plasma total cholesterol concentration. They are broadened to include the measurement of other variables, such as body fatness, blood pressure and diet which, in the light of all the knowledge available at the start of the trial, might be thought to influence the tendency in a given healthy individual to develop IHD. Variables that can be shown to be associated with an increased risk of IHD have come to be known as *risk factors* (Stamler, 1967). In its widest sense, a risk factor may be defined as any characteristic of the host or environment that is associated with an increase (*positive* risk factor) or decrease (*negative* risk factor) in susceptibility to a disease. This definition is arbitrary to the extent that it does not specify the magnitude or time-scale of the change in susceptibility. A factor associated with a 1% change in the 10-year incidence of overt IHD in men aged 80 years would obviously not be worth considering. Stamler (1973) suggests that a positive risk factor for IHD should be defined as one associated with a doubling of the incidence rate before age 65. It may be noted that a risk factor cannot be detected unless its frequency or magnitude can be measured and unless it varies within the population under investigation.

It must be clearly understood that a risk factor for IHD is not necessarily a cause of the disease. Prospective studies cannot reveal the causes of coronary atherosclerosis, but they do provide a short list of candidates for further examination (epidemiological investigation combined with common sense will often take us a long way, but to establish the truth we need evidence of a different kind). In addition to this, they provide information of the kind that is of interest to life-insurance companies, irrespective of its relevance to the cause of IHD. Thus, statistical information on one or more risk factors in a population can be used to estimate the probability that a given individual in that population will develop IHD within a specified time. These estimates may be used to identify members of the population who are 'at risk' and, hence, for whom preventive measures are indicated. They are also essential in the design of primary prevention trials of measures directed against IHD in a well population.

4.4 The plasma cholesterol as a positive risk factor

Shortly after the end of the Second World War, prospective trials of the type discussed in Section 4.2 were initiated in the United States. By 1963, Keys *et al.* (1963) were able to point to four such studies, one of them continued for 15 years before completion and all showing a significantly higher incidence of clinical events in subjects whose plasma cholesterol concentration was above, than in those in whom it was below, the mean or median value at the first examination. Keys *et al.* (1963) drew the further conclusion that the incidence of IHD rose continuously with the initial plasma cholesterol concentration. In the light of these and of other comparable long-term trials, the plasma total cholesterol concentration must now be regarded as a well-established positive risk factor for IHD. Epidemiological studies (see Stamler *et al.*, 1970, for references) have also provided evidence that hypertension, cigarette smoking, hyperglycaemia, hypertriglyceridaemia, obesity, lack of habitual exercise and a diet rich in saturated fat act as positive risk factors for IHD, though the evidence in some cases is open to question. Several of these factors are of interest in relation to the plasma cholesterol because of the possibility that their association with IHD is mediated in part by an effect on the plasma cholesterol concentration.

The results of two North American prospective studies may be mentioned in particular because they have been used to estimate IHD risks on the basis of single or multiple risk factors, including plasma total cholesterol concentration.

In the 'National Cooperative Pooling Project' (1978) the results obtained from several prospective trials carried out in different parts of the United States were pooled to provide information about a total of more than 7000 IHD-free white men, most of whom were aged 30–59 at entry into the trial. The relation between the initial plasma cholesterol measurement and the 10-year incidence of IHD for all age-groups between 30 and 59 is shown in Fig. 13.4A. The risk of developing a first heart attack was significantly higher in men whose plasma cholesterol concentration was between 250 and 274 mg/100 ml than in those in whom it was below 250 mg/100 ml. Moreover, according to Stamler (1973), the risk of a first attack for a man in the lowest quintile (the lowest 20% of the distribution of plasma cholesterol concentrations) was lower than for a man in any of the higher quintiles, and this difference held for men of all ages from 30 to 64 at entry. Stamler (1973) and other epidemiologists have concluded that the relationship between plasma cholesterol concentration and IHD risk. to continuous, with no critical level below which the risk is unrelated to cholesterol concentration, but this is not obvious from Fig. 13.4B.

In the Framingham prospective study, 5127 IHD-free white men and women aged 30–62 living in the New England town of Framingham were recruited in 1949. (See Gordon *et al.*, 1959, for a discussion of the problems associated with the design and execution of this unique trial.) The subjects were examined initially, and subsequently at two-year intervals, for several possible risk factors for IHD, including the plasma concentrations of total cholesterol, β-lipoprotein (S_f 0–20) and pre-β-lipoprotein. Thirty years after the initiation of the trial, survivors of the original population were still

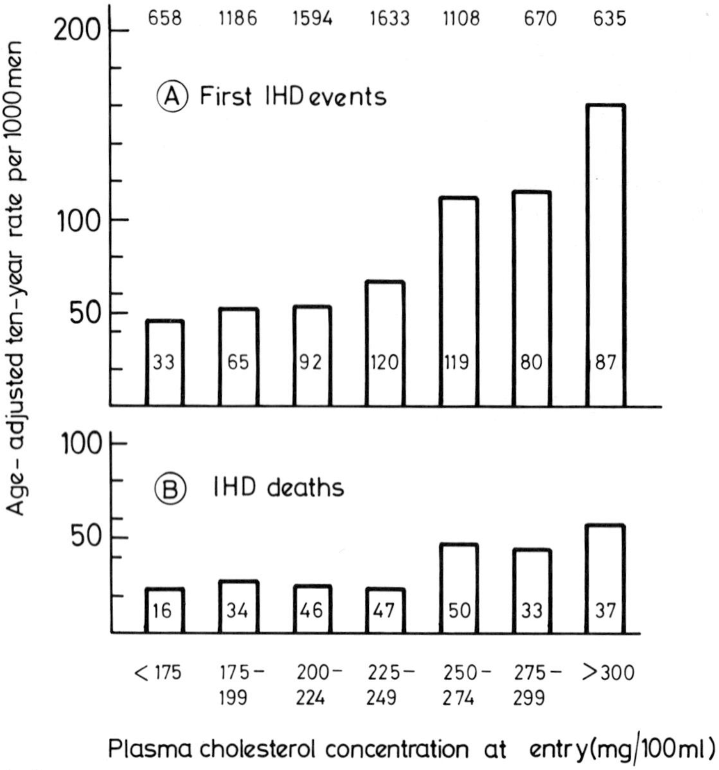

632   The Biology of Cholesterol and Related Steroids

[Figure: Bar chart. Y-axis: Age-adjusted ten-year rate per 1000 men. Numbers above panel A (group sizes): 658, 1186, 1594, 1633, 1108, 670, 635.
Panel A, First IHD events: 33, 65, 92, 120, 119, 80, 87.
Panel B, IHD deaths: 16, 34, 46, 47, 50, 33, 37.
X-axis categories: <175, 175–199, 200–224, 225–249, 250–274, 275–299, >300. Plasma cholesterol concentration at entry (mg/100ml)]

Figure 13.4
The National Co-operative Pooling Project. IHD incidence rate in 7484 normal men aged 30–59 as a function of plasma cholesterol concentration at initial examination. A, ten-year rate for first major coronary events; B, ten-year death rate from IHD. Numbers above A show number of men in each group according to range of plasma cholesterol concentration. Numbers within each rectangle show number of events. (Redrawn from Stamler *et al.*, 1970.)

under observation and their children had also been incorporated into the study. Measurement of plasma HDL cholesterol concentration of the survivors was begun in 1969. The results, which have been reported serially in many publications, show that the risk of developing clinical IHD is proportional to the initial plasma total cholesterol concentration in men aged 30–62 and in women up to age 50 (see Kannel *et al.*, 1961; Kannel *et al.*, 1971; Gordon *et al.*, 1977a). As in the Pooling Project (which included the earlier results of the Framingham study), IHD risk in men appeared to increase continuously from the lowest to the highest cholesterol level in the study population (Fig. 13.5), though it should be noted that risks associated with the lowest cholesterol levels were calculated on the basis of a relatively small absolute number of IHD events. The association was strongest in the younger age-groups in both sexes, and was hardly apparent in women over age 50; this can be seen by comparing the *relative risks* in subjects with high and low antecedent plasma cholesterol concentration at different ages. Table 13.3 shows the ratios of the 14-year incidence rates of IHD at high and low cholesterol levels between ages 35 and 64. In men up to age 44 the risk of developing IHD within 14 years was 5.5 times higher if the initial cholesterol level was 235 mg/100 ml, or greater, than if it was less than

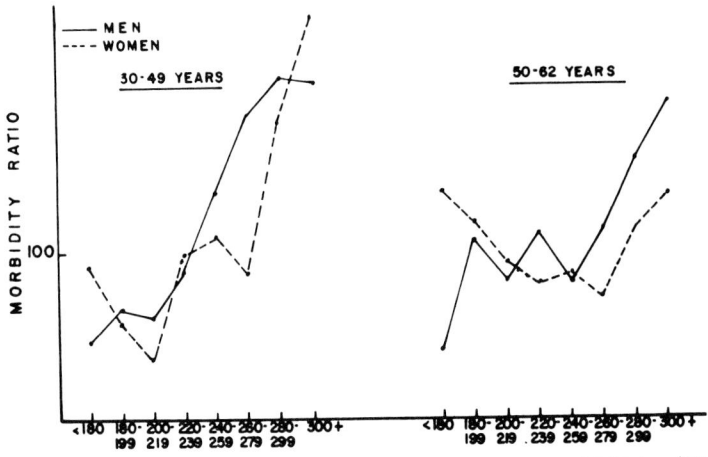

Figure 13.5
Fourteen-year incidence rate of IHD (% of rate in whole populations) in men and women aged 30–62 years as a function of serum cholesterol concentration at entry. (From Kannel *et al.*, 1971.)

Table 13.3
The ratio of the 14-year IHD incidence with high antecedent plasma cholesterol level to that with low antecedent cholesterol level (the relative risk) in men and women

Age (years)	Relative risk Men	Women
35–44	5.5	5.0
45–54	2.4	1.5
55–64	1.7	1.3
All ages	2.5	1.5

High cholesterol level = >265 mg/100 ml.
Low = <220 mg/199 ml.
(From Kannel *et al.*, 1971.)

220 mg/100 ml. In men aged 55 to 64 the relative risk fell to 1.7. In women in each age range the relative risk was lower than in men. The effect of age on the predictive association between IHD and plasma cholesterol may also be seen in Fig. 13.6, in which the antecedent cholesterol concentration is plotted as a function of age in those who developed IHD and in those who did not. The difference between the initial levels in the IHD cases and in whose who remained IHD-free was greater at age 35–49 than at older ages. In other words, the predictive power of plasma total cholesterol concentration for IHD decreases with age.

In addition to these observations on United States populations, a predictive association between plasma cholesterol concentration and IHD has been observed in many other parts of the world (see, for example, Keys *et al.*, 1970, and Medalie *et al.*, 1973). In the 'Seven Countries' inter-population study of Keys *et al.* (1970), the 5-year incidence rate of first attacks of IHD in men aged 40–59 years was shown to be directly related to the initial median plasma cholesterol concentration in populations from seven different countries (Finland, Greece, Holland, Italy, Japan, the United States and Yugoslavia).

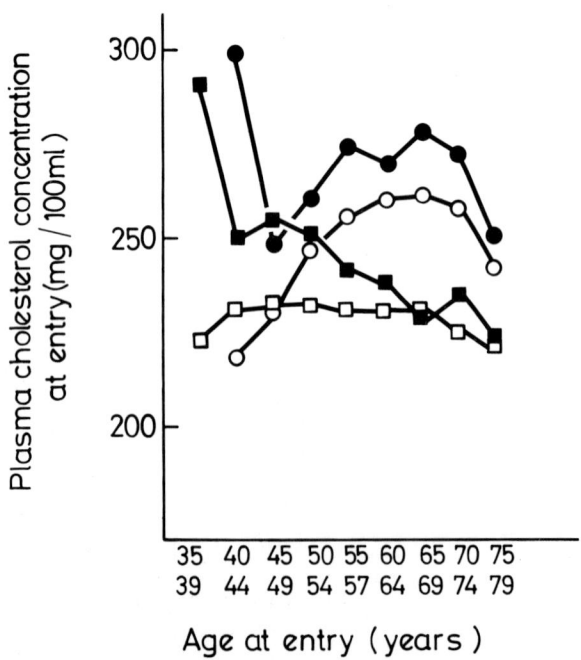

Figure 13.6
The Framingham population. Mean plasma total cholesterol concentration by age and sex of those developing (black symbols) and those not developing (open symbols) IHD within approximately four years of initial cholesterol measurement. Females are circles; males are squares. (From Gordon *et al.*, 1977a.)

Fig. 13.7 shows the IHD death rates as a function of plasma cholesterol level at entry into the study in 13 of the populations investigated by Keys and his international team of workers.

Since LDL is the major carrier of the plasma cholesterol, the plasma LDL concentration should also be a predictor of IHD. This has been shown to be the case in several prospective trials (Stamler, 1973), including the Framingham study, though the predictive power of LDL concentration is no better than that of total cholesterol concentration. In several studies, the plasma VLDL concentration (measured in terms of total triglycerides, S_f 20–400, pre-β-lipoprotein or cholesterol in the VLDL density fraction) was found to be predictive of IHD. In the Framingham study population the association between plasma VLDL concentration and subsequent first attacks of IHD in men at all ages and in women under 50 could be explained by the positive correlation between VLDL and total cholesterol concentrations (Kannel et al., 1971). In a Swedish population, however, plasma triglyceride concentration appeared to be predictive of first IHD attacks in men, even after correction for the effect of the plasma total cholesterol level (Carlson and Böttiger, 1972).

As in several other prospective trials (reviewed in Stamler, 1973), hypertension, cigarette smoking and diabetes were found to be risk factors for IHD in the Framingham study, but plasma cholesterol

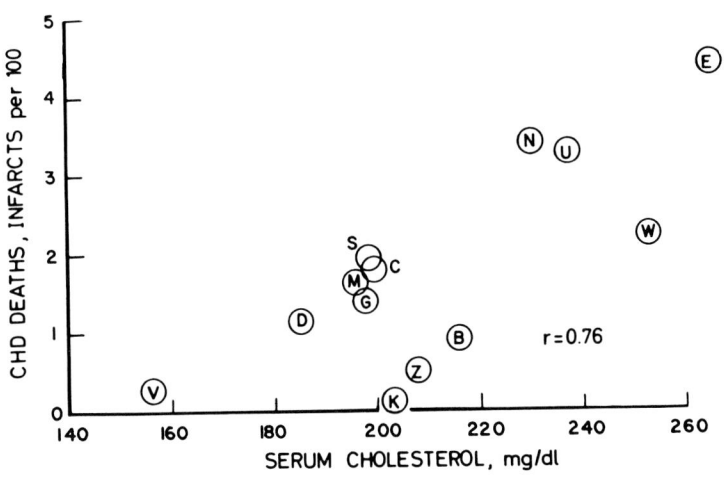

Figure 13.7
Age-standardized 5-year incidence rates of death from ischaemic heart disease (CHD) in IHD-free men aged 30–59 years at entry, from thirteen different populations. B, Belgrade; C, Crevalcore; D, Dalmatia; E, East Finland; G, Corfu; K, Crete; M, Montegiorgio; N, Zutphen; S, Slavonia; U, US railroad; V, Velika Krsna; W, West Finland; Z, Zrenjanin. (From Keys, 1970.)

concentration remained a positive risk factor when the effects of these other variables were eliminated by discriminant analysis. Of paramount importance from the point of view of the prevention of IHD, the Framingham study has confirmed the impression gained from other trials that plasma cholesterol concentration, hypertension and smoking are additive as risk factors (see Rose *et al.*, 1977). Fig. 13.8 shows the ten-year incidence rates (calculated from the results of the Pooling Project) for first attacks of IHD in men with none of these three risk factors, with any one, with any two and with all three. For a man with all three, the chance of experiencing a first attack within ten years (17.1%) is 8.5 times that of a man with none (2.0%). The interaction between plasma cholesterol and the two other risk factors is shown in a different way in Fig. 13.9. IHD risk increases with increasing plasma cholesterol concentration, but at a higher level if the systolic blood pressure is raised and at a still higher level if, in addition to having a raised blood pressure, the subject is a cigarette smoker. Inspection of the risk curves shows that a 45-year-old cigarette smoker with hypertension and a plasma cholesterol concentration of 310 mg/100 ml has nine times the risk of a heart attack within eight years, compared with that of a non-smoker without hypertension and with a plasma cholesterol level of 185 mg/100 ml.

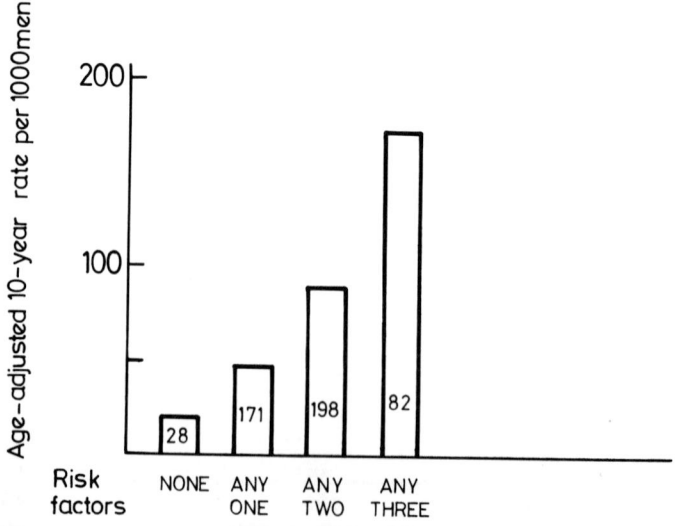

Figure 13.8
The National Co-operative Pooling Project. Ten-year incidence of first attacks of ischaemic heart disease in 7342 normal men aged 30–59, as a function of the number of risk factors at entry into the trial. The three risk factors were: plasma cholesterol concentration ⩾250 mg/100 ml; diastolic blood pressure ⩾90 mm Hg; cigarette smoker. Numbers within each rectangle show number of events. (Redrawn from Stamler *et al.*, 1970.)

Furthermore, for a man with hypertension, the higher the plasma cholesterol level, the greater the risk of developing IHD.

So far, we have considered the plasma cholesterol as a risk factor only for first attacks of IHD, i.e. for heart attacks or other signs of IHD in people with no previous clinical manifestation of disease of the coronary arteries. Evidence from at least one trial (the Coronary Drug Project) suggests, however, that plasma total cholesterol concentration is predictive of death from IHD in men who have already had one or more heart attack (Stamler, 1973).

Since IHD is preceded by the very gradual development of atherosclerosis of the coronaries, it would be reasonable to expect a correlation between the prevalence of risk factors, such as high plasma cholesterol concentration, and the extent of coronary atherosclerosis in the general population. Evidence for or against a relationship between plasma cholesterol concentration and coronary atherosclerosis is difficult to obtain because the state of the coronary arteries is hard to assess accurately in life and because we seldom have adequate information about the plasma cholesterol concentration during life in people who die unexpectedly.

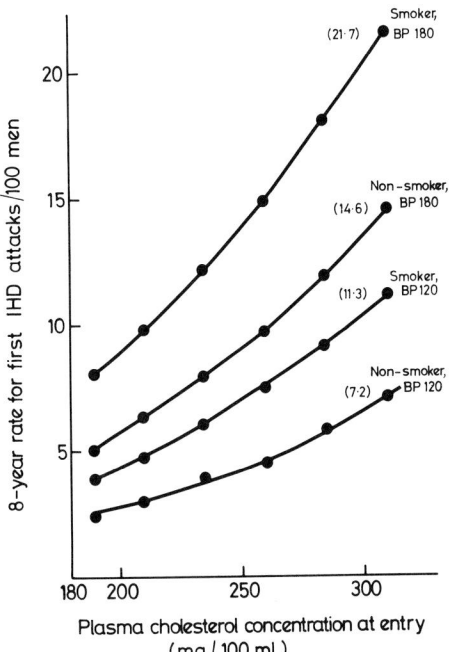

Figure 13.9
The Framingham study. Eight-year incidence of first attacks of ischaemic heart disease in normal 45-year-old men as a function of plasma cholesterol concentration, systolic blood pressure (BP, mm Hg) and cigarette smoking. Values in brackets show eight-year incidence per 100 men. (Constructed from Kannel, 1974.)

One approach to this problem has been to try to relate the extent of atherosclerosis, determined *post mortem*, to the prevalence of a given risk factor in the living population from which the autopsied subjects were derived. This method has been adopted in the International Atherosclerosis Project. The aims, procedures and preliminary results of this study were described in a series of articles on the International Atherosclerosis Project (1968) and the more recent results have been summarized by Strong (1977). In more than 22 000 autopsies of males and females aged 10–69 from 19 populations differing in race or location there was a positive association between the extent of coronary atherosclerosis and the plasma cholesterol level in the population of origin. There was also a positive correlation between coronary atherosclerosis at autopsy and cigarette smoking in the same person (assessed from interviews with surviving relatives), though this has not been confirmed in other studies (Garcia-Palmieri *et al.*, 1977). Population-based studies of the plasma cholesterol in relation to atherosclerosis determined at autopsy are open to many criticisms, discussed fully by those themselves engaged in the International Atherosclerosis Project (McMahon, 1968), but the results of this investigation are at least consistent with the hypothesis that there is a positive association between plasma cholesterol concentration and coronary atherosclerosis in a given person. More direct evidence for this has been obtained by demonstrating a positive association in individuals whose plasma cholesterol concentration has been measured several years before death (Feinleib *et al.*, 1979; Garcia-Palmieri *et al.*, 1977).

Another approach has been to exploit the opportunities afforded by the increasing use of coronary angiography to assess the state of the coronary arteries in life; Lichtlen (1976) has estimated that at least 300 000 such procedures were carried out throughout the world in 1975. Attempts to relate the degree of narrowing of the coronary arteries to the plasma cholesterol concentration in the same person have produced contradictory results. In some cases (Fuster *et al.*, 1975) no significant association was found, whereas in others (Murray *et al.*, 1975, and see this paper for other references) there was a positive relationship between the apparent extent of coronary atherosclerosis and the plasma concentrations of cholesterol and LDL, particularly in the younger subjects. Jenkins *et al.* (1978) have also reported a significant positive correlation between plasma LDL concentration and the extent and severity of coronary atherosclerosis in men and women. However, the value of all these observations is questionable because the *severity* of coronary atherosclerosis is difficult to measure by angiography and because most subjects undergoing coronary angiography have clinical evidence of heart disease. In so far as this is due to relatively advanced atherosclerosis of the coronaries, there may be too little variability in the study population to reveal a graded correlation with plasma cholesterol concentration.

4.5 Plasma cholesterol and the prediction of IHD

The results obtained from prospective studies can be used to calculate risks of first attacks of IHD in individuals of a given age and sex. Thus, for plasma cholesterol concentration as a single positive risk factor, the results of the Pooling Project show that for a man aged 30–59 the risk of a first attack within 10 years is 4.5% if his plasma cholesterol concentration is <175 mg/100 ml, but is 11.2% if it is 250–274 mg/100 ml. In absolute terms, this would represent a massive increase in the total number of first IHD attacks in a population containing millions of men whose cholesterol level was raised from the lower to the higher value. But in relation to the individual it is much less impressive. Thus, although a rise in plasma cholesterol level from 175 to 250 mg/100 ml causes a 2.5-fold increase in 10-year risk, the effect on the chance of remaining IHD-free for 10 years is relatively small (95.5% at the lower, and 88.8% at the higher plasma cholesterol level). The weak predictive power of plasma cholesterol alone was pointed out by Lewis *et al.* in their dissenting opinion in the report by Gofman *et al.* (1956) and is brought out very clearly by comparing the distribution of plasma cholesterol concentrations in the Framingham middle-aged men who developed IHD within 16 years, with those who did not (Fig. 13.10). Though the means of the two distributions are different, in most of the men who subsequently developed IHD the plasma cholesterol concentration was within the range of values of the majority of those who remained IHD-free.

Predictive power can be improved by combining other independent risk factors with the plasma cholesterol concentration to give *multiple risk scores* (see Menotti, 1974). Epstein (1977*a*) has estimated that in several populations in which prospective trials have been carried out, about 50% of first IHD events occur among men with the top 20% of risk scores based on multiple factors, including antecedent plasma cholesterol concentration. This is an improvement on prediction from any single factor, but would still give a high proportion of false negatives (failure to predict those in the lower quintiles of risk score who develop IHD) and false positives (those in the top quintile who remain IHD-free), as shown in the hypothetical example given by Epstein (1977*a*).

Consider 1000 men from a population with a 10% incidence of IHD per 10 years and suppose that we have estimated, by multivariate analysis of the results of a prospective trial, that 50% of new IHD events will occur in the men with the top 20% of risk scores. We can then predict that of the 100 IHD events occurring within 10 years, 50 will occur among the 200 men whom we have identified by their risk scores. We have therefore achieved a 25% rate of correct predictions (50/200), which is only 2.5 times better than the prediction we could have made without any knowledge of risk scores. We have also made 150 false positive predictions and have failed to predict the 50 IHD events occurring among the 800 men in the lower quintiles. We can only increase the number of correct predictions, by including men with lower risk scores, at the cost of increasing the number of false positives. This is simply a reflection of the fact that in any population many people develop IHD in the absence of known risk factors. This has an important practical consequence in relation to community-based prevention of IHD. The possibility of improving our ability to predict IHD in individuals by including HDL cholesterol in the calculation of risk score is considered in the next section.

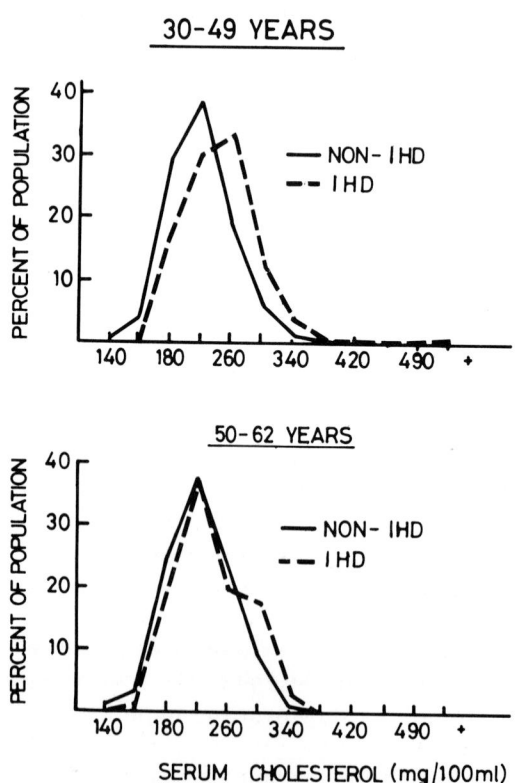

Figure 13.10
The Framingham study. The distribution of serum cholesterol concentrations at entry in men free of IHD who subsequently developed IHD (————) or remained IHD-free (————) during the subsequent 16 years. (From Kannel, 1974.)

4.6 HDL as a negative risk factor

As we have seen (Section 4.2), Barr *et al.* (1951) found that the plasma α-lipoprotein concentration tended to be lower in IHD patients than in subjects who had never had a heart attack. At the same time, they drew attention to the fact that women during the reproductive period, when their susceptibility to IHD is much lower than that of men, have higher plasma α-lipoprotein concentrations than men. These observations were followed by other case-control studies in the 1950's and 1960's (see Wiklund *et al.*, 1975, for references), all showing a negative correlation between IHD and plasma HDL or α-lipoprotein concentration. Additional evidence for this was obtained from the two prospective trials completed in the 1960's. In Keys's study of Minnesota businessmen (Keys *et al.*, 1963) there was a significant negative correlation between the initial plasma α-lipoprotein concentration and the subsequent development of IHD. Gofman *et al.* (1966) also found a negative predictive association between plasma HDL_2 and HDL_3 concentrations (measured in the analytical ultracentrifuge) and IHD in a group of men in the town of Livermore, California.

These observations were largely ignored at the time, possibly because the idea that a cholesterol-carrying lipoprotein might *decrease* susceptibility to IHD could not be reconciled with the then popular view that atherosclerosis is caused by insudation of plasma lipid into the arterial wall. However, in the light of our present understanding of the origin and metabolic role of the plasma HDL (see Chapter 11), these earlier findings, suggesting that HDL may protect against IHD, can now be re-interpreted (Miller and Miller, 1975). This change in angle of vision, together with the development of a simple precipitation method for assaying HDL cholesterol, has given rise to a considerable interest in the associations between plasma HDL, IHD and other risk factors for IHD. It has also led to the current preoccupation in many laboratories with factors that may modify the plasma HDL concentration, and with the question of how HDL might influence the development of atherosclerotic lesions. As a result of this impetus, several retrospective and prospective studies of the relation between plasma HDL and IHD have recently been completed in the United States, Scandinavia and Great Britain, and others are in progress.

In the most extensive of these—the U.S. Co-operative Lipoprotein Phenotyping Study—the prevalence of IHD was shown to be negatively correlated with the plasma HDL cholesterol concentration in men and women, aged 40 years and older, in five U.S. populations (Rhoads *et al.*, 1976; Castelli *et al.*, 1977). This relation between HDL and IHD was apparent over the whole range of plasma HDL cholesterol concentration from <25 mg/100 ml to >44 mg/100 ml and was independent of the positive correlation between IHD prevalence and the plasma concentrations of total and LDL cholesterol. In the U.S. Co-operative Study there was no correlation between IHD prevalence and plasma triglyceride concentration. However, Carlson and Eriksson (1975) found that in Swedish men IHD was more strongly associated with hypertriglyceridaemia than with diminished plasma HDL cholesterol concentration, and that at a given plasma VLDL triglyceride concentration there was no relation between IHD and plasma HDL concentration. They concluded that the negative association between plasma HDL and IHD was secondary to that between HDL and VLDL concentration.

The results of several epidemiological studies on populations in Europe and the American continent have shown that, as well as the association between plasma HDL and VLDL, plasma HDL concentration is negatively correlated with a number of other known or suspected positive risk factors. These include relative body weight, diminished glucose tolerance or clinical diabetes, short sitting or standing height, systolic and diastolic blood pressure, lack of habitual physical activity and cigarette smoking (see, for example, Miller et al., 1976; Gordon et al., 1977a; Nikkilä, 1978; Williams et al., 1979). Some of these associations are weak and not all of them have reached statistical significance in all populations studied. Furthermore, some of them are inter-dependent.

Two prospective trials have shown clearly that plasma HDL cholesterol concentration is a negative risk factor for IHD.

In the most recent extension of the Framingham study, 2470 IHD-free male and female survivors of the original population examined in 1949–1950 were re-examined in 1969–1971 (when they were aged 49–82 years) and were then followed up for 2–8 years; in addition to other lipid and lipoprotein measurements, plasma HDL cholesterol concentration was measured by the heparin/manganese precipitation method. At all ages, plasma HDL cholesterol concentration was higher in the women than in the men. In both sexes and at all age intervals up to 70 years there was a strong negative correlation between initial plasma HDL cholesterol concentration and IHD incidence. There was also some predictive association between plasma triglyceride concentration and IHD in women but not in men. Multivariate analysis showed that the association between HDL and IHD was independent of the plasma VLDL, LDL and total cholesterol concentrations, and of blood pressure, cigarette smoking, relative body weight and glucose tolerance. The relation between the initial plasma HDL cholesterol concentration and the subsequent development of IHD was apparent throughout the range of plasma HDL cholesterol concentration from 25 mg/100 ml to >65 mg/100 ml, the 4-year IHD

Cholesterol and Atherosclerosis   643

incidence in men decreasing from 100/1000 to 25/1000 as the HDL cholesterol concentration increased (Fig. 13.11). As shown in Fig. 13.11, over the range of plasma HDL cholesterol concentration from 35 to 65 mg/100 ml, IHD incidence at a given concentration was lower in women than in men, though only slightly so. This suggests that the difference in IHD risk between men and women in the Framingham population was due largely, though not wholly, to the higher HDL concentration in women at a given age. Gordon et al. (1977b) concluded, from estimates of 'likelihood ratios', that the predictive power of plasma HDL cholesterol concentration for IHD was four times that of LDL cholesterol concentration and eight times that of total cholesterol concentration. They pointed out, however, that in view of the positive predictive correlation between plasma LDL concentration and IHD, and the weak association between HDL and LDL concentration, a factor incorporating both HDL and LDL would be bound to be a better predictor of IHD than either alone.

In a two-year prospective study of more than 6000 men aged 20–49 years living in the Norwegian town of Tromsø, Miller et al. (1977) obtained essentially similar results. Again, there was a strong negative correlation between initial HDL cholesterol concentration and the subsequent incidence of IHD, and this association was independent of

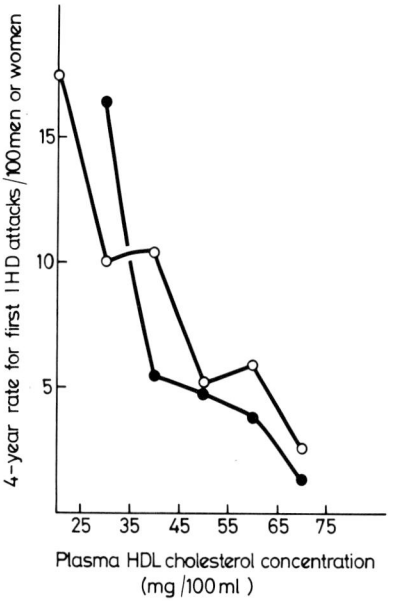

Figure 13.11
The Framingham study. Four-year incidence rate of first attacks of IHD in men (open symbols) and women (closed symbols) as a function of initial plasma HDL cholesterol concentration. (From Gordon et al., 1977b.)

the cholesterol concentration in the d < 1.063 plasma fraction and of various other risk factors for IHD. Miller et al. (1977) estimated that about 85% of the occurrences or non-occurrences of IHD within two years could have been predicted correctly from a factor combining the plasma concentrations of cholesterol in HDL and in the d < 1.063 fraction.

A striking instance of the inverse correlation between plasma HDL concentration and IHD has been reported by Glueck et al. (1975), who have described several families in which some members live into their 80's and 90's without evidence of IHD. In these individuals the plasma HDL cholesterol concentration is usually 75 mg/100 ml or higher. Glueck et al. (1975) suggest that the combination of longevity with increased plasma HDL concentration within families is an inherited abnormality, which they call *familial hyperalphalipoproteinaemia*, and that its inheritance is monogenic. However, although the clustering of very high plasma HDL concentrations in the families investigated by Glueck et al. is consistent with some degree of heritability, the evidence in favour of monogenic inheritance is still incomplete.

The plasma HDL concentration has been reported to be lower in the first-degree relatives of IHD patients than in age-matched control subjects (Pometta et al., 1978). This observation, the complement of that decribed by Glueck et al. (1975), raises the possibility that the well-established aggregation of IHD within families (see Epstein, 1967; Aro, 1973) is mediated in part by a familial clustering of low plasma HDL cholesterol concentrations.

In addition to these population- and family-based studies, there is growing evidence to suggest that IHD prevalence is inversely related to plasma HDL concentration in different populations or racial groups. Examples are the Eskimos (Bang and Dyerberg, 1972) and black South Africans (Walker and Walker, 1978); in both groups the mean plasma HDL cholesterol concentration is higher, and the incidence of IHD is lower, than in whites. However, there are significant differences in the prevalence of IHD in different populations that are not explicable solely by differences in plasma HDL cholesterol concentration. In the Co-operative Phenotyping Study, for example, Japanese men living in Hawaii were found to have a lower IHD prevalence than the Framingham men, but the plasma HDL cholesterol concentrations were similar in the two populations. These inter-population differences in the relative importance of HDL as a risk factor are understandable, since IHD is associated with other risk factors, such as plasma LDL concentration, that are essentially independent of the plasma HDL concentration.

Almost all the epidemiological observations discussed above were based on measurement of cholesterol concentration in the total HDL fraction of plasma (usually the d 1.063—1.21 fraction). However, HDL consists of at least two subfractions which differ in particle size and in lipid and protein composition (see Chapter 11). Hence, the association between IHD and HDL cholesterol concentration may mask a more specific association between IHD and the number or chemical composition of the particles in total HDL or in a particular HDL subclass. Indeed, there is already evidence to suggest that a low HDL_2 concentration is a better predictor of IHD than is a low HDL_3 concentration (Gofman et al., 1966). It should also be noted that the higher plasma HDL cholesterol level in women than in men is due largely to a difference in HDL_2 concentration (Barclay et al., 1963). Moreover, in at least two case-control studies, the plasma concentrations of apoA-I and apoA-II (the major apoproteins of HDL) were found to be lower in IHD patients than in healthy control subjects (Albers et al., 1976; Berg et al., 1976). Future epidemiological studies of IHD risk factors are likely to be designed with a view to examining points such as these in greater detail. It is also to be hoped that simple methods will be developed for assaying HDL-I, the apoE-rich component of human HDL discovered by Mahley et al. (1978), so that its possible relationship to IHD can be explored.

In summary, the limited evidence now available from prospective trials strongly suggests that a combination of the plasma HDL concentration with LDL or total cholesterol concentration gives a more accurate prediction of IHD than does any one of these taken by itself. To this extent, our ability to predict IHD from the plasma lipid or lipoprotein pattern is now distinctly better than that based on plasma cholesterol concentration alone (see Section 4.5). However, a combination of plasma lipid and lipoprotein risk factors which includes HDL concentration is still some way short of a perfect predictor of IHD. Thus, in the Framingham Study (Gordon et al., 1977b, Fig. 2), a substantial proportion of first attacks of IHD in men and woman occurred in the lower quintiles of risk score based on a combination of plasma HDL cholesterol, total cholesterol and triglyceride concentrations. Moreover, in the U.S. Co-operative Study the average difference between plasma HDL cholesterol concentration in IHD cases and controls was only 3–4 mg/100 ml, a difference that is well within the limits of error of a single measurement. Despite this limitation, a measurement of plasma HDL, and perhaps of its subfractions, is certain to be used to an increasing extent in the assessment of IHD risk, both in hospital practice and in epidemiological trials. It is worth noting, however, that accurate measurement of plasma HDL cholesterol concentration requires careful attention to detail and a high standard of quality control, and that a difference of less than 10 mg of HDL cholesterol/100 ml has a significant effect on IHD risk (see Fig. 13.11). The problem of assaying the lipid and protein components of the plasma HDL has been discussed in great depth at an international conference (Lippel, 1979). When we have much more information than is now available on plasma HDL as a risk factor in males and females at all ages, it should be possible to construct multiple risk score tables which incorporate HDL in addition to the other standard risk factors for IHD.

4.7 The significance of plasma cholesterol and HDL as risk factors

4.7.1 General conclusions

The evidence discussed above leaves little doubt that the plasma concentrations of LDL and total cholesterol are positive risk factors for IHD, especially in the younger age groups, and that plasma HDL cholesterol concentration is a negative risk factor at all ages from 20–70 years. Plasma triglyceride concentration may also be an independent risk factor in some populations, but in others the association between triglycerides and IHD seems to be entirely dependent upon the negative correlation between triglyceride and HDL concentration. Several other risk factors, including cigarette smoking and blood pressure, appear to act independently of plasma lipid or lipoprotein concentration and their effects on IHD risk are therefore additive.

The above conclusions with regard to plasma LDL and total cholesterol are based on investigations of human populations living under a wide range of different conditions and are not invalidated by the more recent identification of plasma HDL cholesterol as a negative risk factor. The measurement of plasma total cholesterol concentration is still an essential step in the assessment of IHD risk in the individual subject, particularly in children and young adults, though increasing emphasis is bound to be placed on the lipoprotein pattern, as distinct from the concentration of total cholesterol or total triglyceride. In epidemiological trials, the measurement of plasma total cholesterol may come increasingly to be replaced by that of lipoprotein or apolipoprotein concentrations, as more convenient methods of assay become available. It is likely that additional IHD risk factors will be identified conclusively, and that their interaction with known plasma lipoprotein risk factors will be studied in populations from many parts of the world. Among these newer risk factors, it may well turn out that certain aspects of the clotting mechanism and of platelet behaviour are independent predictors of IHD (see Mitchell, 1978, for discussion and references).

As we have already seen the practical importance of risk factors for IHD is two-fold. First, they make it possible to predict, with varying degrees of accuracy, first attacks of IHD in individuals or populations.

Second, they provide clues to the aetiology and pathogenesis of IHD. As we saw in Section 4.5, the predictive power of plasma total cholesterol concentration (and, by implication, of LDL concentration) for individuals is not very strong. Indeed, if one were to try to predict first attacks of IHD in applicants for a job in which a heart attack could endanger many lives, such as that of railway signal-person or air-line pilot, one would do better to rely on sex alone, since this is a more powerful predictor of IHD than any other known risk factor taken singly or in combination. From the point of view simply of IHD risk, at a given age and in the absence of other information women would be more suitable than men. The relevance of plasma lipid and lipoprotein risk factors to the cause of IHD is considered in the next section.

4.7.2 The plasma cholesterol as a 'cause' of IHD in man

There are several reasons, some of which have already been mentioned in this chapter, for thinking that the predictive association between plasma total or LDL cholesterol concentration and IHD is one of cause and effect. This view is embodied in what is generally known as the *plasma lipid hypothesis*.

(a) Lesions of the coronary arteries, indistinguishable from those responsible for IHD in man, can be induced in non-human primates by feeding diets which raise the plasma cholesterol concentration, mainly in the LDL fraction. On returning the animals to a normal diet, plasma cholesterol concentration falls and the lesions regress (see Sections 3.2 and 3.4).

(b) In human subjects and experimental animals the bulk of the cholesterol present in atherosclerotic lesions is derived from the plasma and is carried into the artery in apo-B-containing lipoproteins. Within the arterial wall, LDL and VLDL particles are taken up by SMC and are bound by proteoglycans in the intima (see Section 2.6).

(c) In intact animals, including non-human primates, experimentally induced hypercholesterolaemia may damage arteries and may also facilitate the development of atherosclerotic lesions in regions of the arterial wall subjected to superficial injury, possibly by interfering with repair. This suggests a mechanism whereby focal areas of spontaneous injury could be converted into atherosclerotic lesions in the presence of hypercholesterolaemia.

(d) Observations on cultured human and animal SMC suggest that plasma LDL stimulates SMC proliferation, an essential feature of the development of atherosclerotic lesions.

(e) The prevalence and incidence of IHD and the extent of coronary atherosclerosis observed *post mortem* are directly related to the plasma cholesterol concentration in different populations (Keys *et al.*, 1970; Epstein, 1971; Stamler, 1973; Strong, 1977). In many populations in which the mean plasma cholesterol concentration is less than 200 mg/100 ml, IHD is almost unknown as a cause of death and fibrous plaques are seldom seen *post mortem* in the coronary arteries of men. Of striking significance in this connection is the very low IHD incidence in some populations in which other risk factors are present. In Japanese men, for example, IHD incidence and mean plasma cholesterol concentration are both very low, despite a high prevalence of hypertension (Kimura, 1977).

(f) In patients with familial hypercholesterolaemia, an inherited disorder due to a mutation at a single gene locus affecting specifically the catabolism of LDL (see Chapter 15), the incidence of IHD is greatly increased.

Taken together, these lines of evidence strongly suggest that a raised plasma cholesterol concentration contributes directly to the development of IHD, and that if the plasma LDL level is high enough, this may be sufficient by itself to initiate coronary atherosclerosis and to lead to death from premature IHD in the absence of other risk factors. The evidence derived from inter-population studies also suggests that the force of certain IHD risk factors is much diminished if the plasma cholesterol concentration falls below about 200 mg/100 ml. Although the conclusion that hypercholesterolaemia is the cause of the premature IHD in familial hypercholesterolaemia seems inescapable, none of the points listed above provides proof that the predictive association between plasma cholesterol concentration and IHD in the *general* population is a causal one. To prove such a relationship it is necessary to show that the incidence of IHD decreases when the plasma total or LDL cholesterol concentration is reduced by some form of controlled intervention in groups of people drawn from the general population who have not had a heart attack (primary prevention trial) or who have already had one or more attacks (secondary prevention trial). Several such trials have now been completed.

Both types of trial present formidable difficulties in design and execution. Owing to the low incidence of clinically detectable IHD in healthy subjects, primary prevention trials require large numbers of control and test subjects and long periods of investigation if the number of IHD events is to be sufficient for statistical evaluation. For example, calculations based on the results of the Framingham trial suggest that in order to demonstrate a significant effect on IHD attack rate by reducing the plasma cholesterol concentration, it would be necessary to achieve a 19% reduction over a 6-year period in a study population of 7000 men aged 45–65 with an initial average plasma cholesterol level of 260 mg/100 ml (Whyte, 1975). Furthermore, even if a significant effect on IHD incidence is achieved, it can usually be argued that the effect was mediated by an influence of the drug or dietary treatment on something other than the plasma cholesterol concentration, such as blood coagulability, platelet behaviour or some property of the arterial wall itself. This applies particularly to trials in which the intervention consists in the addition of polyunsaturated fats to the diet, since dietary linoleic acid appears to diminish platelet activation in man (O'Brien *et al.*, 1976). Several polyunsaturated fatty acids also have complex indirect effects on platelet function by acting as precursors of prostaglandins and of other platelet effectors synthesized within the platelets or by arterial endothelial cells (see Jakubowski and Ardlie, 1978; Gryglewski and Moncada, 1979).

In secondary prevention trials one is faced with the problem of trying to reverse established fibrotic lesions that may have progressed for many years. To judge from the behaviour of experimental atherosclerotic lesions in animals, the time required for regression might be at least as long as the time over which the lesions have developed. In addition to these difficulties, it is not at all easy to achieve a significant and sustained decrease in the plasma cholesterol level in large numbers of free-living subjects for many years; it has certainly not been possible, in any of the trials carried out so far on closed or open populations, to reduce the plasma cholesterol level to anywhere near the levels found in non-industrialized populations with low IHD incidence. Not surprisingly, therefore, the results of intervention trials have been controversial. Indeed, Epstein (1977*b*) has argued that if may never be possible to obtain an unequivocal answer.

In two major primary prevention trials in which diet was used to lower plasma cholesterol level (Dayton *et al.*, 1969; Miettinen *et al.*, 1972), a reduction in the incidence of IHD was observed in the treated group and in the trial of Miettinen *et al.* there was a statistically significant reduction in the death rate from IHD in men. A significant reduction in the incidence of non-fatal IHD was also achieved in the WHO clofibrate trial (Oliver *et al.*, 1978, 1980), and in this trial the effect on IHD incidence was greatest in the men in whom the plasma cholesterol level was reduced to the greatest extent. The results of these trials therefore provide limited support for the plasma lipid hypothesis. However, the design of the two dietary trials mentioned above has been criticized on a number of grounds (see Ahrens (1976) and David and Havlik (1977) for critical discussions of these and other dietary and drug trials of the plasma lipid hypothesis). It should also be noted that the *death rate* from IHD in the WHO clofibrate trial was not affected by the treatment.

Two recent reports suggest that it may be possible to bring about regression of atherosclerosis of the coronary arteries in hypercholesterolaemic patients by drastic reduction of the plasma cholesterol concentration (Buchwald *et al.*, 1974; Thompson *et al.*, 1980). This is at least consistent with the view that the association between plasma cholesterol and atherosclerosis is causal. The incidence of IHD has been reported to be much lower in American Seventh-Day Adventist communities than in the United States as a whole (Wynder *et al.*, 1959). If substantiated, this would also give some support to the plasma lipid hypothesis, since the plasma cholesterol concentration in the members of these communities is lower than in the general population (see Chapter 12, Section 1.3). However, evidence derived from self-selected groups of people can never be conclusive, because self selection may act in favour of other negative or positive risk factors for IHD that are not mediated by the plasma cholesterol level. Thus, a low incidence of IHD in Seventh Day Adventists could be due partly to the presence of a high proportion of non-smokers in these communities.

4.7.3 Does HDL protect against IHD?

The strong inverse correlation between plasma HDL cholesterol concentration and IHD, clearly shown in case-control and prospective studies, suggests that HDL protects against IHD. Our current knowledge of the metabolism of human plasma lipoproteins *in vivo* and *in vitro* suggests two mechanisms by which HDL might counteract the accumulation of cholesterol in the arteries and thus delay the progress of atherosclerosis.

As discussed in Chapter 11, HDL could act as a carrier for transporting cholesterol from extrahepatic tissues, including the arterial wall, to the liver for catabolism and excretion. A high plasma concentration of HDL, particularly of HDL_2, might thus be a consequence of increased clearance of cholesterol from the tissues. It is consistent with this that the extravascular mass of exchangeable cholesterol has been reported to be inversely proportional to the plasma HDL concentration (Miller and Miller, 1975).

The apoE-containing fraction of HDL inhibits the high-affinity uptake and catabolism of LDL by SMC and other human cells in culture. If this occurred *in vivo*, the net effect of a rise in plasma HDL concentration on the intracellular accumulation of cholesterol would be difficult to predict. Increased tissue clearance of cholesterol would be expected to enhance LDL-receptor formation and thus to stimulate LDL uptake. On the other hand, a general inhibition of receptor-mediated uptake of LDL in all cells that have receptors would presumably tend to raise the plasma LDL concentration and hence lead to increased deposition of LDL cholesterol in the arterial wall by the scavenger pathway postulated by Brown and Goldstein (1978).

However, it is conceivable that inhibition is selective and that it is greater in the arterial wall than in other tissues. Selectivity in the inhibition of LDL uptake by HDL could occur if, for example, the degree of inhibition depends on the relative or absolute concentrations of HDL and LDL at the cell surface, and if these values differ from one tissue to another. By a selective mechanism such as this, HDL could decrease receptor-mediated uptake of LDL by artery-wall cells without diminishing the overall rate of LDL catabolism. However, these are rather tenuous speculations. Moreover, it should be noted that there is as yet no evidence that the plasma concentration of apoE-containing HDL is inversely related to the incidence of IHD; in the precipitation method used in epidemiological surveys for assaying HDL cholesterol, the apoE-rich fraction is lost in the precipitate.

There is a tendency on the part of some authors to conclude that the plasma lipid hypothesis of the aetiology of IHD is no longer tenable and that it should be discarded in favour of yet another hypothesis based on the possible protective effect of HDL. However, although the negative association between HDL and IHD is stronger than the positive association between LDL and IHD, the evidence for regarding a low HDL level as a 'cause' of IHD is still largely circumstantial. The association with HDL is predictive and we can point to at least one cellular mechanism that might explain a protective effect of HDL on the arterial wall. Furthermore, it is reasonable to suppose that the protective effect of female sex and, possibly, of habitual strenuous exercise (Morris et al., 1973) is mediated by a relatively high plasma HDL concentration. However, no-one has yet carried out a prospective intervention trial to test whether or not the incidence of IHD can be lowered by raising the plasma HDL concentration. There is also the puzzling anomaly that premature IHD is not an invariable feature of Tangier disease, a condition in which HDL is virtually absent from the plasma. Finally, it should not be forgotten that there is a strong inverse association between plasma HDL and VLDL concentrations and that the metabolism of HDL is closely linked with that of the triglyceride-rich lipoproteins, HDL acting as acceptor for the polar lipids released during the catabolism of VLDL and chylomicrons by endothelial lipoprotein lipase. If triglyceride-rich lipoproteins are atherogenic, then it is possible that in some populations the negative association between plasma HDL level and IHD reflects defective catabolism of VLDL. This does not seem to be the explanation of the predictive power of plasma HDL cholesterol concentration observed in the Framingham study (Gordon et al., 1977b), but it could explain the results of the Swedish study of Carlson and Bottiger (1972) (see Section 4.6).

4.8 The dietary fat hypothesis

The view that a high intake of saturated fat is an important cause of IHD (the dietary fat hypotheses) is sometimes confused with the plasma lipid hypothesis discussed in Section 4.7.2. This confusion seems to have arisen because it was assumed, when the dietary fat hypothesis was first put forward, that the postulated effects of saturated fat on the coronary arteries were mediated by the plasma cholesterol, and that variations in the consumption of saturated fat were the major cause of variability in plasma cholesterol concentration in human populations. Indeed, Bronte-Stewart (1958) wrote of the 'triangular relationship between diet, serum cholesterol level, atherosclerosis and ischaemic heart disease'. However, the plasma lipid hypothesis does not stand or fall on the validity of the belief that an excess of saturated fat in the diet is a cause of IHD. The plasma cholesterol concentration could be causally related to IHD in the absence of a causal relation between dietary fat and IHD, provided that fat intake is not a major cause of variability in plasma cholesterol concentration in free-living populations. To take an extreme instance, the premature IHD of patients with familial hypercholesterolaemia is due to their raised plasma cholesterol level, but this is not caused by dietary fat.

The dietary fat hypothesis was developed as an attempt to explain the fact, clearly recognized soon after the Second World War, that the marked differences in IHD mortality between different populations were largely environmental in origin. This led to a search for factors in the environment that were likely to influence proneness to IHD. It was natural that consideration should be given to the diet, and when it was established that the plasma cholesterol concentration could be altered under experimental conditions by modifying the proportions of animal and vegetable fat in the diet (Groen *et al.*, 1952; Kinsell *et al.*, 1952), comparisons were made between IHD incidence and dietary fat in different populations. It soon became apparent that there was a positive correlation between the consumption of saturated fat and the age-adjusted incidence of IHD in many populations. This led to the proposal that a high intake of saturated fat is a major cause of the high incidence of IHD in affluent industrialized communities (see Bronte-Stewart, 1958). An association between dietary fat and IHD was demonstrated in different racial and economic groups in South Africa (Bronte-Stewart, 1958) and was shown in greatest detail in the Seven Countries Study of Keys *et al.* (1970), who demonstrated a high degree of correlation between the 5-year incidence of first events of IHD and the percentage of total dietary calories taken as saturated fat in 13 populations differing widely in IHD prevalence and incidence. A similar association between saturated fat consumption and IHD has been observed in other inter-population surveys (Masironi, 1970).

In the inter-population study of Keys *et al.* (1970) there was also some association between IHD incidence and the estimated daily intake of cholesterol. However, this could be explained by the association between dietary cholesterol and saturated fat.

Critics of the dietary fat hypothesis have pointed out that estimates of fat consumption based on dietary histories are inaccurate and that those based on national statistics are even more so. Furthermore, several populations have been described in which the incidence of IHD appears to be low despite a high intake of saturated fat (Masironi, 1970). Proponents of the hypothesis suggest that in these populations the high saturated-fat intake is balanced by the absence of other positive risk factors such as cigarette smoking or hypertension, or the presence of negative risk factors such as strenuous physical activity. In view of the multiple aetiology of IHD this seems reasonable. However, a more serious objection to the view that dietary fat has a major influence on IHD is the absence of a consistent relationship between fat intake and IHD *within* any free-living population so far examined. Morris *et al.* (1977) found a negative correlation between first IHD events and the ratio of polyunsaturated to saturated fat in the diet of middle-aged men living in South-East England, but the correlation was not statistically significant; in the Framingham population there was no association between IHD incidence and any dietary constituent (Kannel, 1974); a similar lack of association was noted by Medalie *et al.* (1973) in their Israeli study. It has been suggested that person-to-person variation in fat intake within populations is too small to reveal any association that may exist between IHD incidence and fat intake. It is certainly true that in those populations that have been studied, the variation in fat intake between individuals is far less than that recorded between different populations. Nevertheless, if fat were a major contributor to IHD one would expect to find some evidence of a significant correlation within populations (see also Chapter 12, Section 4.2).

A balanced discussion of the strengths and weaknesses of the dietary fat hypothesis will be found in the review by Kannel (1974). In the debate that is now going on in the medical and lay press, one of the arguments put forward against the hypothesis concerns the possible harmful effects of certain fatty acids, particularly elaidic and other *trans* unsaturated fatty acids, present in partially hydrogenated oils used in the making of margarines rich in polyunsaturated fats. This, however, is not relevant to the question of the causal relation between saturated-fat intake and IHD, though it must be taken into account when one is considering the desirability of an increase in the consumption of these margarines in the general population. For a discussion of the biological effects of hardened or hydrogenated fish and vegetable oils, the reader is referred to the review by Vergroesen and Gottenbos (1975). During the partial hydrogenation of natural oils, *cis-trans* isomerization occurs at the double bonds of mono- and polyunsaturated fatty acids. 'Hardened' soyabean oil, for example, may contain up to 60% of elaidic acid (18:1, ω9 *trans*), the *trans* isomer of oleic acid. There is no evidence that *trans* isomers of 18:1, 18:2 or 18:3 fatty acids have specific harmful biological effects in man or in experimental animals. In human subjects, the effect of elaidic acid on the plasma cholesterol concentration is about the same as that of lauric (12:0) or myristic (14:0) acid. Some of the harmful effects of hydrogenated oils reported in experimental animals may be explained by the fact that hydrogenation causes loss of essential fatty acids, so that diets in which hydrogenated oils are the sole source of fat may be linoleic-acid deficient. The toxic effects of fatty acids containing more than twenty carbon atoms are another matter. Erucic acid (22:1, ω9 *cis*), a constituent of rapeseed oil, causes pathological changes in heart muscle and other tissues, possibly because very-long-chain fatty acids are not oxidized efficiently by the mitochondria (Vles, 1975). It is for this reason that steps are being taken by several governments and by the European Economic Commission to limit the erucic-acid content of edible oils. For references to the pathological effect of polyunsaturated fats in fish oils, see Hornstra *et al.* (1979).

4.9 The plasma cholesterol in relation to total mortality and non-IHD mortality

The epidemiological observations discussed above show that within and between populations there is almost invariably a positive correlation, both prospective and retrospective, between plasma total cholesterol concentration and IHD mortality or incidence. However, there is now enough evidence to hint at the possibility that within populations there is a *negative* correlation between plasma cholesterol concentration and mortality from all causes or, more specifically, from cancer.

In the modified-fat dietary trial of Dayton *et al.* (1969) the decreased IHD mortality in the treated group was balanced by increased mortality from other causes, including cancer at various sites, so that total mortality was not significantly altered by the cholesterol-lowering diet. A similar effect was observed in the W.H.O. co-operative clofibrate trial of Oliver *et al.* (1978, 1980). In this trial, age-standardized death rates from all causes and from causes other than IHD were higher in the clofibrate-treated group (Group I) than in the corresponding control group with high initial plasma cholesterol levels (Group II). Some of the excess mortality in Group I was due to malignant disease at various sites. Oliver *et al.* (1980) suggest that the increased incidence of cancer was due to altered cell-membrane function, caused by loss of cholesterol from cell membranes brought about by the clofibrate-induced fall in plasma cholesterol level. However, if the fall in plasma cholesterol concentration contributed to the increased non-IHD mortality in the clofibrate-treated group, non-IHD mortality should have been higher in the control group with low plasma cholesterol levels (Group III) than in Group II. In fact, mortality from all causes and from causes other than IHD was lowest in Group III, in which the mean plasma cholesterol level remained lower than that in Groups I and II throughout the trial. It seems more likely that the excess mortality in the treated group was due to a toxic effect of the drug, leading to malignancy at some sites, and to hepato-biliary disease induced by increased excretion of tissue cholesterol *via* the liver, a possibility also considered by Oliver *et al.* (1980).

Clinical trials in which the plasma cholesterol level is modified by drugs or by an abnormal diet (as in the trial of Dayton *et al.*, 1969) are unlikely to provide unequivocal evidence about the relation between plasma cholesterol and non-IHD mortality, because it is always difficult to distinguish an effect on mortality mediated by the change in plasma cholesterol level from an effect mediated in some other way. However, several prospective studies of well populations have revealed negative correlations between initial plasma cholesterol level and subsequent mortality from all causes (Shurtleff, 1974), from all causes and from cancer (Beaglehole *et al.*, 1980), from cancer at different sites in different individuals (Kark *et al.*, 1980) and from colon cancer (Rose *et al.*, 1974). Attempts have been made to explain these findings on the assumption that the relation between low plasma cholesterol level and increased mortality from all causes other than IHD, or from cancer, is one of cause and effect. Kark *et al.* (1980), for example, consider the possibility that a low plasma cholesterol concentration reflects a low cholesterol:phospholipid molar ratio in the membranes of certain cells (for the possible relevance of this to malignant transformation, see Chapter 7, Section 4.2).

However, although the association between increased mortality and low plasma cholesterol level was statistically significant in these studies, it is quite unjustifiable to conclude that low plasma cholesterol levels are a cause of increased mortality. Indeed, in some cases the negative correlation may be an artefact due to the presence of undetected disease, causing a lowering of the plasma cholesterol level, in some subjects at the time of their entry into the study. Thus, Rose and Shipley (1980) found that in London civil servants the curve relating total mortality to initial plasma cholesterol concentration was J-shaped, mortality from all causes being higher at the lowest plasma concentrations than at intermediate values. However, when men dying during the first two years after the initial plasma measurement were excluded from the analysis, total mortality was positively correlated with plasma cholesterol level over the whole range of concentrations. This indicates that the high mortality in men with the lowest plasma cholesterol levels at entry was due to the presence, in the population sample, of men with abnormally low cholesterol levels caused by undetected disease. According to Rose and Shipley (1980) the negative correlation between total mortality and plasma cholesterol level observed in the Framingham population (Shurtleff, 1974) can be explained in the same way. It should be noted, however, that the inverse relation between total mortality and plasma cholesterol level in the New Zealand Maoris studied by Beaglehole *et al.* (1980) could not be explained by the presence of undetected disease at entry into the study, although it must be said that the Maoris were exceptional in failing to show the usual positive association between plasma cholesterol concentration and IHD mortality.

The possibility that low plasma cholesterol levels can cause increased total or non-IHD mortality in some populations is clearly one that cannot be dismissed (if established it would have an obvious bearing on the question of the optimal plasma cholesterol concentration in man). Nevertheless, it is difficult to reconcile this with what we know about differences in total mortality *between* populations. Thus, life expectancy for adults is longer in Japan and southern Europe, where plasma cholesterol levels are comparatively low, than in northern Europe and the United States, where the plasma levels are considerably higher; the very low life expectancies in some Asian or Latin American populations, in which plasma cholesterol levels are even lower than in Japan, are readily explained by extreme poverty associated with malnutrition, parasitic infestations and lack of general medical care. In these populations the high total mortality and low plasma cholesterol levels presumably have a common cause. (For a critical discussion of the epidemiological evidence on plasma cholesterol in relation to total mortality, see *Journal of the American Medical Association*, 1980 and Williams *et al.*, 1981).

The relation between colon cancer and plasma cholesterol level affords another example of the discrepancy between results obtained from inter- and intra-population studies. On a world-wide scale, the incidence of colon cancer is *positively* correlated with the dietary intake of fat and cholesterol and with plasma cholesterol concentration, being higher in affluent than in underdeveloped countries (for references, see Cruse *et al.*, 1979). On the other hand, Rose *et al.* (1974) have demonstrated a significant *negative* correlation between initial plasma cholesterol level and subsequent development of colon cancer within six groups of men followed for an average of 11 years, and this association was independent of the interval between initial plasma measurement and diagnosis of the disease. It has been suggested that the relatively high incidence of colon cancer in affluent populations is due to the high cholesterol content of the diet, cholesterol acting as a cocarcinogen (Cruse *et al.*, 1979) or as a precursor of carcinogenic substances formed by bacteria in the intestinal lumen (Hill *et al.*, 1971). However, it is difficult to explain the negative correlation between plasma cholesterol and colon cancer within populations in terms of a carcinogenic or co-carcinogenic effect of dietary cholesterol.

5 THE CLONAL HYPOTHESIS OF ATHEROGENESIS

As an alternative to the orthodox explanation of the pathogenesis of atherosclerotic lesions discussed in Section 3.3, Benditt and Benditt (1973) have suggested that in each human lesion the proliferation of SMC is due to multiplication of a single precursor cell in the arterial wall. The evidence for this view is based on the study of human mosaics that may occur as a consequence of *X-chromosome inactivation*. At an early stage of development in every female mammal, one or other of the two X-chromosomes in each somatic cell is inactivated. The inactivation is random from cell to cell and is inherited by the progeny of the cell, so that only the maternal X-chromosome is functional in all the progeny of a cell in which the paternal X-chromosome was inactivated, and *vice versa*. All females heterozygous for an X-linked gene are therefore mosaics, in the sense that their tissues contain two types of cell differing in genetic expression. If the largest volume of tissue that contains cells of only one genetic type (the *patch size*) is very small, the cells of a mosaic may be used as markers to trace the origin of the cells of a tumour or lesion.

The enzyme glucose-6-phosphate dehydrogenase (G6PD) exists in two forms (A and B) controlled by an X-linked gene. About 40% of black American females are heterozygous for the A and B types and hence are mosaics. These mosaic individuals have been used in the study of the cellular origin of several tumours (Linder and Gartler, 1965, and see Gartler, 1977) and of atherosclerotic fibrous plaques and fatty streaks.

Benditt and Benditt (1973) found that a high proportion of the aortic plaques of G6PD heterozygotes were monotypic; that is, they contained either A-type cells or B-type cells but not both. Since the patch size in adjacent normal arterial wall was less than 10^{-3} mm^3, they concluded that the single-isoenzyme pattern of the plaques could not be due to multiple-cell origin from a clump of cells that happened to be all of the same type. Nor did they regard it as likely that the pattern was due to multiple-cell origin with subsequent selective overgrowth of one or other cell type, since both A-type and B-type plaques occurred in the same artery. They therefore postulated that each plaque was a clone originating from a single cell in which a mutation had occurred; on this view, the human atherosclerotic plaque is analogous to a benign tumour.

If this idea is to be acceptable it must be reconciled with the mass of evidence indicating that environmental factors make a significant contribution to human atherosclerosis. Benditt (1977) suggests that the influence of some environmental risk factors is mediated by the transport of potentially mutagenic substances to the arterial wall by the plasma lipoproteins. The effect of cigarette smoking, for example, could be mediated in this way. However, the monoclonal hypothesis does not provide any obvious explanation as to why an increased plasma concentration of cholesterol-rich lipoproteins is a positive risk factor for coronary atherosclerosis or why HDL is a negative risk factor. Nor is it easy to reconcile with current ideas on the role of repeated cycles of injury and repair in the development of atherosclerotic plaques, since it is unlikely that repair of injured tissue would be initiated by a single cell.

The observation that most human atherosclerotic plaques are monotypic has been confirmed by Pearson *et al.* (1975), who have also shown that a high proportion of fatty streaks contains both A-type and B-type cells. This has been taken as evidence that fatty streaks are not the precursors of fibrous plaques. However, it is by no means certain that monotypic lesions arise from single cells. Thomas *et al.* (1977) have discussed various ways in which a monotypic lesion could develop from a group of cells of both types, without selection based on the A/B difference (so that monotypic lesions of both types could be present in the same artery). They also point out that mixed populations of cells from G6PD mosaics can become monotypic (for A-type *or* B-type cells) when grown in culture. If monotypic lesions do have a multicellular origin, one would expect that fatty streaks, if they represent an early stage in the progress towards fibrous plaques, would tend to be mixtures of the two cell types. Gartler (1977) has also pointed out that a monotypic plaque could result from cyclic injury and repair if many cells at the site of the lesion are senescent, only a few of them being capable of repeated multiplication. Finally, the observation of Pearson *et al.* (1979) that some advanced arterial thrombi in G6PD mosaics are monotypic shows that a monotypic lesion can evolve from what must have begun as a group of cells of mixed type (platelets derived from the circulation).

The development of monotypic lesions by cell selection from a mixed population of A-type and B-type cells would be quite compatible with current views as to how the human fibrous plaque develops and as to how cholesterol-rich plasma lipoproteins act as risk factors for IHD (see Fig. 13.3).

REFERENCES

Abdulla, Y. H., Adams, C. W. M. and Morgan, R. S. (1967). Connective-tissue reaction to implantation of purified sterol, sterol esters, phosphoglycerides, glycerides and free fatty acids. *Journal of Pathology and Bacteriology*, **94**, 63–71.

Adams, C. W. M. (1964). Arteriosclerosis in man, other mammals and birds. *Biological Reviews*, **39**, 372–423.

Adams, C. W. M., Virag, S., Morgan, R. S. and Orton, C. C. (1968). Dissociation of [^{3}H]-cholesterol and ^{125}I-labelled plasma protein influx in normal and atheromatous rabbit aorta. *Journal of Atherosclerosis Research*, **8**, 679–696.

Ahrens, E. H. Jr. (1976). The management of hyperlipidemia: whether, rather than how. *Annals of Internal Medicine*, **85**, 87–93.

Albers, J. J., Wahl, P. W., Cabana, V. G., Hazzard, W. R. and Hoover, J. J. (1976). Quantitation of apolipoprotein A-I of human plasma high density lipoprotein. *Metabolism*, **25**, 633–644.

Anitschkow, N. (1913). Über die Veränderungen der Kaninchenaorta bei experimenteller Cholesterinsteatose. *Beiträge zur pathologischen Anatomie*, **56**, 379.

Anitschkow, N. N. (1928). Über die Rückbildungsvorgänge bei der experimenteller Atherosklerose. *Verk. dtsch. Path. Ges.*, **23**, 473–478.

Armstrong, M. L. Regression of atherosclerosis. In: *Atherosclerosis Review*, Vol. 1. Ed. R. Paoletti and A. M. Gotto. Raven Press, New York, p. 137, 1976.

Armstrong, M. L., Megan, M. B. and Warner, E. D. (1978). The relation of hypercholesterolemic fatty streaks to intimal permeability changes shown by Evans Blue. *Atherosclerosis*, **31**, 443–452.

Armstrong, M. L., Warner, E. D. and Connor, W. E. (1970). Regression of coronary atheromatosis in rhesus monkeys. *Circulation Research*, **27**, 59–67.

Aro, A. (1973). Serum lipids and lipoproteins in first degree relatives of young survivors of myocardial infarction. *Acta Medica Scandinavica*, Supplement **553**, 1–103.

Bang, H. O. and Dyerberg, J. (1972). Plasma lipids and lipoproteins in Greenlandic west coast eskimos. *Acta Medica Scandinavica*, **192**, 85–94.

Barclay, M., Barclay, R. K. and Skipski, V. P. (1963). High-density lipoprotein concentrations in men and women. *Nature*, **200**, 362–363.

Barr, D. P., Russ, E. M. and Eder, H. A. (1951). Protein-lipid relationships in human plasma. II. In atherosclerosis and related conditions. *American Journal of Medicine*, **11**, 480–493.

Beaglehole, R., Foulkes, M. A., Prior, I. A. M. and Eyles, E. F. (1980). Cholesterol and mortality in New Zealand Maoris. *British Medical Journal*, **1**, 285–287.

Benditt, E. P. (1977). Implications of the monoclonal character of human atherosclerotic plaques. *American Journal of Pathology*, **86**, 693–702.

Benditt, E. P. and Benditt, J. M. (1973). Evidence for a monoclonal origin of human atherosclerotic plaques. *Proceedings of the National Academy of Sciences of the USA*, **70**, 1753–1756.

Berg, K., Børresen, A.-L. and Dahlén, G. (1976). Serum-high-density-lipoprotein and atherosclerotic heart-disease. *Lancet*, **1**, 499–500.

Bierman, E. L. and Albers, J. J. (1975). Lipoprotein uptake by cultured human arterial smooth muscle cells. *Biochimica et Biophysica Acta*, **388**, 198–202.

Björkerud, S. Endothelial permeability; interpretations from experimental lesions.

In: *Atherosclerosis III, Proceedings of the Third International Symposium*. Ed. G. Schettler and A. Weizel. Springer-Verlag, Berlin, pp. 14–20, 1974.

Björkerud, S. and Bondjers, G. (1972). Endothelial integrity and viability in the aorta of the normal rabbit and rat as evaluated with dye exclusion tests and interference contrast microscopy. *Atherosclerosis*, **15**, 285–300.

Bond, M. G., Bullock, B. C., Lehner, N. D. M. and Clarkson, T. B. Regression of atherosclerosis at plasma concentrations available to man. In: *Atherosclerosis IV. Proceedings of the Fourth International Symposium*. Ed. G. Schettler, Y. Goto, Y. Hata and G. Klose. Springer-Verlag, Berlin, pp. 278–280, 1977.

Bondjers, G. and Björkerud, S. (1975). HDL-dependent elimination of cholesterol from human arterial tissue. *European Society for Clinical Investigation Abstr.* **9**, 51.

Bronte-Stewart, B. (1958). The effect of dietary fats on the blood lipids and their relation to ischaemic heart disease. *British Medical Bulletin*, **14**, 243–252.

Brown, M. S. and Goldstein, J. L. (1977). Familial hypercholesterolemia: model for genetic receptor disease. *Harvey Lectures*, Series **73**, 163–201.

Buchwald, H., Moore, R. B. and Varco, R. L. (1974). Surgical treatment of hyperlipidemia. *Circulation*, **49**, Supplement I, pp. I-1–I-37.

Carlson, L. A. and Böttiger, L. E. (1972). Ischaemic heart-disease in relation to fasting values of plasma triglycerides and cholesterol. Stockholm prospective study. *Lancet*, **1**, 865–868.

Carlson, L. A. and Eriksson, M. (1975). Quantitative and qualitative serum lipoprotein analysis. 2. Studies in male survivors of myocardial infarction. *Atherosclerosis*, **21**, 435–450.

Carroll, K. K. and Hamilton, R. M. G. (1975). Effects of dietary protein and carbohydrate on plasma cholesterol levels in relaton to atherosclerosis. *Journal of Food Science*, **40**, 18–23.

Casley-Smith, J. R. (1976). The fine structure and functions of blood capillaries, the interstitial tissue and the lymphatics. *Ergebnisse der Angiologie*, **12**, 1–29.

Castelli, W. P., Coorer, G. R., Doyle, J. T., Garcia-Palmieri, M., Gordon, T., Hames, C., Hulley, S. B., Kagan, A., Kuchmak, M., McGee, D. and Vicic, W. J. (1977). Distribution of triglyceride and total, LDL and HDL cholesterol in several populations: a cooperative lipoprotein phenotyping study. *Journal of Chronic Diseases*, **30**, 147–169.

Chobanian, A. V. and Hollander, W. (1962). Body cholesterol metabolism in man. I. The equilibration of serum and tissue cholesterol. *Journal of Clinical Investigation*, **41**, 1732–1737.

Constantinides, P. *Experimental Atherosclerosis*. Elsevier, Amsterdam, 1965.

Cox, G. E., Taylor, C. B., Cox, LaV. G. and Counts, M. A. (1958). Atherosclerosis in rhesus monkeys. I. Hypercholesteremia induced by dietary fat and cholesterol. *Archives of Pathology*, **66**, 32–52.

Cruse, P., Lewin, M. and Clark, C. G. (1979). Dietary cholesterol is co-carcinogenic for human colon cancer. *Lancet*, **1**, 752–755.

Davies, M. J., Fulton, W. F. M. and Robertson, W. B. (1979). The relation of coronary thrombosis to ischaemic myocardial necrosis. *Journal of Pathology*, **127**, 99–110.

Davis, C. E. and Havlik, R. J. Clinical trials of lipid lowering and coronary artery disease prevention. In: *Hyperlipidemia, Diagnosis and Therapy*. Ed. B. M. Rifkind and R. I. Levy. Grune and Stratton, New York, pp. 79–92, 1977.

Day, A. J. and Wilkinson, G. K. (1967). Incorporation of C^{14}-labelled acetate into lipid by isolated foam cells and by atherosclerotic arterial intima. *Circulation Research*, **21**, 593–600.

Dayton, S. and Hashimoto, S. (1966). Movement of labeled cholesterol between plasma lipoprotein and normal arterial wall across the intimal surface. *Circulation Research*, **19**, 1041–1049.

Dayton, S. and Hashimoto, S. (1970). Recent advances in molecular pathology: a review. Cholesterol flux and metabolism in arterial tissue and in atheromata. *Experimental and Molecular Pathology*, **13**, 253–268.
Dayton, S., Pearce, M. L., Hashimoto, S., Dixon, W. J. and Tomiyasu, U. (1969). A controlled clinical trial of a diet high in unsaturated fat in preventing complications of atherosclerosis. *Circulation*, **40**, Supplement 2, 1–63.
Epstein, F. H. (1967). Risk factors in coronary heart disease. Environmental and hereditary influences. *Israel Journal of Medical Sciences*, **3**, 594–607.
Epstein, F. H. (1971). Epidemiologic aspects of atherosclerosis. *Atherosclerosis*, **14**, 1.
Epstein, F. H. (1977a). Highlights of epidemiological research in Western countries. In: *Atherosclerosis IV. Proceedings of the Fourth International Symposium*. Ed. G. Schettler, Y. Goto, Y. Hata and G. Klose. Springer-Verlag, Berlin, pp. 471–478, 1977.
Epstein, F. H. (1977b). Preventive trials and the 'diet-heart' question: wait for results or act now? *Atherosclerosis*, **26**, 515–523.
Feinleib, M., Kannel, W. B., Tedeschi, C. G., Landau, T. K. and Garrison, R. J. (1979). The relation of antemortem characteristics to cardiovascular findings at necropsy. *Atherosclerosis*, **34**, 145–157.
Field, H., Swell, L., Schools, P. E. and Treadwell, C. R. (1960). Dynamic aspects of cholesterol metabolism in different areas of the aorta and other tissues in man and their relationship to atherosclerosis. *Circulation*, **22**, 545–558.
Fischer-Dzoga, K. and Wissler, R. W. Proliferative response of arterial smooth muscle cells to hyperlipemia. In: *Atherosclerosis IV. Proceedings of the Fourth International Symposium*. Ed. G. Schettler, Y. Goto, Y. Hata and G. Klose. Springer-Verlag, Berlin, pp. 624–627, 1977.
Fox, H. Arteriosclerosis in lower mammals and birds: its relation to the disease in man. In: *Arteriosclerosis*. Ed. E. V. Cowdry. MacMillan, New York, pp. 153–193, 1933.
Fuster, V., Frye, R. L., Connolly, D. C., Danielson, M. A., Elveback, L. R. and Kurland, L. T. (1975). Arteriographic patterns early in onset of coronary syndromes. *British Heart Journal*, **37**, 1250–1255.
Garcia-Palmieri, M. R., Castillo, M. I., Oalmann, M. C., Sorlie, P. D. and Costas, R. The relation of ante mortem factors to atherosclerosis at necropsy. In: *Atherosclerosis IV. Proceedings of the Fourth International Symposium*. Springer-Verlag, Berlin, pp. 108–113, 1977.
Gartler, S. M. (1977). Patterns of cellular proliferation in normal and tumor cell populations. *American Journal of Pathology*, **86**, 685–692.
Geer, J. C. and Haust, M. D. *Smooth muscle cells in atherosclerosis*. Monographs on Atherosclerosis, Vol. 2. Karger, Basel, 1972.
Gertler, M. M., Garn, S. M. and Lerman, J. (1950). The interrelationships of serum cholesterol, cholesterol esters and phospholipids in health and in coronary artery disease. *Circulation*, **2**, 205–214.
Glueck, C. J., Fallat, R. W., Millett, F., Gartside, P., Elston, R. C. and Go, R. C. P. (1975). Familial hyper-alpha-lipoproteinemia: studies in eighteen kindreds. *Metabolism*, **24**, 1243–1265.
Gofman, J. W., Hanig, M., Jones, H. B., Lauffer, M. A., Lawry, E. Y., Lewis, L. A., Mann, G. V., Moore, F. E., Olmsted, F. and Yeager, J. F. (1956). Evaluation of serum lipoprotein and cholesterol measurements as predictors of clinical complications of atherosclerosis. *Circulation*, **14**, 691–742.
Gofman, J. W., Lindgren, F., Elliott, H., Mantz, W., Hewitt, J., Strisower, B. and Herring, V. (1950). The role of lipids and lipoproteins in atherosclerosis. *Science*, **111**, 166–171 and 186.
Gofman, J. W., Young, W. and Tandy, R. (1966). Ischemic heart disease, atherosclerosis, and longevity. *Circulation*, **34**, 679–697.

Goldstein, J. L., Anderson, R. G. W., Buja, L. M., Basu, S. K. and Brown, M. S. (1977). Overloading human aortic smooth muscle cells with low density lipoprotein-cholesteryl esters reproduces features of atherosclerosis in vitro. *Journal of Clinical Investigation*, 59, 1196–1202.

Goldstein, J. L. and Brown, M. S. (1978). Familial hypercholesterolemia: pathogenesis of a receptor disease. *The Johns Hopkins Medical Journal*, 143, 8–16.

Gordon, T., Castelli, W. P., Hjortland, M. C., Kannel, W. B. and Dawber, T. R. (1977a). Predicting coronary heart disease in middle-aged and older persons. The Framingham study. *Journal of the American Medical Association*, 238, 497–499.

Gordon, T., Castelli, W. P., Hjortland, M. C., Kannel, W. B. and Dawber, T. R. (1977b). High density lipoprotein as a protective factor against coronary heart disease. *American Journal of Medicine*, 62, 707–714.

Gordon, T., Garcia-Palmieri, M. R., Kagan, A., Kannel, W. B. and Schiffman, J. (1974). Differences in coronary heart disease in Framingham, Honolulu and Puerto Rico. *Journal of Chronic Diseases*, 27, 329–344.

Gordon, T., Moore, F. E., Shurtleff, D. and Dawber, T. R. (1959). Some methodologic problems in the long-term study of cardiovascular disease: observations on the Framingham study. *Journal of Chronic Diseases*, 10, 186–206.

Gould, R. G., Wissler, R. W. and Jones, R. J. The dynamics of lipid deposition in arteries. In: *Evolution of the Atherosclerotic Plaque*. Ed. R. J. Jones. University of Chicago Press, Chicago, pp. 205–214, 1963.

Gresham, G. A. and Howard, A. N. (1960). The independent production of atherosclerosis and thrombosis in the rat. *British Journal of Experimental Pathology*, 41, 395–402.

Gresham, G. A. and Howard, A. N. (1965). Vascular lesions in primates. *Annals of the New York Academy of Sciences*, 127, 694–701.

Groen, J., Tjiong, B. K., Kamming, A. C. E. and Willebrands, A. F. (1952). The influence of nutrition, individuality and some other factors including various forms of stress on the serum cholesterol; an experiment of nine months duration in sixty normal human volunteers. *Voeding*, 13, 556–587.

Gryglewski, R. J. and Moncada, S. (1979). Polyunsaturated fatty acids and thrombosis. *European Journal of Clinical Investigation*, 9, 1–2.

Harker, L. A., Ross, R. and Glomset, J. (1976). Role of the platelét in atherogenesis. *Annals of the New York Academy of Sciences*, 275, 321–329.

Hata, Y., Hower, J. and Insull, W. (1974). Cholesterol ester-rich inclusions from human aortic fatty streak and fibrous plaque lesions of atherosclerosis. *American Journal of Pathology*, 75, 423–456.

Hill, M. J., Crowther, J. S., Drasar, B. S., Hawksworth, G., Aries, V. and Williams, R. E. O. (1971). Bacteria and aetiology of cancer of large bowel. *Lancet*, 1, 95–100.

Hoff, H. F., Jackson, R. L., Mao, S. J. T. and Gotto, A. M. Jr. (1974). Localization of low-density lipoproteins in atherosclerotic lesions from human normolipemics employing a purified fluorescent-labeled antibody. *Biochimica et Biophysica Acta*, 351, 407–415.

Hornstra, G., Haddeman, E. and Ten Hoor, F. (1979). Fish oils, prostaglandins, and arterial thrombosis. *Lancet*, 2, 1080.

Howard, A. N., Patelski, J., Bowyer, D. E. and Gresham, G. A. (1971). Atherosclerosis induced in hypercholesterolaemic baboons by immunological injury; and the effects of intravenous polyunsaturated phosphatidyl choline. *Atherosclerosis*, 14, 17–29.

International Atherosclerosis Project (1968). The geographic pathology of atherosclerosis. *Laboratory Investigation*, 18, 463–653.

Iverius, P. H. (1972). The interaction between human plasma lipoproteins and

connective tissue of glycosaminoglycans. *Journal of Biological Chemistry*, **247**, 2607–2613.
Jakubowski, J. A. and Ardlie, N. G. (1978). Modification of human platelet function by a diet enriched in saturated or polyunsaturated fat. *Atherosclerosis*, **31**, 335–344.
Jenkins, P. J., Harper, R. W. and Nestel, P. J. (1978). Severity of coronary atherosclerosis related to lipoprotein concentration. *British Medical Journal*, **2**, 388–391.
Journal of the American Medical Association (1980). Cholesterol and non-cardiovascular mortality. **244**, 25.
Kannel, W. B. (1974). The role of cholesterol in coronary atherogenesis. *Medical Clinics of North America*, **58**, 363–379.
Kannel, W. B., Castelli, W. P., Gordon, T., McNamara, P. M. (1971). Serum cholesterol, lipoproteins, and the risk of coronary heart disease. *Annals of Internal Medicine*, **74**, 1–12.
Kannel, W. B., Dawber, T. R., Kagan, A., Revotskie, N. and Stokes, J. III (1961). Factors of risk in the development of coronary heart disease—six-year follow-up experience. *Annals of Internal Medicine*, **55**, 33–50.
Kark, J. D., Smith, A. H. and Hames, C. G. (1980). The relationship of serum cholesterol to the incidence of cancer in Evans County, Georgia. *Journal of Chronic Diseases*, **33**, 311–322.
Katz, S. S., Shipley, G. G. and Small, D. M. (1976). Physical chemistry of the lipids of human atherosclerotic lesions. Demonstration of a lesion intermediate between fatty streaks and advanced plaques. *Journal of Clinical Investigation*, **58**, 200–211.
Keys, A. *Coronary heart disease in seven countries*. *Circulation*, Vol. XLI, No. 4, Suppl. 1. Ed. A. Keys. American Heart Association, Monograph No. 29, 1970.
Keys, A., Taylor, H. L., Blackburn, H., Brozek, J., Anderson, J. T. and Simonson, E. (1963). Coronary heart disease among Minnesota business and professional men followed fifteen years. *Circulation*, **28**, 381–395.
Kimura, N. Epidemiological studies of atherosclerotic disease in Japan. In: *Atherosclerosis IV. Proceedings of the Fourth International Symposium*. Ed. G. Schettler, Y. Goto, Y. Hata and G. Klose. Springer-Verlag, Berlin, pp. 462–470, 1977.
Kinsell, L. W., Partridge, J., Boling, L., Margen, S. and Michaels, G. (1952). Dietary modification of serum cholesterol and phospholipid levels. *Journal of Clinical Endocrinology*, **12**, 909–913.
Kramsch, D. M., Huvos, A. and Hollander, W. (1970). A primate model for the study of coronary (atherosclerotic) heart disease. *Circulation*, **42**, Supplement III, 9.
Kritchevsky, D., Tepper, S. A., Vesselinovitch, D. and Wissler, R. W. (1971). Cholesterol vehicle in experimental atherosclerosis. II. Peanut oil. *Atherosclerosis*, **14**, 53–64.
Lehner, N. D. M., Wagner, W. D., Bullock, B. C. and Bond, M. G. Aortic atherosclerosis in primates. In: *Atherosclerosis IV. Proceedings of the Fourth International Symposium*. Ed. G. Schettler, Y. Goto, Y. Hata and G. Klose. Springer-Verlag, Berlin, pp. 280–285, 1977.
Lichtlen, P. Coronary angiography and angina pectoris. *Symposium of the European Society of Cardiology*, Hanover, 1975. Ed. P. R. Lichtlen. Georg Thieme, Stuttgart, 1976.
Linder, D. and Gartler, S. M. (1965). Glucose-6-phosphate dehydrogenase mosaicism: utilization as a cell marker in the study of leiomyomas. *Science*, **150**, 67–69.
Lippel, K. *Report of the High Density Lipoprotein Methodology Workshop*. NIH Publication No. 79-1661, 1979.

Lofland, H. B. and Clarkson, T. B. (1970). The bi-directional transfer of cholesterol in normal aorta, fatty streaks, and atheromatous plaques. *Proceedings of the Society for Experimental Biology and Medicine*, **133**, 1–8.

McGill, H. C. The composition of early lesions. In: *Atherosclerosis III. Proceedings of the Third International Symposium*. Ed. G. Schettler and A. Weizel. Springer-Verlag, Berlin, pp. 27–38, 1974.

McMahan, C. A. (1968). Autopsied cases by age, sex and 'race'. *Laboratory Investigation*, **18**, 468–478.

Mahley, R. W. Alterations in plasma lipoproteins induced by cholesterol feeding in animals including man. In: *Disturbances in Lipid and Lipoprotein Metabolism*. Ed. J. M. Dietschy, A. M. Gotto Jr. and J. A. Ontko. American Physiological Society, Bethesda, pp. 181–197, 1978.

Mahley, R. W., Innerarity, T. L., Bersot, T. P., Lipson, A. and Margolis, S. (1978). Alterations in human high-density lipoproteins, with or without increased plasma-cholesterol, induced by diets high in cholesterol. *Lancet*, **2**, 807–809.

Masironi, R. (1970). Dietary factors and coronary heart disease. *Bulletin of the World Health Organization*, **42**, 103–114.

Medalie, J. H., Kahn, H. A., Neufeld, H. N., Riss, E. and Goldbourt, U. (1973). Five-year myocardial infarction incidence. II. Association of single variables to age and birthplace. *Journal of Chronic Diseases*, **26**, 329–349.

Menotti, A. Multivariate prediction. In: *Atherosclerosis III. Proceedings of the Third International Symposium*. Ed. G. Schettler and A. Weizel. Springer-Verlag, Berlin, pp. 702–705, 1974.

Miettinen, M., Turpeinen, O., Karvonen, M. J., Elosuo, R. and Paavilainen, E. (1972). Effect of cholesterol-lowering diet on mortality from coronary heart-disease and other causes. A twelve-year clinical trial in men and women. *Lancet*, **2**, 835–838.

Miller, G. J. and Miller, N. E. (1975). Plasma-high-density lipoprotein concentration and development of ischaemic heart-disease. *Lancet*, **1**, 16–19.

Miller, G. J., Miller, N. E. and Ashcroft, M. T. (1976). Inverse relationship in Jamaica between plasma high-density lipoprotein cholesterol concentration and coronary-disease risk as predicted by multiple risk-factor status. *Clinical Science and Molecular Medicine*, **51**, 475–482.

Miller, N. E., Førde, O. H., Thelle, D. S. and Mjøs, O. D. (1977). The Tromsø heart-study. High-density lipoprotein and coronary heart-disease: a prospective case-control study. *Lancet*, **1**, 965–968.

Minick, C. R. (1976). Immunologic arterial injury in atherogenesis. *Annals of the New York Academy of Sciences*, **275**, 210–227.

Mitchell, A. The early detection of thrombosis. In: *Very Early Recognition of Coronary Heart Disease*. Ed. L. McDonald, J. Goodwin and L. Resnekov. Excerpta Medica, Amsterdam, pp. 21–26, 1978.

Moore, S., Mustard, J., Packham, M. A. and Kinlough-Rathbone, R. L. Thrombosis and endothelial injury in atherogenesis. In: *Atherosclerosis IV. Proceedings of the Fourth International Symposium*. Ed. G. Schettler, Y. Goto, Y. Hata and G. Klose. Springer-Verlag, Berlin, pp. 601–605, 1977.

Morris, J. N., Chave, S. P. W., Adam, C., Sirey, C., Epstein, L. and Sheehan, D. J. (1973). Vigorous exercise in leisure-time and the incidence of coronary heart-disease. *Lancet*, **1**, 333–339.

Morris, J. N., Marr, J. W. and Clayton, D. G. (1977). Diet and heart: a postscript. *British Medical Journal*, **2**, 1307–1314.

Murray, R. G., Tweddel, A., Third, J. L. H. C., Hutton, I., Hillis, W. S., Lorimer, A. R. and Lawrie, T. D. V. (1975). Relation between extent of coronary artery disease and severity of hyperlipoproteinaemia. *British Heart Journal*, **37**, 1205–1209.

Mustard, J. F., Packham, M. A., Moore, S. and Kinlough-Rathbone, R. L. Thrombosis and atherosclerosis. In: *Atherosclerosis III. Proceedings of the Third International Symposium*. Ed. G. Schettler and A. Weizel. Springer-Verlag, Berlin, pp. 253–267, 1974.

National Cooperative Pooling Project (1978). The pooling project research group. Final report of the pooling project. *Journal of Chronic Diseases*, **31**, 201–306.

Newman, H. A. I. and Zilversmit, D. B. (1962). Quantitative aspects of cholesterol flux in rabbit atheromatous lesions. *Journal of Biological Chemistry*, **237**, 2078–2084.

Nikkilä, E. A. (1978). Metabolic regulation of plasma high density lipoprotein concentrations. *European Journal of Clinical Investigation*, **8**, 111–113.

O'Brien, J. R., Etherington, M. D., Jamieson, S., Vergroesen, A. J. and Ten Hoor, F. (1976). The effect of a diet of polyunsaturated fats on some platelet-function tests. *Lancet*, **2**, 995–997.

Oliver, M. F., Heady, J. A., Morris, J. N. and Cooper, J. (1980). W.H.O. cooperative trial on primary prevention of ischaemic heart disease using clofibrate to lower serum cholesterol: mortality follow-up. *Lancet*, **2**, 379–385.

Oliver, M. F., Heady, J. S., Morris, J. N., Cooper, J., Geizerova, H., Gyarfas, I., Green, K. J. and Strassen, T. (1978). Atromid-S. A co-operative trial in the primary prevention of ischaemic heart disease using clofibrate. Report from the committee of principal investigators. *British Heart Journal*, **40**, 1069–1118.

Pometta, D., Micheli, H., Jornot, C. and Scherrer, J. R. (1978). High density lipoprotein cholesterol (HDL-C) in relatives of coronary patients, relationship to very low density lipoprotein triglycerides (VLDL-Tg). *European Journal of Clinical Investigation*, **8**, 351.

Pearson, T. A., Dillman, J., Solez, K. and Heptinstall, R. H. (1979). Monoclonal characteristics of organising arterial thrombi: significance in the origin and growth of human atherosclerotic plaques. *Lancet*, **1**, 7–11.

Pearson, T. A., Wang, A., Solez, K. and Heptinstall, R. H. (1975). Clonal characteristics of fibrous plaques and fatty streaks from human aortas. *American Journal of Pathology*, **81**, 279–387.

Reichl, D., Myant, N. B., Brown, M. S. and Goldstein, J. L. (1978). Biologically active low density lipoprotein in human peripheral lymph. *Journal of Clinical Investigation*, **61**, 64–71.

Reichl, D., Myant, N. B. and Pflug, J. J. (1977). Concentration of lipoproteins containing apolipoprotein B in human peripheral lymph. *Biochimica et Biophysica Acta*, **489**, 98–105.

Rhoads, G. G., Gulbrandsen, C. L. and Kagan, A. (1976). Serum lipoproteins and coronary heart disease in a population study of Hawaii Japanese men. *New England Journal of Medicine*, **294**, 293–298.

Robertson, T. L., Kato, H., Gordon, T., Kagan, A., Rhoads, G. C., Land, C. E., Worth, R. M., Belsky, J. L., Dock, D. S., Miyanishi, M. and Kawamoto, S. (1977a). Epidemiologic studies of coronary heart disease and stroke in Japanese men living in Japan, Hawaii and California: coronary heart disease risk factors in Japan and Hawaii. *American Journal of Cardiology*, **39**, 244–249.

Robertson, T. L., Kato, H., Rhoads, G. G., Kagan, A., Marmot, M., Syme, S. L., Gordon, T., Worth, R. M., Belsky, J. L., Dock, D. S., Myanishi, M. and Kawamoto, S. (1977b). Epidemiologic studies of coronary heart disease and stroke in Japanese men living in Japan, Hawaii and California. Incidence of myocardial infarction and death from coronary heart disease. *American Journal of Cardiology*, **39**, 239–243.

Rose, G., Blackburn, H., Keys, A., Taylor, H. L., Kannel, W. B., Paul, O., Reid, D. D. and Stamler, J. (1974). Colon cancer and blood-cholesterol. *Lancer*, **1**, 181–183.

Rose, G., Reid, D. D., Hamilton, P. J. S., McCartney, P., Keen, H. and Jarrett, R. J. (1977). Myocardial ischaemia, risk factors and death from coronary heart-disease. *Lancet*, **1**, 105–109.

Rose, G. and Shipley, M. J. (1980). Plasma lipids and mortality: a source of error. *Lancet*, **1**, 523–526.

Ross, R. and Glomset, J. A. (1976). The pathogenesis of atherosclerosis. *New England Journal of Medicine*, **295**, 369–377 and 420–425.

Ross, R. and Harker, L. (1976). Hyperlipidemia and atherosclerosis. Chronic hyperlipidemia initiates and maintains lesions by endothelial cell desquamation and lipid accumulation. *Science*, **193**, 1094–1100.

St. Clair, R. W. (1976). Metabolism of the arterial wall and atherosclerosis. *Atherosclerosis Reviews*, **1**, 61–117.

Schwartz, C. J., Gerrity, R. J., Lewis, L. J., Chisolm, G. M. and Bretherton, K. N. Arterial endothelial permeability to macromolecules. In: *Atherosclerosis IV. Proceedings of the Fourth International Symposium*. Ed. G. Schettler, Y. Goto, Y. Hata and G. Klose. Springer-Verlag, Berlin, pp. 1–11, 1977.

Scott, R. F., Daoud, A. S. and Florentin, R. A. Animal models in atherosclerosis. In: *The pathogenesis of atherosclerosis*. Ed. R. W. Wissler and J. C. Geer. Williams and Wilkins, Baltimore, 1972.

Shimamoto, T. Contraction of endothelial cells as a key mechanism in atherogenesis and treatment of atherosclerosis with endothelial cell relaxants. In: *Atherosclerosis III. Proceedings of the Third International Symposium*. Ed. G. Schettler and A. Weizel. Springer-Verlag, Berlin, pp. 64–82, 1974.

Shurtleff, D. Some characteristics related to the incidence of cardiovascular disease and death: Framingham Study, 18-year follow-up. In: *The Framingham Study: an epidemiological investigation of cardiovascular disease. Section 30*. Ed. W. B. Kannel and T. Gordon. US Government Printing Office, Washington, DC, DHEW publication No. (NIH) 74-599, 1974.

Simionescu, N., Simionescu, M. and Palade, G. E. (1975). Permeability of muscle capillaries to small heme-peptides. Evidence for the existence of patent trans-endothelial channels. *Journal of Cell Biology*, **64**, 586–607.

Simionescu, N., Simionescu, M. and Palade, G. E. (1976). Recent studies on vascular endothelium. *Annals of the New York Academy of Sciences*, **275**, 64–75.

Sirtori, C. R., Ghiselli, G. C. and Lovati, M. R. Dietary effects on lipoprotein composition. In: *The Lipoprotein Molecule*. Ed. H. Peeters. Nato Advanced Study Institute Series, Plenum Press, New York, pp. 261–291, 1978.

Small, D. M. The physical state of lipids of biological importance: cholesteryl esters, cholesterol, triglyceride. In: *Surface Chemistry of Biological Systems*. Ed. M. Blank. Plenum Press, New York, pp. 55–83, 1970.

Smith, E. B. (1974). The relationship between plasma and tissue lipids in human atherosclerosis. *Advances in Lipid Research*, **12**, 1–49.

Smith, E. B. and Slater, R. S. (1972). Relationship between low-density lipoprotein in aortic intima and serum-lipid levels. *Lancet*, **1**, 463–469.

Smith, E. B. and Smith, R. H. Early changes in aortic intima. In: *Atherosclerosis Reviews, Vol. 1*. Ed. R. Paoletti and A. M. Gotto. Raven Press, New York, pp. 119–136, 1976.

Stamler, J. *Lectures on Preventive Cardiology*. Grune & Stratton, New York, 1967.

Stamler, J. (1973). Epidemiology of coronary heart disease. *Medical Clinics of North America*, **57**, 5–46.

Stamler, J., Beard, R. R., Connor, W. E., de Wolfe, V. G., Stokes, J. and Willis, P. W. (1970). Primary prevention of the atherosclerotic diseases. *Circulation*, **42**, A55–A95.

Stary, H. C. (1967). Cell proliferation in the experimental atheroma as revealed by

radioautography after injection of thymidine-H³(P). *Circulation*, **36**, *Supplement II*, p. II–39.
Stary, H. C., Eggen, D. A. and Strong, J. P. The mechanism of atherosclerosis regression. In: *Atherosclerosis IV. Proceedings of the Fourth International Symposium.* Ed. G. Schettler, Y. Goto, Y. Hata and G. Klose. Springer-Verlag, Berlin, pp. 394–404, 1977.
Stein, Y. and Stein, O. Lipid synthesis and degradation and lipoprotein transport in mammalian aorta. In: *Atherogenesis: Initiating Factors. Ciba Symposium 12* (New Series). Elsevier, Amsterdam, pp. 165–179, 1973.
Stenders, S., Christensen, S. and Nyuad, O. (1978). Uptake of labelled free and esterified cholesterol from plasma by the aortic intima-media tissue measured *in vivo* in three animal species. *Atherosclerosis*, **31**, 279–293.
Strong, J. P. An introduction to the epidemiology of atherosclerosis. In: *Atherosclerosis IV. Proceedings of the Fourth International Symposium.* Ed. G. Schettler, Y. Goto, Y. Hata and G. Klose. Springer-Verlag, Berlin, pp. 92–98, 1977.
Strong, J. P., Eggen, D. A. and Oalmann, M. C. The natural history, geographic pathology, and epidemiology of atherosclerosis. In: *The Pathogenesis of Atherosclerosis.* Ed. R. W. Wissler and J. C. Geer. Williams & Wilkins, Baltimore, pp. 20–40, 1972.
Taylor, C. B., Cox, G. E., Manalo-Estrella, P. and Southworth, J. (1962). Atherosclerosis in rhesus monkeys. II. Arterial lesions associated with hypercholesterolemia induced by dietary fat and cholesterol. *Archives of Pathology*, **74**, 16–34.
Taylor, C. B., Manalo-Estrella, P. and Cox, G. E. (1963). Atherosclerosis in rhesus monkeys. V. Marked diet-induced hypercholesteremia with xanthomatosis and severe atherosclerosis. *Archives of Pathology*, **76**, 239–249.
Tejada, C., Strong, J. P., Montenegro, M. A., Restrepo, C. and Solberg, L. A. (1968). Distribution of coronary and aortic atherosclerosis by geographic location, race and sex. *Laboratory Investigation*, **18**, 509–526.
Thomas, W. A., Reiner, J. M., Florentin, R. A., Janakidevi, K. and Lee, K. J. Arterial smooth muscle cells in atherogenesis: births, deaths and clonal phenomena. In: *Atherosclerosis IV. Proceedings of the Fourth International Symposium.* Ed. G. Schettler, Y. Goto, Y. Hata and G. Klose. Springer-Verlag, Berlin, pp. 16–23, 1977.
Thompson, G. R., Myant, N. B., Kilpatrick, D., Oakley, C. M., Raphael, M. J. and Steiner, R. E. (1980). Assessment of long term plasma exchange for familial hypercholesterolaemia. *British Heart Journal*, **43**, 680–688.
Vergroesen, A. J. and Gottenbos, J. J. The role of fats in human nutrition: an introduction. In: *The Role of Fats in Human Nutrition.* Ed. A. J. Vergroesen. Academic Press, London, pp. 1–41, 1975.
Vesselinovitch, D. and Wissler, R. W. (1968). Experimental atherosclerosis in rabbits: the effect of oxygen and/or cholestyramine on its reversibility. *Circulation*, **38**, VI–198.
Vesselinovitch, D. and Wissler, R. W. Requirement for regression studies in animal models. In: *Atherosclerosis IV. Proceedings of the Fourth International Symposium.* Ed. G. Schettler, Y. Goto, Y. Hata and G. Klose. Springer-Verlag, Berlin, pp. 295–363, 1977.
Vles, R. O. Nutritional aspects of rapeseed oil. In: *The Role of Fats in Human Nutrition.* Ed. A. J. Vergroesen. Academic Press, London, pp. 433–477, 1975.
Walker, A. R. P. and Walker, B. F. (1978). High high-density-lipoprotein cholesterol in African children and adults in a population free of coronary heart disease. *British Medical Journal*, **2**, 1336–1337.
Walton, K. W. The role of lipoproteins in human atherosclerosis. In: *The Lipoprotein*

Molecule. Ed. H. Peeters. Nato Advanced Study Institute Series, Plenum Press, New York, pp. 237–244, 1978.

Walton, K. W. and Williamson, N. (1968). Histological and immunofluorescent studies on the evolution of the human atheromatous plaque. *Journal of Atherosclerosis Research*, **8**, 599–624.

Whyte, H. M. (1975). Potential effect on coronary-heart-disease morbidity of lowering the blood-cholesterol. *Lancet*, **1**, 906–910.

Wiklund, O., Gustafson, A. and Wilhelmsen, L. (1975). α-Lipoprotein cholesterol in men after myocardial infarction compared with a population sample. *Artery*, **1**, 399–404.

Williams, P., Robinson, D. and Bailey, A. (1979). High-density lipoprotein and coronary risk factors in normal men. *Lancet*, **1**, 72–75.

Williams, R. R., Sorlie, P. D., Feinleib, M., McNamara, P. M., Kannel, W. B. and Dawber, T. R. (1981). Cancer incidence by levels of cholesterol. *Journal of the American Medical Association*, **245**, 247–252.

Wissler, R. W. and Vesselinovitch, D. Differences between human and animal atherosclerosis. In: *Atherosclerosis III. Proceedings of the Third International Symposium*. Ed. G. Schettler and A. Weizel. Springer-Verlag, Berlin, pp. 319–325, 1974.

Wissler, R. W., Vesselinovitch, D., Hughes, R., Turner, D. and Frazier, L. E. (1971). Atherosclerosis and blood lipids in rhesus monkeys fed human table-prepared diets. *Circulation*, **44**, Supplement II, 11–57.

Woolf, N. and Pilkington, T. R. E. (1965). The immunohistochemical demonstration of lipoproteins in vessel walls. *Journal of Pathology and Bacteriology*, **90**, 459–463.

Wynder, E. L., Lemon, F. R. and Bross, I. J. (1959). Cancer and coronary artery disease among Seventh-day Adventists. *Cancer*, **12**, 1016–1028.

Chapter 14

Disorders of Cholesterol Metabolism: Introduction

1	NOMENCLATURE AND CLASSIFICATION	671
2	DEFINITIONS OF HYPERCHOLESTEROLAEMIA	672
3	THE PLASMA CHOLESTEROL AND COMMUNITY HEALTH	675
3.1	The argument for intervention	675
3.2	Dietary recommendations for the general population	676
3.3	Objections to dietary modification	677
3.4	Outlook for the future	681

BIOCHEMISTRY DEPT.,
WYE COLLEGE
WYE, ASHFORD,
KENT.

Disorders of Cholesterol Metabolism: Introduction

1 NOMENCLATURE AND CLASSIFICATION

Although it is becoming increasingly possible to name and classify disorders of cholesterol metabolism in terms of aetiology, their nomenclature is still determined largely by a combination of historical precedent, presenting symptomatology and methods of detection. For example, 'hypercholesterolaemia' does not refer to any specific disorder, but to an abnormality that is merely a reflection of any one of a number of abnormal plasma lipoprotein patterns with different aetiologies. Nevertheless, this term is too deeply embedded in current usage to be dispensed with and has, indeed, been retained in the name we still use for the disorder of lipoprotein metabolism (familial hypercholesterolaemia) whose basis we probably understand better than that of any other. In this case, the use of an otherwise unsatisfactory name is justified by past usage, and by the fact that detection of hypercholesterolaemia is, and is likely to remain, the most important single step in reaching a diagnosis.

In the remaining chapters of this book, disorders of cholesterol metabolism will be considered under the following headings:

(a) Those in which the underlying disorder is manifested as an abnormality in the plasma lipoprotein pattern. These are subdivided into hyperlipoproteinaemias and lipoprotein deficiencies.
(b) Those in which the major manifestation is an intracellular accumulation of cholesterol-containing lipid; these include Wolman's disease, cholesteryl-ester storage disease, β-sitosterol storage disease and cerebrotendinous xanthomatosis.
(c) Cholesterol gallstones and the formation of supersaturated bile; abnormal lipoprotein patterns due to liver disease.

This classification falls short of the ideal one, which, it may be hoped, will ultimately be based on the underlying cellular or enzymic abnormality responsible for the altered cholesterol metabolism. Moreover, although it provides a convenient scheme for grouping diseases in which there is a primary or secondary disturbance of cholesterol metabolism, it is arbitrary to the extent that the plasma lipoprotein abnormalities grouped under (a) above are often associated with accumulations of cholesterol within cells.

2 DEFINITIONS OF HYPERCHOLESTEROLAEMIA

Before dealing with the hyperlipoproteinaemias in the next chapter, I shall first consider briefly the usefulness of the term 'hypercholesterolaemia' in so far as it implies the presence of a clinical abnormality. As we saw in Chapter 11, the lipids of plasma are components of lipoproteins belonging to several more or less distinct classes, the particles within each class having a characteristic composition, origin and metabolic fate. Hence, we now think of changes in plasma lipid metabolism in terms of changes in the metabolism of one or more of the lipoprotein fractions. However, it would be a mistake to suppose that the concentration of a particular lipid in whole plasma is no longer of any interest to the epidemiologist or the clinician. Extensive information about plasma total cholesterol and total triglyceride concentrations has been collected during the past two or three decades by epidemiologists concerned with the distribution of plasma lipid concentrations in human populations, particularly in relation to IHD (see Chapters 12 and 13), and by clinicians concerned with metabolic diseases affecting the plasma lipoproteins (see Chapters 15, 16 and 18). Much of this information has been supplemented or partly superseded by more detailed studies of the concentrations of lipids in specific lipoprotein fractions; the importance of distinguishing between HDL cholesterol and LDL cholesterol as components of the total cholesterol in plasma has already been stressed in the previous chapter. Nevertheless, the measurement of plasma total cholesterol and total triglyceride concentrations still plays a very important role in epidemiological and genetic investigations of the plasma lipids, in screening for hyperlipoproteinaemia in well populations and in the diagnosis and management of patients with hyperlipoproteinaemia. If we are to interpret the measurements made in these circumstances we need some standard with which to compare the values obtained in a given individual. This problem also arises in relation to plasma lipoprotein concentrations and, for that matter, in relation to any continuous variable (such as blood pressure) that can give rise to overt disease at the extreme limits of its range, but for convenience we shall confine our attention at this point to a consideration of normal standards for plasma cholesterol concentration.

Attempts to define normal ranges for plasma cholesterol concentration in human populations according to age and sex have given rise to a good deal of controversy. This is still largely unresolved, in part because the argument is conducted from two different points of view. Some would hold that for a given age and sex there is a well-defined range of plasma cholesterol concentration compatible with optimal health and that any value above this range signifies disease. The problem then becomes one of ascertaining the limits of the normal range by measuring the plasma cholesterol concentration in random samples of supposedly healthy males and females of different ages. This attitude owes something to the traditional view, implicit in the usual textbook account of human diseases, that it is always possible to make a sharp distinction between health and disease, with the corollary that everyone in the population is either healthy or suffering from one or more disorders which the physician must first diagnose and then treat. Although this concept of disease may be adequate for most occasions, and is certainly the one taken for granted by the patient in his relations with his doctor, there is a growing recognition that it is inappropriate in some contexts.

The distribution of values for plasma cholesterol concentration in human populations is unimodal, without evidence of segregation into two or more modes, and is dependent upon age and sex. Hence, the cut-off point chosen for defining a normal range must be arbitrary and, furthermore, must be adjusted for age and sex. As we saw in Chapter 12, the normal range in any population is usually defined in terms of an age- and sex-adjusted limit set at the upper 90th or 95th percentile, the values corresponding to these percentiles being ascertained by measurement of plasma cholesterol concentration in unbiased samples of the population (exemplified in Table 12.2). Hence, we should say that any individual whose plasma cholesterol concentration is above the chosen cut-off point (adjusted for age and sex) has hypercholesterolaemia. Some such arbitrary definition of hypercholesterolaemia is unavoidable in day-to-day clinical practice, as in the management of a Lipid Clinic, and in the following chapters the upper 95th percentile is taken as the cut-off point.

However, this method of defining hypercholesterolaemia raises two problems. In the first place, there is no reason to suppose that the transition from normocholesterolaemia to hypercholesterolaemia corresponds to what might be called a quantum jump from a state compatible with optimal health to one that is detrimental to health. On the contrary, the epidemiological evidence discussed in Chapters 12 and 13 shows clearly that there is a graded increase in risk of IHD with increasing plasma cholesterol concentration, with no evidence of a risk-free lower limit, and that the risk associated with a given concentration is influenced by the presence of concomitant host or environmental factors such as cigarette smoking and blood pressure.

A further objection to any definition of hypercholesterolaemia framed in this way arises from the fact that the distribution of plasma cholesterol concentrations varies from one geographical region to another and between different economic, racial and social subpopulations within a given region. This means that cut-off points based on values ascertained in a local population cannot have universal validity and, hence, that a given individual could be hypercholesterolaemic in one population but normocholesterolaemic in another if 'local' cut-off points are used.

A partial answer to these anomalies is that the best choice of standards depends to some extent upon the particular circumstances. Experience seems to show that in the diagnosis of the more or less distinct hyperlipoproteinaemias discussed in the next chapter, a cut-off point at the 90th or 95th percentile based on age- and sex-adjusted values from the local population is the most appropriate, though in the case of recent immigrants this may pose a problem as to which is the relevant local population. A different approach is needed in the field of community health, as in screening programmes for the detection of individuals who may be at high risk for IHD, or in attempts to formulate advice to the general population on the avoidance of risk factors. Expert opinion is moving towards the view that any advice given to healthy individuals in relation to plasma cholesterol concentration should ideally be based on multiple risk scores (see Chapter 13), an approach that has something in common with that of a life-insurance company weighting its premiums in accordance with various factors known to influence life expectancy. In the present state of knowledge, multiple risk scores based on plasma cholesterol concentration and other relevant variables can only be calculated in a rough-and-ready manner, nor can we be certain that the scores calculated from prospective studies in one population are valid for other populations. Nevertheless, the use of risk scores, however crude, is at least consistent with the well-established fact that the relation between plasma cholesterol concentration and risk of IHD shows no sharp break between zero risk and high risk. In epidemiological studies, yet other ways of categorizing plasma cholesterol concentrations may be the most appropriate. For example, in the search for correlations between plasma cholesterol level and IHD, or in studies of familial aggregation of cholesterol level, it may be convenient to divide the distribution of values observed in the population into quintiles or quartiles or into values above and below the median.

3 THE PLASMA CHOLESTEROL AND COMMUNITY HEALTH

3.1 The argument for intervention

In this section we shall consider the implications for the community at large of the well-established fact that the plasma cholesterol concentration is a positive risk factor for IHD. This is not the place for a general discussion of atherosclerosis as a public health problem in affluent countries, but we cannot ignore the question 'Should we or should we not advocate intervention to lower the plasma cholesterol level in whole populations or in selected healthy individuals at high risk?' There is no simple answer to this question, which has been at the centre of intense debate in the scientific and lay press for a decade or more. Unfortunately, the debate has been tainted by fanaticism, biased selection of evidence and appeals to irrelevant facts. Both sides have been guilty, but it does sometimes appear that the 'non-interventionists' fail to appreciate the complexity of the evidence that must be taken into consideration if a balanced judgement is to be reached.

As we saw in Chapter 13, the marked differences in IHD incidence that occur between different countries must be due largely to the influence of environmental factors to which whole human communities are exposed. A striking illustration of this is the difference in IHD incidence between groups of genetically similar Japanese men living in Japan, Honolulu (Hawaii) and California. In Japan, the incidence rates of IHD in men are among the lowest recorded anywhere in the world. However, as a consequence of the increasing adoption of an American style of life, the incidence of IHD in Japanese men living in California is now approaching that experienced by native-born white American men living in the same region. This has been demonstrated on several occasions, notably in the 'Ni-Hon-San' study of Robertson *et al.* (1977). In this study it was shown that Japanese men living in San Francisco had a higher incidence of fatal and non-fatal myocardial infarction (3.8/1000 man-years) than those living in Honolulu (3.0/1000 man-years), and that in those living in Honolulu the incidence was higher than in Japanese men living in a representative town in Japan (1.6/1000 man-years). These differences could be correlated with changes in dietary habits and with other aspects of life-style associated with migration across the Pacific from Japan to California (Kagan *et al.*, 1974). In this connection it is worth noting that the differences in incidence rates were highest for the younger men; these would have included a relatively high proportion of second-generation Japanese immigrants exposed to a Hawaian or Californian environment since birth. Furthermore, the higher IHD incidence in Japanese men living in Honolulu than in those living in Japan could be accounted for by the difference in multiple risk score based on a combination of plasma cholesterol concentration, systolic blood pressure and relative body weight, the Framingham prospective observations being used as a basis for the calculations. The difference in risk score between the two populations was due almost entirely to a difference in mean plasma cholesterol concentration; blood pressure was, in fact, higher in men living in Japan than in those living in Honolulu.

The results of the Ni-Hon-San study suggest very strongly that the difference between IHD incidence in American men living in the United States and Japanese men living in Japan is due to factors in the environment, in the broadest sense of the term, that act with greater force in the United States than in Japan to promote coronary atherosclerosis and the subsequent thrombotic changes leading to a heart attack. If this is the case, it follows that if we could identify these environmental factors it should, in principle, be possible to reduce the incidence of IHD in American men to that in Japanese men in Japan. According to the most recent statistics this would mean reducing the IHD death rate in American men aged 35 to 74 to about one-third of its present rate and would result in a net decrease of at least 400 000 in the annual number of fatal myocardial infarctions in American men in this age range.

Considerations such as this have led to the current discussion as to whether or not we have enough evidence about the environmental causes of IHD to justify preventive action of any kind. Although we cannot expect to be able to identify all the environmental causes leading to a high incidence of IHD in a given population, it would be reasonable to assume that at least some of them are mediated by known independent risk factors. In the example discussed at length in the previous paragraphs, the higher incidence of IHD in the Japanese men living in America could be accounted for largely by their increased risk from a high mean plasma cholesterol concentration. A risk factor is not necessarily a cause of IHD. Nevertheless, in view of all the circumstantial evidence for a causal link between plasma cholesterol concentration and IHD (see Chapter 13), it is hard to believe that the environmental contribution to IHD in men living in the United States does not act in part by increasing the plasma cholesterol concentration.

3.2 Dietary recommendations for the general population

The conclusion that some environmental causes of IHD, of which a diet rich in saturated fat and cholesterol may be one, probably act *via* the plasma cholesterol concentration has led authoritative organizations in several countries to recommend modification of the diet on a national scale with the object of lowering the plasma cholesterol level in the population as a whole and of reducing the incidence of obesity. Among these organizations are the Royal College of Physicians of London (Clarke *et al.*, 1976) and the Select Committee on Nutrition and Human Needs, United States Senate (1977). The recommendations of these and other bodies in countries with a high incidence of IHD (see Turpeinen, 1979) are in broad agreement in suggesting that:

> *total dietary calories should not exceed the amount required to maintain normal body weight; total fat intake should be reduced to 30–35% of total calories, mainly by decreasing the consumption of saturated fat, with partial substitution of saturated by polyunsaturated fat; the intake of cholesterol should not exceed 300 mg/day.*

In their recommendations relating to IHD in the general population, several official bodies also advise an increase in the consumption of fibre and a decrease in the consumption of refined sugar. Carrying out all these recommendations requires a knowledge of the composition of foods. General information about the fatty-acid and cholesterol content of foods will be found in the recommendations of the DHSS Committee on Medical Aspects of Food Policy (1974) and in the report of the Royal College of Physicians of London (1976) (Sections 4.9.1 and 16.2); Chapter 3 (Section 2.10) of this book also contains information about cholesterol in foods. Additional information, of the kind required by dietitians in the design of 'plasma-cholesterol lowering' diets for hypercholesterolaemic patients, is given in 'The Composition of Foods' (Paul and Southgate, 1978). Relevant sections of the Royal College of Physicians report are reprinted at the end of this chapter.

The recommendations outlined above are based partly on estimates of the dietary intake of fats and cholesterol in populations with a low incidence of IHD and partly on information about the effects of dietary modification on the plasma cholesterol concentration in open (National Diet—Heart Study Research Group, 1968) or closed (Turpeinen *et al.*, 1968) populations, or in individual subjects tested under experimental conditions (Keys *et al.*, 1965a,b). General advice on the prevention of coronary atherosclerosis in populations with a high incidence of IHD must, of course, take into account the sum total of all known or possible risk factors for IHD, including blood pressure, cigarette smoking, sedentary habit, glucose intolerance, psychological stress and factors related to the clotting mechanism and to platelet behaviour. But we are here concenred only with factors that operate through the plasma cholesterol concentration and that we have some chance of modifying favourably.

3.3 Objections to dietary modification

Although there is widespread support for the view that modification of the diet on a national scale along the lines outlined above would be likely to diminish the incidence of IHD and is therefore desirable, this view has been criticized, mainly on two grounds.

In the first place, it has been argued that the addition of large amounts of polyunsaturated fat to the diet could be detrimental to health by favouring the formation of gallstones and by damaging the myocardium. It is certainly possible that a marked increase in the ratio of polyunsaturated to saturated fat (P/S ratio) in the diet could promote the formation of lithogenic bile in some individuals by increasing the concentration ratio of cholesterol to bile salts and phospholipids in the bile, but the experimental evidence on this point is contradictory. Short-term feeding of polyunsaturated fat has been reported to have no effect on bile composition in normal men (Dam *et al.*, 1967), or in patients who have had gallstones (Watanabe *et al.*, 1962; Sarles *et al.*, 1970) or in Rhesus monkeys (Campbell *et al.*, 1972). On the other hand, Grundy (1975) observed an increase in the lithogenicity of the bile of some hypertriglyceridaemic patients given diets with a high P/S ratio. Of greater relevance to the possible long-term effects of substantial increases in the P/S ratio of diets eaten by large populations is the observation of Sturdevant *et al.* (1973) that in the Los Angeles trial the incidence of gallstones was significantly higher in men who had been given a diet with a high P/S ratio for 5 years than in a control group eating a normal diet. Although Miettinen *et al.*, (1972) did not observe an increased incidence of gallstones in their Finnish hospital patients given a diet with a high P/S ratio, the findings of Sturdevant *et al.* clearly cannot be ignored. However, the P/S ratio in the diets of the treated group studied by Sturdevant *et al.* was about 1.6. This is much higher than the value reported for any known human population, including those with a low incidence of IHD. For example, in Japan, a country with a very low IHD incidence, the P/S ratio estimated from dietary surveys carried out by Keys and his collaborators (Keys *et al.*, 1970) was about 1.0; in no other country has a value as high as this been reported. It is also worth noting that there is no evidence to suggest that the incidence of gallstones is any higher in Japan than in the United States (Redinger and Small, 1972; Heaton, 1973), a country in which the P/S ratio determined by dietary surveys is about 0.3 (Keys *et al.*, 1970).

The results of the Los Angeles trial, together with the results of observations on the short-term effects of polyunsaturated fats on the composition of bile in some hyperlipidaemic subjects, suggest that a marked and sustained increase in the intake of polyunsaturated fat could promote the secretion of lithogenic bile in a significant number of people in a large population, perhaps by stimulating the transfer of cholesterol from the extra-hepatic tissues to the liver for removal *via* the bile. In view of this possibility, it does not seem justifiable to recommend more than a limited increase in polyunsaturated-fat intake in the *general* population. In most official reports on the prevention of IHD, the reason given for recommending an increase in the consumption of polyunsaturated fat is that diets become unpalatable if there is a substantial reduction in saturated fat intake without some substitution by polyunsaturated fats. Thus, an increased intake of polyunsaturated fat is not advocated for its plasma-cholesterol lowering effect, and on this argument there seems no reason why the P/S ratio in the average British diet should be any higher than that in the diets of populations with a low incidence of IHD. This would entail increasing the P/S ratio in Britain from about 0.25 to, say, 0.6 (Shaper and Marr, 1977). There are those who recommend very substantial increases in the intake of polyunsaturated fat in the general population (P/S ratios as high as 2.0 are regarded by some as an ideal at which to aim) on the grounds that 2 g of polyunsaturated fat are required to counteract the effect of every 1 g of saturated fat on the plasma cholesterol concentration in short-term experiments on human subjects (Keys *et al.*, 1965a). In the present state of knowledge this seems unwise, though it may be justifiable, or even desirable, in the treatment of hypercholesterolaemic patients in view of their high risk (see next chapter).

The possibility that some of the commercially available margarines and cooking oils used for increasing the polyunsaturated-fat content of the diet could be injurious to health was mentioned in Chapter 13. Many of these preparations have been hardened by partial hydrogenation, resulting in *cis-trans* isomerization of some double bonds. There is no evidence that unsaturated fatty acids with *trans* double bonds are injurious to man or experimental animals, but the use of vegetable oils rich in erucic acid is potentially harmful. As already mentioned, safeguards to prevent the sale of edible oils with more than a certain percentage of erucic acid are the subject of discussion at international level. It should also be noted that a large number of proprietary brands of margarine is now available in the shops, but that by no means all of them are particularly rich in polyunsaturated fats (see Table 14.1 and appendix to this chapter).

The second ground for criticism of the dietary recommendations put forward on p. 677 is that it has not been proved unequivocally that lowering the plasma cholesterol concentration in the general population would reduce the incidence of first fatal and non-fatal heart attacks. This is undeniable, but it has to be said that the arguments used by those who are opposed to recommending dietary changes in the general population have not always come up to the standards to be expected in a serious scientific debate. The view that a limited change in national dietary habits is desirable has been dismissed by McMichael (1977) as the result of brainwashing 'by propaganda into a widespread acceptance of a fashion'. There may be some truth in this, particularly with regard to those who wish to bring about extreme changes in the intake of polyunsaturated fats in whole populations. However, it can hardly be doubted that the majority of the many experts who have expressed an opinion about an important social problem have done their best to reach what they believe to be the most reasonable working hypothesis on the basis of all the available evidence. As discussed in Chapter 13, the evidence for the plasma lipid hypothesis is derived from several different sources, including epidemiology, experimental atherosclerosis, clinical studies of hyperlipidaemia, observations on pathogenesis at the cellular level and studies of coronary atherosclerosis *post mortem* and *in vivo* in relation to plasma lipid concentrations.

In so far as the plasma lipid hypothesis is accepted, it is reasonable to advocate measures to lower the plasma cholesterol level in populations with high plasma cholesterol concentrations and high incidence of IHD. The argument that those who advocate a selective reduction in the consumption of saturated fat in the general population are influenced by vested interests, apart from its irrelevance to the merits of

Table 14.1

Margarines high in polyunsaturates
(which contain not less than 50% polyunsaturates)

Flora
Marks & Spencers Super Spread Margarine
Co-Op Good Life Margarine
Alfonal Sun O Lat Margarine
Alfonal Snowqueen Margarine
Waitrose Sunflower Oil Margarine
Sainsbury Special Supersoft Margarine
Kraft Golden Corn Oil Margarine

Cooking oils high in polyunsaturates

Tesco Cooking Oil (Mixed Vegetable)
Tesco Corn Oil
Alfonal Sun O Lat
Alfonal Lin O Sat
Alfonal Maizy
Mazola Corn Oil
Co-Op Friary Cooking Oil
Safeway Soya Bean Oil
Safeway Sunflower Seed Oil
Kraft Corn Oil

Margarines and cooking oils high in polyunsaturated fats, obtainable commercially in Britain. The Brands listed in the Table contain not less than 50% of their total fat as polyunsaturated fat. (Information kindly supplied by Miss R. Harrison, Chief Dietician, Hammersmith Hospital).

the case, is double-edged since there are commercial interests that stand to gain from the sale of dairy products rich in saturated fat.

Although the plasma lipid hypothesis has not been proved, no one has put forward an acceptable alternative explanation for the positive association between plasma cholesterol concentration and IHD incidence within and between populations; the explanatory power of the hypothesis, to use Darwin's phrase, is far greater than that of any other. Kaunitz (1961, 1977) has suggested that the raised plasma cholesterol level associated with IHD is a protective response to the development of atherosclerotic lesions rather than a causal factor. In the absence of any suggestion as to how an arterial lesion could cause a change in lipoprotein metabolism that would lead to an increase in plasma cholesterol concentration, this view does not merit serious consideration. There is also the difficulty, though not an insuperable one, that the link between plasma cholesterol level and IHD is predictive. Mann (1977), in a critical review of the dietary fat hypothesis, says categorically that in developed societies with a high incidence of coronary heart disease 'the prevailing hypercholesteremia is contributory and that a major reduction would make a difference in clinical events'. He then draws the erroneous conclusion that the high mean plasma cholesterol concentrations in developed societies must be due to impairment of the conversion of cholesterol into bile acids. There is no evidence for this. In any case, the mechanism he proposes as an explanation for impaired bile-acid formation—the accumulation of oxidation products of cholesterol—would be likely to lead to a *fall* in plasma cholesterol concentration by inhibition of HMG-CoA reductase.

3.4 Outlook for the future

No large-scale primary prevention trial in which dietary modification is the only variable is now being carried out on any human population. Moreover, in view of the huge cost of primary prevention trials on open populations it is likely that the only trials supported in the future will be multifactorial—that is, several risk factors will be altered at the same time, so that if there is a positive outcome it will not be possible to deduce which of several interventions was the effective one. If this is the case, we shall never know the answer to the diet-heart question and we shall have to continue to judge the issue on the basis of incomplete evidence. The medical profession has often had to give advice at a time when the evidence did not amount to proof. Indeed, to be able to base advice on certainty is a luxury often denied to the profession.

Although mortality from IHD in the United States rose progressively from 1946 to the mid-1960's, there has been a striking decrease since about 1968. Between 1968 and 1975 the registered age-adjusted death rate from IHD in the United States fell by 19–35% in white and nonwhite male and female adults (Stamler, 1978), a trend that seems to be beginning in several European countries (Epstein, 1979), including Finland (Salonen *et al.*, 1979) and in Canada and Australia (Havlik and Feinleib, 1979). There is no evidence that coronary death rates are declining in the general population in Great Britain although there has been some improvement in coronary mortality in certain social groups in this region, particularly among doctors (Doll and Peto, 1976). The fall in coronary mortality in the United States is a real one, in the sense that it cannot be explained by changes in the classification or efficiency of *post mortem* registration of the disease, though there is as yet no proof that the prevalence of non-fatal IHD has also declined (Havlik and Feinleib, 1979). Observations on several United States communities in the period 1958–1975 suggest that there has also been a fall in the mean plasma cholesterol concentration in U.S. adults (Beaglehole *et al.*, 1979; Stamler, 1978).

A significant fall in IHD mortality within less than a decade indicates that there has been a decrease in the strength of one or more positive risk factors for IHD. There is no general agreement as to the changes in the life style or environment of Americans that have brought about this decline in mortality; the decline has followed, or coincided with, a decrease in cigarette-smoking among men, an increase in the proportion of polyunsaturated fats in dietary fat and an increase in physical activity among certain classes of Americans, and has been most marked in the higher social classes (Havlik and Feinlieb, 1979). However, the fact that the fall has occurred at a time when there has been a marked change in attitudes towards smoking, exercise and diet among wide sections of the U.S. population gives encouragement to those who believe that measures to counteract known risk factors in the general population are worth attempting. The argument for more intensive intervention in selected members of the general population is discussed in the next chapter. Finally, it remains to be said that whatever opinions we may now hold about risk-factor intervention, our approach to the prevention of IHD is sure to change as we learn more about risk-factors, especially with regard to the influence of diet and other environmental determinants on the plasma HDL concentration and on blood clotting mechanisms.

APPENDIX

Two extracts from *Prevention of Coronary Heart Disease*. Report of a joint working party of the Royal College of Physicians of London and the British Cardiac Society (Clarke *et al.*, 1976).

Disorders of Cholesterol Metabolism: Introduction 683

1. SUMMARY AND RECOMMENDATIONS

1.1 *Introduction*

1. The aim of this Working Party has been to formulate the best possible advice that can at present be given to medical practitioners towards the prevention of coronary heart disease (CHD).

2. There is considerable evidence that the causes of CHD are largely environmental and are rooted in the modern, affluent way of life. CHD risk factors such as cigarette smoking, physical inactivity, obesity and plasma lipid concentrations reflect aspects of our social behaviour. This report is particularly concerned with those risk factors that can be modified.

3. The risk of CHD varies according to the total burden of risk factors present and the recommendations emphasise this multifactorial concept of risk. When dealing with an individual, the overall degree of CHD risk must be considered rather than deciding whether any particular factor has reached a 'critical' level requiring treatment.

4. The measures recommended carry the reasonable hope of conferring some benefit to the community and none of them has a cost that approaches the cost of inaction.

1.2 *Diet*

1. Dietary recommendations for the whole community involve a reduction in the amount of saturated fats and partial substitution by polyunsaturated fats.

2. Where plasma lipid concentrations indicate particularly high risk or where other risk factors are concurrently present, the dietary recommendations should be followed more strictly.

3. Widespread screening for plasma lipid levels is not recommended but estimations should be carried out in certain groups known to be at high risk for CHD.

4. Maintenance of a desirable weight is important as obesity is commonly associated with other more potent risk factors for CHD. Weight reduction should be based on a decrease in all the dietary components; sugar and alcohol are recognised as common sources of excess energy intake. A combination of exercise and diet is strongly recommended.

1.3 *Smoking*

1. Every effort should be made to discourage cigarette smoking, particularly in the young. Doctors and other health workers should set an example.

2. Less harmful methods of smoking should be advised for those who are unwilling to stop.

1.4 *Blood Pressure*

1. Blood pressure should be recorded for every patient, using the opportunities provided by any consultation.

2. In those with even moderatley raised blood pressure, the control of other risk factors (cigarette smoking, diet, physical inactivity) is important.

3. Treatment of raised blood pressure is at present justified on the grounds of reducing the risk of stroke and other implications.Its effect on CHD risk is not yet established.

1.5 *Physical Activity*

1. Physical activity should be encouraged at all ages in both men and women.

2. Few need to consult their doctor before making a graded increase in their physical activity.

1.6 *Stress*

1. While acute stress may occasionally precipitate a heart attack, it is difficult to prove that chronic stress contributes to the development of CHD.

2. The management of stress, whether it be domestic or occupational in origin, is a normal part of medical practice.

2. Initiative, diligence, leadership and hard work, especially in young people, should not be discouraged on the mistaken supposition that these qualities are indicators of future CHD.

1.7 Diabetes Mellitus

1. Reversal of risk factors for CHD should form part of the care of diabetics.
2. Dietary policy for individual diabetics should be determined as much by their plasma lipid concentrations as by the blood sugar response.

1.8 Oral Contraceptives

1. Oral contraceptives constitute a negligible risk in women under the age of 40 years who do not have any risk factors for CHD.
2. They should be used with caution in women over 40 years, those with a family history of premature CHD, and in women who are heavy cigarette-smokers (more than 20 a day) or have other risk factors.

1.9 Children

1. Measures recommended to prevent the development of CHD apply to children as well as to adults since all of the major risk factors found in adult life can occur during childhood. All those concerned with the care of children should be active in the prevention and management of these factors.

1.10 General Practice

1. General practice should provide the main means of identifying those at high risk of CHD.
2. Mass screening for CHD and its associated risk factors is not recommended.
3. The efforts of general practitioners should be supported by a general health education policy that involves hospital and community physicians and their supporting staff.
4. Selective health examinations should be carried out in those groups known to be at high risk for CHD.
5. Interested general practitioners should be encouraged to extend health examinations to other groups of patients where this can be done by the use of existing facilities and services.

1.11 Wider Implications of the Recommendations

1. It was not the purpose of the Working Party to consider the implications of their recommendations for research or for government. However, attention is drawn briefly to areas that may deserve further consideration by other bodies. In the overall allocation of resources the Working Party considered that the achievements of acute coronary care, coronary ambulances and coronary artery surgery could not bring about a major reduction in the overall burden of heart disease in the community. This must come from preventive measures.

2. *Education.* To bring about the recommended changes in behaviour relating to diet, physical activity and cigarette smoking will require the sustained involvement of the community at all levels, aimed particularly at the young. A comprehensive public and professional educational programme will be needed, together with the involvement and co-operation of food manufacturers, educational authorities and the mass media. Apart from formal health education, much can be done by medical practitioners and other health workers who understand the problem and are prepared to provide positive advice to individuals and the community regarding the risk factors for CHD.

3. *Smoking.* The reduction of cigarette smoking will require fiscal measures by the

Disorders of Cholesterol Metabolism: Introduction 685

government and the control of advertising. These measures may be at least as effective as general health education and possibly more so.

4. *Diet.* There are considerable implications in the dietary recommendations for national food policy, for the producers and the manufacturers of food and for the regulations concerning food labelling. Nutritional practices and catering in schools, hospitals, the Armed Forces and other organisations may require to be reviewed.

5. *Physical Activity.* Any improvement in patterns of physical activity can come only from leisure time pursuits. Adequate and convenient recreational facilities are required if the recommendations made are to be effective.

16.2 Dietary Fats

The housewife who buys butter, margarine or lard knows what she means by 'fat'. Cooking oil is a liquid fat. Table fats, cooking oil and the fat on meat are visible fats but there is non-visible fat in most other foods as well, ranking from nearly 40 per cent in many cheeses, potato crisps and chocolate down to only a trace in most fruits and vegetables. The biochemical term 'lipids' covers all the chemical substances included in the housewife's 'fat', such as triglycerides, cholesterol and phospholipids. Cholesterol is present in a number of foods (eggs are the chief source) but it is only a small part of the average dietary fat intake.

The form in which fats chiefly occur both in foods and in the fat depots of the body is the triglycerides composed of fatty acids and glycerol. There are over 40 fatty acids found in nature, accounting for the diversity and specificity of the natural fats. The fatty acids are made up of carbon, hydrogen and oxygen and their properties depend upon the length of the carbon chain and the ability of the carbon chain to combine with additional hydrogen atoms. This latter ability is referred to as the degree of saturation or unsaturation. Fatty acids are classified as saturated, mono-unsaturated, and polyunsaturated. Saturated fatty acids contain as many hydrogen atoms as the carbon chain can hold, e.g. palmitic and stearic acids. Mono-unsaturated fatty acids have two hydrogen atoms missing in the carbon chain, i.e. one double-bond linkage is available; oleic and palmitoleic acids are examples. Polyunsaturated fatty acids (PUFA) may have 2, 3 or 4 more double-bond linkages available, i.e. 4, 6, 8 or more hydrogen atoms are missing in the carbon chain. Examples are linoleic acid (2 double-bonds), linolenic acid (3 double-bonds) and arachidonic (4 double-bonds).

The ratio of dietary polyunsaturated to saturated fatty acids is often abbreviated to the P/S ratio.

Fatty Acid Composition of Food

All the fat-containing foods in our diet consist of a mixture of fatty acids and one should not think of any particular food item as being purely saturated, mono-unsaturated or polyunsaturated. Most foods can, however, be classified as predominantly saturated, mono-unsaturated or polyunsaturated. Saturated fatty acids comprise about 50 per cent of the fatty acids contained in the average British diet and provide about 21 per cent of total energy intake. These are principally the solid fats of animal origin such as those in milk, butter and meat. Some plant products (chocolate and coconut) contain large amounts of the saturated fatty acids. The predominantly unsaturated vegetable and plant fatty acids that have been hardened by hydrogenation become saturated fatty acids. Saturated fatty acids in the diet increase the plasma cholesterol concentration.

Mono-unsaturated fatty acids comprise about 40 per cent of the fatty acids in the average British diet and provide about 16 per cent of the total energy intake. The best example is oleic acid, found in appreciable amounts in most foods. Oleic acid comprises nearly 50 per cent of the fatty content of bacon and about 75 per cent of the fatty acid content of olive oil. These fatty acids have little effect on the plasma cholesterol concentration.

Polyunsaturated fatty acids (PUFA) in the average British diet are much less in quantity than either the saturated or mono-unsaturated fatty acids and they provide slightly less than 5 per cent of the total energy intake. Corn oil and sunflower oil are among the richest food sources of this group of fatty acids. Chicken, fish and many nuts (excluding coconut) are good sources of PUFA. The polyunsaturated fats in the diet tend to lower the plasma cholesterol concentration.

Dietary cholesterol is only part of the body's supply of cholesterol which is derived in two main ways: by synthesis in the tissues, particularly the liver and intestinal wall (endogenous cholesterol) and from the diet (exogenous cholesterol). The body synthesis of cholesterol is several times greater than the dietary intake. There is a feed-back mechanism by which the intake of dietary cholesterol can suppress endogenous cholesterol synthesis but there is considerable variation in this mechanism from one individual to another and possibly from one race to another.

The average British diet contains about 500 mg of cholesterol per day of which 40 to 60 per cent is retained in the body. With higher intakes of cholesterol the percentage absorption falls. The type of dietary fat that accompanies the cholesterol may be a factor in determining the absorption of cholesterol. Fats tending to elevate the plasma cholesterol are the ones in which dietary cholesterol is most soluble. The major dietary sources of cholesterol are egg yolk, liver and kidney. Food from plant sources contains no cholesterol.

Table 6 shows the daily nutrient content and the energy value of the average British diet. Table 7 shows the sources of fat in the average British diet, with major contributions from butter, margarine, cooking fats and meat.

For more detailed information on dietary components refer to *Human Nutrition and Dietetics*, 6th edition by Davidson, Passmore, Brock and Truswell. Churchill-Livingstone, 1975.

Table 6
Nutrient content and energy value of household food. National Food Survey 1973.

		Percentage total calories
Energy kcal	2400	—
Protein g	71	12
Carbohydrate g	293	46
Fat g	111	42
Saturated	52	21
Mono-unsaturated	42	16
Polyunsaturated	12	5
Cholesterol mg	500	—

Table 7
Sources of fat (%) in the British diet. National Food Survey 1973.

	%		%
Butter, margarine and other fats	35	Meats	28
Milk and cream	15	Poultry	1
Cheese	4	Fish	1
		Cakes and biscuit	6
Eggs	3	Other foods	7

REFERENCES

Beaglehole, R., LaRosa, J. C., Heiss, G. E., Davis, C. E., Rifkind, B. M., Muesing, R. M. and Williams, C. D. Secular changes in blood cholesterol and their contribution to the decline in coronary mortality. In: *Proceedings of the Conference on the Decline in Coronary Heart Disease Mortality*. Ed. R. J. Havlik and M. Feinleib. U.S. Department of Health, Education, and Welfare Public Health Service, NIH Publication No. 79-1610, pp. 282–295, 1979.

Campbell, C. B., Cowley, D. J. and Dowling, R. H. (1972). Dietary factors affecting biliary lipid secretion in the Rhesus monkey. A mechanism for the hypocholesterolaemic action of polyunsaturated fat? *European Journal of Clinical Investigation*, **2**, 332–341.

Clarke, C. A., Goodwin, J. F., Shaper, A. G., Ball, K. P., Lloyd, J. K., Oliver, M. F., Rose, G. A., Somerville, W., Truswell, A. S., Turner, R. W. D., McCormick, J. S., Hawthorne, V. M., Ford, G. and Ashley-Miller, M. (1976). Prevention of coronary heart disease. *Journal of the Royal College of Physicians of London*, **10**, 213–275.

Dam, H., Kruse, I., Jensen, M. K. and Kallehauge, H. E. (1967). Studies on human bile. II. Influence of two different fats on the composition of human bile. *Scandinavian Journal of Clinical and Laboratory Investigation*, **19**, 367–378.

Department of Health and Social Security. *Diet and Coronary Heart Disease*. HMSO, London, 1974.

Doll, R. and Peto, R. (1976). Mortality in relation to smoking: 20 years' observations on male British doctors. *British Medical Journal*, **2**, 1525–1536.

Epstein, F. H. *Recent international changes in coronary heart disease*. IFMA Symposium, Brussels, 1979.

Grundy, S. M. (1975). Effects of polyunsaturated fats on lipid metabolism in patients with hypertriglyceridemia. *Journal of Clinical Investigation*, **55**, 269–282.

Havlik, R. J. and Feinleib, M. *Proceedings of the Conference on the Decline in Coronary Heart Disease Mortality*. U.S. Department of Health, Education, and Welfare Public Health Service, NIH Publication No. 79-1610, 1979.

Heaton, K. W. (1973). The epidemiology of gallstones and suggested aetiology. *Clinics in Gastroenterology*, **2**, 67–83.

Kagan, A., Harris, B. R., Winkelstein, W., Johnson, K. G., Kato, H., Syme, S. L., Rhoads, G. G., Gay, M. L., Nichaman, M. Z., Hamilton, H. B. and Tillotson, J. (1974). Epidemiologic studies of coronary heart disease and stroke in Japanese men living in Japan, Hawaii, and California: demographic, physical, dietary and biochemical characteristics. *Journal of Chronic Diseases*, 1974, **27**, 345–364.

Kaunitz, H. (1961). Re-evaluation of some factors in arteriosclerosis. *Nature (London)*, **192**, 9–12.

Kaunitz, H. (1977). Repair function of cholesterol versus the lipid theory of arteriosclerosis. *Chemistry and Industry*, 761–763.

Keys, A. *Coronary heart disease in seven countries*. Circulation, Vol. XLI, No. 4, Supplement 1. Monograph No. 29. Ed. A. Keys. American Heart Association, 1970.

Keys, A., Anderson, J. T. and Grande, F. (1965*a*). Serum cholesterol response to changes in the diet. I. Iodine value of dietary fat versus 2S-P. *Metabolism*, **14**, 747–758.

Keys, A., Anderson, J. T. and Grande, F. (1965*b*). Serum cholesterol response to changes in the diet. II. The effect of cholesterol in the diet. *Metabolism*, **14**, 759–765.

McMichael, J. (1977). Dietetic factors in coronary disease. *European Journal of Cardiology*, **5/6**, 447–452.

Mann, G. V. (1977). Current Concepts. Diet-heart: end of an era. *New England Journal of Medicine*, **297**, 644–650.

Miettinen, M., Turpeinen, O., Karvonen, M. J., Elosuo, R. and Paavilainen, E. (1972). Effect of cholesterol-lowering diet on mortality from coronary heart-disease and other causes. A twelve-year clinical trial in men and women. *Lancet*, **2**, 835–838.

National Diet-Heart Study Research Group (1968). The national diet-heart study final report. *Circulation*, **37**, Supplement 1.

Paul, A. A. and Southgate, D. A. T. McCance and Widdowson's *The Composition of Foods*. Fourth revised and extended edition of MRC Special Report No. 297. HMSO, London, 1978.

Redinger, R. N. and Small, D. M. (1972). Bile composition, bile salt metabolism and gallstones. *Archives of Internal Medicine*, **130**, 618–630.

Robertson, T. L., Kato, H., Rhoads, G. G., Kagan, A., Marmot, M., Syme, S. L., Gordon, T., Worth, R. M., Bersky, J. L., Dock, D. S., Myanishi, M. and Kawamoto, S. (1977). Epidemiologic studies of coronary heart disease and stroke in Japanese men living in Japan, Hawaii and California. Incidence of myocardial infarction and death from coronary heart disease. *American Journal of Cardiology*, **39**, 239–243.

Salonen, J. T., Puska, P. and Mustaniemi, H. (1979). Changes in morbidity and mortality during comprehensive community programme to control cardiovascular diseases during 1972–7 in North Karelia. *British Medical Journal*, **2**, 1178–1183.

Sarles, H., Hauton, J., Planche, N. E., Lafont, H. and Gerolami, A. (1970). Diet, cholesterol gallstones, and composition of the bile. *American Journal of Digestive Diseases*, **15**, 251–260.

Select Committee on Nutrition and Human Needs. United States Senate: *Dietary goals for the United States*. Washington, D.C., 1977.

Shaper, A. G. and Marr, J. W. (1977). Dietary recommendations for the community towards the postponement of coronary heart disease. *British Medical Journal*, **1**, 867–871.

Stamler, J. (1978). Lifestyles, major risk factors, proof and public policy. *Circulation*, **58**, 3–19.

Sturdevant, R. A. L., Pearce, M. L. and Dayton, S. (1973). Increased prevalence of cholelithiasis in men ingesting a serum-cholesterol-lowering diet. *New England Journal of Medicine*, **288**, 24–27.

Turpeinen, O. (1979). Effect of cholesterol-lowering diet on mortality from coronary heart disease and other causes. *Circulation*, **59**, 1–7.

Turpeinen, O., Miettinen, M., Karvonen, M. J., Roine, P., Pekkarinen, M., Lehtosuo, E. J. and Alivirta, P. (1968). Dietary prevention of coronary heart disease: long-term experiment. I. Observations on male subjects. *American Journal of Clinical Nutrition*, **21**, 255–276.

Watanabe, N., Gimbel, N. and Johnston, C. G. (1962). Effect of polyunsaturated and saturated fatty acids on the cholesterol holding capacity of human bile. *Archives of Surgery*, **85**, 136–141.

Chapter 15

Disorders of Cholesterol Metabolism: The Hyperlipoproteinaemias

1	CLASSIFICATION	691
2	PRIMARY AND SECONDARY HYPERLIPOPROTEINAEMIA	692
3	FAMILIAL HYPERCHOLESTEROLAEMIA	693
3.1	Definition and historical background	693
3.2	Clinical and pathological features	695
3.2.1	The homozygous state	695
3.2.2	The heterozygous state	699
3.2.3	FH and the risk of IHD	701
3.2.4	Blood chemistry	703
3.3	Genetic basis	705
3.3.1	Evidence for monogenic inheritance	705
3.3.2	Genetic heterogeneity in FH	708
3.3.3	Distribution and frequency of FH	709
3.4	The metabolic basis of FH	710
3.4.1	Metabolism of cholesterol and LDL *in vivo*	710
3.4.2	LDL-receptor deficiency *in vitro*	714
3.4.3	LDL-receptor deficiency *in vivo*	717
3.4.3.1	Probable significance in FH	717
3.4.3.2	Non-receptor-mediated pathways	718
3.4.3.3	Relative contributions of LDL-receptor and alternative pathways	720
3.4.3.4	Receptor deficiency and cholesterol synthesis *in vivo*	724
3.4.3.5	Direct secretion of LDL	724
3.4.3.6	Summary	724
3.4.4	LDL receptors in hypercholesterolaemia not due to FH	726
3.5	Diagnosis	727
3.5.1	General	727
3.5.2	Early diagnosis	729
3.5.3	The differential diagnosis of FH; familial combined hyperlipidaemia	730
3.5.4	Genetic counselling	731
3.6	Treatment	731
3.6.1	Objectives and indications	731

3.6.2	Diet	733
3.6.3	Drugs	734
3.6.4	Ileal bypass	737
3.6.5	Portacaval anastomosis	738
3.6.6	Coronary artery bypass	739
3.6.7	Plasma exchange	739
4	FAMILIAL TYPE III HYPERLIPOPROTEINAEMIA	742
4.1	Definition and historical background	742
4.2	Abnormalities in the plasma lipids and lipoproteins	745
4.2.1	The hyperlipidaemia	745
4.2.2	β-VLDL	746
4.2.3	ApoE proteins	748
4.3	Clinical features	748
4.4	Genetics	749
4.5	The metabolic basis of Type III hyperlipoproteinaemia	752
4.6	Diagnosis	755
4.7	Treatment	756
5	SECONDARY HYPERCHOLESTEROLAEMIA	756
5.1	Introduction	756
5.2	Diabetes	757
5.3	Hypothyroidism	759
5.4	Renal disease	760
5.5	Other causes of secondary hypercholesterolaemia	762
5.6	The hyperlipidaemia of pregnancy	763

Disorders of Cholesterol Metabolism: The Hyperlipoproteinaemias

1 CLASSIFICATION

Hyperlipidaemia refers to a raised plasma concentration of cholesterol or triglyceride or of both (plasma phospholipid concentrations are not usually considered in routine clinical practice). As explained in the previous chapter, the hyperlipidaemias are defined in terms of arbitrary cut-off points, usually at the upper 95th percentile of plasma lipid concentrations in a random sample of subjects from the local population. The hyperlipidaemias may be subdivided into hypercholesterolaemia, hypertriglyceridaemia and 'mixed' hyperlipidaemia, in which the concentrations of both lipids are raised; the term 'combined hyperlipidaemia' is generally used in the particular sense discussed in Section 3.5.3 and is not synonymous with mixed hyperlipidaemia.

Although measurement of plasma total cholesterol and total triglyceride concentrations is essential as a first step in the diagnosis of a plasma lipid disorder, and may in some cases be adequate as a guide to treatment, it cannot give decisive information about the abnormal plasma lipoprotein pattern responsible for the hyperlipidaemia. It is therefore much more informative to consider a raised plasma lipid concentration as the expression of a raised concentration of one or more plasma lipoprotein fractions (hyperlipoproteinaemia), defined in terms of cut-off points, again, at the upper 95th percentile for each lipoprotein.

The *hyperlipoproteinaemias* are classified in accordance with the recommendations of the World Health Organization (Beaumont *et al.*, 1970) into the six types listed in Table 15.1. This system of classification, based on the proposals put forward by Fredrickson *et al.* in 1967, should be regarded as provisional. It does not include abnormal lipoprotein patterns in which the plasma HDL concen-

Table 15.1
Plasma lipoprotein patterns in the hyperlipoproteinaemias classified according to the WHO system of Beaumont et al. (1970), based on the earlier classification of Fredrickson, Levy and Lees (1967)

Type	Raised lipoprotein concentration	Raised lipid concentration
I	Chylomicrons	Triglycerides, cholesterol
IIa	LDL	Cholesterol (triglycerides normal)
IIb	LDL and VLD	Cholesterol, triglycerides
III	β-VLDL ('floating beta')	Triglycerides, cholesterol
IV	VLDL	Triglycerides (cholesterol normal)
V	Chylomicrons, VLDL	Triglycerides, cholesterol

tration is raised, though hyper-α-lipoproteinaemia is now recognized to be an occasional cause of hypercholesterolaemia. Certain abnormal lipoprotein patterns can usually be diagnosed by measurement of the plasma total cholesterol and triglyceride concentrations. Thus, hypercholesterolaemia in the absence of hypertriglyceridaemia is almost always due to the type IIa pattern (hyper-β-lipoproteinaemia), and hypertriglyceridaemia in the absence of hypercholesterolaemia is usually an indication of the type IV pattern. However, measurement of lipid concentrations without further analysis of the plasma often fails to distinguish the type IIb from the type III pattern.

2 PRIMARY AND SECONDARY HYPERLIPOPROTEINAEMIAS

The abnormal lipoprotein patterns shown in Table 15.1 may be primary, or they may be secondary to one or other of the conditions listed in Table 15.2. A comparison of Table 15.2 with Table 15.1 shows that hypercholesterolaemia, with or without hypertriglyceridaemia, can be caused by several relatively common disorders, particularly hypothyroidism, diabetes and chronic renal disease. The primary hyperlipoproteinaemias may be inherited as single-gene (monogenic) disorders, exhibiting typical Mendelian segregation in families, or they may be due to polygenic or environmental factors. In only a small proportion of hyperlipidaemic individuals in the general population—probably in less than 10%—is the abnormality due to a monogenically inherited hyperlipoproteinaemia. In some instances, the presence of disease may bring to light or exacerbate a monogenically determined predisposition to a specific hyperlipoproteinaemia; a good example is the induction of overt familial type III hyperlipoproteinaemia by myxoedema (see Section 5).

Disorders of Cholesterol Metabolism: The Hyperlipoproteinaemias   693

Table 15.2
Some causes of secondary hyperlipoproteinaemias, including hyper-β-lipoproteinaemia

Lipoprotein pattern	Underlying disease
Type I	Pancreatitis; dysglobulinaemias (including systemic lupus erythematosus); uncontrolled diabetes.
Type IIa	Hypothyroidism; Cushing's syndrome; acute intermittent porphyria; diabetes; nephrotic syndrome; renal transplant; obstructive jaundice.
Type IIb	Oral contraceptives; nephrotic syndrome; diabetes; renal transplant.
Type III	Hypothyroidism; systemic lupus erythematosus; diabetic acidosis.
Type IV	Diabetes; oral contraceptives; alcohol consumption; chronic renal failure; renal dialysis; gout; glycogen storage disease (Von Gierke); lipodystrophy; hypopituitarism; dysglobulinaemias; corticosteroid therapy.
Type V	Diabetes; oral contraceptives; nephrotic syndrome; alcohol consumption.
Hyper-α-lipoproteinaemia	Alcohol consumption; oestrogenic oral contraceptives; habitual strenuous exercise; poisoning with chlorinated hydrocarbons.

In this chapter we shall consider hyperlipoproteinaemia types II and III, the two forms of hyperlipidaemia which are of greatest significance from the point of view of the metabolism of cholesterol, with the main emphasis on the familial forms of these disorders. For a full account of the hyperlipidaemias in general, including their clinical and biochemical features, diagnosis and treatment, the reader is referred to Rifkind (1973), Lewis (1976), Schettler *et al.* (1976) and Fredrickson *et al.* (1978). Some of the conditions leading to secondary hypercholesterolaemia are considered in a separate section at the end of this chapter.

3   FAMILIAL HYPERCHOLESTEROLAEMIA

3.1   Definition and historical background

In the majority of individuals whose plasma cholesterol concentration is above the 95th percentile, their hypercholesterolaemia is caused by polygenic or environmental factors, or by a combination of both. In a small proportion, however, the hypercholesterolaemia is due to a monogenically inherited disorder of plasma LDL metabolism generally known as *familial hypercholesterolaemia* (FH).

FH is characterized by an increased concentration of plasma LDL (hyper-β-lipoproteinaemia or type II hyperlipoproteinaemia), xanthomatous deposits in skin, tendons and arterial walls, premature heart disease and a family history of hypercholesterolaemia, xanthomatosis or heart disease. The FH gene is inherited as an autosomal dominant, the disease being equally frequent in males and females, but those with a double dose of the gene (homozygotes) are more severely affected than heterozygotes. Since LDL is the major carrier of the plasma cholesterol, the hyper-β-lipoproteinaemia of FH almost invariably causes hypercholesterolaemia. However, in a very small number of heterozygous FH patients the plasma total cholesterol concentration is below the age-adjusted upper 95th percentile (Fredrickson et al., 1972; Rifkind, 1973), possibly because the increased plasma LDL cholesterol concentration is balanced by a low HDL or VLDL cholesterol concentration. Hence, paradoxically, FH can occur in the absence of hypercholesterolaemia, though very rarely.

The earliest reference to patients with FH is probably that of Fagge (1873), who described a kindred in which skin xanthomas were transmitted through four generations. By the beginning of the present century there had been several reports of a rare familial disease in which affected members of the family developed skin xanthomas, together with atheromatous plaques in the arteries associated with premature heart disease. In retrospect, these were almost certainly suffering from FH. Shortly after the introduction of simple methods for measuring the plasma cholesterol concentration in the 1920's and 1930's it was shown that these patients were hypercholesterolaemic (Thannhauser, 1958). The disease was therefore called *hypercholesterolaemic xanthomatosis* (Thannhauser, 1940), *essential familial hypercholesterolaemia* (Wilkinson et al., 1948), or *familial hypercholesterolaemia*, the name by which it is now generally known. A further step in the characterization of FH was taken by Gofman et al. (1954) when they showed that the plasma abnormality underlying the hypercholesterolaemia of patients with 'xanthoma tendinosum', most of whom must have been FH heterozygotes, is a selective increase in the concentration of the S_f 0-12 lipoprotein fraction (i.e., LDL). With the simplification of methods for distinguishing specific plasma lipoprotein patterns and the introduction of a rational system for classifying the hyperlipoproteinaemias (Fredrickson et al., 1967), the way was open for the clinical and epidemiological study of FH on a world-wide scale. The elucidation of the genetic basis of FH is dealt with in Section 3.3.

With regard to nomenclature, it should be noted that FH is an unsatisfactory term to the extent that hypercholesterolaemia occurs in other monogenically inherited disorders of lipoprotein metabolism besides FH (see Table 15.1) and that hypercholesterolaemia is not invariably present in all carriers of the FH gene. The terms *familial hyper-β-lipoproteinaemia* or *familial type II hyperlipoproteinaemia* reflect more accurately what is distinctive about FH and would on these grounds be preferable, but are perhaps too cumbersome for everyday use.

3.2 Clinical and pathological features

The clinical signs and symptoms of homozygous and heterozygous FH are sufficiently different to merit separate description. In both, the plasma LDL cholesterol concentration is raised at birth, usually to a degree sufficient to cause an increase in plasma total cholesterol concentration.

3.2.1 The homozygous state

In homozygotes, the plasma total cholesterol concentration is usually above 600 mg/100 ml and may occasionally exceed 1100 mg/100 ml. The hypercholesterolaemia is due to increased LDL concentration, the plasma LDL cholesterol concentration being, on average, nearly six times the normal level (Table 15.3). Xanthomas (Gr. *xanthos*, yellow) are present in the tendons and skin in childhood. The most frequent sites for tendinous lesions are the tendo Achilles and the extensor tendons of the hands. The cutaneous lesions may be planar or tuberous. Common sites for the planar lesions are the buttocks, thighs, elbows, knees and webs of fingers (Fig. 15.1). Less commonly, they may occur in the palmar creases and in the natal cleft. Planar xanthomas may be present at birth; in 50 children with homozygous FH studied by Khachadurian (1972) the median age at which skin xanthomas first appeared was four years. Tuberous lesions (Fig. 15.1) are most frequently seen over the elbows and heels and in the peri-

Table 15.3
Lipid concentrations in fasting plasma in FH, with normal values shown for comparison

		Total cholesterol (mg/100 ml)	LDL	VLDL	HDL
Normal [1] (30–40 years)	Male	201	135	19	43
	Female	190	116	14	60
Heterozygous [2] (30–40 years)	Male	369	299	29	40
	Female	365	296	24	48
	All ages, both sexes	340 (250–500)			
Homozygous [3] (1–19 years)		750 (600–1100)	625	19	34

[1], From various sources; [2], Kwiterovich *et al.*, 1974; [3], Fredrickson *et al.*, 1978.

696 The Biology of Cholesterol and Related Steroids

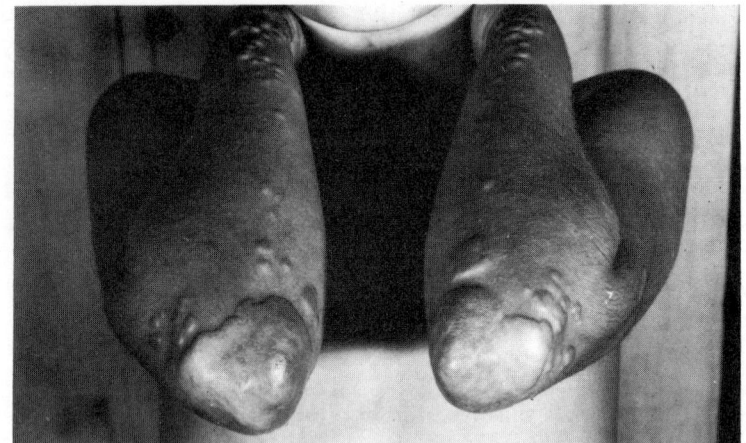

A.

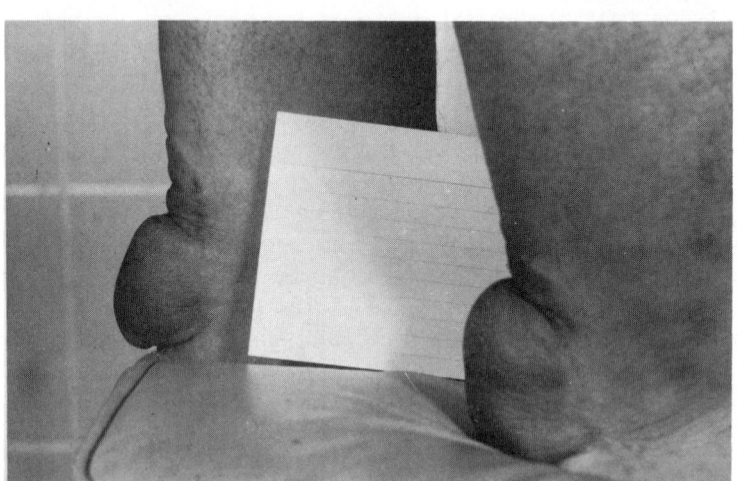

B.

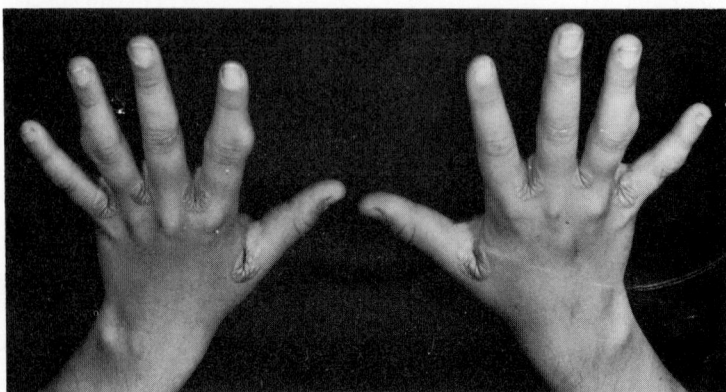

C.

anal region. In young homozygotes, xanthelasmas (cutaneous xanthomas around the eyes) are uncommon, but corneal arcus is present in many children; the presence of arcus in a severely hypercholesterolaemic child is pathognomonic of homozygous FH and is tantamount to a sentence of early death.

Histologically, both tendon and skin xanthomas consist predominantly of accumulations of lipid-filled macrophages (foam-cells) in which the lipid droplets are not surrounded by a membrane (Thannhauser, 1958; Bulkley *et al.*, 1975). In the older lesions and in those in which regression has occurred, the foam cells are surrounded by fibrous tissue and much of the lipid is extracellular. In the more advanced lesions, cholesterol crystals are present in the extracellular lipid. The major lipid in xanthomas is free and esterified cholesterol, with smaller amounts of phospholipid and triglyceride. The fatty-acid composition of the esterified cholesterol differs from that of the plasma esterified cholesterol. Since the cholesterol of xanthomas is thought to be derived from the plasma, probably as LDL cholesteryl ester, this suggests that extensive hydrolysis and re-esterification of the esterified cholesterol takes place within the macrophages.

Ischaemic heart disease usually develops during the first decade of life and progresses to a fatal outcome within a few years. The earliest sign of coronary insufficiency may be a myocardial infarct, sudden death or angina pectoris, usually on exertion but sometimes at rest during an emotional upset. Clinical examination shows electrocardiographic evidence of myocardial ischaemia, often with aortic stenosis and left ventricular hypertrophy. Death from a heart attack may occur in early childhood or, more commonly, in the second decade. Few homozygotes survive beyond the age of 30; in Khachadurian's series the mean age at death was 21 years.

Figure 15.1
Xanthomatous lesions in three patients with familial hypercholesterolaemia in the homozygous form.

A. Plane xanthomas in a 10-year-old girl (A.A-B); plasma total cholesterol concentration, 900–1000 mg/100 ml. Angina was present at age 9 and death from coronary thrombosis occurred at age 11. The parents were first cousins and both had Type II hyperlipoproteinaemia. The genotype of this patient was not ascertained.
B. Tuberous xanthomas in the heels of a 17-year-old girl (P.A.); plasma total cholesterol concentration, 700–750 mg/100 ml. This patient died at age 24 after an operation for aorto-coronary bypass. The parents were first cousins and both had Type II hyperlipoproteinaemia. This patient was receptive-negative (see text).
C. Plane xanthomas in the webs of the fingers of a 12-year-old boy (N.E.); plasma total cholesterol concentration, 600–800 mg/100 ml. The patient died from cardiac failure at age 19. The parents were unrelated. Both had Type II hyperlipoproteinaemia. This patient was receptor-defective (see text).

698 The Biology of Cholesterol and Related Steroids

Post mortem examination shows extensive atherosclerosis of the coronary arteries, with ostial narrowing, and of the thoracic and abdominal aorta. Atherosclerosis may also be present in the pulmonary arteries, the carotids and the larger cerebral arteries. The lesions in the thoracic aorta are especially marked in the basal region adjacent to the aortic valves. When viewed from the luminal aspect, they have the appearance of confluent, xanthoma-like thickenings of the intima extending an inch or more above the aortic orifice (Fig. 15.2). Histologically, these lesions show numerous lipid-filled foam cells, in addition to the other features of typical atheromatous plaques. In some cases, the lesions of the basal aorta extend into the aortic valve cusps, and are accompanied by fibrous thickening and constriction of the aortic root. The unusual intimal thickening at the base of the aorta, characteristic of homozygous FH, may be seen in aortograms during life, as in Fig. 15.3 (see also Stanley *et al.*, 1965).

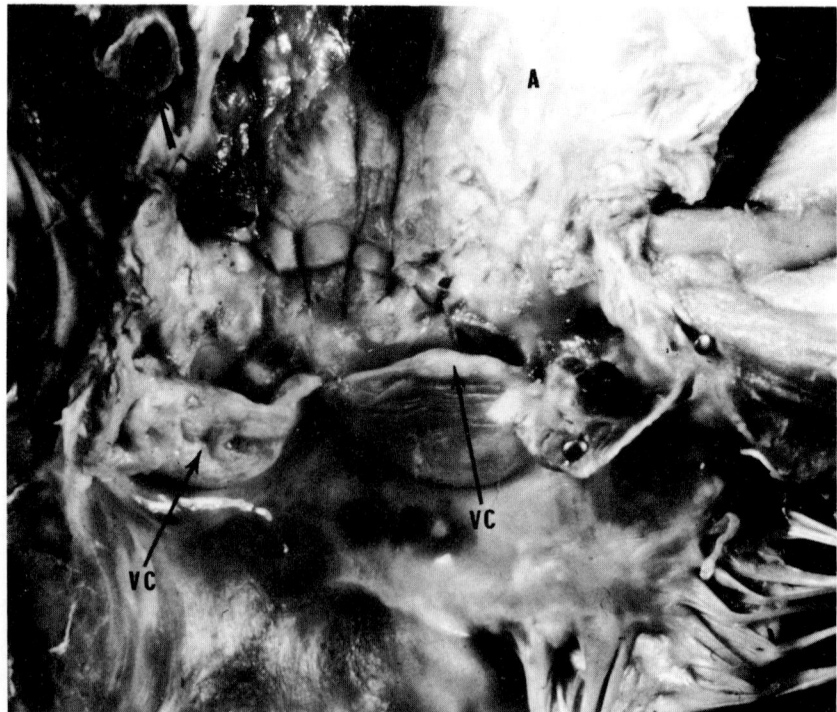

Figure 15.2
Aortic root and valve cusps from the heart of the homozygous FH patient (P.A.) shown in Fig. 15.1B. The luminal surface of the aortic root (A) and parts of the valve cusps (VC) are infiltrated with xanthomatous lipid. Upper arrow shows the cut end of the by-pass tube inserted shortly before the patient's death. Stitches inserted at operation are present above the valve cusps.

According to Khachadurian (1968), about 50% of FH homozygotes experience transient attacks of polyarthritis affecting mainly the knees, ankles and hands. The attacks are accompanied by slight fever and since most FH homozygotes have a precordial systolic murmur and a raised erythrocyte sedimentation rate (Khachadurian and Demirjian, 1967) these attacks are apt to be mistaken for acute rheumatic fever. In the polyarthritis of homozygous FH the antistreptolysin titre is usually normal.

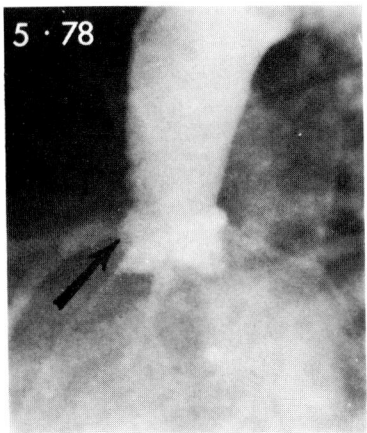

Figure 15.3
Aortogram from a 25-year-old man with FH in the homozygous form, showing the characteristic narrowing and irregularity of the lumen of the aortic root due to infiltration with xanthomatous lipid. Note the right coronary ostial stricture, shown by the arrow. (From Thompson *et al.*, 1980*b*.)

3.2.2 The heterozygous state

In heterozygotes the biochemical and clinical manifestations are much more variable from patient to patient than in homozygotes.

The mean plasma total cholesterol concentration is about twice the age-adjusted mean for normal subjects and is usually within the range 250–500 mg/100 ml. In a group of obligate heterozygotes (parents of homozygotes) studied by Khachadurian (1972) the mean cholesterol concentration was 343 mg/100 ml, compared with 176 mg/100 ml in FH-free subjects from the same population. In a heterozygous man seen at Hammersmith Hospital (Moutafis and Myant, 1969) the plasma cholesterol concentration was about 600 mg/100 ml before treatment and values below the upper 95th percentile are occasionally encountered in patients who, on the basis of their plasma LDL cholesterol concentration and the presence of tendon xanthomas, must be presumed to be carriers of the FH gene. Other aspects of the plasma lipid pattern in heterozygous FH are considered in Section 3.2.4.

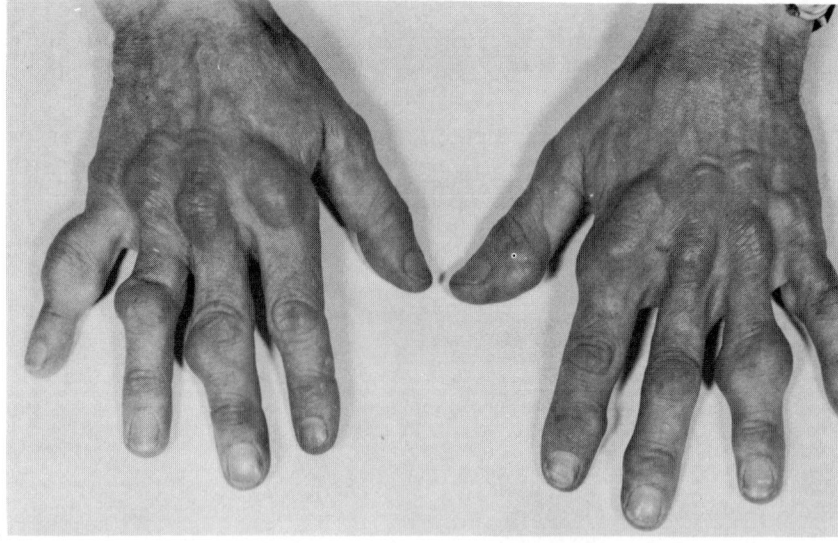

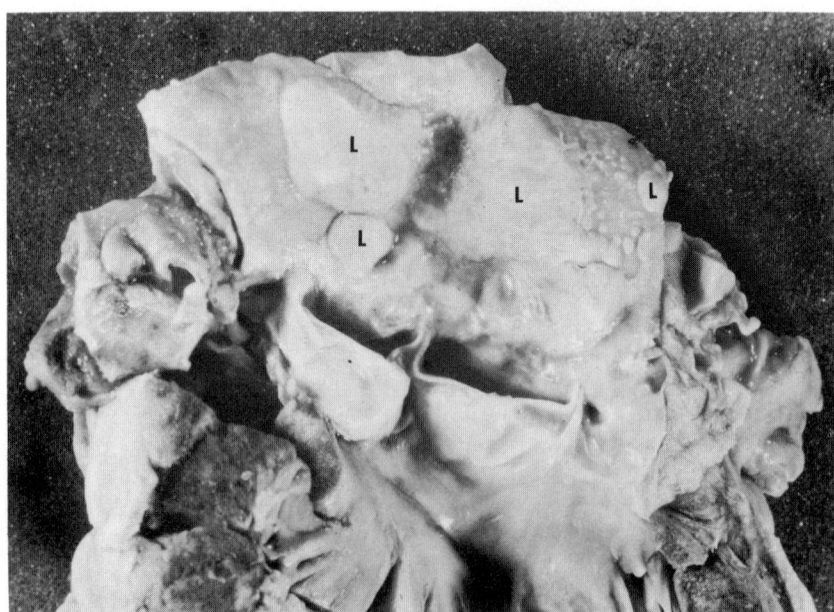

Figure 15.4
A. The hands of a 41-year-old man with FH in the heterozygous form, showing xanthomas in the extensor tendons. X-ray showed small erosions at the base of the proximal phalanx of both index fingers and of the terminal phalanx of the right thumb. Before treament with diet and cholestyramine the plasma total cholesterol concentration was above 600 mg/100 ml. The patient died from coronary thrombosis aged 42. He had a normal daughter.
B. The heart of the same patient, showing subintimal deposits of lipid (L) in the aortic root, without naked-eye involvement of the aortic cusps.

Tendon and skin xanthomas develop in a high proportion of heterozygotes, but at a later age than in homozygotes. Heterozygotes may also develop subperiosteal xanthomas on the tibial tuberosities and the olecranon processes. The tendon xanthomas are similar in distribution to those seen in homozygotes (Fig. 15.4A). The skin lesions are either tuberous xanthomas or xanthelasmas, but it should be borne in mind that xanthelasmas can occur before age 40 in the absence of hyperlipidaemia (Gofman *et al.*, 1954). The planar xanthomas, so characteristic of homozygous state, are seen rarely if ever in heterozygotes. Many adult heterozygotes have corneal arcus, though some normolipidaemic people develop an arcus in their forties or fifties. The recurrent polyarthritis seen in many homozygotes has also been described in heterozygotes (Glueck *et al.*, 1968).

Coronary atherosclerosis with clinical signs of ischaemic heart disease develops sooner or later in most heterozygotes, but at a later age than in homozygotes. The distribution and histological appearance of the atherosclerotic lesions are similar to those in people who have died from IHD without FH; the unusual lesion involving the ascending aorta and aortic valve cusps described in the previous section is uncommon in heterozygotes (Roberts *et al.*, 1973). There may, however, be extensive atheromatous patches in the supravalvular portion of the aorta in the more severely affected heterozygotes; such lesions (Fig. 15.4B) were seen *post mortem* in the patient whose hands are shown in Fig. 15.4A.

The natural history of heterozygous FH has been investigated by examining very large single kindreds, each of which may be assumed to be genetically homogeneous with respect to FH (Harlan *et al.*, 1966; Schrott *et al.*, 1972), or large numbers of patients collected from many different families (Slack, 1969; Stone *et al.*, 1974; Heiberg, 1975). The information obtained from these sources shows that tendon xanthomas are detectable in some patients before the end of the second decade and are present in the majority by the age of 30. Within families, clinical signs of IHD in males tend to be more marked and to appear earlier than in females. Symptoms of IHD may be present before age 30, especially in males, but are usually delayed until the fourth decade. Heterozygous women usually do not develop IHD until the fifth decade and some reach their sixties without clinical evidence of coronary artery disease. In a study of 104 FH heterozygotes, Slack (1969) noted that 51% of the men had had a fatal attack by age 60. By contrast, only 12% of the women had had a myocardial infarct by age 50.

3.2.3 FH and the risk of IHD

The risk of death from IHD in heterozygous FH may be estimated roughly from the cumulative death rates calculated by Slack (1969) and Heiberg (1975). These statistics suggest that the 10-year death rate from IHD in heterozygous men at age 50 is about 30%. This is at least five times the 10-year coronary death rate in middle-aged American men in the general population whose plasma cholesterol concentration is greater than 300 mg/100 ml (Stamler et al., 1970). The higher risk of death from IHD in male heterozygotes than in hypercholesterolaemic men who are not carriers of the FH gene may be due to the fact that the hypercholesterolaemia of FH is present from birth, whereas that in the general population probably develops gradually over the years and is less marked than in many FH patients. Other factors that may contribute to premature atherosclerosis in FH are discussed in Section 3.4.3.

In heterozygous women of a given age, the risk of death from IHD seems to be about the same as that of heterozygous men who are ten years younger. The increased life expectancy in women with FH in the heterozygous form, compared with that in men, is similar to that experienced by women in the general population and is not due to a difference between plasma LDL-cholesterol or total cholesterol concentration in male and female heterozygotes (see Section 3.3).

The contribution of FH to IHD morbidity and mortality in any population will depend, among other things, upon the frequency of the FH gene and the prevalence in the population of risk factors other than FH. Thus, in a country such as Lebanon, where the gene frequency is high and the prevalence of environmental risk factors is low, FH probably makes a greater contribution to IHD than in Western countries. Indirect estimates based on the probable frequency of FH in the population (about 1 in 500 in Britain), together with the risk of coronary death in heterozygotes and the coronary death rate in the general population, suggest that less than 5% of male coronary deaths in Britain are due to FH in the heterozygous state; the contribution of FH in the very rare homozygous state is, of course, negligible. Direct estimates based on ascertainment of FH in unselected members of the general population who have had a heart attack also indicate that in Britain fewer than 5% of all IHD attacks in men are due to FH (Patterson and Slack, 1972). Since environmental risk factors tend to cause IHD relatively late in life, whereas myocardial infarction may occur in male FH heterozygotes in the third and fourth decade, the contribution of FH and IHD is greatest in the younger age groups. Indeed, FH is probably the major cause of myocardial infarction before age 30 in most populations.

It should be noted that although FH is only a minor cause of IHD in the population as a whole, a substantial proportion of men and women with clinical IHD or with angiographic evidence of coronary artery disease have the type II plasma lipoprotein pattern, i.e. a plasma LDL concentration above the upper 95th percentile for the population. Cox *et al.* (1972), for example, found type II hyperlipoproteinaemia in 39% of a group of men who had had a myocardial infarct.

3.2.4 Blood chemistry

Representative values for plasma total- and lipoprotein-cholesterol concentrations in FH are shown in Table 15.3, with normal values included for comparison. Points to note are the similar LDL concentrations in male and female heterozygotes and the low HDL concentration in homozygotes and heterozygous women. A decreased plasma HDL concentration in FH has been reported on several occasions in the United States (see Streja *et al.*, 1978), and in the seven homozygotes seen at Hammersmith Hospital since 1963 the mean HDL-cholesterol concentration was abnormally low (35 ± 12 (SD) mg/100 ml). In a large group of Canadian FH heterozygotes studied by Cagné *et al.* (1979) the plasma HDL concentration was decreased in both sexes and was lower in males than in females. However, in a group of FH patients reported from Japan the plasma HDL concentrations were normal in both heterozygotes and homozygotes (Mabuchi *et al.*, 1979). There is no obvious reason why the underlying defect in FH should lead to a reduced plasma HDL concentration, but there is reason to believe that the negative association between HDL concentration and IHD risk observed in the general population also hold for FH (Streja *et al.*, 1978). It is of considerable interest that mean plasma cholesterol concentrations in FH (heterozygous as well as homozygous) are closely similar in Lebanon and the United States (Khachadurian, 1972; Fredrickson *et al.*, 1978) despite the very different mean cholesterol levels in the two general populations. This indicates that the effect of the FH gene is to swamp the influence of environmental factors on the plasma cholesterol.

The plasma phospholipid concentration is usually raised in FH, a reflection of the increased LDL concentration, but the ratio of esterified to total cholesterol in whole plasma is normal. The plasma triglyceride concentration in FH is usually normal, or may even be at the lower limit of the normal range, particularly in homozygotes. In a few cases, however, there is a moderate increase in triglyceride concentration, with a concomitant increase in VLDL concentration (the type IIb pattern). FH is not associated with any abnormality in plasma glucose or uric acid concentration (Khachadurian, 1972).

The protein of the LDL from FH patients has the same amino acid composition and the same electrophoretic and immunochemical properties as LDL from normal subjects. Moreover, LDL from FH homozygotes is not distinguished from 'normal' LDL by human LDL receptors, since it suppresses HMG-CoA reductase in cultured normal skin fibroblasts at the same concentrations as does normal LDL (Goldstein and Brown, 1973) and is catabolized at the normal rate in the body of a normal subject (Simons *et al.*, 1975). There are, however, several abnormalities in the lipid composition of LDL in FH. These are listed in Table 15.4. Expressed in terms of protein content, there is an increase in free and esterified cholesterol, a decrease in triglyceride and no significant change in the total phospholipid. There is also an increase in the molar ratio of free cholesterol to phospholipid and a change in the composition of the phospholipids, the ratio of lecithin to sphingomyelin being markedly decreased in FH. All these changes are more marked in homozygotes than in heterozygotes. The lipid composition of LDL varies between different normal subjects (Fisher *et al.*, 1972) and within the same subject at different times (Spritz and Mishkel, 1969), especially in response to dietary changes. However, the changes shown in Table 15.4 occur in FH patients irrespective of their diet. The effects of plasma exchange on the lipid composition of LDL in FH suggest that these changes are due to the prolonged stay of LDL molecules in the circulation, resulting from defective catabolism, rather than to a

Table 15.4
The lipid composition of LDL in familial hypercholesterolaemia

Lipid fraction		Normal	Heterozygote	Homozygote
$\dfrac{\text{Total Cholesterol}}{\text{Protein}}$	(W/W)	1.37	1.60	1.91
$\dfrac{\text{Phospholipid}}{\text{Protein}}$	(W/W)	1.00	1.03 (NS)	1.13 (NS)
$\dfrac{\text{Triglyceride}}{\text{Protein}}$	(W/W)	0.28	—	0.10
$\dfrac{\text{Free Cholesterol}}{\text{Phospholipid}}$	(Molar)	0.77	1.03	1.08
$\dfrac{\text{Sphingomyelin}}{\text{Protein}}$	(W/W)	0.26	0.31	0.38
$\dfrac{\text{Lecithin}}{\text{Protein}}$	(W/W)	0.80	0.69	0.62
$\dfrac{\text{Lecithin}}{\text{Sphingomyelin}}$	(Molar)	2.7	2.1	1.4

NS = not significantly different from normal. All other values for FH are significantly different from normal.
Values from Slack and Mills (1970), Shattil *et al.* (1977) and Jadhav and Thompson (1979).

primary abnormality in the newly-formed lipoprotein particles (Jadhav and Thompson, 1979).

The free cholesterol:phospholipid ratio in red-cell membranes is normal in FH but is increased in the membranes of platelets, and this increase is significantly correlated with enhanced sensitivity of the platelets to aggregation by adrenaline and ADP (Shattil et al., 1977).

3.3 Genetic basis

3.3.1 Evidence for monogenic inheritance

We now believe that FH is due to the inheritance of an autosomal dominant mutation at a single gene locus. However, in the absence of a marker by which all carriers of the FH gene can be distinguished from non-carriers, it has been difficult to establish the mode of inheritance of the disease. One reason for this is that in populations with a high mean plasma LDL concentration there is some overlap between the LDL concentration in FH heterozygotes and that in non-carriers of the gene whose LDL concentration is at the upper end of the distribution for the whole population. Hence, there will inevitably be a small proportion of false positive or false negative diagnoses if the diagnosis of FH is based on an arbitrary cut-off point for plasma LDL or plasma total cholesterol concentration. Another difficulty arises from the possibility that FH is genetically heterogeneous in the sense that what appears to be a single clinical disorder may be caused by mutations at different gene loci or by different mutations at the same locus. In other words, 'the FH gene' may, in fact, be several different genes.

In Lebanon, conditions are particularly favourable for studying the genetics of FH. In the first place, the plasma cholesterol concentration in the general population is low by Western standards, so that there is little overlap between the cholesterol levels in non-carriers and carriers of the FH gene. Secondly, the frequency of the FH gene in the Lebanese population is exceptionally high. Thirdly, the incidence of consanguineous marriages, is probably as high as 20% in Lebanon (Dr. V. M. Der Kaloustian, personal communication); hence, an unusually large proportion of carriers of the FH gene have the disease in the unmistakable homozygous form. Finally, since FH in Lebanon is centred mainly in a somewhat isolated and inbred section of the population, it is very probable that all Lebanese patients with FH are carriers of an identical mutation. By taking advantage of this unique opportunity, Khachadurian has been able to establish that FH in Lebanon is a monogenically inherited disorder and that the severe form manifested clinically in childhood represents the homozygous state. Khachadurian (1964, 1972) found that the first-degree relatives of nearly 50 young patients with clinically advanced FH, and with

706 The Biology of Cholesterol and Related Steroids

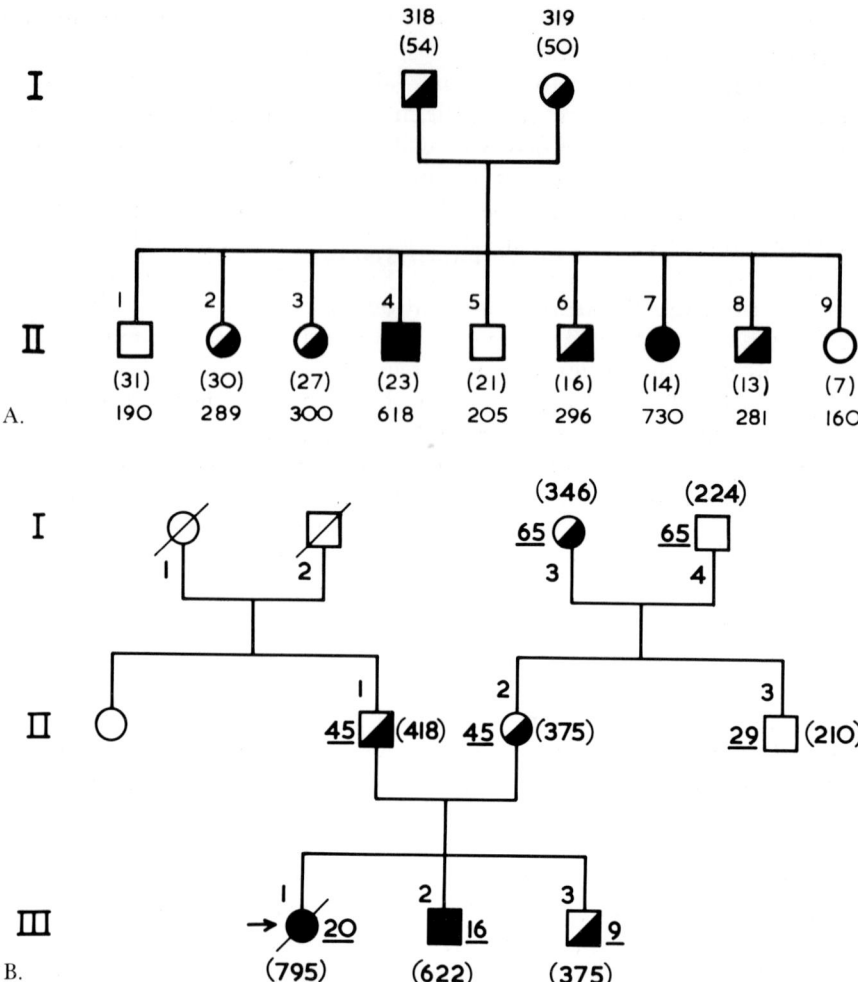

Figure 15.5
A. The pedigree of a Lebanese family illustrating the mode of inheritance of familial hypercholesterolaemia. The parents were first cousins and both are presumed to have FH in the heterozygous form. Subjects II (1), (5) and (9) are presumed normals; subjects II (2), (3), (6) and (8) are presumed heterozygotes; subjects II (4) and (7) had extensive planar and tuberous xanthomas; the father had xanthelasmas. Numbers above parents and below offspring are ages (in parentheses) and plasma total cholesterol concentrations. Modified from Khachadurian (1964).
B. The pedigree of an English family with familial hypercholesterolaemia. White symbols, normal; half black, heterozygous; black, homozygous. The parents of subject II (1) were not examined. Numbers beside symbols are age at examination; numbers in parentheses are plasma total cholesterol concentrations. Subject III (2), the brother of the index patient, is the patient whose aortogram is shown in Fig. 15.3.
(From Myant and Slack (1976), with the permission of Springer-Verlag.)

plasma cholesterol concentrations about four times the mean in normal controls, could be segregated into three groups on the basis of their cholesterol levels: those with levels about four times the normal mean, presumed to be homozygotes; those with levels about twice the normal mean, presumed to be heterozygotes; and those in whom the cholesterol level was within the normal range.

In confirmation of the hypothesis that the index patients were homozygotes, the mean cholesterol level of their parents, all of whom should have been obligate heterozygotes, was about twice the mean value in control subjects. In some of the large families in Khachadurian's study a trimodal distribution of plasma cholesterol concentration could be seen within a single sibship, as in the pedigree shown in Fig. 15.5. Convincing proof that the three modes did indeed represent the homozygous, heterozygous and normal states was obtained by analysis of the sibs of presumptive homozygous index patients, all of whom would, on the single-dominant-gene hypothesis, be the progeny of matings between pairs of heterozygotes. As shown in Table 15.5, the ratio of homozygotes to heterozygotes to normals was very close to the expected Mendelian ratio of 1:2:1.

Using a somewhat different approach, Harlan *et al.* (1966) and Schrott *et al.* (1972) have investigated the inheritance of FH in two very large families comprising several generations, one from North Carolina and the other from Alaska. In view of the geographical isolation of both these families, it may be assumed that within each family all the affected members were carriers of the same mutant gene.

In the family studied by Harlan *et al.* (1966), hypercholesterolaemia (defined as an age- and sex-adjusted plasma cholesterol concentration above the 99th% confidence limit for normal men and women) was inherited as an autosomal dominant trait.

In 92% of the matings from which hypercholesterolaemic progeny were derived, one, and only one, of the putative parents was hypercholesterolaemic, and in the progeny of all matings between hyper-

Table 15.5
Familial hypercholesterolaemia in the sibs of 19 homozygous index patients in Lebanon

	Homozygotes	Heterozygotes	Normal
Observed	17	41	19
Expected	17	34	17

The 'observed' numbers were obtained by removing the 19 homozygous index patients and distributing 9 unexamined sibs among heterozygotes and normals. Taken from Khachadurian (1964, 1972).

cholesterolaemic and normal parents the ratio of affected to unaffected was, again, very close to the Mendelian ratio of 1:1 expected on the assumption that each hypercholesterolaemic parent was heterozygous for a dominant gene. In this study it was clearly established that, contrary to earlier opinions, tendon xanthomas develop in many heterozygotes and are not confined to homozygotes. In the Alaskan family examined by Schrott *et al.* (1972) the distribution of plasma total cholesterol concentrations was bimodal, presumably a consequence of segregation of the values into two distinct populations—those from unaffected individuals (the left-hand population) and those from heterozygotes (the right-hand population). Furthermore, bimodality was evident in the third-degree relatives of the index patient. Taken together, these findings virtually exclude polygenic inheritance, which would give a unimodal distribution displaced to the right of the distribution of values in normal subjects (Carter, 1969). In keeping with inheritance through a single autosomal dominant mutation, analysis of the progeny of all the matings between a normal and a hypercholesterolaemic parent gave the expected 1:1 ratio of normal to hypercholesterolaemic children.

A bimodal distribution of plasma total cholesterol concentration (Nevin and Slack, 1968) or plasma LDL concentration (Fredrickson and Levy, 1972) has also been demonstrated in the first-degree relatives of groups of index patients derived from many families. In the most extensive study of this kind, Kwiterovich *et al.* (1974) observed a bimodal distribution of plasma LDL concentration in the children of 90 matings in which one parent had primary hyper-β-lipoproteinaemia due to FH and the other had not. There were approximately equal numbers of children in the left-hand (unaffected) and right-hand (affected) populations and the mean value of the left-hand population was not significantly different from that of an unrelated group of normal children. These findings demonstrate beyond reasonable doubt that FH was inherited monogenically in the families investigated by Kwiterovich *et al.* (1974).

3.3.2 Genetic heterogeneity in FH

FH is a well-defined disorder with a characteristic clinical picture and plasma lipoprotein pattern. Nevertheless, there is enough variability in the appearance, distribution and age at onset of the xanthomas and in the severity of the accompanying IHD to suggest that the disease is genetically heterogeneous. While it may be assumed that all affected individuals within a given family or within a small isolated population are carrying the same mutant gene, it does not follow that all families with FH are carriers of an identical mutation. There could be different mutant alleles at a single gene locus, giving rise to different defects in the same gene product; this would be analogous to the numerous mutations that occur in the gene coding for the beta chain of haemoglobin. Alternatively, the hyper-β-lipoproteinaemia of FH could be caused by a mutation at any one of a number of genes coding for enzymes or structural proteins, including the apoprotein of LDL, concerned in the regulation of the plasma LDL concentration; a partial analogy to this would be the multiple mutations responsible for the different forms of glycogen storage disease. The study of cultured fibroblasts from FH patients has revealed the existence of three different mutations in homozygotes. All three mutations appear to affect the structure or function of the LDL receptor and it has not yet been shown that the presence of any one of these mutations gives rise to a clinically identifiable form of FH. However, we should continue to keep in mind the possibility that FH can exist in more than one genetically determined clinical form, since this could have important practical consequences. For example, the age at death from IHD in heterozygotes is very variable, ranging from about 30 to more than 70 years, and there is some evidence to suggest that this variability is due partly to the existence of two or more genetically different types of FH, each with a characteristic age at death in the heterozygotes (Heiberg and Slack, 1977). If this turns out to be true, and if we could recognize the two types of FH in heterozygous children, it would be easier to decide whether or not to impose life-long treatment on the patient.

3.3.3 Distribution and frequency of FH

FH is not restricted to any particular race or geographical region. It has been reported in most European countries and in Africa, the Middle East, America, Asia and Australia. A recent report suggests that its frequency in Japan is comparable with that in the United States (Mabuchi *et al.*, 1978). In the absence of a biochemical or clinical marker for identifying heterozygotes, the frequency of carriers in the general population cannot be estimated directly. In the Framingham study of an unbiased sample of 5127 adults from the general population (Kannel *et al.*, 1971), six people with hyper-cholesterolaemia and xanthomatosis were detected, suggesting a minimum heterozygote frequency of about 1:850. However, this is likely to be an underestimate of the true frequency in Framingham, since many adult heterozygotes do not have clinically detectable xanthomas.

Carter *et al.* (1971), using the Hardy-Weinberg equation relating the proportion of homozygotes to heterozygotes in a population in which mating is random, attempted to deduce the frequency of FH heterozygotes in England and Wales on the assumption that there were 50 homozygotes in the whole population. They concluded that the carrier frequency was not greater than 1:200. A more recent calculation, based on the more realistic assumption that there are far fewer than 50 homozygotes in England and Wales, suggests that the carrier frequency is unlikely to be higher than 1:500 (Myant, 1977). This agrees with the conclusion of Goldstein *et al.* (1973) that the minimal heterozygote frequency in Caucasians in the United States is 1:500. In Lebanon, the frequency of heterozygotes may be as high as 1:80 (Myant and Slack, 1976). There is reason to believe that the mutant gene causing FH in Lebanon arose several centuries ago (Myant and Slack, 1976). The FH gene present in the family studied by Harlan *et al.* (1966) is known to have been taken to the United States from Harrogate (England) in 1723 by two affected brothers.

If the frequency of FH heterozygotes in Britain and the United States is, in fact, only about 1:500, it follows that less than 5% of all individuals with the type II lipoprotein pattern (defined in terms of the upper 95th percentile of plasma LDL concentrations) are carriers of the FH gene.

3.4 The metabolic basis of FH

3.4.1 Metabolism of cholesterol and LDL *in vivo*

Numerous observations on cholesterol synthesis and turnover in FH have been made on the supposition that the underlying defect is oversynthesis of cholesterol, but the results have not been consistent, nor have they done much to increase our understanding of the fundamental metabolic abnormality in this disease. In adults with FH in the heterozygous or homozygous form, synthesis in the whole body estimated by the isotopic balance or sterol balance techniques has usually been within the normal range (Lewis and Myant, 1967; Grundy and Ahrens, 1969) or has even been subnormal (Miettinen, 1970). In two homozygous children (Lewis and Myant, 1967; Bilheimer *et al.*, 1975), whole-body synthesis appeared to be increased, though age-matched controls were not available for comparison. On the other hand, in a group of FH children investigated by Martin and Nestel (1979), including a five-year-old homozygote, whole-body synthesis was not significantly higher than that in age-matched normal children. In one homozygous child investigated by Moutafis and Myant (Myant, 1970) and in a group of homozygous children studied by Khachadurian (1969), incorporation of acetate into cholesterol by liver biopsies was increased or was not susceptible to the normal suppression induced by cholesterol feeding. However, Brown *et al.* (1975) found no increase in cholesterol synthesis in skin biopsies from a homozygote. In the light of present knowledge, it seems likely that the absence of a consistent increase in cholesterol synthesis in FH patients, despite the presence of what we now know to be defective regulation of cholesterol synthesis in peripheral tissues *in vitro*, is due to the achievement *in vivo* of a compensated state in which cholesterol synthesis is maintained at the normal level by a raised plasma LDL concentration (see Myant, 1970).

Miettinen *et al.* (1967) have described a family of FH heterozygotes in whom bile-acid synthesis was significantly lower than in control subjects. Others have also reported a diminished rate of synthesis of cholic acid in patients with the type IIa plasma lipoprotein pattern (Einarsson *et al.*, 1974), some of whom were probably heterozygous carriers of the FH gene. However, it seems very unlikely that a reduced capacity for converting cholesterol into bile acids is the cause of the hypercholesterolaemia of FH, since the daily faecal output of total bile acids in homozygotes is normal and, moreover, is stimulated to the normal extent by administration of cholestyramine (Moutafis *et al.*, 1977).

More relevant clues to the metabolic defect in FH have been provided by studies of the metabolism of LDL in heterozygotes and homozygotes. Using the methods described in Chapter 11 (Section 3.6), Langer *et al.* (1972) showed that the fractional catabolic rate of autologous LDL, labelled with ^{125}I in the protein component, is lower in FH heterozygotes than in normal controls. They also showed that labelled LDL from normal subjects and from FH patients is metabolized equally slowly when injected intravenously into the same FH patient. These results suggested that the increased plasma LDL concentration in FH is due to defective catabolism of LDL and that the defect lies in the catabolic mechanism itself, rather than in any abnormality in the LDL of FH patients. These observations were confirmed and extended to homozygotes by Simons *et al.* (1975), who showed that the fractional catabolic rate of autologous LDL in homozygotes is less than half that in normal controls. They also showed that the rate of synthesis of LDL-apoB, determined from the absolute rate of catabolism under steady-state conditions, was considerably increased in homozygous FH.

The main points from these investigations of LDL metabolism in heterozygotes and homozygotes are summarized in Table 15.6. In normal subjects, about half the circulating pool of LDL-apoB is catabolized each day and the half-life of the log-linear phase of the plasma radioactivity curve ($t_{\frac{1}{2}}$) is about 3 days. The fractional catabolic rate decreases and the $t_{\frac{1}{2}}$ increases progressively from normals, to heterozygotes, to homozygotes. The rate of synthesis of LDL-apoB (assumed to be equal to the absolute rate of catabolism) was about the same in the normals and the heterozygotes shown in Table 15.6, but in some other studies (for example, Packard *et al.*, 1976), LDL-apoB synthesis was significantly increased in heterozygotes. By means of the cross-over experiment shown in Fig. 15.6, Simons *et al.* (1975) showed conclusively that the LDL in the plasma of FH

Table 15.6
Metabolism of labelled apoB in LDL in normal subjects and in patients with heterozygous and homozygous FH

Subjects	FCR (fraction/day)	$T_{\frac{1}{2}}$ (days)	Absolute catabolic rate (mg/kg/day)
Normal	0.497 ± 0.90 (SD)	2.9 ± 0.1	17.9 ± 3.3
Heterozygote	0.237 ± 0.04	4.7 ± 0.04	15.0 ± 1.7
Homozygote	0.200 ± 0.013	6.6 ± 0.2	39.3 ± 2.1

FCR, fractional catabolic rate of the plasma LDL-apoB; $T_{\frac{1}{2}}$, half-life of log-linear phase of plasma radioactivity curve; catabolic rate calculated from the FCR and the mass of LDL-apoB in the whole circulation. Values for normals and homozygotes are taken from Simons *et al.* (1975); values for heterozygotes are from Langer *et al.* (1972).

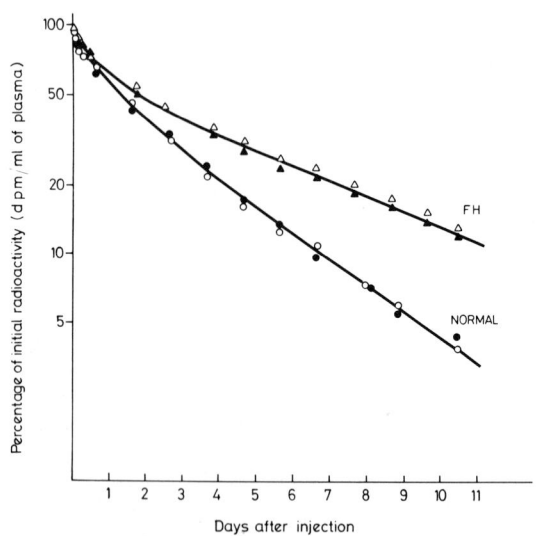

Figure 15.6
Turnover of LDL-apoB in a patient with FH in the homozygous form (upper curve) and in a normal subject (lower curve). Each recipient was given an intravenous injection of a mixture of ^{125}I-labelled LDL from the patient (▲ in upper curve, ● in lower curve) and ^{131}I-labelled LDL from a normal donor (△ in upper curve, ○ in lower curve). Note that the fractional rate of turnover of both samples was lower in the patient than in the normal subject, and that the two samples of LDL behaved identically in the patient and in the normal subject. The FH donor of LDL was the receptor-negative patient whose aorta is shown in Fig. 15.2. (Modified from Reichl *et al.* (1974).)

patients is biologically normal, as suggested earlier by Langer et al. (1972). A mixture of ^{125}I-labelled LDL prepared from a homozygote and ^{131}I-labelled LDL from a normal donor was injected into the homozygote and into a normal subject. The LDL samples from the two sources behaved identically in the bodies of both subjects, showing that the LDL from the homozygote was not distinguished from 'normal' LDL by the tissues of the homozygote or of the normal subject. Thus, it would appear that the abnormal lipid composition of the plasma LDL in FH shown in Table 15.4 does not affect its uptake and catabolism by the tissues *in vivo*. In agreement with this, cultured human fibroblasts respond normally to LDL from homozygotes (see Section 3.2.4).

It was pointed out above that the low fractional catabolic rate of LDL in patients with FH suggests the presence of a defect in the mechanism by which LDL-apoB is catabolized. However, the presence of a very high rate of synthesis of LDL-apoB in homozygotes and of a small increase in some heterozygotes raises the alternative possibility that the low fractional catabolic rate is due to saturation of a normal catabolic mechanism by an increased plasma pool of LDL. If this were so, the fractional catabolic rate should increase when the plasma LDL concentration is lowered by a method that does not itself affect the catabolic mechanism. It is possible to bring about a marked fall in plasma LDL concentration in normal subjects or patients with FH by means of continuous plasma exchange with a plasma fraction containing no cholesterol. The fractional catabolic rate of LDL-apoB can then be determined at different plasma LDL concentrations while the plasma concentration is returning to the pre-exchange level. Using this approach, Thompson *et al.* (1977) showed that the fractional catabolic rate in homozygotes remains abnormally low at plasma LDL concentrations close to the normal range. This indicates clearly that in FH there is a defect in the mechanism for catabolizing LDL-apoB, as well as an increase in LDL synthesis.

The increased synthesis of LDL-apoB in FH is due to direct secretion of pre-formed LDL into the circulation, in addition to that formed by the normal route from VLDL *via* IDL. The evidence for this is twofold. First, the absolute rate of turnover of LDL-apoB in homozygotes is greater than that of VLDL-apoB (Soutar *et al.*, 1977). Second, the relation between the plasma specific activity-time curves for IDL-apoB and LDL-apoB after intravenous injections of radioiodine-labelled VLDL shows that a considerable fraction of the LDL-apoB in the circulation of FH homozygotes is derived from a source other than circulating VLDL (Soutar *et al.*, 1979).

In summary, the metabolic features of FH that have to be explained in terms of a single gene mutation are as follows:

(1) Hypercholesterolaemia due to a selective increase in plasma LDL concentration.
(2) A defect in the mechanism by which LDL-apoB is catabolized in the body, more marked in homozygotes than in heterozygotes.
(3) The absence of any biological abnormality in LDL.
(4) A normal rate of cholesterol synthesis in the whole body, except possibly in some homozygous children, in whom there may be increased synthesis.
(5) An increase in the rate of synthesis of LDL-apoB in homozygotes, accompanied by the direct secretion of pre-formed LDL into the circulation.

Most of these features of FH can be adequately explained in terms of defective or absent LDL receptors. However, as discussed below, it is difficult to predict all the consequences of a receptor defect *in vivo* in the absence of definitive information about the quantitative contribution of receptor-mediated uptake of LDL to the catabolism of LDL in the normal body.

3.4.2 LDL-receptor deficiency *in vitro*

What is almost certainly the primary genetic lesion in FH has been elucidated by biochemical and electron-microscopic studies of cultured cells from normal subjects and FH patients (see Goldstein and Brown, 1977a, 1978). As discussed in Chapter 9, Section 3, cultured skin fibroblasts from normal subjects develop specific surface receptors with high affinity for LDL when incubated in a lipoprotein-free medium. Under similar conditions, cultured fibroblasts from patients with FH diagnosed clinically as homozygous behave in one of three ways with respect to LDL-receptor formation (Goldstein and Brown, 1979).

(1) Cells from the homozygotes from some families develop no receptors and are therefore unable to bind any LDL at all by the specific mechanism; homozygotes possessing these cells are termed *receptor-negative* and the mutant allele coding for the non-functional receptor is designated R^{b^o}, the normal allele being designated R^{b^+}. Fibroblasts from receptor-negative homozygotes, whose genotype is R^{b^o}/R^{b^o}, show no binding of ferritin-labelled LDL at the coated pits when examined by electron microscopy. Absence of LDL receptors has also been demonstrated in cultured arterial smooth-muscle cells and in suspension cultures of lymphocytes from these homozygotes.

(2) The cells from homozygotes from some other families are capable of binding LDL, but only 5–10% of the amount bound by normal fibroblasts. The cells from these homozygotes, termed *receptor-defective*, are thought to develop abnormal receptors with markedly

diminished capacity for high-affinity binding of LDL. The mutant allele coding for the defective receptor is designated R^{b-}.

(3) A third class of homozygote was identified by Goldstein et al. (1977b) in a family in which the index patient, clinically a homozygote, is a genetic compound with two different abnormal alleles at the FH gene locus (see Chapter 8, Section 3.2). One allele ($R^{b+,i0}$) codes for a receptor that can bind LDL but cannot internalize it and the other allele is the R^{b0} mutation described above. The genotype of this patient is therefore $R^{b+,i0}/R^{b0}$. The fibroblasts of this patient are functionally equivalent to those of the R^{b0}/R^{b0} genotype, since they cannot internalize any LDL by the receptor mechanism.

There is as yet no way of distinguishing clinically between the three types of homozygote.

Cultured fibroblasts from heterozygotes develop half the normal number of receptors per cell when they are incubated in a lipoprotein-free medium. The receptors on the fibroblasts of heterozygotes have a normal affinity for LDL and are therefore likely to be the product of the normal allele at the FH gene locus (R^{b+}).

The fibroblasts from FH patients behave in culture in a way that would be predicted from the function of the normal LDL receptor. As shown in Fig. 15.7, the cells from receptor-negative homozygotes show no high-affinity binding and degradation of LDL, and no suppression of HMG-CoA reductase activity or activation of cholesterol esterification when LDL is added to the culture medium. Some LDL is taken up and degraded, but only to a small extent by the low-affinity process discussed in Chapter 9. Since HMG-CoA reductase activity is not suppressed by LDL, receptor-negative fibroblasts in culture synthesize cholesterol at about 50 times the normal rate when LDL is present in the medium. The cells from receptor-defective homozygotes show partial suppression of HMG-CoA reductase activity and detectable activation of cholesterol esterification when LDL is added to the medium. When the cells from heterozygotes are incubated with LDL at a concentration high enough to saturate all the receptors, LDL is degraded at only about half the normal rate. At concentrations below saturation, the interaction between LDL particles and the receptors is such that in the presence of a given LDL concentration in the medium, cells from heterozygotes bind and degrade the same amount of LDL as normal cells incubated in the presence of half the given concentration.

Since the HMG-CoA reductase and ACAT of FH fibroblasts in culture respond normally to intracellular cholesterol or its analogues, cholesterol synthesis is suppressed and cholesterol esterification is stimulated by cholesterol or oxygenated sterols added to the medium in a form in which they can enter the cells by a pathway not mediated

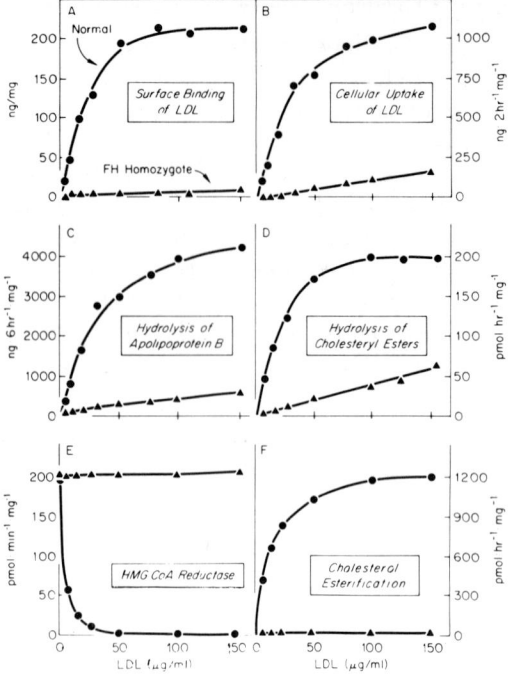

Figure 15.7
Interactions between LDL and LDL-receptors on cultured fibroblasts from a normal subject (●) and a patient with familial hypercholesterolaemia in the homozygous form (▲). After culture for 6 days in a medium containing fetal calf serum, the medium was replaced by medium containing 10% human lipoprotein-deficient serum to induce receptor formation. On day 8 the medium was replaced with 2 ml of fresh medium containing (A to C) ^{125}I-labelled LDL, (D) [^{3}H]cholesteryl linoleate-labelled LDL or (E to F) unlabelled LDL. After incubation with LDL at 37 °C for 2 hours (A and B) or for 6 hours (C to F), the indicated measurements were made.

A and B: Surface binding and cellular uptake of ^{125}I-labelled LDL. Each monolayer was washed six times at 4 °C with an albumin-containing buffer, and a solution containing heparin (10 mg/ml) was added to each dish. The dishes were then incubated at 4 °C for 1 hour. The heparin-containing medium was removed and the amount of ^{125}I-labelled LDL bound to cell surfaces (and hence removable by heparin) was determined. The cells were dissolved in 0.1N NaOH and the amount of ^{125}I-labelled LDL that had entered the cells was determined.

C: Proteolytic hydrolysis of ^{125}I-labelled LDL. The medium was assayed for ^{125}I-labelled trichloroacetic-acid-soluble degradative products formed during the 6-hour incubation.

D: Hydrolysis of LDL-cholesteryl esters. The cellular content of unesterified [^{3}H]cholesterol formed by the hydrolysis of [^{3}H]cholesteryl linoleate-labelled LDL was measured after separation of free from esterified cellular cholesterol.

E: Suppression of HMG-CoA reductase activity. Cells were harvested and enzyme activity determined in detergent-solubilized extracts.

F: Stimulation of cholesteryl [^{14}C]oleate formation, determined from the incorporation of [1-^{14}C]oleate during a 1-hour incubation at 37 °C.

The horizontal axis shows the concentration of LDL (mg of LDL protein/ml of incubation medium) during the experimental incubations on day 8. (From Brown and Goldstein (1976), with the permission of the authors.)

by LDL receptors. Thus, FH cells respond in the same way as do normal cells to ethanolic solutions of cholesterol or oxysterols such as 25-hydroxycholesterol, and to cationized LDL.

3.4.3 LDL-receptor deficiency *in vivo*
3.4.3.1 Probable significance in FH.
While it seems highly probable that the LDL receptor is the product of the normal homologue of the FH gene (the R^{b+} allele), this has yet to be proved. We should therefore keep in mind the possibility, however remote, that the normal allele at the FH locus codes for a protein other than the receptor, for example, a protein component of the plasma membrane that is required for the normal functioning of the receptor and, perhaps, for the normal expression of other properties of the cell surface. In this case, some of the manifestations of FH could be due to abnormalities in a cell-surface component other than the receptor itself. However, in the following discussion I shall assume that the LDL receptor is specified by the R^{b+} allele and, hence, that each and every one of the clinical and biochemical characteristics of FH is explicable ultimately in terms of a deficiency of normal receptors.

A defect in a specific mechanism for catabolizing LDL, revealed by the behaviour of FH cells in culture, provides a very compelling explanation for the selective increase in plasma LDL concentration and the diminished fractional catabolic rate of LDL in FH patients. However, any attempt to transpose the results of observations on cultured cells to cells *in vivo* raises a number of questions to which we have no clear answers. As we saw in Chapter 9, we do not know the extent to which LDL receptors are developed in the cells of the living body. Nor do we know, if receptors are functional *in vivo*, which tissues contribute to receptor-mediated uptake and catabolism of LDL in man; because of the importance of the liver as the final pathway for the exit of plasma cholesterol from the body, it is particularly unfortunate that we cannot yet say whether or not LDL receptors are present on the hepatocytes of human liver.

In view of the presence of a specific defect in the mechanism for catabolizing LDL in FH, it is hard to believe that the receptor pathway does not contribute to LDL catabolism in the normal body. On the other hand, if cells *in vivo* behave like cells in culture with respect to their regulation of receptor activity, one would expect that, at the relatively high concentrations of LDL in human plasma and interstitial fluid, only a small fraction of the maximum number of LDL receptors would be formed under physiological conditions. In agreement with this, lymphocytes freshly isolated from the blood show little or no receptor activity, although they are capable of developing receptors when incubated in a lipoprotein-free medium. For this reason, and for other reasons discussed below, it does not seem likely that the receptor pathway is the sole route for LDL catabolism in the whole body.

3.4.3.2 Non-receptor-mediated pathways.

In FH heterozygotes the absolute rate of catabolism of LDL is normal or increased, although the cells of these patients can form only half the normal number of receptors when maximally expressed. As discussed in Section 3.4.2, at LDL concentrations below saturation, the number of receptors occupied by LDL particles per cell should be normal if the number of binding sites decreases to half-normal but the LDL level is twice normal. Thus, in the presence of a two-fold increase in LDL concentration and a half-normal number of receptors if FH heterozygotes it would be possible to account for a normal absolute catabolic rate, on the assumption that LDL receptors are not saturated *in vivo*. (In the presence of a saturating concentration of LDL, when essentially all the binding sites would be occupied in both normal subjects and FH heterozygotes, LDL-receptor-mediated catabolism in the heterozygotes could not exceed half that in the normals.) However, even if this assumption were valid, we still have to explain why the absolute catabolic rate of LDL in many heterozygotes is considerably greater than that in normal subjects. The discrepancy between the observed rate of catabolism of LDL and the rate attributable to receptor-mediated catabolism is even greater in FH homozygotes, since the absolute rate of catabolism in these patients is at least twice the normal, despite the fact that the cells of receptor-negative homozygotes are almost completely deficient in LDL receptors. Thus, we are driven to the conclusion that the body possesses highly effective mechanisms for catabolizing LDL other than by receptor-mediated uptake. Goldstein and Brown (1977b) have called these alternative routes for LDL catabolism the 'scavenger pathway', on the supposition that it involves macrophages and other phagocytic cells, possibly including arterial smooth-muscle cells.

In principle, non-receptor pathways functioning *in vivo* could include the non-specific, low-affinity uptake and degradation exhibited by cells that also use the receptor-mediated pathway. However, Goldstein *et al.* (1979) have shown that various cells of the macrophage class, including human monocytes, have high-affinity receptors for LDL modified by acetylation but do not possess classical LDL receptors. Thus, it is possible that the non-receptor pathway for LDL catabolism *in vivo* includes both functionally and morphologically distinct entities, the latter involving cell types that catabolize LDL that has been modified in some way during its stay in the plasma or interstitial fluids. It is of considerable interest that the receptors concerned in the uptake and internalization of modified LDL are not subject to regulation. That is to say, they are not switched off when cholesterol accumulates within the cells. Hence, they may continue to accumulate lipoprotein cholesterol *in vitro* until they become foam cells.

There is no evidence that acetylated LDL is, in fact, a normal metabolite of the native LDL present in the circulation. However, LDL fractions whose amino acid composition differs from that of the LDL in the circulation (Hollander *et al.*, 1979), or which are more electronegative than native LDL (Hoff *et al.*, 1979), have been isolated from human aortic wall. Fogelman *et al.* (1980) have also shown that when platelets aggregate in the presence of native LDL, the LDL is converted into an electronegative malondialdehyde-containing product that is readily taken up and internalized by human macrophages in culture.

These observations raise the possibility that modified LDL particles, though not detectable in the circulation, accumulate locally in regions of the arterial intima and are taken up by intimal macrophages by a pathway other than the LDL-receptor pathway, eventually giving rise to foam cells. This would go some way towards reconciling the belief that the foam cells of atherosclerotic lesions derive most of their cholesterol from the plasma LDL with the fact that native LDL, even at high concentrations, will not convert cells in culture into foam cells. However, this suggestion raises the difficulty that the foam cells that are so conspicuous a feature of early lesions are generally held to be derived from smooth-muscle cells (see Chapter 13, Section 2.2), cells which, at least in culture, take up native LDL by the self-limiting LDL-receptor mediated pathway and do not 'recognize' LDL particles that have been made electronegative by acetylation or other means. At present, there seems to be no satisfactory way of resolving this dilemma. Perhaps the view that the foam cells of atherosclerotic lesions are predominantly myogenic should be reconsidered; if they are not derived from smooth-muscle cells this would explain why foam cells develop in the wall of the arteries of FH homozygotes, whose smooth-muscle cells have no LDL receptors. Alternatively, it may turn out that native LDL gives rise to a modified particle (perhaps similar to the *cationized* LDL described by Goldstein *et al.*, 1977a) that can deposit enough lipid within smooth-muscle cells to convert them into foam cells *in vivo*. What does seem clear is that the identification of the LDL species responsible for depositing cholesterol within foam cells in the arterial wall, the nature of these cells and the mechanism by which the lipoprotein is taken up and internalized are central to our understanding of the cellular phase of the development of atherosclerotic lesions.

3.4.3.3 Relative contributions of LDL-receptor and alternative pathways.
The existence of pathways other than the LDL-receptor pathway for the catabolism of LDL *in vivo*, which we may call collectively 'the alternative pathway', raises the question as to the relative contributions of the two routes to total LDL catabolism in the living body under different conditions. In FH homozygotes, 0.15 to 0.20 of the circulating LDL is catabolized per day (Reichl *et al.*, 1974; Bilheimer *et al.*, 1975), whereas normal subjects catabolize about 0.45 per day. On the assumption that the fraction of the circulating LDL catabolized daily by homozygotes (taken as 0.15) represents catabolism by the alternative pathway and that a similar fraction is catabolized by the alternative pathway in normal subjects, Goldstein and Brown (1977b) have argued that in normal subjects the fraction catabolized daily by the LDL-receptor pathway is about 0.3 (0.45–0.15). On this argument, the receptor pathway accounts for about two thirds of the total LDL catabolized in the body of a normal subject. By the same argument, the receptor pathway accounts for about two fifths of the total catabolism in FH heterozygotes (in whom the fractional catabolic rate averages about 0.25/day). A more direct estimate of the magnitude of the LDL-receptor pathway has been attempted by comparing the rate of catabolism *in vivo* of labelled native LDL with that of labelled LDL in which the recognition sites on LDL apoB have been selectively blocked. As discussed in Chapter 9 (Section 3.2), the binding of LDL to the LDL receptors on cultured fibroblasts can be prevented by blocking a limited number of the arginine or lysine residues in apoB- or apoE-containing lipoproteins. Mahley *et al.* (1980) have shown that the rate of catabolism of arginine- or lysine-modified lipoproteins is slower than that of the unmodified native lipoproteins when they are injected intravenously into monkeys and they have concluded that the slower rate of catabolism of the modified lipoproteins is due to deletion of the LDL-receptor pathway.

This approach has been extended to normal human subjects and FH heterozygotes by Shepherd *et al.* (1979) and to receptor-defective FH homozygotes by Thompson *et al.* (1980b). In both investigations the catabolism of autologous ^{125}I-labelled native LDL was compared with that of autologous ^{131}I-labelled LDL treated with 1,2-cyclohexanedione (CHD) to block arginine residues. The results are shown in Figs. 15.8 and 15.9 and are summarized in Table 15.7. In the normal subjects the receptor pathway contributed an average of 32% to the total catabolism of LDL. In the heterozygotes, the absolute catabolic rate of native LDL was increased, but the increase was due entirely to an increase in the rate of catabolism by the alternative pathway. There was a slight decrease in the rate of catabolism by the receptor pathway but this was not statistically significant. In the homozygote, the rate of catabolism of native LDL was doubled, due, again, to an increase in the amount catabolized by the alternative pathway. The rate of catabolism of CHD-LDL was less than that of native LDL (Fig. 15.9), indicating that the capacity for forming a small number of receptors on the cells of this patient may have made a significant contribution to LDL catabolism. In receptor-negative FH homozygotes there should be no difference between the rates of catabolism of native and CHD-treated LDL provided that (1) the reduced rate of catabolism of CHD-LDL in normal subjects is due solely to blocking of receptor-recognition sites by the CHD treatment and (2) CHD-LDL is not distinguished from normal LDL, in either its native or modified form, by the tissues responsible for the alternative pathway.

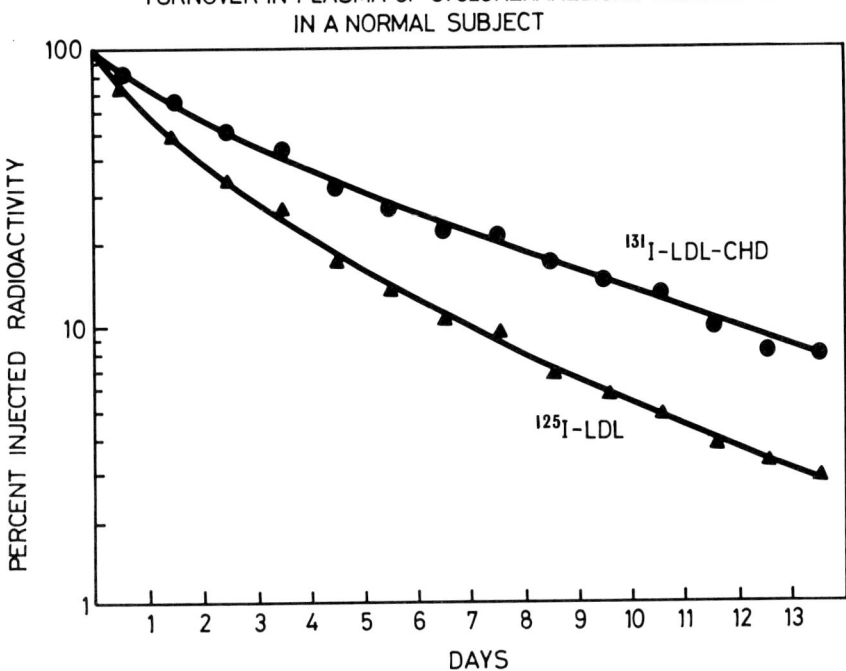

Figure 15.8
The effect of blocking arginine residues of LDL-apoB upon the rate of catabolism of LDL-apoB in a normal human subject. The lower curve (▲) shows the fall in plasma radioactivity after an intravenous injection of ^{125}I-labelled LDL. The upper curve (●) shows the plasma radioactivity curve after intravenous injection of ^{131}I-labelled LDL treated with cyclohexanedione. In this subject, the absolute catabolic rate of the native LDL was 10.9 mg/kg/day and that of the modified LDL was 6.5 mg/kg/day. Therefore the estimated rate of catabolism by the receptor pathway was 4.4 mg/kg/day. (From Shepherd *et al.* (1979), with the permission of the authors.)

The use of autologous LDL in which amino acids required for recognition of LDL receptors have been blocked clearly provides a powerful technique for the quantitative study of the LDL-receptor pathway *in vivo* under a wide variety of conditions. With this technique it should be possible to assess receptor function in the whole body in conditions in which cholesterol metabolism is altered, either in diseases or as a consequence of treatment with drugs or dietary modification. (See Section 3.4.4 for an example of this approach.) It should be noted, however, that the study of the catabolism of modified LDL in the human body cannot, by itself, provide an answer to the important question of the sites of LDL catabolism by the LDL-receptor pathway.

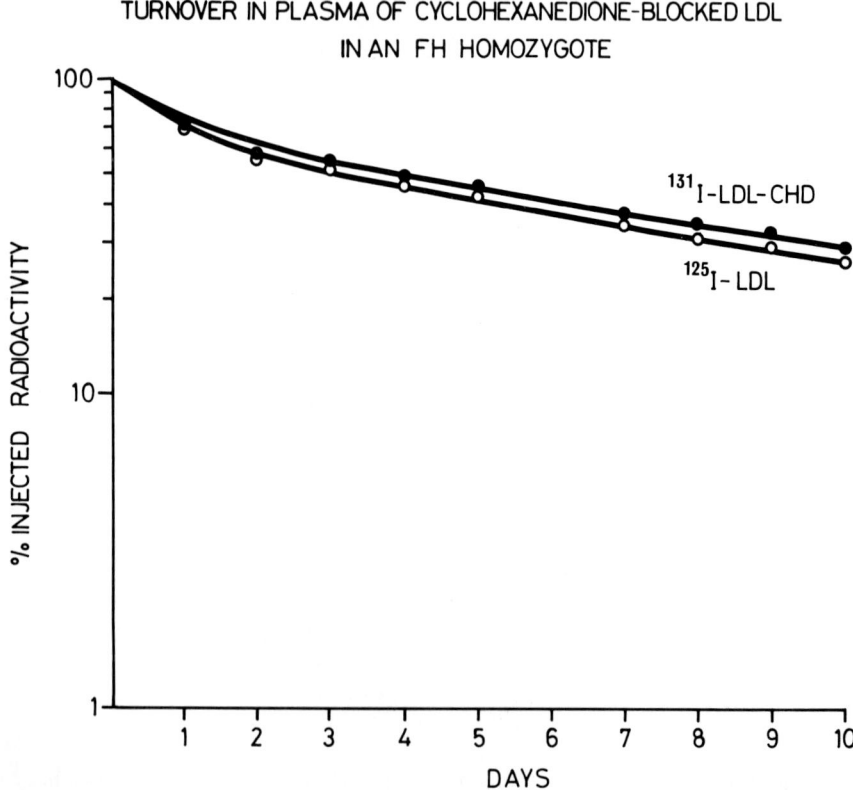

Figure 15.9
The effect of blocking arginine residues of LDL-apoB upon the rate of catabolism of LDL-apoB in a patient with homozygous receptor-defective familial hypercholesterolaemia. Upper curve (●), cyclohexanedione-modified ^{131}I-labelled LDL; lower curve (○), ^{125}I-labelled LDL. For estimates of LDL catabolism by the receptor-mediated and alternative pathways in this subject, see Table 15.7 (homozygote). (From Thompson *et al.* (1980a).)

Table 15.7

Fractional and absolute catabolic rates of the apoprotein of native and cyclohexanedione-treated LDL (CHD-LDL) in normal and FH subjects

	Fractional catabolic rate (fraction/day)			Absolute catabolic rate (mg/kg/day)			Receptor total (%)
	Native LDL	CHD-LDL	Receptor path	Native LDL	CHD-LDL	Receptor path	
Normals	0.333	0.222	0.111	9.5	6.5	3.0	32
Heterozygotes	0.190	0.162	0.028	15.3	12.8	2.5	16
Homozygote	0.134	0.115	0.019	19.9	17.1	2.8	14

Values for normals and heterozygotes are taken from Shepherd et al. (1979). The value for the homozygote is from Thompson et al. (1980b). Values for the receptor pathway are estimated as the difference between the catabolic rates of native LDL and CHD-LDL. Absolute catabolic rates were estimated from the fractional rates calculated by analysis of the plasma disappearance curves of radioactive LDL or CHD-LDL and the total mass of LDL-apoB in the circulation.

3.4.3.4 Receptor deficiency and cholesterol synthesis *in vivo*.
Although LDL suppresses cholesterol synthesis in normal fibroblasts in culture, cultured fibroblasts from FH homozygotes continue to synthesize cholesterol at a high rate when LDL is added to the medium. This indicates that receptor-mediated uptake of LDL is necessary for the suppression of HMG-CoA reductase activity under the conditions in which cells are grown in culture and would lead one to expect that cholesterol synthesis would be increased in FH. However, as discussed in Section 3.4.1, the rate of whole-body synthesis of cholesterol in FH homozygotes differs little, if at all, from that in normal subjects. The explanation for this anomaly may be that, in the long term, cholesterol synthesized within the cells or taken up by the low-affinity process eventually reaches an intracellular concentration at which HMG-CoA reductase activity is fully suppressed. That receptor-mediated uptake of LDL is not required for regulation of cholesterol synthesis in cells *in vivo* is shown by the fact that the synthesis of cholesterol in the whole body (Myant *et al.*, 1978) or in circulating lymphocytes (Reichl *et al.*, 1978) is essentially normal in some patients with familial abetalipoproteinaemia, a condition in which there is no LDL in the plasma or interstitial fluids (see Chapter 16, Section 3 for further discussion of this point).

3.4.3.5 Direct secretion of LDL.
It is not known why the absence of receptors in homozygotes leads to direct secretion of LDL. One possibility is that the plasma LDL normally suppresses its own secretion by the liver by means of a feedback mechanism operating through LDL receptors on liver cells, absence of receptors leading to de-repression of LDL secretion. However, apart from lack of evidence that normal human hepatocytes possess LDL receptors, observations on the effect of plasma exchange on direct secretion of LDL in FH heterozygotes have not provided any support for the above suggestion (Soutar *et al.*, 1979).

3.4.3.6 Summary.
To summarize, most of the symptomatology of FH can be explained by a partial or complete deficiency of receptors if it is supposed (1), that receptor-mediated uptake of LDL normally accounts for a significant fraction, perhaps between one-third and two-thirds, of the total LDL catabolized in the body and (2), that the remaining fraction is removed through a non-saturable clearance mechanism (analogous to renal clearance) by which a constant volume of LDL-containing plasma or interstitial fluid is removed in unit time (Goldstein and Brown, 1977*b*). An additional, saturable mechanism with high and specific affinity for ageing or partially denatured LDL particles may also be concerned in the

uptake and degradation of LDL by macrophages (Goldstein et al., 1979); some such mechanism as this would explain why the fractional catabolic rate of LDL in homozygotes is substantially greater than that of albumin in normal subjects.

On this view, LDL-receptor deficiency leads to a reduced fractional catabolic rate of LDL, with a consequent rise in plasma LDL concentration and an increase in the mean life of LDL particles in the circulation, the latter leading to a change in the lipid composition of LDL. As the plasma LDL concentration rises, the absolute rate of catabolism by the clearance mechanism increases until a new steady state is reached in which the rate of catabolism is equal to the rate of production of LDL.

In homozygotes, the steady state is not achieved until very high plasma LDL concentrations have been reached because, in addition to loss of receptor-mediated catabolism, there is increased production of LDL by direct secretion into the plasma. This increase has yet to be explained in terms of LDL-receptor deficiency.

The development of xanthomas in skin and tendons is readily explained by the accumulation of LDL cholesterol in macrophage-like cells due to uptake of LDL by the non-receptor pathway. Likewise, premature atherosclerosis is explicable by the life-long increase in plasma LDL concentration. This would lead to the pathological changes in the arterial wall described in Chapter 13, including the accumulation of LDL cholesterol in smooth-muscle cells due to receptor-independent uptake of LDL. Thus, there seems no reason to postulate any mechanism for the formation of the characteristic lesions of FH other than a prolonged elevation of plasma LDL concentration caused by defective catabolism of LDL by cells using the receptor pathway. Any peculiarities in the distribution, pathology or age-at-onset of the lesions, compared with those in people with primary hyper-β-lipoproteinaemia but who are not carriers of the FH gene, may reasonably be attributed to the duration and magnitude of the rise in plasma LDL concentration in FH. However, it is worth bearing in mind the possibility that other factors are also involved in the development of the lesions in FH. For example, the prolonged stay of LDL particles in the circulation in FH might modify them in such a way as to make them more atherogenic or more readily taken up by cells of the macrophage system than normal LDL particles. There is also the possibility that the low plasma HDL concentration in many FH patients favours the net accumulation of cholesterol in the cells of some of their tissues, including the arterial wall. Finally, it is conceivable that a deficiency of LDL receptors on the cells of the target tissues in FH modifies their surface properties in a manner that favours their interaction with LDL.

3.4.4 LDL receptors in hypercholesterolaemia not due to FH

The marked effect of a genetically determined deficiency of receptors on the plasma cholesterol concentration raises the question whether, in the absence of FH, variations in the functional activity of the receptor mechanism contribute to the variability in plasma cholesterol concentration in the general population, or to any of the secondary hypercholesterolaemias that occur in disorders of metabolism. Here, it should be noted, we are not considering the genetic potential for synthesizing structurally normal receptors, but the possible influence of such factors as sex, diet and hormones on the ability of cells in the living body to generate receptors and on the efficiency with which these receptors function. Despite its importance, this question seems to have attracted little attention, doubtless owing to the lack of a simple and reliable routine method for assaying LDL receptors *in vitro* and the difficulty of assessing receptor activity *in vivo* (but see Section 3.4.3.3).

In a small sample of normal subjects, Bilheimer *et al.* (1978) could find no significant relation between plasma LDL concentration and the maximal capacity of blood lymphocytes to develop receptors during prolonged incubation in a lipoprotein-free medium. However, this does not exclude the possibility that intrapopulation variability in plasma LDL concentration is mediated to some extent by factors that influence the phenotypic expression of the receptor mechanism *in vivo* by modifying, for example, the production of receptors, the affinity of receptors for LDL, or the rate at which the receptors are internalized.

If diminished receptor function contributes to the development of secondary hypercholesterolaemia, this would be most likely to occur in conditions in which the hypercholesterolaemia is due to the type II lipoprotein pattern, as in some diabetics and some myxoedematous patients. Walton *et al.* (1965) observed a low fractional catabolic rate of LDL in hypothyroid patients. This is consistent with defective receptor function and suggests that the receptor mechanism can be influenced *in vivo* by hormones. In keeping with this, Thompson *et al.* (1981) have shown that receptor-mediated catabolism of LDL is diminished in untreated myxoedema, and that this defect can be reversed by treatment with thyroxine. Chait *et al.* (1978) have also shown that insulin at physiological concentrations increases the high-affinity binding, internalization and catabolism of LDL by cultured skin fibroblasts. Thus, it is possible that diminished receptor function plays some part in the rise in plasma LDL concentration in insulin-dependent diabetes. Diminished receptor function is unlikely to play any part in the pathogenesis of other forms of secondary hyperlipoproteinaemia, since plasma lipoprotein patterns other than type II are not a feature of FH, even in the homozygous form. In view of the very high affinity of LDL receptors for apoE-containing lipoproteins, it is perhaps surprising that β-VLDL does not accumulate in FH. (But see Section 4.5 for an exception to this.)

3.5 Diagnosis

3.5.1 General

FH is usually detected because of premature IHD or xanthoma of tendons or skin, the latter often leading to referral to a skin clinic. Many FH patients are also discovered during the examination of the relatives of index patients. Increasing numbers of symptom-free carriers of the FH gene are now coming to light as a result of the screening of well populations for various purposes and the routine biochemical testing of hospital patients. The diagnosis of FH by examination of cord blood is dealt with below. FH in a suspected carrier of the gene is diagnosed by demonstrating the presence of primary hyper-β-lipoproteinaemia (a plasma LDL concentration above the 95th percentile not secondary to any of the causes listed in Table 15.1) and the presence of hypercholesterolaemia, xanthomatosis or premature IHD in one or more first-degree relatives.

There is no difficulty in diagnosing FH in homozygotes or severely affected heterozygotes. The homozygous state is usually obvious from the early onset of IHD or xanthomatosis, the very high plasma cholesterol concentration in the absence of other metabolic causes, and the characteristic skin lesions. In such cases a diagnosis can be made without the need to measure the plasma LDL concentration, since hypercholesterolaemia of this degree in the absence of marked hypertriglyceridaemia is almost always due to an increased plasma LDL concentration. The more severely affected heterozygotes may occasionally be difficult to distinguish from homozygotes. If the patient has planar skin lesions, the heterozygous state is virtually excluded. The homozygous state is excluded if the patient has a normal parent or child and becomes increasingly unlikely as the age extends beyond 30 years. In doubtful cases a distinction between homozygotes and heterozygotes can be made by examination of fibroblasts cultured from a skin biopsy. In experienced hands this will also permit the differentiation between receptor-negative and receptor-defective homozygotes. From the point of view of prognosis, management and genetic counselling, it is important to establish whether the patient is a homozygote or a heterozygote. In the interests of progress in the understanding of a very rare disease, a complete genotypic diagnosis, based on tissue-culture studies in a competent laboratory, should be attempted in all homozygous patients, especially if more than one homozygote is detected in the same family.

Although the parents and children of a true homozygote are obligate heterozygotes, Morganroth *et al.* (1974) have described two families in each of which the index patient had the biochemical and clinical features of FH in the homozygous form, while both parents and all four grandparents appeared to be normal. The index patients were children (aged 5 and 6 years) with marked primary hypercholesterolaemia due to raised plasma LDL concentrations, together with planar xanthomas in the skin of the hands, knees, elbows and buttocks. Morganroth *et al.* (1974) called this condition 'pseudohomozygous type II hyperlipoproteinemia'. Information about the extent to which LDL receptors can be expressed in cultured fibroblasts from these and any other similar patients would be likely to throw light on this puzzling abnormality.

The diagnosis of the heterozygous state may be difficult if the plasma total cholesterol concentration is only slightly raised, since plasma cholesterol levels in such patients may overlap with the levels in members of the general population whose primary hypercholesterolaemia is multifactorial in origin; as we have seen (Section 3.3.3), less than 5% of people with the type II plasma lipoprotein pattern have FH. In these borderline cases, clearer evidence of the presence of FH may be obtained by direct measurement of plasma LDL concentration, since this gives better separation between heterozygotes and non-carriers of the FH gene (Fredrickson and Levy, 1972). Observations on single large FH families (Schrott *et al.*, 1972) or groups of small families (Fredrickson and Levy, 1972; Kwiterovich *et al.*, 1974) indicate that the number of incorrect diagnoses is minimized if a plasma LDL-cholesterol concentration of about 170 mg/100 ml (164–180 mg/100 ml) is taken as the dividing line between FH carriers and non-carriers of FH who have primary hyper-β-lipoproteinaemia. If the patient has tendon xanthomas or a first-degree relative with hypercholesterolaemia and xanthomatosis, FH is almost certainly present. However, xanthomas do not usually appear in heterozygotes before age 20 and are not always present in older heterozygotes (see Section 3.2).

In the absence of tendon or tuberous xanthomas in the patient or a relative, the diagnosis must remain tentative unless evidence can be obtained by testing his skin fibroblasts or leucocytes *in vitro*. Goldstein *et al.* (1975) found that heterozygotes in whom the diagnosis had already been established could be separated completely from normal subjects and homozygotes by measuring cholesterol esterification in cultured skin fibroblasts, first in the presence of LDL and then in the presence of 25-hydroxycholesterol. This, or an equivalent test, would probably provide decisive diagnostic information in patients with borderline plasma LDL concentrations and without xanthomas. However, in view of the numbers of heterozygotes attending a Lipid Clinic in whom the diagnosis is likely to be doubtful, and the time and skill required for a tissue-culture diagnosis, there is a need for a simpler test that can be adapted for routine use. Fogelman *et al.* (1973, 1975) have shown that when freshly isolated human leucocytes are incubated in a medium containing lipid-free serum, intracellular incorporation of acetate into sterols is considerably enhanced, and that this enhancement is greater with leucocytes from FH heterozygotes than with those from normal subjects. This observation has formed the basis of subsequent attempts by other workers (Betteridge *et al.*, 1975; Bilheimer *et al.*, 1978) to use freshly isolated leucocytes in testing for the presence of FH in the heterozygous form. Bilheimer *et al.* (1978) found that they could separate FH heterozygotes from normal subjects, and from those with hyperlipidaemia not due to FH, by assaying high-affinity degradation of ^{125}I-labelled LDL in lymphocytes incubated for three days in a lipoprotein-free medium. Most of the heterozygotes studied by Bilheimer *et al.* were members of a single large family, from whom both heterozygotes and unaffected normal subjects were drawn. It is to be hoped that the discriminating power of diagnostic tests of this type will be examined in more widely based populations, in which the ratio of normals to heterozygotes would be greater than the 1:1 ratio in a single large FH family.

3.5.2 Early diagnosis

Since the treatment of FH is more likely to be effective if begun at an early age than if delayed until atherosclerosis has started to develop, much attention has been paid to the possibility of diagnosis in infancy. Kwiterovich *et al.* (1973) have shown that FH can be diagnosed in the offspring of known heterozygotes by measuring the plasma LDL-cholesterol concentration in cord blood. While it is clearly important to detect FH carriers among the children of affected parents, the great majority of infants who have FH are not the offspring of parents one of whom is known to have FH. It is therefore very desirable to be able to detect FH by screening unselected infants in the general population.

Glueck *et al.* (1971) examined the cord blood of 1800 consecutive newborn infants and found that plasma total cholesterol concentration exceeded 100 mg/100 ml in 65. However, after examination of the parents and grandparents, only eight of these infants were diagnosed as having FH (Tsang *et al.*, 1974). When these FH infants were re-examined at age 1, five had normal plasma cholesterol concentrations, possibly owing to the effects of diet. Tsang *et al.* concluded that measurement of plasma total cholesterol concentration in cord blood is a useful screening test for FH provided that this is combined with a careful examination of the relatives, but that FH may be masked at age one by the effects of diet. Darmady *et al.* (1972) obtained less encouraging results. They found no evidence of FH among the relatives of any of a group of 302 newborn infants whose plasma total cholesterol concentration in cord blood was above 100 mg/100 ml. Moreover, when re-examined one year later the plasma cholesterol concentrations of these infants were scattered throughout the distribution of values in the whole group. In the only infant diagnosed as having FH at age one year, the cord plasma cholesterol concentration was 85 mg/100 ml. Thus, it appears that the total cholesterol concentration measured in cord blood plasma is not a reliable indicator of the presence of the FH gene in an infant taken at random from the general population.

Since HDL carries a much greater proportion of the total cholesterol in plasma in the newborn than in the adult, variations in HDL-cholesterol concentration may obscure minor increases in LDL-cholesterol concentration and may thus obscure the diagnosis if measurements are restricted to total cholesterol. This suggests that measurement of LDL-cholesterol concentration in cord plasma would provide a better screening test for FH in the newborn than measurement of total cholesterol concentration. In agreement with this, Kwiterovich *et al.* (1973) found that LDL-cholesterol concentration gave better discrimination than total cholesterol concentration in their study of the cord blood of infants born to known heterozygotes.

LDL receptors are present on normal amniotic-fluid cells in culture. Hence, it is possible to diagnose FH in the homozygous state in fetal life. Brown *et al.* (1978) have reported the prenatal diagnosis of homozygous FH in the fetus of a woman who had already had a homozygous son. The amniotic cells from this pregnancy showed an almost complete lack of LDL receptors. On the basis of this finding, the pregnancy was terminated at the 20th week. The diagnosis was confirmed by showing that the plasma cholesterol concentration in the fetus was 279 mg/100 ml.

3.5.3 The differential diagnosis of FH; familial combined hyperlipidaemia

Apart from secondary type II hyperlipoproteinaemias, the commonest condition from which heterozygous FH must be distinguished is the polygenic form of the type II lipoprotein pattern responsible for the primary hypercholesterolaemia of most people whose plasma cholesterol concentration is above the 95th percentile. Within a large FH family it is usually fairly easy to identify the heterozygotes and the normal members on the basis of plasma cholesterol or LDL concentration alone, but in small families or sporadic cases it may be difficult or impossible unless the family history is conclusive or xanthomas are present.

The differential diagnosis of FH is further complicated by the possible existence of another monogenically inherited disorder that may cause the type IIa, type IIb or type IV lipoprotein pattern. The existence of this disorder, termed *familial combined hyperlipidaemia*, was deduced .by Goldstein *et al.* (1973) from the plasma lipoprotein patterns observed in the relatives of hyperlipidaemic survivors of myocardial infarction. According to Goldstein *et al.* (1973), the gene for familial combined hyperlipidaemia may cause hypercholesterolaemia alone, hypertriglyceridaemia alone, or a combination of both, in different members of the same family. This condition can often be excluded in suspected FH patients because it is not expressed in childhood and does not cause tendon xanthomas. However, it would not be easy to exclude familial combined hyperlipidaemia as a cause of primary type II hyperlipoproteinaemia in an adult without xanthomas and with a hypertriglyceridaemic relative. Nikkilä and Aro (1973) have also described families in which two or three different plasma lipoprotein patterns appeared to be present in different relatives of an index patient who had had a myocardial infarct. However, it must be pointed out that the method of genetic analysis used by Goldstein *et al.* (1973) in their study of the relatives of coronary patients has been questioned by others (Patterson and Slack, 1974; Hewitt *et al.*, 1979).

3.5.4 Genetic counselling

Patients in whom a diagnosis of FH has been established may seek genetic counselling if they wish to have children. If one parent of a child is a heterozygote, the child has a 1:2 chance of being a heterozygote and a 1:4 chance of being a heterozygous male, in whom the disease may be severe enough to cause death before age 40. The parents should therefore be advised to have the child tested as soon after the fourth month as possible (the optimal age for early diagnosis). It may then be possible to establish or exclude FH. If both the parents are heterozygotes, each of their offspring has a 1:2 chance of being a heterozygote and a 1:4 chance of being a homozygote. These risks should be explained to prospective parents.

3.6 Treatment

3.6.1 Objectives and indications

Although it has not been proved that lowering the plasma LDL concentration postpones or prevents ischaemic heart disease in FH, there are at least two lines of evidence to suggest that the progress of the atherosclerotic lesions in the coronary arteries can be delayed by cholestyramine treatment (Kuo *et al.*, 1979) or repeated plasma exchange (Thompson *et al.*, 1980a). Whether or not this evidence is confirmed, the assumption that the long-term reversal of the abnormal plasma lipoprotein pattern is beneficial provides the only rational basis for the treatment of this disease. Hence, the problem of treatment is essentially that of finding effective methods of lowering the plasma LDL concentration without unacceptable risk from side-effects. In some inborn errors of metabolism in which the symptoms are due to accumulation of a harmful metabolite, it may be possible to ameliorate the condition by excluding precursors of the metabolite from the diet, or by supplying the missing gene product in a form in which it can reach its normal site of action, or by transplantation of an organ from a normal person. None of these methods is yet feasible in the case of FH, though replacement of an organ in which receptor-mediated catabolism of LDL takes place should be possible in principle. For example, if the normal liver can be shown to possess functioning LDL receptors, liver transplants might be worth considering for the treatment of homozygotes.

Until we are in a position to correct the fundamental metabolic error, we have to rely on dietary, pharmacological and other procedures that lower the plasma cholesterol concentration, often in ways that we do not fully understand. These procedures are considered briefly in this section. More detailed accounts will be found in the reviews by Havel and Kane (1973a), Myant and Slack (1976), Lewis (1976) and Yeshurun and Gotto (1976). The treatment of FH in infants and children is dealt with in the review by Myant and Slack (1976) and in the paper by West et al. (1975).

As regards the indications for treatment, all homozygotes and all moderately or severely affected heterozygotes (those, for example, with tendon xanthomas and a plasma cholesterol concentration above 300 mg/100 ml) should be treated as vigorously as possible once the diagnosis is established. Whether or not all mildly affected heterozygotes should undergo life-long treatment is a matter for argument. Myant and Slack (1976) have suggested that all heterozygous males should be treated as soon as they are detected, preferably in infancy, but that the need to impose treatment on mildly affected female heterozygotes is less compelling, since many heterozygous women live a normal life span without treatment. On the other hand, there are those who argue that anyone whose plasma cholesterol concentration is high enough to cause a significant increase in IHD risk—some would say, anyone with an age-adjusted value above the 95th percentile—should be advised to modify their diet whether or not the raised cholesterol level is due to FH. As discussed in Chapter 13, IHD risk is usually determined by a combination of several factors, of which plasma cholesterol concentration, plasma HDL concentration, blood pressure, cigarette smoking and diabetes are among the most important. The extent to which other risk factors, in addition to hypercholesterolaemia, are present must be taken into consideration in the management of the patient. There is a general impression among clinicians that the risk of IHD varies from one FH family to another. If there is, in fact, a tendency for FH to carry a worse prognosis in some families than in others, the age-at-death from IHD in the patient's relatives should be weighed in the balance when the need for treatment is being considered.

3.6.2 Diet
Modification of the diet to reduce the intake of saturated fat and cholesterol is the basis of all current methods for the treatment of patients with primary hypercholesterolaemia, including those with FH, whichever additional measures are adopted. As discussed in Chapter 11, in normal subjects the plasma cholesterol level falls if the amount of saturated fat as a proportion of total caloric intake is decreased and that of polyunsaturated fat is increased, the fall in plasma total cholesterol concentration being due largely to a fall in LDL concentration. The effect of dietary cholesterol on plasma cholesterol level varies unpredictably from one normal person to another, but in many subjects the level changes in response to relatively small changes in cholesterol intake. As a general rule, therefore, cholesterol intake should be restricted. In most FH heterozygotes, a permanent reduction in plasma total cholesterol concentration of about 15% can be achieved by reducing total fat intake to 30% of total calories and cholesterol intake to less than 300 mg/day, and by increasing the ratio of polyunsaturated to saturated fat to about 1.0. A greater effect on plasma cholesterol level may be achieved by increasing the ratio to higher values, but the possible effects of very large intakes of polyunsaturated fat on gallstone formation (see Chapter 14) suggest that this may be unwise unless the degree of hypercholesterolaemia is high enough to justify the risk involved.

To meet the requirements of a cholesterol-lowering diet, foods rich in cholesterol should be avoided. These include egg yolk (one egg yolk supplying 250–300 mg of cholesterol), shellfish, butter, milk, cream and organ meats (brain, liver, pancreas and heart). Intake of saturated fat should be reduced by reducing the intake of dairy products and by removing visible fat from cuts of meat, by partial substitution of poultry and fish for other meats and by using a suitable polyunsaturated fat for cooking. Modified diets conforming to these general rules may be composed of everyday foods and should have sufficient variety to be palatable to children as well as adults. Once a cholesterol-lowering diet has been prescribed the patient should discuss menus with a dietician. A set of suggestions useful in the conduct of a Lipid Clinic will be found in the review by Myant and Slack (1976). There is usually little difficulty in persuading young children to eat a cholesterol-lowering diet, especially since there will nearly always be other affected members of the family, so that it may be feasible for the whole family to eat the same modified diet. When children are eating a diet low in animal fat, a careful record of growth and development should be kept and the possibility of deficiency of fat-soluble vitamins should be borne in mind.

Treatment by diet alone does not usually bring the plasma cholesterol to within the normal range in heterozygotes and seldom reduces it to below 500 mg/100 ml in homozygotes. Other measures are therefore required in the majority of FH patients.

3.6.3 Drugs

The most effective drugs for the treatment of the hypercholesterolaemia of FH are the non-absorbable exchange resins. The most widely used are cholestyramine and colestipol; DEAE-Sephadex has also been shown to be effective, though it is not yet available on a commercial scale. As discussed in Chapter 11, these drugs act by preventing the reabsorption of bile salts from the lumen of the small intestine and thus enhancing the breakdown of cholesterol to bile acids in the liver. In normal subjects and FH heterozygotes there may also be a slight increase in the fractional catabolic rate of the plasma LDL, with no increase in the rate of production of LDL (Levy and Langer, 1972). When given in combination with a modified diet, maximal effects on the plasma cholesterol concentration are achieved when cholestyramine is given in doses of 20–30 g/day in adults or about 15 g/day in children. When given in these amounts, cholestyramine is without toxic side-effects, though some patients may complain of constipation or flatulence. Malabsorption of fat-soluble vitamins does not occur in adults taking cholestyramine, but should be watched for in children. Folic acid supplements should be given to children taking cholestyramine in maximal doses, since the serum folate level tends to fall (West et al., 1975).

In many heterozygotes, cholestyramine and a low-fat, low-cholesterol diet reduce the plasma cholesterol concentration to within the normal range, but this combination has little effect in homozygotes, though there may be a reduction in the extent of the skin xanthomas, with little or no change in plasma cholesterol level. An additional effect in homozygotes may be obtained by combining cholestyramine with another drug, of which the most effective are clofibrate and nicotinic acid (Moutafis et al., 1971).

Nicotinic acid may be given in doses of up to 10 g/day provided that the daily dose is increased gradually so as to minimize circulatory side-effects. When given alone or together with cholestyramine, nicotinic acid may cause liver damage in some patients. Those undergoing treatment with large doses of nicotinic acid should therefore be tested at three-monthly intervals for signs of damage to liver parenchymal cells (see Myant and Slack (1976) for further details). Figure 15.10 shows the effect of a combination of cholestyramine and nicotinic acid on the plasma cholesterol concentration in a homozygous patient who failed to show any response at all to cholestyramine and a modified diet. There was a rapid and marked fall in the plasma cholesterol level on the addition of nicotinic acid, but this drug was withdrawn when plasma enzyme assays showed evidence of liver damage.

Clofibrate by itself is usually ineffective in heterozygotes or homozygotes, but is probably worth a trial in any heterozygote who fails to respond adequately to diet alone since some patients show a significant fall in plasma cholesterol level when given 1–2 g of clofibrate per day in addition to a modified diet. The main indication for clofibrate in the treatment of FH is as an adjunct to other forms of medical or surgical treatment.

Other drugs that have been found useful in the treatment of FH are β-sitosterol, D-thyroxine and neomycin, a non-absorbable polybasic antibiotic. An account of the use of these and other drugs in the treatment of hypercholesterolaemia will be found in the review by Yeshurun and Gotto (1976). Compactin (ML-236B) formula (**15.1**) is also of potential value in the treatment of FH, though it is not yet

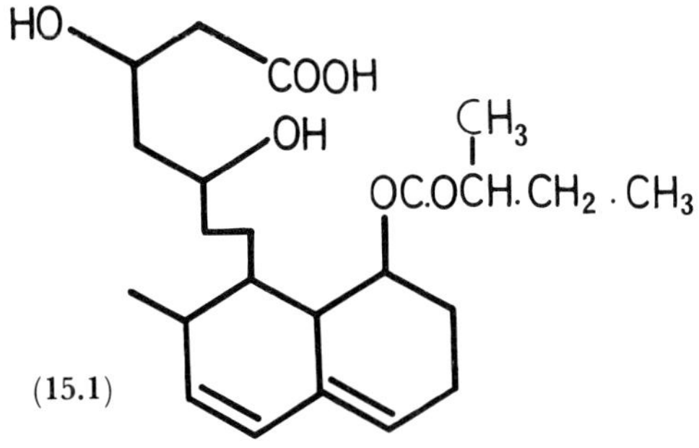

(15.1)

Compactin (ML-236B) in acid form

commercially available. This remarkable substance, isolated by Endo et al. (1976) from the fungus *Penicillium brevicompactum*, is an extremely potent competitive inhibitor of HMG-CoA reductase in microsomal preparations, intact cells or whole animals. The affinity of the enzyme for compactin is about 10 000 times that for HMG-CoA. Preliminary clinical trials (Yamamoto et al., 1980) have shown that the drug brings about a substantial reduction in plasma cholesterol concentration (11–37%) in FH heterozygotes and that it may have a significant effect in homozygotes. Doses that are effective in heterozygotes have had no detectable side-effects during 5-month periods of

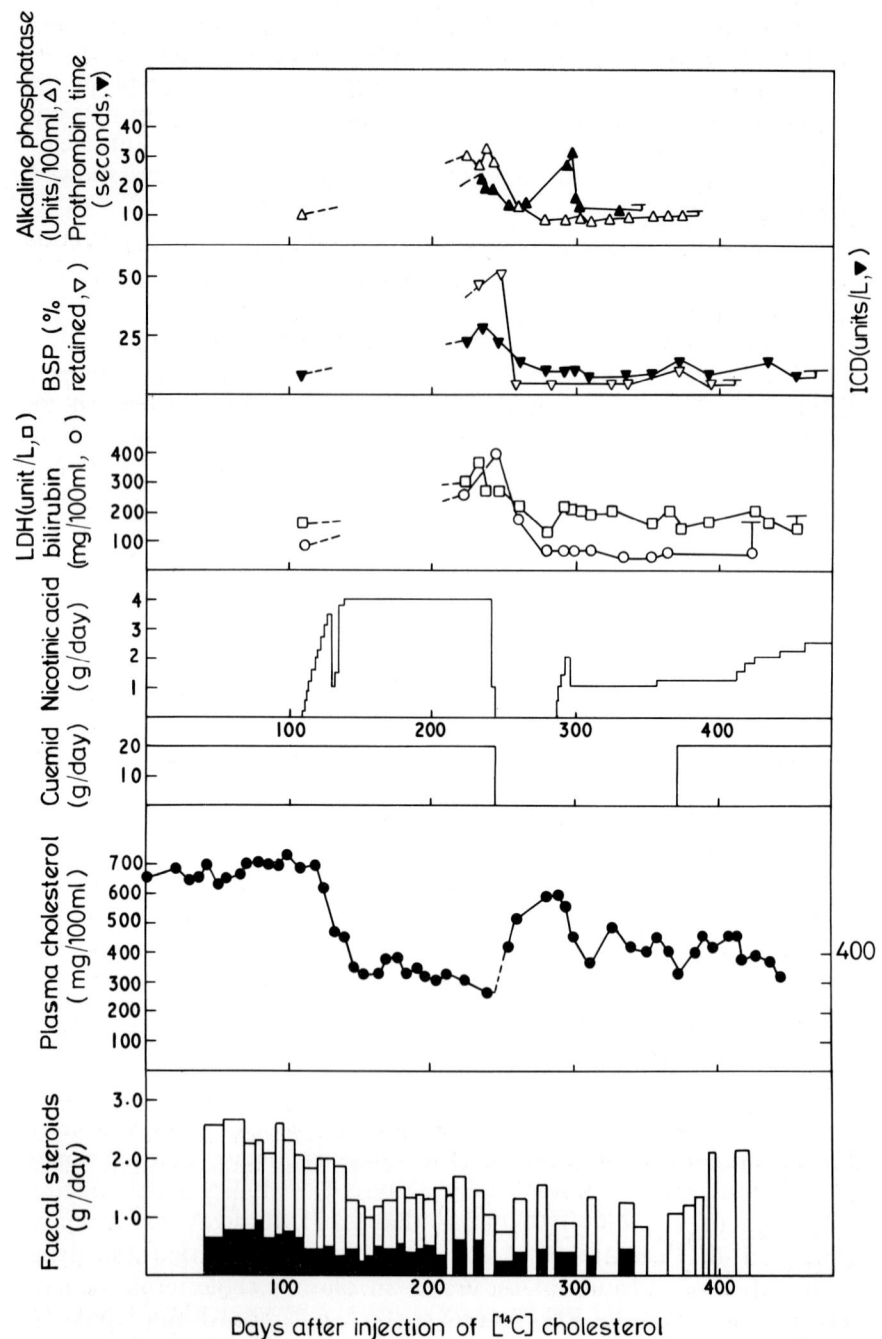

treatment. In principle, the ability of compactin to bring about the selective inhibition of HMG-CoA reductase should make it the ideal drug for use in combination with cholestyramine, since it should counteract the stimulatory effect of cholestyramine on cholesterol synthesis without influencing the increased rate of formation of bile acids.

3.6.4 Ileal bypass

It has long been known that the plasma cholesterol concentration may fall to very low levels in severe disease of the small bowel, or after surgical removal of the ileum or after jejuno-ileal bypass in the treatment of obesity. This led Buchwald (1964) to advocate partial ileal bypass as a method of lowering the plasma cholesterol level in primary hypercholesterolaemia. In Buchwald's hands ileal bypass lowers the plasma cholesterol level in hypercholesterolaemic patients, including FH heterozygotes, by an average of about 40% over and above the effect that can be achieved by modification of the diet alone. Thus, under favourable conditions the combined effect of diet and a bypass operation may be to halve the plasma cholesterol level. Skin and tendon xanthomas may decrease in size or may even disappear, and some patients with angina report improvement in their symptoms. Serial coronary angiography in patients who have undergone an ileal bypass operation suggests non-progression of atherosclerotic lesions over periods of at least two years in a substantial proportion and regression of occlusive lesions in some (Buchwald et al., 1974).

The effect of the operation on the plasma cholesterol is probably due to interference with the reabsorption of bile salts. A bypass operation is thus the surgical equivalent of treatment with an anionic exchange resin. Some of the effects of ileal bypass on cholesterol metabolism in the whole body have been considered in Chapter 10.

The maximal effect on the plasma cholesterol level is achieved within three months and is maintained indefinitely in most patients.

Figure 5.10 (opposite)
Effect of cholestyramine (Cuemid) alone and in combination with nicotinic acid on the plasma cholesterol concentration (●) and faecal steroid output (columns in bottom panel; neutral steroids in black, bile acids in white) in a patient with familial hypercholesterolaemia in the homozygous form. The upper three panels show the effects of nicotinic acid on serum alkaline phosphatase and lactate dehydrogenase (LDH) activities and on hepatic clearance of intravenous bromsulphthalein (BSP). Cholestyramine alone stimulated faecal steroid output to 2–8 g/day but had no effect on plasma cholesterol concentration. When nicotinic acid (4 g/day maximal dose) was given, the plasma cholesterol level fell to 300–350 mg/100 ml within 4 weeks. On withdrawing treatment with both drugs, the plasma cholesterol level rose to 600 mg/100 ml within 6 weeks. The patient was the one whose aorta is shown in Fig. 15.2. From Moutafis and Myant (1971).

A bypass operation has not been proved to be more effective than maximal doses of cholestyramine in the management of primary hypercholesterolaemia, but it may be preferable for patients who are unable or unwilling to take 20–30 g of cholestyramine daily throughout their lives. Ileal bypass seems to be as ineffective as cholestyramine in the treatment of FH homozygotes; in three homozygotes treated by Buchwald *et al.* (1974) the greatest reduction in plasma cholesterol level was only 16% and in the one homozygote treated at Hammersmith Hospital there was no sustained fall (Johnston *et al.*, 1967).

The major side-effect of the operation is severe and persistent diarrhoea, but by no means all patients suffer from this symptom. Since vitamin B_{12} is absorbed from the ileum, this vitamin should be given parenterally to all patients who have undergone the operation, preferably at three-monthly intervals.

3.6.5 Portacaval anastomosis

The use of portacaval anastomosis in the treatment of FH homozygotes arose from a fortuitous observation on patients with glycogen storage disease. It was noted that after an operation to divert dietary glucose from the liver by anastomosing the portal vein to the inferior vena cava, the hyperlipidaemia characteristic of this disease was abolished. Although the reason for this effect of portacaval anastomosis on plasma lipid metabolism has never been convincingly explained, Starzl *et al.* (1973) carried out the operation on a 12-year-old girl with FH in the homozygous form who had failed to respond to treatment and who was suffering from severe and rapidly progressive coronary artery disease with aortic stenosis and angina pectoris. The operation was followed by a fall in plasma cholesterol concentration from about 800 mg/100 ml to less than 300 mg/100 ml, followed later by regression of her skin lesions, cessation of her angina and widening of the lumen of her coronary arteries. Though the patient died within two years of the operation, the results were encouraging enough to suggest that her life would have been prolonged if the operation had been carried out when she was younger. With this in mind, others have carried out this operation on homozygous patients. Upwards of a dozen such operations have now been reported verbally or in published form, but in no case have the results been as striking as those achieved in Starzl's patient.

The response varies widely from one patient to another, but there is no way of predicting how a given patient will respond. In the light of the results that have been achieved so far, it is reasonable to recommend the operation for homozygotes for whom no alternative approach is effective or feasible. The hazards of the procedure are those of a major abdominal operation in a patient who may already be suffering from advanced heart disease, and thrombosis at the site of the anastomosis.

In the patient treated by Starzl, *post mortem* examination of the liver showed a decrease in the amount of endoplasmic reticulum and in the size of the hepatocytes. In a homozygous patient of Bilheimer *et al.* (1975), the synthesis of LDL-apoB was diminished by portacaval anastomosis, suggesting that diversion of portal blood from the liver led to decreased output of VLDL, the precursor of LDL. In support of this, Magide *et al.* (1976) have shown that an operation for portacaval anastomosis in rats decreases the rate of incorporation of [^{14}C]leucine into VLDL protein but not into albumin.

3.6.6 Coronary artery bypass

In FH patients with angina associated with narrowing of the ostia and proximal portions of the coronary arteries, aortocoronary bypass grafts may be indicated. In homozygotes with aortic stenosis due to atheromatous involvement of the aortic valve cusps, replacement of the valves may offer the only means of prolonging the patient's life. Measures to lower the plasma cholesterol concentration should be continued indefinitely after the operation.

3.6.7 Plasma exchange

It has been recognized for several years that it ought to be possible to lower the plasma cholesterol concentration by exchanging the patient's blood or plasma for a substitute deficient in cholesterol. Although plasmapheresis has been used as a short-term treatment in homozygous FH (De Gennes *et al.*, 1967), the technical problem of exchanging a significant fraction of the total plasma volume rapidly and at frequent intervals has only recently been solved by the development of the continuous-flow blood-cell separator. Thompson *et al.* (1975), using the Aminco Celltrifuge, have shown that an exchange of 2–4 l of the patient's plasma with a plasma protein fraction containing essentially no cholesterol brings about an immediate fall in plasma cholesterol concentration to about 30% of the pre-exchange level. After the exchange, the plasma cholesterol level returns to near the baseline value in 2–3 weeks, HDL concentration rising more rapidly than LDL concentration (Fig. 15.11). Thompson *et al.* (1980a) have shown that exchanges at weekly or fortnightly intervals can be carried out in outpatients for periods of two or more years without side-effects and with little inconvenience to the patient. With exchanges at this frequency, the mean plasma cholesterol concentration can be maintained within the normal range in many heterozygotes, and at a level close to the upper limit of the normal in homozygotes, by a combination of diet, drugs and frequent plasma exchanges (Fig. 15.12).

740 The Biology of Cholesterol and Related Steroids

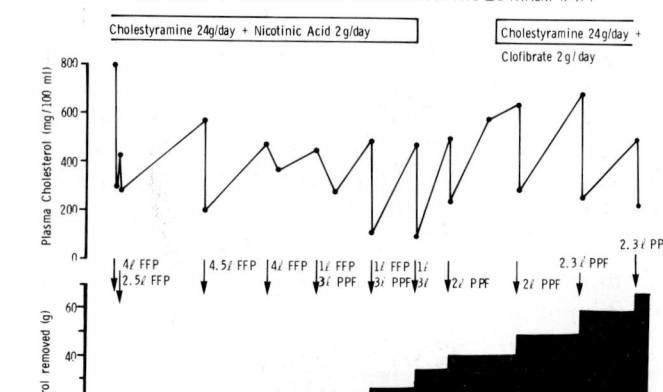

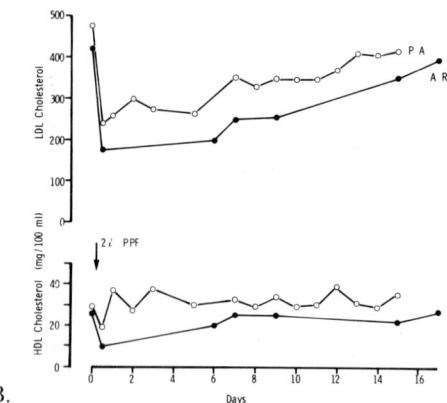

Figure 15.11
Effect of plasma exchange with plasma protein fraction (PPF) or fresh-frozen plasma (FFP) on plasma lipids in familial hypercholesterolaemia in the homozygous form.
A. Effect of repeated exchanges on plasma total cholesterol concentration in a patient with FH in the homozygous form (PA). Arrows show time of each exchange, with volume exchanged. Shaded area shows total amount of cholesterol removed from the patient's body. In this patient, the plasma exchanges were combined with the drug treatments shown at the top of the Figure.
B. Effect of a single 2-litre exchange on plasma LDL- and HDL-cholesterol concentrations in two patients with homozygous familial hypercholesterolaemia (PA and AR).
(From Thompson *et al.* (1975).)

Disorders of Cholesterol Metabolism: The Hyperlipoproteinaemias 741

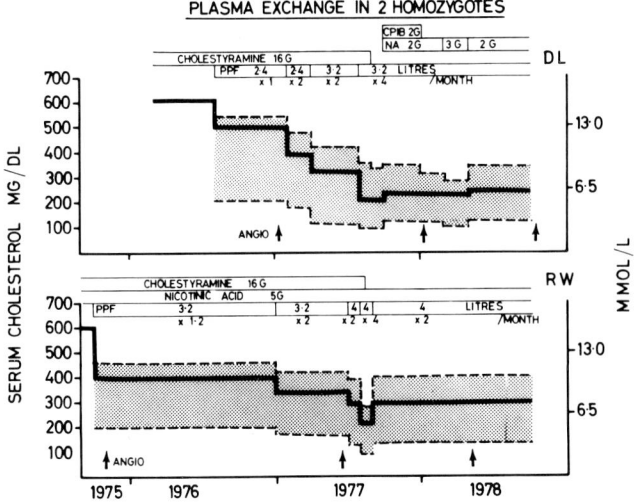

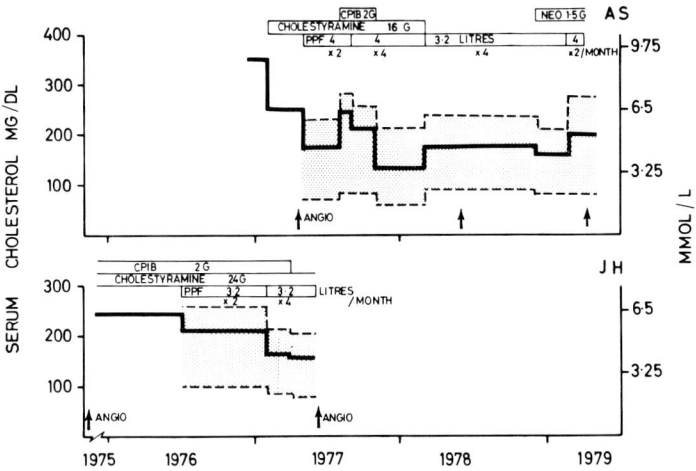

Figure 15.12
Effect of repeated plasma exchanges on the mean (solid line), maximum (upper border of stippled area) and minimum (lower border of stippled area) plasma cholesterol concentration in two FH homozygotes (DL and RW) and two FH heterozygotes (AS and JH). The mean concentration was estimated as the area under the plasma concentration curve between successive exchanges, divided by the time interval. Exchanges were carried out at intervals of 2–3 weeks. Each patient was given drug treatment in addition to the plasma exchanges. CPIB, clofibrate; NA, nicotinic acid; angio, coronary angiogram. The volumes of plasma protein fraction used are shown at the top of each Figure. (From Thompson *et al.* (1980a).)

In a trial of the effects of repeated plasma exchange in a small group of patients, Thompson *et al.* (1980a) have reported a symptomatic improvement in several of those with angina and possible regression of coronary atherosclerosis in one heterozygote. A major limitation to the number of seriously affected FH patients who can be treated effectively by plasma exchange is the availability of a suitable cholesterol-free plasma substitute. This could, in theory, be overcome by a method of selective extra-corporeal removal of LDL from the plasma, so that the patient's own plasma depleted of LDL could be returned to his circulation. This is the principle of a method introduced by Lupien *et al.* (1976), in which LDL is removed from whole blood by heparin-agarose beads, the LDL-depleted blood being reinfused into the patient.

4 FAMILIAL TYPE III HYPERLIPOPROTEINAEMIA

4.1 Definition and historical background

Familial type III hyperlipoproteinaemia, also referred to as *broad beta disease* or *floating beta disease*, is an uncommon disorder characterized by increased concentrations of plasma cholesterol and triglyceride, the presence of one or more abnormal lipoproteins in the plasma, skin xanthomas of a distinctive kind and a tendency to premature atherosclerosis of the coronary and peripheral arteries; the usual features of the family history are dealt with in Section 4.4.

Since this disease was first distinguished from other primary disorders of plasma lipoprotein metabolism by Fredrickson *et al.* (1967), the definition of the type III lipoprotein pattern has changed. There has also been a change of opinion as to the plasma lipid abnormality upon which the diagnosis should be based. The abnormal lipoprotein pattern referred to as type III hyperlipoproteinaemia was first defined in terms of the pattern obtained on paper electrophoresis of whole plasma, together with the lipid composition and electrophoretic behaviour of the VLDL (d <1.006 g/ml). Fredrickson *et al.* (1967) noted that plasma obtained from affected subjects in the fasting state, instead of showing the normal well-separated β and preβ bands, showed a continuous band extending from the β to the preβ zone; hence the name 'broad beta disease'. In addition to this abnormality, the VLDL fraction obtained by separation in the preparative ultracentrifuge was found to have an unusually high cholesterol:triglyceride ratio and to contain a lipoprotein that migrated close to the β zone on paper electrophoresis (Fig. 15.13). This abnormal lipoprotein was designated β-VLDL or floating beta lipoprotein.

Disorders of Cholesterol Metabolism: The Hyperlipoproteinaemias 743

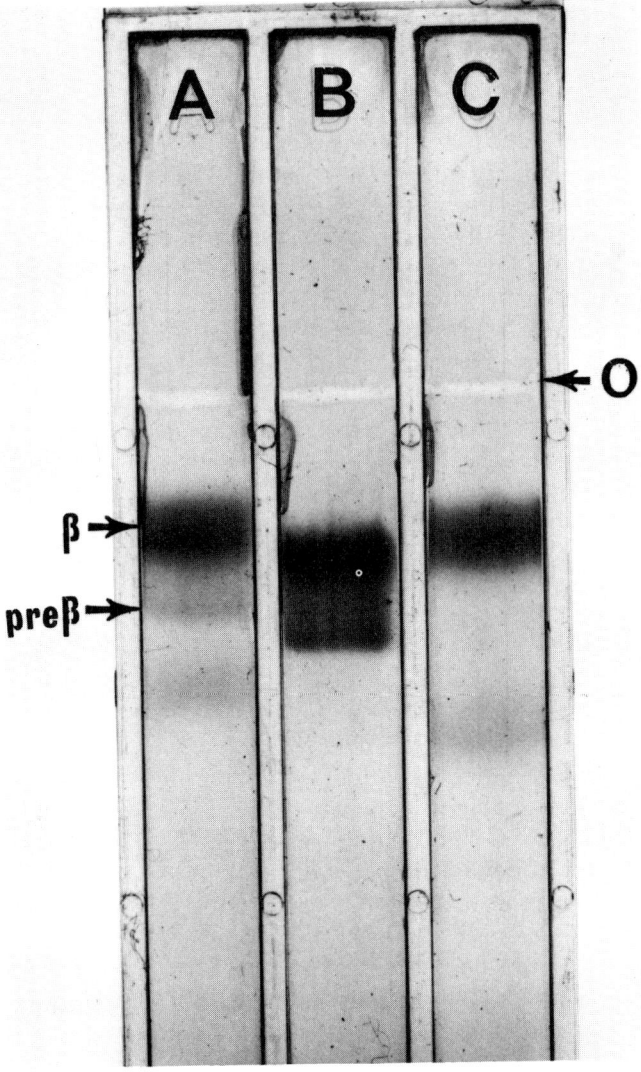

Figure 15.13
Agarose-gel electrophoresis of serum fractions from a 59-year-old man with familial Type III hyperlipoproteinaemia. A, whole serum; B, the serum fraction of density less than 1.006 g/ml, showing the abnormal densely staining band with slightly faster mobility than that of the β band shown in A; C, the serum fraction of d > 1.006 g/ml. O, line of application of the sample. Plasma triglyceride concentration, 334 mg/100 ml, plasma cholesterol concentration, 450 mg/100 ml. The patient had plane xanthomas in the palmar creases and raised xanthomas on the elbows. (With the permission of Dr. J. Slack.)

Quarfordt et al. (1971), using starch-block electrophoresis, separated β-VLDL from the normal preβ-migrating VLDL in the d < 1.006 fraction of plasma from type III patients and showed that the composition of β-VLDL was intermediate between that of normal LDL and normal VLDL (see Section 4.2). Compared with normal VLDL, the β-VLDL was enriched with esterified cholesterol and deficient in both triglyceride and the VLDL apoproteins that react immunologically with antiserum to HDL (presumed to be the apoC proteins). Havel and Kane (1973b) subsequently showed that the protein of β-VLDL was enriched with apoE and was partially depleted of apoC proteins. Since β-VLDL appeared to be a well-defined lipoprotein, present in all patients who had the clinical syndrome of floating beta disease and absent from normal subjects and from most individuals with other forms of hyperlipoproteinaemia, type III hyperlipoproteinaemia came to be defined in terms of the presence of β-VLDL (Fredrickson and Levy, 1972). However, this definition has turned out to have disadvantages as a basis for diagnosing floating beta disease. In particular, β-VLDL may be detectable in plasma in the absence of hyperlipidaemia and in the plasma of some individual who, on other grounds, cannot be regarded as having the disease. In view of these anomalies, definitions based on the cholesterol:triglyceride ratio in the VLDL have been proposed, but there is disagreement as to the ratio that gives the best segregation between affected and normal subjects (compare Hazzard et al., 1972 with Fredrickson et al., 1975). The recent discovery of a discontinuous abnormality in the apoE of patients with floating beta disease has gone some way towards solving the very difficult problem of defining this disorder, but there is still room for disagreement. Furthermore, it now seems that broad beta disease is not inherited monogenically, so that we can no longer hope to be able eventually to define it in terms of the presence of a single abnormal gene product.

Finally, it should be noted that although the type III lipoprotein abnormality has usually been discussed mainly in relation to VLDL, the lipoprotein composition of the d 1.006–1.019 fraction is also abnormal. Indeed, the lipoprotein abnormality extends throughout the range from S_f 12 to S_f 400. This was apparent from observations carried out many years ago by Gofman et al. (1954) on the plasma of a group of patients with tuberous xanthomas who, according to Fredrickson and Levy (1972), were clearly suffering from floating beta disease. When examined in the analytical ultracentrifuge, the plasma from these patients showed a decrease in the S_f 0–12 lipoprotein fraction (d 1.019–1.063) and an increase in the S_f 12–20 (d 1.006–1.019) and S_f 20–400 (d < 1.006) fractions (Fig. 15.14). The presence of an abnormal lipoprotein pattern in the S_f 12–20 fraction in this disease has been confirmed by Patsch et al. (1975), who isolated

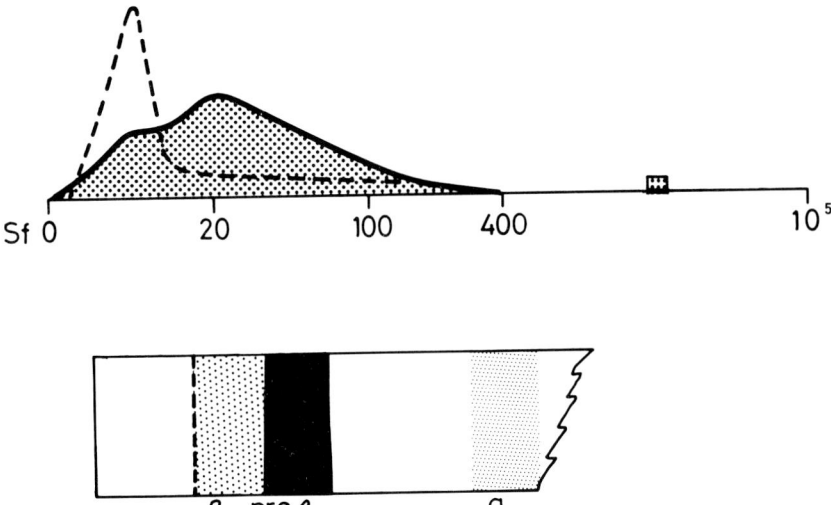

Figure 15.14
Plasma lipoprotein pattern in Type III hyperlipoproteinaemia. The upper section shows the distribution of S_f values obtained in the analytical ultracentrifuge (broken line, normal; shaded area, Type III). The lower section shows a diagrammic representation of the pattern obtained on paper electrophoresis. (From Fredrickson and Levy (1972), with the permission of the authors.)

a well-defined lipoprotein in the S_f 15–20 (d 1.006–1.020) range of the plasma of type III hyperlipoproteinaemic patients by rate-zonal ultracentrifugation. This lipoprotein had a slower electrophoretic mobility and a higher cholesterol:triglyceride ratio than normal VLDL. Since it was not present in normal plasma or in the plasma of patients with other forms of hyperlipoproteinaemia, Patsch *et al.* (1975) concluded that it was distinctive of type III hyperlipoproteinaemia and they therefore called it LP III. Packard *et al.* (1978), using molecular-sieve chromatography, have confirmed the presence of a lipoprotein with the characteristics of Lp III in the plasma of type III hyperlipoproteinaemic patients, but they do not regard it as necessarily belonging to a population of lipoprotein particles distinct from the β-VLDL present throughout the S_f 20–400 range in these patients.

4.2 Abnormalities in the plasma lipids and lipoproteins

4.2.1 The hyperlipidaemia
Plasma lipid concentrations vary markedly in different affected individuals and in the same patient under different dietary conditions. In plasma from patients not undergoing any treatment there is

usually a moderate to marked increase in plasma total cholesterol concentration (300–500 mg/100 ml) and in plasma triglyceride concentration (500–>1000 mg/100ml), the concentration of triglyceride usually exceeding that of cholesterol in whole plasma. The hyperlipidaemia is due to an increase in VLDL and IDL concentrations and is accompanied by a decrease in the concentrations of LDL and HDL (Table 15.8).

Table 15.8

Plasma lipid and lipoprotein concentrations in patients with familial type III hyperlipoproteinaemia

	Cholesterol (mg/100 ml) Total	VLDL	LDL	HDL	Triglyceride (mg/100 ml) Total
All patients	453	287	121	38	699
Normal men (age 30–39)	210	21	143	48	78
Normal women (age 40–49)	217	14	130	62	80

VLDL = d <1.006; LDL = d 1.006–1.063; HDL = d 1.063–1.21 (adapted from values obtained by Morganroth *et al.* (1975) from 49 patients with familial type III hyperlipoproteinaemia.) Note that the 'LDL' fractions included IDL (d = 1.006–1.019).

4.2.2 β-VLDL

As already noted in Section 4.1, the lipid composition of VLDL (d < 1.006) is abnormal, the cholesterol:triglyceride ratio in this fraction usually exceeding 0.3, compared with the normal range of about 0.1 to 0.2. The enrichment of the VLDL fraction with cholesterol is due to the presence of β-VLDL, which, as mentioned above, is richer in esterified cholesterol and poorer in triglyceride than the normal preβ-migrating VLDL that is also present in the plasma of these patients. Table 15.9 shows the lipid and protein composition of β-VLDL, normal VLDL, the IDL fraction (Lp III of Patsch *et al.*, 1975) and normal LDL. There is a progressive increase in the percentages of total cholesterol and protein and a progressive decrease in the percentage of triglyceride in the sequence: normal VLDL, β-VLDL, Lp III and LDL. As discussed below, this is consistent with the view that β-VLDL and Lp III represent stages in the conversion of triglyceride-rich particles into LDL. The ratio of cholesterol to triglyceride in the VLDL in a given patient is presumably a reflection of the relative amounts of β-VLDL and normal VLDL in this fraction.

In parallel with the changes in lipid composition shown in the sequence in Table 15.9, there is a progressive increase in the percentage of apoB and a progressive decrease in that of apoC proteins.

Table 15.9

Lipid and protein composition of β-VLDL and of lipoproteins in the d 1.006–1.020 fraction of plasma from patients with familial type III hyperlipoproteinaemia. Values for normal VLDL and normal LDL are shown for comparison

	Percentage of total weight					Protein composition		
	TG	TC	PL	Protein	apoB (% protein)	apoC (% TMU-soluble protein)	apoE
Normal VLDL	62	15	15	7	40–45	85	14
β-VLDL	39	33	19	10	57	56	44
Lp III	19	36	24	20	—	—	—
Normal LDL	5	45	15	25	>95	Usually absent	

TG, triglyceride; TC, total cholesterol; PL, phospholipid; TMU, tetramethylurea; —, no observation reported.

Values adapted from Quarfordt et al. (1971); Havel and Kane (1973b); Patsch et al. (1975) and from other sources.

These differences are consistent with the known loss of apoC proteins from triglyceride-rich particles during their conversion into LDL. Loss of the polar apoC proteins would explain the decreased electrophoretic mobility of β-VLDL compared with normal VLDL and, hence, the tendency of β-VLDL to overlap with LDL on zonal electrophoresis. The high concentration of apoE in β-VLDL is dealt with below.

4.2.3 ApoE proteins

Table 15.9 shows the marked enrichment of β-VLDL with apoE, already mentioned in Section 4.1. Kushwaha *et al.* (1977) have shown that the concentration of apoE in whole plasma, and in VLDL and other lipoprotein fractions, is higher in patients with type III hyperlipoproteinaemia than in normal subjects or patients with hyperlipidaemias other than that due to the type III abnormality. This suggests that the increased apoE concentration in VLDL is a specific indicator of type III hyperlipoproteinaemia. In addition to an increase in the concentration of immunochemically reactive apoE protein in the VLDL fraction of plasma in these patients, there is an abnormality in the relative amounts of the different apoE subfractions. Utermann *et al.* (1975) have shown that apoE, isolated from normal VLDL protein by preparative polyacrylamide-gel electrophoresis, can be separated by isoelectric focusing into at least three separate components (apoE-I, apoE-II and apoE-III). In all index patients from families with type III hyperlipoproteinaemia, apoE-III is not detectable in VLDL or in any other plasma lipoprotein fraction. The inheritance of this abnormal apoprotein pattern is discussed in Section 4.4.

4.3 Clinical features

Patients with familial type III hyperlipoproteinaemia usually present with skin xanthomas (one of the largest series of patients reported was collected by a dermatologist (Borrie, 1969)) or unexplained hyperlipidaemia. Others may present with symptoms due to premature atherosclerosis of the coronary or peripheral arteries. The clinical symptoms and the combination of hypercholesterolaemia with hypertriglyceridaemia do not usually appear before the end of the second decade, though β-VLDL may be detectable in the plasma of children from affected families.

Typically, the skin xanthomas appear as clusters of raised yellowish lesions with an erythematous base (*tuberoeruptive xanthomas*) on the knees, elbows and buttocks, and deposits of yellow lipid in the creases of the palms (*xanthoma striata palmaris*). Tendon xanthomas may also be present, but are less common than in familial hypercholesterolaemia. Premature ischaemic heart disease has been observed in about a third of the patients in most reports, and premature peripheral vascular disease is almost as common. Thus, the relative frequency of peripheral vascular disease compared with that of coronary artery disease is much higher in floating beta disease than in familial hypercholesterolaemia. Other clinical abnormalities associated with primary type III hyperlipoproteinaemia are hyperuricaemia, glucose intolerance, obesity and diminished thyroid function (Fredrickson and Levy, 1972; Morganroth et al., 1975; Hazzard and Bierman, 1972). The hyperlipidaemia of the type III disorder is exacerbated by hypothyroidism and is decreased by hyperthyroidism.

4.4 Genetics

An obvious familial clustering of the abnormal lipoprotein pattern and clinical manifestations was noted in the earliest descriptions of floating beta disease, suggesting simple Mendelian inheritance. However, the mode of inheritance has been very elusive. This is due not only to the unusual nature of the genetic basis of the disease, but also to its delayed onset and to the problem of finding a satisfactory diagnostic marker that is close enough to the abnormal gene product to be specific.

Studies of the families of many separate index patients (Fredrickson and Levy, 1972; Morganroth et al., 1975) and of a single large family containing four generations (Hazzard, et al., 1975) showed that the disease could manifest itself in parents and their offspring, that it occurred in both sexes and that parental consanguinity was not present. These findings, particularly the presence of the disease in three generations of one family, were consistent with autosomal dominant, rather than autosomal recessive, inheritance. However, several features revealed by these studies could not be reconciled with the view that the type III lipoprotein pattern was determined simply by the presence of a single dominant gene. In the first place, in some families the index patient was found to have two normal parents. To explain this, it was suggested that the mode of inheritance was Mendelian recessive, but that the frequency of the mutant gene in the general population was so high that a significant number of random matings occurred between a homozygote and a heterozygote, giving the appearance of dominant inheritance (*pseudodominance*). A further difficulty arose from the finding that although about half the first-degree relatives of index patients had primary hyperlipoproteinaemia (consistent with the expected 1:1 Mendelian ratio for a dominant gene), in many cases the hyperlipoproteinaemia was not type III. For example, in the families studied by Morganroth et al. (1975) about half the first-degree relatives of index patients had primary hyperlipidaemia, but in nearly half of these the abnormal lipoprotein pattern was type IV and in few was type II or type V. This was explained on the supposition that the presumed dominant gene could express itself phenotypically in more than one way. An alternative suggestion was that the expression of the gene requires the presence of another independently inherited gene (Morganroth et al., 1975), the full clinical syndrome of floating beta disease being a consequence of the coincidence of the gene causing the appearance of β-VLDL and another gene either for type IV hyperlipoproteinaemia or for familial combined hyperlipidaemia (Hazzard et al., 1975), suggestions that have turned out to be not very far from the truth. Moser et al., (1974) also concluded that the inheritance of type III hyperlipoproteinaemia was not monogenic when they failed to find bimodal segregation of the plasma lipoprotein patterns in the first-degree relatives of type III index patients. This confusion has been largely resolved by the investigations of Utermann et al. (1979a,b).

As we saw in Section 4.2, the VLDL apoE of patients with the clinical syndrome of familial type III hyperlipoproteinaemia lacks the apoE-III component. Utermann et al. have shown that this abnormality reflects a genetic polymorphism for apoE proteins in the general population. Three phenotypes can be identified by isoelectric focusing of VLDL apoE: a normal complement of apoE-III (the apoE-N phenotype), complete deficiency of apoE-III (the apoE-D phenotype) and a partial deficiency (the apoE-ND phenotype). Family studies of the segregation of phenotypes have shown that the apoE pattern is determined by two autosomal codominant alleles at the same gene locus, designated $apoE^n$ (the normal gene) and $apoE^d$ (the much rarer mutant gene). Two $apoE^n$ genes give the apoE-N phenotype, two $apoE^d$ genes give the apoE-D phenotype, while the heterozygotes ($apoE^n/apoE^d$) have the apoE-ND phenotype. All patients with familial type III hyperlipoproteinaemia (defined, it should be noted, as hyperlipidaemia together with the presence of β-VLDL in the plasma and a high cholesterol:triglyceride ratio in the VLDL fraction) are homozygous for the $apoE^d$ gene and therefore have the apoE-D phenotype. However, Utermann and his co-workers have shown that the frequency of the apoE-D phenotype in the general population (about 1% in Germany) is many times higher than the incidence of familial type III hyperlipoproteinaemia (about 0.02%). Thus, although the apoE-D phenotype is a necessary condition for the development of type III hyperlipoproteinaemia, less than 5% of all $apoE^d$ homozygotes manifest the disease. In other words, the type III abnormality requires more than a double dose of the $apoE^d$ gene if it is to be expressed.

Studies carried out by Utermann et al. (1979a) on the families of apoE-D index subjects have provided an explanation for this apparent anomaly and, moreover, have revealed an unusual genetic situation that may have wide implications. The results of these studies may be interpreted in the following way.

Everyone, including children, with the apoE-D phenotype has an abnormal plasma lipoprotein pattern characterized by the presence of β-VLDL, increased VLDL concentration and decreased LDL concentration. Utermann *et al.* call this pattern 'primary dysbetalipoproteinaemia'. Since it rarely occurs in heterozygotes (the apoE-ND phenotypes), the abnormality may be regarded as an autosomal recessive trait. In the majority of individuals who have the apoE-D phenotype, there is no hyperlipidaemia and therefore no type III hyperlipoproteinaemia. Indeed, owing to the abnormally low LDL concentration, plasma total cholesterol concentration is subnormal. If, however, some other factor that has an unfavourable effect on plasma lipoprotein metabolism happens to be present, β-VLDL accumulates in sufficient quantity to produce hyperlipoproteinaemia, i.e. the type III abnormality develops. This could explain why so many patients with type III hyperlipoproteinaemia belong to families with a high incidence of hyperlipoproteinaemias other than type III. If, for example an apoE-D individual belonged to a family with a high incidence of the type IV disorder (which could be monogenically or polygenically inherited) and if he happened to inherit the tendency to develop type IV hyperlipoproteinaemia, his primary dysbetalipoproteinaemia would be converted into the type III disorder in his third and fourth decade, and he would then develop the characteristic skin lesions and might also develop premature atherosclerosis. The mechanism by which non-type III forms of hyperlipoproteinaemia enhance the accumulation of β-VLDL in the apoE-D phenotype is discussed in Section 4.5.

In addition to explaining the prevalence of non-type III hyperlipoproteinaemias in the relatives of patients with floating beta disease, these interpretations provide an explanation of another feature of this disorder that has been so baffling. As already noted, vertical transmission has been observed in many families, yet the disease was clearly not inherited as a Mendelian dominant trait since some index patients had two normal parents. Vertical transmission can now be explained in terms of the inheritance of the apoE^d gene. The frequency of this gene in the general population is so high that in some families with familial type III hyperlipoproteinaemia one parent is homozygous (apoE-D) and the other is heterozygous (apoE-ND). In such a mating, 50% of the offspring would be expected to have the apoE-D phenotype. Hence, if homozygous parent and offspring both had the additional factor required to produce the type III disorder, the affected offspring might appear to have inherited the disease from one parent carrying a single dose of a dominant gene.

Type III hyperlipoproteinaemia, as well as occurring in familial form, also occurs sporadically in diabetes, myxoedema, renal disease and systemic lupus erythematosus. It is too early to say whether these secondary forms of the type III disorder can only occur in individuals with the apoE-D phenotype, or whether there are conditions in which a gross abnormality in plasma lipoprotein metabolism can be a sufficient cause of the disorder. Another interesting question for the future is the possible role of the apoE^d gene as a factor influencing plasma cholesterol concentration in the general population. There is also the possibility that this gene is an independent risk factor for IHD, quite apart from its role in the aetiology of familial type III hyperlipoproteinaemia, though it would be difficult to predict whether the combination of low LDL concentration and the presence of β-VLDL would increase or decrease proneness to IHD. This can only be answered by detailed epidemiological investigations.

To summarize this section, individuals who have inherited a double dose of the apoE^d gene develop a 'silent' plasma lipoprotein abnormality in childhood characterized by hypocholesterolaemia, a low plasma LDL concentration and the presence of detectable β-VLDL. If they also inherit a tendency to non-type III hyperlipoproteinaemia, or if they acquire one of several diseases affecting plasma lipoprotein metabolism, their subclinical abnormality is converted into a grossly hyperlipidaemic state characterized by hypercholestrolaemia and hypertriglyceridaemia due to the accumulation of β-VLDL in high concentration, usually leading to the development of skin lesions in adult life and, subsequently, to premature IHD.

4.5 The metabolic basis of type III hyperlipoproteinaemia

Both β-VLDL and the excess of S_f 12–20 lipoproteins in the plasma of patients with floating beta disease are generally considered to be the remnants resulting from the partial degradation of triglyceride-rich particles during the course of their normal catabolism. It is presumed that remnants are not detectable in the plasma of normal subjects because they are rapidly converted into LDL, probably by the liver. In keeping with these ideas, normal VLDL and chylomicrons occur in the plasma of type III patients during fat absorption. Moreover, the lipid and protein composition of β-VLDL is broadly similar to that of the cholesterol-enriched particles that accumulate in the plasma of rats given intravenous injections of chylomicrons or VLDL after exclusion of the liver (Mjøs et al., 1975). On this view, β-VLDL and the S_f 12–20 lipoproteins are essentially normal intermediates that accumulate in plasma in type III hyperlipoproteinaemia because of an imbalance between their rate of production and their rate of conversion into LDL.

This much is still generally accepted, though with the reservation that there may be a crucial abnormality in the protein composition of the remnants in type III. However, there has been disagreement as to whether the primary defect is overproduction of remnant particles leading to saturation of a normal disposal mechanism, or a defect in the mechanisms by which remnants are metabolized. Observations on the catabolism of labelled triglyceride-rich lipoproteins in type III patients have led several groups of workers to conclude that the removal of remnants is impaired (Bilheimer et al., 1971; Hazzard and Bierman, 1971; Quarfordt et al., 1973). However, the more recent studies of Hall et al. (1974), involving compartmental analysis of plasma apoB specific-activity curves obtained after injections of labelled lipoproteins, suggest that in type III there is overproduction of VLDL, together with direct secretion of IDL into the circulation, leading to overloading of the pathway to LDL.

Increased remnant production and an intrinsic defect in remnant removal are not mutually exclusive. Indeed, the genetic studies discussed above are compatible with the view that the pathological accumulation of β-VLDL requires the coincidence of two defects: (1), a structural abnormality in VLDL, perhaps leading to the formation of remnants that cannot be taken up by the liver because they lack a specific protein (apoE-III) essential for their recognition by hepatocytes and (2), a separate abnormality in plasma lipoprotein metabolism, of which type IV hyperlipoproteinaemia is the most frequent. Since the hypertriglyceridaemia of type IV is usually associated with overproduction of VLDL, floating beta disease in a patient belonging to a family with type IV hyperlipoproteinaemia could well be caused by a combination of overproduction of remnants and defective conversion of remnants into LDL by the liver. Certainly, overproduction of remnants would not by itself explain the decreased LDL concentration that is characteristic of the type III disorder, whereas a partial block in the pathway from remnants to LDL would readily explain this. Further evidence for the presence of a block in the metabolism of remnants has recently been obtained by Chait et al. (1977), who demonstrated defective conversion of IDL into LDL in a type III patient and then showed that oestrogens corrected this defect while, at the same time, *stimulating* the production of VLDL. Clearly, the defective formation of LDL observed in the untreated state in this patient was not due to saturation of a normal mechanism by overproduction of VLDL. In the light of these observations, Chait et al. (1977) suggest calling type III hyperlipoproteinaemia 'remnant removal disease'. Increased remnant production, combined with defective conversion of remnants into LDL, would explain the type III disorder observed in many families. A similar combination may also explain the development of secondary forms of type III hyperlipoproteinaemia in various disorders of metabolism, though this point remains to be investigated. The association between type IIa hyperlipoproteinaemia and floating beta disease in some families is more difficult to understand, since there is no reason to suppose that VLDL production is increased in the type IIa disorder.

In keeping with the view that there is a specific defect in the catabolism of remnants in this disease, Havel *et al.* (1980) have shown that the livers of oestrogen-treated rats develop high-affinity receptors for phospholipid particles containing normal human apoE and that these receptors fail to recognize particles containing only the abnormal apoE present in the plasma of patients with floating beta disease. This suggests that the missing apoE component is essential for recognition of remnant particles by the liver. Thus, remnant removal disease may well be a 'remnant recognition disease'.

The possible presence of apoE receptors in normal human liver raises several interesting questions about lipoprotein catabolism in a wider context. The LDL receptor present in many tissues, possibly including the liver (see Chapter 9, Section 3.5), also has high affinity for apoE (probably because apoB and apoE have certain amino-acid sequences in common). If there are apoE receptors in human liver, are they the same as classical LDL receptors and, if so, do they play a significant role in the catabolism of LDL? If hepatic apoE receptors are, in fact, LDL receptors, why is accumulation of remnant particles in the plasma not a constant feature of FH? The alternative possibility—that hepatic apoE receptors are distinct from the LDL receptor—is perhaps more attractive at the present stage of knowledge. On this view, the apoE receptor could recognize a different segment of the apoE protein from that recognized by the LDL receptor.

Occasional reports of an association between FH and floating beta disease (Kwiterovich *et al.*, 1975) can be reconciled with the supposition that apoE receptors and apoB receptors are not identical. Since apoE has such a high affinity for LDL receptors, it is conceivable that under conditions in which the normal pathway for remnant metabolism is partially blocked, some of the β-VLDL that accumulates in the plasma gains access to cells possessing LDL receptors and that receptor-mediated uptake contributes to the total metabolism of remnants. A genetic deficiency of LDL receptors could thus lead to an abnormal accumulation of remnant particles in the plasma in the absence of increased remnant production. Absence of this possible alternative pathway for remnant metabolism may explain the occasional reports of xanthomas in the palmar creases of patients with familial hypercholesterolaemia in the homozygous form. It would be reasonable to look for the presence of β-VLDL and the apoE-D phenotype in such cases. Finally, it is worthwhile recalling the fact that an apoE-rich lipoprotein with many of the characteristics of β-VLDL accumulates in the plasma of cholesterol-fed animals of several species (Mahley, 1978), suggesting that 'remnant' particles tend to accumulate when there is an increased demand for cholesterol transport in the circulation.

4.6 Diagnosis

In severely affected adult patients, type III hyperlipoproteinaemia can be diagnosed without difficulty from the marked increase in plasma cholesterol and triglyceride concentrations and the presence of β-VLDL in the plasma in readily detectable amounts (a broad beta band on zonal electrophoresis of whole plasma is no longer regarded as a reliable diagnostic sign). The diagnosis is favoured by a history of premature atherosclerosis of the peripheral arteries and is reinforced by the presence of tuberoeruptive xanthomas or lipid deposits in the palmar creases, the latter being regarded by some authorities as pathognomonic of the type III disorder. Primary hyperlipoproteinaemia, including type III in the patient's relatives, provides additional evidence for the diagnosis. The differential diagnosis includes type IIb and type IV hyperlipoproteinaemia, both of which are excluded by the absence of β-VLDL in the d < 1.006 fraction of the plasma.

Whether or not it is worth making a distinction between familial and non-familial type III hyperlipoproteinaemia is an arguable point, since all type III is in a sense familial in so far as the disease only manifests itself in people who have inherited a double dose of a rare mutant gene. For this reason, plasma lipid concentrations should be measured in the relatives of all patients found to have the type III disorder in order to detect those at risk for IHD. From the practical point of view, however, it is worth distinguishing between primary type III and type III in which the precipitating cause is an obvious and treatable disorder of metabolism such as diabetes or myxoedema.

When the disease is present in a mild form and there are no overt clinical signs, the diagnosis may be very difficult. Studies of the relatives of patients with unequivocal floating beta disease have shown that a correct diagnosis can usually be made if hypertriglyceridaemia is present and if the ratio of VLDL-cholesterol to total plasma triglyceride exceeds 0.3, a high ratio reflecting the presence of β-VLDL (Fredrickson *et al.*, 1975). Other workers suggest basing the diagnosis on the presence of detectable β-VLDL in the plasma (Hazzard *et al.*, 1975) or on a minimum apoE concentration in whole plasma (Kushwaha *et al.*, 1977). No single diagnostic criterion is free from positive or negative errors; increasing the sensitivity of β-VLDL measurement beyond a certain point merely increases the proportion of false positive diagnoses since β-migrating VLDL is probably present at a finite concentration in normal plasma. According to the current view of the nature of the type III disorder, the diagnosis should not be made in the absence of the apoE-D phenotype, but a diagnosis of the apoE phenotype requires the use of isoelectric focusing, a procedure that is not available in the routine laboratory. Those who find these conclusions depressing may take comfort from the fact that an accurate diagnosis of type III hyperlipoproteinaemia is necessary only in relation to research. In routine clinical practice the treatment of primary mixed hyperlipidaemia is the same whatever the underlying lipoprotein disorder.

4.7 Treatment

Since patients with floating beta disease are at risk for IHD and peripheral vascular disease, they should be given treatment to bring their plasma lipid concentrations to within the normal range. Type III hyperlipoproteinaemia responds to treatment more rapidly and completely than does any other form of hyperlipoproteinaemia. In patients in whom the type III disorder is exacerbated or unmasked by the presence of a recognizable cause such as myxoedema, diabetes, alcoholism or dysglobulinaemia, the appropriate treatment should be given. Patients with 'primary' type III who are overweight, as many of them are, should be given a diet low in calories until ideal body weight is achieved. Cholesterol intake should be reduced to less than 300 mg/day and alcohol consumption should be limited. On this regime, plasma lipid concentrations fall rapidly and in many patients the skin lesions disappear within weeks or months. If dietary modification by itself is not fully effective, the patient should be given clofibrate (2 g/day). This is almost invariably highly effective in lowering plasma lipid levels, possibly by diminishing VLDL production. Cholestyramine is of no value in type III hyperlipoproteinaemia. It will generally be found that β-VLDL is still detectable in the plasma after the lipid concentration has been brought to within the normal range.

5 SECONDARY HYPERCHOLESTEROLAEMIA

5.1 Introduction

The presence of secondary hyperlipidaemia in many systemic diseases has already been referred to in this chapter (see Table 15.2 for a comprehensive list). The abnormal lipoprotein pattern produced by a given metabolic disorder varies considerably from one patient to another and tends to change in the same individual patient under different conditions. For example, in one series of untreated diabetic patients with hyperlipidaemia, types II, III and IV hyperlipoproteinaemia were recorded with roughly equal frequency (Hayes, 1972). Almost by definition, when the underlying metabolic disease responsible for the secondary hyperlipidaemia is treated, the plasma lipoprotein pattern becomes normal. In some cases, however, hyperlipidaemia persists when what appears to be an obvious secondary cause has been successfully treated. In such instances it may be supposed that the disease exacerbates a primary hyperlipoproteinaemia; a possible example of this situation is discussed in Section 5.3.

In many patients with secondary hyperlipidaemia, especially those in whom the underlying cause is alcoholism, acute diabetes or glycogen storage disease, the predominant plasma lipid abnormality is hypertriglyceridaemia due to an increased plasma VLDL concentration or to delayed clearance of chylomicrons. However, some causes of secondary hyperlipidaemia tend to produce hypercholesterolaemia with or without hypertriglyceridaemia. In these cases the plasma lipoprotein pattern resembles that in primary type IIa or type IIb hyperlipoproteinaemia or, more rarely, that seen in floating beta disease. In this chapter we shall consider some of the more interesting aspects of secondary hypercholesterolaemia, with the main emphasis on pathogenesis. The hyperlipidaemia of pregnancy will also be considered here. Abnormal plasma lipid patterns seen in liver disease are dealt with in Chapter 18.

5.2 Diabetes

Most workers agree that a third to a half of all untreated diabetics have hyperlipidaemia. In most cases the increased plasma lipid concentration is confined to the triglycerides and is due to type IV hyperlipoproteinaemia or, less commonly, to chylomicronaemia or to the type V pattern (see Lewis (1976), Chapter 14 for a discussion of the diagnosis, treatment and pathogenesis of diabetic hypertriglyceridaemia). However, in a small proportion of diabetics, particularly in those who are partially controlled by diet and insulin (Schonfeld *et al.*, 1974) or who do not require insulin (Kissebah *et al.*, 1975), hypercholesterolaemia may be the predominant lipid abnormality. For example, in a group of diabetic outpatients investigated by Schonfeld *et al.* (1974), 12% had type IIa hyperlipoproteinaemia. In this study it was also noted that in all the diabetics, whether or not they had hyperlipidaemia, the ratio of triglyceride to cholesterol in LDL was abnormally high. In insulin-deficient diabetics, the plasma

HDL concentration is usually subnormal in the untreated state and in these cases is restored to the normal level when insulin is given (Nikkilä, 1978).

The increase in plasma LDL concentration that occurs in some partially controlled diabetics has not been adequately explained. An important factor in the production of hypertriglyceridaemia in many insulin-deficient diabetics appears to be diminished lipoprotein lipase activity, resulting in the accumulation of triglyceride-rich lipoproteins that would normally be catabolized in the circulation (Nikkilä, 1978). This defect could explain the low plasma HDL concentration observed in many untreated insulin-dependent diabetics, since HDL probably originates in part from the surface components of VLDL and chylomicrons released during their catabolism by lipoprotein lipase (see Chapter 11). However, defective breakdown of triglyceride lipoproteins clearly cannot explain an increase in plasma LDL concentration, since VLDL, and possibly chylomicrons, are obligatory precursors of LDL under normal conditions. On the contrary, defective breakdown of triglyceride-rich lipoproteins would be expected to lead to a fall in plasma LDL concentration, as indeed occurs in familial lipoprotein lipase deficiency and floating beta disease. Two possibilities are worth considering. LDL catabolism may be defective in the diabetic state. There is no direct evidence for this, but it would be consistent with the observation of Chait et al. (1978) that insulin is required for optimal functional activity of LDL receptors *in vitro*. The other possibility is that in some diabetics, in addition to the normal pathway for the production of LDL, some LDL is secreted directly into the circulation (as in homozygous FH). The validity of these speculations could be tested experimentally in diabetic patients with hypercholesterolaemia due to increased plasma LDL concentration.

Since the plasma LDL concentration is influenced by a multiplicity of factors, some of which may have opposing effects, it is hardly surprising that an increased plasma LDL level is an inconstant feature of diabetes and that it occurs only under rather special conditions, notably when the disease is partially controlled by treatment. In addition to causing decreased catabolism of triglyceride-rich lipoproteins, diabetes may also increase VLDL production (Nikkilä and Kekki, 1973). Hence, it is possible that hypercholesterolaemia due to an increase in plasma LDL concentration is the outcome of a balance between increased VLDL production, decreased VLDL catabolism, decreased LDL catabolism and direct secretion of LDL. In diabetic patients with type III hyperlipoproteinaemia (see Stern et al., 1972 and the possible examples of diabetic type III in Hayes, 1972) there may be a defect in the conversion of remnant particles into LDL.

The practical importance of diabetic hyperlipidaemia lies in its possible relevance to the increased risk of IHD and peripheral vascular disease in diabetes. There is good reason to believe that this increase in risk is mediated in some degree by the hypercholesterolaemia or hypertriglyceridaemia that frequently occurs in the diabetic state. For this reason, it is generally agreed that diabetic hyperlipidaemia should be treated when it persists after the hyperglycaemia has been successfully controlled. A discussion of the treatment of diabetic hyperlipidaemia will be found in Lewis (1976).

5.3 Hypothyroidism

Hyperlipidaemia occurs in most hypothyroid patients. It is present in cretinism and juvenile myxoedema, as well as in the myxoedema that develops in adults, either spontaneously or as a complication of surgical or radioiodine 'thyroidectomy' for thyrotoxicosis or angina pectoris. Hyperlipidaemia has also been reported in hypothyroidism secondary to pituitary deficiency. Any of the hyperlipoproteinaemias may occur in hypothyroidism. The abnormal lipoprotein patterns most frequently encountered are those in which the plasma LDL concentration is raised (IIa and IIb), but types III, IV and V may also occur; chylomicronaemia associated with diminished post-heparin lipase activity has been described in myxoedema (Porte et al., 1966).

Hypercholesterolaemia is much commoner than hypertriglyceridaemia in hypothyroidism. In myxoedema the plasma cholesterol concentration may exceed 600 mg/100 ml, but is very variable and bears little relation to the clinical severity of the hypothyroidism (Gildea et al., 1939). When the hypothyroidism is treated successfully, the plasma cholesterol concentration falls rapidly to within the normal range unless there is an underlying primary lipoprotein abnormality, such as FH. Hypercholesterolaemia is so common in hypothyroidism that it is a useful diagnostic sign of this disorder. It is particularly helpful in diagnosis if it is rapidly reversed by small doses of thyroid hormone. This therapeutic response is sometimes useful as a test for distinguishing hypothyroidism from chronic renal disease, a condition in which there may be a reduced basal metabolic rate and a raised plasma cholesterol concentration, the latter failing to respond fully to thyroid hormone.

It has been suggested that some individuals with hypercholesterolaemia, but with no clinical signs of myxoedema, are suffering from a mild deficiency of thyroid hormone sufficient to affect cholesterol or lipoprotein metabolism but not severe enough to cause detectable hypothyroidism (so-called 'preclinical myxoedema'). Bastenie et al. (1971) have claimed that in some of these patients the serum concentration of thyroid auto-antibodies is significantly increased, but the evidence for this is controversial.

Several factors may contribute to the hypercholesterolaemia of human myxoedema. In several animal species, thyroidectomy causes hypercholesterolaemia with a reduced fractional rate of turnover of the plasma cholesterol. One factor responsible for this appears to be a fall in the rate of conversion of cholesterol into total bile acids. In myxoedematous patients the fractional rate of turnover of the plasma cholesterol is also decreased (Kurland *et al.*, 1961). This may be due in part to decreased catabolism of cholesterol in the liver, since treatment with thyroid hormone stimulates cholic-acid synthesis in myxoedema (Hellström and Lindstedt, 1964). However, a more significant effect of thyroid deficiency on human cholesterol metabolism seems to be to diminish the efficiency with which the plasma cholesterol is excreted in the faeces as neutral steroids (Miettinen, 1968). An additional factor that must contribute to hypercholesterolaemia in myxoedema is a diminished fractional catabolic rate of LDL protein (Walton *et al.*, 1965), suggesting that thyroid hormone is required for the efficient catabolism of plasma LDL in the tissues. In support of this, Thompson *et al.* (1981) have reported defective receptor-mediated catabolism of LDL in a myxoedematous patient.

Type III hyperlipoproteinaemia has been reported in myxoedema (Hazzard and Bierman, 1972). In the one case described by Hazzard and Bierman, the hyperlipidaemia was abolished when the hypothyroid state was treated effectively with thyroid hormone, but the β-VLDL and the abnormal cholesterol:triglyceride ratio in the VLDL persisted. This suggests that the myxoedema in this patient had temporarily uncovered an underlying tendency to the type III disorder, dependent, perhaps, upon the presence of the apoE-D phenotype discussed in Section 4.

5.4 Renal disease

It has been known since the early years of the present century that hyperlipidaemia occurs frequently in chronic parenchymatous disease of the kidneys. Some degree of hyperlipidaemia is almost always present in patients with the nephrotic syndrome (see Baxter (1962) for a comprehensive review of the older literature). Hypercholesterolaemia with a normal plasma triglyceride concentration is present in many mildly affected patients and is due to an increased plasma LDL concentration (the type IIa lipoprotein pattern). Hypertriglyceridaemia, with or without an increased plasma cholesterol concentration, is usually present in nephrosis of moderate severity, and in extreme cases the plasma triglyceride concentration may reach values of 3–5 g/ml. In these instances, the hypertriglyceridaemia is due to the type IV pattern or to a combination of chylomicronaemia with increased plasma VLDL concentration (the type V pattern). In chronic renal failure not accompanied by the nephrotic syndrome, type IIa or type IIb hyperlipoproteinaemia may be present, though hypertriglyceridaemia with a normal plasma cholesterol level is a much commoner finding (Brøns et al., 1972), particularly in uraemic patients undergoing repeated haemodialysis (Bagdade et al., 1968).

Since the risk of death from IHD is increased in chronic renal disease, it is desirable to try to remove as many risk factors as possible from these patients. On these grounds hyperlipidaemia, when present, should be treated by the appropriate dietary modification with or without the addition of drugs. A rational approach to treatment would be easier to adopt if we had a clearer understanding of the mechanisms by which renal disease causes hyperlipidaemia. In patients with the nephrotic syndrome, the extent of the hyperlipidaemia is closely related to the extent to which the plasma albumin concentration is reduced by loss of plasma proteins in the urine (Baxter, 1962). This has led to the view that hypoalbuminaemia is a causal factor in the development of hyperlipidaemia in nephrosis. In keeping with this, it has been shown that the hyperlipidaemia of human nephrosis (Baxter et al., 1961) can be reversed by infusing albumin into the circulation. Hyperlipidaemia can also be produced in animals by plasmapheresis repeated on sufficient occasions to cause hypoalbuminaemia, though the effects of plasmapheresis are obviously not confined to the plasma albumin. It has been suggested that proteinuria, an essential feature of the nephrotic syndrome, in some way induces a compensatory increase in the hepatic synthesis of all plasma proteins, including lipoproteins, and that since LDL and VLDL particles are too large to escape into the urine, their concentration in plasma increases, thus causing hyperlipidaemia. In support of these ideas, Marsh and Drabkin (1960) have shown that isolated perfused livers from rats made hypoalbuminaemic by nephrosis, synthesize albumin and the apoproteins of plasma lipoproteins at a greatly increased rate. Clinical studies of the rate of turnover of the plasma triglycerides also suggest that VLDL production is increased in nephrotic patients (McKenzie and Nestel, 1968; Kekki and Nikkilä, 1971). However, this hardly explains why there is usually a greater increase in the plasma concentration of LDL than of VLDL in these patients, unless there is defective catabolism of LDL in addition to the increased production of VLDL.

The hypertriglyceridaemia of patients with chronic renal failure without nephrosis has not been adequately explained. Bagdade et al. (1968) have shown that in some of these patients post-heparin lipase activity is decreased, possibly owing to depletion of tissue stores of lipoprotein lipase by the large doses of heparin used for haemodialysis in the treatment of chronic renal disease.

5.5 Other causes of secondary hypercholesterolaemia

Hyperlipidaemia occurs in some patients with hyperglobulinaemia due to myelomatosis, systemic lupus erythematosus or lymphosarcoma. The globulins usually belong to the IgA or IgG class but may occasionally be IgM. In most cases the hyperlipidaemia is due predominantly to an increased plasma triglyceride concentration, but hypercholesterolaemia may also occur. In some patients with hyperlipidaemia and dysglobulinaemia, auto-antibodies to plasma lipoproteins are present in the circulation (Lennard-Jones, 1960; Lewis and Page, 1965; Beaumont, 1969). Beaumont (1969) has suggested that the formation of a complex between lipoprotein and antibody interferes with the catabolism of the lipoprotein. However, marked hyperlipidaemia can occur in myelomatous patients who have no detectable antibodies to plasma lipoproteins (Roberts-Thomson et al., 1975). Furthermore, the rate of catabolism of plasma lipoproteins may actually be increased by binding to auto-antibodies (Noseda et al., 1972). Glueck et al. (1969) have described three patients, two with lupus erythematosus and one with lymphosarcoma, who had marked chylomicronaemia and hyperglobulinaemia. There was evidence to suggest that the hyperlipidaemia in these patients was due to the presence of auto-antibodies to heparin, leading to diminished lipoprotein-lipase activity. Some patients with systemic lupus erythematosus have hypercholesterolaemia due to type III hyperlipoproteinaemia, together with decreased post-heparin lipase activity, again suggesting the presence of auto-antibodies to heparin (Stern et al., 1972). However, decreased catabolism of triglyceride-rich lipoproteins does not explain the accumulation of β-VLDL in these patients.

Other disorders in which hypercholesterolaemia may occur include acute intermittent porphyria, Cushing's Syndrome, anorexia nervosa, hepatoma and biliary obstruction. Marked increases in plasma HDL-cholesterol concentration have also been observed in men exposed to chlorinated hydrocarbon insecticides such as DDT (Carlson and Kolmodin-Hedman, 1972).

In women under age 40 who are taking oral contraceptives containing an oestrogen, the plasma total cholesterol and triglyceride concentrations are higher than in those not taking contraceptives (Rifkind et al., 1978). The increase in cholesterol concentration is due to a rise in plasma levels of both LDL and VLDL. In older women taking oestrogens for replacement therapy, the plasma total cholesterol concentration is reduced, owing to a substantial fall in the plasma LDL level (Wallace et al., 1979). The plasma HDL-cholesterol concentration in women tends to be increased by oestrogens and to be decreased by progestogens (Bradley et al., 1978).

Hence, the net effect of an oral contraceptive on plasma HDL level will depend upon the relative amounts of oestrogen and progestogen in the contraceptive.

5.6 The hyperlipidaemia of pregnancy

The plasma total cholesterol and triglyceride concentrations rise during the second and third trimesters in most pregnant women. The increase in lipid concentration may amount to a mild or moderate physiological hyperlipidaemia. Lipid concentrations are increased in all three major lipoprotein fractions (VLDL, LDL and HDL) and these increases are accompanied by changes in the composition of LDL and HDL. There is a marked increase in the percentage of triglyceride in LDL and in the ratio of triglyceride to cholesterol in HDL; the increase in VLDL lipids is accompanied by an equivalent rise in VLDL-apoB, without apparent change in VLDL composition (Cramer et al., 1964; Hillman et al., 1975).

Some degree of hyperlipidaemia occurs during pregnancy in most species of laboratory animal, with the interesting exceptions of the rabbit and the guinea-pig. In both these species there is a marked fall in the triglyceride and cholesterol levels in maternal plasma towards the end of pregnancy (Popják, 1954).

REFERENCES

Bagdade, J. D., Porte, D. Jr. and Bierman, E. L. (1968). Hypertriglyceridemia. A metabolic consequence of chronic renal failure. *New England Journal of Medicine*, **279**, 181–185.

Bastenie, P. A., Vanhaelst, L., Bonnyns, M., Rieve, P. and Staquet, M. (1971). Preclinical hypothyroidism: a risk factor for coronary heart disease. *Lancet*, **1**, 203–204.

Baxter, J. H. (1962). Hyperlipoproteinemia in nephrosis. *Archives of Internal Medicine*, **109**, 742–757.

Baxter, J. H., Goodman, H. C. and Allen, J. C. (1961). Effects of infusions of serum albumin on serum lipids and lipoproteins in nephrosis. *Journal of Clinical Investigation*, **40**, 490–498.

Beaumont, J.-L. (1969). Un deuxième type d'auto-anticorps anti-lipoprotéine de myélome- l'IgG anti-Lp Al. Sa. *C. R. Hebdomadaires des Séances de l'Academie des Sciences*, **269**, 107–110.

Beaumont, J. L., Carlson, L. A., Cooper, G. R., Fejfar, Z., Fredrickson, D. S. and Strasser, T. (1970). Classification of hyperlipidaemias and hyperlipoproteinaemias. *Bulletin of the World Health Organization*, **43**, 891–915.

Betteridge, D. J., Higgins, M. J. P. and Galton, D. J. (1975). Regulation of 3-hydroxy-3-methylglutaryl coenzyme-A reductase activity in type II hyperlipoproteinaemia. *British Medical Journal*, **4**, 500–502.

Bilheimer, D. W., Eisenberg, S. and Levy, R. I. (1971). Abnormal metabolism of

very low density lipoproteins (VLDL) in Type III hyperlipoproteinaemia (Type III). *Circulation*, **44**, *Supplement* II, II-56.
Bilheimer, D. W., Goldstein, J. L., Grundy, S. M. and Brown, M. S. (1975). Reduction in cholesterol and low density lipoprotein synthesis after portacaval shunt surgery in a patient with homozygous familial hypercholesterolemia. *Journal of Clinical Investigation*, **56**, 1420–1430.
Bilheimer, D. W., Ho, Y. K., Brown, M. S., Anderson, R. G. W. and Goldstein, J. L. (1978). Genetics of the low density lipoprotein receptor: diminished receptor activity in lymphocytes from heterozygotes with familial hypercholesterolemia. *Journal of Clinical Investigation*, **61**, 678–696.
Borrie, P. (1969). Type III hyperlipoproteinaemia. *British Medical Journal*, **2**, 665.
Bradley, D. D., Wingerd, J., Pettitti, D. A., Krauss, R. M. and Ramcharans, S. (1978). Serum high density-lipoprotein cholesterol in women using oral contraceptives, estrogens and progestins. *New England Journal of Medicine*, **299**, 17.
Brøns, M., Christensen, M. C. and Hørder, M. (1972). Hyperlipoproteinemia in patients with chronic renal failure. *Acta Medica Scandinavica*, **192**, 119–123.
Brown, M. S., Brannan, P. G., Bohmfalk, H. A., Brunschede, G. Y., Dana, S. E., Helgeson, J. and Goldstein, J. L. (1975). Use of mutant fibroblasts in the analysis of the regulation of cholesterol metabolism in human cells. *Journal of Cellular Physiology*, **85**, 425–436.
Brown, M. S. and Goldstein, J. L. (1976). Receptor-mediated control of cholesterol metabolism. *Science*, **191**, 150–154.
Brown, M. S., Kovanen, P. T., Goldstein, J. L., Eeckels, R., Vandenberghe, K., van den Berghe, H., Fryns, J. P. and Cassiman, J. J. (1978). Prenatal diagnosis of homozygous familial hypercholesterolaemia. Expression of a genetic receptor disease *in utero*. *Lancet* **1**, 526–529.
Buchwald, H. (1964). Lowering of cholesterol absorption and blood levels by ileal exclusion. Experimental basis and preliminary clinical report. *Circulation*, **29**, 713–720.
Buchwald, H., Moore, R. B. and Varĉo, R. L. (1974). Surgical treatment of hyperlipidemia. *Circulation*, **49**, *Supplement* I, I-1–I-37.
Bulkley, B. H., Buja, L. M., Ferrans, V. J., Bulkley, G. B. and Roberts, W. C. (1975). Tuberous xanthoma in homozygous type II hyperlipoproteinemia. A histologic, histochemical, and electron microscopical study. *Archives of Pathology*, **99**, 293.
Cagné, C., Moorgani, S., Brun, D., Toussaint, M. and Lupien, P.-J. (1979). Heterozygous familial hypercholesterolemia. Relationship between plasma lipids, lipoproteins, clinical manifestations and ischaemic heart disease in men and women. *Atherosclerosis*, **34**, 13–24.
Carlson, L. A. and Kolmodin-Hedman, B. (1972). Hyper-α-lipoproteinemia in men exposed to chlorinated hydrocarbon pesticides. *Acta Medica Scandinavica*, **192**, 29.
Carter, C. O. An ABC of Medical Genetics. The Lancet Ltd., London, 1969.
Carter, C. O., Slack, J. and Myant, N. B. (1971). Genetics of hyperlipoproteinaemias. *Lancet*, **1**, 400–401.
Chait, A., Bierman, E. L. and Albers, J. J. (1978). Regulatory rôle of insulin in the degradation of low density lipoprotein by cultured human skin fibroblasts. *Biochimica et Biophysica Acta*, **529**, 292–299.
Chait, A., Brunzell, J. D., Albers, J. J. and Hazzard, W. R. (1977). Type-III hyperlipoproteinaemia ("remnant removal disease"). Insight into the pathogenic mechanism. *Lancet*, **1**, 1176–1178.
Cox, F. C., Rifkind, B., Robinson, J., Lawrie, T. D. V. and Morgan, H. G. Primary hyperlipoproteinaemias in myocardial infarction. In: *Protides of the Biological Fluids, Proceedings of the Nineteenth Colloquium*. Ed. H. Peeters. Pergamon Press, Oxford, pp. 279–282, 1972.
Cramér, K., Aurell, M. and Pehrson, S. (1964). Serum lipids and lipoproteins during pregnancy. *Clinica Chimica Acta*, **10**, 470–472.

Darmady, J. M., Fosbrooke, A. S. and Lloyd, J. K. (1972). Prospective study of serum cholesterol levels during first year of life. *British Medical Journal*, **2**, 685–688.
Einarsson, K., Hellström, K. and Kallner, M. (1974). Bile acid kinetics in relation to sex, serum lipids, body weights, and gallbladder disease in patients with various types of hyperlipoproteinemia. *Journal of Clinical Investigation*, **54**, 1301–1311.
Endo, A., Kuroda, M. and Tanzawa, K. (1976). Competitive inhibition of 3-hydroxy-3-methylglutaryl coenzyme A reductase by ML-236A and ML-236B fungal metabolites, having hypocholesterolemic activity. *FEBS Letters*, **72**, 323–326.
Fagge, C. H. (1873). Disease, etc., of the skin. 1. General xanthelasma or vitiligoidea. *Transactions of the Pathology Society of London*, **24**, 242-250.
Fisher, W. R., Hammond, M. G. and Warmke, G. L. (1972). Measurement of the molecular weight variability of plasma low density lipoproteins among normals and subjects with hyper-β-lipoproteinemia. Demonstration of macromolecular heterogeneity. *Biochemistry*, **11**, 519–525.
Fogelman, A. M., Edmond, J., Polito, A. and Popják, G. (1973). Control of lipid metabolism in human leukocytes. *Journal of Biological Chemistry*, **248**, 6928–6929.
Fogelman, A. M., Edmond, J., Seager, J. and Popják, G. (1975). Abnormal induction of 3-hydroxy-3-methylglutaryl coenzyme A reductase in leukocytes from subjects with heterozygous familial hypercholesterolemia. *Journal of Biological Chemistry*, **250**, 2045–2055.
Fogelman, A. M., Shechter, I., Seager, J. Hokom, M., Child, J. S. and Edwards, P. A. (1980). Malonaldehyde alteration of low density lipoproteins leads to cholesteryl ester accumulation in human monocyte-macrophages. *Proceedings of the National Academy of Sciences of the USA*, **77**, 2214–2218.
Fredrickson, D. S., Goldstein, J. L. and Brown, M. S. The familial hyperlipoproteinemias. In: *The Metabolic Basis of Inherited Disease*, 4th edition. Ed. J. B. Stanbury, J. B. Wyngaarden and D. S. Fredrickson. McGraw Hill, New York, pp. 604–655, 1978.
Fredrickson, D. S. and Levy, R. I. Familial hyperlipoproteinemia. In: *The Metabolic Basis of Inherited Disease*, 3rd edition. Ed. J. B. Stanbury, J. B. Wyngaarden and D. S. Fredrickson. McGraw-Hill, New York, pp. 545–614, 1972.
Fredrickson, D. S., Levy, R. I. and Lees, R. S. (1967). Fat transport in lipoproteins—an integrated approach to mechanisms and disorders. *New England Journal of Medicine*, **276**, 34–44, 94–103, 148–156, 215–225, 273–281.
Fredrickson, D. S., Morganroth, J. and Levy, R. I. (1975). Type III hyperlipoproteinemia: an analysis of two contemporary definitions. *Annals of Internal Medicine*, **82**, 150–157.
De Gennes, J.-L., Touraine, R., Maunand, B., Truffert, J. and Laudat, P. (1967). Formes homozygotes cutaneo-tendineuse de xanthomatose hypercholestérolémique dans une observation familiale exemplaire. Essai de plasmaphérèse a titre de traitement héroique. *Bull. Mem. Soc. Hôp. Paris*. **118**, 1377–1402.
Gildea, E. F., Man, E. B. and Peters, J. P. (1939). Serum lipoids and proteins in hypothyroidism. *Journal of Clinical Investigation*, **18**, 739–755.
Glueck, C. J., Heckman, F., Schoenfeld, M., Steiner, P. and Pearce, W. (1971). Neonatal familial Type II hyperlipoproteinemia: cord blood cholesterol in 1800 births. *Metabolism*, **20**, 597–608.
Glueck, C. J., Levy, R. I. and Fredrickson, D. S. (1968). Acute tendinitis and arthritis: A presenting symptom of familial type II hyperlipoproteinemia. *Journal of the American Medical Association*, **206**, 2895–2897.
Glueck, C. J., Levy, R. I., Glueck, H. I., Gralnick, H. R., Greten, H. and Fredrickson, D. S. (1969). Acquired type I hyperlipoproteinemia with systemic lupus erythematosus, dysglobulinemia and heparin resistance. *American Journal of Medicine*, **47**, 318–324.

Gofman, J. W., Rubin, L., McGinley, J. P. and Jones, H. B. (1954). Hyperlipoproteinaemia. *American Journal of Medicine*, **17**, 514–520.

Goldstein, J. L., Anderson, R. G. W., Buja, L. M., Basu, S. K. and Brown, M. S. (1977a). Overloading human aortic smooth muscle cells with low density lipoprotein-cholesteryl esters reproduces features of atherosclerosis *in vitro*. *Journal of Clinical Investigation*, **59**, 1196–1202.

Goldstein, J. L. and Brown, M. S. (1973). Familial hypercholesterolemia: Identification of a defect in the regulation of 3-hydroxy-3-methylglutaryl coenzyme A reductase activity associated with overproduction of cholesterol. *Proceedings of the National Academy of Sciences of the USA*, **70**, 2804–2808.

Goldstein, J. L. and Brown, M. S. (1977a). The low-density lipoprotein pathway and its relation to atherosclerosis. *Annual Review of Biochemistry*, **46**, 897–930.

Goldstein, J. L. and Brown, M. S. (1977b). Atherosclerosis: the low-density lipoprotein receptor hypothesis. *Metabolism*, **26**, 1257–1275.

Goldstein, J. L. and Brown, M. S. (1978). Familial hypercholesterolemia: pathogenesis of a receptor disease. *The Johns Hopkins Medical Journal*, **143**, 8–16.

Goldstein, J. L. and Brown, M. S. (1979). The LDL receptor locus and the genetics of familial hypercholesterolemia. *Annual Review of Genetics*, **13**, 259–289.

Goldstein, J. L., Brown, M. S. and Stone, N. J. (1977b). Genetics of the LDL receptor: evidence that the mutations affecting binding and internalization are allelic. *Cell*, **12**, 629–641.

Goldstein, J. L., Dana, S. E., Brunschede, G. Y. and Brown, M. S. (1975). Genetic heterogeneity in familial hypercholesterolemia: evidence for two different mutations affecting functions of low-density lipoprotein receptor. *Proceedings of the National Academy of Sciences of the USA*, **72**, 1092–1096.

Goldstein, J. L., Hazzard, W. R., Schrott, H. G., Bierman, E. L. and Motulsky, A. G. (1973). Hyperlipidemia in coronary heart disease. I. Lipid levels in 500 survivors of myocardial infarction. *Journal of Clinical Investigation*, **52**, 1533–1543.

Goldstein, J. L., Ho, Y. K., Basu, S. K. and Brown, M. S. (1979). Binding site on macrophages that mediates uptake and degradation of acetylated low density lipoprotein, producing massive cholesterol deposition. *Proceedings of the National Academy of Sciences of the USA*, **76**, 333–337.

Grundy, S. M. and Ahrens, E. H. Jr. (1969). Measurements of cholesterol turnover, synthesis, and absorption in man, carried out by isotope kinetic and sterol balance methods. *Journal of Lipid Research*, **10**, 91–107.

Hall, M. H. III., Bilheimer, D. W., Phair, R. D., Levy, R. I. and Berman, M. A. (1974). A mathematical model for apoprotein kinetics in normal and hyperlipemic patients. *Circulation*, **49–50**, Supplement III, 114.

Harlan, W. R. Jr., Graham, J. B. and Estes, H. E. (1966). Familial hypercholesterolemia: genetic and metabolic study. *Medicine*, **45**, 77–110.

Havel, R. J., Chao, Y.-S., Windler, E. E., Kotite, L. and Guo, L. S. S. (1980). Isoprotein specificity in the hepatic uptake of apolipoprotein E and the pathogenesis of familial dysbetalipoproteinemia. *Proceedings of the National Academy of Sciences of the USA*, **77**, 4349–4353.

Havel, R. J. and Kane, J. P. (1973a). Drugs and lipid metabolism. *Annual Review of Pharmacology*, **13**, 287–308.

Havel, R. J. and Kane, J. P. (1973b). Primary dysbetalipoproteinemia: predominance of a specific apoprotein species in triglyceride-rich lipoproteins. *Proceedings of the National Academy of Sciences of the USA*, **70**, 2015–2019.

Hayes, T. M. (1972). Plasma lipoproteins in adult diabetes. *Clinical Endocrinology*, **1**, 247–251.

Hazzard, W. R. and Bierman, E. L. (1971). Impaired removal of very low density lipoprotein (VLDL) 'remnants' in the pathogenesis of broad-beta disease (type III hyperlipoproteinemia). *Clinical Research*, **19**, 476.

Hazzard, W. R. and Bierman, E. L. (1972). Aggravation of broad-β disease (type 3 hyperlipoproteinemia) by hypothyroidism. *Archives of Internal Medicine*, **130**, 822–828.
Hazzard, W. R., O'Donnell, T. F. and Lee, Y. L. (1975). Broad-β disease (type III hyperlipoproteinemia) in a large kindred. *Annals of Internal Medicine*, **82**, 141.
Hazzard, W. R., Porte, D. Jr. and Bierman, E. L. (1972). Abnormal lipid composition of very low density lipoproteins in diagnosis of broad beta disease (type III hyperlipoproteinemia). *Metabolism*, **21**, 1009–1019.
Heiberg, A. (1975). The risk of atherosclerotic vascular disease in subjects with xanthomatosis. *Acta Medica Scandinavica*, **198**, 249–261.
Heiberg, A. and Slack, J. (1977). Family similarities in the age at coronary death in familial hypercholesterolaemia. *British Medical Journal*, **3**, 493–495.
Hellström, K. and Lindstedt, S. (1964). Cholic-acid turnover and biliary bile-acid composition in humans with abnormal thyroid function. Bile acids and steroids 139. *Journal of Laboratory and Clinical Medicine*, **63**, 666–679.
Hewitt, D., Jones, G. J. L., Goding, J., Wraight, D., Breckenridge, W. C., Little, J. A., Steiner, G. and Mishkel, M. A. (1979). Nature of the familial influence on plasma lipid levels. *Atherosclerosis*, **32**, 381–396.
Hillman, L., Schonfeld, G., Miller, J. P. and Wulff, G. (1975). Apolipoproteins in human pregnancy. *Metabolism*, **24**, 943–952.
Hoff, H. F., Bradley, W. A., Heideman, C. L., Gaubatz, J. W., Karagas, M. D. and Gotto, A. M. (1979). Characterization of low density lipoprotein-like particle in the human aorta from grossly normal and atherosclerotic regions. *Biochimica et Biophysica Acta*, **573**, 361–374.
Hollander, W., Paddock, J. and Colombo, M. (1979). Lipoproteins in human atherosclerotic vessels. I. Biochemical properties of arterial low density lipoproteins, very low density lipoproteins, and high density lipoproteins. *Experimental and Molecular Pathology*, **30**, 144–171.
Jadhav, A. V. and Thompson, G. R. (1979). Reversible abnormalities of low density lipoprotein composition in familial hypercholesterolaemia. *European Journal of Clinical Investigation*, **9**, 63–67.
Johnston, I. D. A., Davis, J. A., Moutafis, C. D. and Myant, N. B. (1967). Ileal bypass in the management of familial hypercholesterolaemia. *Proceedings of the Royal Society of Medicine*, **60**, 746–748.
Kannel, W. B., Castelli, W. P., Gordon, T. and McNamara, P. M. (1971). Serum cholesterol lipoproteins, and the risk of coronary heart disease. *Annals of Internal Medicine*, **74**, 1–12.
Kekki, M. and Nikkilä, E. A. (1971). Plasma triglyceride metabolism in the adult nephrotic syndrome. *European Journal of Clinical Investigation*, **1**, 345–351.
Khachadurian, A. K. (1964). The inheritance of essential familial hypercholesterolemia. *American Journal of Medicine*, **37**, 402–407.
Khachadurian, A. K. (1968). Migratory polyarthritis in familial hypercholesterolemia (Type II hyperlipoproteinemia). *Arthritis and Rheumatism*, **11**, 385–393.
Khachadurian, A. K. (1969). Lack of inhibition of hepatic cholesterol synthesis by dietary cholesterol in cases of familial hypercholesterolaemia. *Lancet*, **2**, 778–780.
Khachadurian, A. K. A general review of clinical and laboratory features of familial hypercholesterolemia (Type II hyperbetalipoproteinemia). In: *Protides of the Biological Fluids, Proceedings of the Nineteenth Colloquium*. Ed. H. Peeters. Pergamon Press, Oxford, pp. 315–318, 1972.
Khachadurian, A. K. and Demirjian, Z. N. (1967). Persistent elevation of the erythrocyte sedimentation rate (ESR) in familial hypercholesterolemia with a preliminary report on the effect of plasma beta-lipoproteins on ESR. *Lebanese Medical Journal*, **20**, 31–43.
Kissebah, A. H., Kohner, E. M., Lewis, B., Siddiq, Y. K., Lowy, C. and Fraser, T.

R. (1975). Plasma-lipids and glucose/insulin relationship in non-insulin-requiring diabetics with and without retinopathy. *Lancet*, **1**, 1104–1108.

Kurland, G. S., Lucas, J. L. and Freedberg, A. S. (1961). The metabolism of intravenously infused C^{14}-labelled cholesterol in euthyroidism and myxedema. *Journal of Laboratory and Clinical Medicine*, **57**, 574–585.

Kuo, P. T., Hayase, K., Kostis, J. B. and Moreyra, A. E. (1979). Use of combined diet and colestipol in long-term $(7-7\frac{1}{2}$ years) treatment of patients with type II hyperlipoproteinemia. *Circulation*, **59**, 199–211.

Kushwaha, R. S., Hazzard, W. R., Wahl, P. W. and Hoover, J. J. (1977). Type III hyperlipoproteinemia: diagnosis in whole plasma by apolipoprotein-E immunoassay. *Annals of Internal Medicine*, **87**, 509–516.

Kwiterovich, P. O., Fredrickson, D. S. and Levy, R. I. (1974). Familial hypercholesterolemia (one form of familial type II hyperlipoproteinemia). *Journal of Clinical Investigation*, **53**, 1237–1249.

Kwiterovich, P. O., Levy, R. I. and Fredrickson, D. S. (1973). Neonatal diagnosis of familial type II hyperlipoproteinaemia. *Lancet*, **1**, 118–122.

Kwiterovich, P. O., Neill, C., Margolis, S., Thamer, M. and Bachorik, P. (1975). Allelism, nonallelism, and genetic compounds in familial hyperlipoproteinemia. *Clinical Research*, **23**, 262A.

Langer, T., Strober, W. and Levy, R. I. (1972). The metabolism of low density lipoprotein in familial type II hyperlipoproteinemia. *Journal of Clinical Investigation*, **51**, 1528–1536.

Lennard-Jones, J. E. (1960). Myelomatosis with lipaemia and xanthomata. *British Medical Journal*, **1**, 781–783.

Levy, R. I. and Langer, T. Hypolipidemic drugs and lipoprotein metabolism. In: *Pharmacological Control of Lipid Metabolism. Proceedings of the Fourth International Symposium on Drugs Affecting Lipid Metabolism, Advances in Experimental Medicine and Biology, Vol. 26*. Ed. W. L. Holmes, R. Paoletti and D. Kritchevsky. Plenum Press, New York, pp. 155–163, 1972.

Lewis, B. *The Hyperlipidaemias. Clinical and Laboratory Practice*. Blackwell, Oxford, 1976.

Lewis, B. and Myant, N. B. (1967). Studies in the metabolism of cholesterol in subjects with normal plasma cholesterol levels and in patients with essential hypercholesterolaemia. *Clinical Science*, **32**, 201–213.

Lewis, L. A. and Page, I. H. (1965). An unusual serum lipoprotein-globulin complex in a patient with hyperlipemia. *American Journal of Medicine*, **38**, 286–297.

Lupien, P.-J., Moorjani, S. and Awad, J. (1976). A new approach to the management of familial hypercholesterolaemia: removal of plasma-cholesterol based on the principle of affinity chromatography. *Lancet*, **1**, 1261–1265.

McKenzie, I. F. C. and Nestel, P. J. (1968). Studies on the turnover of triglyceride and esterified cholesterol in subjects with the nephrotic syndrome. *Journal of Clinical Investigation*, **47**, 1685–1695.

Mabuchi, H., Tatami, R., Haba, T., Veda, K., Veda, R., Kametani, T., Ito, S., Koizumi, J., Ohta, M., Miyamoto, S., Takeda, R. and Takeshita, H. (1978). Homozygous familial hypercholesterolemia in Japan. *American Journal of Medicine*, **65**, 290–297.

Mabuchi, H., Tatami, R., Veda, K., Veda, R., Haba, T., Kametani, T., Watanabe, A., Wakasugi, T., Ito, S., Kuizumi, J., Ohta, M., Miyamoto, S. and Takeda, R. (1979). Serum lipid and lipoprotein levels in Japanese patients with familial hypercholesterolemia. *Atherosclerosis*, **32**, 435–444.

Magide, A., Press, C. M., Myant, N. B., Mitropoulos, K. A. and Balasubramaniam, S. (1976). The effect of portacaval anastomosis on plasma lipoprotein metabolism in rats. *Biochimica et Biophysica Acta*, **441**, 302–307.

Mahley, R. W. Alterations in plasma lipoproteins induced by cholesterol feeding in animals including man. In: *Disturbances in Lipid and Lipoprotein Metabolism*. Ed.

J. M. Dietschy, A. M. Gotto Jr. and J. A. Ontko. American Physiological Society, Bethesda, pp. 181–197, 1978.

Mahley, R. W., Weisgraber, K. H., Melchior, G. W., Innerarity, T. L. and Holcombe, K. S. (1980). Inhibition of receptor-mediated clearance of lysine- and arginine-modified lipoproteins from the plasma of rats and monkeys. *Proceedings of the National Academy of Sciences of the USA*, **77**, 225–229.

Marsh, J. B. and Drabkin, D. L. (1960). Experimental reconstruction of metabolic patterns of lipid nephrosis: key role of hepatic protein synthesis in hyperlipemia. *Metabolism*, **9**, 946–955.

Martin, G. M. and Nestel, P. (1979). Changes in cholesterol metabolism with dietary cholesterol in children with familial hypercholesterolaemia. *Clinical Science*, **56**, 377–380.

Miettinen, T. A. (1968). Mechanism of serum cholesterol reduction by thyroid hormones in hypothyroidism. *Journal of Laboratory and Clinical Medicine*, **71**, 537.

Miettinen, T. A. (1970). Detection of changes in human cholesterol metabolism. *Annals of Clinical Research*, **2**, 300–320.

Miettinen, T. A., Pelkonen, R., Nikkilä, E. A. and Heinonen, O. (1967). Low excretion of fecal bile acids in a family with hypercholesterolemia. *Acta Medica Scandinavica*, **182**, 645–650.

Mjøs, O. D., Faergeman, O., Hamilton, R. L. and Havel, R. J. (1975). Characterization of remnants produced during the metabolism of triglyceride-rich lipoproteins of blood plasma and intestinal lymph in the rat. *Journal of Clinical Investigation*, **56**, 603–615.

Morganroth, J., Levy, R. I. and Fredrickson, D. S. (1975). The biochemical, clinical, and genetic features of type III hyperlipoproteinemia. *Annals of Internal Medicine*, **82**, 158–174.

Morganroth, J., Levy, R. I., McMahon, A. E. and Gotto, A. M. (1974). Pseudo-homozygous type II hyperlipoproteinemia. *Journal of Pediatrics*, **85**, 639–643.

Moser, H., Slack, J. and Borrie, P. Type III hyperlipoproteinemia: A genetic study with an account of the risks of coronary death in first degree relatives. In: *Atherosclerosis III, Proceedings of the Third International Symposium*. Ed. G. Schettler and Z. Weizel. Springer-Verlag, Berlin, p. 845, 1974.

Moutafis, C. D. and Myant, N. B. (1969). The metabolism of cholesterol in two hypercholesterolaemic patients treated with cholestyramine. *Clinical Science*, **37**, 443–454.

Moutafis, C. D. and Myant, N. B. Effects of nicotinic acid, alone or in combination with cholestyramine, on cholesterol metabolism in patients suffering from familial hyperbetalipoproteinaemia in the homozygous form. In: *Metabolic Effects of Nicotinic Acid and Its Derivatives*. Ed. K. F. Gey and L. A. Carlson. Hans Huber, Bern, pp. 659–676, 1971.

Moutafis, C. D., Myant, N. B., Mancini, M. and Oriente, P. (1971). Cholestyramine and nicotinic acid in the treatment of familial hyperbetalipoproteinaemia in the homozygous form. *Atherosclerosis*, **14**, 247–258.

Moutafis, C. D., Simons, L. A., Myant, N. B., Adams, P. W. and Wynn, V. (1977). The effect of cholestyramine on the faecal excretion of bile acids and neutral steroids in familial hypercholesterolaemia. *Atherosclerosis*, **26**, 329–334.

Myant, N. B. The regulation of cholesterol metabolism as related to familial hypercholesterolaemia. In: *The Scientific Basis of Medicine Annual Reviews*. Athlone Press, London, pp. 230–259, 1970.

Myant, N. B. The metabolic lesion in familial hypercholesterolaemia. In: *Cholesterol Metabolism and Lipolytic Enzymes*. Ed. J. Polonovski. Marron Publishing USA, Inc., New York, pp. 39–52, 1977.

Myant, N. B., Reichl, D. and Lloyd, J. K. (1978). Sterol balance in a patient with abetalipoproteinaemia. *Atherosclerosis*, **29**, 509–512.

Myant, N. B. and Slack, J. Type II-hyperlipoproteinemia. In: *Handbuch der inneren Medizin: Fettstoffwechsel.* Ed. G. Schettler, H. Greten, G. Schlierf and D. Seidel. Springer-Verlag, Berlin, pp. 275–300, 1976.

Nevin, N. C. and Slack, J. (1968). Hyperlipidaemic xanthomatosis. II. Mode of inheritance in 55 families with essential hyperlipidaemia and xanthomatosis. *Journal of Medical Genetics,* **5,** 9–28.

Nikkilä, E. A. Metabolic and endocrine control of plasma high density lipoprotein concentration. In: *High Density Lipoproteins and Atherosclerosis.* Ed. A. M. Gotto Jr., N. E. Miller, and M. F. Oliver. Elsevier, Amsterdam, pp. 177–192, 1978.

Nikkilä, E. A. and Aro, A. (1973). Family study of serum lipids and lipoproteins in coronary heart-disease. *Lancet,* **1,** 954–958.

Nikkilä, E. A. and Kekki, M. (1973). Plasma triglyceride transport kinetics in diabetes mellitus. *Metabolism,* **22,** 1–22.

Noseda, G., Riesen, W., Schlumpf, E. and Morell, A. (1972). Hypo-β-lipoproteinaemia associated with auto-antibodies against β-lipoproteins. *European Journal of Clinical Investigation,* **2,** 342–347.

Packard, C. J., Shepherd, J., Third, J. L. H. C., Lorimer, R., Morgan, H. G. and Lawrie, T. D. V. (1976). Low-density-lipoprotein metabolism in Type II hyperlipoproteinaemia. *Biochemical Society Transactions,* **4,** 105–107.

Packard, C. J., Morgan, H. G., Third, J. L. H. C. and Shepherd, J. (1978). An investigation of the defect in type III hyperlipoproteinemia using agarose column chromatography. *Clinica Chimica Acta,* **84,** 33–44.

Patsch, J. R., Sailer, S. and Braunsteiner, H. (1975). Lipoprotein of the density 1.006–1.020 in the plasma of patients with type III hyperlipoproteinaemia in the postabsorptive state. *European Journal of Clinical Investigation,* **5,** 45–55.

Patterson, D. and Slack, J. (1972). Lipid abnormalities in male and female survivors of myocardial infarction and their first-degree relatives. *Lancet,* **1,** 393–399.

Patterson, D. and Slack, J. The inheritance of lipoprotein disorders and the risks of coronary death in first-degree relatives of 193 survivors of myocardial infarction. In: *Atherosclerosis III, Proceedings of the Third International Symposium.* Ed. G. Schettler and A. Weizel. Springer-Verlag, Berlin, pp. 458–463, 1974.

Popják, G. (1954). The origin of fetal lipids. *Cold Spring Harbor Symposia on Quantitative Biology,* **19,** 200–208.

Porte, D. Jr., O'Hara, D. D. and Williams, R. H. (1966). The relation between postheparin lipolytic activity and plasma triglyceride in myxedema. *Metabolism,* **15,** 107–113.

Quarfordt, S., Levy, R. I. and Fredrickson, D. S. (1971). On the lipoprotein abnormality in type III hyperlipoproteinemia. *Journal of Clinical Investigation,* **50,** 754–761.

Quarfordt, S. H., Levy, R. I. and Fredrickson, D. S. (1973). The kinetic properties of very low density lipoprotein triglyceride in type III hyperlipoproteinemia. *Biochimica et Biophysica Acta,* **296,** 572–576.

Reichl, D., Myant, N. B. and Lloyd, J. K. (1978). Surface binding and catabolism of low-density lipoprotein by circulating lymphocytes from patients with abetalipoproteinaemia, with observations on sterol synthesis in lymphocytes from one patient. *Biochimica et Biophysica Acta,* **530,** 124–131.

Reichl, D., Simons, L. A. and Myant, N. B. (1974). The metabolism of low-density lipoprotein in a patient with familial hyperbetalipoproteinaemia. *Clinical Science and Molecular Medicine,* **47,** 635–638.

Rifkind, B. M. (1973). Lipoproteins and hyperlipoproteinaemia. *Clinics in Endocrinology and Metabolism,* **2,** 1–10.

Rifkind, B. M., Tamir, I. and Heiss, G. Preliminary high density lipoprotein findings. The lipid research clinic program. In: *High Density Lipoproteins and*

Atherosclerosis. Ed. A. M. Gotto Jr., N. E. Miller and M. F. Oliver. Elsevier, Amsterdam, pp. 109–119, 1978

Roberts, W. C., Ferrans, V. J., Levy, R. I. and Fredrickson, D. S. (1973). Cardiovascular pathology in hyperlipoproteinemia. Anatomic observations in 42 necropsy patients with normal or abnormal lipoprotein patterns. *American Journal of Cardiology*, **31**, 557–570.

Roberts-Thomson, P. J., Venables, G. S., Onitiri, A. C. and Lewis, B. (1975). Polymeric IgA myeloma, hyperlipidaemia and xanthomatosis: a further case and review. *Postgraduate Medical Journal*, **51**, 44–51.

Schettler, G., Greten, H., Schlierf, G. and Seidel, D. Fettstoffwechsel. In: *Handbuch der inneren Medizin Stoffwechselkrankheiten*, Vol. 4. Springer-Verlag, Berlin, 1976.

Schonfeld, G., Birge, C., Miller, P., Kessler, G. and Santiago, J. (1974). Apolipoprotein B levels and altered lipoprotein composition in diabetes. *Diabetes*, **23**, 827–834.

Schrott, H. G., Goldstein, J. L., Hazzard, W. R., McGoodwin, M. M. and Motulsky, A. G. (1972). Familial hypercholesterolemia in a large kindred. Evidence for a monogenic mechanism. *Annals of Internal Medicine*, **76**, 711–720.

Shattil, S. J., Bennett, J. S., Colman, R. W. and Cooper, R. A. (1977). Abnormalities of cholesterol-phospholipid composition in platelets and low-density lipoproteins of human hyperbetalipoproteinemia. *Journal of Laboratory and Clinical Medicine*, **89**, 341–353.

Shepherd, J., Bicker, S., Lorimer, A. R. and Packard, C. J. (1979). Receptor-mediated low density lipoprotein catabolism in man. *Journal of Lipid Research*, **20**, 999–1006.

Simons, L. A., Reichl, D., Myant, N. B. and Mancini, M. (1975). The metabolism of the apoprotein of plasma low density lipoprotein in familial hyperbetalipoproteinaemia in the homozygous form. *Atherosclerosis*, **21**, 283–298.

Slack, J. (1969). Risks of ischaemic heart-disease in familial hyperlipoproteinaemic states. *Lancet*, **2**, 1380–1382.

Slack, J. and Mills, G. L. (1970). Anomalous low density lipoproteins in familial hyperbetalipoproteinaemia. *Clinica Chimica Acta*, **29**, 15–25.

Soutar, A. K., Myant, N. B. and Thompson, G. R. (1977). Simultaneous measurement of apolipoprotein B turnover in very-low- and low-density lipoproteins in familial hypercholesterolaemia. *Atherosclerosis*, **28**, 247–256.

Soutar, A. K., Myant, N. B. and Thompson, G. R. (1979). Metabolism of apolipoprotein B-containing lipoproteins in familial hypercholesterolaemia. Effects of plasma exchange. *Atherosclerosis*, **32**, 315–325.

Spritz, N. and Mishkel, M. A. (1969). Effects of dietary fats on plasma lipids and lipoproteins: an hypothesis for the lipid-lowering effect of unsaturated fatty acids. *Journal of Clinical Investigation*, **48**, 78–86.

Stamler, J., Beard, R. R., Connor, W. E., de Wolfe, V. G., Stokes, J. and Willis, P. W. (1970). Primary prevention of the atherosclerotic diseases. *Circulation*, **42**, A55–A95.

Stanley, P., Chartrand, C. and Davignon, A. (1965). Acquired aortic stenosis in a twelve-year-old girl with xanthomatosis. *New England Journal of Medicine*, **273**, 1378–1380.

Starzl, T. E., Chase, H. P., Putnam, C. W. and Porter, K. A. (1973). Portacaval shunt in hyperlipoproteinaemia. *Lancet*, **2**, 940–944.

Stern, M. P., Kolterman, O. G., McDevitt, H. and Reaven, G. M. (1972). Acquired type III hyperlipoproteinemia. Report of three cases associated with systemic lupus erythematosus and diabetic ketoacidosis. *Archives of Internal Medicine*, **130**, 817–821.

Stone, N. J., Levy, R. I., Fredrickson, D. S. and Verter, J. (1974). Coronary artery disease in 116 kindred with familial type II hyperlipoproteinemia. *Circulation*, **49**, 476–488.

Streja, D., Steiner, G. and Kwiterovich, P. O. Jr. (1978). Plasma high-density lipoproteins and ischemic heart disease. Studies in a large kindred with familial hypercholesterolemia. *Annals of Internal Medicine*, **89**, 871–880.

Thannhauser, S. J. *Lipidoses*, 1st edition. Oxford University Press, New York, 1940.

Thannhauser, S. J. *Lipidoses. Diseases of the Intracellular Lipid Metabolism*, 3rd edition. Grune & Stratton, New York, 1958.

Thompson, G. R., Lowenthal, R. and Myant, N. B. (1975). Plasma exchange in the management of homozygous familial hypercholesterolaemia. *Lancet*, **1**, 1208.

Thompson, G. R., Myant, N. B., Kilpatrick, D., Oakley, C. M., Raphael, M. J. and Steiner, R. E. (1980*a*). Assessment of long-term plasma exchange for familial hypercholesterolaemia. *British Heart Journal*, **43**, 680–688.

Thompson, G. R., Soutar, A. K., Knight, B. L., Gavigan, S., Myant, N. B. and Shepherd, J. (1980*b*). Evidence for defect of receptor-mediated low-density lipoprotein catabolism in familial hypercholesterolaemia *in vivo*. *Clinical Science*, **58**, 2P-3P.

Thompson, G. R., Soutar, A. K., Spengel, F. A., Jadhav, A., Gavigan, S. and Myant, N. B. (1981). Defects of the receptor-mediated low density lipoprotein catabolism in homozygous familial hypercholesterolemia and hypothyroidism *in vivo*. *Proceedings of the National Academy of Sciences of the USA*, **78**.

Thompson, G. R., Spinks, T., Ranicar, A. and Myant, N. B. (1977). Non-steady-state studies of low-density lipoprotein turnover in familial hypercholesterolaemia. *Clinical Science and Molecular Medicine*, **52**, 361–369.

Tsang, R. C., Fallat, R. W. and Glueck, C. J. (1974). Cholesterol at birth and age 1: comparison of normal and hypercholesterolemic neonates. *Pediatrics*, **53**, 458.

Utermann, G., Jaeschke, M. and Menzel, J. (1975). Familial hyperlipoproteinemia Type III: deficiency of a specific apolipoprotein (apoE-III) in the very-low-density lipoproteins. *FEBS Letters*, **56**, 352–355.

Utermann, G., Pruin, N. and Steinmetz, A. (1979*b*). Polymorphism and apolipoprotein E. III. Effect of a single polymorphic gene locus on plasma lipid levels in man. *Clinical Genetics*, **15**, 63–72.

Utermann, G., Vogelberg, K. H., Steinmetz, A., Schoenborn, W., Pruin, N., Jaeschke, M., Hees, M. and Canzler, H. (1979*a*). Polymorphism of apolipoprotein E. II. Genetics of hyperlipoproteinemia type III. *Clinical Genetics*, **15**, 37–62.

Wallace, R. B., Hoover, J., Barrett-Connor, E., Rifkind, B. M., Hunninghake, D. B., Mackenthun, A. and Heiss, G. (1979). Altered plasma lipid and lipoprotein levels associated with oral contraceptive and oestrogen use. *Lancet*, **2**, 111–114.

Walton, K. W., Scott, P. J., Dykes, P. W. and Davies, J. W. L (1965). The significance of alterations in serum lipids in thyroid dysfunction. II. Alterations of the metabolism and turnover of ^{131}I-low-density lipoproteins in hypothyroidism and thyrotoxicosis. *Clinical Science*, **29**, 217–238.

West, R. J., Fosbrooke, A. S. and Lloyd, J. K. (1975). Treatment of children with familial hypercholesterolaemia. *Postgraduate Medical Journal*, **51**, *Supplement* 8, 82.

Wilkinson, C. F., Hand, E. A. and Fliegelman, M. T. (1948). Essential familial hypercholesterolemia. *Annals of Internal Medicine*, **29**, 671–686.

Yamamoto, A., Sudo, H. and Endo, A. (1980). Therapeutic effects of ML-236B in primary hypercholesterolaemia. *Atherosclerosis*, **35**, 259–266.

Yeshurun, D. and Gotto, A. M. (1976). Drug treatment of hyperlipidemia. *American Journal of Medicine*, **60**, 379–396.

Chapter 16

Disorders of Cholesterol Metabolism: The Hypolipoproteinaemias

1	ACQUIRED HYPOCHOLESTEROLAEMIA	775
2	ABETALIPOPROTEINAEMIA	776
2.1	Characteristic features	776
2.2	Genetics	776
2.3	Pathology	777
2.4	Plasma lipids and lipoproteins	777
2.5	Acanthocytosis	778
2.6	Pathogenesis	781
3	FAMILIAL HYPOBETALIPOPROTEINAEMIA	784
3.1	Distinction from abetalipoproteinaemia	784
3.2	Clinical and biochemical features	785
3.2.1	Heterozygotes	785
3.2.2	Homozygotes	785
3.3	Pathogenesis	785
3.4	Diagnosis	786
4	CHOLESTEROL METABOLISM IN β-LIPOPROTEIN DEFICIENCY	786
5	FAMILIAL HDL DEFICIENCY (TANGIER DISEASE)	788
5.1	Characteristic features	788
5.2	Genetics	789
5.3	Pathology	789
5.4	Plasma lipids and lipoproteins	790
5.4.1	Plasma lipids	790
5.4.2	Plasma lipoproteins	790
5.5	The heterozygous state	791
5.6	Pathogenesis	792
5.6.1	Nature of the gene mutation	792
5.6.2	The lipoprotein abnormalities	794
5.6.3	The intracellular accumulation of cholestrol	794
5.7	Tangier disease and ischaemic heart disease	795

6	FAMILIAL LCAT DEFICIENCY	796
6.1	General remarks	796
6.2	Characteristic features	798
6.3	Genetics	799
6.4	Pathology	801
6.5	Plasma lipids and lipoproteins	801
6.5.1	Lipids	801
6.5.2	Lipoproteins	802
6.6	Red blood cells	805
6.7	Pathogenesis	806
6.7.1	The plasma lipoproteins	806
6.7.2	Lipid deposition in tissues	810

Disorders of Cholesterol Metabolism: The Hypolipoproteinaemias

1 ACQUIRED HYPOCHOLESTEROLAEMIA

The plasma cholesterol concentration may be abnormally low in patients with severe malnutrition, the malabsorption syndrome, malignant disease, parenchymatous disease of the liver, anaemia or myelomatosis. In some instances the degree of hypocholesterolaemia is marked, with plasma cholesterol levels below 100 mg/100 ml in adults.

Hypocholesterolaemia may occur in anaemias of various types, including pernicious anaemia, the microcytic anaemia of iron deficiency, congenital spherocytosis, hereditary sideroblastic anaemia and anaemia secondary to cancer or myeloid leukaemia. In many patients with hypocholesterolaemia associated with anaemia, the plasma cholesterol concentration rises when the anaemia is treated effectively (Rifkind and Gale, 1967). Very low plasma cholesterol levels are often found in patients with hereditary sideroblastic anaemia responsive to large doses of pyridoxine, and the haematological response to pyridoxine may be accompanied by a return of the plasma cholesterol concentration to the normal level (Spitzer *et al.*, 1966). The abnormal erythropoiesis in these patients is probably due to failure to convert pyridoxine into pyridoxal phosphate in the tissues rather than to dietary deficiency of pyridoxine (Spitzer *et al.*, 1966). There is no evidence that the defective pyridoxine metabolism in this disease is responsible for the hypocholesterolaemia, but it is of interest to note that rhesus monkeys fed pyridoxine-deficient diets develop hypocholesterolaemia (Emerson *et al.*, 1960).

As discussed in the previous chapter, hyperglobulinaemia may cause an increase in plasma cholesterol concentration. However, a much more usual finding in patients with myelomatosis or other forms of dysglobulinaemia is a marked fall in plasma cholesterol concentration comparable with that in severe malnutrition or hepatic insufficiency and usually due to a fall in plasma LDL concentration (Lewis and Page, 1954; Burstein and Fine, 1959). The observations of Noseda *et al.* (1972) suggest that in some cases the cause of the hypocholesterolaemia is an increased fractional rate of turnover of the plasma LDL due to the formation of a rapidly degraded LDL-immunoglobulin complex.

In the remaining sections of this chapter we shall consider a group of rare familial disorders characterized by the absence or deficiency of a specific plasma lipoprotein or of a specific enzyme necessary for the formation of normal lipoproteins. The main focus will be on the way in which cholesterol metabolism is altered by these lipoprotein disorders; for fuller accounts of the more clinical aspects the reader is referred to Herbert *et al.* (1978) and to the articles mentioned in Section 6.1.

2 ABETALIPOPROTEINAEMIA

2.1 Characteristic features

The rare inherited disease now generally referred to as abetalipoproteinaemia was first recognized by Bassen and Kornzweig (1950), who described a clinical syndrome characterized by steatorrhoea, retinitis pigmentosa, a progressive neurological disorder resembling Friedreich's ataxia and the presence, in the circulation, of abnormal spiny red cells known as acanthocytes (Gr. *acantha*; a thorn). Ten years later it was discovered that β-lipoprotein is completely absent from the plasma of these patients (Salt *et al.*, 1960; Lamy *et al.*, 1960). Since there is reason to believe that the lipoprotein abnormality is related to the primary genetic lesion more closely than are the clinical manifestations, the designation 'abetalipoproteinaemia' is preferable to the earlier 'Bassen-Kornzweig syndrome'. The malabsorption of dietary fat is accompanied by deficiency of fat-soluble vitamins, reflected in greatly reduced plasma concentrations of vitamins A and E, and by sub-clinical deficiency of essential fatty acids. Many affected children have moderate or marked anaemia but adults with abetalipoproteinaemia usually have normal haemoglobin levels.

2.2 Genetics

What may be called classical abetalipoproteinaemia is inherited as a Mendelian autosomal recessive trait, with no identifiable expression in the heterozygous form, both parents of an affected subject having a normal plasma β-lipoprotein concentration and no detectable clinical signs. In keeping with its inheritance as a rare recessive trait, consanguinity has been noted in the parents of about half the 40 or more patients reported in the world literature and in no case has there been transmission of the clinical disease from parent to offspring. The genetic status of abetalipoproteinaemia is confused by the existence of familial hypobetalipoproteinaemia (see Section 3) which, in its homozygous form, is indistinguishable biochemically from classical abetalipoproteinaemia. Paradoxically, the first patient in whom a total absence of plasma β-lipoprotein was reported was probably suffering from familial hypobetalipoproteinaemia in the homozygous form, since both her parents had an abnormally low plasma LDL concentration (Salt et al., 1960). The first unequivocal description of classical abetalipoproteinaemia was probably that of Lamy et al. (1960), who described this disorder in the offspring (a 7-year-old boy) of an incestuous mating between a brother and his half-sister. The mother of this patient had a normal plasma cholesterol and β-lipoprotein concentration. (The father's plasma lipids were not reported.)

2.3 Pathology

The intestinal villi are normal, in contrast to the atrophy seen in coeliac disease, but the mucosal cells are filled with droplets of fat, many of which are not surrounded by a membrane. The parenchymal cells of the liver also contain numerous fat droplets. In the nervous system, the most striking abnormality is extensive demyelination of nerve fibres in the posterior spinal columns. The abnormal red cells are dealt with in Section 2.5.

2.4 Plasma lipids and lipoproteins

There is a marked reduction in plasma lipid concentrations. Plasma total cholesterol concentration is usually below 50 mg/100 ml and plasma triglycerides are frequently undetectable. The ratio of lecithin to sphingomyelin in the lipids of whole plasma is lower than normal. Plasma vitamin A and vitamin E concentrations are abnormally low and there is a considerable decrease in the ratio of 18:2 and 20:4 to 18:1 and 16:0 fatty acids in the plasma unesterified fatty-acid fraction and in the phospholipids and cholesteryl esters of HDL. In particular, the sphingomyelin of HDL is deficient in linoleate and arachidonate and is enriched with nervonic acid (24:1) (Jones and Ways, 1967).

Examination of whole plasma or serum by zonal electrophoresis or immunochemical methods reveals the complete absence of apoB-containing lipoproteins and, hence, of normal LDL, VLDL and chylomicrons, both in the fasting state and after ingestion of a fatty meal. Electron microscopy of the LDL fraction (d. 1.006–1.063) shows the absence of normal spherical LDL particles of diameter 200–250 Å. However, small amounts of stacked, rectangular particles 100–200 Å long are seen in negatively stained preparations of the 1.006–1.063 density fraction of plasma from abetalipoproteinaemic patients (Forte and Nichols, 1972). These particles are probably abnormal HDL which have acquired the density of normal LDL; they contain the major apoproteins of normal HDL but they have a high free cholesterol:cholesteryl ester ratio (Scanu et al., 1974), a high cholesteryl-ester content (23% instead of the normal 10–15%) and a low protein:lipid ratio (Kostner et al., 1974).

In addition to the abnormal fatty acid pattern of the HDL lipids (see above), the protein component of HDL (d. 1.063–1.21) lacks apoC-III-1, the apoC-III fraction containing only one sialic acid residue per molecule of protein (Gotto et al., 1971). The plasma HDL concentration is usually reduced in abetalipoproteinaemia owing to a relative and absolute decrease in HDL_3 concentration, the HDL_2 level remaining within the normal range (Jones and Ways, 1967).

LCAT activity, determined from the rate of esterification of the plasma free cholesterol in whole plasma *in vitro*, is reduced to about half the normal value in abetalipoproteinaemia and the low rates of esterification are increased by the addition of heat-inactivated normal serum (Cooper and Gulbrandsen, 1971; Scanu et al., 1974; Kostner et al., 1974).

2.5 Acanthocytosis

The acanthocytes present in the blood of abetalipoproteinaemic patients are seen to best advantage when examined by scanning electron microscopy (Fig. 16.1), but they may also be seen in stained smears, or 'wet' preparations of the cells suspended in Dacie's solution. Acanthocytes lack the smooth biconcave discoidal shape of normal erythrocytes (Fig. 16.1A) and appear as globules of variable size with numerous irregular projections. In most patients they comprise 50–100% of the total circulating red-cell population, but they are not present in the marrow. The platelets and the white blood cells are normal in appearance. Abnormal red cells that are morphologically identical with acanthocytes are present in the circulation of some patients with severe non-obstructive liver disease (Smith et al., 1964; McBride and Jacob, 1970). Rather confusingly, these abnormal cells are often referred to as spur cells. As noted below, spur cells differ from acanthocytes in chemical composition. Red cells similar in appearance to the acanthocytes of abetalipoproteinaemia have also been described in patients with a familial neurological disorder but

Disorders of Cholesterol Metabolism: The Hypolipoproteinaemias 779

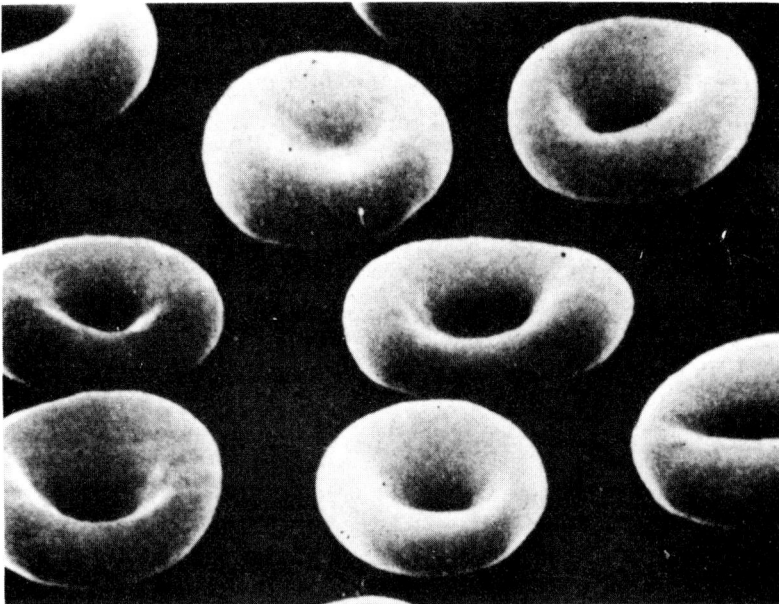

A.

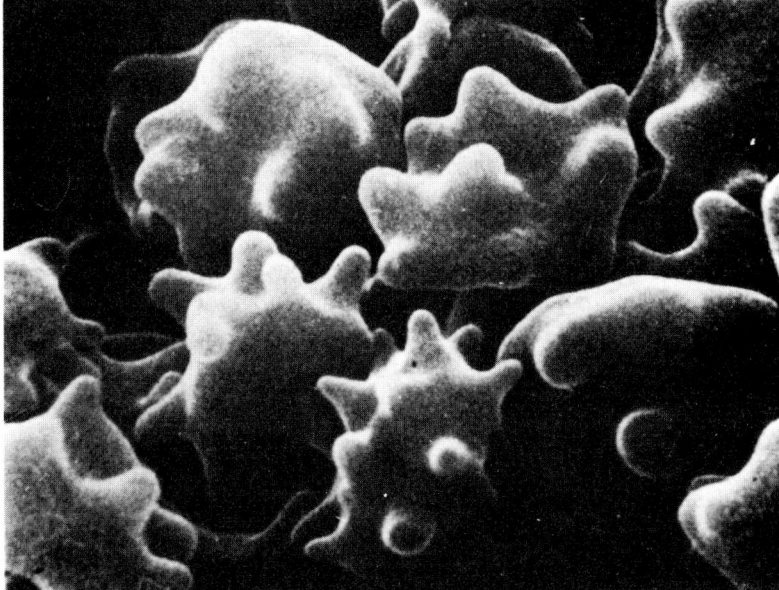

B.

Figure 16.1
Red blood cells fixed in glutaraldehyde and viewed with the scanning electron microscope. A, Normal red cells; B, Acanthocytes from a patient with abetalipoproteinaemia. (From Kayden and Bessis (1970), with the permission of the authors.)

normal plasma LDL concentration (Estes et al., 1967; Critchley et al., 1968). Acanthocytes are readily distinguishable from other abnormally shaped erythrocytes, including microspherocytes, burr cells and the crenated cells produced by washing normal human erythrocytes in physiological saline (Kayden and Bessis, 1970).

The erythrocyte sedimentation rate of whole blood is markedly reduced in abetalipoproteinaemia (0–2 mm/h) owing to failure of the acanthocytes to form rouleaux. The rate of autohaemolysis in defibrinated blood *in vitro* is increased. Osmotic fragility is usually normal, but mechanical fragility is increased. The life-span of the red cells *in vivo* is usually shortened, a change that presumably contributes to the anaemia and the mild reticulocytosis with hyperplastic bone marrow reported in some patients. The abnormal erythrocytes do not revert to the normal shape when they are incubated in normal serum or plasma for up to 24 hours *in vitro* and normal erythrocytes are not converted into acanthocytes when incubated in serum from an abetalipoproteinaemic patient (Lamy et al., 1961; Cooper and Gulbrandsen, 1971). However, when normal blood is infused into the patient, the red cells are converted into acanthocytes within 24 hours (Lamy et al., 1961). The acanthocytes of abetalipoproteinaemia change reversibly to normal biconcave discs when incubated in the presence of 5% albumin solution (Farquhar and Ways, 1966; Khachadurian et al., 1973) or of non-ionic detergents containing oleic acid, but not stearic acid, as the lipophilic group (Switzer and Eder, 1962).

The lipid composition of the acanthocytes of abetalipoproteinaemia exhibits abnormalities qualitatively similar to those observed in the plasma lipoproteins. Total phospholipid per cell is within the normal range but there is a decrease in the content of lecithin and an increase in that of sphingomyelin (Farquhar and Ways, 1966). The fatty acids of the red-cell phospholipids are also markedly deficient in linoleate and arachidonate (Farquhar and Ways, 1966). In view of the importance of unesterified cholesterol as a determinant of the fluidity of biological membranes, there has been much discussion of the cholesterol content of the acanthocytes of abetalipoproteinaemia. McBride and Jacob (1970) found a significant increase in cholesterol content and in free cholesterol:phospholipid molar ratio in the red cells of abetalipoproteinaemic patients, but this has not been generally confirmed. According to other workers, the cholesterol content is near the upper limit of the normal range and the total phospholipid content is near the lower limit, the free cholesterol:phospholipid ratio being slightly, but not significantly, raised (see Herbert and Fredrickson, 1976, Table 6).

2.6 Pathogenesis

The primary defect in abetalipoproteinaemia is generally assumed to be a mutation in the gene coding for apoB. This has not been proved, but an explanation in terms of a failure, at the gene level, to synthesize a specific apolipoprotein is certainly a very appealing one and may well turn out to be true. However, to be fully convincing it must account not only for the hypocholesterolaemia and the absence of apoB-containing lipoproteins in the plasma, but also for all the other manifestations of the disease, including fat malabsorption, an abnormal plasma lipid pattern, the presence of acanthocytes in the circulation, retinitis pigmentosa and a progressive disease of the nervous system.

Deficiency of a protein required for the formation of the polar coat of triglyceride-rich lipoproteins in the gut mucosa and the liver would explain the absence of VLDL, chylomicrons and LDL in the plasma and would also explain the fat malabsorption and the abnormal histology of the intestinal mucosa. During the absorption of fat by the normal intestine, the fatty acids absorbed from the lumen are re-esterified within the mucosal cells to form triglycerides, which appear as cytoplasmic lipid droplets surrounded by rings of increased density, thought to contain the protein of the polar coat material (see Chapter 11). These lipid droplets subsequently appear in the Golgi bodies as nascent triglyceride-rich lipoprotein particles and are then secreted into the intestinal lymphatics. In abetalipoproteinaemia, fatty acids are rapidly absorbed from the intestinal lumen and are esterified in the mucosal cells, giving rise to the lipid droplets seen in osmium-stained preparations of jejunal biopsies (Isselbacher et al., 1964). However, the lipid droplets do not acquire a dense outer coating and do not appear in the Golgi vacuoles as nascent VLDL or chylomicrons (Dobbins, 1966). Thus, the histological appearance of the mucosal cells suggests that the malabsorption of fat is due to failure to assemble triglyceride-rich lipoproteins within the mucosa, rather than to an inability to secrete fully-formed lipoprotein particles into the intestinal lymphatics.

Malabsorption of fat due to failure to form VLDL and chylomicrons in the gut mucosa would be expected to lead to the low plasma concentrations of essential fatty acids and of vitamins A and E seen in abetalipoproteinaemia. However, a high sphingomyelin:lecithin ratio and a high nervonic acid content are not characteristic of the plasma phospholipids in fat malabsorption due to coeliac disease. These abnormal features of the plasma in abetalipoproteinaemia have not been explained.

The low plasma HDL concentration seen in many abetalipoproteinaemic patients may be a consequence of the absence of triglyceride-rich lipoproteins in the plasma, in so far as some HDL is derived from surface components released during their catabolism in the circulation. According to the current view of the origin of the plasma cholesteryl esters, triglyceride-rich lipoproteins are the ultimate source of much of the free cholesterol that acts as substrate for the LCAT reaction on HDL. The absence of triglyceride-rich particles in the plasma in abetalipoproteinaemia may therefore explain the low LCAT activity determined in whole plasma *in vitro* by the method of Stokke and Norum. VLDL is also thought to act as acceptor for esterified cholesterol generated on HDL particles and subsequently transferred from HDL by the cholesteryl-ester exchange protein (see Chapter 11). The absence of acceptor lipoproteins might lead to the formation of a lipid-rich 'HDL' with the density of LDL, though this possibility obviously requires further investigation before it can be considered seriously.

Although the striking appearance of acanthocytes has given rise to a good deal of speculation, the mechanism responsible for their peculiar shape remains unexplained. Presumably, the abnormal shape and increased mechanical fragility are determined by abnormalities in the chemical composition of the plasma membrane. One possibility is that apoB is an integral component of the red-cell membrane and is essential for the maintenance of a normal discoidal conformation. In keeping with this, Langdon (1974) has reported the presence of apoB in normal red-cell ghosts. However, the validity of this observation is open to question (Bjerrum and Lundahl, 1974). An alternative possibility is that when the red cells enter the circulation and come into contact with abetalipoproteinaemic plasma, the lipid composition of the plasma membrane is changed and that as a result of this change the cells are converted into acanthocytes. In favour of the view that the characteristic shape of acanthocytes is acquired after the red cells have entered the circulation, in abetalipoproteinaemia the red cells in the marrow are normal in appearance and, furthermore, normal red cells are converted into acanthocytes in the circulation of an abetalipoproteinaemic patient. However, although it seems very probable that the abnormal lipid composition of the acanthocyte is responsible for its shape, we do not know which of the several lipid abnormalities that have been described is the crucial one.

McBride and Jacob (1970) have suggested that LDL acts as an acceptor for free cholesterol in the red-cell membrane and that in the absence of LDL the membrane becomes overloaded with cholesterol, resulting in an increase in surface area in relation to cell volume. In support of this proposal, they have shown that if rats are made hypobetalipoproteinaemic by treatment with orotic acid, their red blood cells become enriched with cholesterol and assume a shape similar to that of the acanthocytes of human abetalipoproteinaemia. They have also pointed out that in acute liver failure the blood may contain abnormal red cells with a high content of free cholesterol and irregular projections like those of acanthocytes (the so-called 'spur cells'). However, the free-cholesterol content of acanthocytes is often within normal limits and never reaches the level seen in spur cells. Furthermore, in LCAT deficiency, in which the cholesterol content of the red cells may be nearly twice the normal value, the red cells are converted into target cells, which do not have thorn-like projections, rather than into acanthocytes. Thus, it does not seem that an increase in the amount of free cholesterol in the red-cell membrane is sufficient, by itself, to change normal cells into acanthocytes. Nor is it likely that the deficiency of polyunsaturated fatty acids in the red-cell phospholipids causes red cells to become acanthocytes, since acanthocytosis is not a feature of essential-fatty-acid deficiency due to fat malabsorption in the absence of abetalipoproteinaemia.

The high sphingomyelin:lecithin ratio and the high nervonic acid content of the red-cell phospholipids may play some part in the formation of acanthocytes. There is no direct evidence for this, but it is worth noting that Cooper et al. (1977) have shown that the viscosity of artificial liposomal membranes is increased when the sphingomyelin:lecithin ratio is increased. They have also shown that the red-cell membranes in abetalipoproteinaemia have an increased viscosity and have suggested that this change in viscosity is due to their abnormal phospholipid composition and is a cause of the abnormal shape and increased fragility of acanthocytes. Finally, it is conceivable that an essential constituent of the membrane of circulating red cells, yet to be identified, is normally transported into the circulation in association with triglyceride-rich lipoproteins and that in the absence of this constituent the red cells are transformed into acanthocytes.

No satisfactory explanation for the neurological abnormalities in terms of apoB deficiency has yet been put forward. It has been suggested that the progressive demyelination that occurs in abetalipoproteinaemia is due to vitamin E deficiency. In support of this, there is some evidence to suggest that the progress of the neurological disorder can be arrested by adding vitamin E to the diet (Muller et al., 1977). Other possibilities are that the maintenance of a normal myelin sheath in certain regions of the nervous system requires the presence of apoB or of some other component of LDL. The latter might, of course, be cholesterol, but there is no evidence to indicate that the very slow turnover of cholesterol that normally takes place in myelin requires an external source of cholesterol that can only be supplied by the plasma LDL. The pathogenesis of the retinitis pigmentosa in abetalipoproteinaemia is equally obscure.

3 FAMILIAL HYPOBETALIPOPROTEINAEMIA

3.1 Distinction from abetalipoproteinaemia

In addition to abetalipoproteinaemia, the recessive disorder giving rise to complete absence of β-lipoprotein in people who have inherited a double dose of the mutant gene, another, genetically distinct, familial disorder has been described in which there is a *partial* deficiency of plasma β-lipoprotein (see Fredrickson *et al.*, 1972, for an account of the historical background). This is now referred to as *familial hypobetalipoproteinaemia*. Subjects with this condition have abnormally low plasma LDL and total cholesterol concentrations, not attributable to any of the causes considered in Section 1, with at least one similarly affected first-degree relative. Genetic analysis of the families of index subjects indicates that the abnormality is inherited as an autosomal dominant trait, the hypobetalipoproteinaemic members of the family having a single dose of the abnormal gene. Affected individuals differ from subjects who are heterozygous for the mutation causing abetalipoproteinaemia (as defined at present), since the latter have a normal plasma lipoprotein pattern. Thus, both parents of a patient with classical abetalipoproteinaemia (who are presumed to be obligate heterozygotes) have a normal plasma LDL concentration, whereas in several families with familial hypobetalipoproteinaemia it has been possible to demonstrate a diminished plasma LDL concentration in two or more generations, in accordance with the presumed dominant mode of inheritance of the mutation.

Within a few years of the first description of familial hypobetalipoproteinaemia (Van Buchem *et al.*, 1966), families were reported in which some members had hypobetalipoproteinaemia while others had no immunochemically detectable plasma apoB and a clinical syndrome similar to that of patients who had the disorder then called 'abetalipoproteinaemia' (Cottrill *et al.*, 1974; Biemer and McCammon, 1975; Herbert *et al.*, 1978). The abetalipoproteinaemic members of these families are now thought to have a double dose of the mutation causing familial hypobetalipoproteinaemia when present in a single dose. This poses an awkward problem in nomenclature, since we now have to contend with at least two inherited forms of abetalipoproteinaemia that are clinically similar but genetically distinct. One is the so-called classical abetalipoproteinaemia (recessive inheritance); the other, with dominant inheritance, has been called *familial homozygous hypobetalipoproteinaemia*, though this nomenclature will clearly need revision since patients with a double dose of the dominant mutation are abetalipoproteinaemic. To add to the confusion, the first patient to be described with an inherited absence of β-lipoprotein was, as mentioned above, probably carrying a double dose of the mutation for familial hypobetalipoproteinaemia.

3.2 Clinical and biochemical features

3.2.1 Heterozygotes

Most subjects with familial hypobetalipoproteinaemia are symptom-free. Their condition has usually been detected during routine biochemical tests of the plasma lipids or by investigation of the relatives of subjects in whom the diagnosis has already been made. Fat malabsorption is absent or slight, retinitis pigmentosa does not occur and the neurological abnormalities characteristic of abetalipoproteinaemia are either absent or present only in a very mild form. The circulating red blood cells are usually normal in shape and lipid composition, though acanthocytes have been reported in the blood of one affected infant (Biemer and McCammon, 1975).

In most cases the plasma total cholesterol concentration is markedly diminished, but may be within normal limits. Plasma LDL concentration is usually reduced to half or less than half the age-adjusted normal level. There may be some increase in the sphingomyelin:lecithin ratio in the plasma phospholipids, but reports dealing with this point are conflicting.

3.2.2 Homozygotes

In the homozygous state (*familial homozygous hypobetalipoproteinaemia*) malabsorption of fat is marked, chylomicrons do not appear in the blood when fat is fed and jejunal biopsies show fat-loading of the mucosal cells similar to that seen in abetalipoproteinaemia. Retinitis pigmentosa and neurological abnormalities may be present, though the latter are less severe than in abetalipoproteinaemia, and in one patient were barely detectable at age 43 (Biemer and McCammon, 1975). Acanthocytosis is always present.

The pattern of the plasma lipids and lipoproteins is indistinguishable from that in abetalipoproteinaemia. There is a total absence of immunochemically detectable apoB and no apoB-containing lipoproteins can be detected in whole plasma by zonal electrophoresis. As in abetalipoproteinaemia, there is marked hypocholesterolaemia, a reduced HDL concentration and a deficiency of apoC-III-1 in the protein component of HDL.

3.3 Pathogenesis

The low plasma LDL concentration in familial hypobetalipoproteinaemia is due to a decreased rate of synthesis of apoB (Levy *et al.*, 1970) but there are no definite clues as to how the mutation brings about this decrease. The absence or relative mildness of the neurological abnormalities in homozygotes, who have no apoB in their plasma, is of interest from the point of view of pathogenesis, since it raises the possibility that the severe and progressive neurological changes seen in classical abetalipoproteinaemia are not mediated by apoB deficiency. If this were so, we should be obliged to reconsider the assumption that the mutation responsible for classical abetalipoproteinaemia is in the gene coding for apoB.

3.4 Diagnosis

Familial hypobetalipoproteinaemia is diagnosed by demonstrating a primary reduction in plasma LDL concentration to 50% or less of the age-adjusted normal level in the index subject and in at least one first-degree relative. The primary condition is established by excluding the causes of secondary hypobetalipoproteinaemia listed in Section 1. A low plasma total cholesterol concentration is a common presenting sign, but may not be apparent if the low LDL-cholesterol concentration is masked by an increased HDL-cholesterol concentration.

Diagnosis of the homozygous state depends upon the demonstration of abetalipoproteinaemia in the index patient and a reduced plasma total- or LDL-cholesterol concentration in at least one first-degree relative. The diagnosis is excluded if an obligate heterozygote (i.e. a parent or offspring) is found to have a normal plasma LDL concentration. In the light of the information available at present, absence of immunochemically detectable plasma apoB in an adult with no neurological symptoms is more likely to be due to familial homozygous hypobetalipoproteinaemia than to classical abetalipoproteinaemia.

When considering the differential diagnosis in a subject with primary β-lipoprotein deficiency one should bear in mind the possibility that genetic heterogeneity in this condition is greater than has been recognized hitherto. We should not be surprised to come across familial forms of this disorder which cannot be fitted into either of the two genetic patterns discussed in this section.

4 CHOLESTEROL METABOLISM IN β-LIPOPROTEIN DEFICIENCY

Since apoB is an essential constituent of the major cholesterol-carrying lipoprotein of plasma, an inherited deficiency of apoB would be expected to give rise to certain specific abnormalities in the transport and metabolism of cholesterol. Although it would clearly be desirable to test these predictions, there has been surprisingly little attempt at a systematic investigation of cholesterol metabolism in apoB deficiency.

Presumably, the absorption of cholesterol from the lumen of the intestine is defective, since cholesterol transported across the intestinal mucosa is normally secreted into the lymphatics as a component of chylomicrons and VLDL. In agreement with this, Illingworth et al. (1980) observed negligible absorption of oral [^{3}H]cholesterol into the plasma in two abetalipoproteinaemic patients. Hepatic synthesis of cholesterol is generally thought to be regulated by cholesterol absorbed from the intestine and transported to the liver in IDL derived from the triglyceride-rich lipoproteins. Failure to absorb cholesterol would therefore be expected to lead to increased hepatic synthesis of cholesterol by release from feed-back inhibition, and thus to increase the rate of synthesis in the whole body. However, as mentioned below, whole-body synthesis does not seem to be consistently increased in patients with abetalipoproteinaemia. IDL is presumably lacking from the plasma of abetalipoproteinaemic patients.

While it seems likely that bile acids are derived in part from the plasma cholesterol, there is no evidence to suggest that bile-acid synthesis is defective in abetalipoproteinaemia (Kayden, 1978; Myant et al., 1978). The production of adrenal-cortical and gonadal hormones, both of which are derived from cholesterol, has not been investigated in abetalipoproteinaemic patients.

As discussed in Chapter 9, the extra-hepatic tissues in man are thought to satisfy the bulk of their cholesterol requirements by uptake of LDL from the plasma or interstitial fluid. Furthermore, the behaviour of human cells in culture and of human lymphocytes in suspension suggests that in the absence of receptor-mediated uptake of LDL the rate of synthesis of cholesterol is increased to many times the normal rate. If this regulatory mechanism operates *in vivo*, the rate of synthesis of cholesterol in the extra-hepatic tissues of patients with abetalipoproteinaemia should be greatly increased, since there can be no receptor-mediated entry of cholesterol into the cells. The evidence bearing on this question is not entirely consistent, though there is general agreement that in abetalipoproteinaemia cholesterol synthesis in the whole body, or in freshly isolated tissues *in vitro*, is not increased to a degree comparable with that seen in cultured normal cells after pre-incubation in a lipoprotein-free medium or in cultured cells from patients with FH in the homozygous form in the presence of LDL. In an abetalipoproteinaemic adult patient studied by Myant et al. (1978), whole-body synthesis of cholesterol was not increased and acetate incorporation into sterols in freshly isolated lymphocytes *in vitro* was within the normal range (Reichl et al., 1978); a normal rate of whole-body synthesis in an abetalipoproteinaemic adult has also been reported by Kayden (1978). Bilheimer and Grundy (1979), on the other hand, found an increase in sterol synthesis, determined by measurement of sterol balance, in a 12-year-old abetalipoproteinaemic child, and Illingworth et al. (1980) have reported a similar finding in an adult and a child with abetalipoproteinaemia.

Illingworth *et al.* estimated that the observed rise in whole-body sterol synthesis in their patients was just sufficient to compensate for the amount of biliary cholesterol lost in the faeces through failure to reabsorb it. Ho *et al.* (1977) have also reported increased acetate incorporated into sterols of fresh lymphocytes in at least one of two abetalipoproteinaemic patients studied by them.

The absence of a consistent increase in cholesterol synthesis in abetalipoproteinaemia, over and above that to be expected as a response to the non-absorption of intestinal cholesterol, suggests that when there is a life-long deficiency of LDL in the fluid surrounding cells that normally regulate their cholesterol synthesis by the receptor mechanism, alternative regulatory mechanisms are called into play. It is possible, for example, that a steady state is reached in which sterol synthesis is suppressed by cholesterol synthesized within the cell itself rather than by that carried into the cell by LDL. An alternative explanation is suggested by the very high affinity of LDL receptors for apoE. The high-affinity binding of lipoproteins containing apoE is not necessarily followed by their internalization. Nevertheless, it is conceivable that in the absence of competition from LDL, apoE-rich lipoproteins in the plasma transport sufficient cholesterol into circulating lymphocytes to suppress cholesterol synthesis. If apoE-containing lipoproteins can be shown to be present in human interstitial fluid this possibility would also be worth considering in relation to the control of sterol synthesis in the extravascular tissues of abetalipoproteinaemic patients.

This section is a suitable place at which to mention that life expectancy of the members of families with familial hypobetalipoproteinaemia is several years longer than that in the general population, and that the increased longevity is associated with a decrease in proneness to myocardial infarction and a remarkable absence of atheromatous lesions and of intimal proliferation in the coronary arteries (Glueck *et al.*, 1976; Kahn and Glueck, 1978). This is another instance of the predictive association between plasma LDL-cholesterol concentration and ischaemic heart disease, providing further circumstantial evidence for the plasma lipid hypothesis outlined in Chapter 13.

5 FAMILIAL HDL DEFICIENCY

5.1 Characteristic features

Familial HDL deficiency is also known as Tangier disease, after the island in Chesapeake Bay (Virginia) where the first family with this rare disorder was recognized (Fredrickson *et al.*, 1961). The disease is characterized by hypocholesterolaemia, due to absence of normal HDL in the plasma, and extensive deposits of esterified cholesterol in the reticuloendothelial cells of many tissues, particularly the spleen, liver, intestinal wall, skin, thymus and lymph nodes. Lipid deposition causes the tonsils to become enlarged and lobulated, and to assume a characteristic orange-yellow appearance. This abnormality of the tonsils is the commonest presenting clinical sign. Lipid deposits in the cornea have been reported in many adult patients. About half the patients described in the world literature have had clinical signs of peripheral neuropathy, with a variety of neurological signs and symptoms, including loss of various sensory functions, wasting and weakness of muscles and absence of tendon reflexes. In one patient described by Kocen et al. (1967) the neurological abnormalities resembled syringomyelia.

Clinical signs suggestive of coronary atherosclerosis have been reported in at least two patients in their 40's (Herbert et al., 1978), but several patients have survived into the 5th or 6th decade without signs of IHD (see, for example, Utermann et al., 1975). The limited amount of information now available certainly does not allow us to conclude that premature IHD is an inevitable consequence of familial HDL deficiency; this important question is discussed in more detail in Sections 5.3 and 5.7. A fuller account of the clinical features, diagnosis and prognosis of this disease will be found in the article by Herbert et al. (1978).

5.2 Genetics

Genetic analysis of the families of index patients has shown that Tangier disease is due to the inheritance of an autosomal mutation at a single gene locus, affected individuals carrying a double dose of the mutant gene. Since obligate heterozygotes have none of the clinical signs that characterize the homozygous state, the disease is usually classified genetically as autosomal recessive. However, in heterozygotes the plasma HDL cholesterol concentration is usually reduced, sometimes to half the normal level, and foam cells are always present in the rectal mucosa, so that the mode of inheritance could more accurately be described as 'autosomal dominant with incomplete expression in the heterozygous state'. The difference in terminology is, of course, no more than a matter of definition. In the following sections of this chapter, the term 'Tangier disease', when used without qualification, refers to the homozygous state.

5.3 Pathology

The main pathological finding in Tangier disease is the presence of foam cells in many tissues. These foam cells are histiocytes that have become filled with cytoplasmic lipid droplets. The lipid droplets are not bound by a membrane and are therefore histologically different from the intra-lysosomal accumulations of lipid that occur in some other lipid-storage diseases. The lipid in the droplets consists almost entirely of esterified cholesterol in which the predominant fatty acid is oleate. Many of the droplets exhibit birefringence, indicating that the cholesteryl esters are liquid-crystalline at room temperature. In addition to histiocytic foam cells, extensive lipid deposits were noted in the Schwann cells of the peripheral nerves of two patients studied by Kocen *et al.* (1973). Lipid droplets have also been noted in smooth-muscle cells of the muscularis mucosa of the jejunum in patients in whom lipid accumulation had not occurred in the smooth-muscle cells of the arterial walls (Ferrans and Fredrickson, 1975).

Among the tissues in which foam cells accumulate are the tonsils, spleen, lymph nodes, bone marrow, rectal mucosa and submucosa of the small intestine. The cholesteryl ester content of tissues in which foam-cell accumulation occurs may be increased to many times the normal, but there is no significant increase in triglyceride or phospholipid content.

5.4 Plasma lipids and lipoproteins

5.4.1 Plasma lipids

Total plasma cholesterol concentration is reduced, sometimes markedly so. Reported values have usually been between 40 and 100 mg/100 ml. The triglyceride concentration is normal, or may be increased in fat-fed subjects. The phospholipid concentration is less than half the normal level; phospholipid composition in whole plasma may be normal or there may be a slight increase in the lecithin:sphingomyelin ratio. The ratio of esterified to total cholesterol in whole plasma is within the normal range and the fatty-acid composition of the plasma esterified cholesterol is normal, linoleate being the predominant fatty acyl residue. Despite the absence of normal HDL in the plasma, the rate of esterification of the plasma free cholesterol is usually at least half the normal rate and may even be close to the normal range (Assmann, 1978).

5.4.2 Plasma lipoproteins

Zonal electrophoresis of whole plasma shows the complete absence of α-migrating lipoproteins and increased mobility of β-lipoprotein. In whole plasma the apoA-I concentration is decreased to less than 0.5 mg/100 ml (normal, 100–150 mg/100 ml) and the apoA-II concentration is reduced to about 1 mg/100 ml (normal about 30 mg/100 ml). Almost all the apoA-I in the plasma in Tangier disease is in the fraction of density >1.21 g/ml, whereas most of the apoA-II is in the density range corresponding to that of normal HDL (1.063–1.21 g/ml). All the apoA-II in this density fraction is a component of the HDL_T described below. The apoA-I and apoA-II in the plasma of Tangier patients have the same immunochemical and electrophoretic properties and essentially the same amino acid composition as their counterparts in normal plasma.

The plasma fraction isolated in the preparative ultracentrifuge at the density of normal HDL contains measurable amounts of lipoprotein (up to 5 mg of protein/100 ml of plasma), but all of this lipoprotein is grossly abnormal. Electron microscopy shows small spherical particles 60–70 Å in diameter, larger particles 200–250 Å in diameter and other very large particles of irregular shape, together with stacked discs. The small spherical particles have been isolated by gel chromatography of the HDL obtained from very large volumes of plasma from Tangier patients (Assmann *et al.*, 1974). They have α mobility on electrophoresis in polyacrylamide gel but they differ from normal HDL in having apoA-II as their only apoprotein; they contain no immunochemically detectable apoA-I. This subfraction of the HDL in Tangier disease is designated HDL_T (Herbert *et al.*, 1978).

The VLDL in Tangier disease usually has a low content of free and esterified cholesterol and a low apoC content but is normal in other respects. Chylomicrons appear in the circulation after the ingestion of a fatty meal and their clearance from the circulation is usually delayed. Glickman *et al.* (1978) have reported the presence of apoA-I in the plasma chylomicrons of a Tangier patient during alimentary lipaemia. This contrasts with the absence of apoA-I from the circulating chylomicrons of normal subjects. The plasma LDL concentration is often decreased. The triglyceride content of LDL is increased and the cholesteryl ester content is decreased.

5.5 The heterozygous state

The plasma HDL cholesterol concentration in most obligate heterozygotes is decreased to about half the level in normal controls of the same age and sex. However, there is a considerable degree of overlap between plasma HDL levels in the general population and those observed in subjects presumed to have Tangier disease in the heterozygous form. This is partly due to the fact that reduced plasma HDL levels can occur from causes other than a single dose of the Tangier gene. These include primary or secondary hypertriglyceridaemia, familial hyperchylomicronaemia, obstructive or parenchymatous liver disease, and the recently described 'fish-eye disease' (Carlson and Philipson, 1979). These conditions should all be included in the differential diagnosis of heterozygous Tangier disease. In heterozygotes the lipid composition of LDL is normal and the HDL fraction does not contain the abnormal lipoproteins present in the d 1.062–1.21 fraction of the plasma of homozygotes; in particular, HDL_T is not detectable and the molar ratio of apoA-I to apoA-II is normal (Assmann, 1978). The abnormal tonsils, so characteristic of the homozygous state, are not seen in heterozygotes, but an abnormal accumulation of foam cells has been observed in the rectal mucosa of all heterozygotes from whom biopsies have been obtained (Assmann, 1978).

5.6 Pathogenesis

5.6.1 Nature of the gene mutation

Because of the profound decrease in the amount of apoA-I in whole plasma and the absence of apoA-I-containing lipoproteins in the HDL fraction in Tangier disease, it is usually assumed that the primary biochemical lesion is a deficiency of apoA-I, and that this is the cause of all the other clinical and biochemical abnormalities. Since the small amount of apoA-I present in the d > 1.21 fraction of plasma is indistinguishable from normal apoA-I, it has been argued that the mutation is unlikely to be in the structural gene coding for apoA-I and, hence, that the primary genetic abnormality is a defect in the regulation of the production or removal of an apoA-I of normal structure. However, it will not be possible to exclude an abnormality in the structure of 'Tangier' apoA-I until its amino acid sequence has been determined and the sequence compared with that of the normal protein.

A deficiency of apoA-I in the plasma could be due to inadequate synthesis, failure to incorporate the protein into lipoprotein, failure to secrete the appropriate lipoprotein into the circulation, or a selective increase in the catabolism of apoA-I before or after its secretion by the cells in which it is synthesized. In the light of existing knowledge it is not possible to exclude any of these explanations, but the balance of the evidence available suggests that the rate of catabolism of circulating apoA-I is greatly increased.

In favour of this, Schaefer et al. (1976) have shown that the fractional catabolic rate of the protein of ^{125}I-labelled HDL is increased in patients with Tangier disease. Further evidence for a specific enhancement of the catabolism of apoA-I has been obtained from an investigation of the removal of apoA proteins from the circulation of a Tangier patient (see Assmann, 1978). When this patient was given an injection of ^{125}I-labelled normal HDL preceded by a large dose of unlabelled HDL (sufficient to raise the plasma HDL-cholesterol concentration to 25 mg/100 ml), the apoA-I was cleared from the circulation very rapidly, while the apoA-II, which was removed much more slowly, appeared in an abnormal HDL fraction similar to HDL_T. Increased catabolism of apoA-I in the presence of a near-normal plasma HDL-cholesterol concentration certainly suggests the presence of an abnormally active catabolic mechanism for apoA-I. However, a puzzling feature of these observations was the finding that, despite evidence from immunofluorescence studies that in Tangier disease the cells of the jejunal mucosa synthesize apoA-I and secrete it into the intestinal lymphatics, the specific radioactivity of the apoA-I in the 1.006–1.21 density fraction remained constant throughout the experiment. This indicates that none of the newly-synthesized apoA-I molecules were incorporated into lipoproteins of density greater than 1.006 g/ml, and is in agreement with the suggestion of Glickman *et al.* (1978) that in Tangier disease there is a defect in the normal process by which apoA-I in intestinal-lymph chylomicrons is rapidly transferred to HDL before the chylomicrons enter the blood circulation. However, although this could explain the absence of an intestinal contribution to the pool of circulating HDL, it does not explain why in Tangier disease there is no normal apoA-I-containing HDL in the plasma, since the liver is believed to be a major source of the HDL of normal plasma. The finding that, in Tangier patients, jejunal synthesis of apoA-I is detectable in the fasting state and is stimulated by a fatty meal (Glickman *et al.*, 1978) suggests that the gene mutation does not result in loss of the ability to carry out regulated synthesis of apoA-I in those cells in which this normally occurs.

One way of reconciling these findings is to suppose that apoA-I is synthesized in hepatocytes and gut-mucosal cells but cannot be incorporated into HDL particles, and that as a consequence of this failure apoA-I is either discharged directly into the extracellular medium and is then rapidly cleared from the circulation, or is retained in chylomicrons from which it is rapidly released when the chylomicrons are hydrolysed by lipoprotein lipase. In either case, failure to become incorporated into normal long-lived HDL particles could result in very rapid catabolism of apoA-I. However, this explanation raises almost as many questions as it answers. In particular, our limited knowledge of the normal metabolism of apoA-I in man does not allow us to speculate usefully on the nature of the abnormal gene product that would result in failure to incorporate apoA-I into HDL and would also lead to a specific enhancement of its removal from the circulation. One possibility is that the mutation affects the structure of apoA-I in a manner such as to prevent it from interacting with the lipids of an HDL particle, without altering its immunochemical or electrophoretic properties. This might also cause the apoA-I secreted by Tangier cells to be removed rapidly from the circulation. The formation of a structurally abnormal apoA-I is certainly an attractive possibility, but if this is the fundamental defect in Tangier disease one may ask why the apoA-I of normal HDL is also metabolized at an abnormally rapid rate in Tangier patients.

5.6.2 The lipoprotein abnormalities

Whatever view one may hold as to the primary lesion in Tangier disease, most of the lipoprotein abnormalities can reasonably be explained in terms of a gross deficiency of apoA-I in the plasma. The reduced plasma concentration of apoA-II and the presence of small amounts of an apoA-II-containing lipoprotein (HDL_T) in 'Tangier' plasma suggest that in the absence of apoA-I, apoA-II is capable of forming a lipoprotein particle by associating with lipids, but that this abnormal particle is catabolized much more rapidly than is normal HDL; in this connection, it should be noted that apoA-II is capable of forming stable complexes with phospholipids *in vitro* (see Soutar and Myant, 1979). The abnormal large particles present in the HDL fraction are thought to be surface components of VLDL and chylomicrons released during their catabolism in the blood capillaries. Their accumulation in the plasma would be expected in view of the known role of normal HDL in facilitating the disposal of free cholesterol and lecithin derived from the surfaces of triglyceride-rich particles. Since HDL also acts as a reservoir of the apoC taken up by nascent triglyceride-rich particles when they enter the circulation, absence of HDL would explain the low apoC content of VLDL in Tangier disease. Defective catabolism of VLDL may also be the cause of the low plasma LDL concentration. The marked reduction in the cholesteryl-ester content of LDL is consistent with the current view that much of the esterified cholesterol of normal LDL is derived indirectly from the esters generated from free cholesterol in HDL by the LCAT reaction.

The presence, in Tangier plasma, of a normal proportion of esterified cholesterol with a normal fatty acid pattern (indicating that the cholesteryl esters are formed by the LCAT reaction) deserves some comment, since it is generally believed that HDL is the substrate for LCAT and that apoA-I is an essential cofactor for the reaction. Presumably, the small quantities of apoA-I isolated in the $d > 1.21$ fraction of the plasma are sufficient to enable the LCAT reaction to proceed, though at a somewhat reduced rate. The formation of cholesteryl esters by the LCAT reaction in the absence of HDL suggests that VLDL, and possibly LDL, can act as alternative substrates for the enzyme.

5.6.3 The intracellular accumulation of cholesterol

The cholesterol that accumulates in the macrophage-like cells of many tissues is probably derived from the surface components of triglyceride-rich particles. Failure to metabolize these surface components through the normal pathway involving HDL and LCAT results in their phagocytosis by macrophages. The predominance of esterified choleseterol with oleate as the major fatty acid indicates that the esterified cholesterol ingested by macrophages in hydrolysed by the lysosomal ester hydrolase and is then re-esterified by ACAT before it is stored as lipid droplets. The intracellular storage of cholesterol in Tangier disease is similar in certain respects to that occurring in familial LCAT deficiency. In both disorders there is an accumulation of abnormal cholesterol-rich particles in the plasma owing to defective metabolism of the redundant surface material of chylomicrons and VLDL, with subsequent storage of the excess cholesterol in macrophages. However, there are unexplained differences between the biochemical and histological abnormalities in the two conditions, notably with respect to the nature of the abnormal cholesterol-rich lipoproteins and the tissues in which the major accumulations of cholesterol occur (see Section 6.4 of this chapter).

It should be noted that the type of cell in which cholesterol is stored in Tangier disease lends no support to the hypothesis that one of the functions of HDL is to remove cholesterol from cells that have acquired their cholesterol by receptor-mediated uptake of LDL or by synthesis *in situ*. Thus, LDL receptors are not present on macrophages (Goldstein *et al.*, 1979), but they are present on arterial smooth-muscle cells, in which cholesterol storage does not occur in Tangier disease.

5.7 Tangier disease and ischaemic heart disease

The negative association between plasma HDL concentration and incidence of IHD in the general population is generally explained on the supposition that HDL facilitates the removal of cholesterol from the arterial wall and thus counteracts the development of atherosclerosis of the coronary arteries. If this explanation is valid, premature IHD should be a prominent feature of Tangier disease. However, as already mentioned, clinical signs of IHD are by no means the rule in middle-aged Tangier patients and the arterial wall is not one of the tissues in which cholesterol storage occurs. Furthermore, heterozygotes, including those with a marked decrease in plasma HDL concentration, may survive into the 9th decade without evidence of coronary artery disease. Patients with Tangier disease may be protected from IHD to some extent by their low plasma LDL concentration and the low cholesteryl-ester content of their LDL. However, this explanation is not applicable to the heterozygotes, since they have a normal plasma concentration of LDL with normal lipid composition.

6 FAMILIAL LCAT DEFICIENCY

6.1 General remarks

Although hypolipidaemia is not a characteristic feature of familial LCAT deficiency, the plasma of all affected patients is deficient in normal lipoproteins and, moreover, the abnormalities in cholesterol metabolism that result from failure to form normal lipoproteins are similar in several respects to those occurring in familial HDL deficiency. It is therefore appropriate to conclude this chapter with a brief account of familial LCAT deficiency. Less than 30 patients with this disease have been reported in the world literature since its first description in three Norwegian sisters (Norum and Gjone, 1967). Hence, it may justifiably be called 'very rare'. Nevertheless, the intensive study of a mere handful of patients in several laboratories has deepened our understanding of normal human cholesterol metabolism in a way that could not possibly have been foreseen in 1966, when the first patient was diagnosed in Oslo. All of the first nine patients to be investigated in detail were Scandinavian (Table 16.1). Seven of these came from three families living in the same isolated region on the West coast of Norway. In addition to these patients, others have been reported from Germany (two brothers of Sardinian origin), France, England, Canada and Japan. Most recently, LCAT deficiency has been diagnosed at Hammersmith Hospital in three sisters born in County Mayo, Western Ireland (see Table 16.2).

More detailed accounts of the historical background, and of the clinical, pathological and metabolic features of this disease will be found in the review by Gjone *et al.* (1978) and in the symposia edited by Gjone and Norum (1974) and Gjone (1978).

6.2 Characteristic features

Familial LCAT deficiency is characterized by the absence or near-absence of LCAT activity in plasma, a very low plasma cholesteryl-ester concentration, marked abnormalities in the composition and physical properties of the lipoproteins of all density classes, proteinuria frequently associated with renal failure, microcytic anaemia and the presence of corneal opacities.

As shown in Table 16.1, all the Scandinavian patients had corneal opacities, all had anaemia and all but one had proteinuria. LCAT activity was completely absent from the plasma of all the Norwegian patients but was detectable, though at a much reduced level, in patient ML of family II (Table 16.1). The earliest sign of the disease is usually proteinuria, and corneal opacities were noted in childhood or at puberty in four of the Scandinavian patients. General health

Table 16.1
Some clinical and biochemical features of the nine Scandinavian patients with familial LCAT deficiency

Family	Patient	Year of birth	Age detected (years)	Corneal opacity	Anaemia	Proteinuria	Age at renal failure (years)	Total cholesterol	Esterified cholesterol	Triglycerides
I (Norway)	MR (F)	1947	19	+	+	+	—	140	10	130
	IS (F)	1935	31	+	+	+	39	560	60	570
	AR (F)	1933	33	+	+	+	36	300	10	300
II (Sweden)	ML (F)	1921	47	+	+	+	52	340	100	530
	BB (M)	1924	40	+	+	+	40	plasma lipids not reported		
III (Norway)	LG (M)	1932	35	+	+	+	40	235	30	600
	AA (F)	1926	42	+	+	+	53	215	50	900
IV (Norway)	KA (M)	1918	54	+	+	+	54	130	4	250
	DJ (F)	1913	59	+	+	—	—	107	2	105

Plasma lipids (mg/100 ml)

F, female; M, male; —, signifies that the sympton was not reported in 1978.
Note: Patient BB of family II was diagnosed *post mortem*. He died from renal failure at age 40, before the diagnosis had been made in his sister, but was known to have had corneal opacities, anaemia, proteinuria and lipaemic plasma.
(Assembled from Tables 1 and 2 of Gjone *et al.* (1978) and Tables 1 and 2 of Gjone (1974) and from information supplied by K. R. Norum).

appears to be normal until the fourth decade, when signs of renal insufficiency begin to develop, usually leading to renal failure in the 40's or 50's. One patient has died of renal failure and four others have required renal transplants. Neurological symptoms are absent and skin xanthomas are not a feature of the disease. The frequency of premature atherosclerosis is discussed in Section 6.4.

6.3 Genetics

Familial LCAT deficiency is inherited as an autosomal recessive trait, with, usually, no decrease in plasma LCAT activity in the parents of index patients. The mutation is probably very rare in most populations, but in the isolated region in which the Norwegian families were discovered the frequency of carriers has been estimated to be at least 4% (Gjone *et al.*, 1974). Family studies of the Norwegian patients suggest that they are all descended from a common ancestor in whom the mutation occurred at least 250 years ago. Linkage studies indicate that the LCAT locus is situated on the long arm of chromosome 16, near the gene coding for α-haptoglobin. Presumably,

Table 16.2

Total cholesterol concentration, cholesteryl ester : total cholesterol and LCAT activity in the plasma of three LCAT-deficient Irish sisters and their children

Subject	Year of birth	Sex	TC (mg/100 ml)	CE/TC (%)	LCAT activity	Esterification rate
II 1	1924	F	213	16.2	0	0
2	1931	F	193	11.7	0	0
3	1932	F	193	8.5	1.3	0
III 2	1961	F	191	76.4	61	83
3	1964	M	195	65.1	63	90
4	1968	M	238	64.3	63	97
5	1970	F	220	73.9	71	98
6	1972	F	199	76.0	63	79
7	1960	M	218	61.3	64	—
8	1964	M	158	60.1	59	—
Normal control		M	194	77.3	121	110

TC, total cholesterol; CE, esterified cholesterol. II 1, II 2 and II 3 had the clinical and biochemical signs of familial LCAT deficiency described in the text; they were therefore homozygotes and all their children were obligate heterozygotes. III 2 to III 6 were the children of patient II 2; III 7 and III 8 were the children of patient III 3.

LCAT activities (assayed by the method of Glomset and Wright, 1964) and net esterification rates (assayed by the method of Stokke and Norum, 1971) are expressed in μmoles of cholesterol esterified/l of plasma/h.

I am indebted to A. Jadhav and S. Thanabalasingham for the measurements of plasma cholesterol, LCAT activity and esterification rate, and to L. Borysiewicz for the other details.

in those patients who have detectable LCAT activity in their plasma the mutation is different from the one present in the Norwegian families. Genetic heterogeneity is also suggested by the fact that in two Canadian patients (J. Frohlich, personal communication) and in the two Sardinian brothers reported by Utermann *et al.* (1978) immunoreactive LCAT protein was not detectable in the plasma, whereas LCAT has been detected by immuno-assay in the plasma of the Norwegian patients (K. R. Norum, personal communication). There are also differences in the extent to which the abnormal gene is expressed in the obligate heterozygotes from different families. In the parents and children of the Norwegian patients, plasma LCAT activity was normal. However, in the parents of the two Sardinian patients LCAT activity was about half that in control subjects, and in the heterozygous relatives of Frohlich's Canadian patients LCAT activity assayed with an artificial substrate was about 50% of normal. LCAT activity was also significantly below the normal in the children of the three Irish sisters studied at Hammersmith Hospital (Table 16.2). These findings suggest that in some families it may be possible to diagnose the heterozygous state by measuring plasma LCAT activity under conditions in which the enzyme is saturated with substrate.

6.4 Pathology

Examination of biopsy material and of tissues obtained *post mortem* from patients who have developed renal insufficiency has shown the presence of abnormal deposits of lipid in several tissues. The most striking changes are seen in the kidneys (Stokke *et al.*, 1974). The glomeruli are hyalinized and fibrosed, with tubular atrophy and focal necrosis of the capillary endothelium. In the glomeruli there are numerous foam cells and membranous accumulations of lipid in the capillary lumina, in the walls of the capillaries and in the subendothelial and subepithelial layers. The lipid deposits may appear as multilamellar 'myelin figures', as vesicles surrounded by a single bilayer or as membrane-bound granules. The lipid composition of glomeruli isolated by a sieving technique is consistent with the supposition that these abnormal deposits are composed largely of phospholipid:cholesterol bilayers. The renal arteries and arterioles show narrowing of the lumen and thickening of the intima, with foam cells in the subendothelial region and in other layers of the vessel wall. These changes appear to develop very rapidly, as shown by the fact that they were present in a kidney six months after it had been transplanted into a patient.

Foam cells are present in other tissues, including spleen, marrow, liver and the walls of larger arteries. Many phagocytic cells in the spleen, marrow and liver (Kupffer cells) contain lipid granules

800 The Biology of Cholesterol and Related Steroids

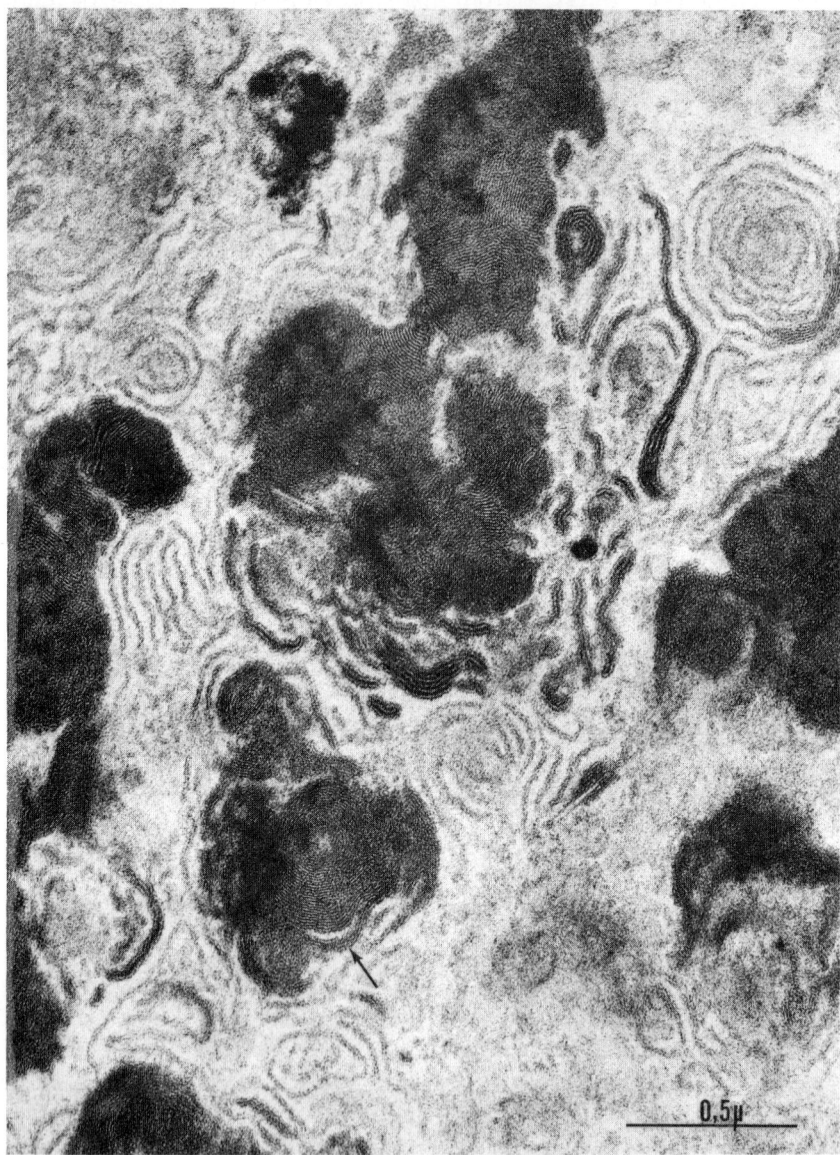

Figure 16.2
Negatively stained electron photomicrograph of cytoplasmic myelin figures in a phagocytic cell from the spleen of a patient with familial LCAT deficiency. (From Hovig and Gjone (1974), with the permission of the authors.)

composed of multiple bilayers in the form of myelin figures (Fig. 16.2). These cells are known as 'sea-blue histiocytes' because of their characteristic staining properties. Extra-cellular deposits of membranous lipid were noted in the perivascular region of the hepatic lobules in a liver biopsy from one patient (Hovig and Gjone, 1974). These histological changes are reflected in a marked increase in the tissue content of unesterified cholesterol. Thus, the free cholesterol content of the spleen of one patient was 90 times that of a normal spleen (Stokke et al., 1974).

The corneal opacities differ in appearance from those seen in any other condition. Minute greyish dots, presumed to be due to deposits of lipid, are present over the whole cornea, giving it a cloudy appearance. At the periphery of the cornea the dots become confluent, forming a ring similar to that seen in *arcus senilis*. In two patients, fundal changes have been observed, with detectable optic atrophy. Loss of visual acuity, however, is not characteristic of familial LCAT deficiency.

Premature atherosclerosis has been demonstrated in several patients. In one female who died at age 40 (AR of family I) atheroma with calcification was noted in the abdominal aorta and other large arteries. However, one of the Norwegian patients (DJ of family IV) had no signs of atherosclerosis at age 65, showing that premature athcrosclerosis is not an inevitable consequence of a total absence of LCAT activity. In the atheromatous lesions in familial LCAT deficiency the ratios both of free to esterified cholesterol and of 18:1 to 18:2 fatty acids in the cholesteryl esters are considerably higher than the corresponding ratios in the atheroma lipids of individuals from the general population. These differences in lipid composition reflect the abnormal composition of the plasma lipids in familial LCAT deficiency (see next section).

6.5 Plasma lipids and lipoproteins

6.5.1 Lipids

Plasma obtained in the fasting state is usually turbid. Total cholesterol concentration is increased in the majority of cases but was below normal in two of the Norwegian patients (family IV, Table 16.1) and was normal in the three Irish patients (Table 16.2). Cholesteryl-ester concentration in whole plasma is always markedly reduced (Table 16.1). The ratio of 18:1 to 18:2 fatty acids in the cholesteryl esters is abnormally high and the ratio of esterified to free cholesterol in the lipoprotein fractions is highest in VLDL and lowest in HDL (the opposite of what is found in normal human plasma). Plasma triglyceride concentration may be normal, but was moderately or markedly increased in five of the Scandinavian patients. Total phospholipid concentration is usually increased, with increased lecithin and decreased sphingomyelin concentrations. Lysolecithin concentration is always markedly reduced.

6.5.2 Lipoproteins

Zonal electrophoresis of whole plasma shows a complete absence of pre-β-migrating lipoproteins and little or no α_1-migrating lipoprotein.

a.

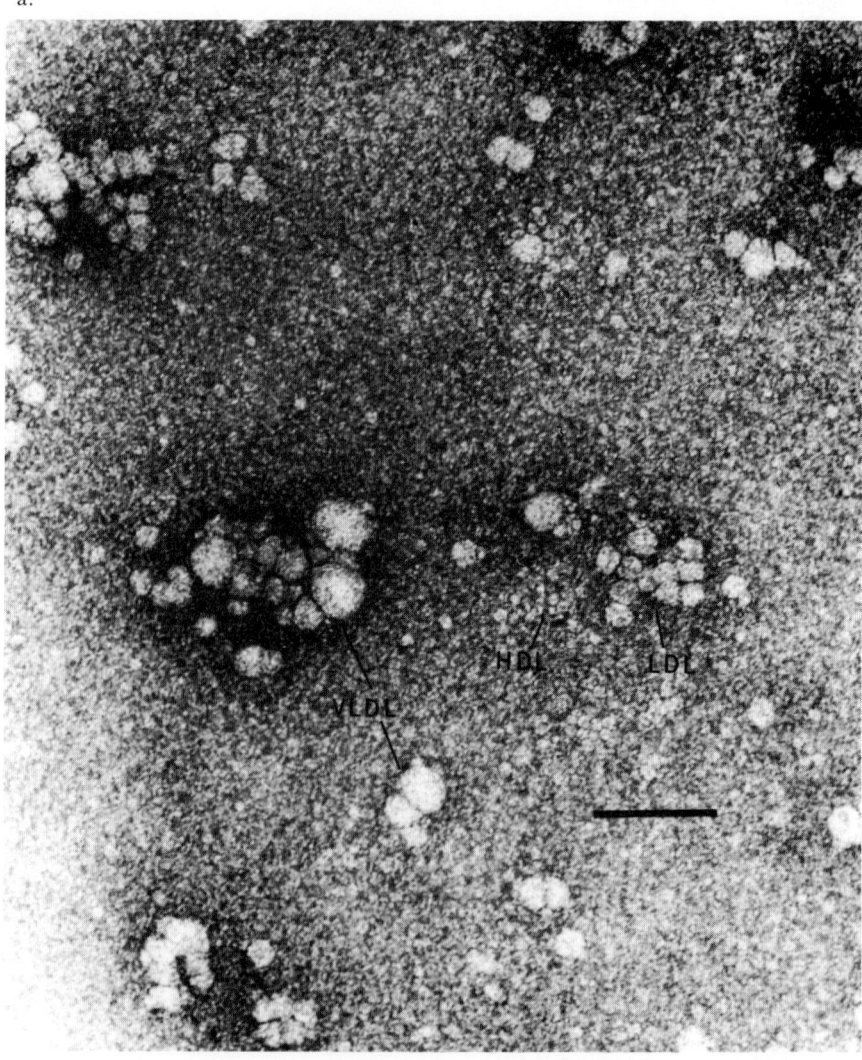

Figure 16.3
Negatively stained electron photomicrograph of whole serum from a normal subject (a) and a patient with familial LCAT deficiency (b), showing normal HDL, LDL

Disorders of Cholesterol Metabolism: The Hypolipoproteinaemias

Electron microscopy of whole plasma shows the presence of particles that are grossly abnormal in size and shape. These include myelin-like multilamellar structures and very large particles with irregular outlines (Fig. 16.3). Examination of the lipoprotein fractions isolated in the preparative ultracentrifuge shows that each fraction is remarkably heterogeneous and is abnormal in chemical composition, electron-microscopic appearance and distribution of particle sizes. In all

b.

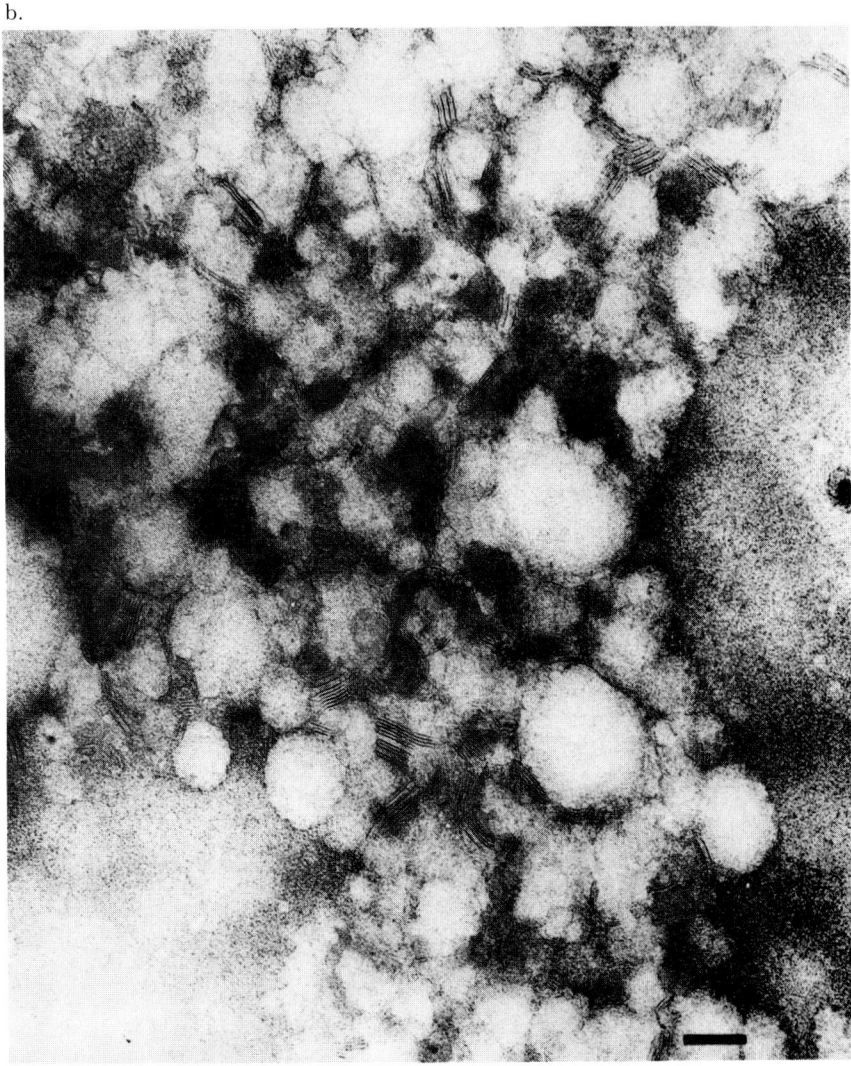

and VLDL particles in (a) and large lipoprotein particles together with myelin figures in (b). (From Forte *et al.* (1974), with the permission of the authors.)

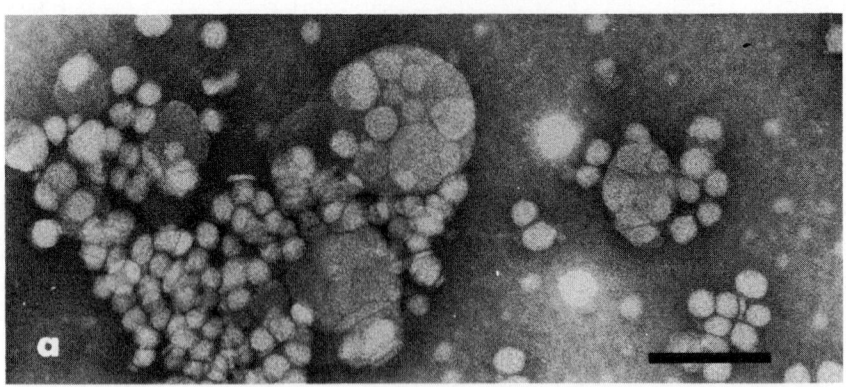
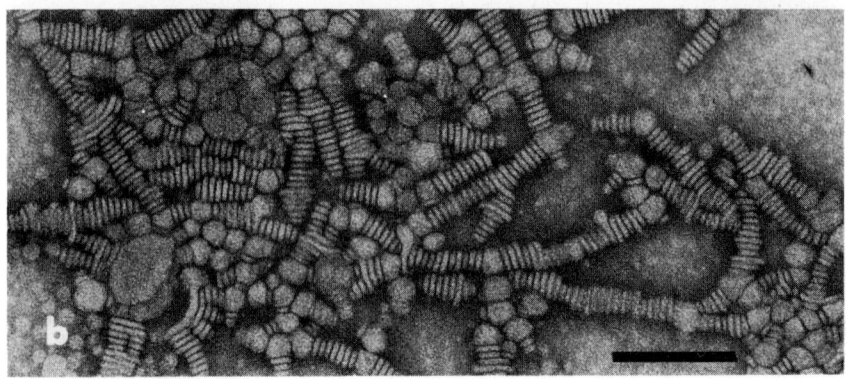
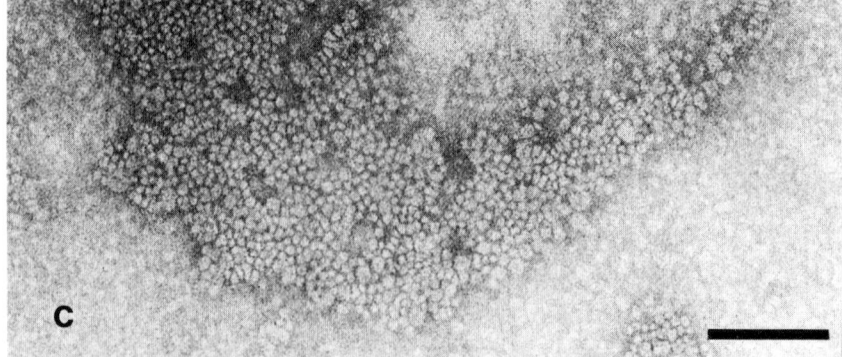

Figure 16.4
Negatively stained electron photomicrograph of the HDL subfraction of the serum of a patient with familial LCAT-deficiency. The subfractions were obtained by gel column chromatography. Fraction (a) contains particles similar to those observed in the LDL fraction. Fraction (b) consists mainly of stacked discs. Fraction (c) consists mainly of small spherical particles 45–80 Å in diameter. Black bars represent 1000 Å. (From Forte *et al.* (1974), with the permission of the authors.)

fractions the ratio of esterified to free cholesterol is greatly reduced and the concentrations of free cholesterol and lecithin are increased.

The VLDL fraction contains large particles with surface indentations, these particles having an electron-microscopic appearance similar to that of triglyceride-rich lipoproteins that have been incubated with lipoprotein lipase, as described by Blanchette-Mackie and Scow (1973). This fraction also contains crescent-shaped particles and whorled bilayers presumed to consist of phospholipid and free cholesterol.

The LDL fraction (d 1.019–1.063) contains three more or less distinct subfractions: (1) large particles (1000 Å in diameter) which appear to be flattened when viewed in the the electron microscope, (2) particles of intermediate size (400–600 Å in diameter) with the appearance and chemical composition of LP-X and (3) particles resembling normal LDL in size and shape, but with less than the normal amount of cholesteryl ester and with a ten-fold increase in triglyceride content. The large flattened particles may be derived from vesicles bounded by single bilayers of phospholipid and free cholesterol.

The HDL fraction is greatly reduced in concentration, and samples isolated by preparative ultracentrifugation have only about a tenth of the normal content of apoA-I. (On the other hand, substantial amounts of apoA-I are recovered in the fraction of d > 1.25 g/ml.) Examination in the electron microscope (Fig. 16.4) shows the presence of disc-shaped particles, 40 Å thick and 150–200 Å in diameter, which tend to form rouleaux and which have a close resemblance to the nascent HDL particles secreted by the perfused rat liver (Hamilton, 1972). In addition to the discoidal particles, the HDL fraction also contains large particles, similar to the large particles present in the LDL fraction, and spherical particles (45–60 Å in diameter) that are considerably smaller than normal HDL. Mitchell et al. (1980) have described the isolation, by affinity chromatography, of an apoE-rich subfraction of HDL from the plasma of patients with familial LCAT deficiency.

6.6 Red blood cells

The lipid composition of the red cells is abnormal (Table 16.3). In particular, the amount of cholesterol per red cell is increased to nearly double the normal. The content of total phospholipid is normal, so that the cholesterol:phospholipid molar ratio is considerably increased. The content of lecithin is increased and that of sphingomyelin is decreased. Target cells (abnormal red cells with increased diameter) are present in peripheral blood and bone

Table 16.3
Lipid composition of red blood cells in familial LCAT deficiency

Lipid	Patients	Normal
Cholesterol (10^{-10} mg/red cell)	1.81	1.11
Total lipid P (10^{-11} mg/red cell)	1.06	1.00
Lecithin (% total PL)	51.0	27.4
Sphingomyelin (% total PL)	14.6	25.9
Phosphatidylethanolamine (% total PL)	19.3	29.0
$\dfrac{\text{Cholesterol}}{\text{Phospholipid}}$ (molar ratio)	1.40	0.89

P, phosphorous; PL, phospholipid. Values for patients are means from six of the Scandinavian patients listed in Table 16.1. (Modified from Gjone *et al.*, 1978.)

marrow. The anaemia present in most patients with familial LCAT deficiency is associated with a reduced life-span of the circulating red cells.

6.7 Pathogenesis

All the clinical and biochemical abnormalities of familial LCAT deficiency can reasonably be explained as the direct or indirect consequences of a deficiency of LCAT in the plasma. Complete deficiency, as in the seven Norwegian patients, is presumably due to a mutation at the LCAT locus such that the liver fails to synthesize any functional enzyme. In patients in whom some enzyme activity is detectable the mutation may cause the synthesis of a structurally abnormal enzyme which retains some catalytic activity. Alternatively, the genetic error in these patients might be a mutation affecting the rate of synthesis of a structurally normal enzyme.

6.7.1 The plasma lipoproteins

The effects of adding LCAT to the plasma of a patient with familial LCAT deficiency are fully consistent with the assumption that all the lipoprotein abnormalities are due to lack of LCAT in the plasma. Furthermore, detailed observations on the changes in the lipid and apolipoprotein composition of the lipoprotein fractions that ensue when LCAT is added to an LCAT-deficient plasma have added considerably to our understanding of the normal intravascular metabolism of lipoproteins (Norum *et al.*, 1975). As Norum and his coworkers have pointed out, one is likely to learn much more about lipoprotein metabolism by seeing what happens when LCAT is added to plasma that has never been in contact with the enzyme, than by studying the effect of adding LCAT to normal plasma, in which the changes induced by the action of the enzyme must already have approached completion. Additional information about the role of LCAT in plasma has also been obtained by observing the effect of reducing the dietary intake of fat in patients with familial LCAT deficiency.

When plasma from an LCAT-deficient patient is incubated with LCAT, the lipoproteins in all density fractions undergo striking changes in chemical composition and structural appearance, all of these modifications reflecting a change towards the normal pattern. (Some of these chemical and structural modifications were mentioned in Chapter 11.)

In the VLDL fraction there is a decrease in the concentrations of free cholesterol, lecithin and apoC-II and -III proteins, an increase in the concentrations of esterified cholesterol, apoC-I and apoE, and a shift in the distribution of particle sizes towards the smaller particles. In the LDL fraction, there is a marked increase in the concentration of esterified cholesterol, especially in the smaller (normal-sized) particles, a decrease in the number of large particles and an increase in the number of smaller particles. There is also a decrease in the triglyceride content of the smaller particles, so that their lipid composition changes towards that of the LDL of normal plasma. The most striking changes occur in the HDL fraction. The concentrations of esterified cholesterol, apoA-I and apoC proteins increase, the concentrations of free cholesterol, lecithin and apoE decrease and there are marked alterations in electron-microscopic appearance, the small spherical particles disappearing and the discoidal particles assuming a spherical shape (Fig. 16.5).

Quantitative analysis of these changes in LCAT-deficient plasma indicates that the bulk of the free cholesterol and lecithin consumed during the incubation is derived from the large VLDL and large LDL particles and that most of the esterified cholesterol formed, presumably on HDL, is ultimately transferred to small VLDL and small (i.e., normal-sized) LDL particles. The net effect of LCAT is, therefore, to bring about the conversion of free into esterified cholesterol, the mass transfer of esterified cholesterol into particles of density < 1.063 g/ml and a redistribution of apoA-I, apoC and apoE. The increased apoA-I content of the HDL fraction after incubation with LCAT may be due either to transfer of apoA-I from the $d > 1.21$ to the d 1.063–1.21 fraction, or to the stabilization of HDL particles, so that they lose less of their apoA-I to the $d > 1.21$ fraction during preparative ultracentrifugation. Thus, the abnormal lipid and apoprotein composition of the lipoprotein fractions of LCAT-deficient plasma are readily understandable in terms of the integrated effects of LCAT on whole plasma.

The effect of LCAT on the HDL discoidal particles is fully in line

808 The Biology of Cholesterol and Related Steroids

with the current view that the HDL secreted by the liver and intestine appear in the plasma as free cholesterol:phospholipid bilayers and that these nascent particles are then converted into spheres by the action of LCAT (see Chapter 11). Thus, at least some of the HDL discs in the plasma of patients with LCAT deficiency may be assumed to be newly-secreted HDL that has not been acted upon by LCAT.

The large cholesterol-rich particles present in the VLDL and LDL

A

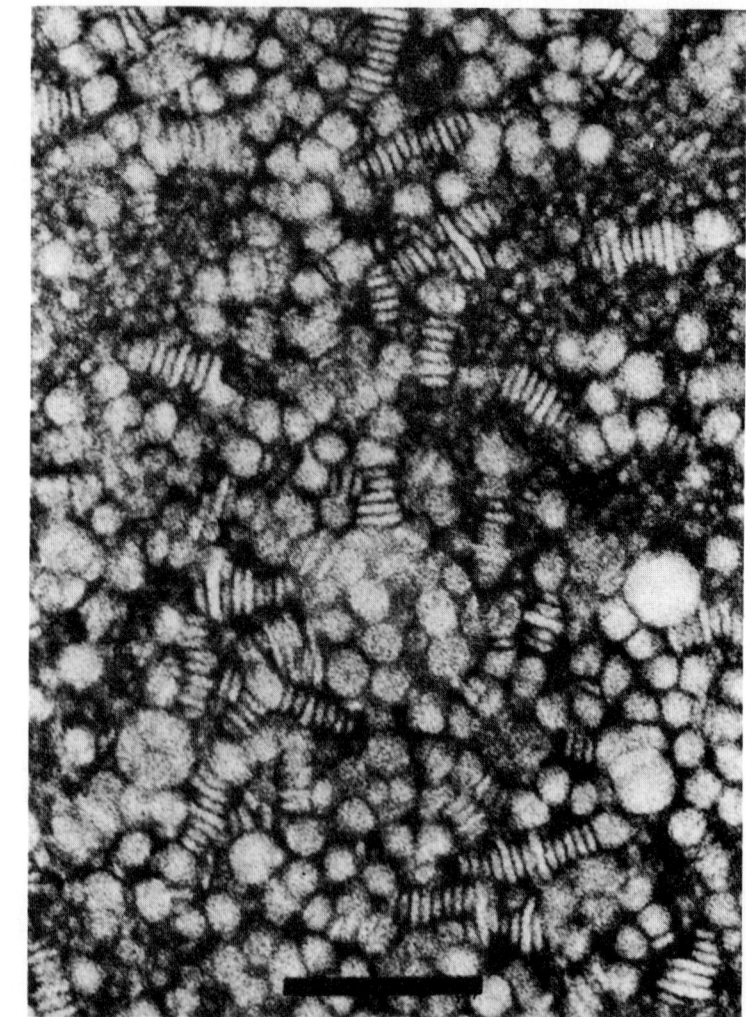

Figure 16.5
Effect of incubating LCAT-deficient plasma HDL in the presence of LCAT from normal human plasma. The LCAT-deficient plasma was obtained from a patient with LCAT deficiency. A shows negatively stained electron photomicrograph of the HDL fraction before incubation with LCAT. Most of the particles are discoidal.

Disorders of Cholesterol Metabolism: The Hypolipoproteinaemias 809

fractions and the small spherical HDL particles are believed to be derived from surface material released from VLDL and chylomicrons during their breakdown by membrane-bound lipoprotein lipase at the luminal surface of the blood capillaries. In keeping with this, when the intestinal secretion of triglyceride-rich lipoproteins is curtailed by withdrawing fat from the diet of a patient with familial LCAT deficiency there is a conspicuous decrease in the concentration of the

B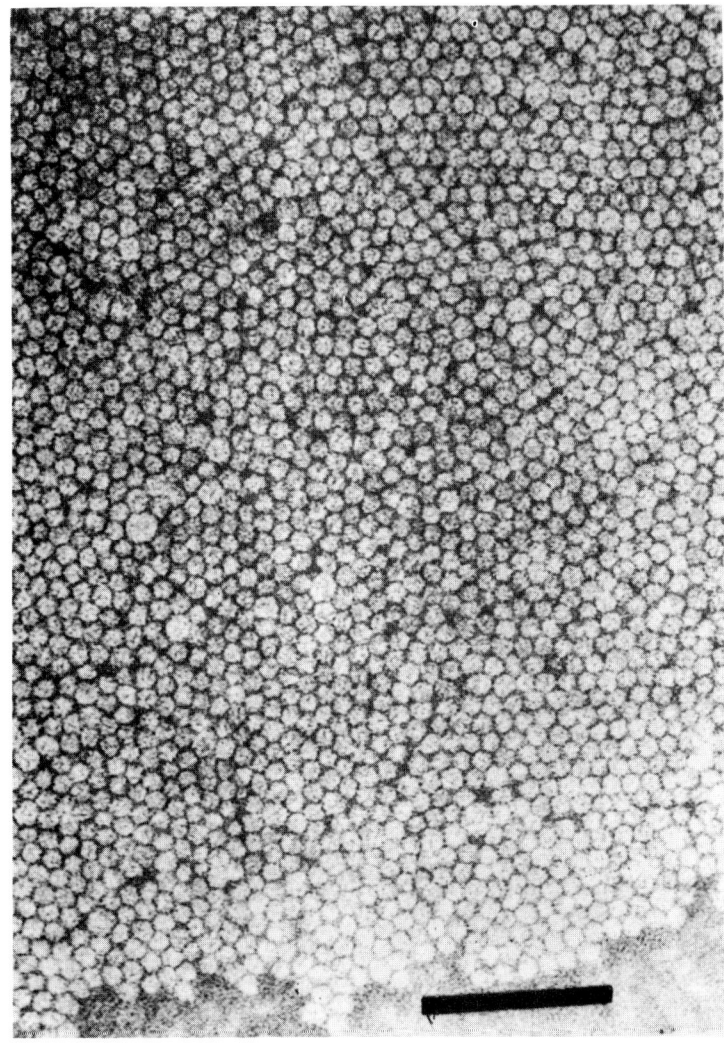

B shows the same HDL fraction after incubation with LCAT at 37 °C. All the particles have been converted into the normal spheres of mature HDL. (× 189 000); bar = 1000 Å. (From Forte et al. (1974), with the permission of the authors.)

large VLDL particles, of the LDL particles of large and intermediate size and of the small spherical HDL particles (Glomset et al., 1975). Thus, it appears that the bilaminar and multilamellar cholesterol-rich structures present in the d < 1.063 lipoproteins are derived from polar surface lipids of triglyceride-rich particles that under normal conditions would be metabolized by LCAT. This conclusion derives some support from the observation that incubation of normal human VLDL in a mixture containing soluble lipoprotein lipase and albumin (but no LCAT) leads to the formation of several types of particle, including large vesicles bounded by a single bilayer (350–800 Å diameter) not unlike some of the abnormal particles present in the d < 1.063 fraction of patients with familial LCAT deficiency (Deckelbaum et al., 1979). Particles consisting mainly of phospholipid and cholesterol and having the density of HDL are also formed from the surface material of VLDL during these incubations. However, these 'HDL' particles are bilaminar discs resembling the discoidal particles, rather than the small spherical particles, seen in the HDL fraction of LCAT-deficient plasma. This raises the interesting possibility that some of the discoidal particles in the HDL of these patients are not nascent HDL secreted by the liver or intestine, but are derived from the surface lipids of VLDL and chylomicrons.

6.7.2 Lipid deposition in tissues

The accumulation of abnormal cholesterol-rich particles in the plasma results in the deposition of membranous lipid material in the cells and extracellular spaces of a variety of tissues. As in Tangier disease, the cells in which lipid accumulates are predominantly macrophages or other elements of the reticuloendothelial system, suggesting that the lipid enters the cells in particulate form by phagocytosis. However, in familial LCAT deficiency much of the cholesterol in the intracellular inclusions is unesterified and is present in myelin-like structures, whereas in Tangier disease the excess of intracellular cholesterol is esterified and is present mainly in the lipid droplets of foam cells. The distribution of the lipid deposits in familial LCAT deficiency also differs in several respects from that in Tangier disease. In LCAT deficiency, cholesterol storage is most marked in the kidneys, spleen, bone marrow and arterial walls; lipid storage in the tonsils, so characteristic of Tangier disease, does not occur and there is no evidence that cholesterol is deposited in the Schwann cells of the nervous system. The characteristic tissue distribution of stored lipid in familial LCAT deficiency explains why renal failure is the outstanding and life-limiting clinical feature of this disease, why it is frequently associated with premature atherosclerosis and why neurological symptoms do not develop. The distribution of the tissues in which lipid storage occurs in familial LCAT deficiency may be a function of the size and physical properties of the cholesterol-rich particles in the plasma and the permeability, to these particles, of the blood vessels in different tissues; it is worth noting that the abnormal lipoproteins in the LDL and VLDL fractions of the plasma in familial LCAT deficiency are not usually present in Tangier disease. There is some evidence to suggest that these particles, particularly the large particles in the d 1.019–1.063 fraction of the plasma, are responsible for the accumulation of membranous lipid in the glomerular tufts, the focal necrosis of the endothelium of the glomerular capillaries and the tendency to premature atherosclerosis (Gjone et al., 1974).

The formation of target cells in the blood of most patients is presumed to be due to expansion of the red-cell surface area by accumulation of excess of cholesterol in the membrane. The abnormal lipid composition of the red cells is probably acquired when the cells are discharged into the circulation and come into contact with abnormal cholesterol-rich lipoproteins in the plasma, since the lipid composition of the red cells of patients with familial LCAT deficiency reverts towards the normal pattern during incubation in normal plasma (Gjone et al., 1978). The shortened life-span of the red cells may be due to increased mechanical fragility caused by the very high ratio of cholesterol to phospholipid in their membranes, but this has yet to be established experimentally. Osmotic fragility of the red cells, at least in some patients, is decreased (Godin et al., 1978).

REFERENCES

Assmann, G. (1978). The metabolic role of high density lipoproteins: perspectives from Tangier disease. In: *High Density Lipoproteins and Atherosclerosis*. Ed. A. M. Gotto, N. E. Miller and M. F. Oliver. Proc. Third Argenteuil Symposium, Elsevier, Amsterdam, pp. 77–89.

Assmann, G., Capurso, A., Smootz, E. and Wellner, U. (1978). Apoprotein A metabolism in Tangier disease. *Atherosclerosis*, **30**, 321–332.

Assmann, G., Fredrickson, D., Herbert, P. N., Forte, T. and Heinen, R. H. (1974). An A-II lipoprotein particle in Tangier disease. *Circulation*, **50**, III–259.

Bassen, F. A. and Kornzweig, A. L. (1950). Malformation of the erythrocytes in a case of atypical retinitis pigmentosa. *Blood*, **5**, 381.

Biemer, J. J. and McCammon, R. E. (1975). The genetic relationship of abetalipoproteinemia and hypobetalipoproteinemia: a report of the occurrence of both diseases within the same family. *Journal of Laboratory and Clinical Medicine*, **85**, 556–565.

Bilheimer, D. W. and Grundy, S. M., personal communication.

Bjerrum, O. J. and Lundahl, P. (1974). Crossed immunoelectrophoresis of human erythrocyte membrane proteins. Immunoprecipitin patterns for fresh and stored samples of membranes extensively solubilized with non-ionic detergents. *Biochimica et Biophysica Acta*, **342**, 69–80.

Blanchette-Mackie, E. J. and Scow, R. O. (1973). Effects of lipoprotein lipase on the structure of chylomicrons. *Journal of Cell Biology*, **58**, 689–708.

Burstein, M. and Fine, J. M. (1959). Sur le taux des β-lipoprotéines dans les myélomes et la macroglobulinémie de Waldenström. *Revue Hématologie*, **14**, 380–383.
Carlson, L. A. and Philipson, B. (1979). Fish-eye disease. A new familial condition with massive corneal opacities and dyslipoproteinaemia. *Lancet*, **2**, 921–923.
Cooper, R. A., Durocher, J. R. and Leslie, M. H. (1977). Decreased fluidity of red cell membrane lipids in abetalipoproteinemia. *Journal of Clinical Investigation*, **60**, 115–121.
Cooper, R. A. and Gulbrandsen, C. L. (1971). The relationship between serum lipoproteins and red cell membranes in abetalipoproteinemia: Deficiency of lecithin:cholesterol acyltransferase. *Journal of Laboratory and Clinical Medicine*, **78**, 323–335.
Cottrill, C., Glueck, C. J., Leuba, V., Nillett, F., Puppione, D. and Brown, W. V. (1974). Familial homozygous hypobetalipoproteinemia. *Metabolism*, **23**, 779–791.
Critchley, E. M. R., Clark, D. and Wikler, A. (196-8). Acanthocytosis and neurological disorder without abetalipoproteinemia. *Archives of Neurology*, **18**, 134–140.
Deckelbaum, R. J., Eisenberg, S., Fainaru, M., Barenholz, Y. and Olivecrona, T. (1979). *In vitro* production of human plasma low density lipoprotein-like particles. A model for very low density lipoprotein catabolism. *Journal of Biological Chemistry*, **254**, 6079–6087.
Dobbins, W. O. (1966). An ultrastructural study of the intestinal mucosa in congenital betalipoprotein deficiency with particular emphasis upon the intestinal absorptive cell. *Gastroenterology*, **50**, 195–210.
Emerson, G. A., Walker, J. B. and Ganapathy, S. N. (1960). Vitamin B_6 and lipid metabolism in monkeys. *American Journal of Clinical Nutrition*, **8**, 424–433.
Estes, J. W., Morley, T. J., Levine, I. M. and Emerson, C. P. (1967). A new hereditary acanthocytosis syndrome. *American Journal of Medicine*, **42**, 868–881.
Farquhar, J. W. and Ways, P. Abetalipoproteinemia. In: *The Metabolic Basis of Inherited Disease*. Ed. J. B. Stanbury, J. B. Wyngaarden and D. S. Fredrickson. McGraw-Hill, New York, 2nd edition, pp. 509–522, 1966.
Ferrans, V. J. and Fredrickson, D. S. (1975). The pathology of Tangier disease: A light and electron microscopic study. *American Journal of Pathology*, **78**, 101.
Forte, T. and Nichols, A. V. (1972). Application of microscopy to the study of plasma lipoprotein structure. *Advances in Lipid Research*, **10**, 1–41.
Forte, T., Nichols, A., Glomset, J. and Norum, K. (1974). The ultrastructure of plasma lipoproteins in lecithin:cholesterol acyltransferase deficiency. *Scandinavian Journal of Clinical and Laboratory Investigation*, **33**, Supplement 137, 121–132.
Fredrickson, D. S., Altrocchi, P. H., Avioli, L. V., Goodman, D. S. and Goodman, H. C. (1961). Tangier disease. *Annals of Internal Medicine*, **55**, 1016–1031.
Fredrickson, D. S., Gotto, A. M. and Levy, R. I. Familial lipoprotein deficiency. In: *The Metabolic Basis of Inherited Disease*. Ed. J. B. Stanbury, J. B. Wyngaarden and D. S. Fredrickson. McGraw-Hill, New York, 3rd edition, pp. 493–530, 1972.
Gjone, E. (1974). Familial lecithin:cholesterol acyltransferase deficiency—a clinical survey. *Scandinavian Journal of Clinical and Laboratory Investigation*, **33**, Supplement 137, 73–82.
Gjone, E. (1978). Recent research on lecithin:cholesterol acyltransferase II. *Scandinavian Journal of Clinical and Laboratory Investigation*, **38**, Supplement 150, 1–232.
Gjone, E. and Norum, K. R. (1974). Recent research on lecithin:cholesterol acyltransferase. *Scandinavian Journal of Clinical and Laboratory Investigation*, **33**, Supplement 137, 7–171.
Gjone, E., Norum, K. R. and Glomset, J. A. Familial lecithin:cholesterol acyltransferase deficiency. In: *The Metabolic Basis of Inherited Disease*. Ed. J. B.

Stanbury, J. B. Wyngaarden and D. S. Fredrickson, McGraw-Hill, New York, 4th edition, pp. 589–603, 1978.

Gjone, E., Skarbövik, A. J., Blomhoff, J. P. and Teisberg, P. (1974). Familial lecithin:cholesterol acyltransferase deficiency. Report of a third Norwegian family with two afflicted members. *Scandinavian Journal of Clinical and Laboratory Investigation*, **33**, Supplement 137, 101–105.

Glickman, R. M., Green, P. H. R., Lees, R. S. and Tall, A. (1978). Apoprotein A-I synthesis in normal intestinal mucosa and in Tangier disease. *New England Journal of Medicine*, **299**, 1424–1427.

Glomset, J. A., Norum, K. R., Nichols, A. V., King, W. C., Mitchell, C. D., Applegate, K. K., Gong, E. L. and Gjone, E. (1975). Plasma lipoproteins in familial lecithin:cholesterol acyltransferase deficiency: effects of dietary manipulation. *Scandinavian Journal of Clinical and Laboratory Investigation*, **35**, Supplement 142, 3–30.

Glomset, J. A. and Wright, J. L. (1964). Some properties of a cholesterol esterifying enzyme in human plasma. *Biochimica et Biophysica Acta*, **89**, 266–276.

Glueck, C. J., Gartside, P., Fallat, R. W., Sielski, J. and Steiner, P. M. (1976). Longevity syndromes: Familial hypobeta and familial hyperalpha lipoproteinemia. *Journal of Laboratory and Clinical Medicine*, **88**, 941–957.

Godin, D. V., Gray, G. R. and Frohlich, J. (1978). Erythrocyte membrane alterations in lecithin:cholesterol acyltransferase deficiency. *Scandinavian Journal of Clinical and Laboratory Investigation*, **38**, Supplement 150, 162–167.

Goldstein, J. L., Ho, Y. K., Basu, S. K. and Brown, M. S. (1979). Binding site on macrophages that mediates uptake and degradation of acetylated low density lipoprotein, producing massive cholesterol deposition. *Proceedings of the National Academy of Sciences of the USA*, **76**, 333–337.

Gotto, A. M., Levy, R. I., John, K. and Fredrickson, D. S. (1971). On the protein defect in abetalipoproteinemia. *New England Journal of Medicine*, **284**, 813–818.

Hamilton, R. L. (1972). Synthesis and secretion of plasma lipoproteins. *Advances in Experimental Medicine and Biology*, **26**, 7–24.

Herbert, P. N. and Fredrickson, D. S. The hypobetalipoproteinemias. In: *Fettstoffwechsel*. Ed. G. Schettler, H. Greten, G. Schlierf and D. Seidel. Springer-Verlag, Berlin, pp. 485–521, 1976.

Herbert, P. N., Gotto, A. M. and Fredrickson, D. S. Familial lipoprotein deficiency. In: *The Metabolic Basis of Inherited Disease*. Ed. J. B. Stanbury, J. B. Wyngaarden and D. S. Fredrickson. McGraw-Hill, New York, 4th edition, pp. 544–588, 1978.

Ho, Y. K., Faust, J. R., Bilheimer, D. W., Brown, M. S. and Goldstein, J. L. (1977). Regulation of cholesterol synthesis by low density lipoprotein in isolated human lymphocytes. Comparison of cells from normal subjects and patients with homozygous familial hypercholesterolemia and abetalipoproteinemia. *Journal of Experimental Medicine*, **145**, 1531–1549.

Hovig, T. and Gjone, E. (1974). Familial lecithin:cholesterol acyltransferase deficiency. Ultrastructural studies on lipid deposition and tissue reactions. *Scandinavian Journal of Clinical and Laboratory Investigation*, **33**, Supplement 137, 135–146.

Illingworth, D. R., Connor, W. E., Lin, D. S. and Diliberti, J. (1980). Lipid metabolism in abetalipoproteinemia: a study of cholesterol absorption and sterol balance in two patients. *Gastroenterology*, **18**, 68–75.

Isselbacher, K. J., Scheig, R., Plotkin, G. R. and Caulfield, J. B. (1964). Congenital β-lipoprotein deficiency: an hereditary disorder involving a defect in the absorption and transport of lipids. *Medicine*, **43**, 347–361.

Jones, J. W. and Ways, P. (1967). Abnormalities of high density lipoproteins in abetalipoproteinemia. *Journal of Clinical Investigation*, **46**, 1151–1161.

Kahn, J. A. and Glueck, C. J. (1978). Familial hypobetalipoproteinemia. Absence of atherosclerosis in a post-mortem study. *Journal of the American Medical Association*, **240**, 47–48.

Kayden, H. J. Abetalipoproteinemia—abnormalities of serum lipoproteins. In: *Protides of the Biological Fluids (Proceedings of the 25th Colloquium, Bruges, 1977)* Pergamon Press, Oxford, p. 271, 1978.

Kayden, H. J. and Bessis, M. (1970). Morphology of normal erythrocyte and acanthocyte using Normarski optics and the scanning electron microscope. *Blood (Journal of Hematology)*, **35**, 427–436.

Khachadurian, A. K., Sha'fi, R. T. and Murad, S. (1973). Studies on the sedimentation rate and membrane permeability of acanthocytes in abetalipoproteinemia. *The Lebanese Medical Journal*, **26**, 425–434.

Kocen, R. S., King, R. H. M., Thomas, P. K. and Haas, L. F. (1973). Nerve biopsy findings in two cases of Tangier disease. *Acta Neuropathologia*, **26**, 317.

Kocen, R. S., Lloyd, J. K., Lascelles, P. T., Fosbrooke, A. S. and Williams, D. (1967). Familial α-lipoprotein deficiency (Tangier disease) with neurological abnormalities. *Lancet*, **i**, 1341–1345.

Kostner, G., Holasek, A., Bohlmann, H. G. and Thiede, H. (1974). Investigation of serum lipoproteins and apoproteins in abetalipoproteinaemia. *Clinical Science and Molecular Medicine*, **46**, 457–468.

Lamy, M., Frézal, J., Polonovski, J. and Rey, J. (1960). L'absence congénitale de β-lipoprotéines. *C.R. Societé Biologie (Paris)*, **154**, 1974–1978.

Lamy, M., Frézal, J., Polonovski, J. and Rey, J. (1961). L'absence congénitale de bêta-lipoprotéines. *La Presse Medicale*, **69**, 1511–1514.

Langdon, R. G. (1974). Serum lipoprotein apoproteins as major protein constituents of the human erythrocyte membrane. *Biochimica et Biophysica Acta*, **342**, 213–228.

Levy, R. I., Langer, T., Gotto, A. M. and Fredrickson, D. S. (1970). Familial hypobetalipoproteinemia, a defect in lipoprotein synthesis. *Clinical Research*, **18**, 539.

Lewis, L. A. and Page, I. H. (1954). Serum proteins and lipoproteins in multiple myelomatosis. *American Journal of Medicine*, **17**, 670–673.

McBride, J. A. and Jacob, H. S. (1970). Abnormal kinetics of red cell membrane cholesterol in acanthocytes: studies in genetic and experimental abetalipoproteinaemia and in spur cell anaemia. *British Journal of Haematology*, **18**, 383–397.

Mitchell, C. D., King, W. C., Applegate, K. R., Forte, T., Glomset, J. A., Norum, K. R. and Gjone, E. (1980). Characterization of apolipoprotein E-rich high density lipoproteins in familial lecithin:cholesterol acyltransferase deficiency. *Journal of Lipid Research*, **21**, 625–634.

Muller, D. P. R., Lloyd, J. K. and Bird, A. C. (1977). Long-term management of abetalipoproteinaemia. Possible rôle for vitamin E. *Archives of Disease in Childhood*, **52**, 209–214.

Myant, N. B., Reichl, D. and Lloyd, J. K. (1978). Sterol balance in a patient with abetalipoproteinaemia. *Atherosclerosis*, **29**, 509–512.

Norum, K. R. and Gjone, E. (1967). Familial plasma lecithin:cholesterol acyltransferase deficiency. Biochemical study of a new inborn error of metabolism. *Scandinavian Journal of Clinical and Laboratory Investigation*, **20**, 231–243.

Norum, K. R., Glomset, J. A., Nichols, A. V., Forte, T., Albers, J. J., King, W. C., Mitchell, C. D., Applegate, K. R., Gong, E. L., Cabana, V. and Gjone, E. (1975). Plasma lipoproteins in familial lecithin:cholesterol acyltransferase deficiency: effects of incubation with lecithin:cholesterol acyltransferase *in vitro*. *Scandinavian Journal of Clinical and Laboratory Investigation*, **35**, Supplement 142, 31–55.

Noseda, G., Riesen, W., Schlumpf, E. and Morell, A. (1972). Hypo-β-lipoproteinaemia associated with auto-antibodies against β-lipoproteins. *European Journal of Clinical Investigation*, **2**, 342–347.

Reichl, D., Myant, N. B. and Lloyd, J. K. (1978). Surface binding and catabolism of low-density lipoprotein by circulating lymphocytes from patients with abetalipoproteinaemia, with observations on sterol synthesis in lymphocytes from one patient. *Biochimica et Biophysica Acta*, **530**, 124–131.

Rifkind, B. M. and Gale, M. (1967). Hypolipidaemia in anaemia. Implications for the epidemiology of ischaemic heart-disease. *Lancet*, **2**, 640–642.

Salt, H. B., Wolff, O. H., Lloyd, J. K., Fosbrooke, A. S., Cameron, A. H. and Hubble, D. V. (1960). On having no beta-lipoprotein. A syndrome comprising a-beta-lipoproteinaemia, acanthocytosis, and steatorrhoea. *Lancet*, **ii**, 325–329.

Scanu, A. M., Aggerbeck, L. P., Kruski, A. W., Lim, C. T. and Kayden, H. J. (1974). A study of the abnormal lipoproteins in abetalipoproteinemia. *Journal of Clinical Investigation*, **53**, 440–453.

Schaefer, E. J., Blum, C. B., Levy, R. I., Goebel, R., Brewer, H. B. and Berman, M. (1976). High density lipoprotein metabolism in Tangier disease. *Circulation*, **54**, Supplement II, II-27.

Smith, J. A., Lonergan, E. T. and Sterling, K. (1964). Spur-cell anemia. Hemolytic anemia with red cells resembling acanthocytes in alcoholic cirrhosis. *New England Journal of Medicine*, **271**, 396–398.

Soutar, A. K. and Myant, N. B. Plasma lipoproteins. In: *Chemistry of Macromolecules IIB. Macromolecular Complexes. International Review of Biochemistry*, Vol. 25, pp. 55–119. Ed. R. E. Offord, University Park Press, Baltimore, 1979.

Spitzer, N., Newcomb, T. F. and Noyes, W. D. (1966). Pyridoxine-responsive hypolipidemia and hypocholesterolemia in a patient with pyridoxine-responsive anemia. *New England Journal of Medicine*, **274**, 772–775.

Stokke, K. T., Bjerve, K. S., Blomhoff, J. P., Öystese, B., Flatmark, A., Norum, K. R. and Gjone, E. (1974). Familial lecithin:cholesterol acyltransferase deficiency. Studies on lipid composition and morphology of tissues. *Scandinavian Journal of Clinical and Laboratory Investigation*, **33**, Supplement 137, 93–100.

Stokke, K. T. and Norum, K. R. (1971). Determination of lecithin:cholesterol acyltransferase in human blood plasma. *Scandinavian Journal of Clinical and Laboratory Investigation*, **27**, 21–27.

Switzer, S. and Eder, H. A. (1962). Interconversion of acanthocytes and normal erythrocytes with detergents. *Journal of Clinical Investigation*, **41**, 1404.

Utermann, G., Dieker, P. and Menzel, H. J. Lecithin-cholesterol acyltransferase deficiency: autosomal recessive transmission in a large kindred. *Proceedings of the 2nd International LCAT Symposium*, Royal Free Hospital, London, p. 47, 1978.

Utermann, G., Menzel, H. J. and Schoenborn, W. (1975). Plasma lipoprotein abnormalities in a case of primary high-density-lipoprotein (HDL) deficiency. *Clinical Genetics*, **8**, 258–268.

Van Buchem, F. S. P., Pol, G., DeGier, J., Böttcher, C. J. F. and Pries, C. (1966). Congenital β-lipoprotein deficiency. *American Journal of Medicine*, **40**, 794.

Chapter 17

Sterol Storage Diseases

1	GENERAL CONSIDERATIONS	819
2	LYSOSOMES AND LIPID STORAGE	820
3	WOLMAN'S DISEASE	823
3.1	Characteristic features	823
3.2	Genetics	823
3.3	Pathology	823
3.4	Enzymology	828
3.5	Diagnosis	828
3.6	Pathogenesis	829
4	CHOLESTERYL ESTER STORAGE DISEASE	831
4.1	Distinction from Wolman's disease: nomenclature	831
4.2	Genetics	831
4.3	Clinical and biochemical features	832
4.4	Pathology	832
4.5	Enzymology	833
4.6	Pathogenesis	833
5	β-SITOSTEROLAEMIA AND XANTHOMATOSIS	835
5.1	Historical background	835
5.2	Clinical and biochemical features	835
5.2.1	Clinical	835
5.2.2	Plasma and tissue lipids	836
5.3	Genetics	836
5.4	Pathogenesis	836
6	CEREBROTENDINOUS XANTHOMATOSIS	837
6.1	Definition and historical background	837
6.2	Clinical and biochemical features	838
6.2.1	Clinical course	838
6.2.2	Plasma lipids	838
6.2.3	Bile	838
6.3	Genetics	839

818 The Biology of Cholesterol and Related Steroids

6.4	Pathology	839
6.4.1	Morphological changes	839
6.4.2	Tissue lipids	840
6.5	Pathogenesis	840
6.5.1	Bile acid metabolism	840
6.5.2	Increased sterol synthesis	843
7	EOSINOPHILIC XANTHOMATOUS GRANULOMA; SCHÜLLER-CHRISTIAN SYNDROME	844
7.1	Historical background and nomenclature	844
7.2	Pathology	845
7.2.1	Histology of the lesions	845
7.2.2	Gross appearance and distribution	846
7.3	Clinical features	846
7.3.1	Schüller-Christian syndrome	846
7.3.2	Xanthoma disseminata	847
7.4	Pathogenesis	848

Sterol Storage Diseases

1 GENERAL CONSIDERATIONS

Intracellular accumulation of cholesterol in certain tissues may occur either when there are excessive amounts of cholesterol-rich lipids or lipoproteins in the plasma, or because of an intrinsic abnormality in the metabolism of lipids in the cells within which cholesterol accumulates.

Examples of the first type of condition are the cholesterol deposits in the histiocytes of xanthomatous lesions in familial hypercholesterolaemia, and the lipid inclusions in foam cells in the tissues of patients with Tangier disease or familial LCAT deficiency. These and other conditions in which deposition of cholesterol is secondary to a disorder of plasma lipoprotein metabolism are not usually classified as storage diseases. They have been dealt with in the two chapters on diseases affecting the plasma lipoproteins (Chapters 15 and 16).

The clearest examples of the second type of condition, in which the primary cause of cholesterol storage lies within the affected cells themselves, are inherited diseases due to deficiency of a specific lysosomal enzyme catalyzing the breakdown of a complex lipid. In several of these hereditary lipidoses, cholesterol accumulates within lipid-laden cells by physical association with the primary stored lipid. In Niemann-Pick disease, for example, the distinctive storage lipid is sphingomyelin, which accumulates within the lysosomes of certain types of cell because of a specific deficiency of lysosomal sphingomyelinase. Nevertheless, cholesterol is a major component of the lipid inclusions and in molar terms may even exceed the amount of sphingomyelin. Comparable accumulations of cholesterol in lipid-filled cells may also occur in other lipidoses in which the primary storage lipid is a sulphatide (metachromatic leucodystrophy) or a ganglioside (Tay-Sachs disease and G_{M1} gangliosidosis). The presence of cholesterol in the lipid inclusions in these diseases may be due partly to the ability of some lipids to dissolve esterified cholesterol and partly to the formation of liquid-crystalline mixtures of free cholesterol and a phospholipid. This is not the place for a detailed account of lipid storage diseases in general (the hereditary lipidoses are dealt with in Hers and Van Hoof (1973) and in Stanbury *et al.* (1978)). However, in Wolman's disease and in cholesteryl ester storage disease the accumulation of cholesteryl ester in the lysosomes seems to be due to deficiency of an esterase responsible for the hydrolysis of esterified cholesterol in normal lysosomes. Both diseases are considered in this chapter. Two other storage diseases, cerebrotendinous xanthomatosis and β-sitosterolaemia, are also considered here, although the pathogenesis of the intracellular accumulation of sterol that occurs in these disorders is not understood. Finally, the Schüller-Christian syndrome is mentioned because of the predominance of cholesterol in the stored lipid.

Before these topics are considered, it may be helpful to deal briefly with some of the more important aspects of lysosomal function in relation to lipid storage.

2 LYSOSOMES AND LIPID STORAGE

The most important function of lysosomes is to digest materials present in endocytotic vacuoles and in portions of the cytoplasm that have become enclosed by membranes to form vacuoles known as autophagosomes. Primary lysosomes fuse with both types of vacuole to form secondary lysosomes, thus enabling the acid hydrolases within lysosomes to digest the large molecules and particulate matter present in the vacuoles. The bilayer membrane surrounding a secondary lysosome is impermeable to the substrates for these enzymes, but the final products of digestion, including free cholesterol released by hydrolysis of cholesteryl esters, diffuse into the cytoplasm and are ultimately removed from the cell. These events are illustrated in Fig. 17.1. The transport of materials from the extracellular medium into the interior of the cell by endocytosis, and the subsequent digestion of the contents of endocytotic vacuoles by lysosomal enzymes, is known as *heterophagy*. The process whereby organelles and other components of the cytoplasm are segregated within membrane-bound vacuoles and are then digested is known as *autophagy*. Heterophagy is a prominent feature of certain types of cell (e.g. macrophages) but in some cells, such as skeletal muscle cells, it occurs only at a very slow rate or not at all. Autophagy probably occurs in all cells and is thought to be responsible for the turnover of many cell constituents.

Under normal conditions, digestion of the contents of secondary lysosomes is complete. If there is a marked increase in the intake of extracellular material by heterophagy there is usually no accumulation of substrate within secondary lysosomes, though the products of digestion may accumulate in extra-lysosomal inclusions. In familial hypercholesterolaemia and Tangier disease, for example, the increased entry of cholesteryl esters into cells in which heterophagy is active does not lead to engorgement of lysosomes, but to the accumulation of cholesteryl ester in extra-lysosomal lipid droplets, the extra-lysosomal cholesteryl ester being formed by esterification of free cholesterol that has diffused out of the lysosomes. There may be some accumulation of lipid within lysosomes, as shown by the occasional finding of membrane-bound lipid inclusions in the foam cells present in the tissues of these patients, but this seems to be the exception

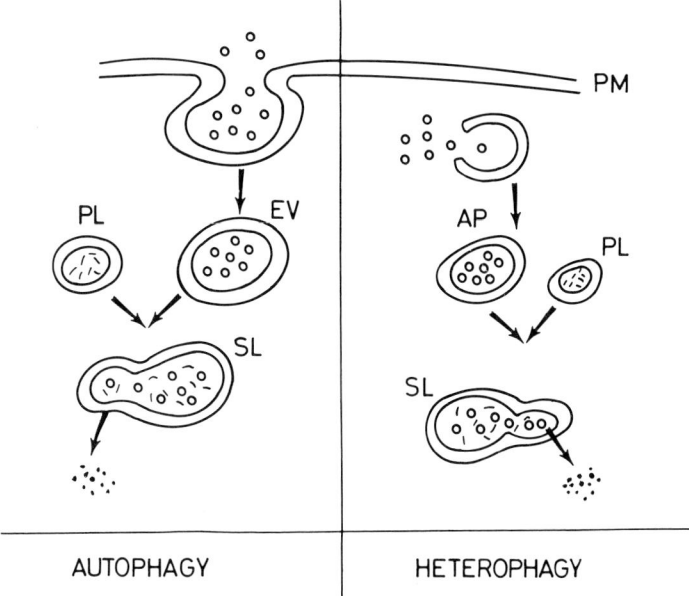

Figure 17.1
Heterophagy and autophagy.
 The left half shows the engulfing of a droplet of extracellular fluid by invagination of a portion of plasma membrane (PM), with the formation of an endocytotic vacuole (EV); the EV fuses with a primary lysosome (PL) to form a secondary lysosome (SL) (or digestive vacuole) in which the contents of the endocytotic vacuole and the primary lysosome are mixed. Digestion of the large molecules engulfed by endocytosis is followed by release of the products of digestion into the cytoplasm. The right half shows the formation of an autophagosome (AP) by enclosure of a portion of the cytoplasm within a membrane not derived from the plasma membrane. Fusion with a primary lysosome to form a secondary lysosome, followed by digestion of the contents, then proceeds as in heterophagy.
 Enzyme molecules, —; large substrate molecules or particles, O.

rather than the rule. Thus, the intracellular accumulation of cholesterol in these diseases is determined largely by overloading of the mechanisms by which the cholesterol of extra-lysosomal cholesteryl ester is removed from the cell, rather than by saturation of the digestive capacity of lysosomes.

The tissue distribution of cholesterol deposition in conditions in which lysosomal function is normal is probably determined by a combination of relative permeability of the regional blood capillaries to the lipids or lipoproteins in which the esterified cholesterol is carried, and the intensity of heterophagy in the cells in which cholesterol accumulates. It is possible that under some conditions the incoming load of substrate is sufficient to saturate a lysosomal enzyme, so that accumulation occurs mainly within lysosomes. This seems to happen, for example, in cholesterol-fed rabbits. When rabbits are given a cholesterol-rich diet, the lysosomes in aortic smooth-muscle cells become engorged with cholesteryl esters derived from the hyperlipidaemic plasma (Peters and de Duve, 1974). This, however, is a very abnormal situation and may have little or no relevance to what happens during the natural development of atherosclerotic lesions in man.

In the inherited lysosomal diseases the situation is very different. Here the abnormality is a partial or complete deficiency of a specific hydrolytic enzyme due to a mutation at a single gene locus. Several of the consequences of a mutation in a gene coding for a lysosomal enzyme were predicted by Hers (1965) and are worth considering in this section, particularly in relation to cholesterol storage.

Since the lysosomal membrane is generally impermeable to all but the final products of digestion by acid hydrolases, the substance whose further metabolism is blocked, owing to lack of the necessary enzyme, remains within lysosomes. Hence, the stored material is largely intra-lysosomal, the lysosomes becoming greatly enlarged. Indeed, the hallmark of an inherited lysosomal disease is the presence of abnormal cytoplasmic inclusions surrounded by bilayer membranes. If engorged lysosomes are disrupted *in vivo*, some of the stored material may be extra-lysosomal, but this seems to be relatively uncommon.

Although only one enzyme is genetically deficient, more than one substance may accumulate in the lysosomes. This may be because the missing enzyme is normally responsible for the hydrolysis of two or more substrates, as in Wolman's disease, in which absence of an ester hydrolase leads to accumulation of triglyceride as well as cholesteryl ester. Heterogeneity of stored material may also be due to physical association between the primary storage substance and other substances, as in the accumulation of cholesterol in the lipid inclusions in Niemann-Pick disease, or it may be due to inhibition of other enzymes by the primary storage substance.

As far as we know, lysosomes in all cells contain the same complement of acid hydrolases and in all inherited lysosomal diseases the enzyme in question is deficient in every cell in the body. Hence, the tissue distribution of stored material in a given disease must depend largely upon the nature of the deficient enzyme. If the stored material or its precursor is present in plasma and interstitial fluid it will reach the lysosomes of cells in which heterophagy occurs. In Gaucher's disease, for example, the cerebroside stored in histiocytes of the reticuloendothelial system originates in the plasma membranes of defunct blood cells ingested by endocytosis. If the stored material is not present in the extracellular medium it must reach lysosomes by autophagy. In this case, a cell will only accumulate a substance in its lysosomes if that substance (or its precursor) is normally synthesized within the cell. In some lysosomal storage diseases such as Wolman's disease, and, to a lesser degree, Niemann-Pick disease, the stored material is present in a wide variety of cell types. It is conceivable that in these cases the stored material reaches the lysosomes by both autophagy and heterophagy.

3 WOLMAN'S DISEASE

3.1 Characteristic features

Wolman's disease (Abramov *et al.*, 1956; Wolman *et al.*, 1961) is a rare inherited disorder of cholesterol metabolism characterized clinically by marked enlargement of the liver and spleen, calcification of the adrenals and severe gastro-intestinal symptoms leading to death from cachexia, usually within the first six months of life. The underlying lesion is the widespread intracellular accumulation of cholesteryl ester and triglyceride.

3.2 Genetics

Wolman's disease is inherited as an autosomal recessive trait. In three of the 15 families listed by Patrick and Lake (1973) the parents were first cousins. Heterozygotes are clinically normal but have reduced cholesteryl-ester hydrolase activity in their leucocytes. About a third of the patients reported were from Israel, but others have been identified in Europe and North America and two have been reported from Japan.

3.3 Pathology

An abnormal accumulation of lipid is present in virtually every organ in the body and is most marked in the liver, spleen, bone marrow and lymphoid tissue. Chemical and histochemical analysis shows that the major lipids present in excess are esterified cholesterol and triglyceride. In liver and spleen the cholesteryl-ester content of fresh tissue is increased up to 100-fold and the triglyceride content may be 20 times normal. There is a small but consistent increase in the content of free cholesterol; the total phospholipid content of the tissues is normal. Representative values for the lipid content of liver and spleen in patients with Wolman's disease are shown in Table 17.1. In all the patients from whom this Table was compiled, the triglyceride content of the liver and spleen was markedly increased. However, Lough *et al.* (1970) have described one patient in whom the spleen and adrenals contained normal amounts of triglyceride, with greatly increased amounts of cholesteryl ester.

Light microscopy shows the presence of numerous histiocytic foam cells filled with Sudanophilic cytoplasmic vacuoles in most organs. The distribution of these lipid-filled histiocytes is extremely widespread. They are very numerous in the spleen, liver, bone marrow and lymphoid tissue but are also present in the small intestine, adrenals, ovary, testis, thyroid, renal glomeruli and pulmonary alveoli, and in the leptomeninges and the connective tissue of the choroid plexus. In addition to the presence of histiocytic foam cells throughout the body, lipid droplets are present in the Kupffer cells and in the parenchymal cells of the liver (Fig. 17.2) and adrenal cortex, in the mucosal cells of the small intestine, the ganglion cells of Auerbach's plexus, Meissner's plexus and the thoracic sympathetic chain and in cardiac muscle cells and the smooth-muscle cells of the intestine. Lipid vacuoles are also present in the endothelial cells of the arterial wall, in the circulating lymphocytes and in some polymorphonuclear leucocytes. The staining properties of the lipid inclusions are consistent with the presence of cholesteryl esters and triglyceride, and many of the foam cells contain crystals of cholesteryl ester.

Electron microscopy shows that the cytoplasmic lipid vacuoles are surrounded by single bilayer membranes (Fig. 17.2) and that acid-phosphatase activity is intense at the outer margins of the vacuoles (Fig. 17.3).

The lesions in the adrenals are almost pathognomonic of Wolman's disease and are of sufficient interest to warrant further mention in this section. (Detailed descriptions of the pathology of other organs will be found in the two case reports of Wolman *et al.* (1961) and in the reviews of Patrick and Lake (1973) and Frederickson and Ferrans (1978)).

The adrenal glands are greatly enlarged, sometimes to three times the normal weight, and in cut sections multiple focal areas of calcification are seen in the inner regions of the cortex. The presence of calcified areas in the adrenals is usually detectable by radio-

Table 17.1
Lipid content of the liver and spleen in Wolman's disease (all values expressed in g/100 g fresh weight)

		Esterified cholesterol	Free cholesterol	Triglyceride	Phospholipid
Liver	Wolman's disease	0.68–5.90	0.56–3.80	12.0–20.8	1.0–2.8
	Controls	0.08–0.15	0.35	0.26–1.30	1.4–2.5
Spleen	Wolman's disease	0.39–1.56	0.45–1.01	0.5–2.9	1.0–3.0
	Controls	0.03–0.08	0.21–0.35	0.03–0.08	1.0–2.0

Adapted from Patrick and Lake (1973).

826 The Biology of Cholesterol and Related Steroids

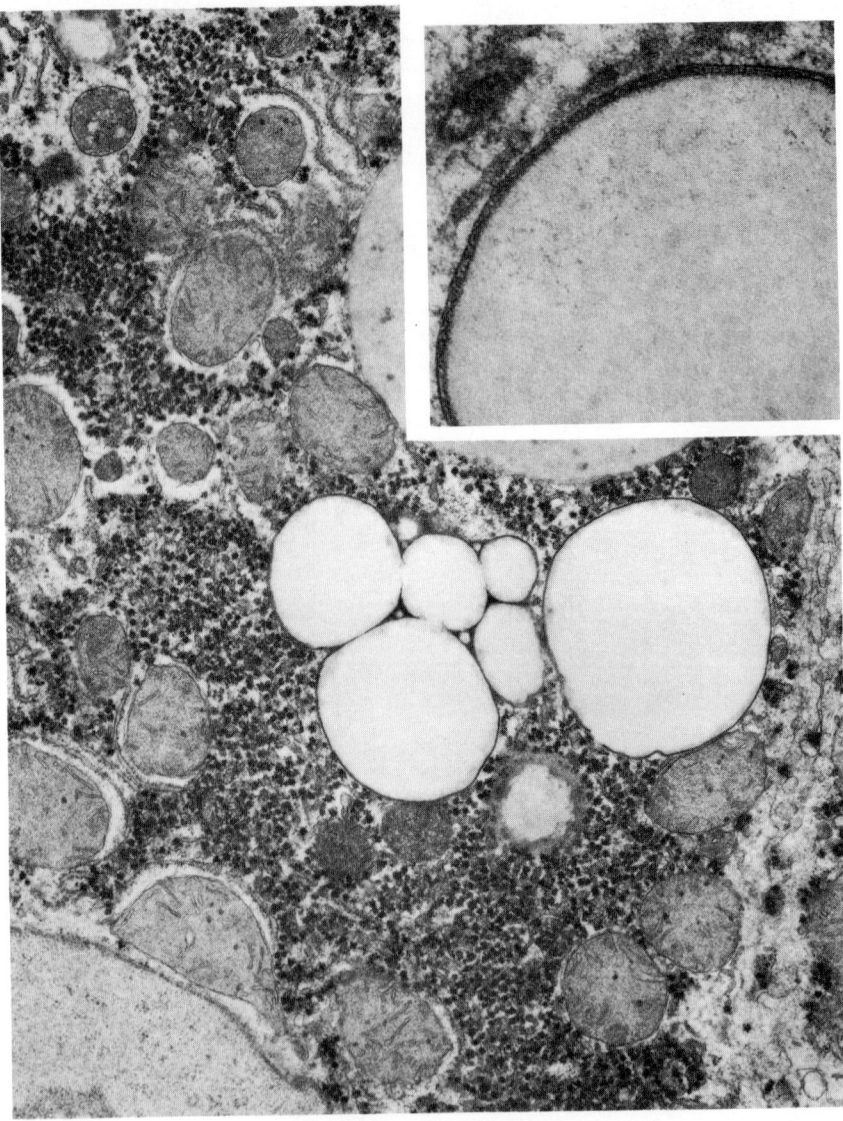

Figure 17.2
Electronphotomicrograph of part of a liver cell from a patient with Wolman's disease, showing a collection of lipid droplets with well-defined membranes and (inset) part of a lipid droplet enclosed by a bilayer membrane. Main picture, ×17 000: inset, ×80 000. (From Patrick and Lake (1973), with the permission of the authors and of Academic Press.)

graphic examination within the first weeks of life and has been detected at autopsy in a fetus estimated to be 14 weeks old (Lake, 1977). Histological sections show more or less normal architecture of the zona glomerulosa and zona fasciculata, but many of the parenchymal cells are enlarged and contain lipid-filled vacuoles. In the region corresponding to the fetal cortex and the zona reticularis the cells have lost their normal arrangement and many are enlarged and have a vacuolated cytoplasm or are necrotic. This region of the cortex contains histiocytic foam cells, many of which contain crystals of cholesteryl ester, and large foci of amorphous extracellular material staining positively for calcium. The cholesterol content of the adrenals is greatly increased; in one of two patients reported by Wolman *et al.* (1961) cholesterol, mainly esterified, accounted for 18% of the wet

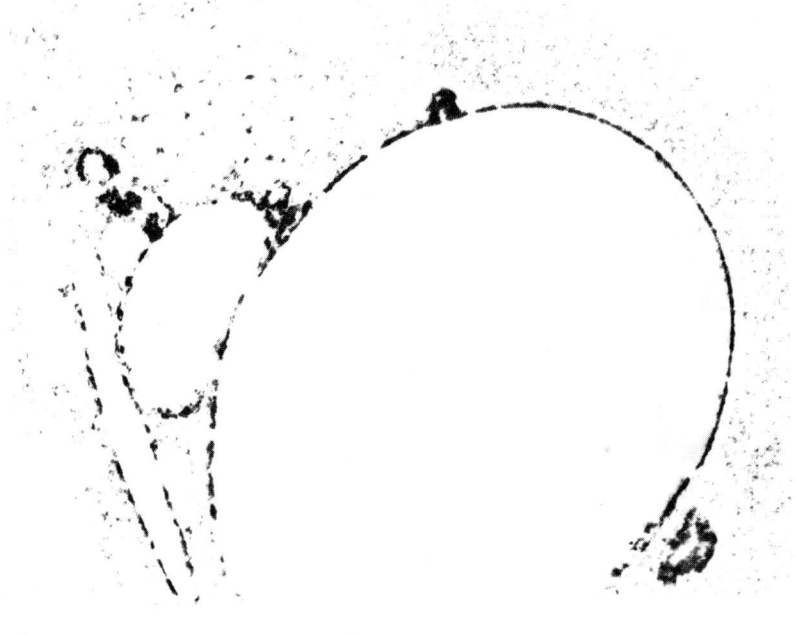

Figure 17.3
Electronphotomicrograph of a lipid droplet in a liver cell from a patient with Wolman's disease, showing the presence of acid phosphatase activity at the outer aspect of the droplet (shown by black deposits). × 26 500. Before electronmicroscopy, sections of the tissue were exposed to a buffer containing α-glycerophosphate and lead acetate. The black dots in the picture are due to the presence of a lead phosphate complex formed from lead acetate and the phosphate released locally by the action of acid phosphatase on the substrate. (From Patrick and Lake (1973), with the permission of the authors and of Academic Press.)

weight of the adrenals, compared with 1% in the adrenals of normal infants.

The plasma lipid and lipoprotein patterns are usually normal, but increased concentrations of VLDL and decreased concentrations of HDL have been reported in a few patients. In an atypical patient reported by Eto and Kitagawa (1970) the plasma LDL concentration was very low and acanthocytes were present in the circulation.

3.4 Enzymology

Normal human tissues hydrolyse emulsions of triglyceride and cholesteryl ester at pH 4.4 and this hydrolase activity is resistant to inhibition by E600, a compound that inhibits microsomal ester hydrolase activity at neutral pH. Since human lysosomes contain cholesteryl ester hydrolase with optimal activity at acid pH (Kothari et al., 1970), the acid hydrolase activity in whole homogenates of human tissue is assumed to be lysosomal. Patrick and Lake (see Patrick and Lake, 1973) have shown that E600-resistant acid hydrolase activity, with triglyceride or cholesteryl ester as substrate, is not detectable in liver, spleen or leucocytes from patients with Wolman's disease, but that the tissues of these patients have normal E600-sensitive hydrolase activity at neutral pH. Deficiency of acid ester hydrolase has also been described in cultured skin fibroblasts from patients with Wolman's disease (Kyriakides et al., 1972). Patrick and Lake conclude from these observations that the intracellular accumulation of cholesteryl ester and triglycerides in Wolman's disease is due to a deficiency of a single lysosomal acid hydrolase responsible for the hydrolysis of both cholesteryl ester and triglycerides in the lysosomes of normal tissues.

3.5 Diagnosis

The earliest symptoms are usually persistent vomiting and diarrhoea beginning within a few weeks of birth. A physical examination shows abdominal distension due to gross enlargement of the liver and spleen. An X-ray of the abdomen shows calcification of the adrenals, numerous Sudanophilic foam cells are seen in bone-marrow aspirates and a blood film shows the presence of vacuolated lymphocytes. The diagnosis is confirmed by demonstrating the absence or near-total deficiency of acid ester hydrolase in circulating leucocytes tested against a fatty acid ester of p-nitrophenol as substrate. Diagnosis of the heterozygous state in the patient's relatives, of obvious importance in genetic counselling, can be made with a high degree of probability by assaying acid ester hydrolase activity in the leucocytes, using values obtained from age-matched controls as the standard. The activity in the leucocytes of heterozygous relatives is usually about half that in the leucocytes of the index patient (Patrick and Lake, 1973).

3.6 Pathogenesis

The demonstration that the lipid inclusions are bounded by membranes associated with an acid hydrolase, coupled with the evidence for a monogenically inherited deficiency of a lysosomal ester hydrolase which uses the stored lipid as substrate, shows beyond reasonable doubt that Wolman's disease is an inborn lysosomal disease, as defined by Hers (1965). The accumulation of esterified cholesterol in the lysosomes of a wide variety of cells is readily explained by deficiency of a cholesteryl-ester hydrolase normally present in the lysosomes of all tissues. The presumption that cholesteryl esters within lysosomes normally undergo hydrolysis is also in keeping with the observation of Brown et al. (1975) that the hydrolysis of LDL cholesteryl esters taken up by normal cultured fibroblasts is inhibited by chloroquine, a general inhibitor of lysosomal enzymes.

The presence of large amounts of triglyceride in the lipid inclusions is usually explained on the assumption that the deficient ester hydrolase catalyzes the hydrolysis of the ester bond in triglyceride as well as in esterified cholesterol. In agreement with this, the tissues in Wolman's disease are deficient in acid hydrolytic activity against dispersions of triglycerides and cholesteryl esters (Patrick and Lake, 1969). However, proof of the existence of a single human lysosomal enzyme capable of using both substrates would require the purification of the proposed enzyme so that its properties, especially its substrate specificity, can be examined. An alternative explanation of the presence of triglyceride in the storage lipid is that triglycerides accumulate in the lipid inclusions merely by physical association with the stored cholesteryl ester. This cannot be excluded, but it does not explain why in some tissues the amount of triglyceride stored may exceed that of cholesteryl ester. Nor does it explain the absence of acid triglyceride hydrolase activity in the tissues in Wolman's disease.

The pathogenesis of Wolman's disease raises the two interrelated questions of the origin of the cholesteryl esters in the storage granules and the distribution of the tissues in which storage occurs. These questions also apply to the similar but less acute disease known as cholesteryl ester storage disease (see next section) and are touched on again in Section 4.6. As discussed in Chapter 9, many cells in the human body are capable of developing receptors which mediate the uptake of LDL, including its cholesteryl esters, by endocytosis, with the subsequent hydrolysis of the apoprotein and cholesteryl esters by lysosomal enzymes. Clearly, the cholesteryl esters of LDL are a potential source of the stored lipid in Wolman's disease. Indeed, it is conceivable that heterophagy of plasma LDL particles is essentially the only route by which esterified cholesterol enters lysosomes. If this were the case, it would raise the intriguing possibility that the tissue distribution of storage lipid in Wolman's disease reflects the distribution of tissues responsible for the uptake and degradation of LDL *in vivo* at normal plasma LDL concentrations. Wolman's disease would then be the perfect natural experiment for observing the sites of LDL degradation in the whole body. It is perhaps significant that the cells in which LDL receptors have been demonstrated (vascular endothelial and smooth-muscle cells, fibroblasts and lymphocytes) are not those in which storage of cholesteryl ester is most conspicuous in Wolman's disease. It is also possible that some of the lipid-filled cells acquire their cholesteryl ester by uptake of a modified form of LDL *via* a pathway not involving LDL receptors (see Chapter 9, Section 2.2.3).

LDL uptake, both receptor-mediated and receptor-independent, may well be the major source of lysosomal cholesteryl ester, but it would be difficult to exclude the existence of other sources. Some cholesteryl ester may reach lysosomes by endocytosis of plasma lipoproteins other than LDL. It is also possible that cholesterol esterified by ACAT within the cell itself is taken into lysosomes by autophagy. With this possibility in mind, Lough *et al.* (1970) have pointed out that cholesteryl ester synthesis is most marked in several of the tissues (liver, adrenal cortex and small intestine) in which lipid storage in Wolman's disease is most prominent. It should be possible to get some idea of the origin of lysosomal cholesteryl esters in Wolman's disease by determining their fatty acid composition. A predominance of linoleate would suggest plasma lipoproteins as the major source, whereas if these esters are synthesized by microsomal ACAT and are then introduced into lysosomes by autophagy, oleate should be the major fatty acid. Unfortunately, the few observations that have been made on the fatty acid composition of the cholesteryl esters in whole tissues in Wolman's disease are contradictory and difficult to interpret. What is needed is a careful analysis of the cholesteryl-ester fatty acids in isolated lysosomes from a variety of tissues from Wolman patients.

It is not clear why the changes in the adrenal cortex should be so marked. In the newborn human infant the most conspicuous region of the adrenal cortex is the inner layer known as the fetal zone. After birth, this layer degenerates rapidly. Konno *et al.* (1966) have suggested that accumulation of lipid in the cells of the fetal zone in some way interferes with normal involution and promotes conditions in which calcification occurs. This rather imprecise proposal is difficult to reconcile with the finding of calcification in the adrenals of a fetus with Wolman's disease (Lake, 1977).

4 CHOLESTERYL ESTER STORAGE DISEASE

4.1 Distinction from Wolman's disease: nomenclature

The name *cholesteryl ester storage disease* (CESD) refers to a rare inherited disorder of lipid metabolism, resembling Wolman's disease in that the underlying lesion in both conditions is the lysosomal storage of cholesteryl ester and triglyceride in many tissues, but differing from the latter disease in several important respects. In particular, the clinical course in CESD is relatively benign, in contrast to the rapid downhill course leading to death in infancy in patients with Wolman's disease. The clinical picture and biochemical and pathological findings in all the patients reported as having Wolman's disease conform so closely to the findings in the 3 affected siblings originally described by Wolman *et al.* (1961) that the assumption that this disease is genetically homogeneous seems justified. In CESD, on the other hand, there is enough variability in the clinical and biochemical features in different families to suggest genetic heterogeneity. In the first reported patient with CESD (Fredrickson, 1963), a 12-year-old girl whose deceased twin was also believed to have been affected, the major physical sign was enlargement of the liver, and massive accumulation of cholesteryl ester was noted in a biopsy of liver. The newly discovered disorder was therefore referred to as *familial hepatic cholesterol ester storage disease*. When the study of other patients with this disease showed that storage of cholesteryl ester occurs in other tissues besides the liver (Partin and Schubert, 1969), the less specific name CESD was adopted and is now in general use. This nomenclature is not entirely satisfactory because a generalized storage of cholesteryl ester, not confined to the liver, is common to Wolman's disease and CESD. However, both names have become established by usage, though CESD could perhaps be regarded as a juvenile or adult form of Wolman's disease, by analogy with the juvenile and infantile forms of Gaucher's disease. Young and Patrick (1970) have proposed that the general term *acid lipase deficiency* should be used and that the term *Wolman's disease* should refer only to the acute infantile form.

4.2 Genetics

In the dozen or so patients reported in the world literature, the majority were female, but the patient of Lageron *et al.* (1967) and one of the two fully-affected members of the family described by Schiff *et al.* (1968) were males. Since CESD is almost certainly genetically heterogeneous, it is not justifiable to group all the reported families for combined genetic analysis. In at least one family, both parents were normal, indicating a recessive mode of inheritance. However, in the family of 7 siblings described by Schiff *et al.* (1968), 4 younger siblings of the index patient had enlargement of the liver with increased serum bile acid concentration, but in three of those from whom liver biopsies were obtained, liver histology was normal by light microscopy. This suggests dominant inheritance with partial expression in the heterozygous state in this family. Measurement of acid cholesteryl-ester hydrolase activity in the leucocytes of first-degree relatives of index patients may permit the detection of heterozygous carriers.

4.3 Clinical and biochemical features

The presenting symptom in CESD is usually enlargement of the liver, which may be noted in early childhood but in some patients was not reported until adult life. The clinical course is very mild compared with that in Wolman's disease. The severe gastrointestinal symptoms that are a major cause of death in infancy in Wolman's disease are not a feature of CESD. An enlarged spleen and cirrhosis of the liver with signs of oesophageal varices have been reported in some patients. Premature atherosclerosis of the coronaries and other arteries has been demonstrated *post mortem* in two patients, but clinical symptoms or signs attributable to coronary atherosclerosis have not been reported. Calcification of the adrenals was noted in only one patient and the peculiar enlargement of the tonsils so characteristic of Tangier disease is not seen in CESD. Most patients with CESD have hypercholesterolaemia due to an increased plasma LDL concentration and several have had a marked reduction in plasma HDL concentration. An increased concentration of serum bile acids was noted in 7 members of the CESD family described by Schiff *et al.* (1968), but this abnormality has not been reported in other affected families.

4.4 Pathology

On naked-eye inspection the liver is seen to be markedly enlarged and to have a butter-yellow colour due to massive infiltration with lipid (Fredrickson *et al.*, 1972). The spleen and adrenals may also be enlarged. Chemical analysis of the lipids of whole liver shows that the major lipid present in excess is cholesteryl ester, which may account for as much as 18% of the fresh weight of the tissue, and that there is a significant increase in triglyceride content. An increase in cholesteryl-ester content has also been reported in spleen, lymph nodes, small intestine and lesion-free aortic wall.

Microscopic examination of the liver shows the presence of numerous Sudanophilic vacuoles in the hepatocytes and Kupffer cells, with crystals of cholesteryl ester in the lipid droplets. Interlobular fibrosis is usually present and the fibrous tissue is infiltrated with histiocytic foam cells containing lipid and an autofluorescent material with the staining properties of ceroid (an ill-defined substance thought to be formed within lysosomes by the slow autoxidation and cross-polymerization of neutral lipids in biological materials). Electron-microscopy shows that the lipid inclusions are surrounded by bilayer membranes. Lipid-filled vacuoles are also present in histiocytes and other cells in the spleen, bone marrow, lymph nodes, adrenals, small intestine, smooth muscle and thymus. Birefringent lipid inclusions, indicative of the presence of esterified cholesterol, have also been observed in cultured skin fibroblasts from a patient with CESD.

Skin xanthomas are not seen in CESD, but extensive atheromatous plaques were observed *post mortem* in the coronaries and other arteries of one patient who died at age 21, and atheroma was present in the ascending aorta of another patient who died at age 9 (Fredrickson and Ferrans, 1978).

4.5 Enzymology

A marked or total deficiency of acid hydrolase activity towards dispersions of cholesteryl ester and triglyceride has been demonstrated in various tissues and in leucocytes and cultured skin fibroblasts from patients with CESD (Burke and Schubert, 1971; Fredrickson *et al.*, 1972). The degree of enzyme deficiency in CESD appears to be no less marked than in Wolman's disease. Thus, in one of the patients from the family described by Schiff *et al.* (1968), acid hydrolase activity was not detectable in the liver (Burke and Schubert, 1971) and in the patient studied by Fredrickson *et al.* (1972) acid hydrolase activity towards cholesteryl oleate and glyceryl trioleate was reported to be 'practically absent'.

4.6 Pathogenesis

The evidence from chemical and enzymic analysis of the tissues and from the histological and electron-microscopic appearance of the lipid-filled cells indicates clearly that the underlying metabolic lesion, as in Wolman's disease, is a specific deficiency of a lysosomal acid hydrolase. Although the mode of inheritance is not as clear as in Wolman's disease, family studies leave little doubt that CESD is monogenically inherited. CESD may therefore be regarded as another inborn lysosomal storage disease. Many of the differences between CESD and Wolman's disease can be explained by the comparatively slow rate of accumulation of lipid in the tissues of patients with CESD. This would explain the generally benign course of the disease, especially the absence of early gastro-intestinal signs and of calcification of the adrenals; the longer life-span of CESD patients would also give time for the development of atherosclerosis and hepatic fibrosis. Inability to hydrolyse cholesteryl esters in the cells of the arterial wall, thus delaying the normal removal of cellular esterified cholesterol as free cholesterol, may contribute to the formation of atherosclerotic lesions in the arteries. Additional factors may be the hypercholesterolaemia and the low plasma HDL concentration in many patients, though it is possible that the low HDL concentration is a consequence of the failure of tissue cells to release free cholesterol for uptake by HDL, as discussed in Chapter 9.

Goldstein *et al.* (1975) have shown that cultured fibroblasts from CESD patients hydrolyse cholesteryl ester carried in LDL at about 30% of the normal rate and that this defect leads to delay in the suppression of HMG-CoA reductase activity on addition of LDL to the culture medium. Cultured CESD fibroblasts, on the other hand, hydrolyse endogenously synthesized cholesteryl ester at the normal rate. The decreased rate of hydrolysis of LDL cholesteryl esters (in which linoleate is the major fatty acid) leads to intracellular accumulation of cholesteryl esters (mainly 18:2) when LDL is added to the medium. These findings suggest that heterophagy of LDL is the major source of lysosomal esterified cholesterol in CESD, at least in fibroblasts, but do not exclude the possibility that autophagy of endogenous cholesteryl ester makes an additional contribution to the storage material in other cells. Analysis of the fatty-acid pattern of the cholesteryl ester of whole tissues in CESD patients has not provided any consistent information as to the origin of the stored cholesteryl ester.

The enzymological studies referred to in Section 4.5 suggest that the deficiency of acid ester hydrolase activity in CESD is as complete as it seems to be in Wolman's disease. Patrick and Lake (1973), for example, found an almost total deficiency of acid hydrolase activity towards *p*-nitrophenyl ester in infants with Wolman's disease and in three patients (presumably with CESD) aged 3, 8 and 10 years. How are we to explain the much slower rate of deposition of cholesteryl ester in CESD than in Wolman's disease if the underlying enzyme defect is virtually complete in both disorders? One possibility is that enzyme activity assayed wtih detergent-solubilized substrates does not reflect accurately the activity of the enzyme towards its natural substrates within lysosomes. It is conceivable, for example, that the cells of CESD patients produce an abnormal acid hydrolase that has some residual activity in its natural environment but none when tested against an artificial substrate, whereas in Wolman's disease there is no functional activity against natural or unnatural substrates. The possibility that the enzyme defect is not the same in the two diseases is supported by the observation of Fredrickson *et al.* (1972) that an artificial substrate (hexadecanyl-1,2-dioleate) was hydrolysed at acid pH much more rapidly by liver from a patient with CESD than by liver from an infant with Wolman's disease. A discrepancy between acid hydrolytic activity in the intact cell compared with that towards artificial substrates is also suggested by the observations of Goldstein *et al.* (1975) on the fibroblasts of a CESD patient. Whereas the ability of cell-free extracts of the cultured fibroblasts to hydrolyse an artificial substrate at acid pH was reduced to less than 5% of the normal, chloroquine-sensitive hydrolysis of LDL cholesteryl esters by the intact fibroblasts was as high as 30% of normal

5 β-SITOSTEROLAEMIA AND XANTHOMATOSIS

5.1 Historical background

In 1974, Bhattacharyya and Connor described what appeared to be a new familial sterol storage disease in two sisters. The presenting symptoms were tuberous and tendon xanthomas, known to have been present since childhood. Laboratory investigation showed normal plasma cholesterol concentrations, but substantial amounts of plant sterols were found in the plasma, red blood cells, adipose tissue, skin surface lipids and xanthomatous lesions. Both patients ate the usual American diet, which supplies up to 250 mg of plant sterol per day. An additional 8 patients from four families have since been reported (Shulman *et al.*, 1976; Khachadurian, 1978; Khachadurian and Clancy, 1978; Miettinen, 1980). In their initial description of this disease Bhattacharyya and Connor referred to it as *β-sitosterolaemia and xanthomatosis*.

5.2 Clinical and biochemical features

5.2.1 Clinical

Tendon xanthomas are usually present on the Achilles and patellar tendons and on the extensor tendons of the hands. The most frequent sites for the tuberous lesions of the skin are the buttocks and elbows. Xanthelasmas were also present in the 31-year-old patient of Shulman *et al.* (1976). The xanthomas appear in childhood, and in one patient a skin xanthoma was known to have been present at the age of $1\frac{1}{2}$ years. Clinical signs of ischaemic heart disease were not reported in any of the patients from the first three families, but Miettinen's patient had premature coronary artery disease, with anginal pain at age 17.

Diagnosis and treatment are considered in the review by Bhattacharyya and Connor (1978).

5.2.2 Plasma and tissue lipids

Plasma total cholesterol concentration was within normal limits in all but one patient, who had a moderate increase in plasma LDL concentration. The plasma concentration of total plant sterols is increased from the usual very low values in normal adults (<1 mg/100 ml) to values ranging from 20 to more than 30 mg/100 ml, so that plant sterols may account for up to 20% of the total sterols in plasma. The major plant sterol in the plasma is β-sitosterol, but small amounts of campesterol and traces of stigmasterol are also present. About 60% of the plasma β-sitosterol is esterified with long-chain fatty acids. The plant sterols as a whole are carried mainly in LDL, but significant amounts are also carried in HDL.

Plant sterols are present in unesterified form in the membranes of red blood cells and the ratio of β-sitosterol to cholesterol is similar in red cells and plasma, suggesting that plasma and red-cell plant sterols are in complete exchange equilibrium.

In the xanthomas, about 20% of the total sterol is plant sterol, of which the major component is β-sitosterol; the remaining 70–80% is accounted for by cholesterol. Both cholesterol and the plant sterols of xanthomas are largely in unesterified form. As in the xanthomas of familial hypercholesterolaemia, much of the sterol in the xanthomas of these patients is intracellular, presumably as lipid droplets in histiocytic cells.

5.3 Genetics

The number of affected families that have been discovered is so small that no definite conclusions can be drawn as to the mode of inheritance. The disease is certainly familial—in one of the families reported by Khachadurian (1978) all five siblings had β-sitosterolaemia—and is presumably genetic. Since it occurs in both sexes and since β-sitosterolaemia has not been found in the parents of any index patient, the most probable mode of inheritance is autosomal recessive.

5.4 Pathogenesis

Since animal tissues lack the ability to alkylate the sterol side-chain at C-24, the plasma and tissue plant sterols (all three of which contain an alkyl group at C-24) must be derived from vegetable matter in the diet. In keeping with this, Bhattacharyya and Connor (1978) have shown that the plasma β-sitosterol concentration in β-sitosterolaemic patients decreases markedly when the dietary intake of β-sitosterol is minimized.

Bhattacharyya and Connor (1974) have shown that in patients with β-sitosterolaemia the absorption of a single oral dose of β-

sitosterol is increased from a normal value of less than 5% to about 30% of the dose, without a corresponding increase in cholesterol absorption. Thus, it seems likely that the accumulation of plant sterols in the plasma and tissues is due to loss of the normal mechanisms responsible for selectivity in the intestinal absorption of sterols. There is no evidence to indicate whether this defect is in the membranes at the luminal surfaces of the mucosal cells or whether it concerns one of the several steps involved in the transport and secretion of sterol once it has entered the mucosal cells. Until we understand why the normal human intestine does not absorb plant sterols, there seems little to be gained by speculating about the reasons for the partial loss of the ability to discriminate between cholesterol and plant sterols in patients with β-sitosterolaemia. Equally puzzling is the formation of xanthomatous lesions, in which 70–80% of the total sterol is cholesterol, at an early age despite a normal or near-normal plasma cholesterol concentration. A useful step towards an understanding of this would be to determine the extent to which the cholesterol in the lesions is derived from the plasma or from synthesis *in situ*.

6 CEREBROTENDINOUS XANTHOMATOSIS

6.1 Definition and historical background

Cerebrotendinous xanthomatosis (CTX) is a rare familial sterol storage disease characterized by (1) the presence of xanthomas in the central nervous system, lungs and tendons, in the absence of hypercholesterolaemia; (2) dementia, cataracts and a progressive neurological disorder involving especially the cerebellum and the corticospinal tracts.

The first unequivocal description of a patient with CTX was that of van Bogaert *et al.* (1937). This patient (a male) developed ataxia and slurred speech before age 20 and later developed bulbar paralysis and weakness of the limbs with muscle wasting; he also had bilateral cataracts and xanthomas in the Achilles tendons. He died at age 40 from pulmonary disease secondary to bulbar paralysis. Throughout the course of his illness his plasma cholesterol concentration remained within normal limits. At autopsy, numerous xanthomatous deposits containing cholesterol crystals were found in the brain, especially in the grey matter of the cerebellum, and demyelination was noted in the spinal cord.

Since the original description of van Bogaert *et al.*, more than twenty other patients, including the female paternal cousin of the first patient, have been reported in the world literature. Van Bogaert *et al.* (1937) drew attention to the presence of cholesterol in the xanthomas, but Menkes *et al.* (1968) later showed that 5α-cholestanol was also present in very large amounts in the brain lesions. Subsequently, 5α-cholestanol was demonstrated in excessive amounts in the tendon xanthomas and plasma (Philippart and van Bogaert, 1969) and in a wide variety of other tissues (Salen, 1971).

6.2 Clinical and biochemical features

6.2.1 Clinical course

Typically, retardation of mental development begins in childhood, followed by mental deterioration progressing to dementia in adolescence. Signs of neurological involvement, including ataxia, spasticity and muscle weakness, are usually apparent by the end of the second decade. The neurological signs increase progressively, and in some patients death, which in the majority of cases has occurred in the fifth or sixth decade, was attributable to spinal cord paralysis. Xanthomas, not usually noticeable until the third decade, occur most frequently in the Achilles tendons but may also be present in the extensor tendons of the fingers and in other tendons. Tuberous xanthomas and xanthelasmas have also been noted but are less common than tendon xanthomas. Cataracts, often present by the mid-twenties, have been reported in almost every patient. Signs or symptoms of coronary atherosclerosis have been reported in several patients and four have died from acute myocardial infarction, one at age 36 (Salen, 1971). Pulmonary insufficiency has been reported as a relatively late manifestation of CTX.

6.2.2 Plasma lipids

The plasma cholesterol and triglyceride concentrations are usually within normal limits, though moderate hypercholesterolaemia has been reported in a few patients. The plasma 5α-cholestanol concentration has been found to be markedly increased in all CTX patients in whom it has been measured; in 5 patients studied by Salen (1971) it was increased to about 10 times the mean value of 0.24 mg/100 ml in unaffected relatives. The distribution of 5α-cholestanol between the different plasma lipoprotein fractions is similar to that of cholesterol, the bulk of the total being carried in LDL. The 5α-cholestanol in plasma is present partly in esterified form, esterification by the plasma LCAT occurring at a rate comparable with that of cholesterol (Salen and Grundy, 1973). The red-cell content of cholesterol is normal, but 5α-cholestanol is present in the red-cell membranes at a 5α-cholestanol:cholesterol ratio similar to that in plasma.

6.2.3 Bile

The composition of duodenal bile is abnormal with respect to bile acids and neutral sterols (Salen, 1971; Salen *et al.*, 1977). In normal human bile, cholic acid and chenodeoxycholic acid are present in roughly equal amounts and together comprise about 90% of the total bile acids. In CTX there is a marked reduction in the amount of chenodeoxycholic acid in the bile, the proportion of cholic acid increasing to about 80% of the total bile acids. In addition to the abnormal cholic acid:chenodeoxycholic acid ratio, the bile of CTX patients contains significant amounts of allocholic acid and of C_{27} alcohols with the hydroxylated ring system of cholic acid and the C_8 side-chain skeleton of cholestane, but with hydroxyl groups at C-23, 24 and 25 (see Section 6.5).

In the neutral sterol fraction of the bile, up to 10% of the total sterol is 5α-cholestanol. Hence, the ratio of 5α-cholestanol to cholesterol in bile is much higher than the corresponding ratio in plasma. Substantial quantities of the cholesterol precursors, lanosterol and lathosterol (cholest-7-en-3β-ol), are also present in the bile in CTX.

6.3 Genetics

Analysis of the pedigrees of all known CTX families strongly suggests that the disorder is inherited as an autosomal recessive trait. Most of the index patients reported have had at least one affected brother or sister, in two of the first four families described the parents were first cousins, and in no family has an examined parent of an index patient had clinical signs of CTX or an increased plasma 5α-cholestanol concentration.

6.4 Pathology

6.4.1 Morphological changes

The most striking visible changes are seen in the central nervous system and are most conspicuous in the cerebellum. Multiple xanthomas are present in the cerebellar white matter, with atrophy of the adjacent cerebellar grey matter. Light microscopy of the lesions shows extensive demyelination with cystic areas of necrosis and the presence of large foam cells with lipid-filled vacuoles in their cytoplasm. Numerous birefringent cholesterol crystals, mainly extracellular, are seen in frozen sections of lesions examined under polarized light. Similar xanthomatous lesions are present in many other areas of the brain, including the cerebral and cerebellar peduncles, the basal ganglia and the lentiform nucleus. Focal areas of demyelination and collections of histiocytic foam cells around the blood vessels are widely scattered throughout the spinal cord. The peripheral nerves are unaffected.

Xanthomas have also been described in the lungs, femur and

vertebral bodies. The gross and microscopic appearance of the tendon lesions is similar to that of the tendon xanthomas of familial hypercholesterolaemia.

6.4.2 Tissue lipids

The cholesterol content of the brain is significantly increased, due mainly to an increase in esterified cholesterol (Menkes et al., 1968). Much more striking, however, is the massive increase in free and esterified 5α-cholestanol. In normal brain, 5α-cholestanol is present only in traces. In the brains of CTX patients, 20–30% of the total sterol may be due to 5α-cholestanol, both free and esterified (Menkes et al., 1968). Similar excessive amounts of 5α-cholestanol are present in histologically normal regions of the cerebrum and cerebellum, as well as in the brain xanthomas. 5α-Cholestanol also accounts for about 20% of the total sterols of peripheral nerve.

The sterols of the tendon lesions may contain up to 10% of 5α-cholestanol in free and esterified form. In some CTX patients there appears to be a generalized storage of 5α-cholestanol (though not to the degree seen in the central nervous system) in a wide variety of histologically normal tissues. Thus, Salen (1971) found up to 2.7% of 5α-cholestanol in the sterols of 11 apparently normal tissues obtained at autopsy, including kidney, adipose tissue and aorta. Bhattacharyya and Connor (1978) also found up to 5% of 5α-cholestanol in the skin of a CTX patient.

6.5 Pathogenesis

6.5.1 Bile acid metabolism

From the point of view of the pathogenesis of CTX, the metabolic abnormalities of greatest interest are those related to bile acid synthesis. However, early hopes that the study of bile acid metabolism in CTX would disclose a single enzyme defect that could explain every abnormal feature of this disease have not been fulfilled.

The marked reduction in the amount of chenodeoxycholic acid in the bile, referred to in Section 6.2, is associated with a decrease in the daily output of total bile acids (Salen and Grundy, 1973). The synthesis of both the primary bile acids is depressed, but that of chenodeoxycholic acid is reduced to a much greater extent than is that of cholic acid (Salen et al., 1979). In addition to synthesizing reduced amounts of primary bile acids, patients with CTX excrete large amounts of abnormal C_{27} alcohols in their bile and faeces, as already mentioned in Section 6.2 above and in Chapter 5. About 100 mg of the 25-hydroxy sterols, 5β-cholestane-3α,7α,12α,25-tetrol, 5β-cholestane-3α,7α,12α,23ξ,25-pentol and 5β-cholestane-3α,7α,12α,24α,25-pentol are excreted daily by these patients

(Setoguchi et al., 1974; Shefer et al., 1975). The structural formulae of these compounds are shown in Fig. 17.4.

The observation that sterol alcohols hydroxylated at C-25 accumulate in CTX patients has led Salen et al. (1977) to suggest that the major pathway for bile acid synthesis in man differs from that in rats, in which the initial step in side-chain cleavage is the 26-hydroxylation of 5β-cholestane-3α,7α-diol and of 5β-cholestane-

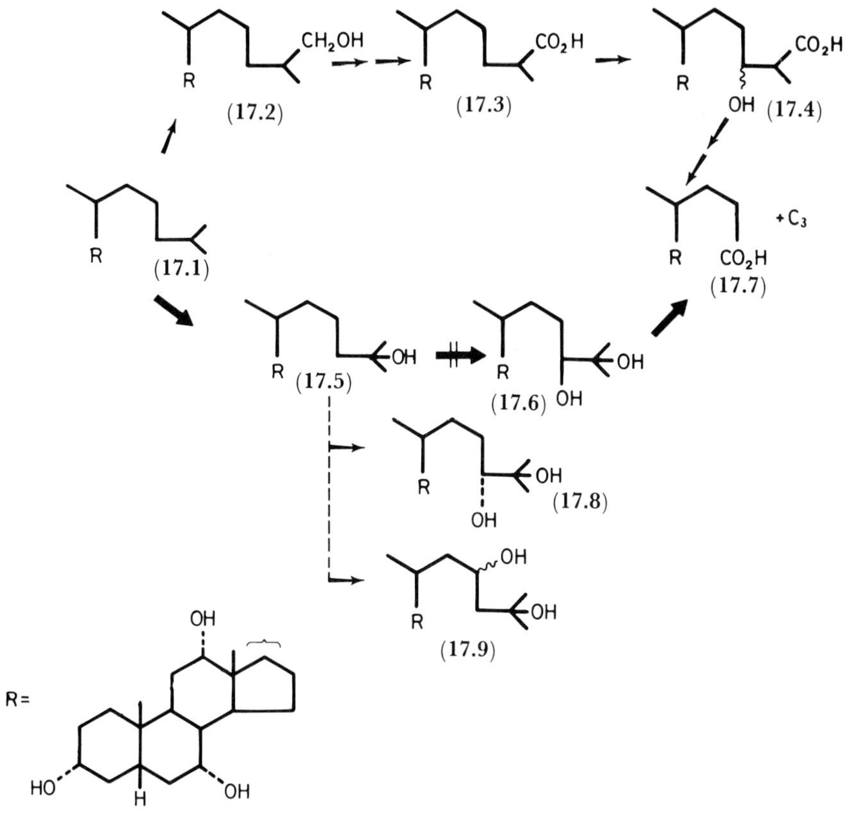

Figure 17.4
Proposed alternative route for the formation of cholic acid *via* 25-hydroxylation of the side-chain of 5β-cholestane-3α,7α,12α-triol. The upper sequence shows the classical pathway *via* 26-hydroxylation. The middle sequence (**17.1** → **17.7**) shows the proposed 25-hydroxylation pathway. Partial block of 24β-hydroxylation of (**17.5**) leads to accumulation of (**17.5**) and of the two abnormal pentols (**17.8**) and (**17.9**).

(**17.1**), 5β-cholestane-3α,7α,12α-triol; (**17.2**), 5β-cholestane-3α,7α,12α,26-tetrol; (**17.3**), 3α,7α,12α-trihydroxy-5β-cholestan-26-oic acid; (**17.4**), 3α,7α,12α,24ξ-tetrahydroxy-5β-cholestan-26-oic acid; (**17.5**), 5β-cholestane-3α,7α,12α,25-tetrol; (**17.6**), 5β-cholestane-3α,7α,12α,25-pentol; (**17.7**), cholic acid; (**17.8**), 5β-cholestane-3α,7α,12α,24α,25-pentol; (**17.9**), 5β-cholestane-3α,7α,12α,23ξ,25-pentol.

Note: (**17.6**) is (24*S*) and (**17.8**) is (24*R*).

3α,7α,12α-triol (see Chapter 5 for an account of the classical pathway). Salen *et al.* suggest that in human liver the cleavage of the side-chain is initiated by a microsomal hydroxylation at C-25, followed by β-hydroxylation at C-24, leading to cleavage at C-24 to give the C_{24} primary bile acid and acetone (Fig. 17.4). They propose that in CTX there is a partial block in the 24β-hydroxylation of the 25-hydroxy tetrol (**17.5**), resulting in the accumulation of this compound and of the two abnormal pentols (**17.8**) and (**17.9**) formed by the further enzymic hydroxylation of (**17.5**). In support of these proposals, Björkhem *et al.* (1975) have shown that human liver microsomes contain an efficient enzyme system for the 25-hydroxylation of 5β-cholestane-3α,7α,12α-triol. Furthermore, Setoguchi *et al.* (1974) have demonstrated the presence of radioactive compound (**17.5**) and radioactive 25-hydroxy pentols in the bile of CTX patients given intravenous injections of [^{14}C]cholesterol. Salen *et al.* (1977) have also shown that radioactive 5β-cholestane-3α,7α,12α,25-tetrol is converted into cholic acid in normal human subjects and CTX patients, but that the rate of conversion into cholic acid is considerably slower in CTX than in normal subjects. Finally, Shefer *et al.* (1976) have demonstrated the presence of a microsomal enzyme in human liver that catalyzes the 24β-hydroxylation of 5β-cholestane-3α,7α,12α,25-tetrol (step (**17.5**) → (**17.6**), Fig. 17.4) and have reported decreased activity of this enzyme in the liver microsomes of two CTX patients.

All these observations are consistent with the possibility that the 25-hydroxylation pathway is the major route for cholic acid synthesis in man and that 25-hydroxylated C_{27} sterols accumulate in CTX because of a block in the further metabolism of 5β-cholestane-3α,7α,12α,25-tetrol (**17.5**). This would explain the decreased synthesis of total bile acids and could also account for the relatively marked depression of chenodeoxycholic acid synthesis if it is supposed that the slow turnover of intermediates behind the block allows time for the 12α-hydroxylation of 5β-cholestane-3α,7α-diol and thus diverts this precursor of chenodeoxycholic acid into the pathway leading to cholic acid. Salen *et al.* (1979) have pointed out that the 12α-hydroxylation of 5β-cholestane-3α,7α-diol would also provide an explanation for the failure of 25-hydroxylated precursors of chenodeoxycholic acid to accumulate in CTX.

However, although a block in the 24β-hydroxylation of (**17.5**) provides a possible explanation of the abnormal bile acid metabolism in CTX, the supposition that human bile acids are synthesized predominantly by the 25-hydroxylation pathway is in conflict with evidence to indicate that the major pathway in man is essentially the same as that in rats. As discussed in Chapter 5, the presence of trihydroxycholestanoic acid ((**17.3**), Fig. 17.4) in normal human bile and the observation that the isopropyl unit of the side-chain is removed as propionate (not acetone) in bile acid formation in human liver indicate that the major pathway in man involves a 26-hydroxylation, presumably by the 26-hydroxylase demonstrated in human liver mitochondria by Björkhem *et al.* (1975). Furthermore, Hanson *et al.* (1979) have shown that (25R)-5β-cholestane-3α,7α,12α,26-tetrol (the natural stereoisomer in man) is converted into cholic acid about six times as efficiently as 5β-cholestane-3α,7α,12α,25-tetrol when the two ring-labelled compounds are injected into normal human subjects. An additional objection to the 25-hydroxylation pathway is its failure to explain the formation of chenodeoxycholic acid in normal man, since Björkhem *et al.* (1975) have shown that the microsomal 25-hydroxylase in human liver is virtually inactive towards 5β-cholestane-3α,7α-diol, whereas the microsomal 26-hydroxylase is very active towards this substrate.

An alternative explanation for the accumulation of 25-hydroxylated alcohols in CTX, not ruled out by Setoguchi *et al.* (1974), is that side-chain cleavage in man proceeds through the classical pathway, beginning with hydroxylation at C-26, and that the mitochondrial 26-hydroxylase is deficient in this disease. A block at this step could divert bile acid precursors into a minor or quiescent pathway involving 25-hydroxylation. This would account equally well for the presence of the C_{27} bile alcohols discovered by Setoguchi *et al.* (1974) and, at the same time, would be consistent with all the evidence pointing to 26-hydroxylation as a normal step in human bile acid formation. On this view, the slower incorporation of a tracer dose of radioactive 5β-cholestane-3α,7α,12α,25-tetrol into cholic acid in CTX patients than in normal subjects could be due to the increased load of endogenous 25-hydroxylated intermediates in CTX.

In view of this alternative possibility, information about the activity of the mitochondrial 26-hydroxylase in the livers of CTX patients would be of considerable interest.

6.5.2 Increased sterol synthesis

Whatever explanation may be favoured as to the enzymic basis of the abnormal bile acid metabolism in CTX, we still have to account for the massive accumulation of sterol, particularly 5α-cholestanol, in the tissues. Moreover, since CTX is monogenically inherited, the abnormalities in bile acid and sterol metabolism must be explained in terms of a single mutation.

Salen and Grundy (1973) observed a 60% increase in whole-body synthesis of cholesterol and a 3-fold increase in that of 5α-cholestanol in 3 CTX patients. Nicolau *et al.* (1974) have also reported abnormally high hepatic HMG-CoA reductase activity in one CTX patient. In view of these findings, Salen *et al.* (1977) have suggested that a decrease in bile-acid synthesis, which they assume to be the primary defect in CTX, leads to increased hepatic synthesis of cholesterol, accompanied by increased hepatic synthesis of 5α-cholestanol, due to release of HMG-CoA reductase from the normal feed-back inhibition by bile acids. On this view, the liver is the source of the 5α-cholestanol in brain and other tissues. However, other workers (Muckenhausen *et al.*, 1968; Bhattacharyya and Connor, 1978) have been unable to detect increased whole-body synthesis of cholesterol in CTX. Moreover, the hypothesis of Salen *et al.* (1977) fails to explain why a moderate increase in cholesterol synthesis in the livers of CTX patients should lead to a marked increase in 5α-cholestanol synthesis, particularly since the much greater increase in cholesterol synthesis that occurs in cholestyramine-treated human subjects is not known to be accompanied by overproduction of 5α-cholestanol. In this connection, it would be of interest to test the assumption that the 5α-cholestanol in the xanthomas of CTX patients is derived from the plasma rather than from synthesis *in situ*. Finally, there is the question as to why cholesterol, which accounts for up to 80% of the total sterols in the xanthomas, accumulates in tissues in the presence of a normal plasma cholesterol concentration. This problem is analogous to that discussed in the section on β-sitosterolaemia, a disease in which there is also accumulation of cholesterol and of an abnormal sterol in xanthomatous lesions in the presence of a normal plasma cholesterol concentration.

7 EOSINOPHILIC XANTHOMATOUS GRANULOMA; SCHÜLLER-CHRISTIAN SYNDROME

7.1 Historical background and nomenclature

The term *Schüller-Christian syndrome* refers to a triad of abnormalities comprising diabetes insipidus, exophthalmos and focal lesions of membrane bone. The first patient in whom the syndrome was described was a 16-year-old boy reported by Schüller in 1915; the second was a 5-year-old girl described by Christian in 1919. The cellular pathology of this syndrome is now considered to be common to a wide spectrum of disorders characterized by the presence of granulomatous lesions which at some stage of their evolution contain eosinophils, reticulum cells and cholesterol-rich foam cells, the presence of foam cells giving the lesions the appearance of xanthomas. The nomenclature of these disorders, sometimes grouped together under the general term *histiocytosis*, is confusing and controversial and is still overloaded with terms introduced at a time when different manifestations of what later turned out to be a single disease were given separate, usually latinized, names.

Classification of the xanthomatous disorders considered in this chapter was greatly simplified when Thannhauser and Magendantz (1938) postulated the existence of a single disease characterized by the presence of *eosinophilic xanthomatous granulomas* that could involve various organs (particularly bone, brain, lungs and skin) and in which the lesions could occur singly or in various combinations in different organs, giving rise to a multiplicity of apparently distinct clinical entities. On this view, the Schüller-Christian syndrome may be regarded as an eosinophilic xanthomatous granulomatosis in which the site of the lesions is such as to cause diabetes insipidus and exophthalmos, while in the skin disease called *xanthoma disseminata* (see below) the lesions are present predominantly in the skin.

The hallmark of all these disorders is the presence of the characteristic granulomas, with an essentially normal plasma lipid pattern; hence the older term *essential xanthomatosis of the normocholesterolaemic type*. To some extent, the different clinical manifestations of eosinophilic xanthomatous granulomatosis may represent stages in the progress of a single disease. For example, patients in whom the initial clinical signs are confined to the Schüller-Christian triad may later develop xanthoma disseminata, or this sequence may be reversed. There is also reason to believe that the granulomas evolve according to a well-defined pattern, beginning with the accumulation of histiocytes, progressing through a stage in which foam cells are prominent and ending with a quiescent stage in which the foam cells disappear (see below). The idea that the xanthomatous granuloma represents one stage in an evolving lesion has led to the proposal that the ill-defined disorder that is characterized by the early and rapid development of widespread histiocytic granulomas *without* foam cells and that usually leads to death in infancy (the *Letterer-Siwe syndrome*) represents a rapidly progressive form of eosinophilic xanthomatous granulomatosis from which the patient dies before xanthoma cells have had time to develop. Further discussion of the classification of the group of disorders to which the Schüller-Christian syndrome belongs will be found in Thannhauser (1958) and Newton and Hamoudi (1973). In this section we shall consider the pathology and major clinical features of the more benign forms of histiocytosis in which the predominant lesion is an eosinophilic granuloma with cholesterol-rich foam cells.

7.2 Pathology

7.2.1 Histology of the lesions
The lesion begins with the peri-vascular accumulation of capillary endothelial cells, eosinophils and histiocytes. Subsequently, numerous cholesterol-rich lipid droplets appear in the cytoplasm of the histiocytes, converting them into foam cells. This is the stage in the

progress of the lesion corresponding to the xanthomatous granuloma. In some lesions, particularly those in skin and brain tissue, extracellular cholesterol crystals, possibly released from dead foam cells, may be present in large numbers. This stage is often followed by a healing phase in which the foam cells disappear and the proliferative components of the lesion are replaced by fibrous tissue. Lesions at all stages of development may be seen at the same time in a given patient. In skin and brain tissue the xanthomatous phase tends to appear early in the life-history of the lesion.

7.2.2 Gross appearance and distribution

The xanthomas in bone usually appear on X-ray examination as sharply defined osteolytic lesions, 1–2 cm in diameter, similar to those seen in fibrocystic bone disease. Occasionally, however, the lesions are small and diffusely scattered, giving rise to a mottled appearance not unlike that of the bones in Gaucher's disease. When the lesions are present in long bones, the X-ray picture may show evidence of spontaneous fractures. When the skull is involved, X-ray examination usually shows irregular, punched-out cystic areas encroaching on the inner and outer tables. Naked-eye examination of systemic xanthomas obtained from bone, brain, lung or other organs shows yellowish rubbery masses. The gross appearance of the skin xanthomas is described in Section 7.3. Chemical analysis of xanthomatous portions of tissue shows a 10- to 20-fold increase in cholesterol content.

The commoner sites in which the xanthomas occur are the bones, the lungs, the brain and the skin, but in the more rapidly progressive forms of histiocytosis, widespread lesions are found in the liver, spleen and lymph nodes, as well as in the more commonly affected organs. Almost any part of the skeleton may be involved, but the most frequently affected sites are the skull, the pelvis and the upper part of the femur. Small xanthomas may develop in the jaws, particularly in the tooth sockets, leading to erosion of the roots and loosening of the teeth.

The anatomical sites of lesions responsible for diabetes insipidus is variable. Pituitary function may be interfered with if a lesion develops in the dura mater or cranial bones at a site where it compresses the pituitary stalk or the subthalamic region of the brain. Alternatively, the lesion may be in the brain substance itself. Bilateral exophthalmos is due to the presence of granulomatous xanthomas in the orbital cavities or in the bone lining the cavities.

7.3 Clinical features

7.3.1 Schüller-Christian syndrome

As discussed in Section 7.1, the triad of abnormalities named after

Schüller and Christian is one manifestation of a general disorder that can be expressed in different clinical forms. The syndrome occurs most commonly in infants and children, but its appearance may be delayed until adult life. The development of diabetes insipidus with bilateral exophthalmos is often preceded by the appearance of skin xanthomas or overt bone disease, the latter sometimes causing visible deformities of the skull and of the long bones, as in the 51-year-old male patient described by Thannhauser (1958). The exophthalmos may be extreme and has been described as 'frog-like'.

The clinical course is very variable. Often, the disease appears to be self-limiting, the patient reaching a stable state or even progressing to a permanent remission; the bone lesions in Schüller's patient eventually became smaller and almost disappeared, while Christian's patient recovered spontaneously. More commonly, however, replacement therapy for diabetes insipidus is required throughout the life of the patient. The bone lesions may also become progressively larger and more widespread over the course of years, leading to a variety of symptoms, including nerve deafness, disorganization of large joints and spontaneous fractures. Neurological symptoms are not a common feature of the syndrome and the mental faculties usually remain unimpaired.

Although the Schüller-Christian syndrome should always be excluded in young patients with diabetes insipidus, it is responsible for only a small fraction of all patients who have diabetes insipidus. The diagnosis is suggested by the presence of polyuria in a patient who has skin xanthomas of the type described in Section 7.3.2 and a normal plasma cholesterol concentration. Occasionally, the presenting symptom is bone pain or limitation of movement, especially if there is a bone xanthoma involving a joint. X-ray examination shows the typical bone lesions. If the lungs are involved, the X-ray shows numerous small opacities, giving an appearance similar to that seen in miliary tuberculosis. The diagnosis is confirmed by microscopy and lipid analysis of biopsy specimens, showing the characteristic histological appearance and a greatly increased cholesterol content.

The differential diagnosis includes familial hypercholesterolaemia, osteolytic bone disease due to causes other than eosinophilic granulomatosis, and diabetes insipidus not associated with granulomas of the Schüller-Christian syndrome. The bone lesions usually respond to local X-irradiation.

7.3.2 Xanthoma disseminata

Xanthomatous lesions, similar in their histopathology to that of the eosinophilic granulomas of bone and other organs, also occur in skin and mucous membranes and are known as *xanthoma disseminata*. They may occur alone or in association with systemic granulomas elsewhere in the body. As mentioned in the previous section, xanthoma disseminata is often associated with the Schüller-Christian syndrome. The lesions differ in distribution and appearance from the skin xanthomas of familial hypercholesterolaemia and other hyperlipidaemias. Common sites are the axilla, the eyelids, the folds of the neck, the scrotum and the groins. They may also occur on the elbows but, unlike the planar and tuberous lesions of familial hypercholesterolaemia, are commoner on the flexor than the extensor surfaces. When present in skin, the lesions tend to be arranged in lines along the skin-folds. Other sites are the cornea and sclera and the mucous membranes of the mouth, epiglottis, larynx and bronchus. The skin lesions are slightly raised, smooth patches, their colour ranging from lemon yellow to dark brown.

7.4 Pathogenesis

Eosinophilic xanthomatous granulomatosis does not appear to be genetic in origin. Although there are occasional reports of the occurrence of the disorder in sibs, Thannhauser (1958) has referred to a pair of identical twins, one of whom had bone lesions, while the other was normal. The early localization of the lesions around blood capillaries and the prominence of eosinophils suggests an autoimmune component in the pathogenesis, but this has not been demonstrated. The reason for the accumulation of cholesterol in the histiocytic cells in the xanthomatous stage of the lesions is not known. Thannhauser (1958) concluded that the cholesterol in the foam cells must be synthesized *in situ* since the plasma cholesterol concentration is not increased. However, there is no experimental evidence for this.

REFERENCES

Abramov, A., Schorr, S. and Wolman, M. (1956). Generalized xanthomatosis with calcified adrenals. *American Journal of Diseases of Children*, **91**, 282–286.

Bhattacharyya, A. K. and Connor, W. E. (1974). β-Sitosterolemia and xanthomatosis. A newly described lipid storage disease in two sisters. *Journal of Clinical Investigation*, **53**, 1033–1043.

Bhattacharyya, A. K. and Connor, W. E. β-Sitosterolemia and xanthomatosis. In: *The Metabolic Basis of Inherited Disease*. Ed. J. B. Stanbury, J. B. Wyngaarden and D. S. Fredrickson. McGraw-Hill, New York, 4th edition, pp. 663–669, 1978.

Björkhem, I., Gustafsson, J., Johansson, G. and Persson, B. (1975). Biosynthesis of bile acids in man. Hydroxylation of the C_{27}-steroid side chain. *Journal of Clinical Investigation*, **55**, 478–486.

Brown, M. S., Dana, S. E. and Goldstein, J. L. (1975). Receptor-dependent hydrolysis of cholesteryl esters contained in plasma low density lipoprotein. *Proceedings of the National Academy of Sciences of the U.S.A.*, **72**, 2925–2929.

Burke, J. A. and Schubert, W. K. (1972). Deficient activity of hepatic acid lipase in cholesterol ester storage disease. *Science*, **176**, 309–310.
Christian, H. A. (1919). Defects in membranous bones, exophthalmos and diabetes insipidus; an unusual syndrome of dyspituitarism. A clinical study. *Contributions to Medical and Biological Research*, **1**, 391–401.
Eto, Y. and Kitagawa, T. (1970). Wolman's disease with hypolipoproteinemia and acanthocytosis: Clinical and biochemical observations. *Journal of Pediatrics*, **77**, 862–867.
Fredrickson, D. S. (1963). Newly recognised disorders of cholesterol metabolism. *Annals of Internal Medicine*, **58**, 718 (A).
Fredrickson, D. S. and Ferrans, V. J. Acid cholesteryl ester hydrolase deficiency (Wolman's disease and cholesteryl ester storage disease). In: *The Metabolic Basis of Inherited Disease*, Chapter 32. Ed. J. B. Stanbury, J. B. Wyngaarden and D. S. Fredrickson. McGraw-Hill, New York, 1978.
Fredrickson, D. S., Sloan, H. R., Ferrans, V. J. and Demosky, S. J. Jr. (1972). Cholesteryl ester storage disease: A most unusual manifestation of deficiency of two lysosomal enzyme activities. *Transactions of the Association of American Physicians*, **85**, 109–119.
Goldstein, J. L., Dana, S. E., Faust, J. R., Beaudet, A. L. and Brown, M. S. (1975). Role of lysosomal acid lipase in the metabolism of plasma low density lipoprotein: Observations in cultured fibroblasts from a patient with cholesteryl ester storage disease. *Journal of Biological Chemistry*, **250**, 8487–8495.
Hanson, R. F., Staples, A. B. and Williams, G. C. (1979). Metabolism of 5β-cholestane-3α,7α,12α,26-tetrol and 5β-cholestane-3α,7α,12α,25-tetrol into cholic acid in normal human subjects. *Journal of Lipid Research*, **20**, 489–493.
Hers, H. G. (1965). Inborn lysosomal diseases. *Gastroenterology*, **48**, 625–633.
Hers, H. G. and Van Hoof, F. *Lysosomes and Storage Diseases*. Ed. H. G. Hers and F. Van Hoof. Academic Press, New York, 1973.
Khachadurian, A. β-Sitosterolemia and xanthomatosis. Quoted in Bhattacharyya, A. K. and Connor, W. E. *The Metabolic Basis of Inherited Disease*, Chapter 31. p. 669, 1978.
Khachadurian, A. K. and Clancy, K. F. (1978). Familial phytosterolemia (β-sitosterolemia): report of five cases and studies in cultured skin fibroblasts. *Clinical Research*, **26**, 329A.
Konno, T., Fujii, M., Watanuki, T. and Koizumi, K. (1966). Wolman's disease: The first case in Japan. *Tohoku Journal of Experimental Medicine*, **90**, 375–385.
Kothari, H. V., Bonner, M. J. and Miller, B. F. (1970). Cholesterol ester hydrolase in homogenates and lysosomal fractions of human aorta. *Biochimica et Biophysica Acta*, **202**, 325–331.
Kyriakides, E. C., Paul, B. and Balint, J. A. (1972). Lipid accumulation and acid lipase deficiency in fibroblasts from a family with Wolman's disease, and their apparent correction *in vitro*. *Journal of Laboratory and Clinical Medicine*, **80**, 810–816.
Lageron, A., Caroli, J., Stralin, H. and Barbier, P. (1967). Polycorie cholestérolique de l'adulte. I. Étude clinique, électronique, histochimique. *Presse Medicale (Paris)*, **75**, 2785–2790.
Lake, B. D. (1977). Histochemical and ultrastructural studies in the diagnosis of inborn errors of metabolism. *Records of the Adelaide Children's Hospital*, **1**, 337–345.
Lough, J., Fawcett, J. and Wiegensberg, B. (1970). Wolman's disease. An electron microscopic, histochemical and biochemical study. *Archives of Pathology*, **89**, 103–110.
Menkes, J. H., Schimschock, J. R. and Swanson, P. C. (1968). Cerebrotendinous xanthomatosis: the storage of cholestanol within the nervous system. *Archives of Neurology*, **19**, 47–53.

Miettinen, T. A. (1980). Phytosterolaemia, Xanthomatosis and premature atherosclerotic arterial disease: a case with high plant sterol absorption, impaired sterol elimination and low cholesterol synthesis. *European Journal of Clinical Investigation*, **10**, 27–35.

Muckenhausen, C., Derby, B. M. and Moser, H. W. (1968). Conversion of C[14] cholesterol to cholestanol in cerebrotendinous xanthomatosis. *Federation Proceedings*, **28**, 882.

Newton, W. A. Jr. and Hamoudi, A. B. Histiocytosis: A histologic classification with clinical correlation. In: *Perspectives in Pediatric Pathology*, Volume 1. Ed. H. S. Rosenberg and R. P. Bolande. Year Book Medical Publishers, Chicago, pp. 251–283, 1973.

Nicolau, G., Shefer, S., Salen, G. and Mosbach, E. H. (1974). Determination of hepatic 3-hydroxy-3-methylglutaryl CoA reductase activity in man. *Journal of Lipid Research*, **15**, 94–98.

Partin, J. C. and Schubert, W. K. (1969). Small intestinal mucosa in cholesterol ester storage disease. A light and electron microscope study. *Gastroenterology*, **57**, 542–558.

Patrick, A. D. and Lake, B. D. (1969). An acid lipase deficiency in Wolman's disease. *Biochemical Journal*, **112**, 29P.

Patrick, A. D. and Lake, B. D. Wolman's disease. In: *Lysosomes and Storage Diseases*. Ed. H. G. Hers and F. Van Hoof. Academic Press, New York, Chapter 18, 1973.

Peters, T. J. and de Duve, C. (1974). Lysosomes of the arterial wall. II. Subcellular fractionation of aortic cells from rabbits with experimental atheroma. *Experimental and Molecular Pathology*, **20**, 228–256.

Philippart, M. and van Bogaert, L. (1969). Cholestanolosis (cerebrotendinous xanthomatosis): a follow-up study on the original family. *Archives of Neurology*, **21**, 603–610.

Salen, G. (1971). Cholestanol deposition in cerebrotendinous xanthomatosis: a possible mechanism. *Annals of Internal Medicine*, **75**, 843–851.

Salen, G. and Grundy, S. M. (1973). The metabolism of cholestanol, cholesterol, and bile acids in cerebrotendinous xanthomatosis. *Journal of Clinical Investigation*, **52**, 2822–2835.

Salen, G., Shefer, S., Zaki, F. G. and Mosbach, E. H. Inborn errors in bile acid synthesis. In: *Clinics in Gastroenterology*, **6**, No. 1. Ed. G. Paumgartner, 1977.

Salen, G., Shefer, S., Mosbach, E. H., Hauser, S., Cohen, B. I. and Nicolau, G. (1979). Metabolism of potential precursors of chenodeoxycholic acid in cerebrotendinous xanthomatosis (CTX). *Journal of Lipid Research*, **20**, 22–30.

Schiff, L., Schubert, W. K., McAdams, A. J., Spiegel, E. L. and O'Donnell, J. F. (1968). Hepatic cholesterol ester storage disease, a familial disorder. I. Clinical aspects. *American Journal of Medicine*, **44**, 538–546.

Schüller, A. (1915–1916). Über eigenartige Schädeldefekte im Jugendalter. *Fortschritte auf dem Gebiete der Röntgenstrahlen*, **23**, 12–18.

Setoguchi, T., Salen, G., Tint, S. and Mosbach, E. H. (1974). A biochemical abnormality in cerebrotendinous xanthomatosis. Impairment of bile acid synthesis associated with incomplete degradation of the cholesterol side chain. *Journal of Clinical Investigation*, **53**, 1393–1401.

Shefer, S., Cheng, F. W., Dayal, B., Hauser, S., Tint, G. S., Salen, G. and Mosbach, E. H. (1976). A 25-hydroxylation pathway of cholic acid biosynthesis in man and rat. *Journal of Clinical Investigation*, **57**, 897–903.

Shefer, S., Dayal, B., Tint, G. S., Salen, G. and Mosbach, E. H. (1975). Identification of pentahydroxy bile alcohols in cerebrotendinous xanthomatosis: characterization of 5β-cholestane-$3\alpha,7\alpha,12\alpha,24\xi,25$-pentol and 5β-cholestane-$3\alpha,7\alpha,12\alpha,23\xi,25$-pentol. *Journal of Lipid Research*, **16**, 280–286.

Shulman, R. S., Bhattacharyya, A. K., Connor, W. E. and Fredrickson, D. S. (1976).

β-Sitosterolemia and xanthomatosis. *New England Journal of Medicine*, **294**, 482–483.
Stanbury, J. B., Wyngaarden, J. B. and Fredrickson, D. S. (Eds.). *The Metabolic Basis of Inherited Disease*, 4th edition. McGraw-Hill Book Company, New York, 1978.
Thannhauser, S. J. *Lipidoses. Diseases of the Intracellular Lipid Metabolism*, 3rd edition. Grune and Stratton, New York, 1958.
Thannhauser, S. J. and Magendantz, H. (1938). The different clinical groups of xanthomatous diseases; a clinical physiological study of 22 cases. *Annals of Internal Medicine*, **11**, 1662–1746.
Van Bogaert, L., Scherer, H. J. and Epstein, E. *Une forme cérébrale de la cholestérinose généralisée*. Masson et Cie., (Eds.), Paris, France, 1937.
Wolman, M., Sterk, V. V., Gatt, S. and Frenkel, M. (1961). Primary familial xanthomatosis with involvement and calcification of the adrenals: Report of two more cases in siblings of a previously described infant. *Pediatrics*, **28**, 742–757.
Young, E. P. and Patrick, A. D. (1970). Deficiency of acid esterase activity in Wolman's disease. *Archives of Disease in Childhood*, **45**, 664–668.

Chapter 18

Cholesterol Gallstones; Plasma Cholesterol in Liver Disease

1	CHOLESTEROL GALLSTONES	855
1.1	Epidemiology and clinical associations	855
1.1.1	Prevalence	855
1.1.2	Age, sex and other associations	857
1.2	Solubilization of cholesterol	857
1.3	Conditions required for the formation of cholesterol stones	859
1.3.1	Bile supersaturated with cholesterol	859
1.3.2	Origin of the biliary lipids	862
1.3.3	The pathogenesis of supersaturated bile	863
1.3.3.1	Diminished bile-salt pools	863
1.3.3.2	Secretion rates of biliary lipids	864
1.3.3.3	Effect of removing the gallbladder	867
1.4	Medical treatment of gallstones	868
1.4.1	Background	868
1.4.2	Dissolution of cholesterol stones by chenodeoxycholic acid	869
1.4.2.1	The clinical response	869
1.4.2.2	The mechanism of action of chenotherapy	870
1.4.3	Other forms of medical treatment	871
1.5	Experimental gallstones in animals	872
2	THE PLASMA CHOLESTEROL IN LIVER DISEASE	874
2.1	Biliary obstruction	874
2.1.1	The plasma lipids and lipoproteins	874
2.1.2	The cause of the hypercholesterolaemia	876
2.1.3	The lipid composition of blood cells	878
2.1.4	Xanthomas in biliary obstruction	880
2.2	Parenchymatous liver disease	881
2.2.1	Plasma lipids and lipoproteins	881
2.2.2	The lipid composition of blood cells	881

Cholesterol Gallstones; Plasma Cholesterol in Liver Disease

In this chapter we consider two aspects of cholesterol metabolism in diseases of the liver and biliary system: (1) the formation of cholesterol gallstones and (2) the abnormal plasma lipoprotein patterns associated with obstructive or parenchymatous liver disease.

1 CHOLESTEROL GALLSTONES

1.1 Epidemiology and clinical associations

1.1.1 Prevalence

The prevalence of gallstones is difficult to assess accurately in any community because at least 50% of all gallstone disease is asymptomatic throughout life. In this respect the problem is analogous to that of estimating the prevalence of coronary atherosclerosis in life. The best available estimates of the age-related frequency of gallstones in different populations are probably those derived from extensive *post mortem* surveys, but this information is accurate only in so far as the autopsies are representative of the whole population under investigation. In underdeveloped countries, where autopsies are usually infrequent, estimates of prevalence must be less accurate than in communities in which the autopsy rate may approach 100%. Useful information may also be obtained from the recorded numbers of cholecystectomies in large general hospitals, and from cholecystographic surveys of people chosen at random from defined populations. The latter approach is particularly valuable in the study of small communities with an unusually high incidence of gallstones, such as the American Indians of the Southwest of the United States (Comess *et al.*, 1966). Finally, observations on the 'lithogenicity' of bile (deduced from its lipid composition) in randomly chosen subjects may help in the prediction of the prevalence of cholesterol gallstones within a population.

Information combined from these various sources (see Redinger and Small, 1972; Heaton, 1973) shows that in the affluent communities of Western Europe and North America the prevalence of gallstones is very high—more than 20% in some autopsy surveys of adults—and is much greater than the prevalence in the rural communities of underdeveloped countries and in Asian populations in general, including Japan. Within these broad regions there are considerable variations and some anomalies. For example, the prevalence in Sweden is far higher than that recorded in any other European country, and several surveys of Indian tribes living in Arizona and New Mexico have revealed prevalences of over 50% in young women. At the other extreme, gallstones are very rare in most rural African communities.

The great majority of gallstones in affluent communities and in American Indians are radiolucent cholesterol stones, consisting mainly of cholesterol monohydrate in crystalline form, together with small amounts of calcium salts, pigment, protein and other amorphous solids. In the rural communities of underdeveloped countries, gallstones are usually pigment stones, often associated with persistent haemolysis due to infestation with blood-borne parasites.

The reasons for the marked regional variations in gallstone prevalence are not known. Differences in diet have, of course, been suggested as contributory causes, especially in view of the ease with which cholesterol gallstones can be produced in animals of some species by changing their diet (see Section 1.5). Although a correlation between gallstones and a high caloric intake has been reported in European women (Sarles *et al.*, 1970), changes in the fatty acid content of the diet have been found to have little effect on the lipid composition of bile in short-term experiments on human subjects (Dam, 1971). However, the addition of moderate amounts of cholesterol to the diet increases the lithogenicity of the bile in normal human subjects (Den Besten *et al.*, 1973). Pomare and Heaton (1973) have drawn attention to the fact that gallstone prevalence tends to be high in populations consuming fibre-depleted diets rich in refined sugar and they have shown that the addition of bran to the diet of human subjects markedly increases the proportion of chenodeoxycholate in the bile. In view of the favourable effect of exogenous chenodeoxycholic acid on the lithogenicity of human bile (see Section 1.4), this observation raises the possibility that the low fibre content of some Western diets contributes to the development of gallstones by helping to tip the balance towards the formation of lithogenic bile.

1.1.2 Age, sex and other associations

Cholesterol gallstones are rare before puberty. Thereafter, their frequency increases with age at least until the seventh decade. In countries where gallstone disease is due mainly to cholesterol stones, the incidence in women is two to three times that in men and the frequency of gallstones is higher in women who have borne children than in those who have not. The incidence of gallstones is significantly increased in young women taking oral contraceptives, an association that may be explained by the observation of Pertsemlidis et al. (1974) that the administration of oestrogen with progestin increases the saturation of their bile with cholesterol. There is also an association between obesity and gallstones. The incidence of gallstones is increased in diabetes and in diseases of the small bowel, including ileal resection and Crohn's disease. In so far as cholesterol gallstones and ischaemic heart disease are both prevalent in affluent countries there is a general association between the two diseases. However, an association within populations has not been demonstrated. Furthermore, apart from age, the known risk factors for IHD do not predispose to cholesterol gallstones. In particular, there is no association between hypercholesterolaemia and gallstones, and female sex is a negative risk factor for IHD but a positive risk factor for cholesterol gallstones. As discussed in Chapter 14, a significant increase in the incidence of gallstones has been reported in healthy subjects who ate polyunsaturated-fat diets (Sturdevant et al., 1973) or who took clofibrate (Oliver et al., 1978) continuously for several years while participating in primary IHD-prevention trials. Cholestyramine, a drug that resembles ileal disease in its ability to interfere with the reabsorption of bile acids, has not been reported to cause gallstones in man.

1.2 Solubilization of cholesterol

Although free cholesterol is almost completely insoluble in water, the cholesterol of normal human bile is held in solution by the formation of mixed micelles with bile salts and lecithin, the major phospholipid of bile. The maximum amount of free cholesterol that can be maintained in micellar solution in an aqueous medium containing cholesterol, bile salts and lecithin is determined largely by the proportions of bile salt and lecithin in the mixture. To a first approximation this holds true for concentrations of total solid ranging from 5% to 20% by weight, a range that includes the lower and upper limits of solute concentration found in human gallbladder bile (Admirand and Small, 1968).

The molar percentages of cholesterol, bile salts and lecithin present in mixtures of the three components in an aqueous medium may be represented graphically by plotting the values on triangular coordinates. In the triangular phase diagram shown in Fig. 18.1 the point M represents a mixture containing 5 moles % of cholesterol, 15 moles % of lecithin and 80 moles % of bile salt. The solubility of cholesterol as a function of the molar percentages of lecithin and bile salt is represented by a continuous line, as shown in Fig. 18.1. In any mixture whose composition lies below the line, cholesterol will be in stable micellar solution (the 'micellar zone'); thus, the point M represents a mixture in which all the cholesterol is present in micellar solution. Points lying along the line represent mixtures saturated with cholesterol. In all mixtures shown by points above the line, some cholesterol is present in crystalline or liquid-crystalline form, or in unstable supersaturated micelles from which cholesterol will eventually precipitate.

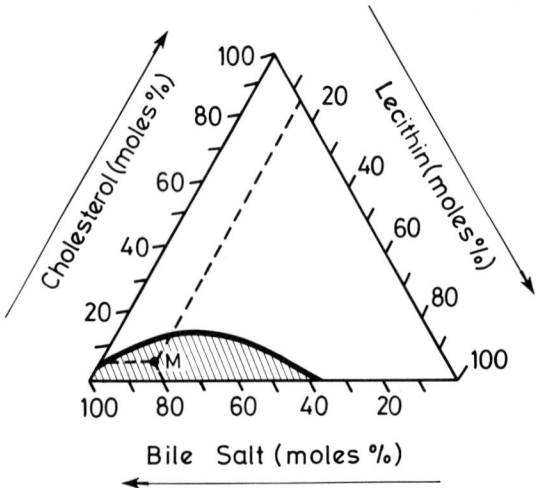

Figure 18.1
Triangular phase diagram for displaying the composition, in molar percentages, of mixtures of cholesterol, bile salts and lecithin in an aqueous medium containing a fixed proportion of total solids. The point M corresponds to a mixture containing 5 moles % of cholesterol, 15 moles % of lecithin and 80 moles % of bile salt. The curve drawn with a continuous line (the 'saturation curve') shows the maximum solubility of cholesterol in mixtures containing variable molar ratios of bile salt to lecithin. All points lying on the curve correspond to mixtures that are just saturated with cholesterol; points above the curve correspond to mixtures containing more cholesterol than the amount required to saturate the mixture; those below the curve lie within the micellar zone and correspond to mixtures that are unsaturated with cholesterol. Note that the concentration of water, the fourth component in the system, is invariable and is not shown in the diagram. The saturation curve shown in this diagram indicates the maximum solubility of cholesterol in mixtures containing 10% by weight of total solids. A family of saturation curves could be drawn, corresponding to a series of different concentrations of total solid, but the curves would be very similar for concentrations between 5% and 20%. (Adapted from Redinger and Small, 1972.)

Although there is broad agreement as to the maximum solubility of cholesterol in artificial bile-salt/lecithin mixtures, solubilities reported by Hegardt and Dam (1971) and by Mufson *et al.* (1974) are lower than those reported by Admirand and Small (1968). As Carey and Small (1975) have pointed out, minor differences in the position of the line demarcating the micellar zone determined by different workers are to be expected in view of the difficulty in achieving true equilibrium solubility within a reasonable time; under some conditions complete equilibration between cholesterol in the solid and micellar phases may take up to 30 days. In addition to this, the solubility of cholesterol in bile-salt/lecithin mixtures is influenced by temperature and by the presence of ions in the aqueous medium. The nature of the bile salts in the mixture seems to have little influence on cholesterol solubility in the three-component mixture in water (Carey and Small, 1975).

While triangular phase diagrams provide a clear and informative way of showing the composition of a mixture in which the proportions of three components vary, there is also a need for a numerical index indicating, in terms of a single number, the extent to which a given bile sample or artificial mixture is saturated with cholesterol. Metzger *et al.* (1972) have proposed the use of the term 'lithogenic index', which may be defined as the ratio of the *actual amount of cholesterol* present in a given mixture of cholesterol, bile salt and lecithin in water or bile, to the *maximum amount of cholesterol* that could be dissolved in the mixture. Thus, samples with a lithogenic index of 1.0 are just saturated with cholesterol, while those with a lithogenic index greater or less than 1.0 are supersaturated or unsaturated, respectively. Metzger *et al.* (1972) calculated the lithogenic index from the observed composition of the sample and the saturation curve determined by Admirand and Small (1968) from artificial mixtures of cholesterol, bile salt and lecithin in water containing 10% of total solids. As mentioned above, there is some disagreement as to the exact position of the saturation curve for cholesterol. To this extent, there is a degree of arbitrariness in the calculated lithogenic index. However, it is quite legitimate to compare the lithogenic indices of two samples, calculated on the basis of the same saturation curve. Thus, one may say that one sample of bile is more lithogenic than another if it has a higher lithogenic index.

1.3 Conditions required for the formation of cholesterol stones

1.3.1 Bile supersaturated with cholesterol

Cholesterol stones form in the gallbladder when conditions are such that cholesterol in the bile cannot be held in micellar solution by the combined detergent action of lecithin and bile salts. This leads to the precipitation of cholesterol as microcrystals, which eventually coalesce to form macroscopic stones. The sequence of events that leads to the formation of cholesterol stones in the bile is still not fully understood, but there is general agreement that a necessary condition is the presence, in the gallbladder, of bile that is saturated or supersaturated with cholesterol.

The first clear indication for this view was provided by Isaksson (1954), who compared the solubility of cholesterol in artificial bile salt/lecithin mixtures with the composition of gallbladder bile from normal subjects and from patients with cholesterol gallstones. Isaksson showed that cholesterol precipitated from solution if the mass ratio of cholesterol to bile salt plus lecithin was greater than 1:11 and that in the bile of most of his patients this ratio was exceeded, whereas in most normal biles the ratio was less than 1:11. In Isaksson's series of subjects some normal biles had ratios above this value and in some gallstone biles the ratios were normal. However, this is not surprising since the solubility of cholesterol in mixtures of cholesterol, bile salt and lecithin is determined, not by the sum of the concentrations of bile salt and lecithin, but by the proportions of the three components in the mixture, as may be seen by inspection of Fig. 18.1.

Extending these observations, Admirand and Small (1968) determined the composition of uncentrifuged bile obtained at operation from the gallbladders of subjects without gallbladder disease and from those with cholesterol gallstones. When the molar percentages of cholesterol, bile salt and lecithin were plotted as single points on triangular co-ordinates (as in Fig. 18.1), there was complete separation between the normal biles and the biles of gallstone patients. Furthermore, all the normal biles had compositions within the micellar zone determined in artificial mixtures and all the 'gallstone' biles had compositions at or above the limit of the micellar zone. Many of the abnormal biles whose composition was outside the micellar zone contained microcrystals of cholesterol. Admirand and Small concluded that in bile from their patients with cholesterol gallstones the concentration of cholesterol in relation to the concentrations of bile salts and lecithin was such as to produce a supersaturated bile from which cholesterol had precipitated in the gallbladder. Subsequently, Small and Rapo (1970) showed that *hepatic* bile of American Indians with cholesterol gallstones was supersaturated with cholesterol. When these abnormal biles (which were translucent when fresh) were frozen and thawed, cholesterol was precipitated in crystalline form. Small and Rapo concluded that the bile responsible for the formation of cholesterol stones in the gallbladder is produced by the liver and is not formed by modification of normal hepatic bile in the gallbladder. In agreement with this, the hepatic bile of age-matched white subjects without cholesterol stones is unsaturated with cholesterol (Redinger and Small, 1972).

These findings have led Small to put forward the view that the primary event in the production of cholesterol gallstones is the hepatic secretion of bile supersaturated with cholesterol (see Small, 1970 and Redinger and Small, 1972). In addition to the above evidence, based on the study of individual subjects with and without gallstones, Redinger and Small (1972) have pointed out that in different animal species the tendency to form cholesterol gallstones, either spontaneously or under experimental conditions, can be predicted from the concentration of cholesterol relative to the concentrations of bile salts and lecithin in gallbladder bile. Thus, in dogs and pigs, which do not form gallstones, the lithogenic index of the bile is very low. On the other hand, the bile of baboons, a species in which cholesterol stones occur spontaneously, is usually saturated with cholesterol. Epidemiological investigations have also shown that there is a close correlation between the lithogenic index of gallbladder bile and the prevalence of cholesterol gallstones in different populations throughout the world. For example, the Masai, in whom cholesterol gallstones are never found, secrete bile with a lithogenic index of less than 0.5 (Biss et al., 1971), whereas the bile of Swedish and North American Indian women (who have exceptionally high prevalences of cholesterol gallstones) is usually saturated or even supersaturated (Nakayama and Van der Linden, 1971; Thistle and Schoenfield, 1971a).

Although there can be little doubt that the secretion of supersaturated bile is a necessary condition for the precipitation of cholesterol crystals in the gallbladder, the association between gallstone formation and a high lithogenic index determined in a single sample of bile is not invariable. Thus, Dam and Hegardt (1971) could not distinguish gallstone patients from healthy subjects on the basis of the lipid composition of bile, and there are several reports of patients with cholesterol gallstones whose bile, obtained on a single occasion in the fasting state, was not saturated with cholesterol (see, for example, Danzinger et al., 1972). Conversely, in some populations, notably Swedish women and young North American Indian women, a high proportion of subjects without gallstones secrete a bile that is supersaturated with cholesterol. Holzbach et al. (1973) have also reported the frequent occurrence of supersaturated bile in the gallbladders of white Americans without gallstones.

Some of these discrepancies may be due to the fact that the composition of human bile varies throughout the 24-hour cycle. Metzger et al. (1973) have shown that both hepatic bile and gallbladder bile of healthy American white women tend to become saturated with cholesterol after a 12-hour fast and then to become unsaturated when a meal is infused into the duodenum. If the formation of cholesterol crystals in the gallbladder requires the presence of a supersaturated bile for a minimum period of time during the 24-hour cycle, some people may secrete supersaturated bile for short periods without forming gallstones. Another possibility, suggested by Redinger and Small (1972), is that cholesterol stones may take several years to grow to a detectable size and that some individuals with supersaturated gallbladder bile but no evidence of stones may, in fact, be 'incubating' stones. This is probably the explanation of the very high prevalence of supersaturated biles in young American Indian women without evidence of gallstones, since nearly 70% of this population eventually develop stones. Variations in the lithogenicity of bile over the 24 hours, and perhaps over much longer periods, may also explain why samples of normal bile can sometimes be obtained from patients with cholesterol stones.

It should be noted that the frequency of supersaturated bile in some populations with normal biliary tracts, such as the American subjects studied by Holzbach *et al.* (1973), is high enough to raise the suspicion that gallstone formation requires, in addition to a supersaturated bile, the presence of some other factor necessary for the precipitation of cholesterol crystals from metastable micelles, or the absence of a factor that normally maintains the cholesterol of supersaturated bile in micellar solution. This interesting possibility has been discussed by Holzbach *et al.* (1973).

Though not strictly relevant to the present argument, the physiological basis of diurnal variation in bile composition is worth considering at this point. Metzger *et al.* (1973) have suggested that the bile salts secreted during the fasting state are stored in the gallbladder and, hence, are not available for reabsorption from the ileum, and that this results in a reduced rate of secretion of bile salts without a concomitant fall in the rate of hepatic secretion of cholesterol. In agreement with this interpretation, it has been shown that the saturation of bile with cholesterol is inversely related to the rate of secretion of bile salts in monkeys (Dowling *et al.*, 1971) and human subjects (Northfield and Hofmann, 1975). In both species, the bile becomes supersaturated with cholesterol when the rate of secretion of bile salts falls below about 10 μmoles/kg/hour.

1.3.2 Origin of the biliary lipids

Variability in the composition of bile is of interest in relation to the hypothesis that the free cholesterol and phospholipids of bile are derived from the plasma membranes of the cells lining the canaliculi and are washed into the bile by the solvent action of the bile salts (see Small, 1970). In favour of this view, the ratio of free cholesterol to phospholipid remains constant when the rate of secretion of the biliary lipids in bile-fistula rats is varied by infusing bile salts at different rates (Hardison and Francis, 1969). The molar ratio of cholesterol to phospholipid in normal human bile is usually about 0.3, a ratio similar to that found in the plasma membranes of some cells. However, the ratio in human bile varies quite widely during the normal 24-hour cycle. Thus, Metzger *et al.* (1973) have shown that there is a two- to three-fold rise in the cholesterol:phospholipid ratio in the bile of normal and gallstone human subjects during a 6-hour fast. This is difficult to reconcile with the view that the biliary cholesterol and phospholipid are derived from a specific plasma membrane. A further difficulty arises from the fact that lecithin is virtually the only phospholipid of human bile, whereas plasma membranes contain considerable amounts of other phospholipids, particularly sphingomyelin and phosphatidylethanolamine. However, it could be argued that the lipid mixture removed from the plasma membrane by bile salts is not representative of the plasma membrane as a whole. For example, it is conceivable that only the outer leaflet of the bilaminar membrane on the luminal surface of the canalicular cells is exposed to the leaching action of the aqueous solution of bile salts flowing down the canaliculus, and that this portion of the membrane is relatively rich in lecithin. See Evans (1980) for a discussion of heterogeneity in the distribution of phospholipids in hepatocyte plasma membranes.

These speculations concern only the *immediate* origin of the biliary lipids. Gregory *et al.* (1975) have shown that the lipids secreted in the bile of rats are not synthesized in the walls of the canaliculi but are derived from specific compartments of the pools of lecithin and cholesterol in hepatic microsomes; transport of both lipids from the microsomes to the canalicular membrane appears to be very rapid and may possibly be mediated by a cytoplasmic carrier. It should be noted that any hypothesis as to the derivation of the biliary lipids must explain why human bile sometimes becomes supersaturated with cholesterol.

1.3.3 The pathogenesis of supersaturated bile
Secretion of an abnormal bile supersaturated with cholesterol could be due to increased hepatic secretion of cholesterol, decreased hepatic secretion of bile salts or phospholipids, or a combination of each of these abnormalities. Despite the efforts of many investigators over the past decade, there is no general agreement as to the relative importance of these factors in the production of gallstones in man. This is due partly to inconsistencies in the observations reported from different laboratories.

1.3.3.1 **Diminished bile-salt pools.** In patients with choles-

terol gallstones the total amount of bile salt in the enterohepatic circulation is significantly diminished. This was first shown by Vlahcevic et al. (1970), who found that the total bile-salt pool in a group of white American men with gallstones was only about half that in control men without stones. Decreased bile-salt pools have since been reported in other white subjects with cholesterol gallstones (Swell et al., 1970; Danzinger et al., 1973; Pomare and Heaton, 1973) and in North American Indian women with cholesterol stones or with supersaturated bile but no stones (Vlahcevic et al., 1972). It is now generally accepted that the bile-salt pool is almost invariably diminished in patients with cholesterol stones and a functioning gallbladder, though there is disagreement as to the cause of this abnormality.

In the American Indian women with gallstones studied by Vlahcevic et al. (1972) the fractional rates of turnover of the pools of cholic acid and chenodeoxycholic acid were markedly increased. Since the fractional rate of turnover of a bile-salt pool is a function of the fraction lost by excretion at each enterohepatic cycle and the number of cycles per day, Vlahcevic et al. concluded (on the reasonable assumption that the cycling frequency was normal in their patients) that the efficiency of reabsorption of bile salts from the ileum is decreased in patients with cholesterol gallstones. Defective reabsorption of bile salts from the intestine would be expected to lead to a compensatory increase in bile-acid synthesis, as in patients with ileal disease or in those given cholestyramine. However, bile-acid synthesis was normal in American Indian women with gallstones and was decreased in the American men with gallstones investigated by Vlahcevic et al. They therefore concluded (Vlahcevic et al., 1972) that the decreased bile-salt pool in their gallstone patients was due to the presence of two abnormalities—defective ileal reabsorption of bile salts and an inability on the part of the liver to increase bile-acid synthesis to a rate sufficient to compensate for increased excretion. This combination of abnormalities would lead to a steady state in which the mass of bile salt in the enterohepatic circulation was decreased. On this interpretation, feedback inhibition of bile-acid synthesis in the liver of the gallstone patient comes into play at an abnormally low bile-salt pool size; there is no question of an intrinsic incapacity of the liver to make bile acids at the normal rate, since the maximal capacity for bile-acid synthesis during complete interruption of the enterohepatic circulation is normal in patients with gallstones (Small et al., 1972).

1.3.3.2 Secretion rates of biliary lipids. Essentially the same conclusions were reached by Grundy et al. (1972) on the basis of observations on the secretion of biliary lipids in women with and without cholesterol stones. Grundy and his coworkers found that in

American Indian women with cholesterol stones, the hourly secretion of bile salts into the duodenum was decreased and the hourly secretion of cholesterol was increased, in comparison with the corresponding rates of secretion in white women without stones. Obesity (known to be associated with increased biliary secretion of cholesterol) was more frequent in the Indian women than in the white women, but these differences were significant even when the rates were expressed in terms of a standard body weight. Grundy et al. (1972) concluded that the formation of a highly lithogenic bile in Indian women with cholesterol stones is due to a combination of decreased bile-salt secretion and increased cholesterol secretion in the bile.

Sterol balance measurements showed that in the Indian women with gallstones, whole-body synthesis of cholesterol was increased, while bile-acid synthesis was normal. The daily faecal output of bile acids in the Indian women was equal to, or greater than, that in the white women without stones. Since the flux of bile salts into the intestine was reduced in the Indian women, their ability to reabsorb bile salts must have been impaired. Thus, the sterol balance measurements agreed with the earlier findings of Vlahcevic et al. (1972) in pointing to a diminished capacity of the liver to compensate for diminished reabsorption of bile salts by the intestine. Grundy et al. suggested that the increased biliary secretion of cholesterol was due to increased hepatic synthesis. In keeping with this, there is evidence to suggest that HMG-CoA reductase activity in the livers of patients with cholesterol gallstones is greater than that in the livers of normal subjects (Salen et al., 1975; Coyne et al., 1976; Maton et al., 1979). It has also been reported that the activity of cholesterol 7α-hydroxylase is decreased in the livers of gallstone patients (Nicolau et al., 1974; Coyne et al., 1976). However, this is difficult to reconcile with the lack of consistent evidence for an absolute decrease in the rate of bile-acid synthesis in gallstone patients.

These observations suggested that the formation of lithogenic bile in patients with gallstones is brought about by a reduction in the biliary secretion of bile salts secondary to a fall in the total mass of bile salts in the enterohepatic circulation, combined with an increase in cholesterol secretion in the bile, due possibly to increased hepatic synthesis of cholesterol. The inference that a reduction in the bile-salt pool would favour the formation of lithogenic bile was based on experimental observations on animals and human subjects showing that a controlled decrease in the availability of bile salts in the enterohepatic circulation led to a decrease in the biliary secretion of bile salts and phospholipids without a proportionate decrease in cholesterol secretion (Thureborn, 1962; Swell and Bell, 1968; Scherstén et al., 1971; Small et al., 1972).

With regard to the mechanisms responsible for the small bile-salt pool in patients with cholesterol gallstones, it should be noted that a minor impairment in the reabsorption of bile salts, such as that observed by Grundy *et al.* (1972) in American Indian women with gallstones, would not, by itself, be enough to affect the size of the pool in normal subjects, since the increased loss of bile salts would be balanced by increased bile-acid synthesis. This may be seen from the fact that cholestyramine does not diminish the size of the bile-salt pool (Kenney and Garbutt, 1970) and does not promote the secretion of lithogenic bile (Wood *et al.*, 1972) in normal human subjects; it is only when there is severe malabsorption of bile salts, as in ileal disease, that the reduction in the bile-salt pool is sufficient to cause gallstones (Pomare and Heaton, 1973). For this reason it has generally been assumed that in patients with cholesterol gallstones without overt disease of the small bowel the regulation of bile-acid synthesis by feedback inhibition is abnormal. This assumption seems reasonable, but it has never been tested experimentally.

The view that decreased biliary secretion of bile salts is an essential factor in the formation of lithogenic bile in gallstone patients has been challenged by Northfield and Hofmann (1975), who found normal rates of secretion of all three biliary lipids in a group of white men and women with cholesterol gallstones and functioning gallbladders. In these patients, the cycling frequency of the bile salts in the enterohepatic circulation was inversely proportional to the size of the bile-salt pool, so that the rate of secretion of bile salts remained more or less constant despite variability in pool size. Northfield and Hofmann (1975) suggested that a major determinant of the small bile-salt pool in patients with cholesterol stones is an increased cycling frequency of the pool, due possibly to overactive emptying of the gallbladder in response to meals. This, they argued, would produce a steady state in which the pool size was diminished but hepatic synthesis of bile acids was normal (since the absolute rate at which bile salts returned to the liver would be normal). On this view, the major functional abnormality in the gallstone patient lies in the gallbladder rather than the liver. Northfield and Hofmann suggested that the difference between their observations and those of Grundy *et al.* (1972) was due to a difference in the racial origin of the two groups of patients and the presence of obesity in the American Indian women, the latter providing an adequate explanation for increased biliary secretion of cholesterol.

Although more recent work has, in general, confirmed the importance of a functioning gallbladder in the genesis of cholesterol stones, it now seems clear that bile-salt secretion rates are, in fact, significantly decreased in non-obese white patients with cholesterol stones. On the other hand, in obese subjects (who are unusually prone to gallstone formation) the biliary secretion of cholesterol is markedly increased, while that of bile salts is decreased only when expressed in terms of body weight (Shaffer and Small, 1977). Furthermore, in contrast to the findings of Northfield and Hofmann (1975), Shaffer and Small (1977) found normal cycling frequencies of the bile salt pool in patients with cholesterol stones and in obese subjects with lithogenic bile but no gallstones.

These findings suggest that the immediate cause of the secretion of lithogenic bile is not the same in all groups of subjects. In non-obese whites, lithogenicity is usually associated with decreased secretion of bile salts and lecithin, whereas in obese subjects, including American Indian women, the major abnormality seems to be increased secretion of cholesterol. The increased biliary secretion of cholesterol in obese subjects is presumably a reflection of increased hepatic synthesis of cholesterol, but we still require an explanation of the decreased secretion of bile salts in those patients in whom this is the cause of the lithogenic bile. Thus, in the light of current knowledge, cholesterol gallstone disease may be classified tentatively in terms of functional abnormalities of the enterohepatic circulation, as shown in Table 18.1.

1.3.3.3 Effect of removing the gallbladder. A possible clue to the cause of decreased bile-salt secretion is provided by the effect of surgical removal of the gallbladder on the lipid composition of the bile in non-obese patients with cholesterol stones. Shaffer and Small (1977) have shown that in these patients cholecystectomy increases the rate of secretion of bile salt and phospholipid, without causing a significant change in cholesterol secretion. The net result is therefore

Table 18.1
Possible abnormalities underlying the secretion of lithogenic bile

Change in biliary secretion	Associated or underlying abnormality
1. Primary decrease in bile-salt secretion.	Small bile-salt pool. Possibly due to faulty feedback control of bile-acid synthesis.
2. Secondary decrease in bile-salt secretion.	Small bile-salt pool due to malabsorption caused by ileal disease.
3. Primary increase in cholesterol secretion.	Common in obesity. Possibly due to oversynthesis of cholesterol in the liver.
4. Combined 1 and 3.	? Genetic, as in American Indian women.
5. Secondary increase in cholesterol secretion.	Mobilization of excess stores of tissue cholesterol during treatment with clofibrate or diets with very high P/S fat ratio.

P/S = polyunsaturated/saturated (see Chapter 14, Section 3.3.)

a marked decrease in the lithogenic index of hepatic bile. The increased rate of secretion of bile salts and phospholipid is due to an increased cycling frequency of the bile-salt pool. This suggests that in the presence of a functioning gallbladder the cycling frequency of the bile salts is maintained at the normal, relatively low rate, owing to retention of bile in the gallbladder during periods of fasting. Since the bile-salt pool is reduced, perhaps because of an abnormality in the regulation of bile-acid synthesis, secretion of bile salts is also reduced. When the storage effect of the gallbladder is abolished by cholecystectomy, the cycling frequency increases so that the effect of the small pool on bile-salt secretion rate is largely nullified. This interpretation of the effects of removal of the gallbladder on the composition of the bile is supported by the observation that the lithogenicity of the bile of patients with cholesterol stones decreases when the gallbladder becomes non-functional (Redinger, 1976).

1.4 Medical treatment of gallstones

1.4.1 Background

The idea that gallstones might be dissolved within the gallbladder by changing the composition of the bile has been discussed from time to time since the beginning of the present century, but it is only recently that this possibility has been explored systematically. Rewbridge (1937) succeeded in bringing about the disappearance (presumably by dissolution) of cholesterol stones in two patients by the daily administration of a bile-salt mixture. However, apart from a few sporadic observations, such as the demonstration that human cholesterol stones would dissolve if they were put into the gall bladders of dogs and other animals (see Johnston and Nakayama (1957) for a review of the relevant literature), Rewbridge's observation was largely ignored for many years. Interest in the problem was reawakened when it became clear that the formation of cholesterol stones requires the presence of supersaturated bile in the gallbladder, with the corollary that it should be possible to dissolve the stones *in vivo* by making the bile unsaturated with cholesterol. Using this new approach, Thistle and Schoenfield (1971*b*) showed that the oral administration of chenodeoxycholic acid, but not of cholic acid, decreased the lithogenicity of the bile of women with cholesterol stones. Needless to say, the patients on whom this trial was carried out were symptom-free and therefore did not necessarily require surgical removal of their gallbladders.

1.4.2 Dissolution of cholesterol stones by chenodeoxycholic acid

1.4.2.1 The clinical response. The observation that chenodeoxycholic acid would cause the bile of gallstone patients to become unsaturated with cholesterol was quickly followed by the demonstration that chenodeoxycholate, given in large daily doses for many months, brings about the partial or complete dissolution of cholesterol stones in a high proportion of patients (Danzinger et al., 1972; Bell et al., 1972).

More extensive clinical trials have since shown that chenodeoxycholic acid in doses of 15 mg/kg/day will dissolve cholesterol stones in most patients in whom the gallbladder functions normally (Dowling, 1977). Cholic acid, on the other hand, appears to have no effect on cholesterol stones (Thistle and Hofmann, 1973). Dissolution of gallstones by chenodeoxycholic acid usually takes at least six months and may take up to two years. Judged from the results of 'chenotherapy' in patients who have been treated for at least two years, chenodeoxycholic acid is without serious side-effects when given in the doses required for gallstone dissolution. However, it remains to be shown that the treatment would be without harmful effects on the liver and intestinal mucosa if it was continued throughout the life of the patient. Many patients have dose-related diarrhoea during chenotherapy and in some there is a mild, but usually transient, rise in liver enzymes in the serum. In experimental animals, including baboons (Morrissey et al., 1975) and monkeys (Webster et al., 1975), chenodeoxycholic acid in doses similar to those used for gallstone dissolution in human subjects is toxic to the liver. This is due to the effect of lithocholic acid formed by the bacterial 7α-dehydroxylation of chenodeoxycholate in the animal intestine. Lithocholic acid is also formed from chenodeoxycholic acid in man, but is rapidly converted into the sulphate ester and, in this form, is excreted in the faeces (Allan et al., 1976). Thus, the lack of toxicity of chenodeoxycholic acid in man, in contrast to its marked toxicity in non-human primates, seems to be due to the presence of a more efficient system for sulphating lithocholate in the human body than in animals.

Bile salts absorbed from the intestine suppress the conversion of cholesterol into bile acid by inhibiting cholesterol 7α-hydroxylase (see Chapter 5). As discussed below, chenodeoxycholate also decreases the rate of secretion of cholesterol in the bile. These effects might be expected to favour the accumulation of cholesterol in the plasma and tissues of patients undergoing chenotherapy. However, no increases in plasma cholesterol concentration or in the mass of exchangeable cholesterol in the whole body have been observed in patients treated with chenodeoxycholic acid for periods of up to six months (Thistle *et al.*, 1973; Pedersen *et al.*, 1974). The possibility that chenotherapy may have an unfavourable effect on whole-body metabolism of cholesterol when continued for many years obviously cannot be excluded by these negative observations.

Owing to its effectiveness in dissolving cholesterol gallstones and its comparative safety (at least in the short term), chenotherapy provides an alternative to surgery in the treatment of selected forms of gallstone disease. As yet, there is no general agreement as to the indications for this form of treatment (see Dowling, 1977). One important question that needs to be answered is that of the speed and frequency of recurrence of gallstones that have been dissolved by chenotherapy. If recurrence is the rule rather than the exception, then it may be necessary to maintain the treatment throughout the life of the patient. In this case, one would need to balance the disadvantages of life-long medical treatment against the potential hazards of surgery.

1.4.2.2 The mechanism of action of chenotherapy.

When chenodeoxycholic acid is administered to gallstone patients in therapeutic doses, the biliary cholic and deoxycholic acids are almost completely replaced by chenodeoxycholate, and substantial amounts of sulphated lithocholic and ursodeoxycholic acids appear in the bile (Danzinger *et al.*, 1973; Salen *et al.*, 1974); ursodeoxycholate (the 7β-epimer of chenodeoxycholate) is a metabolite of chenodeoxycholate and is probably derived from its precursor *via* the formation of 7-ketolithocholic acid by bacteria in the intestine (Fig. 18.2). In addition to these changes in the composition of the bile, there is an increase in the size of the pool of chenodeoxycholic acid and a decrease in the pool size of cholic and deoxycholic acids, the net effect being an increase in the pool of total bile salts in the enterohepatic circulation. The increase in the size of the bile-salt pool may contribute to the decreased lithogenicity of the bile, already referred to (Section 1.3.3), but it cannot be the whole explanation, since the administration of cholic acid to patients with cholesterol stones also increases the bile-salt pool (La Russo *et al.*, 1975) but has no effect on the lithogenic index of the bile (Thistle and Schoenfield, 1971*b*) and does not promote the dissolution of gallstones (Thistle and Hofmann, 1973). The explanation for the specific effect of chenodeoxycholate on the lithogenicity of the bile in gallstone patients seems to be that it decreases the rate of secretion of cholesterol in the bile without a corresponding fall in bile-salt or phospholipid secretion, whereas cholic acid has no effect on cholesterol secretion (La Russo *et al.*, 1975). It has been suggested that chenodeoxycholic acid decreases the biliary secretion of cholesterol by inhibiting hepatic HMG-CoA reductase (Coyne *et al.*, 1976). However, it has yet to be shown that this enzyme in human liver is more readily inhibited by chenodeoxycholic acid than by cholic acid.

1.4.3 Other forms of medical treatment

Other attempts to dissolve cholesterol stones in man include the use of phenobarbital, ursodeoxycholic acid and wheat-bran.

Phenobarbital has been reported to diminish the lithogenic index of the bile in monkeys (Redinger and Small, 1973), possibly by stimulating the synthesis of bile acids. However, phenobarbital does not have a favourable effect on the lithogenic index of human bile (Mok and Dowling, quoted in Mok et al., 1974).

Like chenodeoxycholic acid, ursodeoxycholic acid (see Fig. 18.2) decreases the lithogenicity of the bile in human subjects and dissolves cholesterol gallstones (Makino et al., 1975). It appears to have several

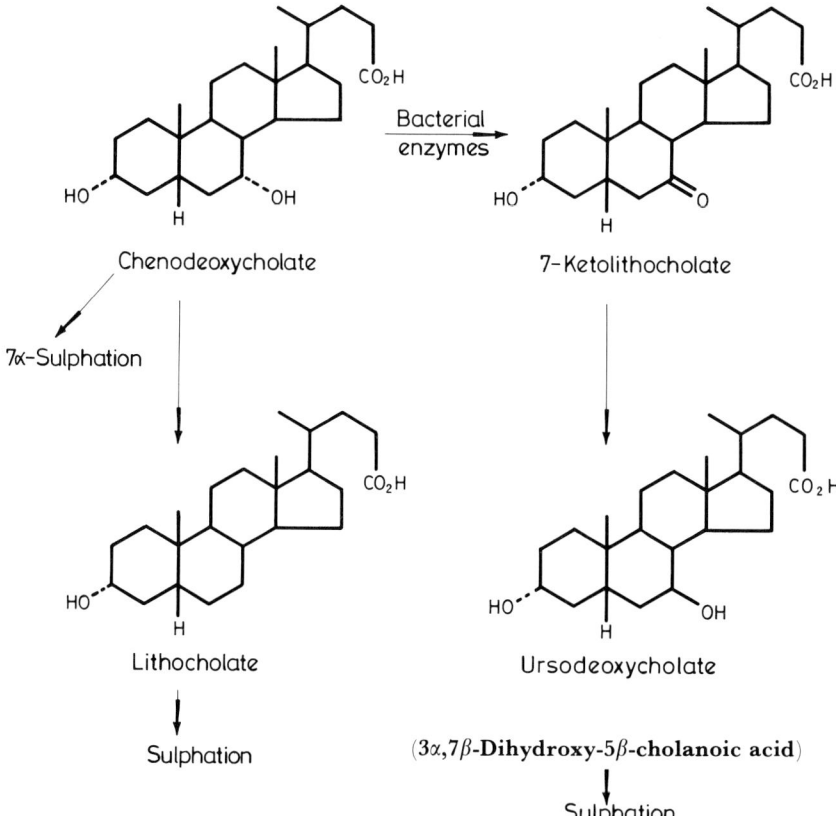

Figure 18.2
Products of the metabolism of chenodeoxycholic acid in patients treated by 'chenotherapy' for cholesterol gallstones. Conjugation is ignored in this Fig.

advantages over chenodeoxycholate as a therapeutic agent. In particular, it is effective in smaller doses, it takes less time to dissolve gallstones (Nakagawa et al., 1977), it does not cause the release of liver enzymes into the plasma and it has less tendency than chenodeoxycholic acid to cause diarrhoea. In keeping with its milder effect on lower-bowel function, Chadwick et al. (1979) have shown that ursodeoxycholic acid, unlike chenodeoxycholic acid, does not damage the rabbit's colonic mucosa. If these apparent advantages are confirmed by more prolonged and extensive clinical trials than have yet been carried out, ursodeoxycholic acid could well become the bile acid of choice for the medical treatment of cholesterol stones. However, the cost of manufacturing ursodeoxycholic acid is at present such that its use in the treatment of gallstones is more expensive than that of chenodeoxycholic acid. Why ursodeoxycholic acid should be more efficient than chenodeoxycholic acid in the dissolution of cholesterol stones is a question that has been much discussed but has not yet been resolved. Experiments in vitro suggest that ursodeoxycholate is not as efficient as chenodeoxycholate in forming a micellar solution of cholesterol in the presence of lecithin (Carey et al., 1977). This raises the possibility that the reason for the greater therapeutic efficiency of ursodeoxycholic is that it has a more favourable effect on some physiological factor such as bile-salt pool size or hepatic synthesis of cholesterol.

Pomare et al. (1975) have shown that the feeding of very large amounts of wheat-bran to patients with radiolucent gallstones decreases the degree of saturation of the bile with cholesterol. Bran has not been shown to dissolve gallstones, but Pomare et al. suggest that it might help to prevent the recurrence of stones after chenotherapy.

1.5 Experimental gallstones in animals

A great deal of work has been done on the production of cholesterol gallstones in animals by the feeding of abnormal diets or the administration of drugs in the expectation that this would throw light on the mechanisms responsible for the spontaneous formation of gallstones in man. Although the results of this work have not been without relevance to the gallstone problem, it must be admitted that most of what we know about the formation of human gallstones and about the conditions required for their dissolution has been derived from clinical studies. An account of the experimental production of cholesterol gallstones in nonhuman primates will be found in the review by Portman et al. (1975); Dam has also discussed gallstone formation in nonprimates, particularly in the hamster, a species on which he and his associates have worked for many years (Dam, 1971).

As we have already seen, the molar concentration of cholesterol in animal bile varies very widely between different species. For example, in guinea-pig bile there is virtually no cholesterol, whereas the lithogenic index of the bile of baboons is close to the saturation curve of Admirand and Small (1968). Corresponding to these differences, there are considerable species differences in the ease with which cholesterol stones can be produced by experimental means. In general, spontaneous cholesterol gallstones are rare in animals, whether in the wild state or in captivity, or living under domestication. The exception to this general rule seems to be the baboon. Cholesterol stones have been reported in *Papio anubis* and *P. cynocephalus* and in a high proportion of captive female baboons (McSherry et al., 1972).

Cholesterol stones have been produced in many species of monkey, usually by feeding semipurified diets with a high content of saturated fat and enriched with cholesterol. Portman et al. (1975), for example, were able to produce cholesterol stones in about 50% of adult squirrel monkeys by feeding a butter-fat diet containing 1% of cholesterol for 6 months. Cholesterol gallstones have also been produced by dietary means in hamsters, dogs, prairie dogs, mice and rabbits (see Portman et al., 1975).

Certain aspects of gallstone formation in hamsters and rabbits are worth mentioning briefly. Dam et al. (see Dam, 1971) have shown that it is possible to produce cholesterol stones in the gallbladders of 80–100% of young hamsters by feeding them a diet containing no polyunsaturated fat and a high proportion of glucose or sucrose. The addition of cholesterol to diets is not necessary for gallstone formation in hamsters; indeed, Dam et al. (1968) found that when the diet was enriched with cholesterol, the incidence of gallstone formation was diminished. This paradoxical effect may be due to inhibition of the hepatic synthesis of cholesterol by the fed cholesterol (Dam, 1971). Gallstones containing a high proportion of cholesterol can be produced in rabbits by feeding them diets containing 40% of casein, but the stones produced by dietary manipulation in rabbits tend to contain high percentages of allo bile acids. Of particular interest is the observation of Hofmann and Mosbach (1964) that rabbits fed 5α-cholestanol form gallstones consisting almost entirely of allodeoxycholic acid conjugated with glycine.

Cholestyramine induces the formation of cholesterol stones in guinea-pigs fed a pellet diet (Schoenfield and Sjövall, 1966). However, when cholestyramine is added to a fat-free glucose diet fed to young hamsters, the incidence of cholesterol-rich gallstones is reduced and stones that have already formed are dissolved (Bergman and Van der Linden, 1967). Clofibrate inhibits the formation of diet-induced cholesterol stones in young hamsters, possibly by suppressing cholesterol synthesis in the liver (Dam, 1971).

In general, diets that produce cholesterol gallstones in animals of a given species also increase the lithogenic index of gallbladder bile, usually by increasing the molar percentage of cholesterol without changing the ratio of phospholipids to bile salts (Dam, 1971). Osuga and Portman (1972) have demonstrated a close correlation between the lithogenic index of gallbladder bile, the presence of microcrystals of cholesterol in the bile and the incidence of cholesterol stones in individual squirrel monkeys fed lithogenic diets.

2 THE PLASMA CHOLESTEROL IN LIVER DISEASE

The presence of abnormal lipoproteins and of an abnormal lipid pattern in the plasma of patients with liver disease has been mentioned in Chapters 11 and 16. In this section I shall deal more fully with the effects of obstructive and parenchymatous disease of the liver on cholesterol metabolism, especially in relation to the plasma and the blood cells.

2.1 Biliary obstruction

2.1.1 The plasma lipids and lipoproteins

Biliary obstruction, whether intrahepatic or extrahepatic, is often accompanied by hypercholesterolaemia and an increased plasma phospholipid concentration. The plasma triglyceride concentration may be normal or slightly increased. Hyperphospholipidaemia is due to the presence of increased amounts of lecithin, with no consistent changes in the plasma concentrations of other phospholipids (Petersen, 1953); the hypercholesterolaemia is due largely to a rise in plasma free cholesterol concentration. There is usually a fall in the ratio of esterified to free cholesterol in the plasma, but changes in the absolute concentration of plasma cholesteryl ester are variable. If the degree of obstruction is mild, the concentration remains normal or may even increase. However, in severe chronic obstruction the cholesteryl ester concentration falls, leading to a marked decrease in the ratio of esterified to total cholesterol in the plasma (Table 18.2).

The fall in plasma cholesteryl ester concentration in severe biliary obstruction is thought to be due to decreased plasma LCAT activity resulting from damage to the liver cells responsible for the synthesis and secretion of the enzyme (Gjone and Norum, 1970; McIntyre *et al.*, 1975). The suggestion that diminished cholesterol-esterifying activity in the plasma of some patients with obstruction is due to an inhibitory effect of bile salts in the plasma on the esterification reaction (Cooper and Jandl, 1968) has not been substantiated (Gjone and Blomhoff, 1970).

The low plasma LCAT activity in severe biliary obstruction, in

Table 18.2
Plasma lipid concentrations in obstructive and parenchymatous liver disease

	Cholesterol (mg/100 ml)				Phospholipid (mg/100 ml)		Triglyceride (mg/100 ml)
	Total	Free	Esterified	% Esterified	Total	Lecithin	
Normal	200–250	60	165	73	150–300	70–100	30–150
Biliary obstruction	250–600	110–500	30–150	20–70	300–700	200–600	100–300
Chronic parenchymatous	120–400	25–150	75–200	5–50	150–350	100–200	50–250

(Values assembled from Gjone and Norum (1970) and other sources.)

addition to causing a fall in plasma cholesteryl ester concentration, also results in the appearance of abnormal lipoproteins in the plasma similar to those seen in familial LCAT deficiency (see Chapter 16). The most striking of these are the lipoprotein particles known as LP-X (Seidel et al., 1969). Under the electron microscope these particles appear as discoidal structures 400–600 Å in diameter and about 100 Å thick (Hamilton et al., 1971); they are thought to exist in the plasma as vesicles enclosed by continuous bilayers of equimolar amounts of free cholesterol and phospholipid in association with small quantities of protein, triglyceride and esterified cholesterol. The precise conditions necessary for the appearance of LP-X in obstructive jaundice are not entirely clear. Although LP-X particles are detectable in the plasma of most patients with obstruction, they are not present in all such patients (Magnani and Alaupovic, 1976). Moreover, Ritland et al. (1973) have shown that LP-X may appear in the plasma of obstructed patients in whom plasma LCAT activity is normal. Possibly, LP-X forms in the plasma when there is a relative deficiency of LCAT, due either to decreased LCAT activity, or to a very marked increase in the entry of free cholesterol and lecithin into the plasma, or to a combination of both.

Patients with LCAT deficiency secondary to biliary obstruction have low plasma HDL concentrations, and electron microscopy of the HDL density fraction may reveal the presence of abnormal stacked bilaminar discs 150–250 Å in diameter and 40 Å thick, similar to the nascent HDL particles discussed in Chapter 11 (Forte et al., 1974).

2.1.2 The cause of the hypercholesterolaemia

Several explanations have been suggested for the hypercholesterolaemia of biliary obstruction. They may all contain an element of the truth.

The marked deficiency of LCAT in severely obstructed patients almost certainly contributes to the increased plasma concentration of free cholesterol and phospholipid in these patients, but it cannot be the whole explanation, since the degree of hypercholesterolaemia in biliary obstruction may greatly exceed that in familial LCAT deficiency, a condition in which there is usually a total absence of LCAT. Moreover, hypercholesterolaemia may be present in some patients with obstruction in whom LCAT activity is normal (Ritland et al., 1973).

Epstein (1932) suggested many years ago that a major factor in causing the hypercholesterolaemia is the reflux of cholesterol from ruptured bile canaliculi into the plasma. Backflow of biliary lipid into the plasma may well be a necessary event in the development of hypercholesterolaemia in human biliary obstruction, but the idea that the excess of lipid in the plasma is due simply to the addition of the biliary lipid mixture to the plasma must be an oversimplification, since the ratio of excess cholesterol to phospholipid in the plasma of obstructed patients is much greater than the cholesterol:phospholipid ratio in human bile. A more plausible explanation is suggested by the observation that intravenous infusions of lecithin into experimental animals cause hypercholesterolaemia and increased hepatic synthesis of cholesterol (Friedman and Byers, 1957; Jakoi and Quarfordt, 1974). The hypercholesterolaemia induced by intravenous lecithin is probably due to withdrawal of free cholesterol from the plasma membranes of tissue cells into the bilayers of phospholipid vesicles present in the lecithin emulsions; stimulation of cholesterol synthesis in the liver may be a response to withdrawal of cholesterol from the hepatocytes (Jakoi and Quarfordt, 1974).

On the basis of these observations it is reasonable to suppose that when the biliary tree is obstructed, biliary lecithin and free cholesterol enter the circulation and that the lecithin and cholesterol form particles which take up more cholesterol from the tissues until the cholesterol:phospholipid molar ratio is approximately 1.0, i.e. the particles acquire the lipid composition of LP-X. This explanation is in keeping with the fact that lecithin is the major phospholipid in human bile and is also the major phospholipid present in excess in the plasma patients with obstructive jaundice. Increased hepatic synthesis of cholesterol may also contribute to the hypercholesterolaemia, though there is little direct evidence to suggest that cholesterol synthesis in the liver is increased in human biliary obstruction. With regard to the mechanism by which LP-X is formed from biliary lipids, the above hypothesis implies that the lipid composition of the fully-formed particle is determined by events taking place within the plasma. However, Manzato *et al.* (1976) have isolated from human bile an albumin-containing lipoprotein that contains free cholesterol and phospholipid in a ratio closely similar to that in LP-X. They suggest that this lipoprotein is a precursor of LP-X and that in biliary obstruction the LP-X precursor enters the bloodstream, where it is converted into LP-X by uptake of additional protein from the plasma.

Whatever the mechanism by which reflux of biliary lipids contributes to the formation of LP-X, the leaching out of cholesterol from cell membranes by phospholipid clearly cannot be the sole source of the excess of plasma free cholesterol in obstructive liver disease, since the cholesterol content of red blood cells, and probably of other cells (see next section), is *increased* rather than *decreased*. Even if the initial events involve a shift of cholesterol from cell membranes into plasma, in established obstructive jaundice there must be a net increase in the amount of free cholesterol in the plasma-cell membrane system owing to failure to dispose of lipids derived from surface material of triglyceride-rich particles in the presence of LCAT deficiency. An additional source of free cholesterol may be increased synthesis in the tissues in response to withdrawal of cholesterol into the plasma.

2.1.3 The lipid composition of blood cells

In many patients with obstructive liver disease the lipid composition of the red cells is abnormal (Table 18.3). The amounts of cholesterol and lecithin per red cell increase without a significant change in the red-cell content of other phospholipids. The percentage increase in cholesterol exceeds that in lecithin, so that the molar ratio of cholesterol to phospholipid is increased. The increase in cholesterol content of the red-cell membrane leads to an increase in surface area without change in cell volume. The expanded surface area of the red cells decreases their osmotic fragility and causes them to adopt an abnormal shape. In wet preparations the cells appear bowl-shaped and in dried smears they have an increased diameter and are 'targeted'; hence the name 'target cells'.

These changes in lipid composition and appearance are reversed when the biliary obstruction is relieved. Cooper and Jandl (1968) have also shown that normal red cells take up free cholesterol and are converted into target cells when they are incubated *in vitro* with serum from a patient with biliary obstruction. These observations suggest that the abnormal red cells in patients with obstructive jaundice acquire their excess of cholesterol and lecithin by reversible uptake from the plasma lipoproteins, analogous to the changes in composition of red-cell lipids that can be brought about by incubating normal red cells in the presence of cholesterol/phospholipid vesicles containing varying proportions of cholesterol (Cooper *et al.*, 1975). However, the conditions required for the production of target cells in obstructed patients are not fully understood. Nor is it clear why some patients with liver disease have target cells in their blood while others have the cholesterol-enriched spur cells discussed in Section 2.2.

As discussed above, many patients with obstructive jaundice have diminished plasma LCAT activity, and this is likely to be an important factor in promoting the transfer of free cholesterol and lecithin to the red-cell membrane, possibly *via* the formation of LP-X. In support of this, Verkleij *et al.* (1976) have shown that LP-X particles fuse with red cells and thus increase their membrane surface area. Cooper *et al.* (1972) failed to find a significant negative correlation between LCAT activity and the cholesterol content of red cells in biliary obstruction. However, it is arguable that what matters is not the absolute level of LCAT activity in the plasma, but the presence of a *relative* deficiency sufficient to permit the accumulation of lipoproteins in the plasma with an abnormally high free cholesterol:phospholipid ratio when there is a pathological influx of free cholesterol and lecithin into the circulation. Nevertheless, the

Table 18.3
Lipid composition of abnormal red cells in liver disease

	Lipid content (μg/10⁸ cells)				Molar ratio	
	Cholesterol	Phospholipid (total)	Lecithin	Other phospholipid	Cholesterol / Phospholipid	Cholesterol / Lecithin
Normal RBC	12.2	29.6	9.5	20.1	0.83	2.59
Target cells in biliary obstruction	18.1	37.0	16.7	20.3	0.98	2.17
Spur cells in non-obstructive liver disease	20.9	32.2	11.5	20.7	1.30	3.64

'Other phospholipid' includes sphingomyelin, phosphatidyl ethanolamine and phosphatidyl serine. Reported normal values differ slightly from one laboratory to another. (Assembled from Cooper, 1970.)

presence of LP-X cannot be essential for the formation of red cells with an abnormally high cholesterol content, because spur cells, which have even more cholesterol than target cells (Table 18.3), can appear in the circulation in the absence of LP-X.

Cooper and Jandl (1968) have suggested that an additional factor in the enrichment of red cells with cholesterol in obstructive liver disease is the ability of bile salts to promote the bulk transfer of free cholesterol from serum lipoproteins to red cells. However, it seems unlikely that the plasma bile-salt concentration in many obstructed patients is high enough to influence the partition of cholesterol between plasma and red cells (Cooper *et al.*, 1975).

In addition to changes in the lipid composition of the red-cell membrane in obstructive liver disease, qualitatively similarly changes may occur in the total lipids of the platelets in peripheral blood (Owen *et al.*, 1978). There is an increase in the cholesterol:phospholipid molar ratio and in the lecithin:sphingomyelin ratio. The possible effects of these changes on platelet membrane function and on platelet aggregation in response to adrenaline and ADP *in vitro* have been discussed by Owen *et al.* (1978).

2.1.4 Xanthomas in biliary obstruction

In severe biliary obstruction associated with marked hyperlipidaemia, xanthomas may appear in the skin. They may be quite limited in distribution, occurring mainly around the eyelids. However, in the acute attacks of primary biliary cirrhosis (a condition associated with generalized inflammation of the bile canaliculi) and in congenital atresia of the bile ducts, the skin lesions may be widespread (Ahrens and Kunkel, 1949). In these conditions, the patient may develop planar, tuberous and tubero-eruptive xanthomas, especially on the trunk, elbows, knees, buttocks and palms. The palmar lesions may include xanthomatous nodules distributed along the creases. Xanthomas in the peripheral nerves have also been described in patients with primary biliary cirrhosis (Thomas and Walker, 1965).

The plasma lipoprotein fraction responsible for the development of skin xanthomas in biliary obstruction is not known. In a study of 18 patients with primary biliary cirrhosis, Ahrens and Kunkel (1949) found that in all of those who developed xanthomas the plasma free-cholesterol and phospholipid concentrations were raised. However, it seems unlikely that LP-X is involved in xanthoma formation, since skin xanthomas do not occur in the presence of the high plasma LP-X concentrations seen in familial LCAT deficiency.

2.2 Parenchymatous liver disease

2.2.1 Plasma lipids and lipoproteins

In patients with parenchymatous liver disease the plasma total cholesterol concentration tends to be low and the plasma lipoprotein pattern is often abnormal. Table 18.2 shows representative values for plasma lipid concentrations in non-obstructive liver disease, compiled mainly from reports of patients in whom the disease was chronic.

In the presence of acute hepatocellular damage due to alcohol, drug poisoning or viral hepatitis the plasma cholesteryl ester concentration usually falls to very low levels, esterified cholesterol sometimes comprising less than 5% of the total cholesterol in plasma. The plasma phospholipid and free cholesterol concentrations may be normal or increased. Plasma triglyceride concentrations are variable but are usually increased; the very marked hypertriglyceridaemia that sometimes occurs in acute alcoholism is not necessarily a consequence of hepatocellular injury.

In chronic parenchymatous disease of the liver, similar but less marked changes are usually seen. Some of these changes are illustrated in Table 18.2.

The low plasma cholesteryl ester concentration is associated with diminished LCAT activity, presumably a consequence of failure of the damaged hepatocytes to synthesize the enzyme (Simon and Sheig, 1970). During recovery from acute alcoholic hepatitis there is a parallel rise in plasma LCAT activity and cholesteryl ester concentration (Ragland et al., 1978).

Changes in the plasma lipoprotein pattern include a reduction in VLDL concentration, a low cholesteryl-ester concentration in all lipoproteins obtained in the fasting state and the presence of stacked bilaminar discs in the HDL density fraction similar to those present in the plasma of patients with familial LCAT deficiency (Ragland et al., 1978). Despite the very low levels of LCAT activity in parenchymatous liver disease, LP-X is seldom detectable in the plasma.

2.2.2 The lipid composition of blood cells

The lipid composition of the red cells is altered in many patients with non-obstructive liver disease. The cholesterol content of the cells increases, without a concomitant change in total phospholipid content (Table 18.3). This results in a marked increase in free cholesterol:phospholipid molar ratio to values approaching those in the red cells of patients with familial LCAT deficiency. In severe alcoholic cirrhosis the increased cholesterol content of the red-cell membrane may cause the cells to assume an abnormal shape resembling that of the acanthocytes present in the blood of abetalipoproteinaemic patients. These abnormal red cells are known as 'spur cells'. Though they are indistinguishable from acanthocytes in appearance they differ from them with respect to the lipid composition of the cell membrane. Acanthocytes have an essentially normal cholesterol and phospholipid content, but the percentage of lecithin in the phospholipids is decreased (see Chapter 16). The presence of spur cells in the blood is usually accompanied by a marked haemolytic anaemia (Smith et al., 1964). This may be due to increased viscosity of the plasma membrane, resulting in increased mechanical fragility.

Normal red cells take up cholesterol and develop spurs when they are incubated with plasma from a patient with spur-cell anaemia (Smith et al., 1964) and spur cells lose cholesterol to the medium when incubated with normal human serum (Cooper et al., 1972). These observations suggest that, like target cells, spur cells are formed as a result of the reversible transfer of lipid from the plasma to the red-cell membrane under conditions in which the lipid composition of the plasma is grossly abnormal. A marked reduction in plasma LCAT activity is probably a necessary condition for the formation of spur cells. However, this cannot be the only factor, since spur cells are not present in familial LCAT deficiency.

REFERENCES

Admirand, W. H. and Small, D. M. (1968). The physicochemical basis of cholesterol gallstone formation in man. *Journal of Clinical Investigation*, **47**, 1043–1052.

Ahrens, E. H. and Kunkel, H. G. (1949). The relationship between serum lipids and skin xanthomata in eighteen patients with primary biliary cirrhosis. *Journal of Clinical Investigation*, **28**, 1565–1574.

Allan, R. N., Thistle, J. L. and Hofmann, A. F. (1976). Lithocholate metabolism during chenotherapy for gallstone dissolution. 2. Absorption and sulphation. *Gut*, **17**, 413–419.

Bell, G. D., Whitney, B. and Dowling, R. H. (1972). Gallstone dissolution in man using chenodeoxycholic acid. *Lancet*, **2**, 1213–1216.

Bergman, F. and Van der Linden, W. (1967). Diet-induced cholesterol gallstones in hamsters: prevention and dissolution by cholestyramine. *Gastroenterology*, **53**, 418–421.

Biss, K., Ho, K.-J., Mikkelson, B., Lewis, L. and Taylor, C. B. (1971). Some unique biologic characteristics of the Masai of East Africa. *New England Journal of Medicine*, **284**, 694–699.

Carey, M. C., Mazer, N. A. and Benedek, G. B. (1977). Novel physical-chemical properties of ursodeoxycholic acid (UDCA) and its conjugates: relevance to gallstone dissolution in man. *Gastroenterology*, **72**, 1036.

Carey, M. C. and Small, D. M. Solubility of cholesterol in bile. In: *Advances in Bile Acid Research, 3rd Bile Acid Meeting*, Freiburg. Eds. S. Matern, J. Hackenschmidt, P. Back and W. Gerok. F. K. Schattauer Verlag, Stuttgart, pp. 277–283, 1975.

Chadwick, V. S., Gaginella, T. S., Carlson, G. L., Debongnie, J.-C., Phillips, S. F. and Hofmann, A. F. (1979). Defective molecular structure on bile acid induced alterations in absorptive function, permeability and morphology in the perfused rabbit colon. *Journal of Clinical Medicine*, **94**, 661–674.

Comess, L. J., Bennett, P. H. and Burch, T. A. (1966). Clinical gallbladder disease in Pima Indians. Its high prevalence in contrast to Framingham. *New England Journal of Medicine*, **17**, 894–898.

Cooper, R. A. (1970). Lipids of human red cell membrane: normal composition and variability in disease. *Seminars in Hematology*, **7**, 296–322.

Cooper, R. A., Arner, E. C., Wiley, J. S. and Shattil, S. J. (1975). Modification of red cell membrane structure by cholesterol-rich lipid dispersions. A model for the primary spur cell defect. *Journal of Clinical Investigation*, **55**, 115–126.

Cooper, R. A., Diloy-Puray, M., Lando, P. and Greenberg, M. S. (1972). An analysis of lipoproteins, bile acids, and red cell membranes associated with target cells and spur cells in patients with liver disease. *Journal of Clinical Investigation*, **51**, 3182–3192.

Cooper, R. A. and Jandl, J. H. (1968). Bile salts and cholesterol in the pathogenesis of target cells in obstructive jaundice. *Journal of Clinical Investigation*, **47**, 809–822.

Coyne, M. J., Bonorris, G. G., Goldstein, L. I. and Schoenfield, L. J. (1976). Effect of chenodeoxycholic acid and phenobarbital on the rate-limiting enzymes of hepatic cholesterol and bile acid synthesis in patients with gallstones. *Journal of Laboratory and Clinical Medicine*, **87**, 281–291.

Dam, H. (1971). Determinants of cholesterol cholelithiasis in man and animals. *American Journal of Medicine*, **51**, 596–613.

Dam, H., Prange, I. and Søndergaard, E. (1968). Alimentary production of gallstones in hamsters. 20. Influence of dietary cholesterol on gallstone formation. *Zeitschrift für Ernährungswissenschaft*, **9**, 43–48.

Dam, H. and Hegardt, F. G. (1971). The relation between formation of gallstones rich in cholesterol and the solubility of cholesterol in aqueous solutions of bile salts and lecithin. *Zeitschrift für Ernährungswissenschaft*, **10**, 239–252.

Danzinger, R. G., Hofmann, A. F., Schoenfield, L. J. and Thistle, J. L. (1972). Dissolution of cholesterol gallstones by chenodeoxycholic acid. *New England Journal of Medicine*, **286**, 1–8.

Danzinger, R. G., Hofmann, A. F., Thistle, J. L. and Schoenfield, L. J. (1973). Effect of oral chenodeoxycholic acid on bile acid kinetics and biliary lipid composition in women with cholelithiasis. *Journal of Clinical Investigation*, **52**, 2809–2821.

Den Besten, L., Connor, W. E. and Bell, S. (1973). The effect of dietary cholesterol on the composition of human bile. *Surgery*, **73**, 266–273.

Dowling, R. H. (1977). Chenodeoxycholic acid therapy of gallstones. *Clinics in Gastroenterology*, **6**, 141–163.

Dowling, R. H., Hofmann, A. F. and Barbara, L. (Eds.). *Workshop on Ursodeoxycholic Acid*. Held in Cortina d'Ampezzo, Italy, March 1978. MTP Press, Lancaster, 1978.

Dowling, R. H., Mack, E. and Small, D. M. (1971). Biliary lipid secretion and bile composition after acute and chronic interruption of the enterohepatic circulation in the Rhesus monkey. IV. Primate biliary physiology. *Journal of Clinical Investigation*, **50**, 1917–1926.

Epstein, E. Z. (1932). Cholesterol of the blood plasma in hepatic and biliary diseases. *Archives of Internal Medicine*, **50**, 203–222.

Evans, W. H. (1980). A biochemical dissection of the functional polarity of the plasma membrane of the hepatocyte. *Biochimica et Biophysica Acta*, **604**, 27–64.

Forte, T., Nichols, A., Glomset, J. and Norum, K. R. (1974). The ultrastructure of plasma lipoproteins in lecithin:cholesterol acyltransferase deficiency. *Scandinavian Journal of Clinical and Laboratory Investigation*, **33**, Supplement 137, 121–132.

Friedman, M. and Byers, S. (1957). Interrelationship of plasma cholate and phospholipid concentrations and their resultant effect on plasma cholesterol in biliary obstruction. *American Journal of Physiology*, **188**, 337–341.

Gjone, E. and Blomhoff, J. P. (1970). Plasma lecithin-cholesterol acyltransferase in obstructive jaundice. *Scandinavian Journal of Gastroenterology*, **5**, 305–308.

Gjone, E. and Norum, K. R. (1970). Plasma lecithin-cholesterol acyltransferase and erythrocyte lipids in liver disease. *Acta Medica Scandinavica*, **187**, 153–161.

Gregory, D. H., Vlahcevic, Z. R., Schatzki, P. and Swell, L. (1975). Mechanism of secretion of biliary lipids. I. Role of bile canalicular and microsomal membranes in the synthesis and transport of biliary lecithin and cholesterol. *Journal of Clinical Investigation*, **55**, 105–114.

Grundy, S. M., Metzger, A. L. and Adler, R. D. (1972). Mechanisms of lithogenic bile formation in American Indian women with cholesterol gallstones. *Journal of Clinical Investigation*, **51**, 3026–3043.

Hamilton, R. L., Havel, R. J., Kane, J. P., Blaurock, A. E. and Sata, T. (1971). Cholestasis: lamellar structure of the abnormal human serum lipoprotein. *Science*, **172**, 475–478.

Hardison, W. G. M. and Francis, T. I. (1969). The mechanism of cholesterol and phospholipid excretion in bile. *Gastroenterology*, **56**, 1164 (Abstract).

Heaton, K. W. (1973). The epidemiology of gallstones and suggested aetiology. *Clinics in Gastroenterology*, **2**, 67–83.

Hegardt, F. G. and Dam, H. (1971). The solubility of cholesterol in aqueous solutions of bile salts and lecithin. *Zeitschrift für Ernährungswissenschaft*, **10**, 223–233.

Hofmann, A. F. and Mosbach, E. H. (1964). Identification of allodeoxycholic acid as the major component of gallstones induced in the rabbit by 5α-cholestan-3β-ol. *Journal of Biological Chemistry*, **239**, 2813–2821.

Holzbach, R. T., Marsh, M., Olszewski, M. and Holan, K. (1973). Cholesterol solubility in bile. Evidence that supersaturated bile is frequent in healthy man. *Journal of Clinical Investigation*, **52**, 1467–1479.

Isaksson, B. (1954). On the lipid constituents of bile from human gallbladder containing cholesterol gallstones. A comparison with normal human bladder bile. *Acta Societatis Medicorum Upsaliensis*, **59**, 277–295.

Jakoi, L. and Quarfordt, S. H. (1974). The induction of hepatic cholesterol synthesis in the rat by lecithin mesophase infusions. *Journal of Biological Chemistry*, **249**, 5840–5844.

Johnston, C. G. and Nakayama, A. F. (1957). Solubility of cholesterol and gallstones in metabolic material. *Archives of Surgery*, **75**, 436–442.

Kenney, T. J. and Garbutt, J. T. (1970). Effect of cholestyramine on bile acid metabolism in normal man. *Gastroenterology*, **58**, 966 (Abstract).

La Russo, N. F., Hoffman, N. E., Hofmann, A. F., Northfield, T. C. and Thistle, J. L. (1975). Effect of primary bile acid ingestion on bile acid metabolism and biliary lipid secretion in gallstone patients. *Gastroenterology*, **69**, 1301–1314.

McIntyre, N., Harry, D. S. and Pearson, A. J. G. (1975). The hypercholesterolaemia of obstructive jaundice. *Gut*, **16**, 379–391.

McSherry, C. K., Morrisey, K. P., Javitt, N. B., May, P. and Glenn, F. Gallstone research in baboons. In: *Medical Primatology*, Part II, 1972. Ed. E. I. Goldsmith and J. Moor-Jankowski, S. Karger. Basel, pp. 16–28.

Magnani, H. N. and Alaupovic, P. (1976). Utilization of the quantitative assay of lipoprotein X in the differential diagnosis of extrahepatic obstructive jaundice and intrahepatic disease. *Gastroenterology*, **71**, 87–93.

Makino, I., Shinozaki, K., Yoshimo, K. and Makagawa, S. (1975). Dissolution of cholesterol gallstones by ursodeoxycholic acid. *Japanese Journal of Gastroenterology*, **72**, 690–702.

Manzato, E., Fellin, R., Baggio, G., Walch, S., Neubeck, W. and Seidel, D. (1976).

Formation of lipoprotein-X. Its relationship to bile compounds. *Journal of Clinical Investigation*, **57**, 1248–1260.

Maton, P. N., Reuben, A., Ellis, H. J. and Dowling, R. H. (1979). Hepatic cholesterol synthesis in cholelithiasis: role of HMGCoA reductase in determining biliary cholesterol secretion. *Clinical Science and Molecular Medicine*, **56**, 15P.

Metzger, A. L., Adler, R., Heymsfield, S. and Grundy, S. M. (1973). Diurnal variation in biliary lipid composition. Possible role in cholesterol gallstone formation. *New England Journal of Medicine*, **288**, 333–336.

Metzger, A. L., Heymsfield, S. and Grundy, S. M. (1972). The lithogenic index—a numerical expression for the relative lithogenicity of bile. *Gastroenterology*, **62**, 499–500.

Mok, H. Y. I., Perry, P. M. and Dowling, R. H. (1974). The control of bile acid pool size: effect of jejunal resection and phenobarbitone on bile acid metabolism in the rat. *Gut*, **15**, 247–253.

Morrissey, K. P., McSherry, C. K., Swarm, R. L., Nieman, W. H. and Deitrick, J. E. (1975). Toxicity of chenodeoxycholic acid in the nonhuman primate. *Surgery*, **77**, 851–860.

Mufson, D., Triyanond, D., Zarembo, J. E. and Ravin, J. (1974). Cholesterol solubility in model bile systems: implications in cholelithiasis. *Journal of Pharmacological Science*, **63**, 327–332.

Nakagawa, S., Makino, I., Ishizaki, T. and Dohi, I. (1977). Dissolution of cholesterol gallstones by ursodeoxycholic acid. *Lancet*, **2**, 367–369.

Nakayama, F. and Van der Linden, W. (1971). Bile composition: Sweden versus Japan. Its possible significance in the difference in gallstone incidence. *American Journal of Surgery*, **122**, 8–12.

Nicolau, G., Shefer, S., Salen, G. and Mosbach, E. H. (1974). Determination of hepatic 3-hydroxy-3-methylglutaryl CoA reductase activity in man. *Journal of Lipid Research*, **15**, 94–98.

Northfield, T. C. and Hofmann, A. F. (1975). Biliary lipid output during three meals and an overnight fast. I. Relationship to bile acid pool size and cholesterol saturation of bile in gallstone and control subjects. *Gut*, **16**, 1–11.

Oliver, M. F., Heady, J. A., Morris, J. N., Cooper, J., Geizerova, H., Gyarfas, I., Green, K. J. and Strassen, T. (1978). Atromid-S. A co-operative trial in the primary prevention of ischaemic heart disease using clofibrate. Report from the committee of principal investigators. *British Heart Journal*, **40**, 1069–1118.

Osuga, T. and Portman, O. W. (1972). Relationship between bile composition and gallstone formation in squirrel monkeys. *Gastroenterology*, **63**, 122–133.

Owen, J. S., Hutton, R. A., Hope, M. J., Harry, D. S., Bruckdorfer, K. R., Day, R. S., McIntyre, N. and Lucy, J. A. (1978). Lecithin:cholesterol acyltransferase deficiency and cell membrane lipids and function in human liver disease. *Scandinavian Journal of Clinical and Laboratory Investigation*, **38**, Supplement 150, 228.

Pedersen, L., Arnfred, T. and Thaysen, E. H. (1974). Cholesterol kinetics in patients with cholesterol gallstones before and during chenodeoxycholic acid treatment. *Scandinavian Journal of Gastroenterology*, **9**, 787–791.

Pertsemlidis, D., Panveliwalla, D. and Ahrens, E. H. Jr. (1974). Effects of clofibrate and of an estrogen-progestin combination on fasting biliary lipids and cholic acid kinetics in man. *Gastroenterology*, **66**, 565–573.

Petersen, V. P. (1953). The individual plasma phospholipids in obstructive jaundice. *Acta Medica Scandinavica*, **144**, 345–353.

Pomare, E. W. and Heaton, K. W. (1973). Bile salt metabolism in patients with gallstones in functioning gall bladders. *Gut*, **14**, 885–890.

Pomare, E. W., Low-Beer, T. S. and Heaton, K. W. The effect of wheat-bran on bile salt metabolism and bile composition. In: *Advances in Bile and Research*. Ed. S.

Matern, J. Hackenschmidt, P. Black and W. Gerok. F. K. Schattauer Verlag, Stuttgart, pp. 355–360, 1975.

Portman, O. W., Osuga, T. and Alexander, M. Nutritional influences on gallstones, bile lipids, and arterial lipids. In: *Atherosclerosis III, Proceedings of the 3rd International Symposium*. Ed. G. Schettler and A. Weizel. Springer-Verlag, Berlin, pp. 389–392, 1974.

Portman, O. W., Osuga, T. and Tanaka, N. (1975). Biliary lipids and cholesterol gallstone formation. *Advances in Lipid Research*, **13**, 135–194.

Ragland, J. B., Heppner, C. and Sabesin, S. M. (1978). The role of lecithin:cholesterol acyltransferase deficiency in the apoprotein metabolism of alcoholic hepatitis. *Scandinavian Journal of Clinical and Laboratory Investigation*, **38**, Supplement 150, 208–213.

Redinger, R. N. (1976). The effect of loss of gallbladder function on biliary lipid composition in subjects with cholesterol gallstones. *Gastroenterology*, **71**, 470–474.

Redinger, R. N. and Small, D. M. (1972). Bile composition, bile salt metabolism and gallstones. *Archives of Internal Medicine*, **130**, 618–630.

Redinger, R. N. and Small, D. M. (1973). Primate biliary physiology VIII. The effect of phenobarbital upon bile salt synthesis and pool size, biliary lipid secretion, and bile composition. *Journal of Clinical Investigation*, **52**, 161–172.

Rewbridge, A. G. (1937). The disappearance of gallstone shadows following the prolonged administration of bile salts. *Surgery*, **1**, 395–400.

Ritland, S., Blomhoff, J. P. and Gjone, E. (1973). Lecithin:cholesterol acyltransferase and lipoprotein-X in liver disease. *Clinica Chimica Acta*, **49**, 251–259.

Salen, G., Nicolau, G., Shefer, S. and Mosbach, E. H. (1975). Hepatic cholesterol metabolism in patients with gallstones. *Gastroenterology*, **69**, 676–684.

Salen, G., Tint, G. S., Eliav, B., Deering, N. and Mosbach, E. H. (1974). Increased formation of ursodeoxycholic acid in patients treated with chenodeoxycholic acid. *Journal of Clinical Investigation*, **53**, 612–621.

Sarles, H., Hauton, J., Planche, N. E., Lafont, H. and Gerolami, A. (1970). Diet, cholesterol gallstones and composition of bile. *American Journal of Digestive Diseases*, **15**, 251–260.

Scherstén, T., Nilsson, S., Carlin, E., Filipson, M. and Brodin-Persson, G. (1971). Relationship between the biliary excretion of bile acids and the excretion of water, lecithin and cholesterol in man. *European Journal of Clinical Investigation*, **1**, 242–247.

Schoenfield, L. J. and Sjövall, J. (1966). Bile acids and cholesterol in guinea pigs with induced gallstones. *American Journal of Physiology*, **211**, 1069–1074.

Seidel, D., Alaupovic, P. and Furman, R. H. (1969). A lipoprotein characterizing obstructive jaundice. I. Method for quantitative separation and identification of lipoproteins in jaundiced subjects. *Journal of Clinical Investigation*, **48**, 1211–1223.

Shaffer, E. A. and Small, D. M. (1977). Biliary lipid secretion in cholesterol gallstone disease: the effect of cholecystectomy and obesity. *Journal of Clinical Investigation*, **59**, 828–840.

Simon, J. B. and Scheig, R. (1970). Serum cholesterol esterification in liver disease. Importance of lecithin-cholesterol acyltransferase. *New England Journal of Medicine*, **283**, 841–846.

Small, D. M. (1970). The formation of gallstones. *Advances in Internal Medicine*, **16**, 243–264.

Small, D. M. and Rapo, S. (1970). Source of abnormal bile in patients with cholesterol gallstones. *New England Journal of Medicine*, **283**, 51–57.

Small, D. M., Shaffer, E. A. and Braasch, J. W. Bile composition at and after surgery in normals, pigment stone patients and cholesterol stone patients. In: *Bile Acids in Human Disease, 2nd Bile Acid Meeting, Freiburg*. Ed. P. Back and W. Gerok. Schattauer Verlag, Stuttgart, p. 177, 1972.

Smith, J. A., Lonergan, E. T. and Sterling, K. (1964). Spur-cell anemia. Hemolytic anemia with red cells resembling acanthocytes in alcoholic cirrhosis. *New England Journal of Medicine*, **271**, 396–398.

Sturdevant, R. A. L., Pearce, M. L. and Dayton, S. (1973). Increased prevalence of cholelithiasis in men ingesting a serum-cholesterol-lowering diet. *New England Journal of Medicine*, **288**, 24–27.

Swell, L. and Bell, C. C. (1968). Influence of bile acids on biliary lipid excretion in man. Implications in gallstone formation. *American Journal of Digestive Diseases*, **13**, 1077–1080.

Swell, L., Bell, C. C. and Vlahcevic, Z. R. (1970). Relationship of bile acid pool size to biliary lipid excretion and the formation of lithogenic bile in man. *Gastroenterology*, **61**, 716–722.

Thistle, J. L. and Hofmann, A. F. (1973). Efficacy and specificity of chenodeoxycholic acid therapy for dissolving gallstones. *New England Journal of Medicine*, **289**, 655–659.

Thistle, J. L., Hoffman, N. E. and Hofmann, A. F. (1973). Effect of bile acid administration on cholesterol kinetics in patients with radiolucent gallstones. *Gastroenterology*, **65**, 572 (Abstract).

Thistle, J. L. and Schoenfield, L. J. (1971a). Lithogenic bile among young Indian women. Lithogenic potential decreased with chenodeoxycholic acid. *New England Journal of Medicine*, **284**, 177–181.

Thistle, J. L. and Schoenfield, L. J. (1971b). Induced alterations in composition of bile of persons having cholelithiasis. *Gastroenterology*, **61**, 488–496.

Thomas, P. K. and Walker, J. G. (1965). Xanthomatous neuropathy in primary biliary cirrhosis. *Brain*, **88**, 1079–1088.

Thureborn, E. (1962). Human hepatic bile: composition changes due to altered enterohepatic circulation. *Acta Chirurgia Scandinavica Supplement*, **303**, 63pp.

Verkleij, A. J., Nauta, I. L. D., Werre, J. M., Mandersloot, J. G., Reinders, B., Ververgaert, P. H. J. Th., De Gier, J. (1976). The fusion of abnormal plasma lipoprotein (LP-X) and the erythrocyte membrane in patients with cholestasis studied by electronmicroscopy. *Biochimica et Biophysica Acta*, **436**, 366–376.

Vlahcevic, Z. R., Bell, C. C., Buhag, I., Farrar, J. T. and Swell, L. (1970). Diminished bile acid pool size in patients with gallstones. *Gastroenterology*, **59**, 165–173.

Vlahcevic, Z. R., Bell, C. C., Gregory, D. H., Buker, G., Juttijudata, P. and Swell, L. (1972). Relationship of bile acid pool size to the formation of lithogenic bile in female Indians of the Southwest. *Gastroenterology*, **62**, 73–83.

Webster, K. H., Lancaster, M. C., Hofmann, A. F., Wease, D. F. and Baggenstoss, A. H. (1975). Influence of primary bile acid feeding on cholesterol metabolism and hepatic function in the rhesus monkey. *Mayo Clinic Proceedings*, **50**, 134–138.

Wood, P. D., Shioda, R., Estrich, D. L. and Splitter, S. D. (1972). Effect of cholestyramine on composition of duodenal bile in obese human subjects. *Metabolism, Clinical and Experimental*, **21**, 107–116.

Index

The index should be used in conjunction with the summaries of contents in the text. For steroid names, the letters in the main part of the name take precedence over numbers or Greek letters denoting position or configuration, e.g. cholestane-11β-12α-diol precedes cholest-7-en-3β-ol but 25-hydroxycholesterol precedes 26-hydroxycholesterol.

A

Abetalipoproteinaemia,
  acanthocytes, 778–780
  cholesterol absorption, 788
  cholesterol synthesis, 724, 787
  LCAT activity, 778
  lymphocytes, 787
  neurological abnormalities, 783
  red cells, 783
  sterol balance, 787
Acansterol,
  starfish, 146, 147
Acanthocytes (see Abetalipoproteinaemia)
ACAT (acyl-CoA:cholesterol O-acyltransferase),
  absorption of cholesterol, 470–471
  activation by LDL uptake, 274, 425
  distribution in tissues, 274
  effect of cholesterol feeding, 274
  FH fibroblasts, 715
  LDL receptor pathway, 425
  reaction catalyzed, 273
  substrate specificity, 274
[^{14}C]Acetate,
  dilution of pool, 344
  sterol synthesis, 344
Acetate thiokinase (see Acetyl-CoA synthase)
Acetyl-CoA,
  origin from citrate, 185
Acetyl-CoA synthase,
  rate-limiting, 344
  reaction catalyzed by, 185
Acetyl-LDL,
  macrophage uptake, 407–408, 718–719
ACTH,
  glucocorticoid synthesis, 270
  HMG-CoA reductase activity, 271
  hydrolysis of cholesteryl ester, 270
  side-chain cleavage, 270

Acyl-CoA:cholesterol O-acyltransferase (see ACAT)
Addition,
  antiparallel, 165, 199, 200
  sterol biosynthesis, in, 165
Adenosine 3'-phosphate 5'-sulphatophosphate,
  donor for sterol sulphation, 287
Adipose tissue,
  cholesterol and ageing, 133
  LDL receptors in, 427
  nicotinic acid, effect on, 495
Adrenal glands, see also ACTH
  calcification in Wolman's disease, 823, 824–828, 830
  cholesteryl ester hydrolase, 284
  cholesteryl esters, 138
  cholesteryl sulphate, 138
  sterol content, 138
Adrenodoxin,
  mitochondrial side-chain cleavage, 267
Aglycone,
  definition, 143
Agnosterol,
  systematic name, 27
  wool fat, in, 132
Aldosterone,
  formation from corticosterone, 263
Alligator mississippiensis,
  bile acids in, 238
Allo-,
  use as prefix, 27
Allo bile acids,
  biosynthetic routes to, 241–242
  gallstones, in, 873
Allocholic acid (3α,7α,12α-trihydroxy-5α-cholan-24-oic acid),
  CTX bile, 839
  human faeces, 241
  iguana bile, 242
  leopard-seal bile, 241

890 Index

Allodeoxycholic acid (3α,12α-dihydroxy-
    5α-cholan-24-oic acid),
    5α-cholestanol-fed rabbit, 241, 873
Allolithocholic acid (3α-hydroxy-5α-cholan-
    24-oic acid),
    mobility on TLC, 32
4-Aminopyrazolopyrimidine (see 4-APP)
Amphipathic helices,
    apolipoproteins, in, 517
Anaemia,
    hypocholesterolaemia, 775
    LCAT deficiency, in, 796
    liver disease, in, 882
Androstenedione,
    precursor of sex hormones, 263
Antiparallel (antiplanar) addition,
    double-bond saturation, in, 165
    squalene cyclization, in, 199
Aorta,
    FH, in, 698
    LCAT deficiency, in, 801
ApoA-I,
    acceptor for cholesterol, 439
    cofactor for LCAT, 277
    lipoprotein distribution, 512
    polyunsaturated fat, effect of, 536
    Tangier disease, 790–791
ApoA-II,
    catabolism in Tangier disease, 794
    HDL protein, 513
    HDL_T, in Tangier disease, 791
ApoA-IV,
    lipoprotein distribution, 512
    lipoproteins in chyluria, 524
    rat plasma, 513
    triglyceride-rich lipoproteins, 524
ApoB,
    cyclohexanedione, 419
    heterogeneity, 520
    receptor recognition, 418, 419
ApoC-I,
    HDL as reservoir, 527
    VLDL and chylomicron metabolism, 524–525
ApoC-II,
    activator for lipoprotein lipase, 525
    HDL as reservoir, 527
    VLDL and chylomicron metabolism, 524–525
ApoC-III,
    apoE antagonist, 526
    HDL as reservoir, 527
    HDL in abetalipoproteinaemia, 778
    VLDL and chylomicron metabolism, 525
ApoD,
    distribution, 512
ApoE (arginine-rich protein),
    cyclohexanedione, 419
    genetic abnormalities, 750–752
    HDL_c, 515

nascent HDL, 523
hepatic receptor for, 526, 754
IDL, 514
LCAT-deficient HDL, in, 805
LDL receptor, 419
β-VLDL, 514
Apolipoproteins (see ApoA-I, etc.)
4-APP (4-aminopyrazolopyrimidine),
    HMG-CoA reductase, 388
    LDL receptor, 432–433
    plasma cholesterol, 388
Arcus,
    familial LCAT deficiency, 796, 801
    FH, in, 697, 701
    fish-eye disease, 791
    Tangier disease, 789
Arginine-rich protein (see ApoE)
Artery,
    ACAT activity in, 274
    cholesterol changes with age, 134
    cholesteryl ester hydrolase in, 283, 284
    free and esterified cholesterol, 134, 136
    non-cholesterol sterols in, 136
    sterol synthesis, 342, 356
Asterosaponin A,
    starfish, 147
Asterosterol,
    starfish, 146
Atheroma, see also Fatty streaks, Plaques
    cholesterol, origin of, 611
    lipoproteins in, 612–613
Atherosclerosis,
    CTX, in, 838–839
    experimental,
        endothelial permeability and, 624
        fatty streaks, 618–619
        hypercholesterolaemia, 623
        non-human primates, 618–621
        role of injury, 622
    FH, in, 697–703
    LCAT deficiency, in, 801, 811
    regression,
        biochemical reversal, 627
        cholestyramine, 731
        ileal bypass, 737–738
        plasma exchange, 731, 742
        prevention trials, 649
        removal of collagen, 627
    Tangier disease, in, 651, 789, 795
Δ^5-Avenasterol (stigmasta-5,Z-24(28)-dien-
    3β-ol) (see 28-Isofucosterol)
Δ^7-Avenasterol (stigmasta-7,Z-24(28)-dien-
    3β-ol),
    sunflower seeds, in, 150
Axial conformation,
    reactivity of substituents, effect on, 31, 32
AY-9944,
    Δ^7-reductase inhibitor, 172
Ayrton,
    mirror imaging, interest in, 9

Azasteroids, see also Solasodine
  plants, presence in, 154

B

Bacteria,
  bile-acid metabolism, 235
  enzymic assays, 104–105, 109–110
  inability to synthesize sterols, 220
  polyprenols, synthesis of, 220
Bassen-Kornzweig syndrome (see Abetalipo-proteinaemia)
Bilayer,
  cholesterol and permeability, 327
  membrane structure, 318
Bile, see also Gallstones
  cholesterol in, 127, 130
  gallbladder cholesterol, 130
  hepatic, 860
  lithogenic, 860
  non-cholesterol sterols in, 127
  origin of lipids, 862–863
Bile acids, see also Allo bile acids
  assay,
    enzymic, 109–110
    radioimmuno-, 113–114
  bacterial modifications, 235
  biliary cholesterol, solubilization of, 857–859
  conjugated, hydrolysis of, 56
  micelles, required for, 468–469
  pool size, chenodeoxycholate, effect on, 870
    different species, in, 245
    gallstone disease, in, 864 et seq.
  R_f, prediction of, 63
  separation of 5α and 5β, 64
  serum, in, 113
  sterol absorption, required for, 468
  sulphates,
    bile, urine and faeces, in, 114
    biosynthesis, 243
    meconium, in, 304
  synthesis,
    5α-cholestanol, from, 287
    cholestyramine, effect on, 254, 492–493
    corticosteroids, effect on, 253
    CTX, in, 842–843
    dietary cholesterol, effect on, 482
    fetal, 304
    FH, in, 711
    germ-free animals, in, 256
    hypercholesterolaemia, in, 491
    hypertriglyceridaemia, in, 491
    pathways in man, 234–235, 238
    phenobarbital, effect on, 253
    β-sitosterol, from, 472
    thyroid, effect on, 253–254
  turnover and secretion,
    bile fistula, effect on, 249
    cholestyramine, effect on, 249
    ileal resection, effect on, 249
    rates, 246–248
Bile fistula,
  bile acid synthesis, effect on, 249
Bimolecular nucleophilic substitution,
  geranyl PP, in formation of, 194–195
  mechanism, 166
Boat and chair,
  conformations of steroid rings, 29–30
  cyclization of squalene, during, 201–202
Brassicasterol (24β-methylcholesta-5,22-dien-3β-ol),
  formula, 152
  rapeseed, presence in, 152
Bufogenins,
  esterification with suberylarginine, 143
  formula, 144
  toad poisons, presence in, 143
Bufotoxins (see Bufogenins)

C

CAMP (see Cyclic AMP)
Campesterol ((24R)-24-methylcholest-5-en-3β-ol),
  absorption, 471
  biosynthesis, 216
  formula, 152
  separation from β-sitosterol, 62, 70
  β-sitosterolaemia, 836
Cancer,
  colon and dietary cholesterol, 657
  plasma cholesterol, and, 655–656
Cardenolides (see Cardiotonic steroids)
Cardiotonic steroids, see also Bufogenins
  anti-microbial action, 155
  higher plants, presence in, 154
  synthesis from cholesterol, 216–217
Cataract,
  CTX, in, 837, 838
Cell line,
  established, 399
  L-strain, 400–401, 404
  primary, 399
Centrifugation,
  density-gradient, 140
Cerebrotendinous xanthomatosis (see CTX)
Ceroid,
  cholesteryl ester sorage disease, in, 833
Chalinasterol (24-methylenecholesterol)
  pollen, presence in, 150, 153
Chemical shift, definition, 85
Chenodeoxycholic acid (3α,7α-dihydroxy-5β-cholan-24-oic acid),
  assay, enzymic, 110
  biosynthesis, 233
  CTX bile, in, 839
  gallstone therapy, use in, 869–871
  measurement of turnover, 109

892 Index

Chenodeoxycholic acid—*contd.*
  β-sitosterol, formation from, 472
  sulphate ester, 114
Chirality,
  definition, 6
  evolutionary origin, 9
Chiroptical effects (see CD and ORD)
p-Chlorophenoxyisobutyrate (see Clofibrate)
Cholane,
  stereochemical formula, 22
Cholanic acid,
  systematic name, 27
5β-Cholan-24-oic acid,
  trivial name, 27
5,6-*cis*-Cholecalciferol (see Vitamin D$_3$)
Cholesta-5,8(14)-diene,
  formula, 25
Cholesta-5,7-dien-3β-ol (see 7-Dehydrocholesterol)
Cholesta-5,24-dien-3β-ol (see Desmosterol)
5α-Cholesta-8,24-dien-3β-ol (see Zymosterol)
Cholestane (5α-cholestane),
  GLC standard, use as, 75–76, 103, 111
  mass spectrometry, 89
  stereochemical formula, 22, 24, 27
5β-Cholestane (coprostane),
  nomenclature, 27
  structural formula, 24
5α-Cholestane-3β,7α-diol,
  formula, 26
5β-Cholestane-3α,7α-diol,
  chenodeoxycholic acid synthesis, in, 233, 843
5β-Cholestane-3α,7α,12α,23ξ,25-pentol,
  CTX, presence in bile, 98, 840–841
5β-Cholestane-3α,7α,12α,24α,25-pentol,
  CTX, presence in bile, 98, 234, 840–843
5β-Cholestane-3α,7α,12α,25-tetrol,
  CTX, presence in bile, 97, 234, 840–843
5β-Cholestane-3α,7α,12α,26-tetrol,
  bile acid synthesis, in, 233, 843
Cholestane-3β,5α,6β-triol,
  oxidation of cholesterol, 45
5β-Cholestane-3α,7α,12α-triol,
  cholic acid synthesis, in, 231
Cholestanol (5α-cholestan-3β-ol),
  absorption, 472
  assay by GLC, 104
  biosynthesis, 287
  configuration, 38
  contaminant of cholesterol, 101
  conversion to allo bile acids, 241–242
  conversion to allodeoxycholate in rabbits, 241
  conversion to bile acids, 287
  CTX, brain and xanthomas, 838
    plasma concentration, 838
    red cells, 838
  digitonide formation, 44

  esterified, 132, 287, 838
  faeces, 137
  higher algae, 156
  liver, presence in, 127
  nerve, 132
  separation from isomers, 62, 68, 70, 106, 108
  smegma, 132
  structural formula, 25
  TMS ether on GLC, 72
5α-Cholestan-3α-ol (see Epicholestanol)
5α-Cholestan-3β-ol (see Cholestanol)
5β-Cholestan-3α-ol (see Epicoprostanol)
5α-Cholestan-7α-ol,
  absolute configuration at C-7, 39
5β-Cholestan-3β-ol (see Coprostanol)
Cholestanone (5α-cholestan-3-one),
  5α-cholestanol, precursor of, 286
  formula, 39
5α-Cholestan-3-one (see Cholestanone)
5β-Cholestan-3-one (see Coprostanone)
Cholesta-5,7,9(11)-trien-3β-ol,
  UV spectrum, 81
Cholest-5-ene-3β,4β-diol,
  formation of digitonide, 44
Cholest-5-ene-3β,6β-diol,
  Lifschütz reaction, in, 48
Cholest-5-ene-3β,7α-diol (see 7α-Hydroxycholesterol)
Cholest-5-ene-3β,7β-diol (see 7β-Hydroxycholesterol)
Cholest-5-ene-3β,25-diol (see 25-Hydroxycholesterol)
Cholest-5-ene-3β,26-diol (see 26-Hydroxycholesterol)
Cholest-4-ene-3β-ol,
  Lifschütz reaction, 48
Cholest-5-en-3α-ol (epicholesterol),
  intestinal absorption, 472
Cholest-5-en-3β-ol (see Cholesterol)
5α-Cholest-7-en-3β-ol (see Lathosterol)
5α-Cholest-8-en-3β-ol,
  cholesterol synthesis, intermediate in, 208
5α-Cholest-14-en-3β-ol,
  absolute configuration at C-20, 39–40
Cholest-4-en-3-one (see Cholestenone)
Cholestenone (cholest-4-en-3-one),
  5α-cholestanol, biosynthetic intermediate, 287
  enzymic formation, 104
  formula, 38
Cholesterol,
  absolute configuration,
    elucidation of, 39–40
  adipocytes, content, 133
  algae, presence in, 156
  arterial wall, content, 134–135
  bile, content, 127, 678–679
  biological membranes, role in, 317

birefringence of liquid crystals, 42, 518, 609, 790, 824, 833, 839
Δ^5 bond,' effect on shape, 34
colour reactions, 46–48
condensing effect, 321
configuration at C-20, 18
contaminants in standards, 101
dibromide, 45
dietary cholesterol,
  bile-acid synthesis, effect on, 482
  cholesterol synthesis, effect on, 371–375, 481–483
diffusion in membranes, 332
digitonide, 43
distribution in body, 127
exchangeable mass,
  human, size in, 457
  hypercholesterolaemia, effect of, 491
  isotopic equilibrium, 450
  multiple pools, 450
  three-pool model, 458
  two-pool model, 455–456
excretion by cells, 405–406
fetal tissues, 301
flip-flop, 332
foods, content, 141–142, 677
free and esterified in tissues, 127
functions, biological, 126
H atoms, origin of, 213, 348
insects, requirement for, 145, 146
intestinal absorption,
  abetalipoproteinaemia, in, 788
  animals, 478
  bile salts required for, 468
  esterification during, 470–471
  human, 476–477
  micelles, required for, 468–472
  plant sterols, effect of, 479
  polyunsaturated fat, effect of, 479
  sites of, 467
  sterol specificity, 471–472
intestine, content, 136
IR spectrum, 82
liver, content, 127, 129
mevalonate carbon, distribution of, 183, 213
mevalonate hydrogen, distribution of, 213
myelin, content, 309
oxidation by O_2, 45–46
phase transition temperature, effect on, 322–325
physical constants, 41
plasma (see Plasma cholesterol)
pregnenolone, conversion into, 261
protozoa, presence in, 125
separation by chromatography, 62, 67, 70, 106
skin, content, 131
solubilization in bile, 857–859
sources of, for steroid hormones, 271
stereochemistry, 32–34
steroid hormones, precursor of, 261
sulphate (see Cholesteryl sulphate)
synthesis, see also LDL receptor
  abetalipoproteinaemia, in, 724, 787–788
  absolute measurement, 349
  artery, 356
  brain, 310–311
  cells in culture, in, 408–411
  cholestyramine, effect of, 492–493
  dietary cholesterol, effect of, 371–375, 481–483
  dietary fat, effect of, 379
  enterohepatic circulation and, 379–381
  fasting, effect of, 378
  feedback inhibition, 371–375
  fetus, 302–304, 309–310
  FH, in, 710–711
  hepatomas, in, 412
  human, 463, 466
  intravenous lecithin, effect of, 384
  invertebrates, 220
  liver, 353–354
  plants, 216
  squalene method, 462–463
  sterol analogues, effect on, 411
  tissue contributions to, 352–357
  whole-body, in, 459–463
  TMS ether, in GLC, 72
  in mass spectrometer, 89
turnover,
  definition, 454
  plasma specific activity, 455
  production rate, 454
  sterol balance, 454
Cholesterol esterase (see Cholesteryl ester hydrolase)
Cholesterol 7α-hydroxylase,
  changes in activity, 257–259
  cofactor requirements, 232, 235
  compartmentation of substrate, 236
  diurnal rhythm, 259
  parallel with HMG-CoA reductase, 257, 363
  rate-limiting step, 256–257
  reaction mechanism, 235–236
Cholesterol 7α-monooxygenase (see Cholesterol 7α-hydroxylase)
Cholesterol oxidase,
  cholesterol assay, use in, 104
Cholesteryl ester,
  adrenals, gonads and placenta, 138, 270–271
  animal tissues, 127, 129, 134, 136
  biliary obstruction, in, 874
  cholesterol absorption, role in, 470–471
  cholesterol feeding, effect on, 129
  cholesteryl ester storage disease, in, 831, 832

Cholesteryl ester—*contd.*
  enzymic hydrolysis,
    adrenals and gonads, in, 284
    artery, in, 283–284
    foam cells, in, 607–609
  exchange proteins, 554–555
  fatty streaks, in, 607–608
  fibrous plaques, in, 609–610
  Liebermann-Burchard reaction, 47
  liver disease, in, 881
  lysosomal hydrolysis, 282, 283, 285, 829
  plasma,
    dietary fat, effect of, 509
    fatty acids, in, 509
    origin in LCAT reaction, 538–539
    turnover, 540–547, 555–558
  skin, in, 131
  Tangier disease, 789, 790
  Wolman's disease, 824, 829–830
  xanthomas, in, 697
Cholesteryl ester hydrolase,
  arterial wall, 283–284, 614
  cholesterol assay, in, 105
  distribution, 275
  pH optima, 275
  reaction, 275
Cholesteryl ester storage disease,
  bile acids in serum, 832
  cholesteryl ester, 831, 832
  cholesteryl ester hydrolase in, 833
  HDL concentration, 832, 834
  IHD, 832–833
  lysosomes in, 834
Cholesteryl sulphate,
  distribution in animal tissues, 125–126
  human faeces, in, 287
  precursor of steroid hormones, 287–288
  synthesis, 287
Cholestyramine,
  atherosclerosis, regression, 731
  bile acids, 249, 254, 492
  cholesterol 7α-hydroxylase, 257–259
  experimental gallstones, in, 873
  FH,
    heterozygotes and homozygotes, 734
  HMG-CoA reductase, 379
  intestinal wall, effect on, 492
  LDL turnover, 532
  plasma cholesterol, 492–493
  skin xanthomas, resolution of, 492
  VLDL, 493
Cholic acid, see also Chapter 5
  measurement of turnover, 109
  β-sitosterol, formation from, 472
  systematic name, 27
Cholyl-CoA,
  bile-acid synthesis, in, 233
Chromatography,
  column, 58
  gas-liquid (see GLC)
  high-pressure (high performance) liquid, 59
  thin-layer (see TLC)
Chrysanthemyl alcohol,
  structure, 93
Chylomicrons,
  composition, 512–513
  lipoprotein lipase, 524–525
  remnant uptake, hepatic, 435
  sterol synthesis, effect on, 377
Circular dichroism (CD),
  determination of stereochemistry, use in, 90
cis/*trans* Ring junction (see Ring junction)
cis-trans Isomerization,
  fatty acid, of, 654, 679
Citrate,
  cytosolic acetyl-CoA, source of, 185
Citrate-ATP lyase,
  formation of cytosolic acetyl-CoA, 185
Citrate cleavage enzyme (see Citrate-ATP lyase)
Citronellal,
  structure determination of cholesterol, 40
Clathrin,
  coated pits, in, 420
Clerosterol (24β-ethylcholesta-5,25-dien-3β-ol),
  formula, 152
  verbenaceae, in, 152
Clofibrate (*p*-chlorophenoxyisobutyrate),
  biliary cholesterol, 494, 655
  cholesterol metabolism, 495
  FH, 735
  floating beta disease, 756
  LDL turnover, 533
  plasma cholesterol, 494
  tissue cholesterol excretion, 655
  WHO trial, 649, 654
Coated pits,
  clathrin in, 420–421
  endocytosis, 435
  LDL receptor, 420
Collagen,
  arterial intima, in, 607
  regression, after, 627
Compactin,
  FH treatment, 735–736
  HMG-CoA reductase, 425, 735
Concerted reaction,
  cyclization of squalene, in, 199
  definition, 165
Condensing effect,
  structural features required for, 321
Configuration,
  definition, 6
  relative and absolute, 11
  rules for designation, 13

Conformation,
  definition, 10
  studied with NMR, 86
Co-ordinate induction/repression,
  cholesterol feeding, 363
  fasting, 363, 378
  HMG-CoA reductase, 363
  mammals, 359
Coprolites,
  steroids in, 137
Coprostane (see 5β-Cholestane)
Coprostanol (coprosterol) (5β-cholestan-3β-ol),
  absorption, 472
  discovery, 34
  elucidation of configuration, 38
  faeces, in, 137
  Liebermann-Burchard reaction, in, 47
  separation, 70
  systematic name, 27
  upper intestine, in, 137
Coprostanone (5β-cholestan-3-one),
  faeces, in, 112, 137
  formula, 38
  systematic name, 27
Coprosterol (see Coprostanol)
Corals,
  gorgosterol in, 147
Cord plasma,
  cholesterol concentration, 577–578, 595
Coronary angiography,
  FH, 698
  IHD, 638
Coronary heart disease (see IHD)
Corpus luteum,
  HMG-CoA reductase in, 305
  sterols in, 138
Corticosteroids,
  bile-acid synthesis, effect on, 253
  β-sitosterol, synthesis from, 472
Corticosterone,
  diurnal rhythm, 370
  rats, mice and rabbits, 261
Cortisol,
  man and other species, formation in, 261
Cracking pattern (fragmentation pattern),
  bile alcohols, 97
  5α-cholestane, 89
  cholesterol TMS ether, 89
  presqualene alcohol, 92
CTX,
  bile, abnormal composition, 839
    alcohols, 840–843
      in faeces, 97, 98
  cataracts, 837
  5α-cholestanol, 838 et seq.
  cholesterol synthesis in, 842–843
  HMG-CoA reductase, 843
  IHD, 838
  xanthomas, 838, 839

Culture (cell),
  cholesteryl ester, 402
  definition, 399
  HDL in medium, 405
  sterol,
    excretion, 404–406
    requirement, 401
    synthesis, 408–411
    uptake, 404
Cyclic AMP,
  cholesteryl ester hydrolase, effect on, 270
  HMG-CoA reductase, 364–367, 413
Cycloartenol,
  biosynthesis, 215
  conversion to cholesterol, 216
  conversion to phytosterols, 216
  formula, 150
Cycloeucalenol,
  formula, 151
Cyclohexane,
  boat and chair forms, 29
Cyclohexanedione,
  apoE, 419
  scavenger pathway, 720
  LDL, 419, 427
  LDL catabolism in vivo, 533
Cytochrome P450,
  adrenal-cortex mitochondria, in, 267
  14α-demethylation, 209
  7α-hydroxylation, 232, 235–236, 259
  11β-hydroxylase, 267
  12α-hydroxylation, 232
  17α-hydroxylase, 268
  18-hydroxylase, 267
  21-hydroxylase, 268
  17–20 lyase, 268
  20–22 lyase, 267

D

Dammarenediol,
  stereochemistry of cyclization to, 201
7-Dehydrocholesterol (cholesta-5,7-dien-3β-ol),
  accumulation by AY-9944, 172
  contaminant of cholesterol, 101
  conversion to vitamin D_3, 289
  formation of digitonide, 44
  gut mucosa, presence in, 136
  insects, presence in, 145
  intestinal absorption, 472
  separation from cholesterol, 45, 108
  skin, presence in, 131, 132
  systematic name, 27
Dehydroepiandrosterone (3β-hydroxyandrost-5-en-17-one),
  formation of digitonide, 44
  precursor of sex hormones, 263–266
  synthesis in placenta, 305

Deity,
  achiral nature of, 10
14α-Demethylase,
  hamster ovary, genetic deficiency, 401
  sterol synthesis, in, 207
Deoxycholic acid (3α,12α-dihydroxy-5β-cholan-24-oic acid), see also Chapter 5
  elucidation of structure, 37–38
Deoxycorticosterone (21-hydroxyprogesterone),
  11β-hydroxylation, 267
  precursor of corticosterone, 263
14α-Desmethyllanosterol (4,4-Dimethyl-5α-cholesta-8,24-dien-3β-ol),
  enzymic formation, 209–211
  formula, 209
  nerve tissue, presence in, 132
  sterol biosynthesis, in, 78, 207–209
Desmosterol (cholesta-5,24-dien-3β-ol),
  accumulation with triparanol, 172
  barnacles and molluscs, presence in, 149
  brain myelin, presence in, 309
  chick embryos, presence in, 131
  GLC separation from cholesterol, 71, 108
  higher algae, presence in, 156
  intermediate in sterol formation, 207
  L-strain fibroblasts, synthesis, 401
  rat brain, presence in, 132
  skin, presence in, 131
  systematic name, 27
Dexamethasone,
  HMG-CoA reductase, effect on, 413
Diabetes (see Insulin)
Diabetes insipidus,
  bone lesions in, 846
  Schüller-Christian syndrome, 847
5α,6β-Dibromocholestan-3β-ol,
  purification of cholesterol, use in, 45
Diet, see also Polyunsaturated fat, Fibre
  cholesterol in, 141–142, 677
  dietary fat and IHD, 652–654
  experimental atherosclerosis, 617 et seq.
  HDL, effect on, 581
  cis-trans isomerization of fat, 654
  LCAT deficiency, fat-free, 809
  plasma cholesterol, effect on, 479, 483–484, 487–491, 576, 577, 597
  recommendations, 677
Digitogenin,
  formula, 154
Digitonide,
  step in identification, 78
  sterol biosynthesis, study of, 45, 342
  structural requirements for, 44
  use in purification of steroids, 44
Digitonin,
  association with cholesterol, 43
  sterol analysis, in, 78

Digitoxigenin,
  formula, 154
Digoxigenin,
  higher plants, in, 154
Digoxin,
  higher plants, in, 154
Dihydrobrassicasterol (24β-methylcholest-5-en-3β-ol),
  ferns, in, 152
  formula, 152
24:25-Dihydrolanosterol,
  intermediate in sterol formation, 207
Dihydroparkeol,
  non-enzymic formation, 206
10,11-Dihydrosqualene,
  substrate for squalene epoxidase, 198
Dihydrotachysterol,
  biological activity, 291–292
  structural formula, 291
3α,7α-Dihydroxy-5β-cholan-24-oic acid
  (see Chenodeoxycholic acid)
3α,7β-Dihydroxy-5β-cholan-24-oic acid
  (see Ursodeoxycholic acid)
3α,12α-Dihydroxy-5β-cholan-24-oic acid
  (see Deoxycholic acid)
7α,12α-Dihydroxycholest-4-en-3-one,
  cholic acid synthesis, in, 231
20,22-Dihydroxycholesterol,
  precursor of pregnenolone, 261
(20S)-20,22ξ-Dihydroxycholesterol,
  meconium, presence in, 137
(20R)-20,26-Dihydroxyecdysone,
  insects, presence in, 145
3α,7α-Dihydroxy-12-keta-5β-cholanoic acid,
  standard in bile-acid assay, 111
1α,25-Dihydroxyvitamin D_3,
  biological activity, 290
  formation in kidneys, 290
β,β-Dimethylacrylate,
  as sterol precursor, 180
Dimethylallyl pyrophosphate,
  formula, 191
4,4-Dimethyl-5α-cholesta-8,24-dien-3β-ol
  (see 14α-Desmethyllanosterol)
4,4-Dimethyl-5α-cholest-7-en-3β-ol,
  separation by TLC, 62
4,4-Dimethyl-5α-cholest-8(9)-en-3β-ol,
  separation by TLC, 62
4,4-Dimethyl-5α-cholest-8(14)-en-3β-ol,
  separation by TLC, 62
Diurnal rhythm,
  fetal liver, 304
  hepatoma, 368
  HMG-CoA reductase activity, 368
  HMG-CoA synthase activity, 271
  7α-hydroxylase activity, 259
  mechanisms, 369–371
  plasma corticosterone, 259
D_2O,
  assay of cholesterol synthesis, use in, 346

developing brain, incorporation into, 310, 350
sterol precursor, 301–302
Dolichol,
biosynthesis from mevalonic acid, 214–215
formula, 214

E

α-Ecdysone (ecdysone) ((22R)-2β,3β,14α,22,25-pentahydroxy-5β-cholest-7-en-6-one),
biosynthesis, 219
glucosides in faeces, 145
insects, in, 145
plants, in, 146, 154
sulphate esters in faeces, 145
Elaidic acid (18:1, ω9 trans),
soyabean oil, in hardened, 654
Electron spin resonance (ESR),
steroid analysis, use in, 87
Electrophilic reagent,
definition, 165
Elimination,
sterol biosynthesis, in, 165
Enantiomer,
definition, 7
Endocytotic vesicles,
cholesteryl esters, 425
coated pits, 420
LDL receptor, 421
lysosomes, 425
Endoplasmic reticulum,
cholesterol in, 140
Enterohepatic circulation,
bile acids, 249
cholesterol 7α-hydroxylase, 259
cholestyramine, 249, 254
HMG-CoA reductase, effect of interruption, 279
Eosinophilic xanthomatous granuloma (see Schüller-Christian syndrome)
Epi-,
use as prefix, 27
Epicholestanol (5α-cholestan-3α-ol),
configuration, 39
IR spectrum, 83
separation from isomers, 62, 70
systematic name, 27
Epicoprostanol (5β-cholestan-3α-ol),
configuration, 38
IR spectrum, 83
systematic name, 27
Epimerization,
definition, 28
Epicoprostanol (see 5β-Cholestan-3α-ol)
Equatorial conformation,
effect of reactivity of substituents, 31–32
5,6-cis-Ergocalciferol (see Vitamin D$_2$)

Ergostanol,
side-chain, 21
Ergosterol,
conversion to vitamin D$_2$, 288
discovery, 3
formation of digitonide, 44
insects, in, 145
regulated synthesis, 359
side-chain, 14, 21
synthesis from lanosterol, 218
UV spectrum, 81
Erucic acid (22:1, ω9),
mitochondrial oxidation, 654
rapeseed oil, in, 654
toxic effects, 654, 679
Erythrocytes (see Red Cells)
(24S)-24-Ethylcholesta-5,22-dien-3β-ol (also 24α-Ethylcholesta-5,22-dien-3β-ol) (see Stigmasterol)
24β-Ethylcholesta-5,25-dien-3β-ol (see Clerosterol)
24α-Ethylcholesta-7,22-dien-3β-ol (see α-Spinasterol)
(24R)-24-Ethylcholest-5-en-3β-ol (also 24α-Ethylcholest-5-en-3β-ol) (see β-Sitosterol)
24-Ethylidenelophenol,
precursor of plant sterols, 216
Euphol,
stereochemistry of cyclization to, 201
Exophthalmos,
Schüller-Christian syndrome, in, 847

F

Faeces,
cholesteryl sulphate, 137
germ-free, 137
new-born humans, 137
non-cholesterol steroids in, 137
steryl sulphates in insect, 145
Familial abetalipoproteinaemia (see Abetalipoproteinaemia)
Familial combined hyperlipidaemia,
definition, 731
Familial HDL deficiency (see Tangier disease)
Familial hyperalphalipoproteinaemia,
IHD incidence in, 644
Familial hypercholesterolaemia (see FH)
Familial hypobetalipoproteinaemia,
acanthocytosis, 785
cholesterol synthesis, 787
first description, 777
increased life expectancy, 788
neurological abnormalities, 785
Familial LCAT deficiency,
anaemia, 796
arcus, 796, 801
fat-free diet, 809

Familial LCAT deficiency—*contd.*
  foam cells, 799
  genetic heterogeneity, 799
  HDL abnormalities, 805
  IHD, 801, 811
  LCAT activity, 799, 807–810
  LCAT,
    effect of *in vitro*, 807–810
  LDL abnormalities, 805
  LPX, 805
  macrophages, 799–800
  myelin figures, 799, 803
  red cell composition, 805
  renal disease, 796, 799
  sea-blue histiocytes, 801
Familial type III hyperlipoproteinaemia
    (see Floating beta disease)
Farnesyl pyrophosphate,
  conversion into presqualene pyrophosphate, 90, 191, 196
  formation from geranyl PP, 194
  formula, 191
Fat (see also Adipose tissue, Polyunsaturated)
  dietary, 509, 653
  trans isomers, 654
Fatty streaks,
  cholesterol content, 134, 608
  cholesteryl ester, 607, 609
  histology, 607
  normal arteries, in, 610–611
Fetus,
  adrenal synthesis of 16α-hydroxydehydroepiandrosterone, 266
  bile acids formed by, 304
  cholesterol synthesis in, 302–304
  HMG-CoA reductase activity in, 303–304
  maternal cholesterol in, 301–302
  non-cholesterol sterols in brain, 310
  plasma cholesterol in, 301
  synthesis of brain cholesterol, 307–310
  synthesis of dehydroepiandrosterone, 305
FH (familial hypercholesterolaemia),
  aorta in, 698
  arcus in, 697, 701
  bile-acid synthesis in, 711
  cholesterol synthesis in, 710–711, 724
  diagnosis,
    leucocytes, 729
    newborn, in, 729–730
  gene frequency, 709–710
  HDL concentration, 703
  IHD in, 697, 701–703
  LDL,
    biological normality, 711
    composition and concentration, 703–704
    metabolism, 711–713, 722
    oversynthesis, 711

LDL-receptor,
  defects *in vitro*, 714–717
  internalization defect, 715
  receptor-defective, 714
  receptor-negative, 714
monogenic,
  evidence for, 705–708
  plasma cholesterol, 695, 699
  platelets, 705
  polyarthritis in, 699, 701
  red cells, 705
scavenger pathway,
  cell types responsible for, 718
  CHD-blocked LDL, 722
  measurement with cyclohexanedione, 720
treatment,
  cholestyramine, 734
  compactin, 735
  diet, 733
  nicotinic acid, 734
  plasma exchange, 739
  surgery, 737–739
xanthomas,
  presence in, 695, 697, 699–701, 754
Fibre,
  bile-acid metabolism, effect on, 253
  cholesterol absorption, 479
  plasma cholesterol, 488–490
Fingerprint region,
  IR spectroscopy, in, 84
Fish-eye disease, 791
Flip-flop (see Membranes, Red cells, Lecithin, Cholesterol)
Floating beta disease (familial type III hyperlipoproteinaemia),
  apoE abnormality, 748
  cholesterol:triglyceride ratio, 755
  clofibrate, 756
  FH, associated with, 754
  genetic basis, 750–752
  inheritance, 749
  LP III, 745
  remnant-recognition disease, 754
  β-VLDL in, 743–745
Floating β-lipoprotein (see β-VLDL)
Foam cells,
  acetyl-LDL, 408
  cationized LDL, 614, 719
  fatty streaks, in, 607
  LCAT deficiency, 799–800, 810
  liquid-crystalline cholesterol, 608, 790
  macrophage uptake, 408
  Schüller-Christian syndrome, 845
  smooth-muscle cells, 607, 719
  Tangier disease, 790, 794–795
  xanthomas, in, 697
Foetus (see Fetus)
Framingham,
  diet as risk factor, 653

HDL as risk factor, 642–643
LDL as risk factor, 634
plasma cholesterol, 634
prospective study, 631
Fucosterol (stigmasta-5,E-24(28)-dien-3β-ol),
brown algae, in, 156
formula, 153
Fungi,
lanosterol synthesis, 218
typical sterols in, 156
zymosterol in, 218
Fungisterol,
formula, 156
Fur licking,
ingestion of sterols in, 137
Fusidic acid,
relation to protosterol, 169, 205
Fusidium coccineum,
source of fusidic acid, 169

G

Gallstones,
American Indians, 855, 861
chenotherapy, 869–871
decreased bile-salt secretion, 864–866
dietary, 873
discovery of cholesterol, 3
hepatic HMG-CoA reductase, 865
obesity, 866
pathogenesis, 864–867
polyunsaturated fat and, 678–679
prevalence, 855
rabbits, 873
solubilization of cholesterol, 859–861
species differences, 861
ursodeoxycholic acid, 871–872
Gamabufogenin (gamabufotalin),
formula, 144
Ganglioside,
G_{M1} in Tay-Sachs disease, 819
Gas-liquid chromatography (see GLC)
Genetic relatedness,
definition, 586
twins, 589
Geranylgeranyl pyrophosphate,
carotenoid synthesis, in, 217
Geranyl pyrophosphate,
formation, 195
formula, 191
Geranyl transferase,
formation of farnesyl pyrophosphate, in, 197
reaction mechanism, 195
yeast, in, 192
Germ-free animals,
bile-acid synthesis in, 256
faecal steroids in, 137

GLC,
liquid phases for, 66–67
mass spectrometry combined with, 88
methods of detection in, 65
quantitative, 74–76
radioassay combined with, 76–77
R_T of bile acids, 72–74
R_T of sterols, 69–72
separation of cholesterol, for, 67, 70
Glucagon,
free fatty acids and, 382
HMG-CoA reductase, effect on, 413
Glucocorticoids,
diurnal rhythm, role in, 370
HMG-CoA reductase, effect on, 413
synthesis, 261–263
Glucose-6-phosphate dehydrogenase,
mosaics, 657
Glucuronides,
bile salts, 243
Glycosaminoglycans (see Mucopolysaccharides)
Golgi apparatus,
free cholesterol in, 140
Gonadotrophic hormones,
pregnenolone synthesis, effect on, 273
Gonads,
sterol content, 138
Gorgosterol,
corals, presence in, 147

H

Hamster,
gallstones in, 873
HDL (high-density lipoprotein),
adrenal uptake, 435
assay, 645–646
biliary obstruction, 876
catabolism,
apoE receptors and, 537
hepatic and extra-hepatic, 536–537
cholesteryl ester storage disease, 832, 834
discs, 523, 804–805
FH,
concentration in, 703
functions, 528
HDL_2 and HDL_3, 437–438, 513, 584, 641, 645
heritability, 644
IHD sex ratio, 643
LCAT,
substrate for, 437–439, 522
LDL receptor, 433–434
nascent, 523, 805, 876, 881
negative risk factor for IHD, 572, 641–643, 650–651
oestrogens, effect on, 762
plasma cholesterol, 508, 512
progestogens, effect on, 762

Index 899

HDL—*contd.*
  reverse cholesterol transport, 436–439, 559
  sterol excretion from cells, 405
  sterol synthesis, 411
  structure, 517
HDL-I,
  apoE-rich component, 645
HDL$_c$,
  cholesterol feeding, after, 515
  LDL receptor, binding by, 419
HDL$_T$,
  apoA-II content, 791
  heterozygotes, absence from, 792
  Tangier disease, in, 791, 793
Hepatoma,
  diurnal rhythm in, 368
  feedback inhibition, 371–372
  HMG-CoA reductase in, 412
Heritability,
  definition, 589
  plasma cholesterol concentration, 589, 590–591
  variation with time and space, 590
High-density lipoprotein (see HDL)
Histiocytosis (see Schüller-Christian syndrome)
HMG-CoA (see β-Hydroxy-β-methyl-glutaryl-CoA)
HMG-CoA lyase,
  mitochondria, in, 354
  subcellular distribution, 181
HMG-CoA reductase,
  activation energy, 375
  4-APP, 388
  CAMP, effect on, 364–367
  cholesterol feeding, effect on, 361, 371–378
  cold-inactivation, 364
  CTX, in, 844
  distribution, M.W. and properties, 187
  enterohepatic circulation, 379–381
  fasting, effect on, 361
  feedback inhibition, 372
  fetal tissues, in, 303
  half-life, 369
  hormones, 382–383
  LDL receptor, control by, 425, 715–717
  membrane fluidity, effect on, 375–376
  parallel with 7α-hydroxylase activity, 257, 363
  phosphorylation-dephosphorylation, 364–367
  rabbit ovary, in, 305
  rate-limiting, 360
  reaction mechanism, 187
  Triton WR-1339, 384
  X-irradiation, 383–384
HMG-CoA synthase,
  discovery, 181
  diurnal rhythm in adrenals, 271
  HMG-CoA reductase, 363

  iso-enzymes of, 364
  microsomes and mitochondria, in, 181
  M.W. and properties, 186
  plasma-cholesterol depletion and, 271
  reaction mechanism, 186
[^{3}H]H$_2$O,
  assay of sterol synthesis, in, 346
  diurnal rhythm, 350
  sterol incorporation of H, 346–349
Holothurins,
  sea cucumbers, presence in, 148
Homogenization,
  mechanical methods, 56–57
3β-Hydroxyandrost-5-en-17-one
  (see Dehydroepiandrosterone)
3α-Hydroxy-5α-cholan-24-oic acid
  (see Allolithocholic acid)
3α-Hydroxy-5β-cholan-24-oic acid
  (see Lithocholic acid)
3β-Hydroxychol-5-enoic acid,
  human urine, presence in, 234
  precursor of chenodeoxycholic acid, 234
  sulphate ester in meconium, 304
3β-Hydroxy-5α-cholestan-6-one,
  formation of digitonide, 44
3β-Hydroxy-5α-cholestan-7-one,
  formation of digitonide, 44
3β-Hydroxycholest-5-en-7-one
  (see 7-Ketocholesterol)
7α-Hydroxycholest-4-en-3-one,
  bile-acid synthesis, in, 231
7α-Hydroxycholesterol (cholest-5-ene-3β,7α-diol),
  bile-acid synthesis, in, 231
  inhibition of sterol synthesis, 411
  oxidation of cholesterol, from, 45
  systematic name, 27
7β-Hydroxycholesterol (cholest-5-ene-3β,7β-diol),
  inhibition of sterol synthesis, 411
  Lifschütz reaction, 48
  oxidation of cholesterol, from, 45
(22R)-22-Hydroxycholesterol,
  meconium, presence in, 137
25-Hydroxycholesterol (cholest-5-ene-3β,25-diol),
  inhibition of sterol synthesis, 411
  oxidation of cholesterol, 45
26-Hydroxycholesterol (cholest-5-ene-3β,26-diol),
  atheroma, presence in, 36
  bile-acid formation, in, 233
  nervous tissue, presence in, 132
  nomenclature, 239
16α-Hydroxydehydroepiandrosterone,
  fetal adrenals, in, 266
  precursor of oestriol, 267
(20R)-20-Hydroxyecdysone,
  insects, in, 145

11β-Hydroxylase,
  corticosterone formation, in, 267
12α-Hydroxylase,
  cofactor requirements, 232, 237
  substrate specificity, 234, 237
17α-Hydroxylase,
  requirement for P450, 268
18-Hydroxylase,
  aldosterone formation, in, 267
21-Hydroxylase,
  requirement for P450, 268
25-Hydroxylase,
  bile-acid formation, in, 234, 843
26-Hydroxylase,
  CTX, in, 843
  stereospecificity of different enzymes, 238–240
  subcellular distribution, 237–238
7α-Hydroxylation, see also Cholesterol 7α-hydroxylase
  deoxycholic acid, of, 244
26-Hydroxylation,
  side-chain cleavage, in, 233
  stereochemistry, 237–238
β-Hydroxy-β-methylglutaryl-CoA (HMG-CoA),
  biosynthesis from leucine, 180
  cleavage by HMG-CoA lyase, 181
  HMG-CoA synthase, 181
  mechanism of synthesis, 186
17α-Hydroxyprogesterone,
  steroid hormone formation, in, 263
3-Hydroxysteroid dehydrogenase,
  bile-acid assay, in, 109
7α-Hydroxysteroid dehydrogenase,
  assay of chenodeoxycholate, use in, 110
3α-Hydroxysteroid ketoreductase,
  bile-acid formation, in, 232
  reaction mechanism, 237
Δ^5-3β-Hydroxysteroid oxidoreductase,
  cofactor requirements, 232
  subcellular distribution, 237
3β-Hydroxysteroid sulphotransferase,
  sterol sulphation, in, 287
25-Hydroxyvitamin D$_3$,
  biological activity, 290
  formation in liver, 290
Hypercholesterolaemia, see also Chapter 15
  bile-acid output in, 491
  biliary obstruction, in, 874
  cholesterol synthesis in, 491
  exchangeable mass in, 491
Hypertriglyceridaemia,
  bile-acid output in, 491
  cholesterol turnover in, 491
Hypocholesterolaemia,
  abetalipoproteinaemia, in, 777
  anaemia, in, 775
  LCAT deficiency, in, 796
  liver disease, in, 881
  malabsorption, in, 775
  myelomatosis, in, 775
  pyridoxine deficiency, in, 775
  Tangier disease, in, 790

I

IDL (intermediate-density lipoprotein),
  apoE, 525
  liver uptake, 559
  β-VLDL, 514
  VLDL and chylomicron remnants, 525
Iguana (green),
  synthesis of allocholic acid, 242
IHD,
  apoA-I and apoA-II, 645
  atherosclerosis, role in, 610, 628, 637
  cholesteryl ester storage disease, 832–833
  coronary angiography, 638
  CTX, 838
  fall in mortality, 681–862
  FH, age at, 697
  genetic influences, 588, 592
  HDL as negative risk factor, 572, 641–643
  HDL$_2$ concentration, 645
  hypobetalipoproteinaemia, in, 788
  LCAT deficiency, in, 801
  LDL as risk factor, 572, 635, 788
  Maoris, in, 656
  plasma cholesterol and, 631 et seq.
  plasma exchange, 731, 739–742
  platelet behaviour, 646, 649
  β-sitosterolaemia, 835
  Tangier disease, in, 651, 789
  VLDL as risk factor, 635, 642, 651
Ileal resection (or bypass),
  bile acids, effect on, 249
  bile-acid synthesis, 496
  cholesterol absorption, 480
  FH treatment, 737
  plasma cholesterol, 496
  regression of atherosclerosis, 737
Inhibitor 1,
  phosphatase inhibitor, 365
Insects,
  demethylation of side-chain, 218
  formation of C$_{21}$ and C$_{19}$ steroids, 219
  hormones in, 219
  inability to synthesize sterols, 219
Insulin,
  cholesterol synthesis, effect on, 413
  diurnal rhythm, 370
  free fatty acids, mobilization of, 382
  HMG-CoA reductase, 382, 413
  hyperlipoproteinaemia in diabetes, 758
  LDL-receptor function, 726
Intermediate-density lipoprotein (see IDL)
Intestine,
  non-cholesterol sterols in, 136, 137

Intestine—*contd.*
  sterol synthesis,
    bile salts, effect of, 385
    diurnal rhythm, 368
    mucosa, in, 355
    villi, in, 355
IRIS,
  Infrared Information Search, 84
IR spectroscopy,
  fingerprint region, 84
  principle, 82–84
Ischaemic heart disease (see IHD)
28-Isofucosterol (stigmasta-5,Z-24(28)-dien-3β-ol),
  higher plants, in, 153
Δ^7-Δ^8-Isomerase,
  reaction mechanism, 211, 212
Isopentenyl pyrophosphate,
  biosynthesis from mevalonate, 188
  formula, 191
  precursor of carotenoids, 217
  sterol building block, role as, 191 *et seq.*
Isopentenyl pyrophosphate isomerase,
  inhibition by iodoacetamide, 172
  reaction mechanism, 193–195
Isoprene,
  biogenetic rule, 167
  structure, 167
Isoprenoid unit,
  definition, 167
  sterol synthesis, role in, 176, 179
  unit in terpenoids, 167
Isotopic labelling,
  nomenclature, 28–29
Isovalerate,
  sterol precursor, role as, 180

J

Jelly-fish,
  sterols in, 149

K

Kant,
  on chirality, 9
Kelvin,
  on chirality, 9
β-Ketoacyl thiolase,
  M.W. and properties, 185
7-Ketocholesterol (3β-hydroxycholest-5-en-7-one),
  atheroma, in, 36
  inhibition of sterol synthesis, 411
  oxidation of cholesterol, from, 45
Δ^5-3-Ketosteroid isomerase,
  bile-acid formation, in, 232
  reaction mechanism, 237
3-Ketosteroid reductase,
  4-demethylations, in, 211

Δ^4-3-Ketosteroid-5α-reductase,
  formation of allo bile acids, in, 242
Δ^4-3-Ketosteroid-5β-reductase,
  bile-acid formation, in, 232
  reaction mechanism, 237
  subcellular distribution, 237
Kupffer cells,
  acetyl-LDL, uptake of, 407

L

Lanostane,
  structural formula, 23
5α-Lanosta-8,24-diene-3β,32-diol,
  14α-demethylation, in, 210
5α-Lanost-9(11)-en-3β-ol (see Dihydroparkeol)
Lanthanide shift reagent,
  definition, 86
Lanosterol,
  CTX bile, in, 839
  cyclization of 2,3-oxidosqualene, from, 199–201
  hamster ovary, in, 401
  liver, presence in, 127
  not fully isoprenoid, 168
  skin, presence in, 131
  synthesis in fungi, 218
  systematic names, 27
Lathosterol (5α-Cholest-7-en-3β-ol),
  absorption, 472
  contaminant of cholesterol, 101
  CTX bile, in, 839
  digitonide, formation of, 44
  fur licking, ingestion from, 137
  GLC separation from cholesterol, 71, 108
  intermediate in sterol formation, 207, 208
  intestine, presence in, 136
  IR spectrum, 82
  liver, presence in, 127
  molluscs, in, 149
  rat faeces, in, 137
  sebum, presence in, 132
  skin,
    presence in, 131
  synthesis in invertebrates, 220
  systematic name, 27
LCAT (lecithin : cholesterol acyltransferase),
  abetalipoproteinaemia, 778
  apoA-I and cholesterol uptake, 439
  assay, 279
  biliary obstruction, 874, 878
  cofactor requirements, 277
  distribution, 277
  LCAT deficiency, 799, 807–810
  liver disease, 881–882
  nascent HDL, 522, 807
  reaction and properties, 276–279
  reverse cholesterol transport, in, 437–439
  Tangier disease, 794

LCAT deficiency (see Familial LCAT deficiency)
LDL (low-density lipoprotein), see also LDL receptor
  apoB heterogeneity, 520
  catabolism,
    cyclohexanedione, effect of, 419
    hepatic and extra-hepatic, 429, 535
    cationized, 614, 719
  FH,
    composition, 704
    metabolism, 711 et seq.
    scavenger pathway for, 718–722
  inhibition of sterol synthesis, 412
  LCAT deficiency, abnormal in, 805
  liquid-crystalline, 518–519
  lymph concentration, 431
  plasma cholesterol, 508, 511
  platelet aggregation, modified by, 719
  risk factor for IHD, 572, 635, 788
  structure, 517–520
  Tangier disease, abnormal in, 791
  turnover,
    cholestyramine, 532
    clofibrate, 533
    diet, 532
    measurement, 528–529
    nicotinic acid, 532
    rates in man, 530–532
    sex hormones, 533
    thyroid, 533
LDL receptor,
  ACAT, 425
  4-APP, 432–433
  cationized LDL, 426
  cell types, in, 424, 427
  coated pits, 420
  FH,
    defects in vitro, 415, 714–717
    receptor-defective, 714
    receptor-negative, 714
    scavenger pathway, 718
  HDL interaction, with, 433–434
  induction-repression, 420, 426
  LDL catabolism in vivo, 430–432, 720
  liver, 429
  lymphocytes, 427
  lysosomal hydrolysis, 425
  myxoedema, defective in, 726
  non-genetic variations, 726
  plasma membrane, in, 421
  properties, 418–420
  subcellular membranes, in, 421
  uptake and degradation of LDL, 416–417
Lecithin,
  biliary obstruction, 874
  cholesterol synthesis after intravenous, 384, 877
  flip-flop, 332

lateral diffusion, 332
membrane, 318
spur cells, in, 882
substrate for LCAT, 276–279
target cells, in, 805, 878–879
Lecithin:cholesterol acyltransferase (see LCAT)
Leonardo da Vinci,
  interest in mirror images, 9
Liebermann-Burchard reaction,
  cholesterol assay, use in, 102
  description, 46
Lifschütz reaction,
  description, 47
Lipoprotein lipase,
  apoC-II as cofactor, 525
  hydrolysis in vitro, 525
  VLDL and chylomicrons, 524–525
Liquid crystals, see also Membranes
  cholesterol, 42
  cholesteryl ester storage, 833
  CTX, 839
  foam cells, 609
  LDL, 518–519
  Tangier disease, 790
  Wolman's disease, 824, 827
Lithocholic acid (3α-hydroxy-5β-cholan-24-oic acid),
  alkaline hydrolysis, effect of, 56
  mobility on TLC, 32
  sulphate, 115
Lithogenic index,
  chenodeoxycholic acid, effect on, 868
  definition, 859
  gallstone formation, 860–861
Liver,
  apoE receptors, 537, 754
  cholesterol feeding, 371–378
  cholesterol in, 127
  diurnal rhythm, 368–371
  HDL catabolism, 536–537
  human, 354
  LDL catabolism, 429–430, 534–535
  LDL receptors, 429, 717, 732
  non-cholesterol sterols, 127
  squalene content, 129
  sterol synthesis, 353–354
Low-density lipoprotein (see LDL)
Lophenol (see Methostenol)
Lp-X,
  biliary obstruction, 876–878
  electron microscopy, 514, 876
  LCAT deficiency, 805
  xanthomas, and, 880
L-strain (see Cell line)
17–20 Lyase,
  formation of C_{19} steroids, in, 268
  requirement for P450, 268
20–22 Lyase,
  reaction mechanism, 267

Lymphocytes,
  cholesterol synthesis in abetalipoprotein-
      aemia, 787
  LDL receptor in, 428
  sterol synthesis in, 342, 357
  synthesis in culture, 357
  Wolman's disease, 824
Lysosomes,
  artery, 283–284, 822
  chloroquine, 425
  cholesteryl ester hydrolase, 282, 425, 821,
      828
  heterophagy and autophagy, 820–821
  LDL receptor, 425
  proteolysis, 425
  storage diseases, 820–823

M

Macdougallin,
  formula, 151
Macrophages,
  acetyl-LDL, 407–408
  excretion of cholesterol, 406–407
  foam cells, 408, 607
  LCAT deficiency, 810
  scavenger pathway for LDL, 718
  Tangier disease, 794–795
  uptake of cholesterol, 406
Malabsorption,
  abetalipoproteinaemia, in, 776, 781
  hypocholesterolaemia due to, 775
Malondialdehyde,
  effect on LDL, 719
Maoris,
  IHD and plasma cholesterol, 656
Masai,
  cholesterol metabolism in, 483–484
Mass spectrometry,
  combined with GLC, 88
  cracking pattern, 87
  principle, 87
  steroid identification, 87
Meconium,
  bile acids in, 304
  cholesteryl sulphate in, 137
  disulphate esters in, 137
  sulphate esters in, 304
Membranes,
  asymmetry of bilayer, 318
  cancer, 655
  cholesterol in, 317–318
  condensing effect, 321
  diffusion in, 331–332
  enzymes in, 326, 330, 375
  flip-flop, 332
  fluidity, 321–325, 329–330, 375–376
  permeability, 327–329
  phase changes, 321–325
  red cells, 318, 328

  trans-membrane transport, 330
  white cells, 328
MER 29 (see Triparanol)
Methionine,
  alkylation of side-chain, in, 216
Methostenol (4α-methyl-5α-cholest-8-en-3β-
      ol),
  rat skin, presence in, 131
  structural formula, 151
  systematic name, 27
4α-Methyl-5α-cholest-8-en-3β-ol (see
      Methostenol)
(24R)-24-Methylcholest-5-en-3β-ol (see
      Campesterol)
24β-Methylcholest-5-en-3β-ol (see
      Dihydrobrassicasterol)
24-Methylenecholesterol (see
      Chalinasterol)
24-Methylenecycloartenol,
  precursor of plant sterols, 216
24-Methylenelophenol,
  precursor of plant sterols, 216
trans-Methylglutaconate shunt,
  kidney, operation in, 191, 357
  measurement, 358
  route for MVA metabolism, 190
β-Methylglutaconyl-CoA,
  precursor of HMG-CoA, 180
Mevaldate reductase,
  labelling of mevalonic acid, use in, 188
Mevaldic acid,
  conversion of mevalonic acid, 188
Mevalonate kinase,
  isopentenyl pyrophosphate synthesis, 188
Mevalonic acid,
  C atoms in squalene and cholesterol, 183
      213
  ^{13}C-NMR spectrum, 86
  discovery, 181
  H atoms in lanosterol and cholesterol, 213
  labelling with ^{2}H, ^{3}H and ^{14}C, 173
  metabolism via trans-methylglutaconate
      shunt, 190, 357
  precursor of carotenoids, 217
  prochiral centres, 8
  prochiral H atoms, 19
Micelles,
  bile, in, 857–859
  intestinal, 468
  β-sitosterol, 472
Microsomes, see also ACAT, Cholesterol
      7α-hydroxylase, HMG-CoA re-
      ductase
  enzymes in bile-acid synthesis, 232, 235–
      237
  enzymes in steroid-hormone synthesis, 268
  operational definition, 140
  origin of cholesterol in, 140
Milk,
  cholesterol distribution in, 138

diet and cholesterol content, 139
inhibitor of sterol synthesis in, 303, 367
plant sterols in, 139
Mitochondria,
adrenodoxin in, 267
enzymes in steroid-hormone formation, 267–268
oxidation of erucic acid, 654
source of acetyl units, 185
Mixed-function oxidase,
bile-acid formation, in, 235
steroid-hormone formation, in, 267
Monocytes,
acetyl-LDL, 407
scavenger pathway for LDL, 718
sterol synthesis in, 357
Mucopolysaccharides (glycosaminoglycans),
arterial wall, 607
LDL binding, 607
negative charges, 607
Multiple risk score,
prediction of IHD, 639
α-Muricholic acid (3α,6β,7α-trihydroxy-5β-cholanoic acid),
chenodeoxycholic acid from, 234
β-Muricholic acid (3α,6β,7β-trihydroxy-5β-cholanoic acid),
chenodeoxycholic acid from, 234
MVA (see Mevalonic acid)
Mycoplasma mycoides,
membrane fluidity in, 329
Myelin,
cholesterol incorporation into, 311
developmental changes, 309
figures, in multilamellae, 318, 799, 803
formation in brain, 307
regulation of deposition, 358
Myelomatosis,
hypocholesterolaemia in, 775

N

Nervonic acid (24:1),
abetalipoproteinaemia, in, 777
Nervous tissue,
cholesterol synthesis in, 307–310
non-cholesterol sterols in, 132
Nicotinic acid,
fatty-acid mobilization, 495
FH treatment, 734
hepatic cholesterol synthesis, 495
LDL turnover, 532
plasma cholesterol, 495
skin cholesterol, 496
Nuclear magnetic resonance (NMR),
^1H, ^{13}C and ^{31}P signals, 86
lanthanide shift reagents, 86
[^{13}C]mevalonic acid, 86
presqualene alcohol, 94

principle, 84–85
steroid conformation, 86
Nucleophilic reagent,
definition, 165

O

Obtusifoliol,
precursor of plant sterols, 216
[^{14}C]Octanoate,
assay of sterol synthesis, 345
cytosolic acetyl-CoA, 345
Oestradiol,
formation from testosterone, 266
synthesis in placenta, 305
Oestriol,
formation in placenta, 267, 305
Oestrogen,
plasma cholesterol, effect on, 583, 762
plasma HDL, effect on, 762–763
Oestrone,
formation by aromatization, 266
Optical rotatory dispersion (ORD),
determination of absolute configuration, 88
Ostreasterol (see Chalinasterol)
2,3-Oxidosqualene,
cyclization to protosterol, 199–201
formation from squalene, 198
2,3-Oxidosqualene cyclase,
cycloartenol-cyclase in *Ochromonas malhamensis*, 215
lanosterol-cyclase, 205
M.W. and properties, 205–206
Oxycholesterol,
Lifschütz reaction, in, 47

P

Parent steroids,
basis for steroid nomenclature, 20–23
stereochemistry of, 23
Parkeol,
formula, 151
Pasteur,
interest in mirror images, 9
Peak shift,
steroid analysis, in, 98–99
Pectin (see Fibre)
(22R)-2β,3β,14α,22,25-Pentahydroxy-5β-cholest-7-en-6-one (see α-Ecdysone)
Phase transition temperature (T_c),
cholesterol, effect on, 323–325
fatty acyl chains, 322
natural membranes, 329
Phenobarbital,
bile-acid synthesis, 255
HMG-CoA reductase, 384
intestine, sterol synthesis in, 385

Pheromones,
  MVA as precursor, 218
Phospholipid, see also Lecithin, Sphingomyelin
  cholesterol interaction, 320–321
  lateral membrane diffusion, 331–332
  membrane constituent, 318
  phase transition temperature, 322
5-Phosphomevalonate,
  from mevalonate, 188
Phosphomevalonate decarboxylase,
  reaction mechanism, 189
Phosphomevalonate kinase,
  formation of isopentenyl PP, 188
Phosphoprotein phosphatase,
  reaction catalyzed, 365
Phytoene,
  carotenoid synthesis, in, 217
Phytosterols (see Plant sterols)
Placenta,
  esterified cholesterol in, 138
  formation of,
    oestradiol and oestriol, 305
    oestriol, 267
    pregnenolone and progesterone, 305
  inability to synthesise cholesterol, 305
  uptake of maternal cholesterol, 302
Placosterol,
  in sponges, 148
Plant sterols,
  absorption, 471–472, 836–837
  animal tissues, in, 126
  cycloartenol, in synthesis of, 215
  esterified, 836
  faeces, in, 137
  gut mucosa, in, 136
  higher plants, in, 150
  LDL, in, 836
  milk, in, 139
  plasma concentration,
    normal, 836
    β-sitosterolaemia, 836
  red cells, in, 836
  β-sitosterolaemia, 835
Plaques,
  lipid composition, 610
  monotypic in mosaics, 658
Plasma cholesterol,
  carbohydrate, 488
  cholesteryl ester exchange proteins, 554–555
  cholestyramine, 492–493
  clofibrate, 494
  colon cancer, 655
  dietary cholesterol, 480, 484, 577
  dietary protein, 487
  esterified,
    composition, 509
  exchange between lipoproteins, 549–550
  exchange with red cells, 547–549, 550–552

exercise, 581
FH, 695, 699
fibre, 488–490
habitual diet,
  lack of effect, 576
heritability, 588–590, 592–593
ileal resection, 496
infarct, effect on, 573
mortality, all causes, 654
neomycin, 496
nicotinic acid, 495
oral contraceptives, 583, 763
perinatal, 578
plant sterols, 490
polymorphic antigens, 594
polyunsaturated fat, 484
portacaval anastomosis, 496–497
risk factor for IHD, 572, 631 et seq., 639–640
seasonal variation, 577
serum cholesterol, difference between, 574
specific activity curves, 449–450, 455, 493
sugar, 488
trace elements and vitamins, 491
Plasma exchange,
  atherosclerosis, 731, 742
  FH treatment, 739–742
  LDL catabolism, after, 713
Plasma lipid hypothesis,
  definition, 647
  evidence for, 647–650
  prevention trials, 648–650
Plasmalemmal vesicles,
  capillary endothelium, in, 614–616
Plasma lipoproteins,
  animals, 515
  atherogenic, 616
  cholesterol distribution in, 508, 511
  cholesterol-feeding, 515
  diabetes, 757
  oral contraceptives, 762–763
  pregnancy, 763
  renal disease, 760–761
  thyroid, 759
Platelets,
  ADP,
    aggregation, 880
  biliary obstruction, 880
  FH, composition in, 705
  IHD, in, 646, 647
  LDL,
    effect of aggregation, 719
    polyunsaturated fat, effect on, 649
    prostaglandins, effect on, 649
Polyarthritis,
  FH, in, 699, 701
Polyprenols,
  bacteria, in, 214, 220
Polyunsaturated fat,
  bile-acid synthesis, 485–487

bile composition, effect on, 678
cholesterol absorption, 479
cis-trans isomerization, 654, 679
gallstones, 487, 678–679
HDL, effect on, 536
IHD prevalence, 653
optimal dietary, 679
plasma cholesterol, 484
toxicity in margarines, 653–654
Ponasterone A,
plants, in, 154
Poriferasterol,
separation by GLC, 70
sponges, in, 148
Portacaval anastomosis,
7α-hydroxylase activity after, 258
lipoprotein metabolism, effect on, 497, 739
plasma cholesterol, 496–497
Precursor,
criteria for, 171
Pregnancy,
hypercholesterolaemia in, 763
Pregnane,
formula, 22
5α-Pregnan-3β-ol,
formation of digitonide, 44
Pregnenolone,
ACTH on formation, 270
conversion to progesterone, 263
formation from cholesterol, 261, 267
17α-hydroxylation, 263
precursor of cardenolides, 217
precursor of steroid hormones, 261
role of 20-22 lyase, 267
Presqualene alcohol,
determination of structure, 91 *et seq.*
NMR spectrum, 94
Presqualene pyrophosphate,
absolute configuration, 96
determination of structure, 90–97
farnesyl pyrophosphate, formation from, 191, 197
Prevention trials, 648–649, 650
Previtamin D_2 (6,7-*cis*-tachysterol),
formation from ergosterol, 288
Primary intermediate,
definition, 163
Prochirality,
definition, 7
Production rate (see Cholesterol, turnover)
Progesterone,
formation in placenta, 266
precursor of cardenolides, 217
precursor of steroid hormones, 261–265
Propionyl-CoA,
side-chain cleavage, in, 233
Prostaglandins,
platelets, 649
sterol synthesis, effect on, 414

Protosterol,
cycloartenol synthesis, in, 215
fusidic acid, similarity to, 205
product of squalene cyclization, 199–201
variety of rearrangements, 201–202
Provitamin D (see Ergosterol, 7-Dehydrocholesterol)
Pseudodominance,
floating beta disease, in, 749
Pseudohomozygous type II hyperlipoproteinaemia,
description, 728
Pyridoxine deficiency,
hypocholesterolaemia in, 775
5-Pyrophosphomevalonate,
MVA, formation from, 188

R

Rate-limiting step,
HMG-CoA reduction, 359
Rearrangement,
sterol biosynthesis, in, 165
Receptor defective,
FH genotype, 714
Receptor negative,
FH genotype, 714
Red cells,
abetalipoproteinaemia, 780
biliary obstruction, 878–880
5α-cholestanol in, 838
cholesterol exchanges, 547–552
cholesterol in, 318, 328, 331, 550, 551, 780, 879
FH, composition, 705
flip-flop in, 332
fluidity of membrane, 329
LCAT deficiency, 805–806
liver disease, 881–882
LPX, fusion with, 878
plant sterols in, 836
spur cells, 878, 881–882
target cells, 805, 878
Δ^7-Reductase,
inhibition by AY-9944, 172
reaction mechanism, 212
Δ^{24}-Reductase,
inhibition by triparanol, 172
mechanism, 211
Reductase kinase,
HMG-CoA reductase, 365
regulation of, 367
Reductase kinase kinase,
microsomal, 365
Rembrandt,
Anatomy lesson of Dr. Tulp, 9
Renal disease,
haemodialysis in, 761

Renal disease—*contd.*
  LCAT deficiency, 796
  plasma lipoprotein abnormalities, 760–761
Reverse cholesterol transport,
  acceptors, 435
  apoA-I, 439
  HDL, 436–439, 559
  LCAT, role in, 437–439
Ring junctions,
  cis/trans configuration, 23
  influence of configuration on, 32
Rosenheim reaction,
  ergosterol and, 48
R/S notation (see Sequence-rule)
Ružička,
  biogenetic isoprene rule, 168
  cyclization hypothesis, 183–184, 202–205

S

Sapogenins,
  plants in, 154
  synthesis from MVA, 216
Saponification,
  methods for, 56
Saponins,
  plants, in, 154
Schüller-Christian syndrome,
  bone lesions, 846
  diabetes insipidus, 846, 847
  exophthalmos, 847
  xanthomas, 843–846
Sea-blue histiocytes,
  LCAT deficiency, in, 801
Sea cucumbers,
  sterols in, 146
Sea urchins,
  sterols in, 146
Sebaceous glands,
  secretion of sebum, 130
  squalene synthesis, 355
Sebum,
  agnosterol in, 132
  5α-cholestanol in, 132
  lanosterol in, 132
  squalene in human, 132
Sequence-rule,
  disadvantages, 20
  use in nomenclature, 15–20
Serendipity,
  definition, 182
1,2 Shift,
  evidence for, in sterol synthesis, 202–204
  lanosterol synthesis, in, 199
  sterol rearrangement, in, 166
Side-chain,
  alkylation by transmethylation, 216

cleavage in bile-acid formation, 231, 233, 240
  effect on R_f, 62
  nomenclature, 13
  position established, 36
β-Sitosterol ((24R)-24-ethylcholest-5-en-3β-ol),
  absorption, 471, 836–837
  animal tissues, in, 126
  bile acid formation from, 472
  biosynthesis, 216
  cholesterol absorption, effect on, 479
  cholesterol 7α-hydroxylase, effect on, 258
  corticosteroid, conversion to, 472
  esterification, 836
  formula, 152
  metabolism, 472
  plasma concentration, 836
  separation by GLC, 70
  separation by TLC, 62
  side-chain configuration, 21
β-Sitosterolaemia,
  IHD, 835
  plant sterols, 835, 836, 837
  xanthomas, 835
Skin, see also Sebaceous glands, Sebum
  squalene synthesis, 355
  sterol precursors in, 55, 130, 131
  sterols in human, 127, 131
  sterols in rat, 130, 131
Smooth-muscle cells,
  arterial intima, 606
  fatty streaks, in, 607
  foam cells from cataionized LDL, 614, 719
  LDL receptors, 427–428
Solasodine,
  formula, 155
Sphingomyelin,
  abetalipoproteinaemia, 777, 780
  FH-LDL, in, 704
  LCAT deficiency, 802
  Niemann-Pick disease, 819
  Tangier disease, 790
α-Spinasterol (24α-ethylcholesta-7,22-dien-3β-ol),
  formula, 153
  spinach, in, 153
Sponges,
  sterols in, 148
Squalene,
  cyclization,
    Robinson scheme, 175
    Ružička mechanism, 199–201
    Woodward and Bloch scheme, 177–179
  epoxidation, 198
  epoxide (see 2,3-Oxidosqualene)
  fish liver, in, 129
  foods, in, 143
  formation from presqualene PP, 197

function in sharks, 129
human sebum, in, 132
mevalonate carbon in, 183
plasma, in, 462
steps in biosynthesis, 192
synthesis in skin, 355
tissue concentration, 142–143
whole-body sterol synthesis, 462
Squalene epoxidase,
cofactor requirements, 198
substrate specificity, 198
Squalene monooxygenase (see Squalene epoxidase)
Squalene synthetase,
liver and yeast, in, 193
reaction mechanism, 197–198
Starfish,
sterols in, 146, 147
Steady state,
definition, 454
LDL turnover in, 530
Sterol,
definition, 4
Stereoisomer,
definition, 6
Stereospecific,
enzyme activity, 8
Steroid,
definition, 4
nomenclature of substituents, 11, 24–25
numbering, 12
Sterols,
evolutionary age, 317
evolution in membranes, 317, 333–334
function in invertebrates, 144
inhibitory analogues, 411–413
insects, in, 145
Stigmasta-5,E-24(28)-dien-3β-ol (see Fucosterol)
Stigmasta-5,Z-24(28)-dien-3β-ol (see 28-Isofucosterol)
Stigmasta-7,Z-24(28)-dien-3β-ol (see Δ⁷-Avenasterol)
Stigmasterol (24α-ethylcholesta-5,22-dien-3β-ol),
absorption, 471
discovery, 3
formula, 153
side-chain, 14, 21
β-sitosterolaemia, 836
Suberylarginine,
bufogenins, in, 143
Substitution,
sterol biosynthesis, in, 165
Sulphate esters,
bile acids, 114
cholesterol, 125, 126

T

6,7-cis-Tachysterol (see Previtamin D_2)
Tangier disease (familial HDL deficiency),
apoA-I,
catabolism, 792–793
chylomicrons, 791
d > 1.21, 792
structure, 791
synthesis in intestine, 793
arcus, 789
cholesterol esterification, 790
cholesteryl ester deposits, 789–790
foam cells, in, 790
HDL_T, 791
hypocholesterolaemia, 790
IHD in, 651, 789, 795
LCAT activity, 790, 794
LDL, 791, 795
tonsils in, 789
VLDL, 791
Tay-Sachs disease,
ganglioside, 819
T_c (see Phase transition temperature)
Terpene,
definition, 167
Testosterone,
formation from androstenedione, 266
Tetrahymena pyriformis,
tetrahymanol in, 202
Tetrahymanol,
stereochemistry of cyclization to, 202
Thin-layer chromatography (see TLC)
Thyroid,
bile-acid synthesis, 253, 494
cholesterol synthesis, 494
hypercholesterolaemia, 760
LDL catabolism, 533, 760
LDL-receptor function, 726, 760
plasma lipoproteins, 759
TLC,
argentation chromatography, 63, 108
derivatization, after, 59
methods of detection, 60–61
methyl sterols, 63
preparative, 59
R_f of bile acids, 63–64
R_f of sterols, 61–63
Toad poisons (see Bufogenins)
Tonsils,
Tangier disease, in, 789
Triglyceride, see also VLDL
formation of remnants, 525
LCAT deficiency, 801
LDL core lipids, 520
lipoprotein lipase, 524
mass transfer, 554
risk factor for IHD, 635, 642
β-VLDL, 514
VLDL and chylomicrons, 509, 513

3α,7α,12α-Trihydroxy-5β-cholan-24-oic acid (see Cholic acid)
3α,6β,7α-Trihydroxy-5β-cholanoic acid (see α-Muricholic acid)
3α,6β,7β-Trihydroxy-5β-cholanoic acid (see β-Muricholic acid)
3α,7β,12α-Trihydroxy-5β-cholanoic acid, identification by peak shift, 99
3α,7α,12α-Trihydroxy-5β-cholestanoic acid, alligator bile, in, 238
 conversion to cholic acid *in vivo*, 234
 human bile, in, 234
 stereoisomers of, 238
4,4,14-Trimethyl-5α-cholesta-7,9(11),24-trien-3β-ol (see Agnosterol)
Trimethylsilyl ether (TMS ether), GLC, in, 70–72
Triparanol,
 inhibition of Δ^{24}-reductase, 172
Triton WR-1339,
 HMG-CoA reductase, 384, 385
Tschugaeff reaction,
 description of, 48
Twins,
 genetic relatedness, 586
 heritability, in study of, 589
 mirror imaging in, 9

U

Unstirred layer,
 sterol absorption, in, 468–469
Ursodeoxycholic acid (3α,7β-dihydroxy-5β-cholan-24-oic acid),
 gallstone therapy, 871–872
 sulphate, 114
UV spectroscopy,
 conjugated double bonds, 81
 provitamin D, 81

V

Velásquez,
 interest in mirror images, 9
Very-low-density lipoprotein (see VLDL)
Vitamin D$_2$ (5,6-*cis*-ergocalciferol),
 conformation, 289
 formation from ergosterol, 288
Vitamin D$_3$ (5,6-*cis*-cholecalciferol),
 active analogues, 291–292
 active metabolites, 290–291
 formation from 7-dehydrocholesterol, 289
 hydroxylations, 290
 intestinal absorption, 472
5,6-*trans*-Vitamin D$_3$,
 biological activity, 291
VLDL (very-low-density lipoprotein), see also Triglyceride
 hydrolysis, 524
 LCAT deficiency, abnormal in, 801
 nascent, 525
 portacaval anastomosis, effect on, 739
 remnants, 524–525
 risk factor for IHD, 635, 642, 651
 structure, 520
 Tangier disease, abnormal in, 791
β-VLDL (floating β-lipoprotein),
 cholesterol-feeding, 515
 occurrence, 514
 type III hyperlipoproteinaemia, in, 742 *et seq.*

W

Walpole, Horace,
 writer, 182
Wheat bran (see Fibre)
White cells,
 membranes in leukaemia, 328, 331
 sterol synthesis, in, 342, 356
Wolman's disease,
 acanthocytes, 828
 adrenals, 823, 824–828, 830
 cholesteryl ester, 824, 829–830
 cholesteryl ester hydrolase, 828–830
 foam cells, 824
 lymphocytes, 824, 828
 lysosomes, 828

X

Xanthelasma,
 FH, in, 697, 701
 β-sitosterolaemia, in, 835
Xanthomas,
 biliary obstruction, in, 880
 cholestyramine, effect on, 492
 CTX, 838–840
 disseminata, 845, 847–848
 FH, in, 695, 697, 699–701
 lipids in, 697
 peripheral nerves, in, 880
 Schüller-Christian syndrome, 845–846
 β-sitosterolaemia, 835
 striata palmaris, 748, 754
 tuberoeruptive, 748, 880
X-chromosome inactivation,
 mammalian cells, in, 657
 mosaics, in females, 657
X-irradiation,
 HMG-CoA reductase, effect on, 384

Z

Zymosterol (5α-cholesta-8,24-dien-3β-ol),
 formula, 156
 intermediate in sterol formation, 207
 liver, in, 127
 systematic name, 27